Vitreoretinal Surgery

Thomas H. Williamson

Vitreoretinal Surgery

Third Edition

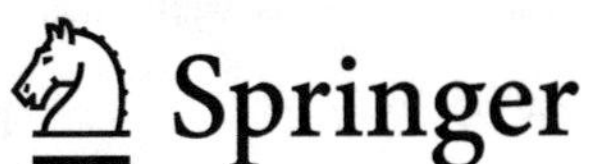

Thomas H. Williamson
Department of Ophthalmology
St. Thomas' Hospital
London
UK

ISBN 978-3-030-68771-7 ISBN 978-3-030-68769-4 (eBook)
https://doi.org/10.1007/978-3-030-68769-4

This Springer imprint is published by the registered company Springer Nature Switzerland AG
The registered company address is: Gewerbestrasse 11, 6330 Cham, Switzerland

Preface

Readers of the first and second editions will know that the purpose of this textbook is to provide a cohesive approach to vitreoretinal diagnosis and surgery. The book has been deliberately written single handedly by the author to prevent the duplication that makes multi-author texts often unwieldy and contradictory. The text is a condensation of the knowledge I have built up over 25 years in vitreoretinal surgery in a tertiary referral unit in central London in the UK. The surgical methods provide an effective way of dealing with almost all vitreoretinal problems.

Surgical technique is in constant development, a reflection of the excitement that surrounds this great speciality. Even in the short time from publication of the first edition in 2008, and the second edition in 2012, there have been major changes in methodology such as the adoption of small gauge vitrectomy in nearly all centres. This edition brings the subject up to date yet again, and therefore should be beneficial to existing users of the book and to new.

The text has been extensively overhauled and expanded, and the figures increased from 600 in the first edition, to 1000 in the second, and to 1225 in the third. The text provides the essential information to diagnose vitreoretinal disorders and perform surgery. The figures are used to illustrate clinical features and describe surgical methods.

To provide the reader with an alternative viewpoint on surgery, 16 international experts have provided completely new surgical *Pearls of Wisdom*. These are scattered through the text and have been an extremely popular addition in the past. I am incredibly grateful to the contribution of these surgeons to the book.

For the first time, I have included finite element analysis of vitreoretinal conditions provided by Mahmut Dogramaci, who is a vitreoretinal surgeon in the UK. These provide an engineer's look at the physics of vitreoretinal surgery.

Finally, my thanks go to all the trainees and surgeons who have been kind enough to provide me with feedback on the book and for their compliments and support.

As a new initiative, I will be providing web-based seminar teaching based on the book through Medsales Academy, UK. Look out for this and join in the courses for direct access to live teaching with me, the author.

I hope you enjoy the third edition; any feedback will be gratefully received. If you wish to give feedback, you can find my contact details on www.retinasurgery.co.uk.

London, UK Thomas H. Williamson

Contents

Contributors

Surgical Pearls

Mahmut Dogramaci, England, UK

Kimberley Drenser, MI, USA

Moto Kamei, Aichi, Japan

Ferenc Kuhn, AL, USA

D. Alistair H. Laidlaw, London, UK

Kenneth K. W. Li, Hongkong, China

Tamer Mahmoud, MI, USA

Zofia Michalewska, Lodz, Poland

Manish Nagpal, Gujarat, India

Jerzy Nawrocki, Lodz, Poland

Stanislao Rizzo, Rome, Italy

Mario Romano, Milano, Italy

Alfonso Savastano, Rome, Italy

Mano Shunmugam, Kuala Lumpur, Malaysia

David Steel, Sunderland, UK

Louisa Wickham, London, UK

George A. Williams, MI, USA

List of Figures

List of Tables

Anatomy and Clinical Examination of the Eye

1

Contents

Introduction

Surgical Anatomy of the Retina and Vitreous

The Vitreous

Embryology

During early development, the invaginated optic vesicle (optic cup) contains the primary vitreous, a vascularised tissue supplying the lens and retina (both of which have an ectodermal origin). During the third month of gestation, the primary vitreous gradually loses its vascularity and is replaced by the secondary vitreous derived mainly from the anterior retina and ciliary body. The principal remnants of the primary vitreous are Cloquet's canal and some epipapillary gliosis. A mild exaggeration of the latter is seen in Bergmeister's papilla (fibrous tuft) on the optic nerve head, while a Mittendorf's dot is a primary vitreous remnant on the posterior capsule of the lens. The hyaloid artery may occasionally persist as a vascular channel growing into the central gel from the optic disc or as a glial plaque on the posterior lens capsule (see Chap. 13).

The Anatomy

The vitreous cavity is the space within the eye bounded anteriorly by the lens and its zonular fibres, and more posteriorly by the ciliary body, retina, and optic disc. Its volume is usually about 4 ml, though this may increase to as much as 10 ml in highly myopic eyes. Normally, the space is entirely occupied by vitreous gel, a virtually acellular viscous fluid with 99% water content. Its low molecular and cellular content is essential for the maintenance of transparency. The major molecular constituents of the vitreous gel are hyaluronic acid and type 2 collagen fibrils. The cortical part of the vitreous gel has a higher content of hyaluronic acid and collagen compared with the less dense central gel. In addition, the gel exhibits "condensations" both within its substance and along its boundaries. The boundary condensations are termed the anterior and posterior hyaloid membranes. A central tubular condensation called Cloquet's canal is a remnant of the primary vitreous, stretching sinuously between the lens anteriorly and the optic disc posteriorly. The gel is unimportant in maintaining the shape or structure of the eye. Indeed, apart from its role in oculogenesis, the vitreous has no well-substantiated function. An eye devoid of gel is not adversely

T. H. Williamson, *Vitreoretinal Surgery*, https://doi.org/10.1007/978-3-030-68769-4_1

affected apart from a poorly understood increased risk of nuclear sclerotic cataract. The pO_2 of the vitreous is relatively low and it has been suggested that the vitreous may act to reduce oxidative stress on the lens fibres thereby reducing cataractogenesis [1]. The vitreous gel is, however, primarily implicated in the pathogenesis of a variety of sight-threatening conditions.

Anatomical Attachments of the Vitreous to the Surrounding Structures

The posterior hyaloid membrane adheres to the internal limiting membrane of the retina by the insertion of vitreous gel fibrils. The internal limiting membrane has type 4 collagen and is the basement membrane of the Muller's cells. The potential space between the internal limiting membrane and the posterior hyaloid membrane is the plane of cleavage of the gel from the retina in posterior vitreous detachment.

The vitreous possesses various sites of increased adhesion to the surrounding structures. These attachments form the basis of much vitreoretinal pathology.

The vitreous base is an annular zone of adhesion some 3–4 mm wide, which straddles the ora serrata. Its anterior border is the site of insertion of the anterior hyaloid membrane. The posterior border of the vitreous base is surgically important because this is the anterior limit of potential separation between the gel and the retina and a common site for retinal tear formation. Adhesion of the vitreous base to the retina and the pars plana is difficult to break even with severe trauma.

Weigert's ligament is a circular zone of adhesion, 8–9 mm in diameter, between the gel and the posterior lens capsule. It is the junction between the anterior hyaloid membrane and the expanded anterior portion of Cloquet's canal.

The posterior hyaloid membrane and the slightly expanded posterior limit of Cloquet's canal meet around the margin of the optic disc and produce another ring of adhesion. During posterior vitreous detachment, gliotic tissue is avulsed from the edge of the nerve head to produce the Weiss's ring, which can be used as an indicator of posterior vitreous detachment.

A circle of relatively increased adhesion to the retina may be present in the parafoveal area and implicated in macular hole formation (Figs. 1.1, 1.2, 1.3).

Exaggerated vitreoretinal adhesions are also present in lattice degeneration, which comprises oval or elongated areas of thinning and vascular sclerosis in the peripheral retina with overlying degenerative vitreous gel. The lesions are generally orientated circumferentially but may be radially directed along the post-equatorial course of retinal veins. Lattice degeneration is found in approximately 7% of normal eyes and is frequently associated with tearing of the retina. The surgeon can experience the adhesion of the vitreous to lattice during induced vitreous separation in macular hole surgery (see Chap. 8). Trying to pull the vitreous off lattice will result in tearing of the retina. Some eyes also demonstrate abnormally strong vitreoretinal adhesions along the course

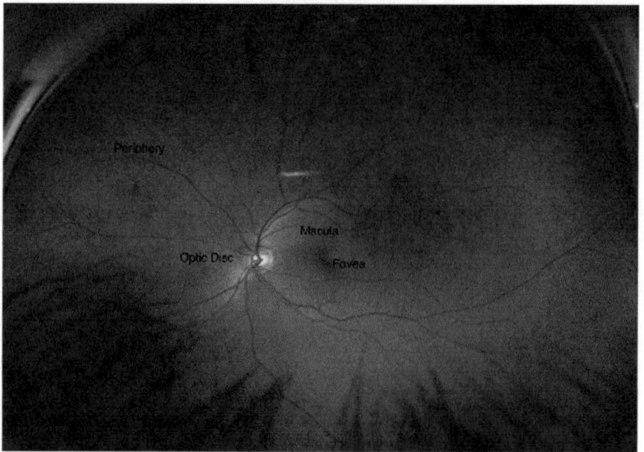

Fig. 1.1 Normal retinal features

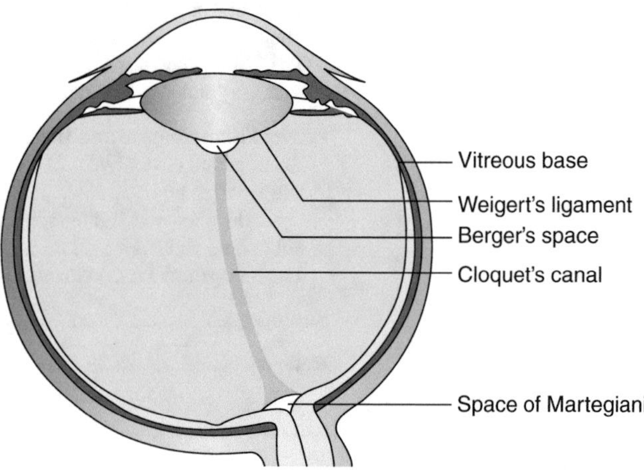

Fig. 1.2 The macroscopic anatomical landmarks are shown

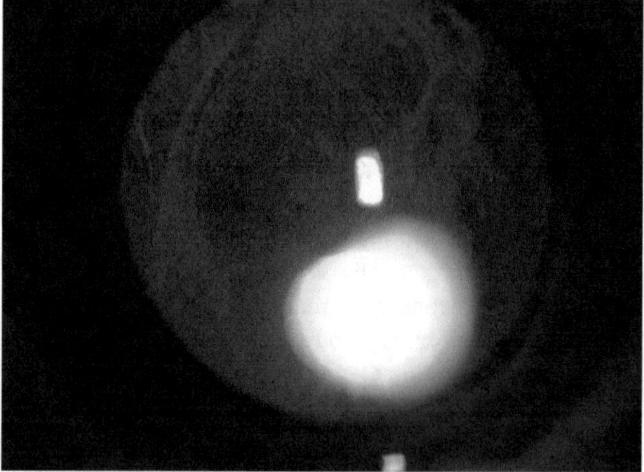

Fig. 1.3 Using retro illumination Weigert's ligament on the back of the lens can be seen in this patient with mild vitreous haemorrhage

of the retinal veins (paravascular adhesions) which may result in retinal tear formation (Figs. 1.4 and 1.5).

The Retina

Embryology

The optic cup develops from the optic vesicle at 6–7 weeks of gestation and consists of two layers of ectoderm the outer becoming the retinal pigment epithelium (RPE) and the inner the neurosensory retina. The space between the two layers is the same as the "subretinal" space in retinal detachment. The retina develops as two neuroblastic layers, inner and outer, which differentiate into the various cells of the retina. The receptor cells are the last to appear at approximately 13 weeks. At 5.5 months, the adult arrangement can be seen but the retina is not completely developed until 3–4 months after birth when the macula is formed. The retinal pigment epithelium becomes pigmented from 6 weeks to 3 months of gestation.

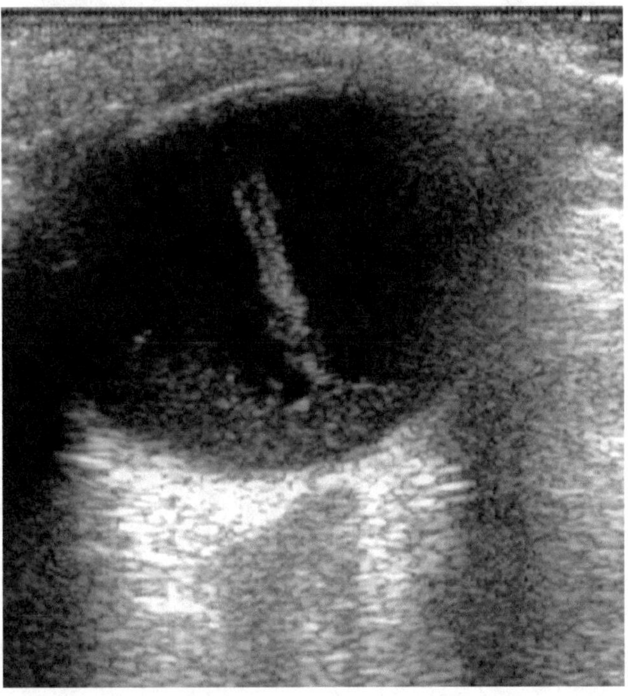

Fig. 1.4 An ultrasound of vitreous haemorrhage (seen especially in the retrohyaloid space) shows Cloquet's canal delineated by the haemorrhage

Anatomy

The retina is divided into regions with the macula consisting of the area between the temporal vascular arcades, serving approximately 20° of visual field. The fovea is the central darkened area with a pit called the foveola. The cones are densest at the fovea, at 15,000/mm^2, with 4000–5000/mm^2 in the macula. There are six million cones and 120 million rods in total.

Cones provide high resolution, colour vision in photopic conditions. They react quickly and recover rapidly to different light stimuli. Three types of cone photoreceptors exist in the human eye with different opsin proteins bound to a common chromophore (11-*cis*-retinal). The three types provide sensitivities that peak at different light wavelengths short S cones at 420 nm (blue), middle M cones at 530 nm (green), long L cones at 560 nm (red).

The retina is organised into four layers of cells and two layers of neuronal connection. The retina has a structural cell called the Muller cell, which extends through all the layers. These cells are specialised glial cells that hold a sink of ions during depolarisation of receptors and are essential for the physiology of the eye. They may also have functions in:

- Cone neuroprotection
- Control of vascular permeability and haemostasis
- Pigment recycling

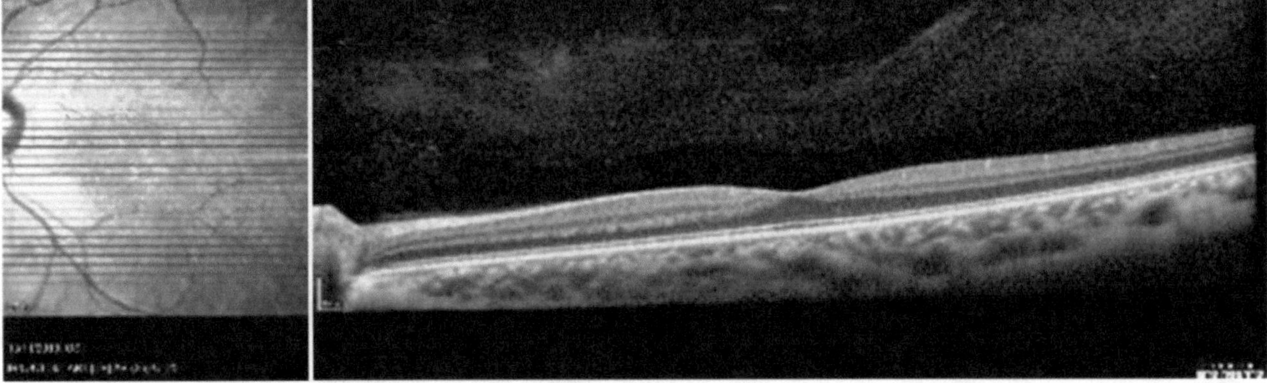

Fig. 1.5 Premacular bursa. The reason for this feature in the vitreous is unclear

There are astrocytes and microglial cells in addition to the retina.

The retinal layers are, from outer to inner retina.

Retinal Pigment Epithelium

A single layer of pigmented cuboidal epithelial cells, which look after the function of the receptors by:

- Absorbing stray light (using melanin pigment)
- Transporting metabolites between the receptors and the choroid
- Providing a blood–retinal barrier
- Regenerating the visual pigments
- Phagocytosing the receptor outer segments leading to lipofuscin production (Figs. 1.6 and 1.7).

Photoreceptor Layer

The photoreceptor transduces light into neuronal signals. The action of light closes gated cation channels leading to hyperpolarisation of the cell. Two types of photoreceptors exist, the rods predominantly in the periphery and absent from the fovea and the cones concentrated at the macula. They are made up of:

Outer Segments

Light is absorbed by the visual pigments that are contained in stacked discs. The discs are separate in the rods (1000 in number) but are interconnected in the cones. These join to the inner segment by the cilium.

Inner Segments

These consist of an inner myoid which contains the Golgi apparatus and ribosomes for making cell structures and an outer ellipsoid which contains mitochondria for energy production. These connect to the nucleus by the outer connecting fibre. The inner connecting fibre connects to the synaptic region. The latter has synapses arranged as triads with connections to one bipolar cell and two horizontal cells. In cones, there may be up to 20 triads whereas the rods have only one.

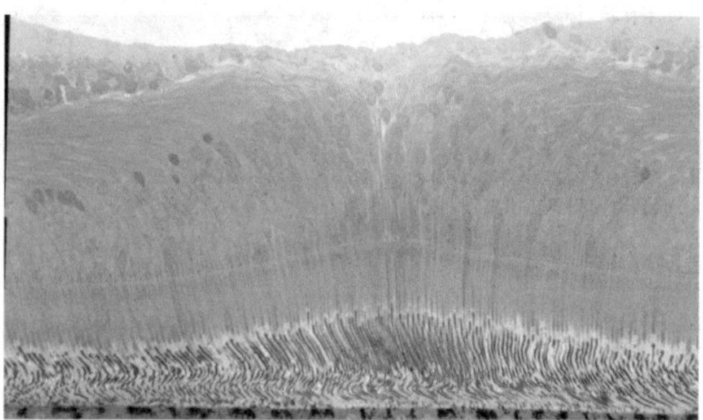

Fig. 1.6 The foveal anatomy showing increased numbers of cones and absence of the nerve fibre layer

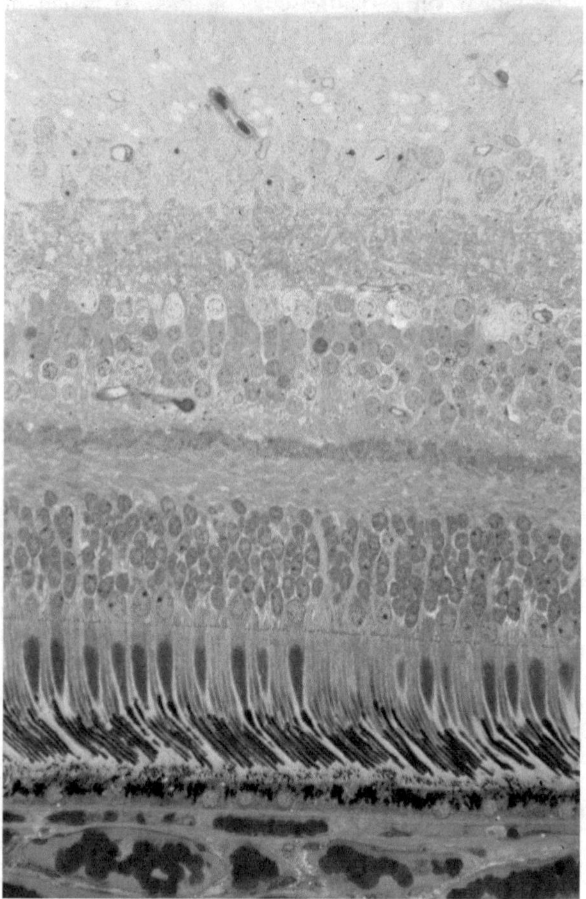

Fig. 1.7 The normal stratified structure of the retina

Outer Limiting Layer

This consists of junctional complexes from the Muller cells and photoreceptors and is located at the inner connecting fibres.

Outer Plexiform Layer

The cell processes of the horizontal cells and bipolar cells synapse with the receptors (Fig. 1.8).

Intermediary Neurones

Inner Nuclear Layer

This contains the cell bodies of the bipolar cells, the Muller cells, Amacrine cells, and horizontal cells.

Inner Plexiform Layer

The bipolar cells' axons pass through, synapsing with the Amacrine cells which help process the neuronal signals to the ganglion cells.

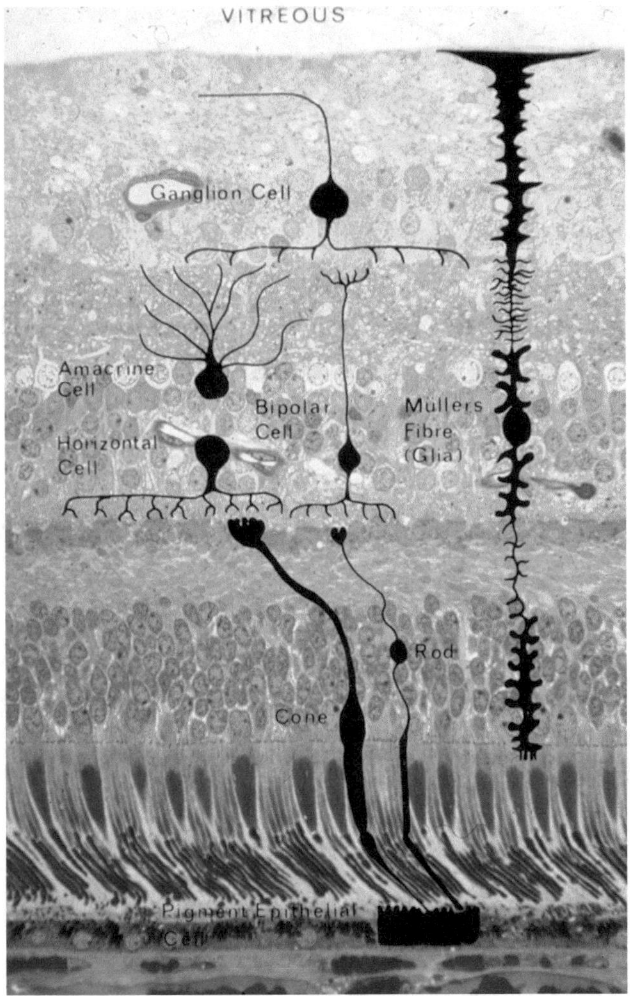

Fig. 1.8 The cell types are shown and their position in the retina are indicated (courtesy of John Marshall)

Ganglion Cells

Ganglion Cell Layer

The cell bodies of the ganglion cells are found here. These cells have gathered pre-processed information from the other retinal cells. The cells receive different visual information such as a sustained response to light, transient response, or response to movement. At the macula, there is 1 ganglion cell to 1 receptor but on average in the whole retina there is 1 for 130 receptors.

Nerve Fibre Layer

The nerve fibres of the ganglion cells on the inner surface of the retina pass tangentially towards the optic nerve.

Inner Limiting Membrane

Note: The internal limiting membrane (ILM) is a tough membrane laid down by the Muller cells with connections to the hyaloid membrane of the vitreous.

Retinal Blood Vessels

The central retinal artery supplies the neural retina except for the photoreceptors, which are supplied by the choriocapillaris. This is an end artery system with a single draining vessel, the central retinal vein. Both vessels have four main branches which divide at the optic disc to supply nasal and temporal quadrants. At the posterior pole, there is a capillary network at the level of the nerve fibre layer and the outer plexiform layer. In the periphery, there is one capillary network at the inner nuclear layer. The capillary endothelium forms the inner retinal blood–retina barrier by having tight intercellular junctions.

Other Fundal Structures

Bruch's Membrane

A pentilaminar structure partly representing the basement membranes of the RPE and the choriocapillaris. It is of ectodermal and mesodermal origin. Accumulation of damage in Bruch's is seen in age-related macular degeneration.

Choroid

This is a vascular layer (large vessels are outer, and the capillaries are inner) with a high relative blood flow and low oxygen utilisation (3%). It supplies the RPE and photoreceptors. The highly anastomotic and fenestrated capillaries are arranged into lobules and are supplied by the posterior ciliary arteries and drained by the vortex veins.

The Physiology of the Vitreous

The physiology of the vitreous is not well understood. It is thought that molecules can move in the gel because of diffusion and convection and by the effects of saccades on the fluid component of the gel. Diffusion is most important for animals with smaller eyes, whereas convection is more important for larger eyes such as human eyes. Molecules with an anionic charge move more easily in the gel. Small soluble molecules like fluorescein move at a similar rate to aqueous, larger molecules like albumin may move 30–50% less rapidly than aqueous [2]. Convection is estimated to account for 30% of movement of molecules in the vitreous because there is a pressure differential from the anterior ingress of aqueous, to the posterior egress of fluid through the retina by the RPE pump. The saccadic movement of the eyes induces convection currents in the anterior vitreous which circulate around the vitreous base because of the effect of the indentation of the lens into the vitreous cavity [3].

The measured viscosity of the vitreous depends on the technique used with estimates saying from 5 to 2000 mPas (aqueous = 1 mPas). It is non-Newtonian, i.e. a non-linear relationship and bimodal probably because there is a micro and macro viscosity component. The vitreous is relatively hypoxic (pO_2 of 30–40 mmHg) in comparison to air, (150 mmHg), and arterial blood (100 mmHg) [4]. The relatively small proportion of ocular blood supply to the retina (2–3%) has a profound effect on the vitreal PO_2 [5, 6]. There are oxygen gradients in the vitreous with higher PO_2 in the anterior vitreous than the posterior. Ascorbate concentrations are high in the vitreous; the ascorbate may react with oxygen to reduce the PO_2 [6].

The reason for low PO_2 in the vitreous is unknown but it may be to protect the lens proteins from oxidation [7]. Removal of the vitreous by vitrectomy causes nuclear sclerotic cataracts except in ischemic eyes such as diabetic retinopathy and retinal vein occlusion [8]. Inserting tamponade agents such as silicone oil into the vitreous cavity increases the concentration of ions, e.g. K^+, Ca^+ in the remaining aqueous layer in the cavity [9].

Anatomy and Physiology and the Vitreoretinal Surgeon

There are certain features of the anatomy and physiology that the surgeon should remember whilst operating.

At the ora serrata the non-pigmented epithelium is continuous with the neurosensory retina and therefore retinal detachments can extend anteriorly through the ora on rare occasions. Ultimately the ciliary body may be detached causing reduction in intraocular pressure (IOP) and even hypotony and choroidal effusion.

The posterior attachment of the vitreous base to the retina moves more posteriorly in the elderly [10].

The nerve fibre layer orientation is especially important whilst working on the surface of the retina where damage to the nerve fibres might occur, e.g. in macular hole surgery (Chap. 8).

The fovea is the thinnest part of the retina and is therefore prone to dehiscence and hole formation during retinal elevation, e.g. in macular surgery.

The force required to cause a retinal detachment has been put at approximately 200 dynes/cm^2 (approximately 0.27 mmHg, i.e. not very much) in primates. Several mechanisms have been implicated in keeping the retina attached:

The retinal pigment epithelium applies forces to the retina: through ionic flow as calcium and magnesium move across the RPE, hydrostatic forces from the intraocular pressure and flow of fluid out of the eye. The RPE pump works against the relative resistance to fluid flow of the retina and has been estimated at 0.3 ml/h/mm^2.

Increased osmotic pressure exerted by the increased protein content in the choroidal circulation also encourages fluid flow across the retina.

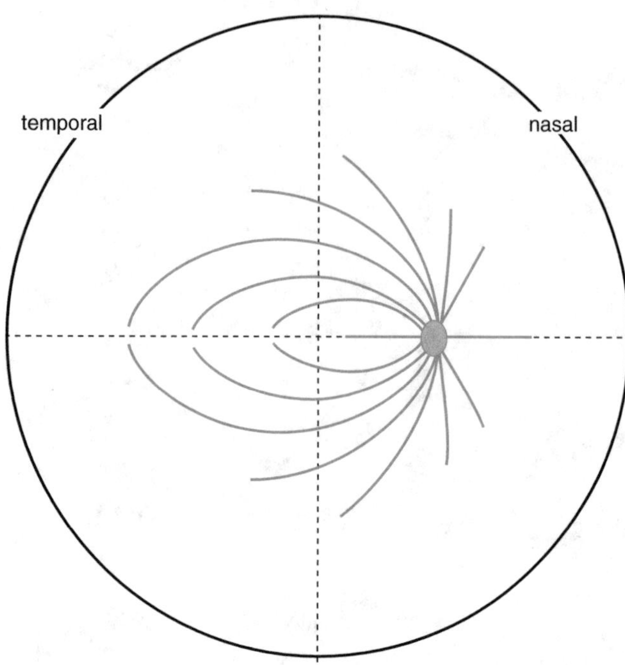

Fig. 1.9 Always consider in which direction the nerve fibres run on the surface of the retina when operating so as to minimise damage to the fibres. Try to cut or scrape along the direction of the nerve fibres rather than perpendicular to their direction

In addition, there are intercellular components aiding adhesion of the retina to the RPE such as the interphotoreceptor matrix, and interdigitation of rod outer segments with RPE microvilli (Fig. 1.9).

Interestingly evidence of vitreous collagen metabolism (C-propeptide levels of type II pro-collagen) [11] is found in the vitreous cavity of vitrectomised eyes although hyaluronan levels are reduced (Figs. 1.10 and 1.11).

Clinical Examination and Investigation

Examination of the Eye

Examination Technique

Visual Acuity

LogMar values are recommended for the ease of analysis of data for surgical audit and governance. This can be measured by Snellen chart or EDTRS chart but requires full refractive correction.

The Slit Lamp

The vitreoretinal surgeon must be able to use the slit lamp, Goldman tonometry, and various contact lenses, or three mirrors contact lens and be able to visualise the vitreous by looking behind the posterior lens. The vitreous must be inspected for clarity, cellular infiltration and, by asking the

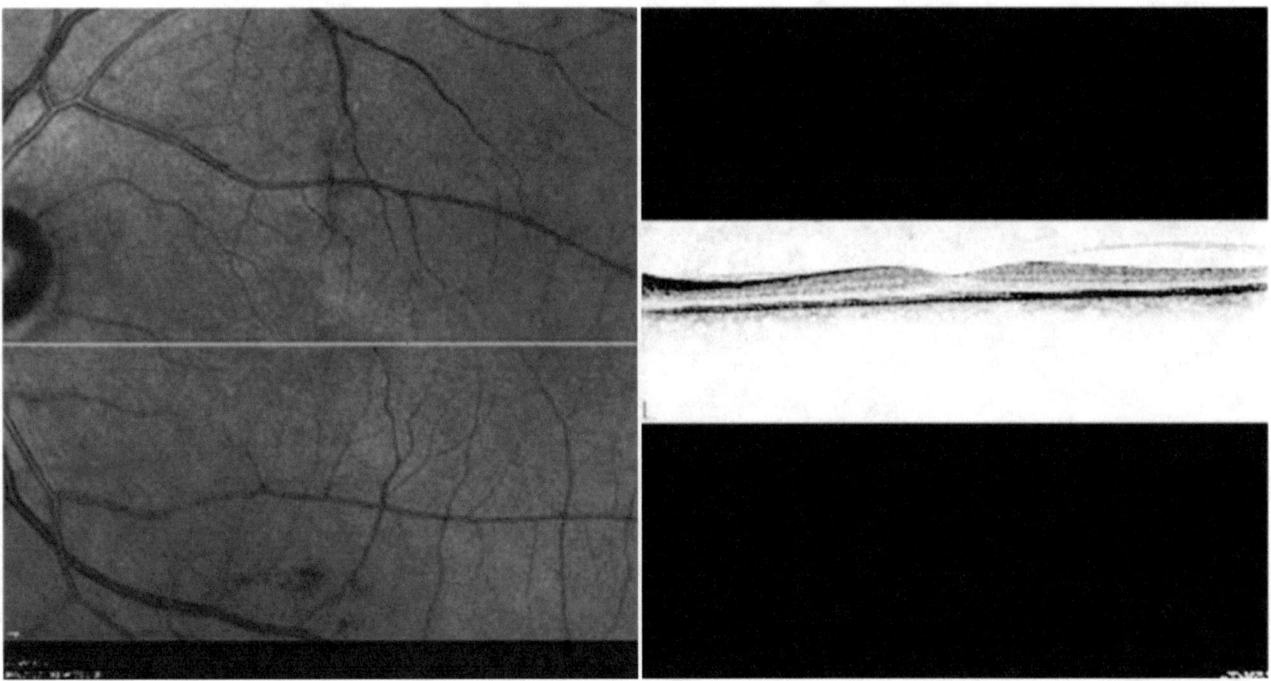

Fig. 1.10 The vitreous is more strongly attached to the fovea. The posterior hyaloid membrane can be seen detached from the temporal retina but still attached at the fovea and nasal to the fovea on optical coherence tomography (OCT)

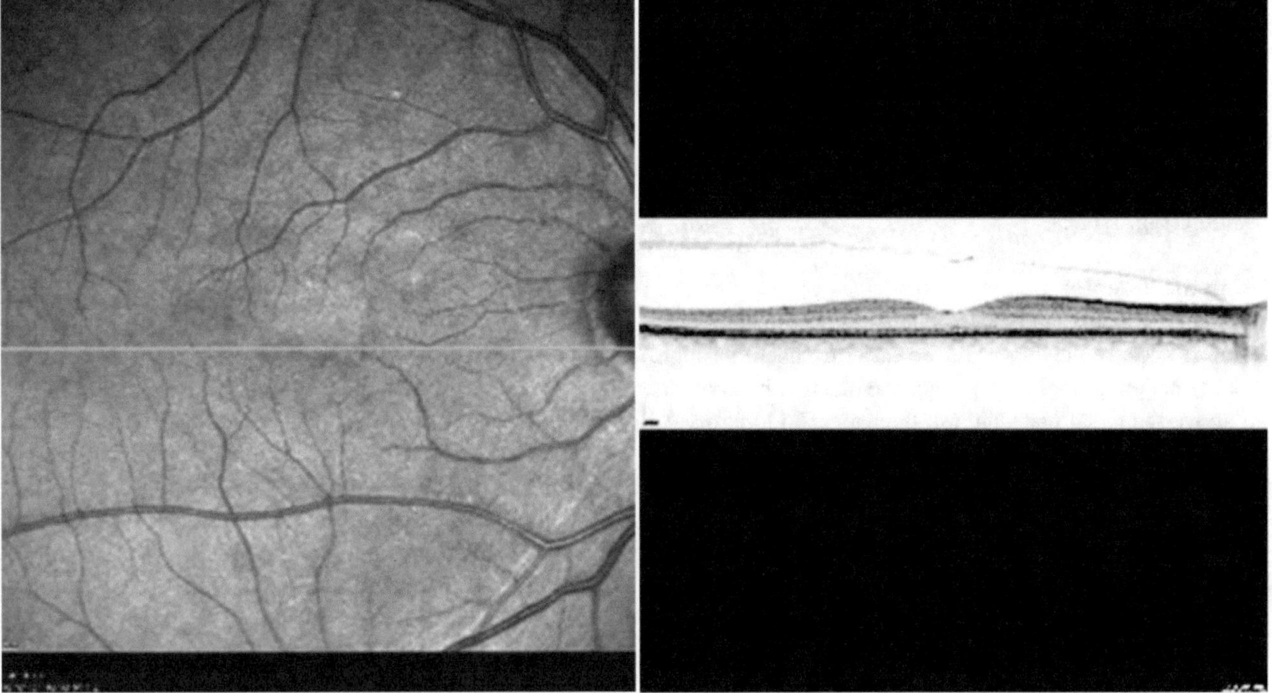

Fig. 1.11 The vitreous is more adherent to the optic nerve head. The posterior hyaloid membrane can be seen separated from the retina but attached to the optic nerve head

patient to move the eye to inspect the mobility of the vitreous. The slit lamp allows the use of specialised lenses for the examination of the vitreous and retina, e.g. super-field, 90D or 60D lenses non-contact lenses (Table 1.1).

Binocular Indirect Ophthalmoscope

A principle extra skill required is the use of the binocular indirect ophthalmoscope with indentation of peripheral retina [12].

Table 1.1 Various lenses and their characteristics

Lens	Slit lamp or BIO	Field of view	Magnification	Depth perception	Uses	Periphery
20D	Bio	Good	Fair	Fair	Peripheral	Far periphery
28D	Bio	Very good	Poor	Poor	Small pupil or paediatric	Far periphery
90D	Slit lamp	Poor	Good	Fair	Small pupil	Posterior to the equator
Super field	Slit lamp	Good	Good	Fair	General	Equator
60D	Slit lamp	Poor	Very good	Good	Macula	Not for the periphery
Goldman three mirror	Slit lamp	Poor	Very good	Good	General	Equator
Hruby lens	Slit lamp	Poor	Very good	Very good	Macula	Nil
Rodenstock	Slit lamp	Very good	Poor	Poor	Panretinal photo coagulation	Equator

Method: Examine in a systematic manner. Always lay the patient flat on an examination couch preferably with no pillow.

Note: Commence examination standing at the patient's side whilst examining the 12 o'clock position of the retina and move around the head of the patient to the other side of the patient systematically examining the whole of the peripheral retina returning to the 12 o'clock position.

Remember the patient looks in the direction of the retina that the observer wishes to see, e.g. if examining the superonasal retina the patient looks superonasally. Initially examine the eye without indentation thereby orientating to the distribution of subretinal fluid (SRF) and to provide a clue to localisation of features such as retinal breaks according to Lincoff's rules (described in Chap. 5). Using indentation to examine the retina, move around the patient's head in the opposite direction finally returning to the original starting position (Fig. 1.12).

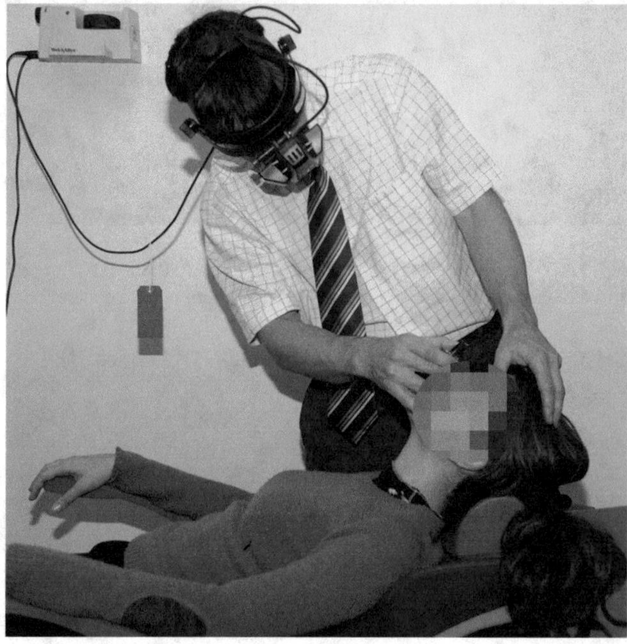

Fig. 1.12 Notice the sideways lean when examining with the indirect ophthalmoscope in order to avoid backache

Using the Indenter

The superior retina (and the temporal side) is often easier to examine because the upper lids are easier to indent through. Ask the patient to look down, place the indenter head on the lid above the tarsal plate and ask the patient to look up. As they do this, rotate the indenter superiorly and apply pressure in the globe aiming towards the centre of the eye.

Note: Get the feel for the required pressure to apply to the globe by pressing the indenter gently on your thumb just enough to depress the skin of the tip of your thumb. Try not to push back into the orbit which only succeeds in indenting the orbital septum and causing the patient discomfort.

Observe the indent on the retina whilst gliding the indenter back and forward or from side to side. Watching the movement of the retina facilitates retinal tear detection. Aim to be able to examine the retina right up to the ora serrata, small anteriorly placed holes can be difficult to find and will cause failure of surgery if undetected. When examining the inferior retina ask the patient to look up, place the indenter below the inferior tarsus and then ask the patient to look inferiorly. The horizontal positions are difficult to see because the canthal tendons and caruncle make indentation uncomfortable. Orientate the indenter vertically, place the indenter above or below these structures and move it sideways to move them out of the way for indentation.

Use a metal indenter either the modified thimble variety or the pen-sized stick.

Ultrasonography

Ultrasound is essential for the examination of the eye with medial opacities (Figs. 1.13 and 1.14).

Note: Learn to perform this technique. Ultrasound is a dynamic examination from which information can be rapidly obtained in the clinical setting.

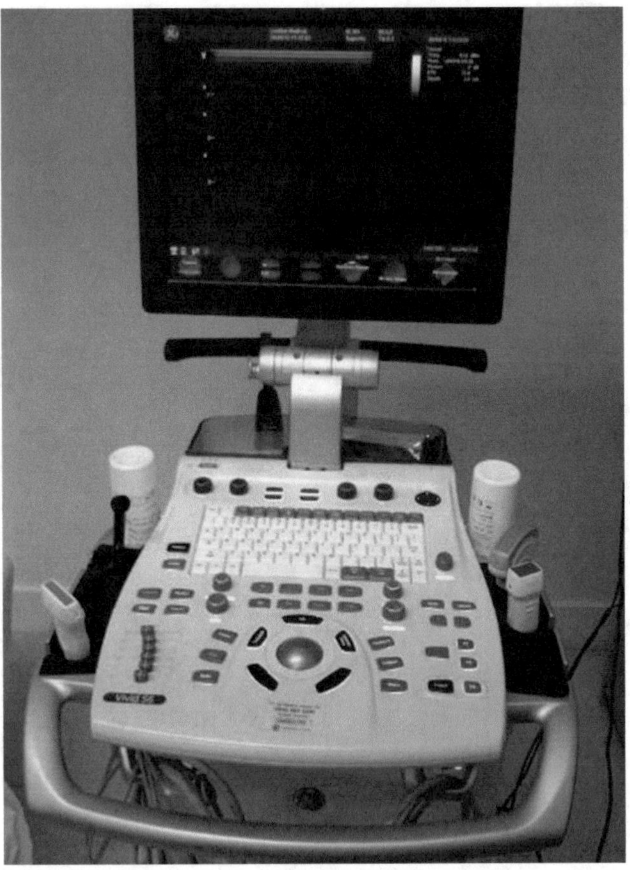

Fig. 1.13 B-scan ultrasound is essential for the running of a vitreoretinal clinic and should be present in every clinic and operated primarily by the vitreoretinal surgeon himself for interpretation of the dynamic signs in the eye

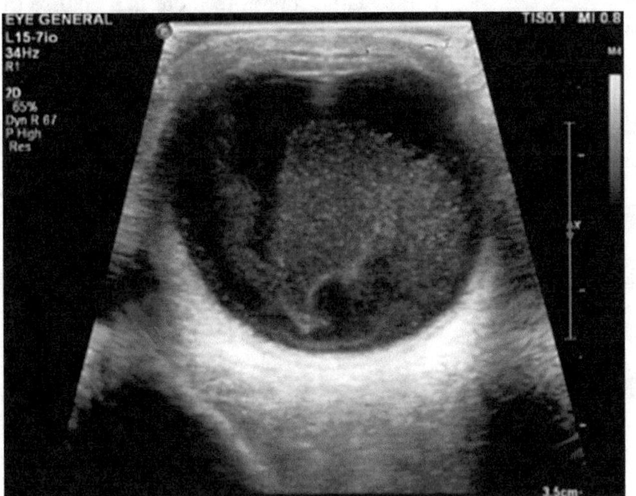

Fig. 1.14 Diffuse vitreous haemorrhage

Ultrasound has a frequency, number of cycles per second of 20 hertz (Hz) which is inaudible to human ears. The higher the frequency of the ultrasound (the shorter the wavelength) the higher is the resolution but at the cost of less penetration into tissues.

Appropriate frequencies for ophthalmology vary from 7.5 MHz to 10 MHz for the posterior segment and with 20–50 MHz for the anterior segment.

Sound travels faster through solids than liquids, e.g. through both aqueous and vitreous at 1500 meters/second (m/s) and through the cornea and lens at 1650 m/s. Therefore, clear images are readily available from the eye and orbit.

Sound is reflected when it encounters an interface of different tissue densities resulting in an echo whose strength relates to the difference in the densities. The signal is highest when the interface is perpendicular to the ultrasound beam.

In B-scan ultrasonography, an oscillating sound beam is emitted, and the signal is reconstructed to produce a 2D image of the tissue.

Some tissues will absorb the sound waves (e.g. a dense cataract) reducing the signal from more posteriorly placed tissues.

Normally the vitreous is echo lucent.

When performing the scan, the operator should be seated and facing the patient and the machinery. For a short scan, the patient may be seated but if a prolonged scan is proposed the supine positioning of the patient is recommended to avoid fatigue of the observer's arm. The examiner should hold the probe in the dominant hand and place the lead around the shoulders to support the weight of the ultrasound cable during the examination. Perform the scan with contact jelly on the closed eyelids of the patient. Increase the gain to allow visualisation of the vitreous but without producing artefacts. Detect the lens (two-bracket shaped echoes anteriorly) and the optic nerve (an echo lucent band extending from the posterior pole) to check your alignment and to orientate yourself in the eye. Perform horizontal scans asking the patient to look right and left to detect the dynamic properties of the tissues and then vertical scans with eye movements up and down. To inspect a particular region of the eye ask the patient to look in the direction of the region of interest, e.g. up and left for the superotemporal area of the left eye. With this dynamic technique, information can quickly be gathered regarding the anatomy and pathology of the vitreous, retina, and choroid. Furthermore, colour Doppler ultrasound can be used to detect blood vessels in the retina in suspected retinal detachment in complex cases such as trauma [13] (Fig. 1.15).

Abnormalities are seen in.

Asteroid hyalosis	Multiple small, highly reflective vitreous opacities

Vitreous Haemorrhage

Diffuse fine echoes or clumps of organised clots are seen in the vitreous cavity often with diffuse haemorrhage behind the posterior hyaloid (subhyaloid haemorrhage). Clot on the posterior cortex, especially inferiorly can be mistaken for retina. If no attachment to the disc is seen this will usually rule out retinal detachment, however, sometimes there are

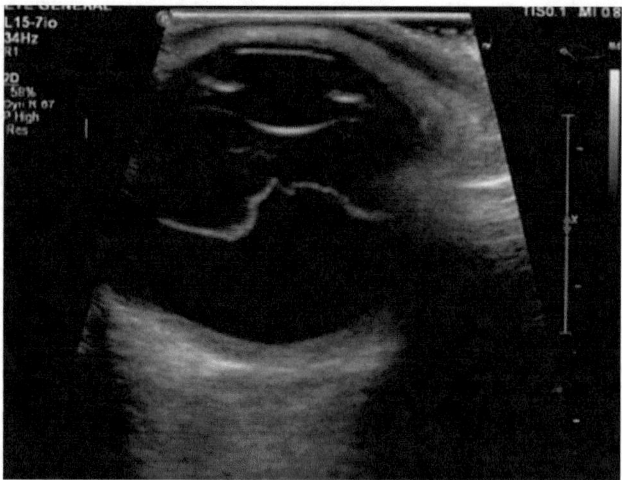

Fig. 1.15 A posterior vitreous detachment on US

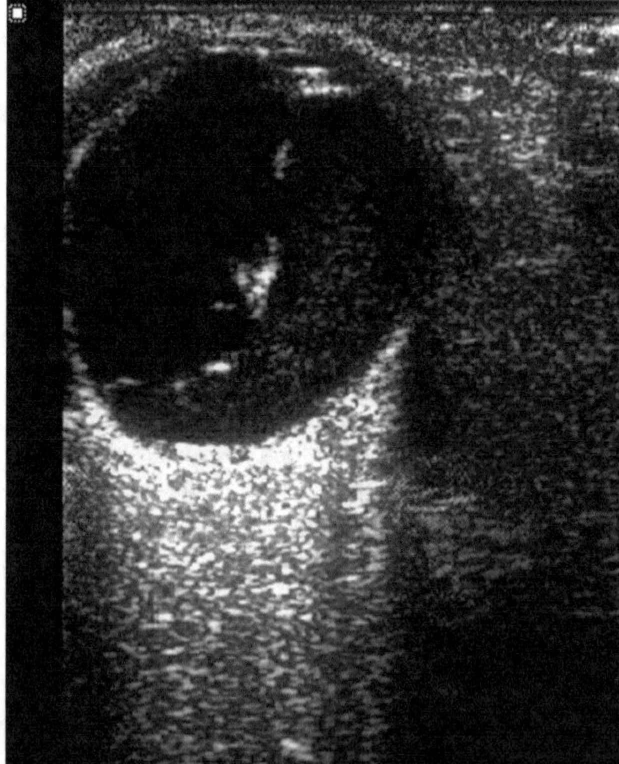

Fig. 1.16 Moving the eye from side to side shows mobility of the vitreous in this patient with subhyaloid haemorrhage

disc attachments of the vitreous to disc new vessels (Figs. 1.16 and 1.17).

Posterior Vitreous Detachment

The posterior hyaloid membrane is seen as a low continuous and sinuous echo, which whips around the eye with eye movements (Fig. 1.18).

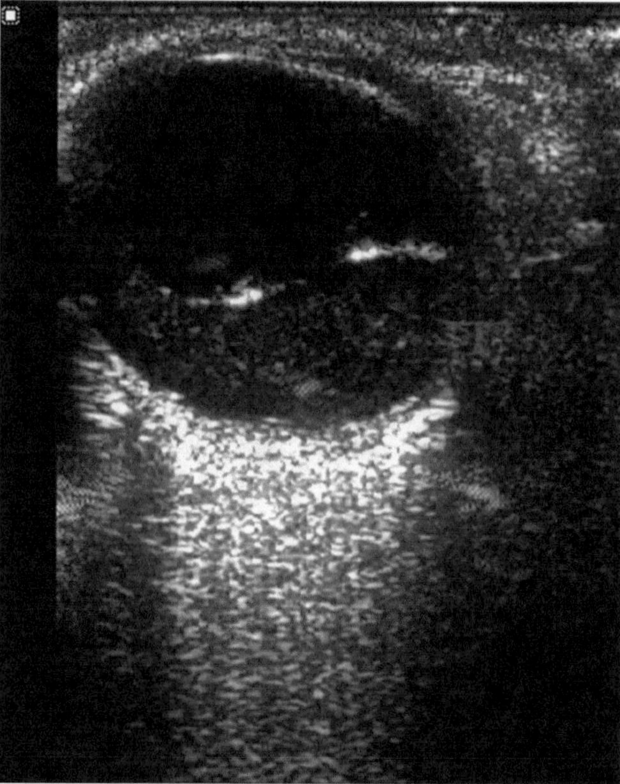

Fig. 1.17 Ultrasound left

Retinal tear	the flap of a retinal tear may be seen in a patient with vitreous haemorrhage and posterior vitreous detachment. Most tears that produce haemorrhage are large therefore there is a chance of seeing the break on ultrasound. However, it is not safe to assume that there is no break if none is detected on ultrasound.
Retinal detachment	a highly reflective, undulating membrane from the ora serrata anteriorly and the optic nerve posteriorly indicates retinal detachment. Initially the retina is mobile but will stiffen and shorten with the development of proliferative vitreoretinopathy (PVR) (Figs. 1.19, 1.20, 1.21, 1.22).

Subretinal Haemorrhage

Often seen in choroidal neovascularisation (CNV) is vitreous haemorrhage with a craggy mass of subretinal blood in the macula.

Retinoschisis	This is smooth, dome-shaped, less mobile, and thinner than rhegmatogenous retinal detachment (RRD).

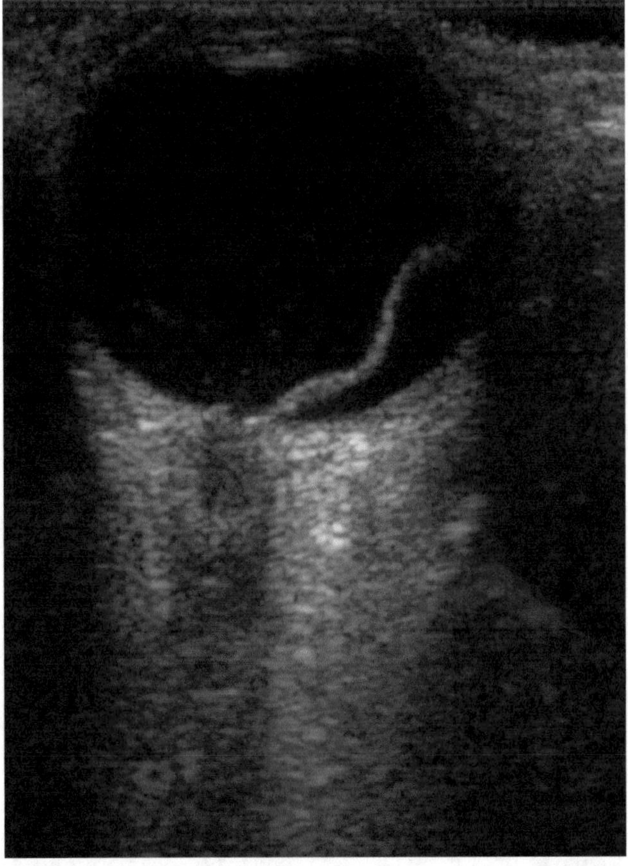

Fig. 1.18 The sinuous shape of a recent onset retinal detachment. Notice how the retina attaches into the optic nerve head and the vitreous can be seen anteriorly

Fig. 1.19 Retinal detachments have a sinuous mobility on ultrasound and an attachment at the optic disc

Choroidal Elevation — Choroidal effusions are smooth, dome-shaped, immobile, and thick with a high signal. If haemorrhage is present the suprachoroidal fluid is diffusely echogenic. Tumours have a vascular circulation on colour Doppler.

Trauma — The above features can be discriminated to determine the degree of injury in a blood-filled eye. In addition, features such as intraocular foreign bodies can be detected as a high reflection with shadow. Even eyes with scleral rupture can be examined. Use plenty of contact jelly so that the probe can be placed on the eye with no pressure applied to the globe (Figs. 1.23, 1.24, 1.25).

Optical Coherence Tomography

Optical Coherence Tomography (OCT), first developed for ophthalmic imaging in the 1990s [14], is invaluable in the retinal clinic. OCT scanning provides 2-dimensional cross-sections of the retina from which 3D dimensional reconstructions can be created [15] (Figs. 1.26, 1.27, 1.28).

The first-generation (TD-)OCTs were only capable of resolutions between 10 and 20 μm because they relied on the mechanical movement of a mirror to measure the time taken for light to be reflected and were therefore relatively slow to perform. These have been superseded by spectral domain OCT (SD-OCT) that is able to simultaneously measure multiple wavelengths of reflected light and have a reported resolution of up to 5–6 μm. With higher resolution scanning a cross-sectional B-scan can reveal most layers within the neurosensory retina [16]. A few histological studies have correlated the OCT appearance with histological sections of human and animal retinas [17, 18]. Further studies have correlated the segmentation (bands) on an OCT with retinal layers by sequential ablation of these layers surgically [19, 20]. The outer red line is frequently assumed to represent the RPE alone but corresponds with the highly reflective chorio-retinal complex.

Time-Domain OCT

Conceptually, OCT operates on the same physical principles as an ultrasound scan except it uses light as the carrier signal. As such, the spatial resolution of an OCT is

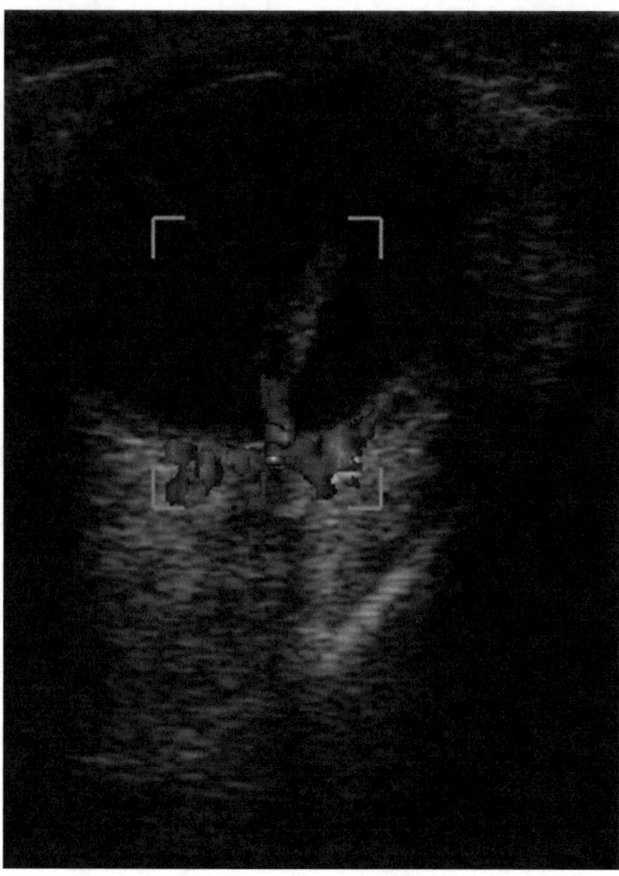

Fig. 1.20 Colour Doppler imaging can be used to detect blood vessels to confirm that an echo is representative of the retina

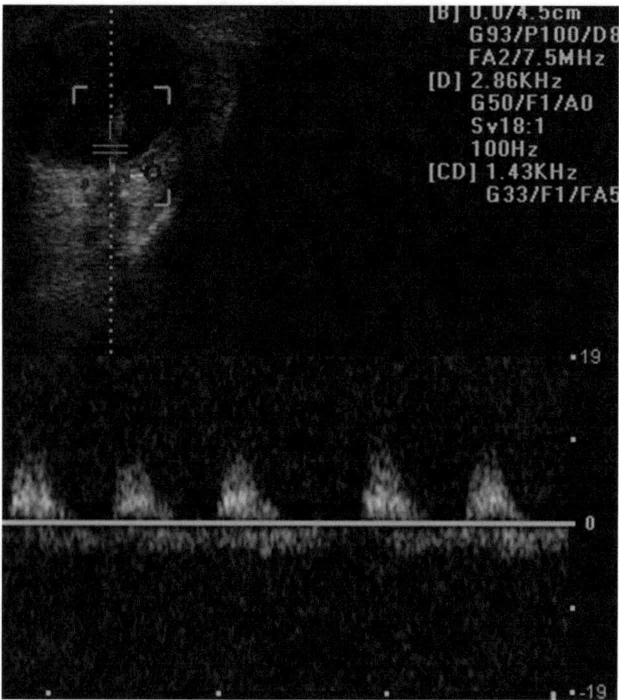

Fig. 1.21 Colour Doppler imaging can be used to detect blood vessels to confirm that an echo is representative of the retina

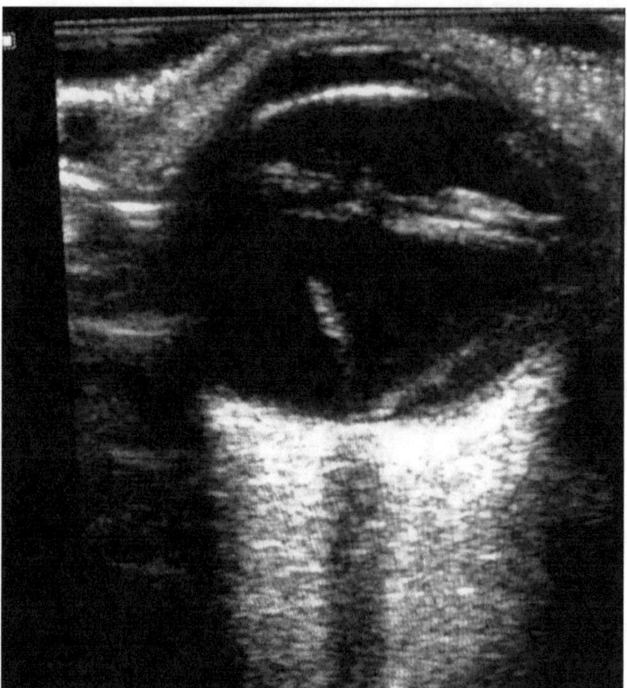

Fig. 1.22 A contracted vitreous and stiff RRD on US

much higher than conventional 10–20 MHz ultrasound because of the naturally shorter wavelength of light. The source of light in an OCT is produced by a superluminescent diode, femtosecond laser or more recently using white light [21].

OCT works by splitting a beam of light into 2 arms—a reference arm and a sampling arm. First-generation OCTs are time-domain OCT (TD-OCT) so named because the length of the reference arm is varied with time, to correlate with the back-reflected sample arm. This is achieved with the use of an adjustable mirror of known distance within the device. The sample arm is focused onto the retina with the use of an in-built 78D lens. The sample beam is reflected off the structures in the eye and is recombined with the reference beam by using a Michaelson interferometer within the unit. A single cycle of this process yields 1 A-scan. This single scan comprises data on the distance the sample arm has travelled and the back-reflectance and back-scatter of the beam. Tissue layers at varying depths and optical characteristics produce differing reflective intensities. As in an ultrasound scan, to produce a B-scan image, multiple A-scans are obtained in rapid succession across the area of interest. Software combines this information to produce a 2-dimensional image either in greyscale or with arbitrary false colouring. The result is a cross-sectional scan, a reconstructed 3-dimensional topographical image, quantitative thickness measurements or more recently, z-plane or coronal scans [21].

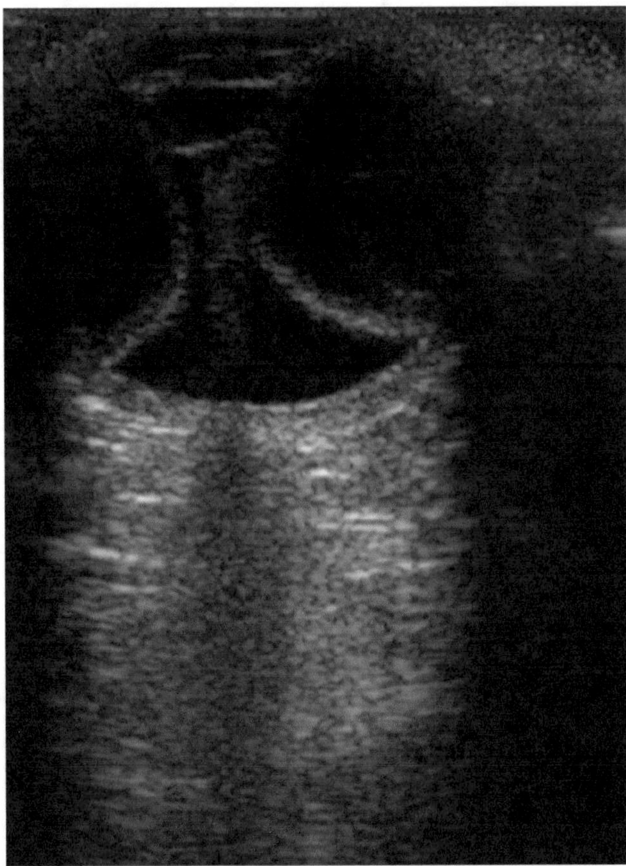

Fig. 1.23 On ultrasound choroidal effusions have a smooth dome-shaped outline. The choroidal effusions can touch centrally, "kissing choroidals", surgically these can be separated (they are sometimes mildly adherent) but initially you may need to infuse through the anterior chamber because there is no space to insert the pars plana infusion until the choroidals are drained

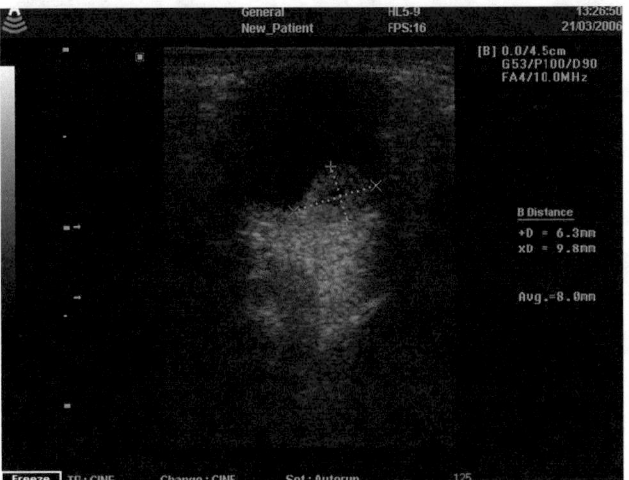

Fig. 1.24 Ultrasound reveals a choroidal haemorrhage which can be measured

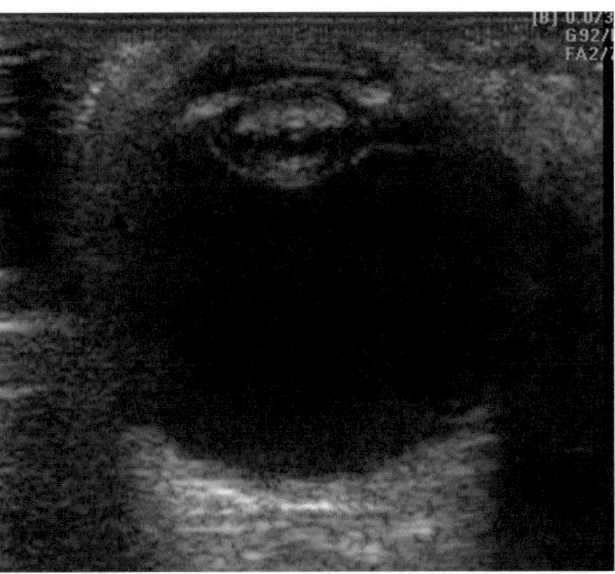

Fig. 1.25 The cataract in this patient is clearly seen and can attenuate the signal from more posteriorly

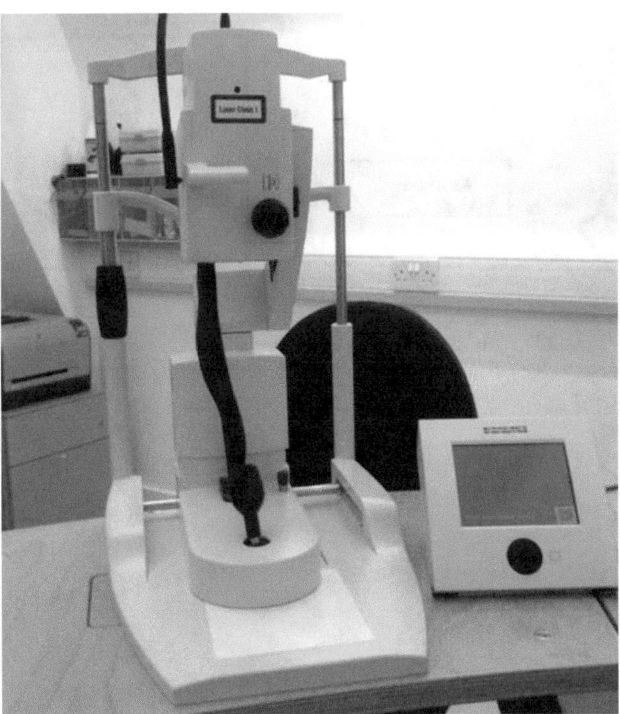

Fig. 1.26 OCT machinery has now become commonplace in vitreoretinal clinics and is extremely useful for discriminating different types of macular pathology

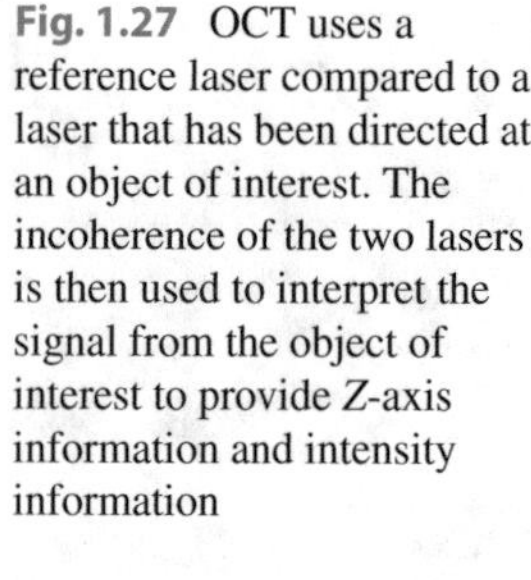

Fig. 1.27 OCT uses a reference laser compared to a laser that has been directed at an object of interest. The incoherence of the two lasers is then used to interpret the signal from the object of interest to provide *Z*-axis information and intensity information

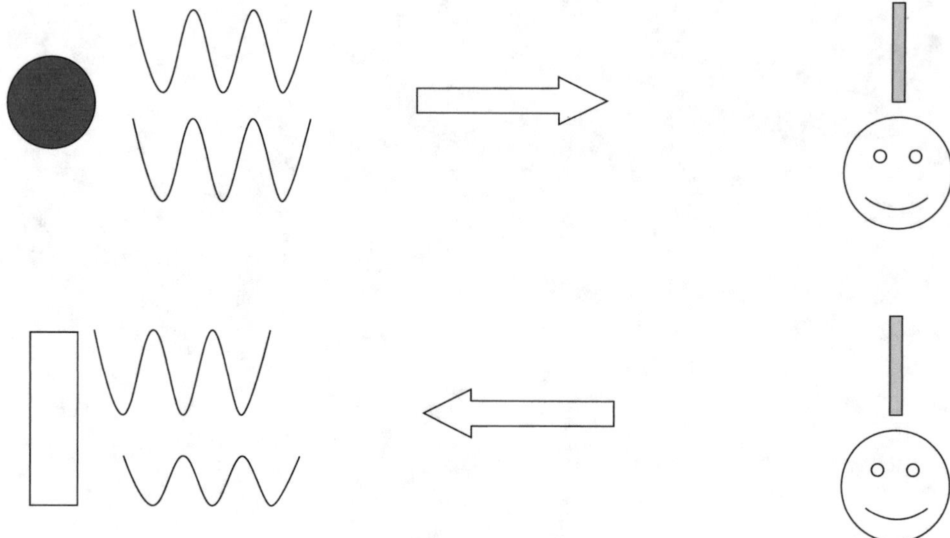

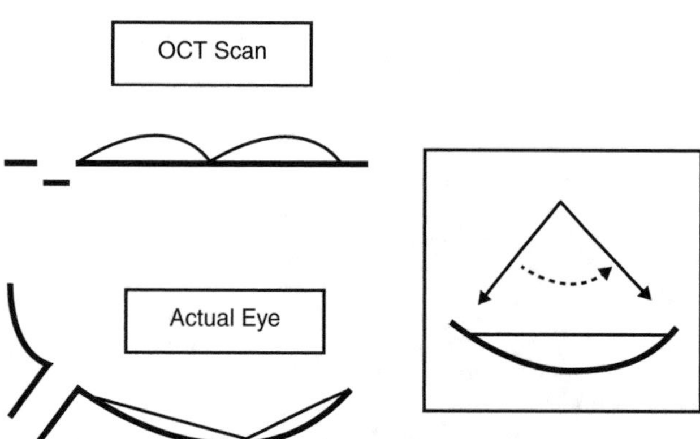

Fig. 1.28 With most OCT scanners the posterior pole of the eye has been falsely flattened, the images should be interpreted with this in mind

Colour Coding (Fig. 1.29)

Fig. 1.29 OCT provides a cross-sectional scan of the macula which provides essential information to diagnose disorders and plan surgery. Colour coding has been replaced by greyscale which is regarded as having better resolution

Fig. 1.29 (continued)

Reflection	
Nil	Black
Low	Green
Mod	Red
High	White

Device	Manufacturer	Technology	Signal wavelength	Scan Speed (A-scans/s)	Axial resolution (µm)	Transverse resolution (µm)	Scanning field	Macular depth range	Focus range (D)
STRATUS OCT™ Optical Coherence Tomography (for comparison)	Carl Zeiss Meditec, Inc.	TD-OCT	820 nm	400	≤10	20	26° × 20.5°	2 mm	
iVue	Optovue	SD-OCT	840 nm	26,000	5	15	21° × 21°	2.3 mm	−15 to 12
Cirrus™ 6000 OCT Optical Coherence Tomography Instrument	Carl Zeiss Meditec, Inc.	SD-OCT	840 nm	100,000	5	15	36° × 30°	2.9 mm	−20 to 20
SPECTRALIS® OCT 2	Heidelberg Engineering, Inc.	SD-OCT	820 nm and 870 nm	85,000		6	55°		
3D OCT-2000	Topcon Medical Systems	SD-OCT	840 nm	50,000	6		12 mm × 9 mm	2.3 mm	−13 to 12
Revo FC	Optopol Technology	SD-OCT	830 nm	80,000	2.6	12–18	5 mm × 12 mm	2.4 mm	−25 to 25
Envisu C2300	Leica	SD-OCT	870 nm	32,000	3		70°	2 mm	
Mirante	Nidek	SD-OCT	880 nm	85,000	7	20	16.5 mm × 12 mm (89°)		−15 to 15

Scan of Normal Features

Frequency-Domain OCT

Unlike TD-OCT, frequency-domain OCT (FD-OCT) generates the axial scan by Fourier transformation of the acquired spectral interference fringes generated by the interaction of the reference and sample arms. Therefore, the reference arm in an FD-OCT does not have to move, allowing dramatically quicker scan acquisition speeds than is possible by TD-OCT.

Spectral-Domain OCT (SD-OCT), also known as Fourier-Domain OCT is based upon the underlying principle of FD-OCT but SD-OCT is able to extract more information in a single scan as it distributes several optical frequencies onto a detector stripe [22].

Time-encoded FD-OCT, also known as Swept-Source OCT (SS-OCT) is again based on FD-OCT. However, unlike Fourier-domain OCT which emits multiple optical frequencies all at once, the Swept-Source OCT emits multiple frequencies in single successive steps. SS-OCT is at present not commercially available but has shown promise in recent studies which have demonstrated significantly improved resolution and image-penetration for imaging structures and pathology deep to the retina because it operates in the 1050 nm wavelength range [23, 24] (Fig. 1.30).

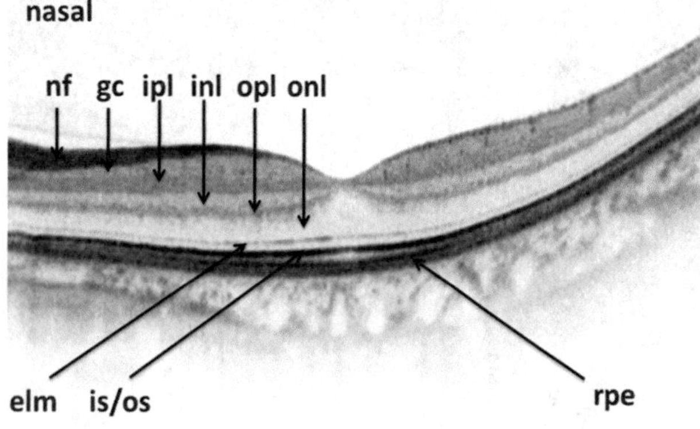

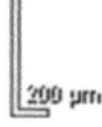

Fig. 1.30 With high-resolution OCT B-scan image of the normal human macula the individual layers of the retina can be seen. Note resolution is usually better with greyscale rendering. *NF* Nerve Fibre Layer, *GC* Ganglion Cell Layer, *IPL* Inner Plexiform Layer, *INL* Inner Nuclear Layer, *OPL* Outer Plexiform Layer, *ONL* Outer Nuclear Layer, *ELM* External Limiting Membrane, *IS/OS* Photoreceptor Inner Segment & Outer Segment Junction (ellipsoid layer); *RPE* Retinal Pigment Epithelium and Inner Choroidal layers

Full-Field OCT

The latest generation OCT is the Full-field OCT (FF-OCT), another version of the TD-OCT, which uses a broadband (white) light source instead of a laser or superluminescent diode [21]. Also known as T-scan (transverse) OCT or en face OCT, it acquires tomographic data by acquiring multiple coronal scans instead of the usual axial scans (A-scans) of previously described TD-OCT [25]. SS-OCT is also capable of this scanning Scheme [26]. The advantage of this method is that it is not only possible to generate B-scans but also C-scans (coronal) alongside a simultaneous, conventional fundus image (coronal plane).

Scan Resolution

Obtaining a scan requires sequential scanning in the form of multiple A-scans for TD-OCT and SD-OCT and C-scans for FF-OCT. The volume of information obtained can be measured in volumetric pixels (voxels) [26]. Increasing the number of voxels captured can be achieved by either increasing the scanning frequency rate, using multiple detector arrays or both [22, 26]. Commercially available SD-OCT scanners became available in early 2006 and most have imaging speeds of 25,000 axial scans per second with an axial resolution of between 5 and 7 microns. Technological optimisation of these variables has produced OCT scanners that achieve up to 250,000 axial scans per second whilst maintaining axial resolution at 8–9 microns thus yielding more than 100 megavoxels [26]. Clinically, this translates into a high-resolution macular scan in 1.3 s or even the potential to measure blood flow velocities in vessels as narrow as 13.64 μm [27, 28]. Higher scanning speeds are less likely to suffer from motion artefact [29]. Signal strength is the measure of the amount of reflected light received by the scanner. It is graded to serve as a proxy measure of scan quality. A signal strength of at least 7 should be aimed for in order to obtain consistently accurate results [30, 31]. High scan rates can reduce signal strengths to below this number [26].

Images and Measurements

Software-controlled scanning protocols translate voxel datasets into clinically representative images and are numerous. Post-scan software processing also determines surface segmentations like the internal limiting membrane (ILM) and retinal pigment epithelium (RPE) amongst others and assigns a false colour to each layer depending on the signal reflectance. However, grayscale and proportion-corrected OCT images reveal a finer gradation of signal reflectance and can be used to demonstrate additional information not present in false-colour images [32]. Software outlining of the ILM is necessary for calculation of retinal thickness, however, it has been shown to be inaccurate in up to 19% of scans [33]. Hence new algorithms are being constantly developed to overcome these short-falls [33–35]. Results depended more on the algorithm used than the hardware, emphasizing the need for robust software [36]. The clinician should check the image used in analysis because artefacts exist (43.2% in one study, with 30% requiring manual remeasurement due to spurious central point thickness (CPT)) [37].

Performing the Scan

The rapid, non-contact, non-invasive nature of OCT scanning lends itself to the busy vitreoretinal clinic.

- Obtaining an OCT image requires mydriasis to ensure an artefact-free scan. Non-mydriatic scanning is possible but may result in vignetting of the macular scan as the edges of the sample beam are clipped by the pupillary margin. If it is not possible to dilate the patient, then scanning in a dark environment would reduce this phenomenon as most OCT scanners use near-infrared light which does not induce papillary constriction.
- The macula is visualised on the monitor and the area of interest aligned with the aid of fixation targets. It is useful to ensure the patient blinks several times prior to acquiring the scan to ensure an even tear film. Even the presence of contact lenses can affect retinal nerve fibre layer thickness measurements [38]. Dense media opacities will degrade image quality though OCT is able to quite effectively penetrate most cataracts, asteroid hyalosis, and vitritis. Mathematical models have been developed to improve the quality of these degraded images [39], however, the experienced examiner is usually still able to discern sufficient detail in most cases.

Macular Scan Patterns

- Radial scans, "spokes of a wheel" centred on the fovea.
- Raster, parallel lines creating a "square".
- Single high-resolution line scans.

On the "fast-macular thickness map" protocol with TD-OCT scanning, 6 radial sampling scans of the macula are acquired, and a macular topographical colour-coded map of the macula is produced. The software interpolates adjacent thickness values in the interspersing macular areas which lie between the 6 radial scans. Clinicians should therefore be aware of small lesions suspected to lie within these areas as they may fail to be picked up with this protocol. This is not an issue with the newer SD-OCT, which acquires a raster series of high-resolution images [29].

Central Retinal Thickness

Central retinal thickness, CRT, is the simplest measure to use and has been quoted in numerous studies. CRT was compared between 6 commercially available OCT scanners in a study involving healthy eyes and a variation of between 0.45% and 3.33% was found. The discrepancies were explained by the slightly different segmentation algorithms employed by each device [40]. In effect, this means that the line which the software uses to determine the outer retinal boundary differs and so different OCT systems should not be used interchangeably [40, 41].

Inner Segment and Outer Segment Junction and External Limiting Membrane

The predominant contribution to this "outer red line" is by the Bruch's membrane and inner choroid with a smaller contribution by the RPE [20]. Of particular interest is the band correlating to the junction of the inner and outer segments (IS/OS) of the photoreceptors. This is better visualised as a red line just inner to the outer red line (ORL) on the higher resolution SD-OCT. The IS/OS band is a high-reflectance signal at this junction resulting from the abrupt change in the refractive index stemming from the highly organised stacks of membranous disks in the photoreceptor outer segments [16]. Optical coherence tomographic changes in this area have been studied in a number of conditions and visual acuity has been significantly correlated with OCT detection of the IS/OS junction in retinitis pigmentosa [42], macula-off retinal detachments [43], full-thickness macular holes [44–46], central serous chorioretinopathy [47], age-related macular degeneration [41], and macular oedema associated with branch retinal vein occlusions [48, 49].

The external limiting membrane (ELM) appears to show prognostic promise [43]. In a series of consecutive retinal detachments (RD), IS/OS disruption was observed in macula-off eyes. As predicted, postoperative VA was significantly correlated with IS/OS integrity. None of the eyes with preoperative disruption of ELM and IS/OS regained postoperative IS/OS integrity. In contrast, 7 of 11 eyes that had intact ELM on OCT preoperatively regained the IS/OS junction during follow-up [43].

The inner retina has moderate reflectance, receptors low reflectance, and the RPE shows high scatter from melanin. The laser is thereafter blocked and no information from the choroid is usually obtained. Measurements of the tissues in the z-axis are possible to quantify retinal thickness and volume.

OCT is useful for a variety of macular disorders such as macular holes, cystoid macular oedema, epiretinal membranes, and choroidal neovascular membranes and in retinoschisis in myopes and optic disc anomalies. In macular holes, OCT is used for detection, differentiation from pseudo and lamellar holes, and for staging. OCT can be used for detection and monitoring of the cystoid macular oedema (CMO) in diabetes, retinal vein occlusion, and in uveitis, and for identifying vitreomacular traction (Figs. 1.31 and 1.32).

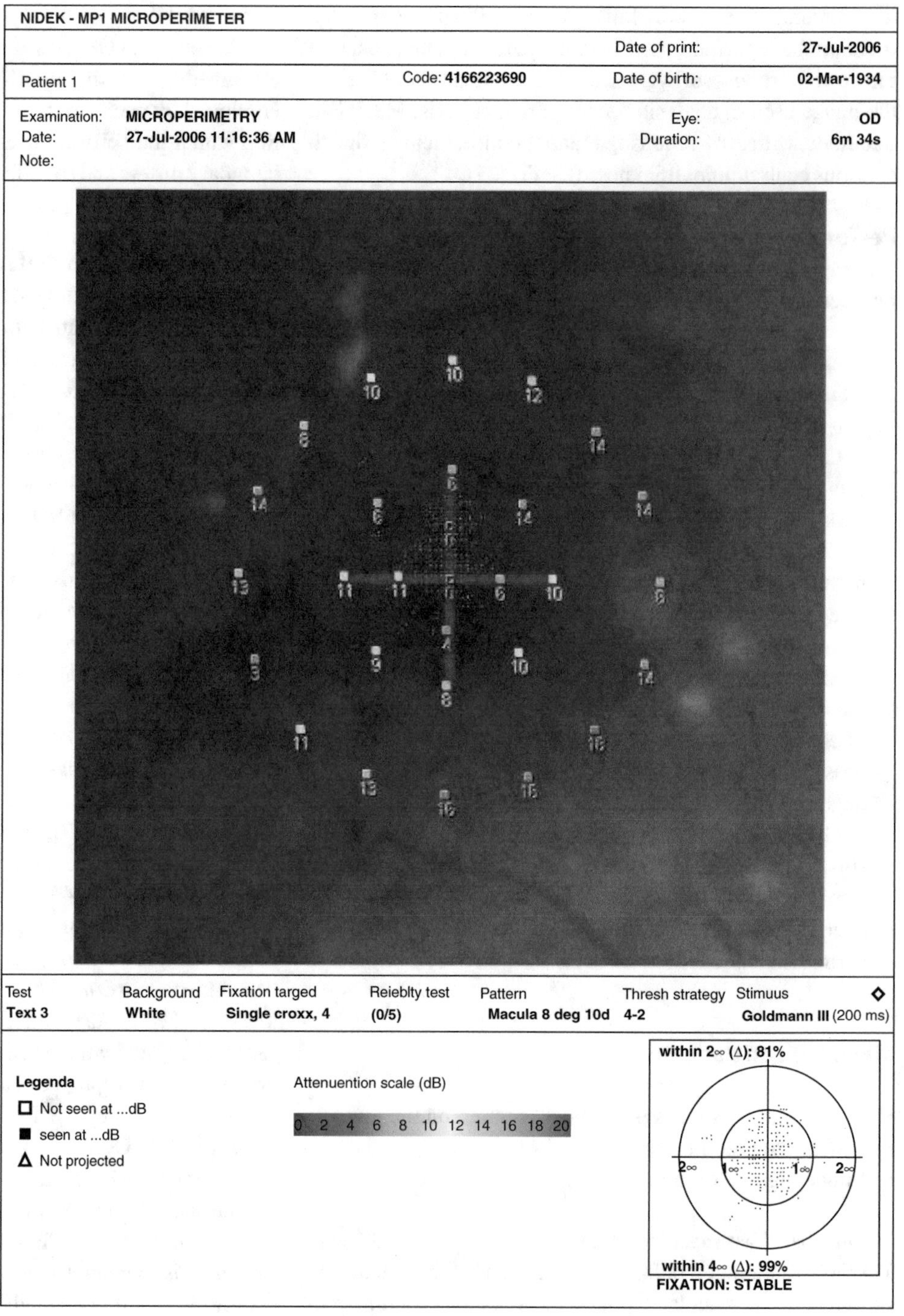

Fig. 1.31 Microperimetry is a useful tool to determine the fixation of the eye and detect localised loss of vision in the macula

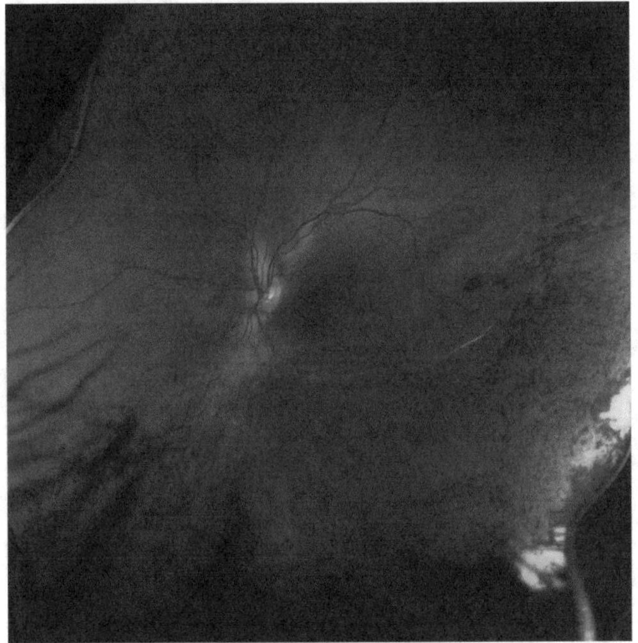

Fig. 1.32 In primary care wide-angle laser imaging systems are sometimes used to view the retina. There are pigmentary changes in the periphery where a retinal detachment has reattached

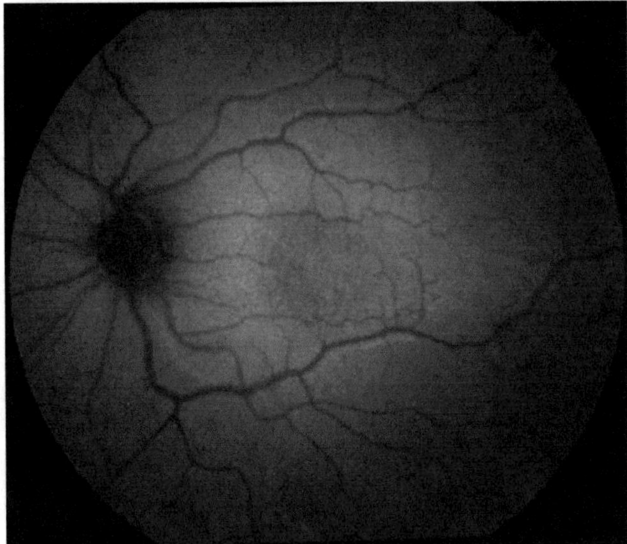

Fig. 1.33 Shift of the retina seen on autofluorescence

Subjective Tests

The vitreoretinal patient often complains of symptoms that are related to the dysfunction of the macula such as distortion and change in image size. At present the methods available to assess these are limited. Amsler charts can be used at the most basic level to determine distortion. The Watzke Allen test (see Chap. 8) is used to discriminate macular holes from pseudo holes or partial-thickness holes in the fovea (Fig. 1.33).

The Preoperative Assessment

Every patient should be thoroughly examined before surgery, at most two weeks before surgery. The situation with vitreoretinal conditions can change rapidly, e.g. the development of proliferative vitreoretinopathy in rhegmatogenous retinal detachment. Make sure you know the status of the vitreous preoperatively, i.e. is it attached or detached (perform ultrasound when there are medial opacities). Biometry for lens implantation is useful in case a cataract extraction is required unexpectedly during surgery. Use information sheets (see DVD for examples). Make sure the patient is realistic about outcomes and the risks for reoperation. Help them with the choice of anaesthesia. Mark the forehead on the side of the eye to be operated upon on the day of surgery with an indelible marker pen (Table 1.2).

Table 1.2 Advantages and disadvantages of anaesthesia

Types of anaesthesia		Advantages	Disadvantages
General		Complete control of the eye during surgery No peroperative stress for the patient Allows peroperative examination of the fellow eye Patient does not hear surgeons' conversation during training	Risk to general health Longer recovery for the patient postoperatively May require inpatient admission
Local anaesthesia	All	Day case surgery Minimal risk to general health	Patient stress levels Patient aware of conversations during training
	Peribulbar	Minimal soft tissue injury More effective anaesthesia and akinesia	Risk of globe perforation Difficult to top up during surgery Patient may see an instrument close to the retina if the optic nerve is not blocked
	Subtenon's cannula	Minimal risk of globe rupture Can be applied after draping Can be topped up Projects anteriorly deep-set globes for easier surgical access	Less effective anaesthesia and akinesia Poor application leads to conjunctival chemosis

Summary

A working knowledge of the anatomy of the retina is of great importance to the surgeon. Learn to examine the eye to a high standard and obtain the basic investigational skills of ocular ultrasonography and optical coherence tomography.

References

1. Stefansson E, Landers MB III, Wolbarsht ML. Vitrectomy, lensectomy, and ocular oxygenation. Retina. 1982;2(3):159–66.
2. Xu J, Heys JJ, Barocas VH, Randolph TW. Permeability and diffusion in vitreous humor: implications for drug delivery. Pharm Res. 2000;17(6):664–9.
3. Repetto R, Siggers JH, Stocchino A. Mathematical model of flow in the vitreous humor induced by saccadic eye rotations: effect of geometry. Biomech Model Mechanobiol. 2010;9(1):65–76. https://doi.org/10.1007/s10237-009-0159-0.
4. Stefansson E. Ocular oxygenation and the treatment of diabetic retinopathy. Surv Ophthalmol. 2006;51(4):364–80. S0039-6257(06)00078-6 [pii]. https://doi.org/10.1016/j.survophthal.2006.04.005.
5. Williamson TH, Harris A. Ocular blood flow measurement. Br J Ophthalmol. 1994;78(12):939–45.
6. Shui YB, Holekamp NM, Kramer BC, Crowley JR, Wilkins MA, Chu F, et al. The gel state of the vitreous and ascorbate-dependent oxygen consumption: relationship to the etiology of nuclear cataracts. Arch Ophthalmol. 2009;127(4):475–82. 127/4/475 [pii]. https://doi.org/10.1001/archophthalmol.2008.621.
7. Holekamp NM, Shui YB, Beebe DC. Vitrectomy surgery increases oxygen exposure to the lens: a possible mechanism for nuclear cataract formation. Am J Ophthalmol. 2005;139(2):302–10. S0002-9394(04)01147-X [pii]. https://doi.org/10.1016/j.ajo.2004.09.046.
8. Holekamp NM, Shui YB, Beebe D. Lower intraocular oxygen tension in diabetic patients: possible contribution to decreased incidence of nuclear sclerotic cataract. Am J Ophthalmol. 2006;141(6):1027–32.
9. Winter M, Eberhardt W, Scholz C, Reichenbach A. Failure of potassium siphoning by Muller cells: a new hypothesis of perfluorocarbon liquid-induced retinopathy. Invest Ophthalmol Vis Sci. 2000;41(1):256–61.
10. Bishop PN, Holmes DF, Kadler KE, McLeod D, Bos KJ. Age-related changes on the surface of vitreous collagen fibrils. Invest Ophthalmol Vis Sci. 2004;45(4):1041–6.
11. Itakura H, Kishi S, Kotajima N, Murakami M. Vitreous collagen metabolism before and after vitrectomy. Graefes Arch Clin Exp Ophthalmol. 2005;243(10):994–8. https://doi.org/10.1007/s00417-005-1150-9.
12. Schepens CL. A new ophthalmoscope demonstration. Trans Am Ophthalmol Soc. 1947;51:298–304.
13. Wong AD, Cooperberg PL, Ross WH, Araki DN. Differentiation of detached retina and vitreous membrane with color flow Doppler. Radiology. 1991;178(2):429–31.
14. Huang D, Swanson EA, Lin CP, Schuman JS, Stinson WG, Chang W, et al. Optical coherence tomography. Science. 1991;254(5035):1178–81.
15. Hee MR, Izatt JA, Swanson EA, Huang D, Schuman JS, Lin CP, et al. Optical coherence tomography of the human retina. Arch Ophthalmol. 1995;113(3):325–32.
16. Chan A, Duker JS, Ishikawa H, Ko TH, Schuman JS, Fujimoto JG. Quantification of photoreceptor layer thickness in normal eyes using optical coherence tomography. Retina. 2006;26(6):655–60. 00006982-200607000-00011 [pii]. https://doi.org/10.1097/01.iae.0000236468.33325.74.
17. Hoang QV, Linsenmeier RA, Chung CK, Curcio CA. Photoreceptor inner segments in monkey and human retina: mitochondrial density, optics, and regional variation. Vis Neurosci. 2002;19(4):395–407.
18. Gloesmann M, Hermann B, Schubert C, Sattmann H, Ahnelt PK, Drexler W. Histologic correlation of pig retina radial stratification with ultrahigh-resolution optical coherence tomography. Invest Ophthalmol Vis Sci. 2003;44(4):1696–703.
19. Chauhan DS, Marshall J. The interpretation of optical coherence tomography images of the retina. Invest Ophthalmol Vis Sci. 1999;40(10):2332–42.
20. Ghazi NG, Dibernardo C, Ying HS, Mori K, Gehlbach PL. Optical coherence tomography of enucleated human eye specimens with histological correlation: origin of the outer "red line". Am J Ophthalmol. 2006;141(4):719–26. S0002-9394(05)01106-2 [pii]. https://doi.org/10.1016/j.ajo.2005.10.019.
21. Sacchet D, Moreau J, Georges P, Dubois A. Simultaneous dual-band ultra-high resolution full-field optical coherence tomography. Opt Express. 2008;16(24):19434–46. 174457 [pii]
22. Bourquin S, Seitz P, Salathe RP. Optical coherence topography based on a two-dimensional smart detector array. Opt Lett. 2001;26(8):512–4. 63959 [pii]
23. Yasuno Y, Miura M, Kawana K, Makita S, Sato M, Okamoto F, et al. Visualization of sub-retinal pigment epithelium morphologies of exudative macular diseases by high-penetration optical coherence tomography. Invest Ophthalmol Vis Sci. 2009;50(1):405–13. iovs.08-2272 [pii]. https://doi.org/10.1167/iovs.08-2272.
24. Srinivasan VJ, Adler DC, Chen Y, Gorczynska I, Huber R, Duker JS, et al. Ultrahigh-speed optical coherence tomography for three-dimensional and en face imaging of the retina and optic nerve head. Invest Ophthalmol Vis Sci. 2008;49(11):5103–10. iovs.08-2127 [pii]. https://doi.org/10.1167/iovs.08-2127.
25. Rosen RB, Hathaway M, Rogers J, Pedro J, Garcia P, Laissue P, et al. Multidimensional en-face OCT imaging of the retina. Opt Express. 2009;17(5):4112–33. 177004 [pii]
26. Potsaid B, Gorczynska I, Srinivasan VJ, Chen Y, Jiang J, Cable A, et al. Ultrahigh speed spectral/Fourier domain OCT ophthalmic imaging at 70,000 to 312,500 axial scans per second. Opt Express. 2008;16(19):15149–69. 171960 [pii]
27. Wang RK, An L. Doppler optical micro-angiography for volumetric imaging of vascular perfusion in vivo. Opt Express. 2009;17(11):8926–40. 179889 [pii]
28. Tao YK, Kennedy KM, Izatt JA. Velocity-resolved 3D retinal microvessel imaging using single-pass flow imaging spectral domain optical coherence tomography. Opt Express. 2009;17(5):4177–88. 177008 [pii]
29. Srinivasan VJ, Wojtkowski M, Witkin AJ, Duker JS, Ko TH, Carvalho M, et al. High-definition and 3-dimensional imaging of macular pathologies with high-speed ultrahigh-resolution optical coherence tomography. Ophthalmology. 2006;113(11):2054 e1–14. S0161-6420(06)00731-7 [pii]. https://doi.org/10.1016/j.ophtha.2006.05.046.
30. Wu Z, Vazeen M, Varma R, Chopra V, Walsh AC, LaBree LD, et al. Factors associated with variability in retinal nerve fiber layer thickness measurements obtained by optical coherence tomography. Ophthalmology. 2007;114(8):1505–12. S0161-6420(06)01600-9 [pii]. https://doi.org/10.1016/j.ophtha.2006.10.061.
31. Wu Z, Huang J, Dustin L, Sadda SR. Signal strength is an important determinant of accuracy of nerve fiber layer thickness measurement by optical coherence tomography. J Glaucoma. 2009;18(3):213–6.

https://doi.org/10.1097/IJG.0b013e31817eee20. 00061198-200903000-00010 [pii]

32. Ishikawa H, Gurses-Ozden R, Hoh ST, Dou HL, Liebmann JM, Ritch R. Grayscale and proportion-corrected optical coherence tomography images. Ophthalmic Surg Lasers. 2000;31(3):223–8.
33. Haeker M, Abramoff M, Kardon R, Sonka M. Segmentation of the surfaces of the retinal layer from OCT images. Med Image Comput Comput Assist Interv. 2006;9(Pt 1):800–7.
34. Garvin M, Abramoff M, Wu X, Russell S, Burns T, Sonka M. Automated 3-D intraretinal layer segmentation of macular spectral-domain optical coherence tomography images. IEEE Trans Med Imaging. 2009;28(9):1436–47. https://doi.org/10.1109/TMI.2009.2016958.
35. Sadda SR, Joeres S, Wu Z, Updike P, Romano P, Collins AT, et al. Error correction and quantitative subanalysis of optical coherence tomography data using computer-assisted grading. Invest Ophthalmol Vis Sci. 2007;48(2):839–48. 48/2/839 [pii]. https://doi.org/10.1167/iovs.06-0554.
36. Hood DC, Raza AS, Kay KY, Sandler SF, Xin D, Ritch R, et al. A comparison of retinal nerve fiber layer (RNFL) thickness obtained with frequency and time domain optical coherence tomography (OCT). Opt Express. 2009;17(5):3997–4003. 176995 [pii]
37. Domalpally A, Danis RP, Zhang B, Myers D, Kruse CN. Quality issues in interpretation of optical coherence tomograms in macular diseases. Retina. 2009;29(6):775–81. https://doi.org/10.1097/IAE.0b013e3181a0848b.
38. Youm DJ, Kim JM, Park KH, Choi CY. The effect of soft contact lenses during the measurement of retinal nerve fiber layer thickness using optical coherence tomography. Curr Eye Res. 2009;34(1):78–83. 908191255 [pii]. https://doi.org/10.1080/02713680802579188.
39. Tappeiner C, Barthelmes D, Abegg MH, Wolf S, Fleischhauer JC. Impact of optic media opacities and image compression on quantitative analysis of optical coherence tomography. Invest Ophthalmol Vis Sci. 2008;49(4):1609–14. 49/4/1609 [pii]. https://doi.org/10.1167/iovs.07-1264.
40. Wolf-Schnurrbusch UE, Ceklic L, Brinkmann CK, Iliev ME, Frey M, Rothenbuehler SP, et al. Macular thickness measurements in healthy eyes using six different optical coherence tomography instruments. Invest Ophthalmol Vis Sci. 2009;50(7):3432–7. iovs.08-2970 [pii]. https://doi.org/10.1167/iovs.08-2970.
41. Sayanagi K, Sharma S, Yamamoto T, Kaiser PK. Comparison of spectral-domain versus time-domain optical coherence tomography in management of age-related macular degeneration with ranibizumab. Ophthalmology. 2009;116(5):947–55. S0161-6420(08)01143-3 [pii]. https://doi.org/10.1016/j.ophtha.2008.11.002.
42. Aizawa S, Mitamura Y, Baba T, Hagiwara A, Ogata K, Yamamoto S. Correlation between visual function and photoreceptor inner/outer segment junction in patients with retinitis pigmentosa. Eye. 2009;23(2):304–8. 6703076 [pii]. https://doi.org/10.1038/sj.eye.6703076.
43. Wakabayashi T, Oshima Y, Fujimoto H, Murakami Y, Sakaguchi H, Kusaka S, et al. Foveal microstructure and visual acuity after retinal detachment repair: imaging analysis by Fourier-domain optical coherence tomography. Ophthalmology. 2009;116(3):519–28. S0161-6420(08)01021-X [pii]. https://doi.org/10.1016/j.ophtha.2008.10.001.
44. Sano M, Shimoda Y, Hashimoto H, Kishi S. Restored photoreceptor outer segment and visual recovery after macular hole closure. Am J Ophthalmol. 2009;147(2):313–8 e1. S0002-9394(08)00618-1 [pii]. https://doi.org/10.1016/j.ajo.2008.08.002.
45. Baba T, Yamamoto S, Arai M, Arai E, Sugawara T, Mitamura Y, et al. Correlation of visual recovery and presence of photoreceptor inner/outer segment junction in optical coherence images after successful macular hole repair. Retina. 2008;28(3):453–8. https://doi.org/10.1097/IAE.0b013e3181571398. 00006982-200803000-00009 [pii]
46. Inoue M, Watanabe Y, Arakawa A, Sato S, Kobayashi S, Kadonosono K. Spectral-domain optical coherence tomography images of inner/outer segment junctions and macular hole surgery outcomes. Graefes Arch Clin Exp Ophthalmol. 2009;247(3):325–30. https://doi.org/10.1007/s00417-008-0999-9.
47. Piccolino FC, de la Longrais RR, Ravera G, Eandi CM, Ventre L, Abdollahi A, et al. The foveal photoreceptor layer and visual acuity loss in central serous chorioretinopathy. Am J Ophthalmol. 2005;139(1):87–99. S0002-9394(04)01006-2 [pii]. https://doi.org/10.1016/j.ajo.2004.08.037.
48. Ota M, Tsujikawa A, Murakami T, Yamaike N, Sakamoto A, Kotera Y, et al. Foveal photoreceptor layer in eyes with persistent cystoid macular edema associated with branch retinal vein occlusion. Am J Ophthalmol. 2008;145(2):273–80. S0002-9394(07)00829-X [pii]. https://doi.org/10.1016/j.ajo.2007.09.019.
49. Murakami T, Tsujikawa A, Ohta M, Miyamoto K, Kita M, Watanabe D, et al. Photoreceptor status after resolved macular edema in branch retinal vein occlusion treated with tissue plasminogen activator. Am J Ophthalmol. 2007;143(1):171–3. S0002-9394(06)01014-2 [pii]. https://doi.org/10.1016/j.ajo.2006.08.030.

2 Introduction to Vitreoretinal Surgery 1

Contents

T. H. Williamson, *Vitreoretinal Surgery*, https://doi.org/10.1007/978-3-030-68769-4_2

Introduction

A variety of surgical techniques exist to treat vitreoretinal disorders and the choice of method depends upon the individual surgeon. Pars plana vitrectomy is, however, the most versatile methodology available [1]. Technological advances have improved the applicability of the operation extending its role in ophthalmology [2] (Figs. 2.1, 2.2, 2.3).

Before starting the operation run through the usual surgical preoperative checks:

Do you have the correct patient?	Check the notes and the patient
Do you have the correct operation?	Check the notes for the pathology, intended operation, and the dates of the clinical entries.
Do you have the correct eye?	Check the notes and the eye to be operated upon, tape down the other eye (some surgeons like to put a plastic eye shield over the fellow eye to avoid putting pressure on this eye during surgery) and check the preoperative marking for the eye to be operated.

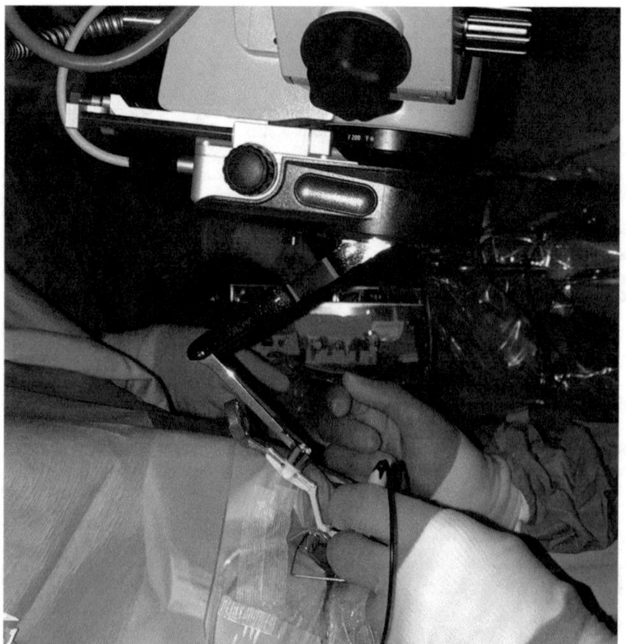

Fig. 2.1 A typical set up for an IVS for surgery

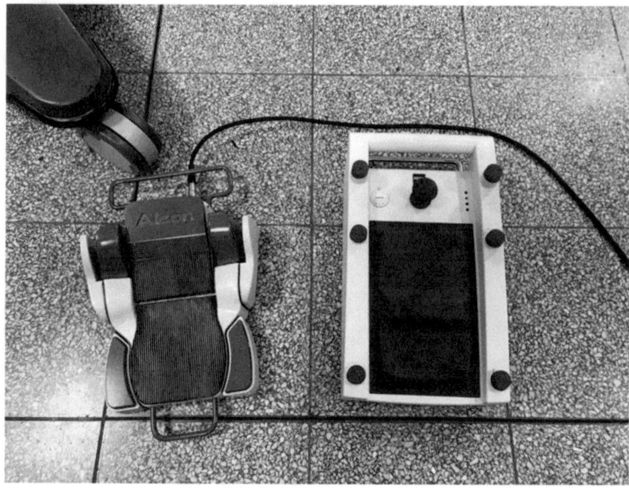

Fig. 2.2 A footpedal set up for surgery

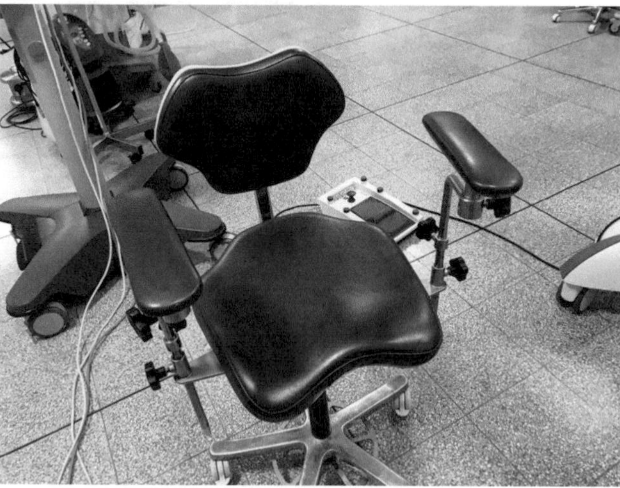

Fig. 2.3 Use a seat with armrests at the correct height for you to rest your elbows on

Confirm the pupils have been dilated. Warn the theatre staff of the need for any special instrumentation or medications. Now, look at the set-up of the operating table and the position of the patient on it.

Note: I previously used wrist rests but had the experience of one slipping and my hand moving and the instrument touching the retina. Now I tend to rest my elbows on the arms of a chair. In that case if the arm of the chair slips, I have time to react and prevent movement of the intraocular instrument.

Keep the eye as close to your body as possible during surgery preventing any leaning on your part which leads to backache. Adjust the operator's seat height to allow a straight back and legs bent under the table in comfortable reach of the foot pedals, weight resting on the heels to allow easy mobility of the forefoot. Use elbow rests, especially when embarking on long operating sessions.

I prefer the microscope pedal on the dominant foot as the X–Y control is the most actively used function during surgery. This leaves the vitrectomy pedal on the other foot. Set up the vitrectomy equipment with 300–600 mmHg vacuum, 5000–15,000 cuts per minute vitrectomy, and the infusion pressure 25–35 mmHg. Smaller gauge instrumentation is now routinely used in many institutions. There are subtle differences in surgical technique with these methods, which will be described later in the chapter.

If you are using a 3D television set up such as the Ngenuity then you can relax more in the chair though there are problems with twisting to see the screen.

Choice of Anaesthesia

The anaesthesia for the operation is down to personal preference and circumstance but both general anaesthesia and local anaesthesia are appropriate. To minimise conjunctival manipulation, I favour peribulbar anaesthesia (extraconal sharp needle injection) before draping (with a top up of subtenon's anaesthesia if the conjunctiva has been opened). In 23, 25, and 27 gauge where the conjunctiva is not opened using peribulbar anaesthesia avoids any significant conjunctival wounds. I inject 6 mls of Lidocaine 2% without Adrenaline (you can mix with Bupivacaine 0.75% for a longer-lasting effect). The site of injection is 2/3 of the way laterally from the inner canthus. Insert the needle percutaneously trying to follow the orbital floor without hitting the periosteum. I slightly waggle the needle tip as I go and watch the eye for any movement. This is to check that I am not hitting Sclera. You must make sure you are deep enough to penetrate the orbital septum. Drawback to make sure you are not in a blood vessel and then inject. If the effect is not reaching the superior rectus an additional injection of 2 mls can be made supero nasally. Be careful of the nasociliary artery which passes in this area and is the continuation of the ophthalmic artery.

General advice is not to do a sharp injection on eyes with 26 mm or more axial length. In that case, do a Subtenon's injection. This is performed inferonasally with a cut down with spring scissors through conjunctiva and Tenons. Insert a blunt curved cannula, follow the sclera back into the intraconal space and inject 3–4 mls of anaesthesia.

A good retrobulbar (sharp needle injection into the intraconal space) gives incredibly good anaesthesia and immobilisation of the eye and is still used in many centres but does run an increased risk of globe perforation.

The patient may be given sedation intravenously under anaesthetic supervision to block out memory of the procedure and to reduce anxiety. This runs the risk, however, that the patient falls asleep and on awakening may move their head, which is potentially problematic if you are starting an internal limiting membrane (ILM) peel or other delicate procedure. In most circumstances local anaesthesia is satisfactory; however, some patients do not enjoy the experience. Anaesthetic blockade of the relatively large optic nerve is not consistent so that some patients may visualise instrumentation in the eye during surgery, especially when it is close to the retina and therefore in focus with only 10% having a total loss of vision [3]. Most patients find this experience interesting rather than frightening (6% the latter).

Note: With local anaesthesia, I tape the forehead of the patient to the headrest to prevent upward movement of the patient and minimise rotation of the head. Patients instinctively turn their heads away from the side of the operated eye. This can lead to pooling of fluid in the nasal conjunctiva and poorer visualisation during surgery. Taping acts as a physical reminder to the patient that they need to stay still.

General anaesthesia is useful for very prolonged operations, when training surgeons, for young patients or patients with anxiety and those with poor communication.

Patients can be treated as a day case without overnight stay. Many surgeons will review the next day although same day review has been described [4]. Next day review is primarily for measuring the intraocular pressure either high from the gas bubble or low from small incision surgery. A few will review in 2 weeks only. I prefer to see either on the next day or within the first 5 days depending on the severity of the case. A phone call on the first day is helpful for informing the patient about the operation, e.g. gas insertion, and for communication of any postoperative instructions (Fig. 2.4).

Pars Plana Vitrectomy

Prepare the eye with dilute povidone-iodine and topical anaesthetic onto the conjunctiva:

1. Drape and insert a lid speculum.
2. Incise the sclerotomies (with the trochars on the stents) at 45 degrees circumferential to the corneo-scleral limbus and remove the stents.
3. Secure the infusion cannula and check its penetration into the vitreous cavity.
4. Insert the endo-illumination and focus on the viewing system.

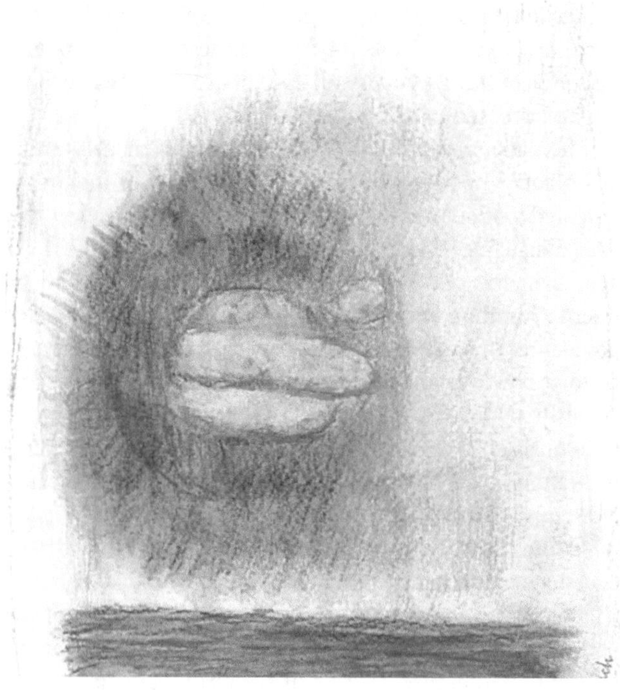

Fig. 2.4 A patients drawing of their visual experience during vitrectomy surgery under local anaesthesia for macular hole

Table 2.1 Typical vitrectomy cutter settings

Modality	Low-speed cutter	High-speed cutter
Infusion	20–30 mmHg (26–39 cmH_2O)	20–30 mmHg (26–39 cmH_2O)
Cutter rate	5000 cpm	15,000 cpm
Vacuum	300 mmHg	600 mmHg

5. Insert vitrectomy cutter and excise the vitreous.
6. Take as much vitreous as possible.
7. Search the retina for iatrogenic or pre-existing breaks with endo-illumination and indentation.
8. Remove the superior trochars, rub down the sclerotomies to seal them.
9. Check for leaks.
10. Remove the infusion trochar, rub down and check for a leak.

This is the most performed operation in modern vitreoretinal practice and the second commonest intra-ocular ophthalmic operation in the USA. Variations in technique with different gauge instrumentation will be described later in the chapter. The basic operation is described here with additional manoeuvres explained in the following chapters. In most centres, a three-port approach is used, one sclerotomy for an infusion cannula and two used alternately for a light pipe and a surgical instrument of varying sorts.

For draping and sterility follow the usual processes. A lid speculum is inserted (Table 2.1).

Sclerotomies

Where to Place the Trochars?

The trochars should be placed 4 mm from the corneo-scleral limbus in the phakic eye and 3.5 mm in the aphakic or pseudophakic eye. None of the trochars should be placed on the horizontal meridian where they would damage the long ciliary arteries and nerves.

Start with the infusion sclerotomy. This is created in the inferotemporal quadrant just below the horizontal meridian. This sclerotomy should not be too inferior where it will tend to knock against the lid speculum restricting movement of the eye inferiorly during searches of the retina. Theoretically, the incisions are best made circumferentially to the limbus because of the orientation of the scleral collagen fibres. The trochars are best inserted at a shallow angle to the surface for 2 mm to allow a self-sealing wound at the end of surgery (Figs. 2.5 and 2.6).

Creating a Self-Sealing Sclerotomy

Wounds and Tissue Manipulation

The surgeon should carefully consider certain principles when creating an incision. Wounds can be created in relatively stiff tissues or in relatively soft and malleable tissues: different principles may apply.

A wound perpendicular to the surface of the tissue in any rigid structure is inherently unstable because pressure on any of the surfaces of the tissue will allow sliding of the wound causing an opening to appear. Most wounds in the eye are required to maintain the intraocular fluid contents, therefore any opening risks leakage of the intraocular fluids, causing a drop in intraocular pressure and risking complications. By sloping the wound, 2 of the surfaces become more stable, in addition, a greater surface area is created within the wound producing more friction and prevent sliding. This configuration, however, is still open to instability from pressure on the 2 remaining surfaces. We will see later how the use of a narrow wound can be used to make a sloped wound stable. A partially angled and vertical wound may also incur the same advantages and disadvantages. However, by using a partial vertical profile the length of the wound can be shortened whilst still obtaining the advantage of some stability (Figs. 2.7, 2.8, 2.9).

A Chevron wound, sloping in two different directions is inherently stable, because pressure on all 4 surfaces cannot open the wound. In addition, the cross-sectional area of the wound is again increased whilst keeping the overall area of tissue disruption to a minimum. A disadvantage is that these wounds are difficult to suture satisfactorily should some instability be found (Fig. 2.10).

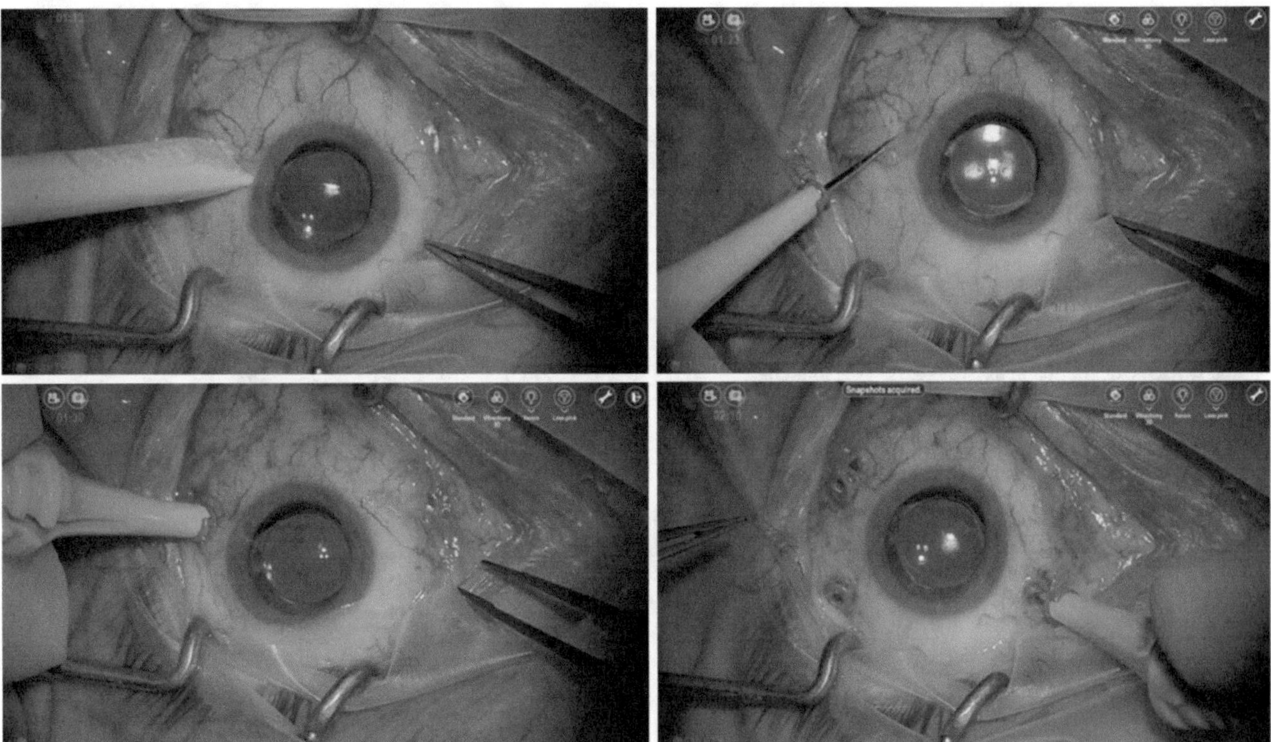

Fig. 2.5 Insert the inferotemporal trochar first, measuring 3.5–4 mm from the limbus. Angle at 45 degrees to create a sloped wound. With valved trochars, all three can be inserted before attaching the infusion line

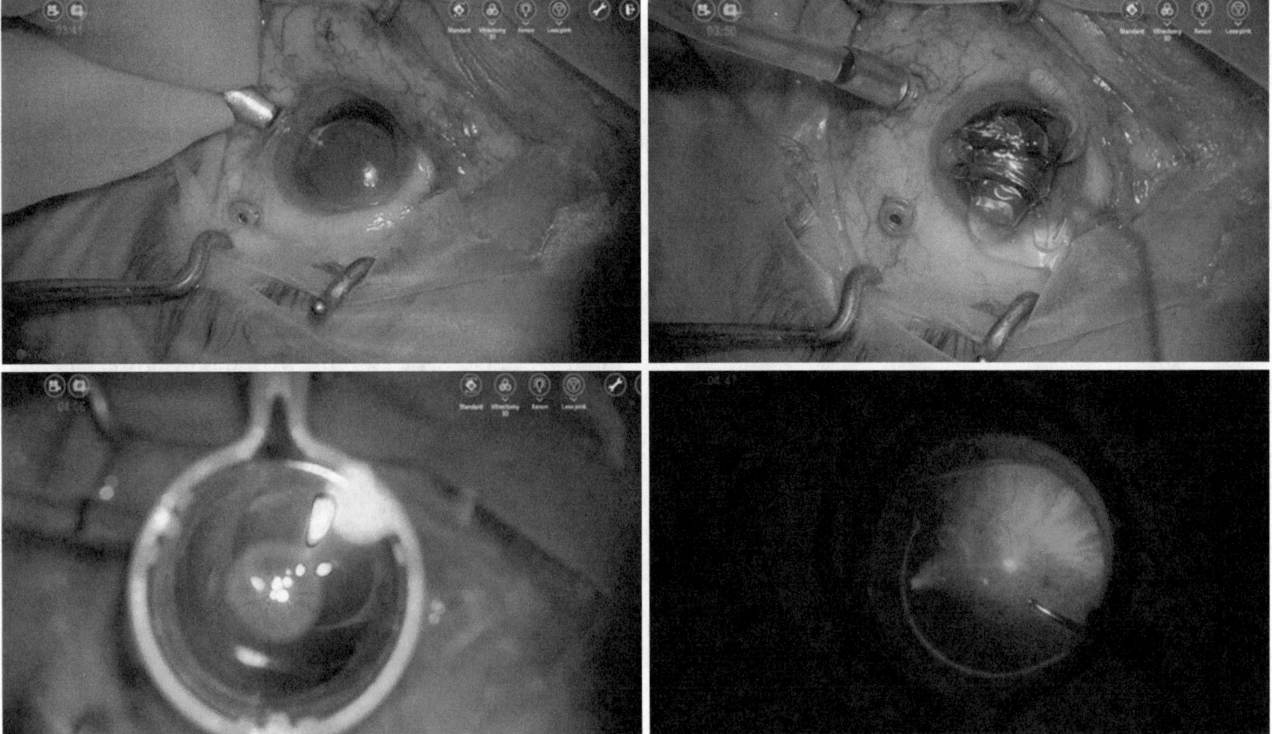

Fig. 2.6 Check the infusion needle has penetrated all of the layers of the eye-wall. Apply Hydroxymethlycellulose (HPMC) to the cornea, rotate in the IVS lens, insert the light fibre-optic, focus, and commence the vitrectomy

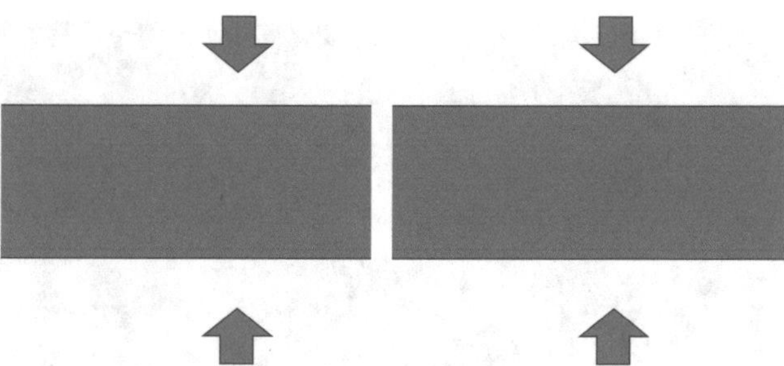

Fig. 2.7 A vertical perpendicular wound is unstable because pressure on 4 locations (arrows) can cause movement and because the area of the wound surface (for friction in the wound) is at the minimum

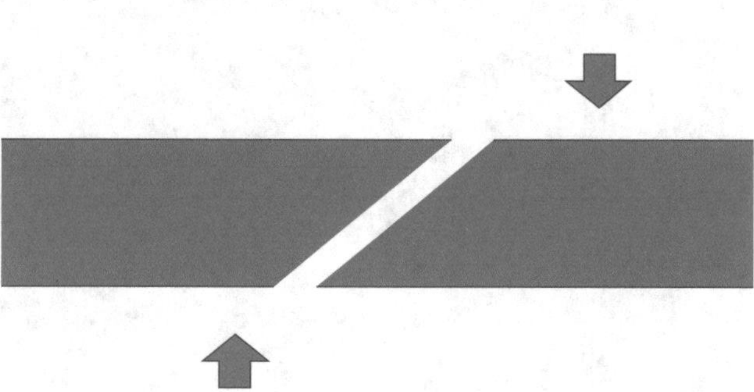

Fig. 2.8 A diagonal wound is only destabilised by pressure on two locations and increases the surface area of the wound

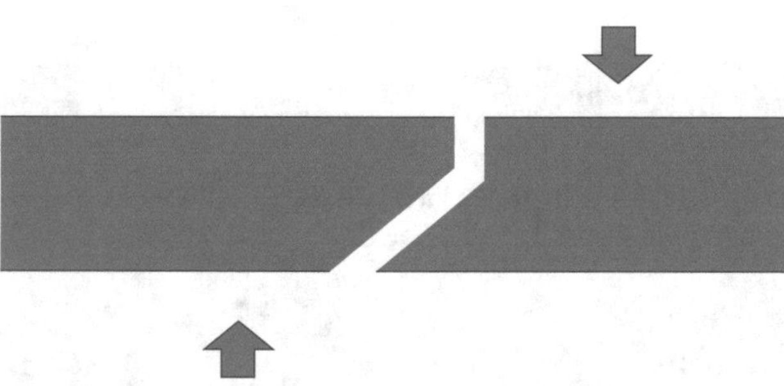

Fig. 2.9 A partially sloped wound can achieve some of the advantages of sloped wound and may be easier to suture

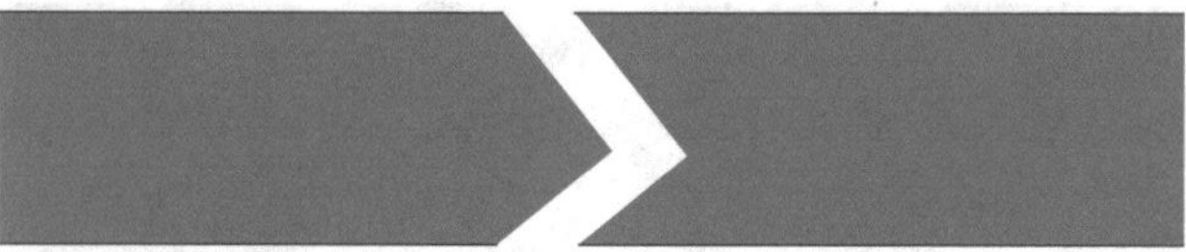

Fig. 2.10 A chevron-shaped wound is stable in all directions

When dealing with the eye most of the surfaces are not flat but are curved. Despite this, essentially the same principles apply with instability of wounds perpendicular to the curve and increased stability when the wounds are shelved into the curve (Figs. 2.11 and 2.12).

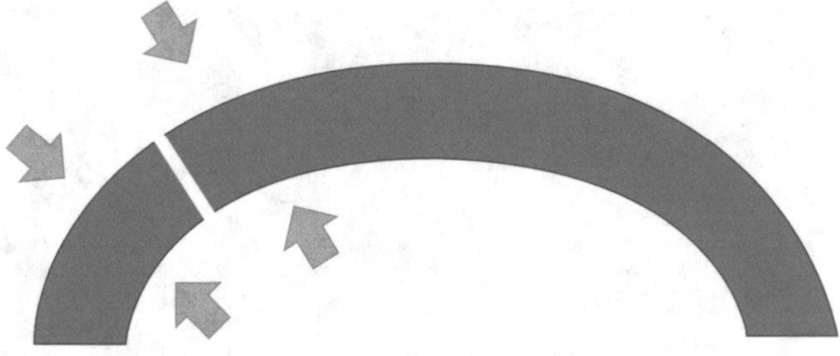

Fig. 2.11 The perpendicular wound is unstable in a curved tissue

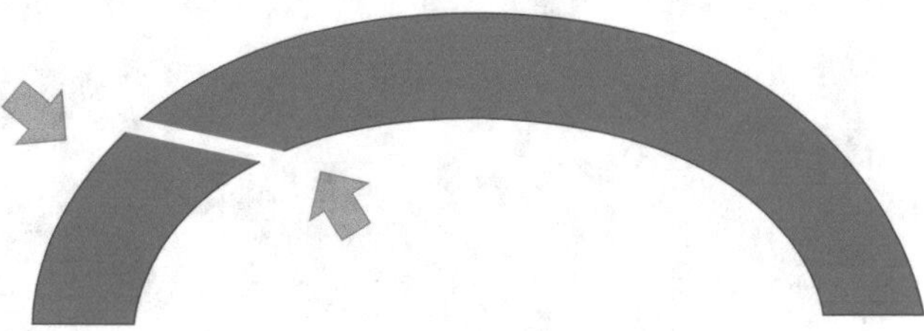

Fig. 2.12 The sloped wound is more stable

Wounds, however, do not exist only in 2 dimensions, and the 3D profile of the wound also affects its stability. A simple shelved wound is often used in anterior segment surgery. This will not usually require suturing. Note that an incision, which you believe is straight, may in fact be curved because of the way the tissue moves ahead of the blade in the tissue, following the spherical shape of the structures of the eye.

There are two orifices, which must open, internal and external. A tangential line can be drawn from the fixed ends of the wound at the external orifice when looking at the wound *en face*, if this line does not cross the internal orifice, it is very difficult for the internal and external orifices to open simultaneously without an external force (e.g. the surgeon actively opening the wound). Therefore, a narrow, long-shelved wound in a spherical object is very stable, explaining why anterior segment wounds can be left unsutured in cataract surgery. If the wound is made too wide and not long enough, the tangential line from the fixed points of the external curve will cross the internal curve and it is very easy for the wound to separate opening the internal orifice and leaking intraocular fluids. We will see later how a simple suturing technique will reposition the tangential line and re-stabilise the wound (Figs. 2.13, 2.14, 2.15, 2.16, 2.17, 2.18, 2.19, 2.20, 2.21, 2.22, 2.23, 2.24).

Securing the Infusion Cannula

Once inserted make sure that the infusion cannula is secure and unlikely to disengage or move position because movement of the cannula can cause several problems:

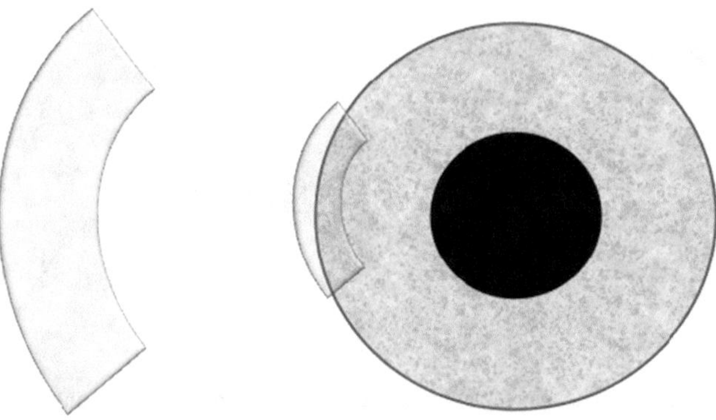

Fig. 2.13 Wounds in the eye are also influenced by their width and length

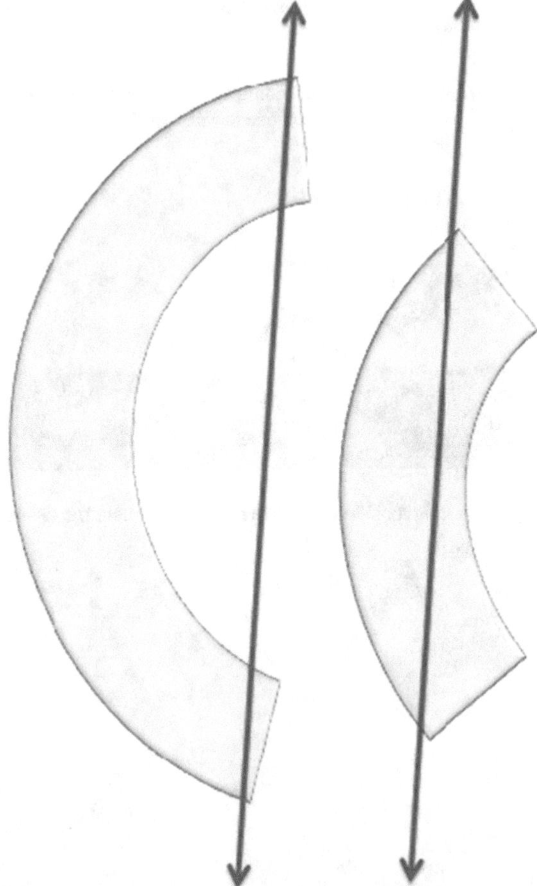

Fig. 2.14 A wound needs to rotate along a line from the corners of its outer incision to open. If the line crosses within the arc of the inner incision (left) the wound will leak. If the line does not cross within the inner arc it will be secure. Sloped, tangential wounds are often used in the globe. The angle of the slope can be varied but the curvature of the eye must be considered. If the angle is too shallow there is a risk that the incision will not enter the eye. Even if the eye is entered, the long track of the incision risks injury to delicate intraocular structures. A steeper incision, however, risks creating a wound, which is less stable. Therefore, a short wound is hard to seal but has a low chance of tissue injury whereas a long wound is easy to seal but has a high chance of tissue injury. In fact, an angled wound may have a curved profile and not a straight one because of its interaction with the tissue during its creation. Be careful about rotating, an instrument within the tissue to increase the angle, because this may tear the tissue internally and any structures within. Therefore, any change in angulation of an instrument while still in the tissue should be kept to a minimum

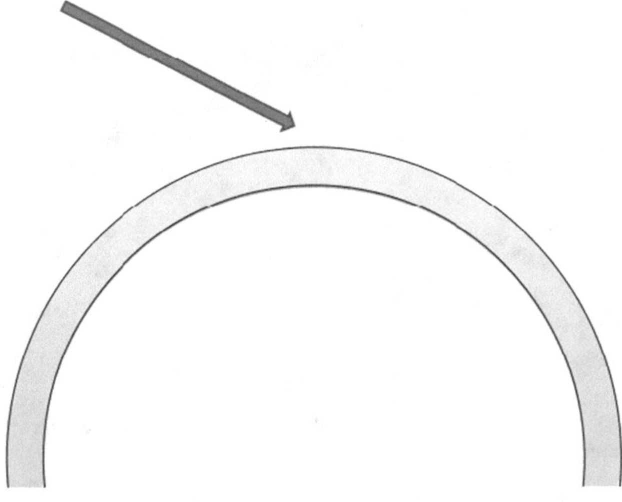

Fig. 2.15 If the angle of insertion is to shallow there is a risk that the blade not to penetrate the eye, see below

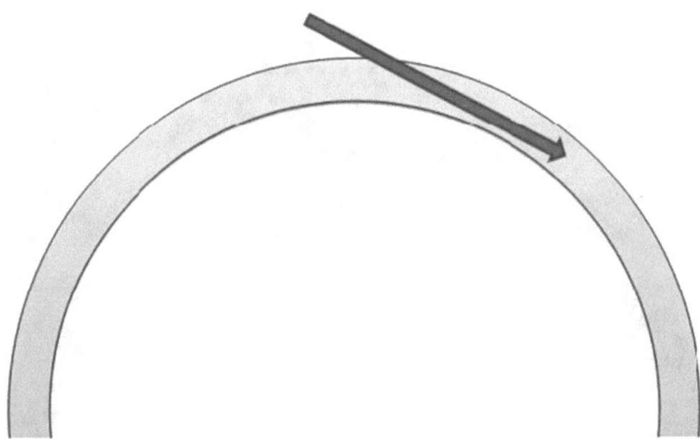

Fig. 2.16 The blade remains in the sclera

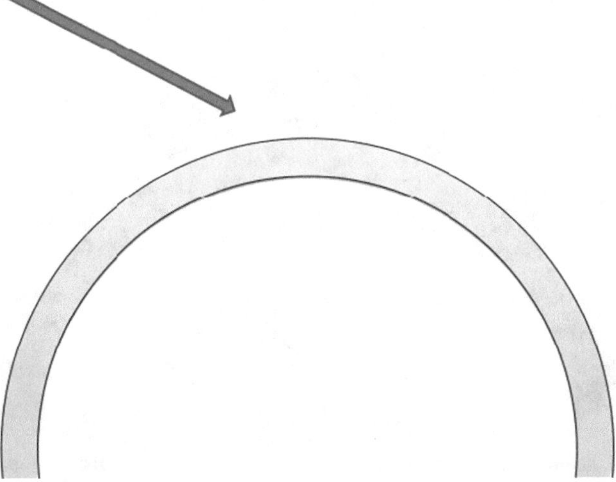

Fig. 2.17 Care has been taken to avoid damage to the internal curvature of the structure by inserting the instrument too far

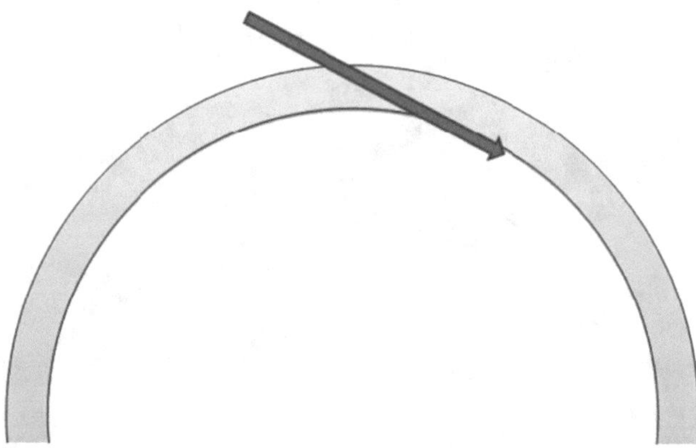

Fig. 2.18 The blade penetrates the sclera but can damage internal structures

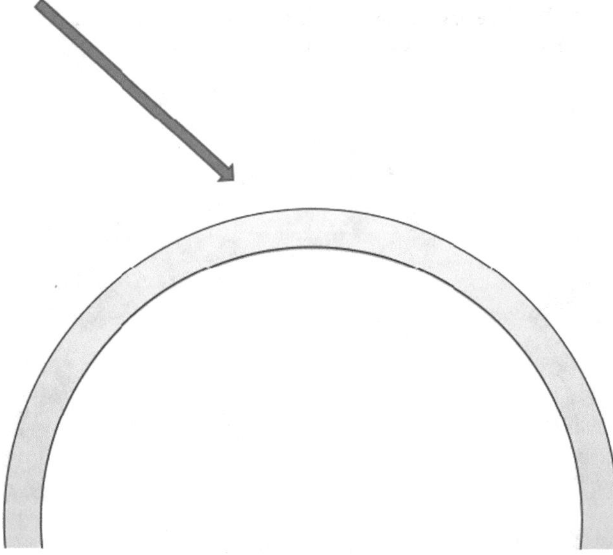

Fig. 2.19 A steeper insertion avoid internal injury but leads to a shortened wound less likely to self-seal

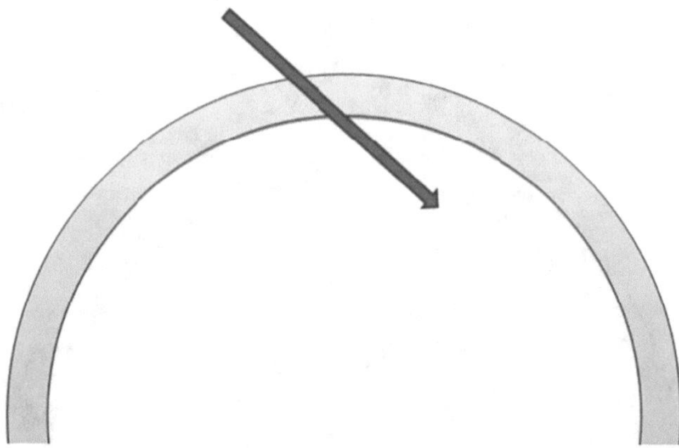

Fig. 2.20 The sort passage through the sclera is likely to risk postoperative leakage

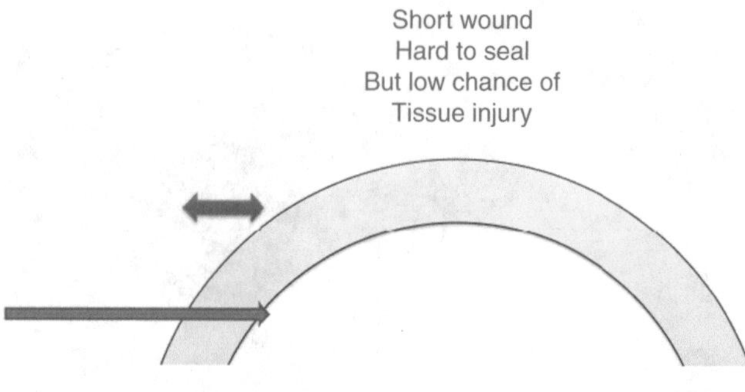

Fig. 2.21 The short wound reduces the risk of injury but increases the chance of instability

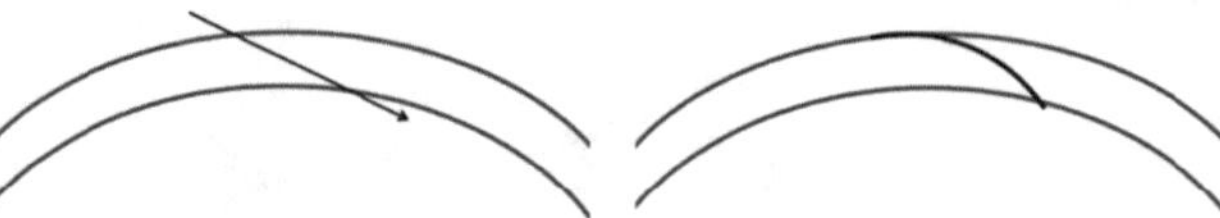

Fig. 2.22 We may think we are going to create a straight wound but could, in fact, be creating a curved one because of the movement of the tissue

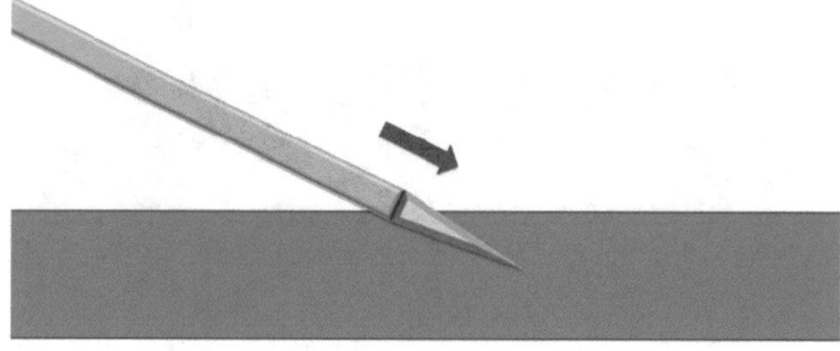

Fig. 2.23 Rotating a blade within the structure can tear the tissue

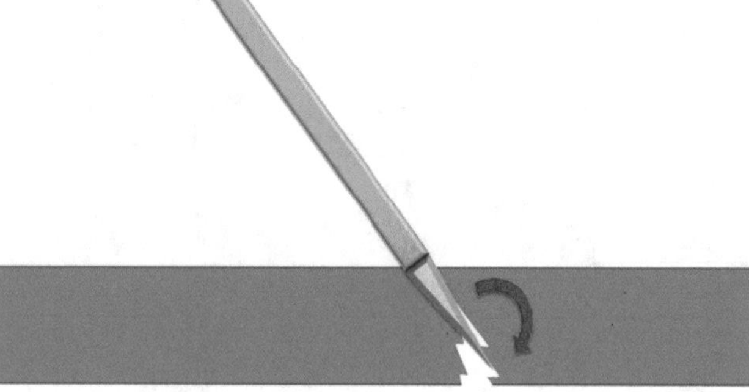

Fig. 2.24 Inner arc the tissues are still apposed, and the wound will not leak

1. Damage to the peripheral posterior lens capsule or lens zonule.
2. Incarceration of the vitreous base preventing fluid infusion and causing peroperative hypotony.
3. Retinal tear formation.
4. Misdirection of tamponade agents, e.g. gas or oil into the anterior chamber or even into the subretinal or suprachoroidal spaces.

Tape the infusion line to the drape about 5 cm from the eye and at 6–7 o'clock (right eye). This allows a circumferential movement of the internal trochar if the infusion line is moved during eye manipulations. If you tape the infusion line at 8–9 o'clock then any movements make the trochar rotate radially and anteriorly into the zonule risking damage to the zonule and air in the anterior chamber.

Checking the Infusion

Now check that the cannula has penetrated the choroid and will infuse into the vitreous cavity. To do this, view the cannula tip in the eye from the side and with the naked eye (use the light pipe, positioned supranasally, to illuminate the tip). A glistening metallic tip should be seen. If so, switch on the infusion. If the tip has a dull brown appearance the choroid may have been pushed inwards but not penetrated. Do not switch on the infusion. The end of the cannula must be cleared otherwise the infusion fluid will enter the suprachoroidal space causing a choroidal effusion. If an effusion is created this will usually resolve quickly if the cannula penetration into the vitreous cavity is achieved and fluid allowed to perfuse the cavity.

Note: Small gauge trochars can be quite long, in time the infusion cannula check can be dropped, however, be careful in eyes with total retinal detachment, anterior proliferative vitreoretinopathy, or choroidal effusions where the inner structures can be lifted away from the sclera increasing the risk of non-penetration.

In the circumstances where rigid tissues are opposed to elastic tissues, the 2 tissues may react differently to the instrumentation. A blade inserted into a rigid tissue will cut this tissue but may push elastic and mobile tissue away from the blade tip without penetrating it. This feature is classically used in neurosurgery to create a burr hole in the skull. The burr oscillates rather than rotating only in one direction. This means that the burr can drill into the rigid bone of the skull, but should it encounter the elastic dura mater, the dura will be able to move with the blade back and forward without being penetrated or torn. In the eye, the same phenomenon is seen when inserting a blade through the sclera, and into the choroid. The choroid is elastic and will move away from the blade so that a large wound is found in the sclera but only a small penetration is found in the choroid (Figs. 2.25 and 2.26).

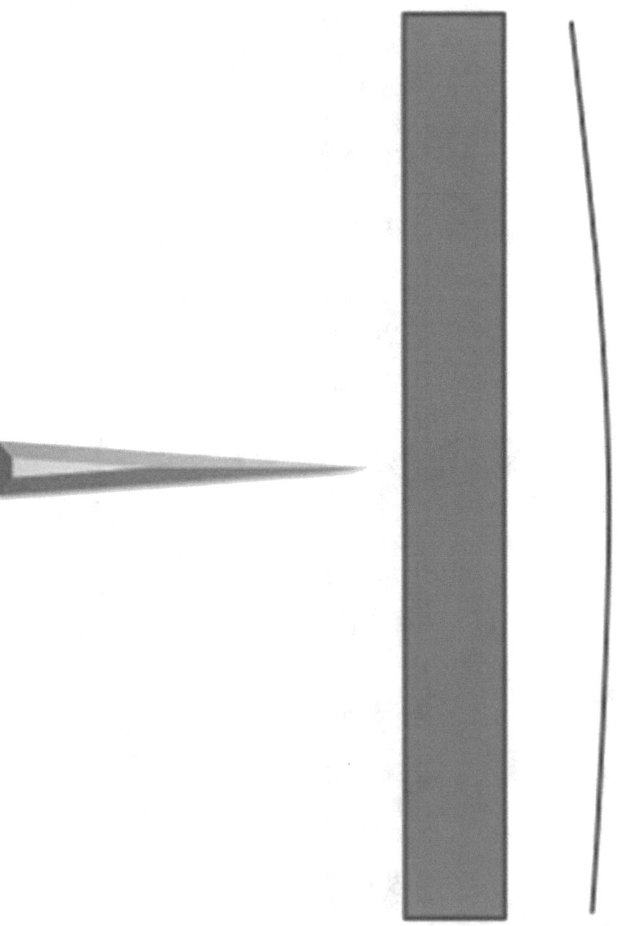

Fig. 2.25 Blades inserted through rigid tissues may create an incision, however, the blade may push an underlying malleable tissue away from the blade tip and not create an incision in the second tissue

How to Clear the End of Non-Penetrating Infusion Cannula?

In an aphake or pseudophake make the superonasal sclerotomy and insert the cutter and push against the end of the cannula to clear the choroid away. In a phakic patient insert the vitreous cutter and remove some of the vitreous whilst pressing the infusion cannula into the eye to allow apposition of the cutter tip to the cannula without touching the lens. This allows clearance of the choroid by scraping the cannula tip onto the cutter. Turn the infusion on before releasing the indentation of the cannula:

To allow the pressure to rise in a controlled fashion.

To prevent movement of the infusion tip back under the choroid before the flow of fluid has commenced.

Thinking in Compartments

The eye to maintain its shape as a spheroid is required to exist at a pressure higher than the atmospheric pressure (10–21 mmHg). Therefore, surgery on the eye often requires the employment of infusion fluids to maintain the pressure. The effects of any infusion cannula will vary depending upon which compartment the infusion is inserted into. Care must be taken that the infusion does not switch between compartments, as the effects of the infusion will be changed. The external tubing attached to an infusion can alter the angulation of the infusion. Therefore, simply by angling the eye for examination the infusion may be inad-

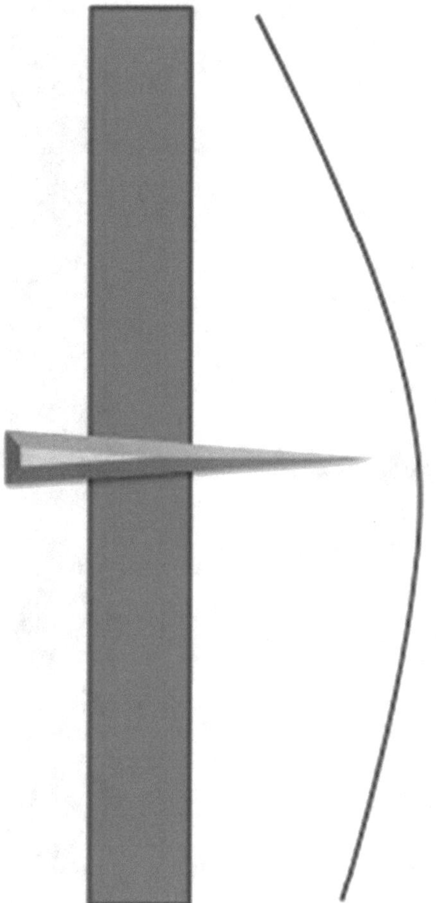

Fig. 2.26 The elastic tissue moves with the blade

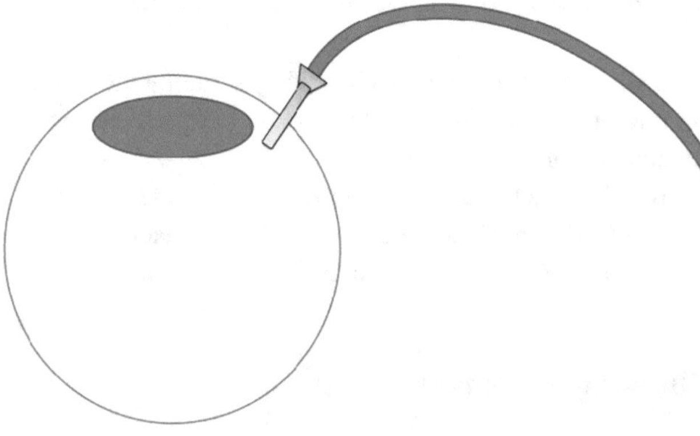

Fig. 2.27 Instruments that have fixed point outside of the eye can rotate and change position on movement of the eye

vertently relocated into a different compartment, potentially displacing the membrane that divides the two compartments. Disorders of the eye such as retinal detachment or choroidal effusion will create yet more compartments, into which an infusion may erroneously be inserted with subsequent consequences for that compartment (Figs. 2.27, 2.28, 2.29, 2.30, 2.31, 2.32).

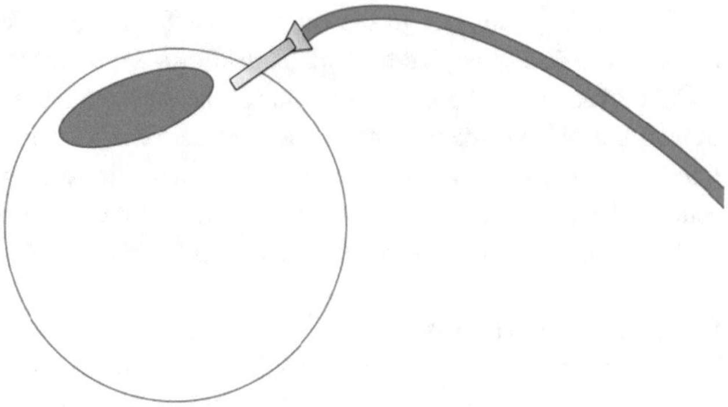

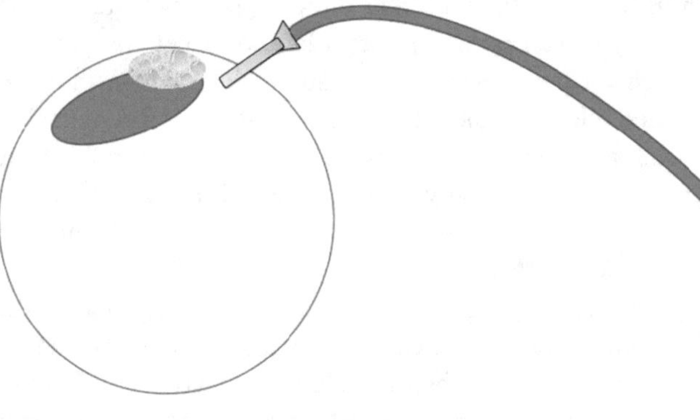

Fig. 2.28 This movement may move the instrument from one compartment to another

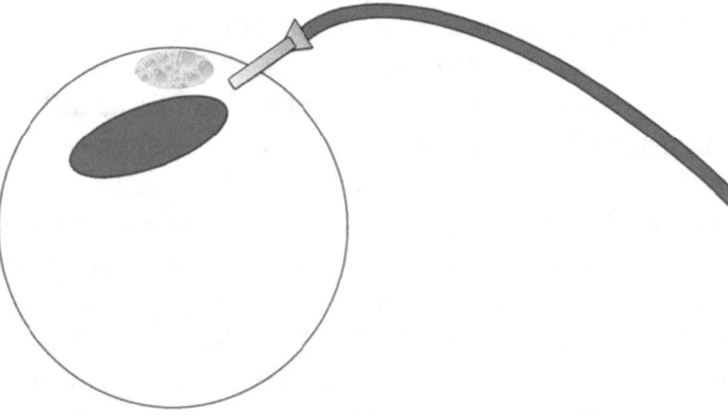

Fig. 2.29 This can involve infusion, e.g. gas, into the wrong compartment

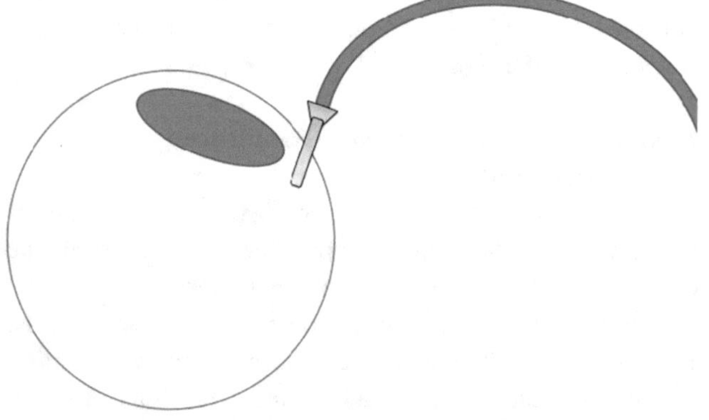

Fig. 2.30 This may distort the compartment membrane

Fig. 2.31 The infusion may move posteriorly

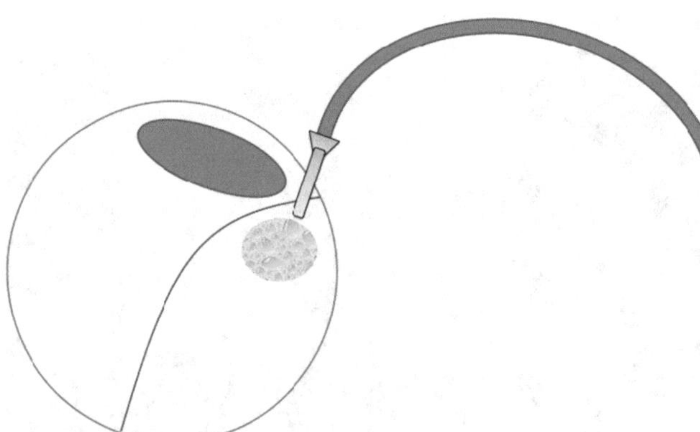

Fig. 2.32 This may cause infusion into the subretinal compartment

The Superior Trochars

Where to Place

Insert the two superior trochars one in the superotemporal quadrant and one in the superonasal quadrant. Place these approximately 150° apart. If the trochars are too close together they will force the surgeon's hands close together and reduce manoeuvrability. Too far apart and the movement of the eye becomes difficult. When one trochar is being used during indentation a trochar on the horizontal will tend to cause circumferential rotation of the eye instead of a movement in the superior to inferior plane.

Surgical Tip

Subconsciously the surgeon uses the force of the instruments on the trochars to move the eye around to aid visualisation of the different parts of the retina when operating, for example to move a slightly depressed eye superiorly to allow direct viewing of the macula, or to move the eye superiorly to see the superior retina. Placing the trochars too close to the horizontal creates difficulty with manipulation of the eye in this way.

Wash the eye with balanced salt solution to clear any blot clots and apply hydroxymethylcellulose (HPMC) to the cornea.

Note: During small gauge surgery, insert the light pipe second using its illumination to find the exterior portion of the trochar for insertion of the instrument, e.g. cutter.

Checking the View

Insert the light pipe into one trochar, rotate in the indirect viewing system (IVS) and dim the room lights. With the BIOM system set the focus wheel to ¼ from the top of its range of adjustment. Invert the image (a stereo image inverter is required) and using the XY control of the microscope to obtain a red reflex in the lens. Increase the magnification to higher than is anticipated during the surgery and focus onto the optic disc by adjusting the IVS lens.

Note: Using high magnification at this stage ensures that the focus at lower magnifications is maintained for later in the operation. Time is not wasted later by refocusing during crucial manoeuvres in the operation. This is important if using a digital display such as the Ngenuity.

Lower the IVS lens until it reaches the lowest point that the optic disc remains in focus. This results in a focal range that is anterior to the optic disc and will allow a focused image from the disc to the ora serrata throughout surgery in all but highly myopic eyes. There is no point in the focal plane existing posterior to the disc, i.e. into the invisible tissue in the orbit!

Most IVS now have motorised focussing, which greatly improves the ease of surgery. The systems can be integrated into the microscope with automated inversion and focus on the foot pedal (Figs. 2.33 and 2.34).

The Independent Viewing System [5]

1. To focus anteriorly, the IVS lens goes down and to focus posteriorly the lens goes up.
2. The IVS is easier to use when it is further away from the cornea.

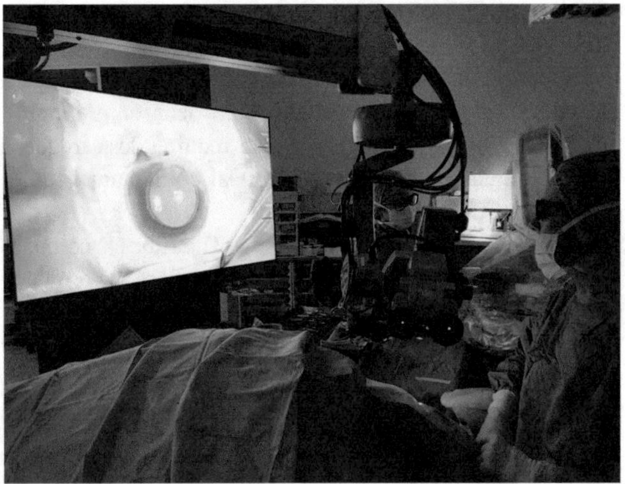

Fig. 2.33 Digital 3D visualisation has been introduced. This uses two digital cameras and polarised filters to view a high-definition television screen. This provides some improvements in ergonomics for surgery. Displacement of the images can be increased to give enhanced depth perception for macular work. At present, there is reduced resolution and artefacts in the image which make searching for small peripheral retinal breaks less effective. Observers can see the surgical field in 3D by wearing polarised spectacles. This is very useful for training

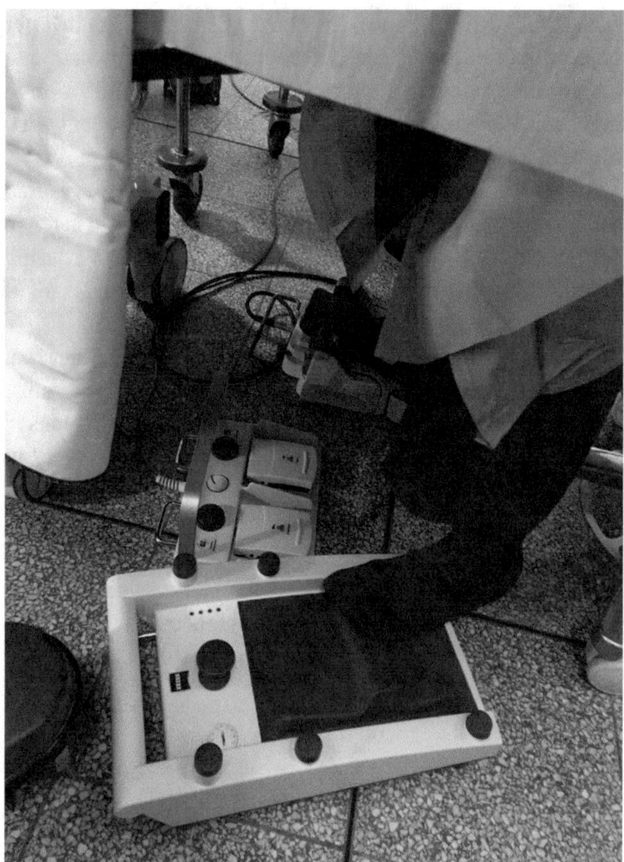

Fig. 2.34 3D imaging requires another footpedal to allow changing of settings, e.g. inversion of the image

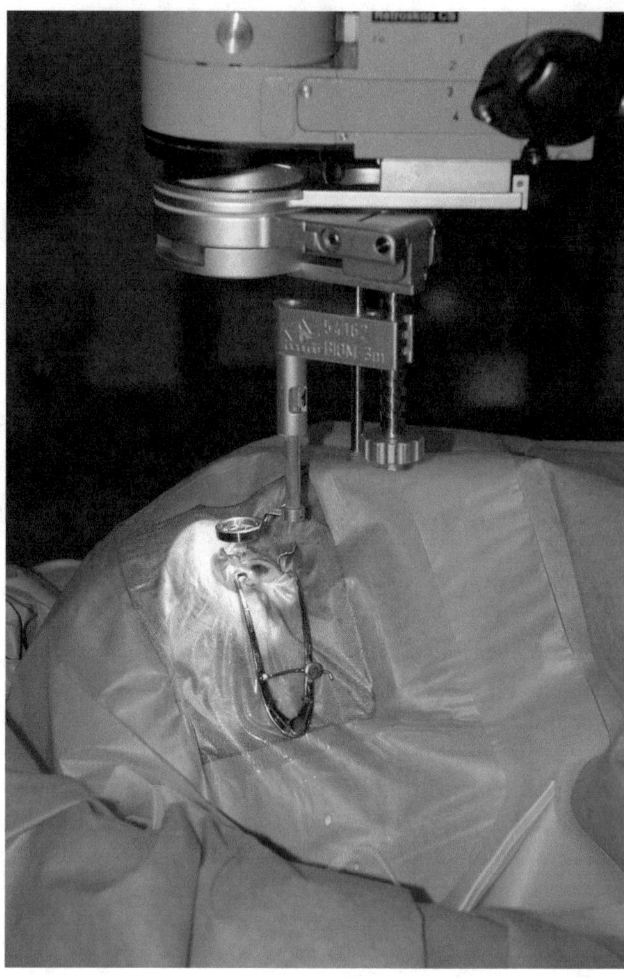

Fig. 2.35 The IVS (in this case a BIOM system) is attached to the microscope allowing visualisation of the posterior segment without a contact lens

3. The field of view is increased when the lens is closer to the cornea (Fig. 2.35).

The assistant should use a straight bore cannula to irrigate the cornea to help avoid splashing the lens or preferably place HPMC onto the cornea which requires less frequent application and helps keep the corneal epithelium healthy (Figs. 2.36, 2.37, 2.38, 2.39, 2.40).

There are now several IVS systems. The Eibos is compact and easy to focus with a fingertip during surgery but provides a smaller field of view than the BIOM (Oculus). It is covered with a sterilised sleeve and so requires only one system per operating theatre. The BIOM is sterilised in total requiring at least two or three systems per theatre. It is more difficult to focus peroperatively unless a motorised unit is purchased. The view is, however, superior and is therefore the system favoured by this surgeon. The Zeiss system has an even wider field of view and a useful focussing system in the +2D objective lens. Most come with a wide-angle lens for peripheral retina and a high magnification lens for the macula. The IVS provides reduced depth perception compared with contact lenses. Using the latter can be helpful for macular membrane peels.

Surgical Pearl

Optimising Use of the Wide-Angle Viewing System

It is not easy to obtain the best possible view of the retinal periphery and anterior vitreous when using indirect vitrectomy viewing systems such as the Zeiss Resight, Oculus Biom, or Volk Merlin. The best view entails almost restless use of the foot pedal to adjust the position of the hanging lens in both the *XY* plane and *z*-axis.

XY plane: The anterior limit of the retinal view is dependent on the degree of eye roll, the greater the roll the further out you can see. The microscope has, however, to be adjusted to match this maximum possible eye roll. It is common to see the eye rolled a long way, but then rolled back to match a partly adjusted microscope position. The microscope must constantly catch up with the eye position, not vice versa.

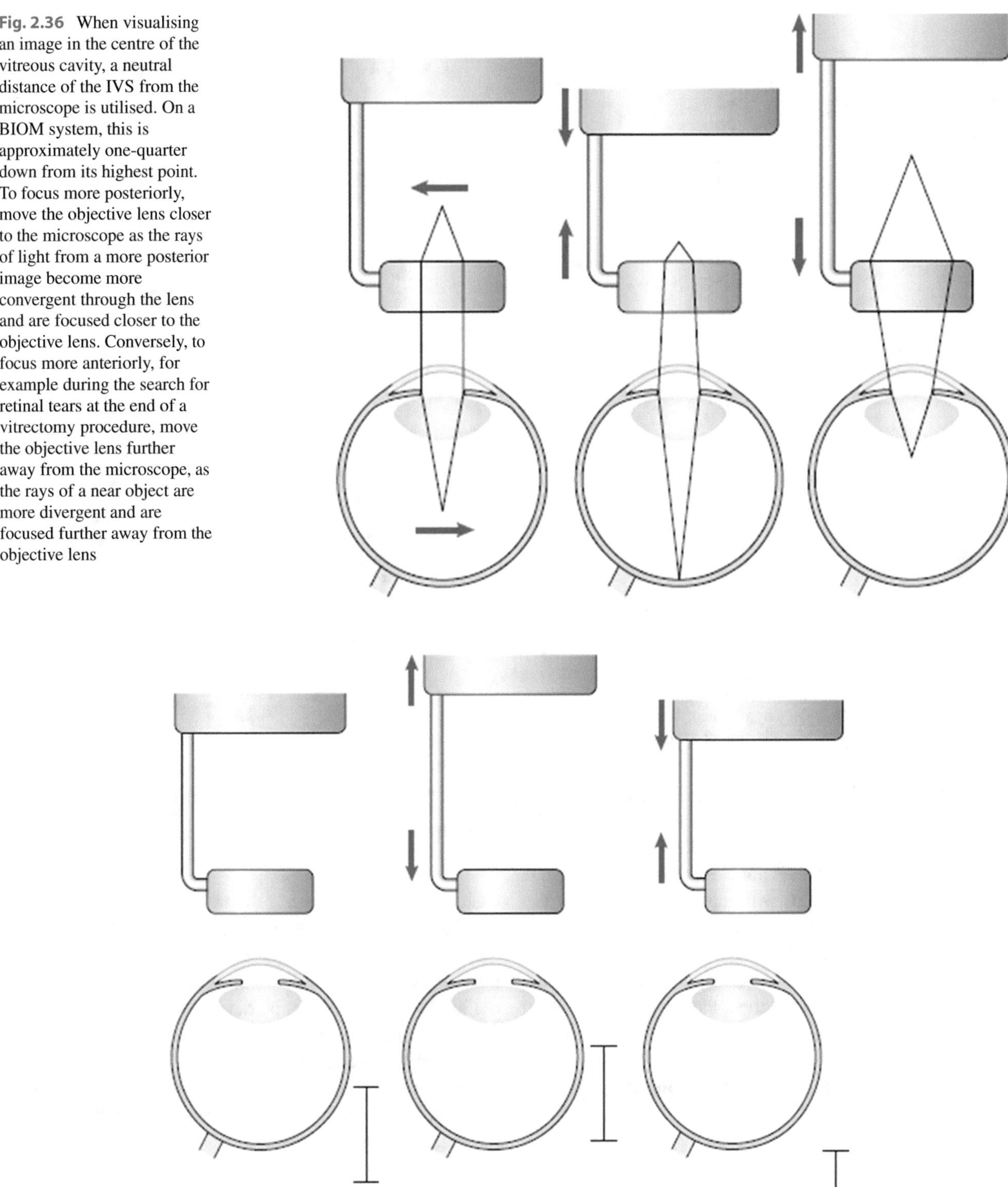

Fig. 2.36 When visualising an image in the centre of the vitreous cavity, a neutral distance of the IVS from the microscope is utilised. On a BIOM system, this is approximately one-quarter down from its highest point. To focus more posteriorly, move the objective lens closer to the microscope as the rays of light from a more posterior image become more convergent through the lens and are focused closer to the objective lens. Conversely, to focus more anteriorly, for example during the search for retinal tears at the end of a vitrectomy procedure, move the objective lens further away from the microscope, as the rays of a near object are more divergent and are focused further away from the objective lens

Fig. 2.37 When finding the optimal focal range for use at the beginning of the operation, increase the magnification of vision and focus on the disc. Increasing the magnification in this way ensures that there is a fine focus on the back of the eye. Because there is a focal range for the lens system (analogous to that used in photography), employ this focal range during the surgery. With the focal range in the mid position, it is possible to focus in the mid-vitreous without the disadvantage of focal range going into the invisible tissues of the orbit behind the eye. By moving the objective lens further away from the microscope, until focus is just retained in the posterior pole or the optic disc, a focal range going from the optic disc, anteriorly to as far as the ora serrata is possible in most eyes. This will allow visualisation of the whole retina throughout the surgery without having to re-focus or re-adjust the lens. This manoeuvre at the beginning of the operation will save time later on avoiding re-adjusting focus throughout points of the surgery where delay is not advantageous. On the other hand, focusing onto the optic disc with the objective lens too close to the microscope, will only allow focus on the optic disc and the rest of the focal range will be going into the orbit, forcing you to refocus during surgery

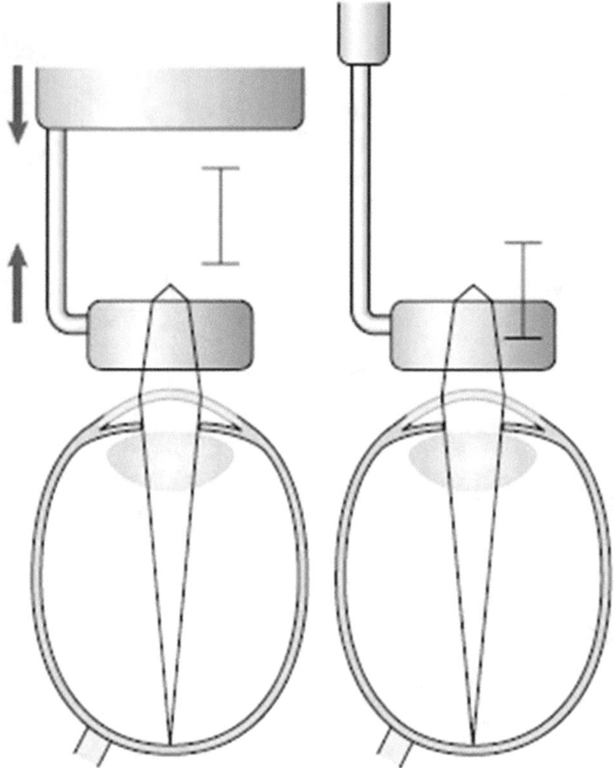

Fig. 2.38 In a highly myopic eye, it may not be possible to bring the virtual image into focus when the +2 lens is inserted between the microscope and the objective lens. Only by removing this lens will the focal range for the system to allow visualisation of the image

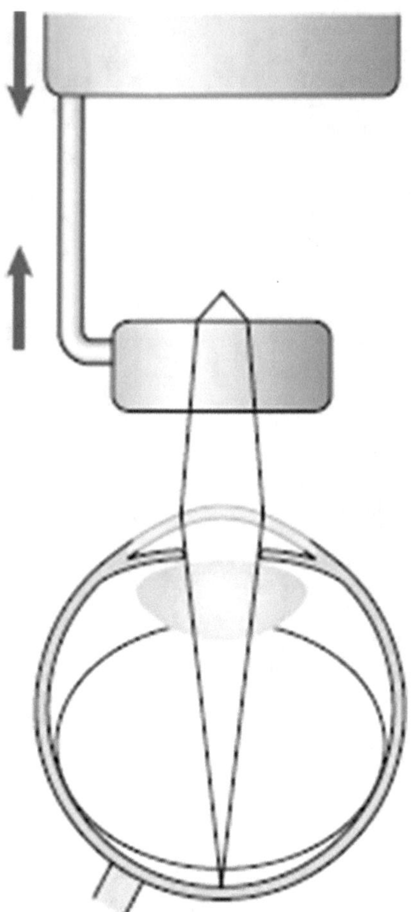

Fig. 2.39 The reduced refractive index of air causes a myopic shift on the back of an intraocular lens or phakic lens by producing convergence of the rays of light from an image, thereby, producing an image closer to the objective lens of the IVS. Therefore, the lens needs to be elevated relative to the microscope to overcome this and retain focus

Z-axis: Maximising the angle of retina which can be seen at any one time is dependent on optically coinciding the edges of the hanging lens and the patient's pupil. If peripheral iris can be seen the lens is not close enough to the eye. If it is too close, a grey patch will appear in the view or the hanging lens will touch the cornea.

The eye retracts when rolled so constant attention to the *z*-axis as well as *XY* plane is required. Co-ordinating hands and feet in this way takes practice, the reward is, however, being able to see much more anterior retina and vitreous.

Mr. D Alistair H Laidlaw, St Thomas Hospital, London, UK

Removing the Vitreous

Complex machinery is used in ophthalmic surgery. They consist of a computer, pumps, and instrument devices in the body of the machine and foot pedals to control the functions. In vitrectomy, the devices include guillotine cutters driven by electronic motors or by compressed gas (Fig. 2.41).

In most circumstances, the machinery is connected to the eye by tubing. This creates two compartments connected to each other, i.e. the eye and the machine. The utilisation of machinery creates the need to understand the flow of fluid in the tubes and pumps. A major function of the machinery is to provide a constant pressure in the globe to maintain safety of the intraocular structures, particularly the vascular network. Sudden drops in intraocular pressure risk rupture of blood vessel walls and resultant haemorrhage. The eye is connected to the machinery by tubing, which provides a flow of fluid into the eye. The tubing provides a resistance to flow according to the Hagan Poiseuille law.

Hagan Poiseuille Law

$$\text{Volume Flow Rate}(Q) = \frac{\pi d^4 (\text{Pa} - \text{Pb})}{\text{L}\,8\,\text{n}}$$

d diameter of the tube
Pa-Pb pressure difference between ends of the tube
L length of the tube

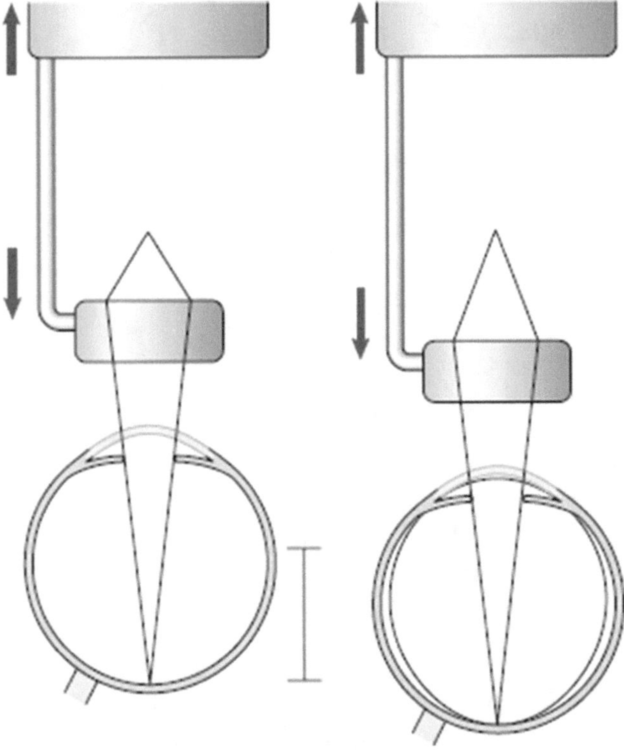

Fig. 2.40 The loss of the intraocular lens causes light to diverge from the eye. The virtual image then is further away from the objective lens and the lens needs to be moved further away from the microscope to retain focus. When air is inserted, having contact either with the cornea or bulging through the pupil, the light diverges further and the vitreal image is then further away from the objective lens and there must be more distance produced between the objective lens and the microscope

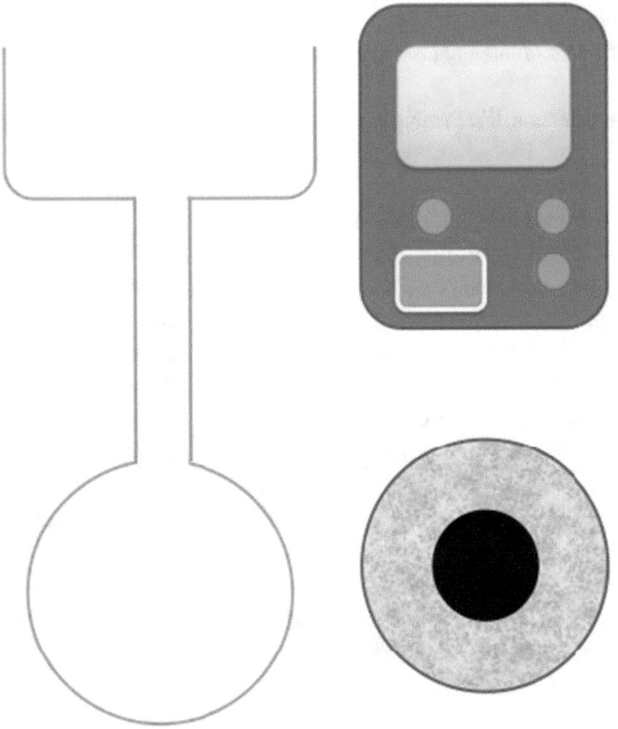

Fig. 2.41 Connecting a piece of machinery to the eye introduces the physics of two compartments joined by a tubing system

n viscosity

Therefore, the flow rate is reduced by reduction in the diameter of the tube, by the increased length of the tubing, and by increased viscosity of the fluid. The flow is increased by the pressure differential at the ends of the tube, for example:

- Increasing the pressure by raising the height of an infusion bottle relative to the eye or increasing the pump pressure.
- Reducing the pressure in the eye by wound leakage or aspiration of fluid.

Another way to envisage the flow of fluid between the compartments is to consider resistance to flow in the system. There is a resistance to inflow from the tubing. There is a resistance to outflow from the eye usually at a wound. Resistance at the wound is reduced when the cross-sectional opening of the wound, is largest. A circle provides the largest cross-sectional area for a given perimeter therefore a large circular wound has low resistance. Resistance will be reduced by active aspiration of liquid by the action of aspiration pumps. If the resistance to outflow from the globe is greater than the resistance to inflow through the tubing, then the pressure in the globe will be maintained. If the resistance at the wound is less than the resistance in the tubing, the pressure in the globe will drop and the structure of the eye collapse (Fig. 2.42, 2.43).

Flow rate = Velocity × Cross - sectional Area of the tube

In addition, manipulations of the globe will affect movement of the fluid between the machine and the eye. For example, indentation of the globe will cause a temporary pressure rise, until fluid can flow either up the tube or out through the wound. Conversely, release of any indentation will cause a temporary drop in pressure until fluid can be replaced by the inflow. Therefore, the rate of change of the globe shape should be performed slowly to allow these adjustments to occur, thereby avoiding sudden changes in pressure. The sphere has the maximal volume for a surface area and therefore any deviation from the spherical shape causes a reduction in volume and potential pressure rises (Fig. 2.44).

Fluids can be allowed to enter the eye passively, for example by connection to an infusion bottle, in which case the bottle height will relate to the infusion pressure. The height must be measured between the vertical position of the eye and the fluid chamber feeding the infusion line. This can be converted from mmH_2O to mmHg to allow an estimation of the IOP.

Infusion Heights14 mm H_2O = 1 mmHg

Alternatively, fluids can be allowed to enter using pumps. More commonly, however, pumps are used to control fluid egress through instrumentation, for example during the phacoemulsification tip in cataract surgery or the cutter in

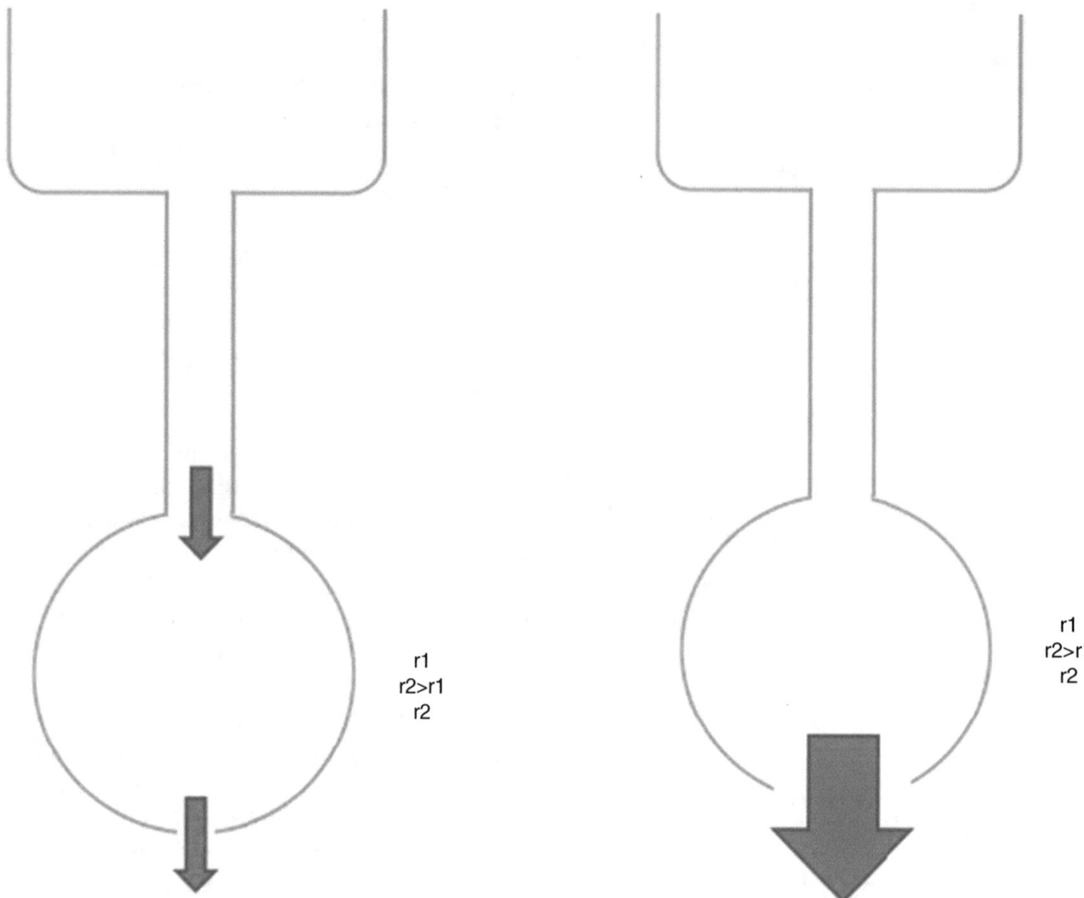

Fig. 2.42 The ocular compartment being a sphere need to maintain a pressure above atmospheric pressure. As long as the resistance to inflow of fluid (r1) is less than the resistance to outflow (r2, e.g. a wound) the pressure is maintained

Fig. 2.43 If the resistance to outflow is lower than the resistance to inflow the sphere will collapse

vitrectomy. Two common types of pumps are utilised. The peristaltic pump involves the production of indentations directly onto the tube enclosing the fluid. These indentions are rotated to move the fluid along the tube. In this type of pump flow is controlled by the rate of rotation of the pump. Increasing the rotations increases the flow of fluid. Vacuum may be created in the tube if the flow is high and there is a blockage in the tube preventing flow further down the tubing system. It is important that the tubing cannot collapse as this will lead to a rapid negative pressure on re-expansion of the tube when the blockage is released (Fig. 2.45).

The second type of pump involves flow of gas along a tubing mechanism. The gas passes along a wide portion of tubing at which point there is a high pressure but low velocity of the gas according to Bernoulli's principle. The introduction of a constriction in the tubing increases the velocity of the gas and consequently, the pressure is reduced. At this point, the tubing is connected to a compartment and the low pressure created (vacuum) is used to draw fluid into the pump compartment. This type of pump is vacuum controlled, and flow is created secondary to the vacuum.

- Bernoulli's Principle states that as the speed of a moving fluid increases, the pressure within the fluid decreases.

Pressure × velocity = k

The flow of fluids into the active end of the instrument in the eye creates certain effects. In general, flow is highest in the centre of the tube of an instrument. Liquid at the periphery of the tube is slowed down because of its contact with the wall of the tube. This creates areas of fluid flow around the tip with high velocity (in the centre of the flow) and low velocity (at the periphery). Once again Bernoulli's equation is important because at the border of the tip where the velocity is low the pressure is high, whereas in the centre where the velocity is high the pressure is low. Therefore, if the tip is close to a malleable tissue there is the potential for drawing the tissue from the high-pressure area to the low-pressure area and therefore into the instrument creating injury (Figs. 2.46 and 2.47).

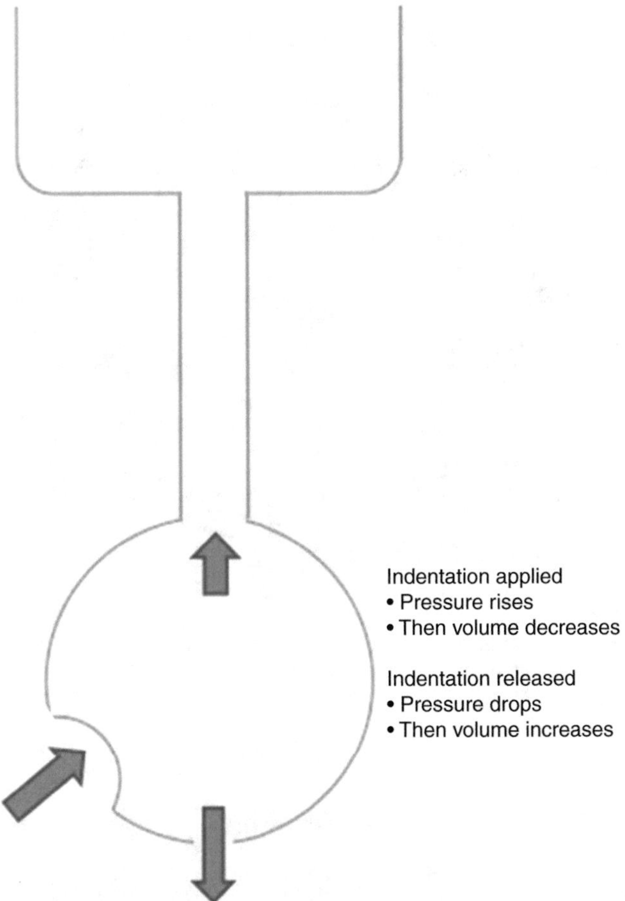

Fig. 2.44 Indentation of the eye increases the pressure before volume is lost up the tubing or out of the wound. Releasing the indentation drops the pressure before the volume is regained from the second compartment via the tubing

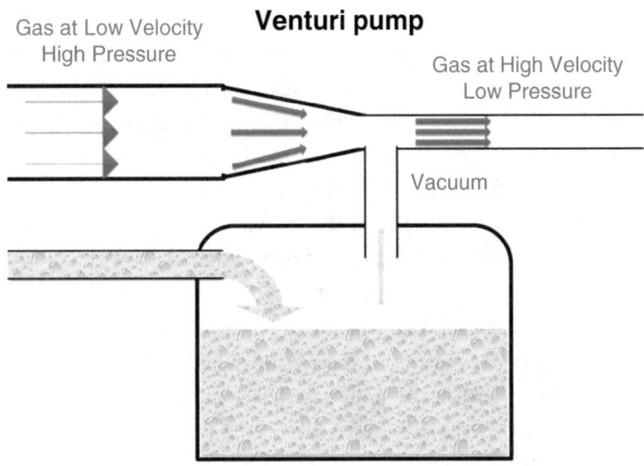

Fig. 2.46 The venturi pump creates a vacuum in a chamber which move the fluid towards the chamber creating flow in the tubing

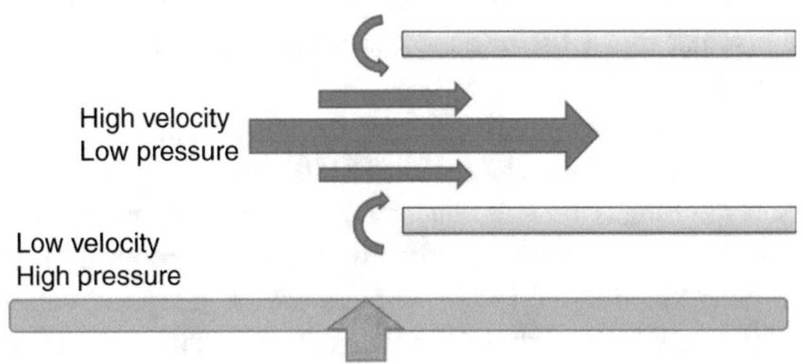

Fig. 2.47 Flow of fluid into an aspiration port has higher velocity centrally (low pressure) and lower velocity peripherally (high pressure). The pressure difference can risk engaging tissue close to the orifice into the port

Fig. 2.45 A peristaltic pump creates flow by the action of indentations on the tubing

The same principle can be seen in surgical wounds in which there is flow of fluid. The centre of the wound will have high flow and the edge of the wound low flow. The pressure differential created can draw tissue into the wound, for example retina into a trochar.

Duty cycle is a measure of the effectiveness of an instrument. It is determined by the time that the function of the instrument is active over the period of the function. There may be conditions that maximise the duty cycle for an instrument such as port size, speed of oscillations or cutter blades, or the time in which a cutter blade is open or closed.

$D = \tau/T$

- D is the duty cycle.
- τ is the duration that the function is active.
- T is the period of the function.

For vitrectomy cutters the larger the calibre of the cutter and the larger the size of the port on the cutter tip, the higher the flow rates that can be achieved. However, this is at the cost of a larger wound size for insertion of the instrument. The calibre of cutters is often reduced to 23–27 G to reduce the wound size. Therefore, the efficiency of the guillotine becomes more important with increased rates of cuts, e.g.

5000 cuts per minute. It is important that there is more time when the orifice is open to aid flow rates and improve the duty cycle. If cut rates are too slow the tissue is less effectively cut because the velocity of the guillotine is less. If the cut rate is too high, the orifice is closed more often than open reducing the flow rate [6–8] (Fig. 2.48).

Keep the fingers light on the instruments to ease any tension and to improve manoeuvrability. The surgeon can apply forces to the trochars via the instrument shafts to rotate and manoeuvre the globe into position for maximal visualisation of the peripheral retina (a technique which is lost with the use of some flexible 27 gauge instruments for which manufacturers are trying to achieve more stiffness). The light pipe shines onto the active instrument or behind it to retro illuminate.

Note: Be aware of where the light pipe is in the eye. Ignoring the position of the light pipe is a common reason for touching the lens. Also, any drift into the eye could result in a macular injury because the instruments are pointing at the macula.

As with any surgery perform the easiest moves first so that if a complication arises from a difficult part of the operation the effects on subsequent manoeuvres are minimised. Therefore, when removing the vitreous excise centrally first to clear some space in the vitreous cavity. Keep the cutter orifice in view during the vitreous clearance but also angled towards the vitreous you are removing. Then take the "easy" vitreous on the same side of the eye as the cutter and away from any hazards, e.g. a bullous retinal detachment. Finally, remove vitreous from the hazardous areas (Figs. 2.49 and 2.50).

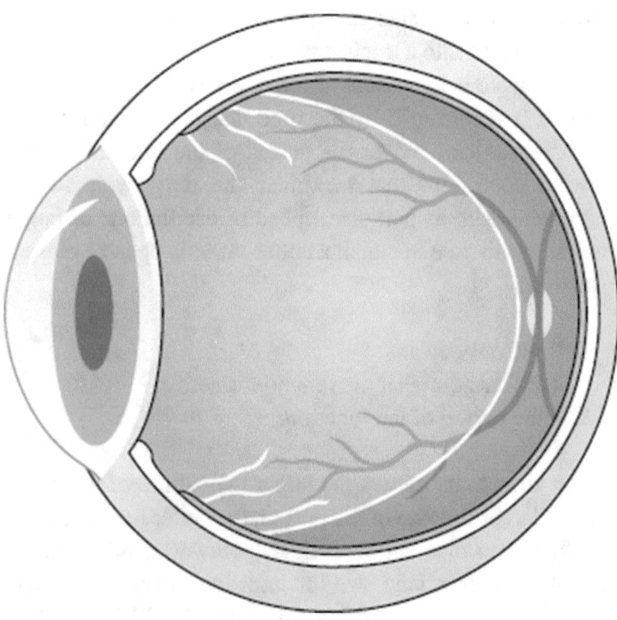

Fig. 2.48 A typical vitreous detached from the back of the eye but still attached at the vitreous base

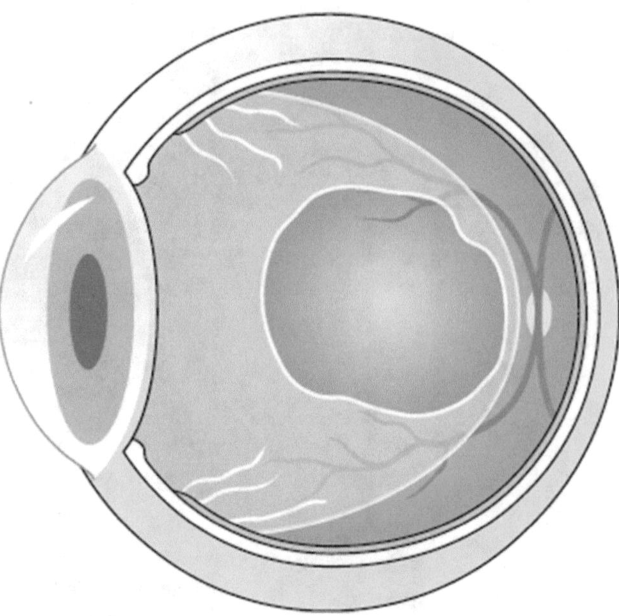

Fig. 2.49 At the commencement of the PPV remove the central vitreous to create space for the instruments

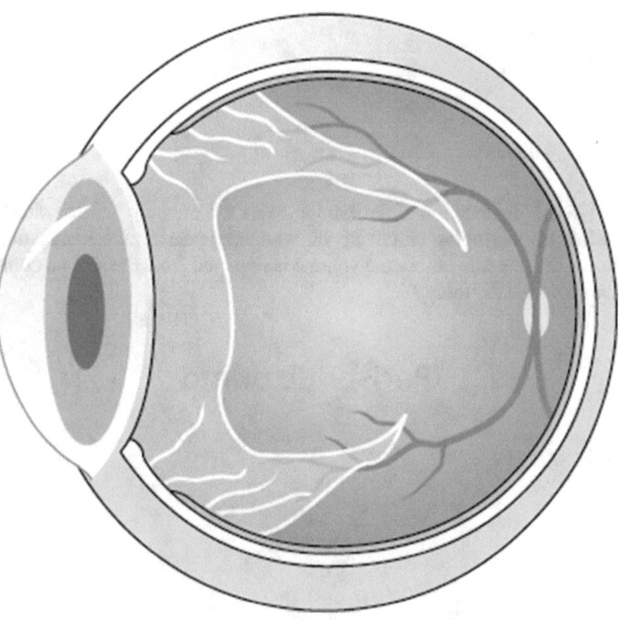

Fig. 2.50 Gradually work towards the peripheral gel then remove this as close to the vitreous base as possible

The vitreous cutter should be moved only minimally in the eye. Try keeping it in one place letting the vitreous come to the tip, which the gel will do especially if it is detached. Remember the vitreous is anchored at the vitreous base so that just posteriorly to the base is a good place to have the cutter tip. Work around the periphery systematically so that the same areas are not gone over twice. In a phakic eye you may proceed from 2 o'clock to 6 o'clock. Change the instruments over to the opposite hands (a good vitreoretinal surgeon can use both hands with ease) and do the other side from 10 o'clock to 6 o'clock. The 2 o'clock to 10 o'clock vitreous can be taken from either side.

Note: Think of the space around the periphery of the lens as a circular channel in which it is safe to pass instruments. The walls of the channel are the posterior bulge of the lens and the pars plana.

This avoids the risk of a "lens touch" which is an indentation on the posterior capsule and cortex of the lens from contact with the shaft of an instrument (in pseudophakic and aphakic eyes you do not need to change hands). Keep away from the back of the lens by passing the cutter around the periphery and letting the vitreous come anteriorly towards the tip. Be aware of the position of the light pipe, it is too easy only to concentrate on the cutter and forget about the light pipe.

Note: Avoid a "lazy" right foot, i.e. make sure you actively use the XY control of the microscope to maximise your view during the surgery.

You should become good enough that the maximum vacuum and cut rates are used throughout ("left foot flat to the floor"), slower vacuum is only required when close to mobile and detached retina. Some prefer a so-called 3D setting where the cutter has a lower cut rate and higher vacuum as you progress the foot pedal depression (Fig. 2.51).

Remember in eyes with attached gel (e.g. macular holes, see Chap. 8) you will need to induce a vitreous detachment and often these eyes have more vitreous volume to remove (therefore more time is required for vitreous removal) than an eye with a shrunken detached gel (e.g. rhegmatogenous retinal detachment). Take as much vitreous as possible, especially at the site of the trochars and the infusion site to minimise the chance of problems such as:

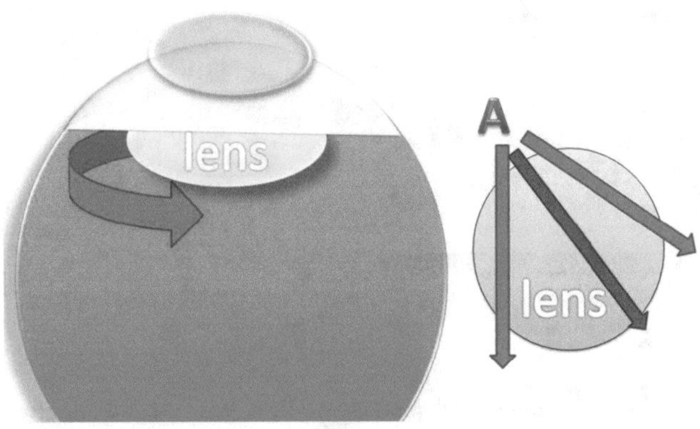

Fig. 2.51 The surgeon can go more anteriorly in the circular "channel" around the periphery of the lens than is possible across the posterior of the lens. Therefore, from sclerotomy (A) instruments can be safely passed across the periphery of the lens (blue arrows) but not across the middle (red arrow)

1. Vitreous incarceration into trochars or the infusion cannula precedes retinal incarceration. Too much vitreous left around the trochars allows the vitreous to be drawn into the trochar by the flow of infusion fluid. This causes traction on the retina and can pull retina into the trochar, especially if the retina is detached near the trochar.
2. Non-penetration of instruments through the vitreous base during insertion running a risk of giant retinal tear. By pushing the vitreous base into the centre of the eye the traction on the retina can tear the retina causing a giant retinal tear.
3. Clogging of flute needles during aspiration procedures, e.g. when draining subretinal fluid from a retinal break. If too much vitreous is left near a retinal break it enters the flute needle preventing SRF drainage. Excise the vitreous with the cutter and continue the drainage with the cutter or the flute.
4. Minimising the risk of postoperative entry site breaks. Incarcerated vitreous in the sclerotomies may gradually contract to cause retinal traction and retinal break formation postoperatively. This seems to be much less common since small-gauge instrumentation has been introduced.

The next stage is to perform the vitreoretinal procedures explained elsewhere in the appropriate chapters.

Vitrectomy Cutters

Most cutters work by guillotine action either driven by electric motor or by pneumatic action with a spring return. An electric motor in the handpiece tends to be bulky, a pneumatic spring return system produces small handpieces, but surgery is reliant on a compressed gas cylinder, which may run out of pressure in the middle of surgery.

Conventionally to increase the flow rate of the vitreous (the volume of vitreous extracted per unit of time) through the cutter slower cut rates (more time for the vitreous to enter the cutter tip), higher vacuums, and larger ports (the orifice on the cutter) are required. This will produce large bites of vitreous at each cut. Large bites, however, allow a larger transfer of forces to the gel and may secondarily cause forces on the retina. Therefore, equipment has been designed to allow smaller bites at a higher speed to maintain flow rates of vitreous and to overcome the reduction in gauge of many new instruments. With extremely high-speed cutting there is not enough time to engage the vitreous. Therefore, higher vacuums are required but multiple small bites = less action on retina. This in turn may lead to less tractional retinal tears. The movement of the vitreous becomes smoother and more predictable allowing cutting closer to the retina. One paper has described less GFAP upregulation, a sign of Muller cell "stress", with high-speed cutters in an animal model [9].

Gauge [10]	Diameter	Inner tube areas (mm^2)	Port areas (mm^2)
20	0.9 mm	0.350–0.352	0.254–0.306
23	0.6 mm	0.169–0.196	0.122–0.173
25	0.5 mm	0.128–0.129	0.066–0.125

The position of the port has been moved nearer to the end of the shaft with modern cutters allowing alterations in surgical technique. The efficiency of the cutter depends on the duty cycle $D = \tau/T$ where τ is the duration that the function is active, and T is the period of the function. Modern cutters maintain their duty cycles even at high cut rates thereby maintaining vitreous flow rates [11–13]. Different settings can be used but I find proportional vacuum (the cut rate is at maximum and the vacuum increases with pedal pressure) satisfactory although I will reduce the cut rate of some high-speed cutters because their duty cycles are not efficient at the higher settings, e.g. reduce from manufacturer's claimed cut rate of 7500 rpm to 5000 rpm (Fig. 2.52).

Common vitrectomy cutter settings with increased pedal pressure	Cut rate	Vacuum
Proportional vacuum	Constant	Increased
Dual linear	Increased	Increased
3D vitrectomy	Reduced	Increased

Handling the Light Pipe

The natural tendency is for the surgeon to let the instruments drift into the eye during periods of loss of concentration. Remember the maxim "if in doubt pull out". Damage is unlikely from inadvertently removing an instrument from the eye but possible if it goes too far in and contacts the retina. This is, especially important when waiting for a change of instrument to be handled by the assistant when the light pipe is still in the eye; therefore, developing the habit of always pulling back on the instrument during any delays in the procedure is recommended.

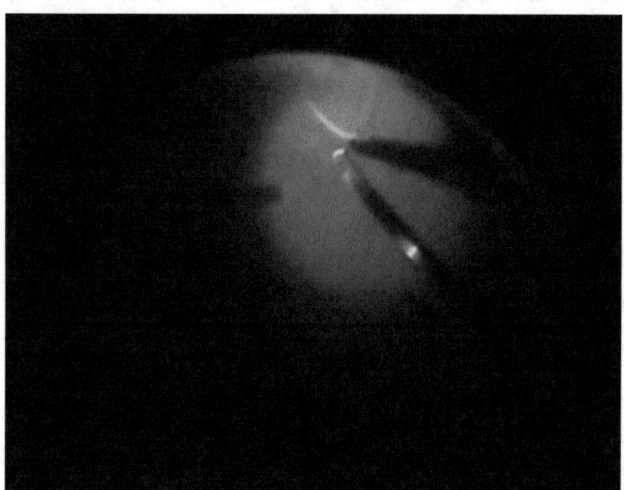

Fig. 2.52 The white line shows an elevated ridge of retina. This indicates traction on the retina from the vitreous during cutting with the vitrector

The light pipe does not need to be pointed at the active instrument in fact illumination is often more satisfactory if the light is shone onto the posterior pole of the eye. A beginner's tendency to want to shine straight onto the instrument tip rotates the light pipe anteriorly bringing the shaft dangerously close to the lens.

Insert the light pipe only far enough to provide illumination, minimising the presentation of the bare fibre optic into the view. This avoids glare, especially with tapered fibre-optic tips (Fig. 2.53).

Note: Avoid light toxicity by removing the light pipe periodically or at least by pointing the illumination away from the macula. Experimentally the likelihood of toxicity increases severely after 13 min. 10 min is a rough amount of maximal exposure of the retina during surgery after which illumination of the retina should cease for a period of 30 s (Fig. 2.54).

Note: Occasionally, the tapered light tip (fibre optic protruding from end of sheath) will cause glare, for example when the eye is air filled. In this case, cut the protruding end of the fibre optic off with scissors to minimise the exposed fibre optic.

The HD camera systems like Ngenuity allow lower illumination levels for surgery than conventional microscopes.

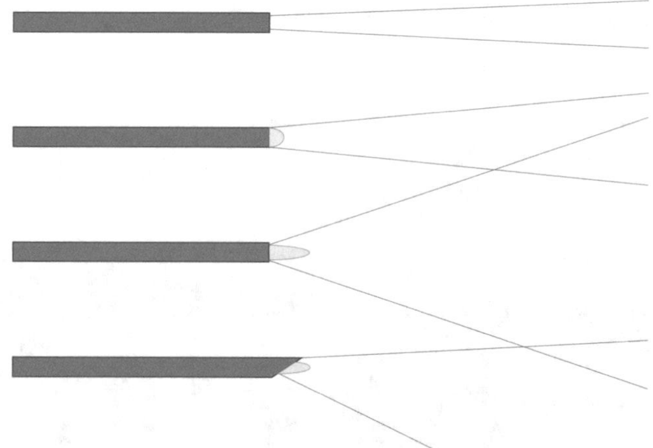

Fig. 2.53 Different configurations of light pipe provide different widths and direction of illumination. A non-protruding fibre optic provides a narrow beam, the width of illumination is increased as the fibre optic protrudes from the sleeve. The bottom example has the sleeve extended at one meridian to prevent glare from the light pipe towards the surgeon whilst illuminating the retina

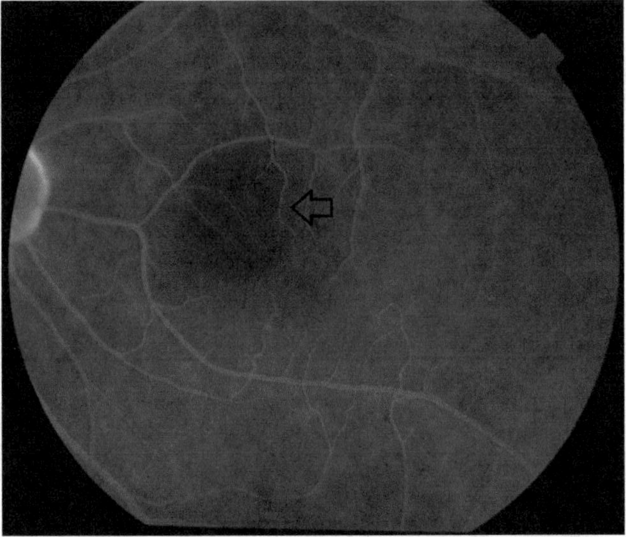

Fig. 2.54 A suspected area of light toxicity from endo-illumination. Be particularly wary of Xenon light sources, which decay as the bulb ages. The surgeon, therefore, needs to increase the power of the illumination with time. If the bulb is changed, the light settings must be reduced or the illumination can reach excessive levels

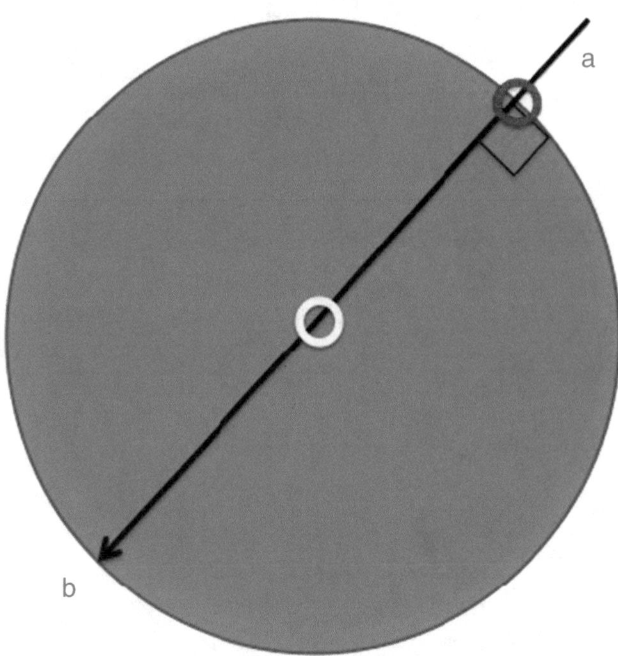

Fig. 2.55 Most instruments in the eye (controlled from a) are restricted in their movement by the wound through which they are inserted (red circle). The furthest the instrument can be inserted is through the centre of the sphere. If in this position, the instrument cannot be moved laterally without touching the wall of the sphere (b)

Intraocular Instruments, Arc of Safety

Inserting instruments into the internal volume of sphere creates certain dynamics, which should be understood. In most circumstances in intraocular surgery, the instrument is anchored in its movement at its point of insertion into the globe. This influences how the instrument can be moved around within the sphere. The maximum insertion of the instrument is when the instrument passes through the centre of the sphere, and any movement from this position risks impact of the instrument on the interior wall of the sphere. The surgeon, therefore, needs to make a compensating retraction of the instrument. Elongated eyes with long axial length may require more adjustment of the insertion of the instrument when moving anteriorly and less adjustment when moving posteriorly. Small globes will require a more rapid adjustment on the instrument (Figs. 2.55, 2.56, 2.57, 2.58, 2.59, 2.60, 2.61).

The instrument rotates around the point of insertion, and therefore an arc of safety can be described centred on the insertion point. When the instrument tip is a certain distance away from the surface of the inside of the globe, movement of the instrument is safe along an arc. In a smaller eye, the arc has a smaller radius, in a larger eye it has a larger radius. In a spheroidal eye with elongated axial length the arc of safety demonstrates the asymmetry causing a higher risk of instrument contact going anteriorly than posteriorly (Figs. 2.62, 2.63, 2.64, 2.65, 2.66, 2.67, 2.68).

Obstructions in the compartment can affect the arc, for example an instrument in the vitreous cavity anteriorly placed behind the lens has a small arc of safety because the posterior curvature of the lens protrudes into the compartment. The arc is small adjacent to the lens and disappears when the instrument is extended beyond the lens border, but a larger arc of safety is available near the wound itself (Figs. 2.69, 2.70, 2.71, 2.72).

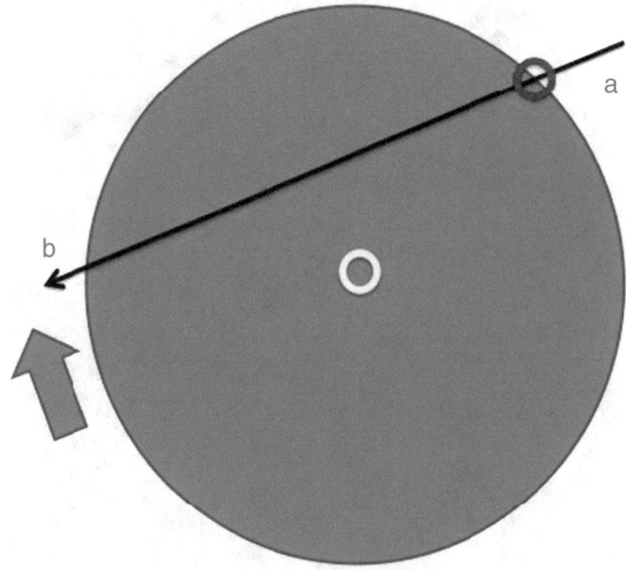

Fig. 2.56 Movement laterally allows the instrument to touch the wall of the eye

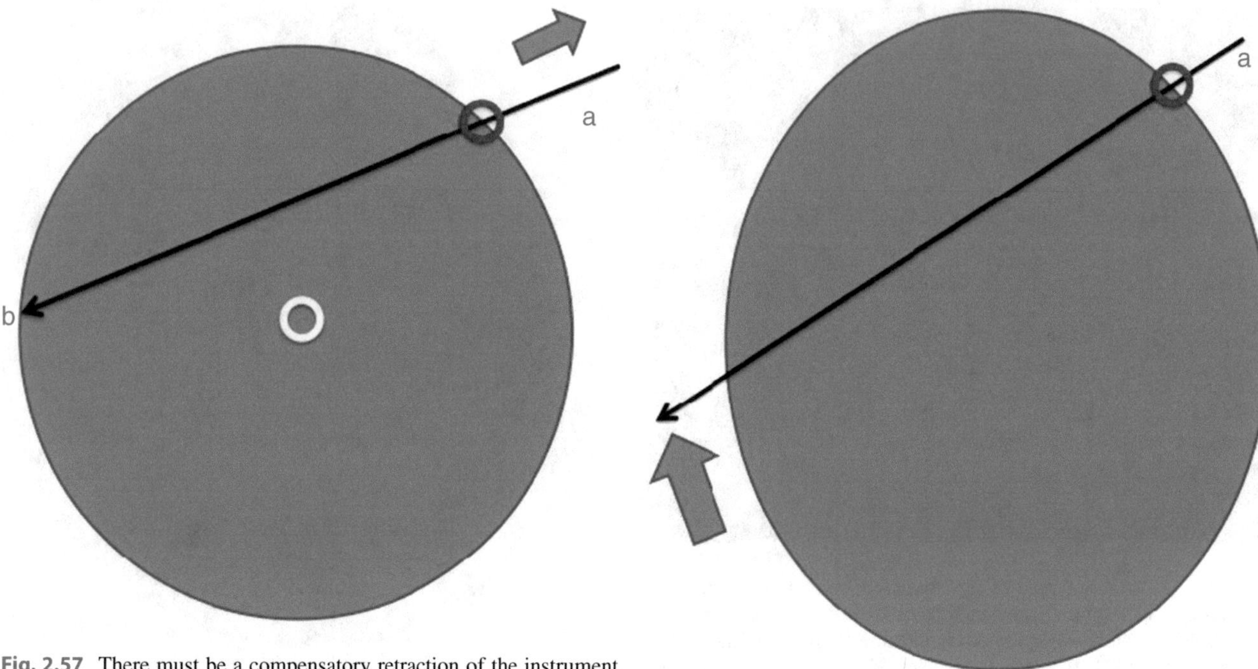

Fig. 2.57 There must be a compensatory retraction of the instrument to allow it to be moved

Fig. 2.59 Anterior movement is more restricted

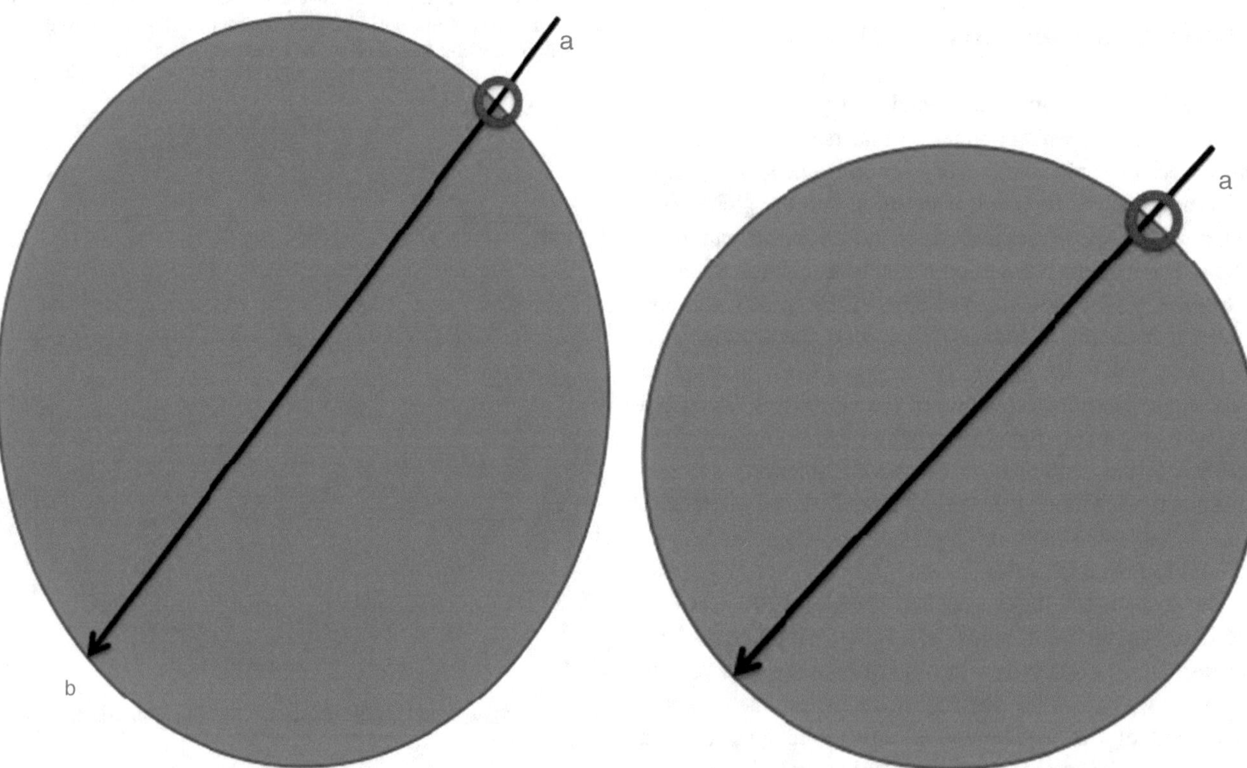

Fig. 2.58 In an oblong eye the safe movement of the instrument is asymmetrical

Fig. 2.60 In smaller eyes the movement of the instrument is further restricted

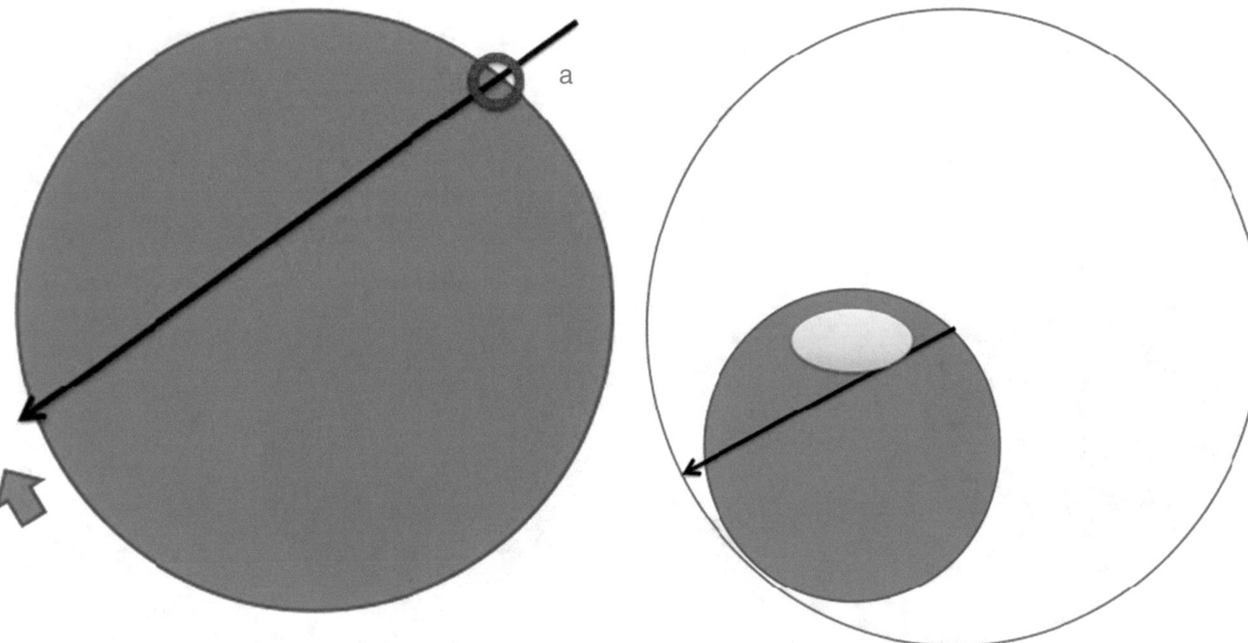

Fig. 2.61 Smaller movements risk injury

Fig. 2.63 It indicates how the tip moves relative to other structures

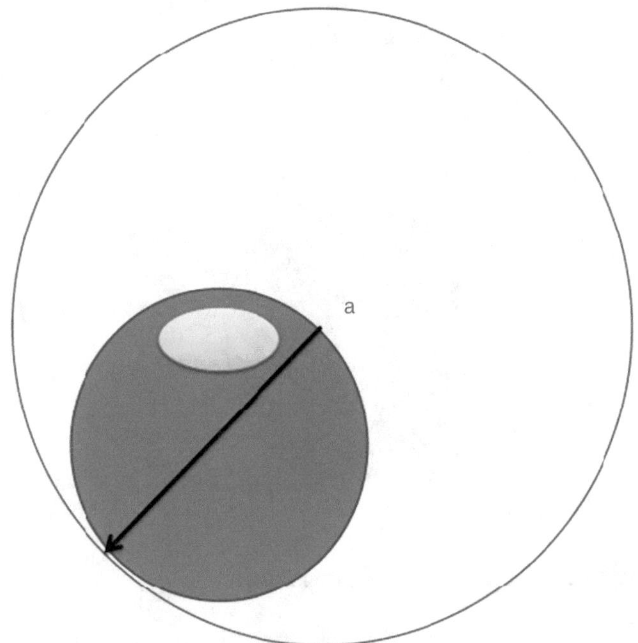

Fig. 2.62 An arc of safety rotating around the wound can be drawn. This arc varies with the size of the eye

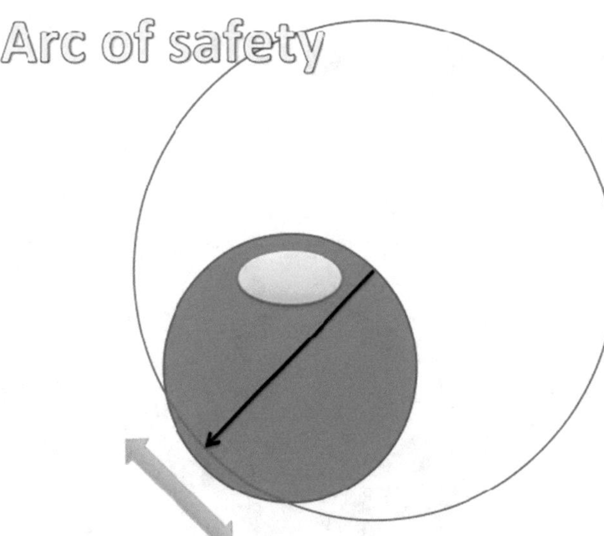

Fig. 2.64 If the arc is kept within the sphere of the eye, there is a safe range of movement for the instrument

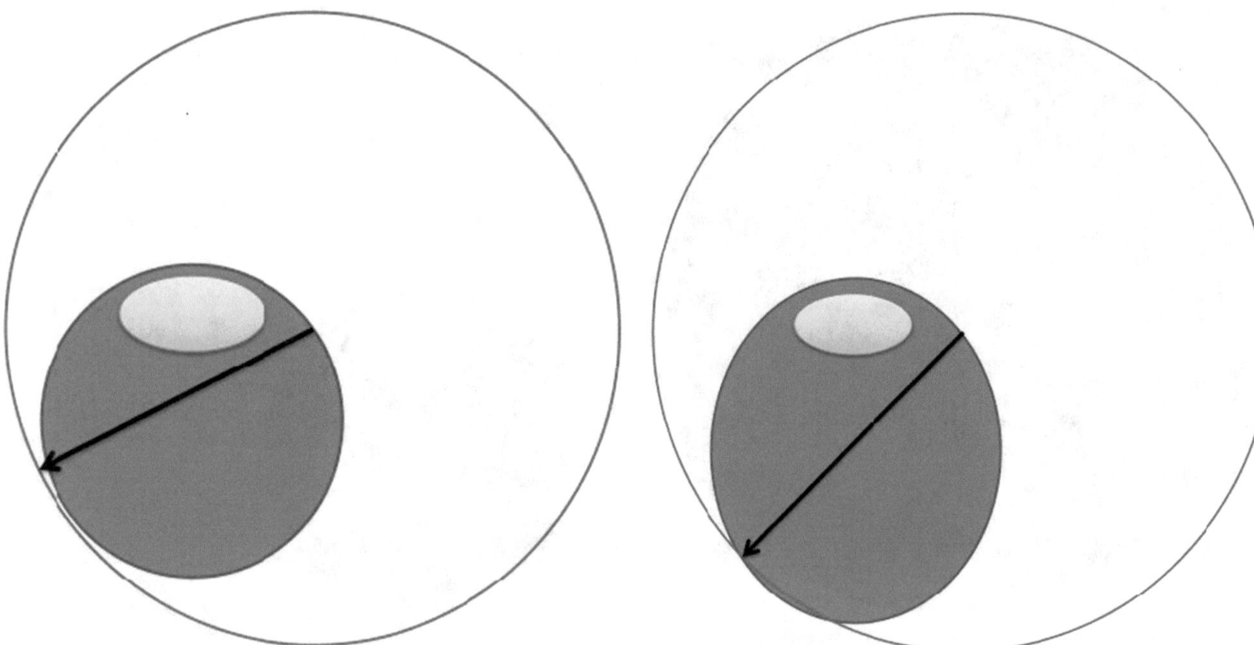

Fig. 2.65 In a smaller eye the instrument will need to be retracted further to achieve the same range of safe usage. The arc of safety has a reduced radius

Fig. 2.67 Large oblong eyes will have a larger radius of arc of safety, but the arc is more posteriorly placed in the eye

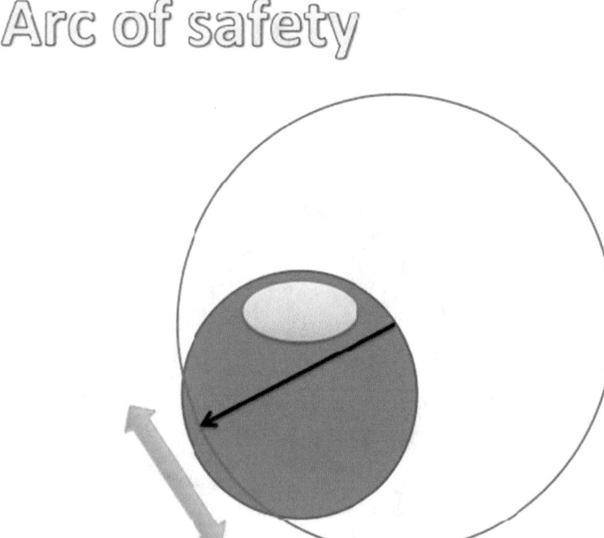

Fig. 2.66 Use the arc of safety to determine where you can move safely within the eye

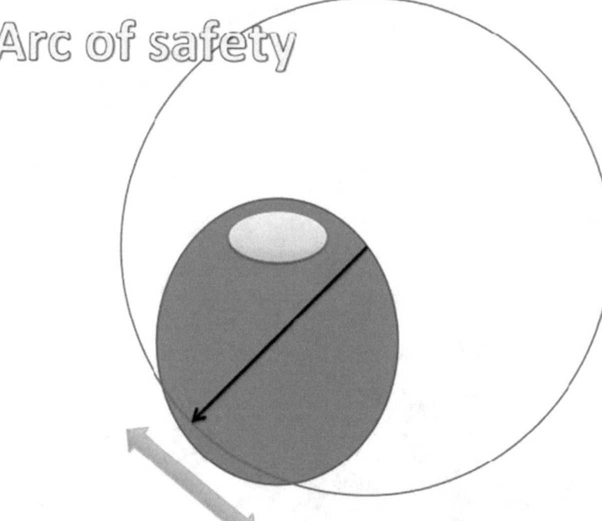

Fig. 2.68 The safe arc may be asymmetrical

The Internal Search (Figs. 2.73 and 2.74)

This is one of the most crucial parts of the vitrectomy and will be required in almost all patients. The IVS makes this part much more attainable but still requires some development of technique. The aim is to see the entire retina not directly visible, i.e. up to the ora serrata. In rhegmatogenous retinal detachment, the search is for the detection of pre-existing breaks and so the procedure is performed early in the operation. In all other conditions, the search is performed at the end of the operation to check if a retinal break has been created during a manoeuvre, e.g. tearing the retina during surgical peeling of the posterior hyaloid membrane. The search gives the opportunity to fix the mistake whilst still in the eye. Never ignore a problem. In vitreous surgery, the surgeon will not get away with it. Always "check and treat" if a problem has been created. It does not feel good to have a straightforward macular procedure return with a detached retina two weeks later.

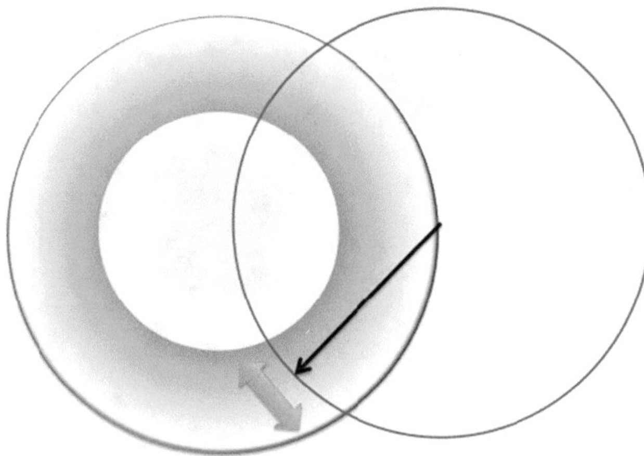

Fig. 2.69 Sometimes a compartment is restricted by another object, e.g. the lens in the anterior vitreous cavity. The arc of safety is influenced by the extra object and will vary

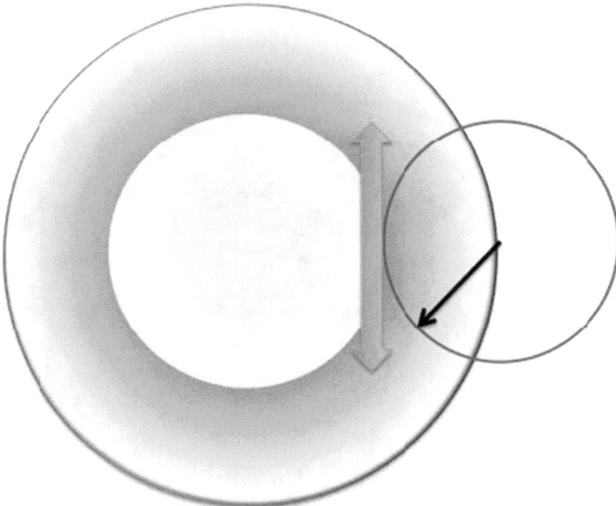

Fig. 2.70 Close to the wound the arc is the largest

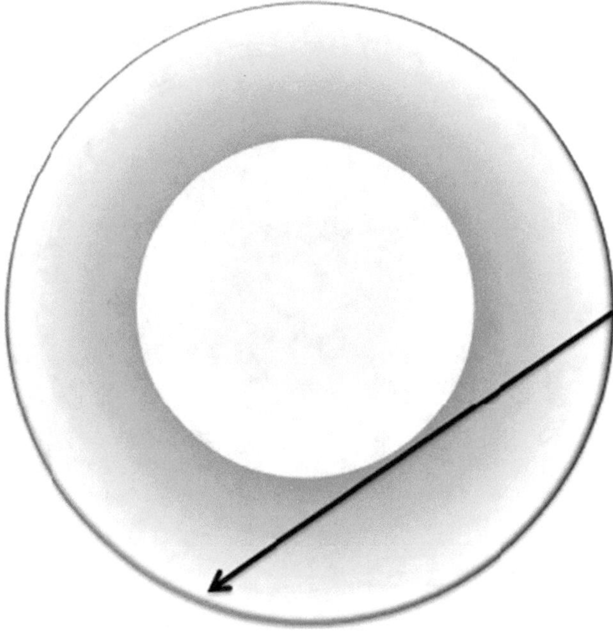

Fig. 2.71 Reaching past the object (e.g. posterior lens) severely restricts mobility

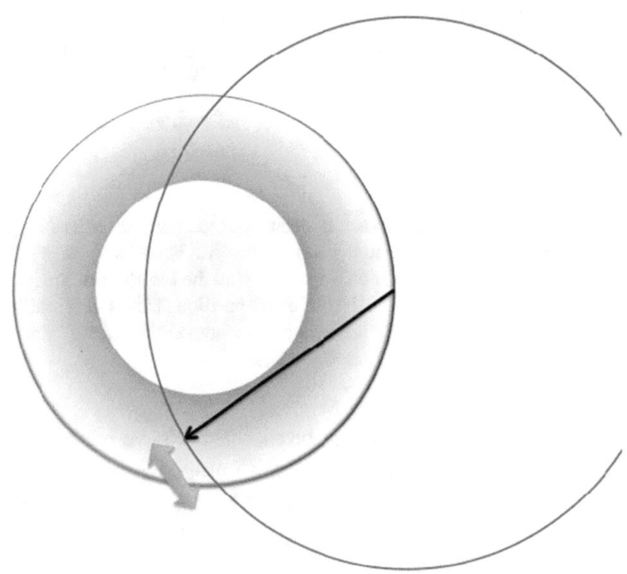

Fig. 2.72 The shaft of the instrument restricts movement

Again, a systematic approach should be followed. Usually, you will do one side and then the other. It is useful to have a specialised indentor for this so that the conjunctiva is not torn and the angel of the indentor allows easy passage around the IVS system and lens. In most patients, you can indent on the surface of the conjunctiva. Apply gentle pressure towards the centre of the eye to produce a ridge that can be seen internally with the IVS. This brings the peripheral retina into view. Observe the retina on the ridge whilst moving the indentor posteriorly and watch for any abnormalities whilst moving around the clock hours of the eye. Movements should be gentle and smooth. Inspect the retina during the movement of the ridge from the ora serrata to just posterior to the equator.

Most breaks appear at the posterior border of the vitreous base, but some may be more posterior, e.g. retinal scrapes from instruments or operculated holes. Be wary of anatomical variations, in some patients the posterior attachment of the vitreous is abnormally far back, e.g. some myopes. As the retina moves dynamically there is a good chance to spot a problem. Work up to 12 o'clock and then examine the other side of the eye. Overlap at 12 and 6 o'clock to make sure the entire retina has been seen. Remember in younger patients the posterior border of the vitreous base is more anterior.

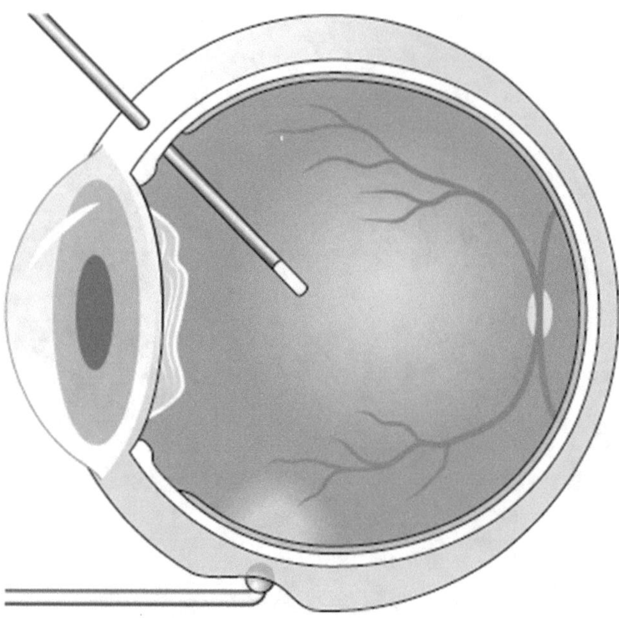

Fig. 2.73 Searching the retina by indentation should be routinely performed in all PPVs

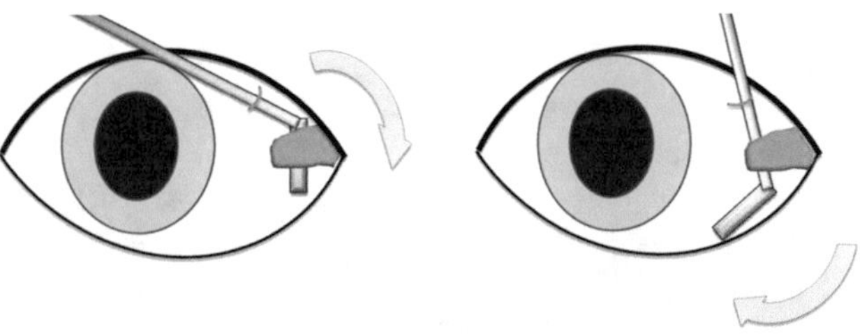

Fig. 2.74 If the conjunctiva has been opened over the sclerotomy superiorly, allowing access to the subconjunctival space, a squint hook can be passed into the subtenon's space behind the insertion of the rectus muscle and down towards the 6 o'clock position. This is very useful on the nasal side where the shortened conjunctival fornix may make trans conjunctival indentation less adequate

You may find pre-existing breaks which have been present for months or years. These are unlikely to detach but should be treated in any case. An air bubble will be enough to support these low-risk breaks postoperatively.

Thinking in Compartments

Forces on a compartment will influence a secondary membrane such as a retinal detachment. For example, indentation of the sclera within the elevation of a retinal detachment will have a small effect on movement of the retinal detachment. However, if indentation is applied at the junction of the membrane to the wall of the eye and then a much larger movement of the membrane is induced (Figs. 2.75 and 2.76).

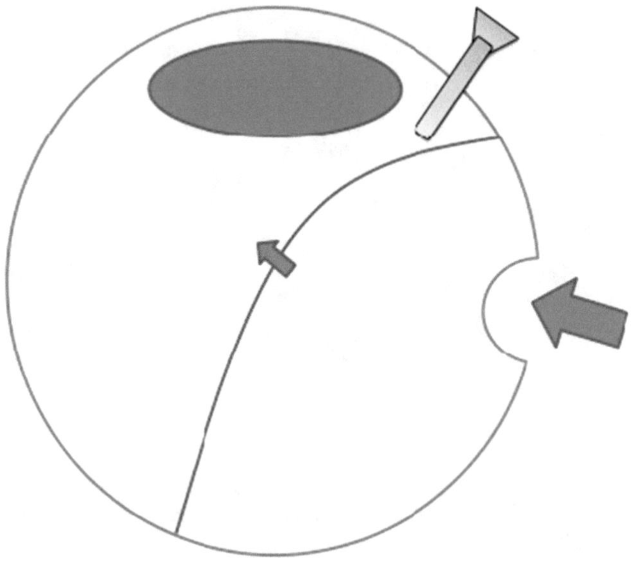

Fig. 2.75 Pressure on a compartment wall that is far away from the insertion of the diaphragm (retina in this case) causes minimal movement of the diaphragm

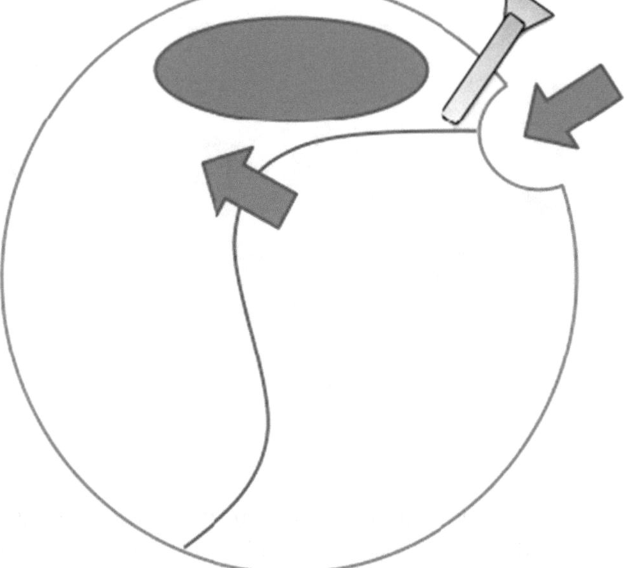

Fig. 2.76 Indentation near the insertion of the diaphragm causes a large movement in the diaphragm risking complications

Manipulation of one compartment causes pressure rises in that compartment, which are usually compensated for by egress of fluid from a wound or passage of fluid into an infusion port. To minimise pressure fluctuations and ingress and egress of fluid, indentations should be kept constant but can be moved around the wall of the globe whilst maintaining the pressure. In other words, it is better to move an instrument whilst maintaining pressure rather than releasing and reapplying pressure excessively (Figs. 2.77 and 2.78).

Light and Laser Properties

The commonest source of illumination for ocular surgery is the microscope light. Systems may employ Halogen, Xenon, or LED sources of light.

Visualisation can be influenced by the field of view provided by the equipment and the quality of the image (dependent upon the degradation of the image by the optical elements of the instrument). Field of view is reduced when increased magnification is used. If magnification is increased, then field of view is decreased. The advantages to a surgical manoeuvre from the introduction of high magnification can be lost because the reduced field of view creates other problems such as the potential for unnoticed damage to peripheral tissues. Manoeuvres may be performed best with a balance of magnification and field of view.

If a variable aperture is available this should be adjusted until the smallest aperture is reached at which the illumination is not noticeably reduced. This will maximise the depth of focus of the image in the same way that the photographer uses a small aperture to increase the depth of focus in a photograph.

During illumination from the operating microscope, retro-illumination of structures is provided by a co-axial light (or light slightly angled at 2°), which shines through the pupil of the eye. This provides better contrast for certain manoeuvres during surgery.

Light hazard to the retina varies with wavelength of the light with shorter wavelengths more hazardous. Filters may be used in the light source to remove the blue or ultraviolet spectrum. Tissue damage increases with illumination and duration of exposure to light in addition therefore lower illumination and shorter duration of surgery are both useful.

Laser is an acronym for "light amplification by stimulated emission of radiation". It is the coherence of the light from the laser both temporally and spatially, which gives it the properties allowing aiming and focussing of the light energy.

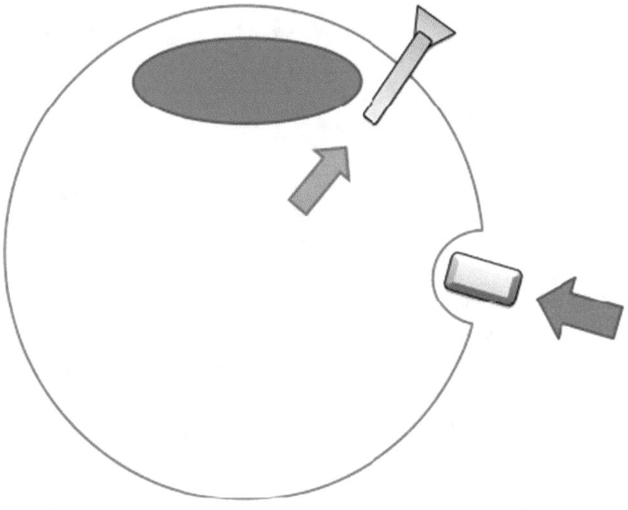

Fig. 2.77 When pressure by indentation is applied there is an initial reduction in the volume of the cavity

Types of Laser in Ophthalmology

- Argon is a laser with ionised argon as the active medium and with a beam in the blue and green visible light spectrum; used for photocoagulation.
- Excimer laser (excited dimer) is a laser with rare gas halides as the active medium. The laser is in the ultraviolet spectrum. Its effect is to break chemical bonds without heat and with minimal penetration of tissues.
- Neodymium: yttrium-aluminium-garnet (Nd: YAG) laser has a medium of a crystal of yttrium, aluminium, and garnet doped with neodymium ions. The laser is near-infrared spectrum at approximately 1060 nm and can be used for photocoagulation and photoablation.

Argon lasers (514 nm wavelength), double frequency YAG lasers (532 nm), dye lasers (577–630 nm), diode pumped solid-

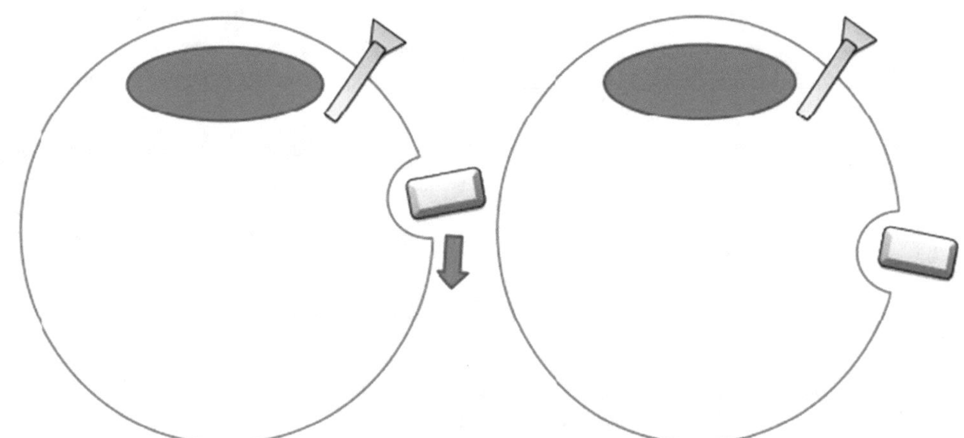

Fig. 2.78 By maintaining the pressure whilst moving the indentation no further volumetric changes are required and the cavity is stable

state lasers (532 nm), and diode lasers are available. Argon provides wavelengths in the blue and green spectra but has been recently superseded by others such as double frequency YAG laser (producing a 532 nm wavelength from a YAG tube, normally 1064 nm), partly because manufacturers can produce smaller more portable equipment of higher reliability.

Laser is focussed to achieve the desired effect usually a thermal burn. The thermal burn consists of protein denaturation and coagulation at 60 °C seen as blanching of the tissue (photocoagulation). It can be difficult to titrate the dose of irradiation as the desired effect is non-linear. A threshold must be reached before the desired effect can be seen. Therefore, the surgeon must gradually increase the laser parameters until the minimum is reached to achieve an effect. The lowest power to achieve a visible effect indicates to the user the threshold at which an effect is gained without side effects. If the temperature is raised too high, to 100 °C, the water in the tissue boils, expanding into a gas. This creates cavitation and cell rupture. Loss of the water creates a rapid temperature rise and at 300 °C the tissue can carbonise.

The photons from laser scatter within the biological tissues and create a spheroidal spread. Therefore, the burn produced is wider than the diameter of the laser light and there is a scatter of energy anteriorly and even more so posteriorly from the point of focus of the laser. Short duration, high power laser application creates a long narrow area of damage from scattering. Long duration, low power laser application creates a shallower but wider area of damage and the thermal energy has time to spread by conduction (Figs. 2.79 and 2.80).

Different wavelengths of laser have different effects on tissue. As wavelength shortens the absorption increases and the scatter decreases. On the retina, in the green spectrum a thermal burn is produced in the retinal pigment epithelium, easily identified by whitening of the tissue. It is therefore easy to adjust the dosage to produce the minimum burn necessary for adhesion or controlled damage of the retina without damaging superficial retinal nerve fibres causing further visual loss. Yellow lasers (561 nm) are available which may have advantages around the macula because of reduced absorption by Xanthophyll. Diode lasers are available which produce a wavelength of 810 nm (infrared), these burn deep into the retina and choroid without a visible burn on the retina until a large burn has occurred in the choroid. Care must be taken when using diode lasers that choroidal ischemia is not created.

As the tissue is altered by the thermal energy the absorption and scattering properties are changed. The initial burn may increase posterior scattering until the tissue carbonises when anterior scattering increases.

Most often laser is applied using a slit lamp and various contact lenses. The optics of these lenses may alter the effects of the laser by magnification.

Lens	Viewing (Image) Magnification	Laser spot magnification
Ocular Mainster PRP 165	×0.51	×1.96
Volk SuperQuad 160	×0.5	×2.0
Volk Equator Plus	×0.44	×2.27
Goldmann 3-mirror	×1.06	~ ×0.94

Laser may also be applied peroperatively via fibre-optic instruments (Table 2.2).

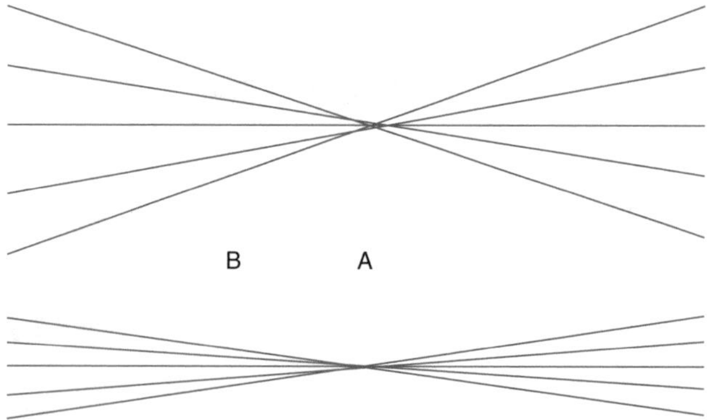

Fig. 2.79 For laser to create a burn the laser is focused at point A. The more diffuse the spread of laser before or after the focal point the less chance of tissue effects away from the focal point, B

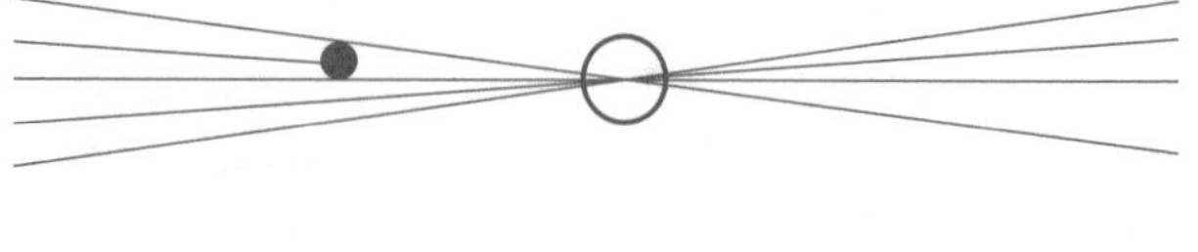

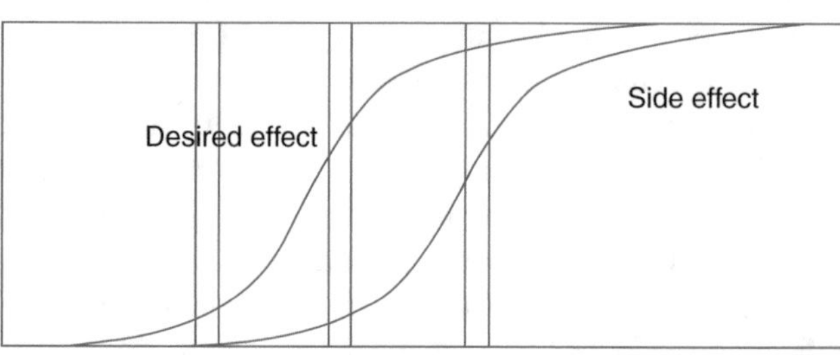

Fig. 2.80 Laser creates its thermal effect when a threshold of energy is reached. The surgeon needs to gradually increase the energy until the effect is seen but is not provided with information from the tissue reaction until that point. Starting with a high energy setting risks moving into the side effect portion of the treatment profile

Table 2.2 Absorption of laser wavelengths

	Laser wavelength		
Chromophore	Green (514–532 nm)	Yellow (560–580 nm)	Red (620–676)
Melanin	High	High	Moderate
Oxygenated haemoglobin	High	High	Low
Reduced haemoglobin	High	High	Moderate
Xanthophyll	Minimal	Negligible	Negligible

Endolaser (Figs. 2.81, 2.82, 2.83)

Laser is applied internally during the PPV via a fibre optic. It is used for retinopexy or for retinal ablation in diabetes [14]. Argon lasers (514 nm wavelength), double frequency YAG lasers (532 nm), dye lasers (577–630 nm), diode-pumped solid-state lasers (532 nm) and diode lasers are available. Argon provides wavelengths in the blue and green spectra but has been recently superseded by others such as double frequency YAG laser (producing a 532-nm wavelength from a YAG tube, normally 1064 nm), partly because manufacturers can produce smaller more portable equipment of higher reliability.

In the green spectrum, a thermal burn is produced in the retina, identified by a whitening of the retina. It is therefore easy to adjust the dosage to produce the minimum burn necessary for adhesion of the retina without damaging superficial retinal nerve fibres causing further visual loss.

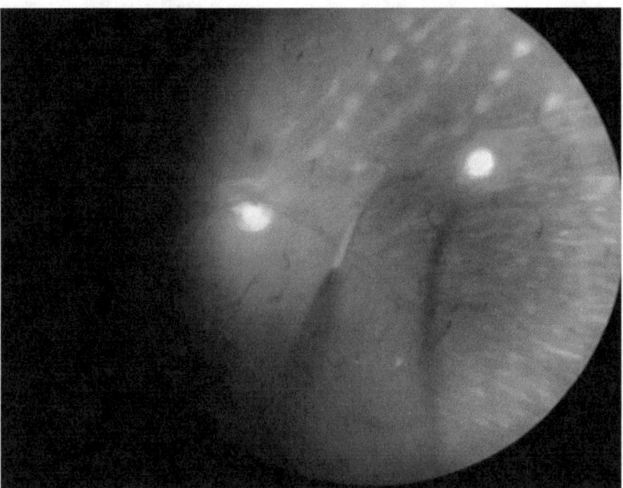

Fig. 2.81 Applying laser to the retina

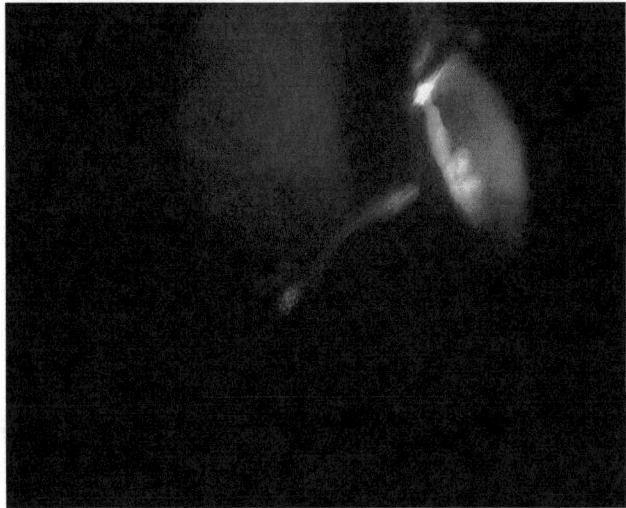

Fig. 2.82 Laser can be applied peripherally by asking the assistant to indent the eye

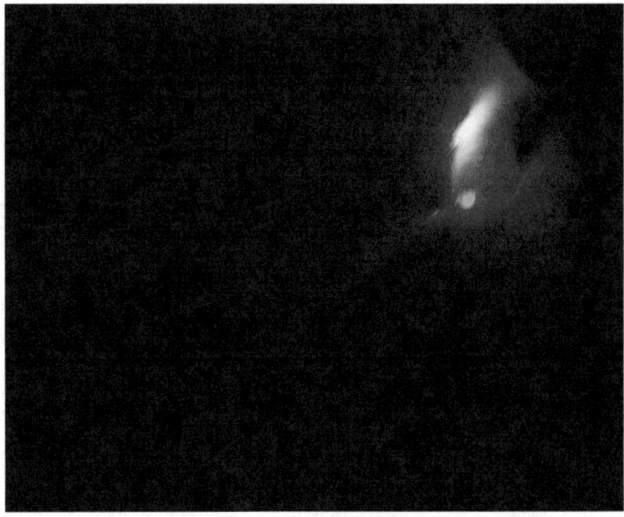

Fig. 2.83 Alternatively, the fibre optic can be placed externally to the eye and used to indent and transilluminate the retina for peripheral laser application

Yellow lasers (561 nm) are available which may have advantages around the macula because of reduced absorption by Xanthophyll.

Diode lasers are available which produce a wavelength of 810 nm (infrared), these burn deep into the retina and choroid without a visible burn on the retina until a large burn has occurred in the choroid. Care must be taken when using diode lasers that choroidal ischemia is not created.

The adhesion of the retina from laser has been described as early as 24 h after application [15]. Use a curved endolaser probe in phakic eyes to avoid the shaft of the laser contacting the lens. The curve can also be used to aid application of laser to the pre-equatorial retina as the tip can be kept more perpendicular to the retinal surface. Straight probes must approach some peripheral retina at an oblique angle risking a scrape of the retina.

Standard settings are 200 mW, 0.1 second burn duration, and 0.1 second interval between burns on repeat. Continuous burns are used by some surgeons, but this runs the risk of an excessive burn during delays in change of direction of the laser probe. It is hard to keep the rate of movement of your instrument constant over the retina. If the instrument is slowed down, for example during a change of direction you will increase the burn in that area. Short rapid repeated burns avoid this problem (Fig. 2.84).

Increase the intensity of the burns by:

1. Increasing the power
2. Increasing the duration
3. Going closer to the retina

Avoid lasering onto preretinal, retinal, or subretinal haemorrhage if possible. Lasering haemorrhage causes a burn in a layer of the retina that is undesirable and may not produce the adhesion between retinal and RPE and choroid that is necessary or the destruction of ischaemic outer retina that is desired.

Always check and recheck the position of the macula if you are applying pan-retinal photocoagulation (PRP) so that you do not drift into that area. Put a line of laser on the temporal edge of the macula to indicate the posterior extent of PRP in that meridian.

Fibre-optic instruments can be used to provide light inside the sphere of the eye. The tips of the fibre optic can be varied to provide different angles of illumination (Fig. 2.85, 2.86, 2.87, 2.88, 2.89, 2.90).

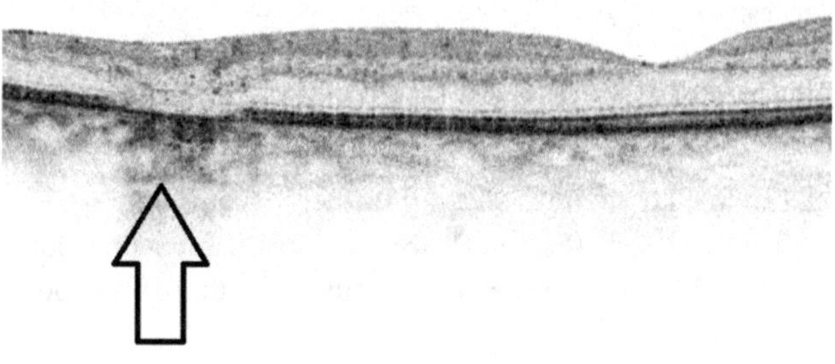

Fig. 2.84 A laser burn (arrow) showing fusion of the layers of the retina

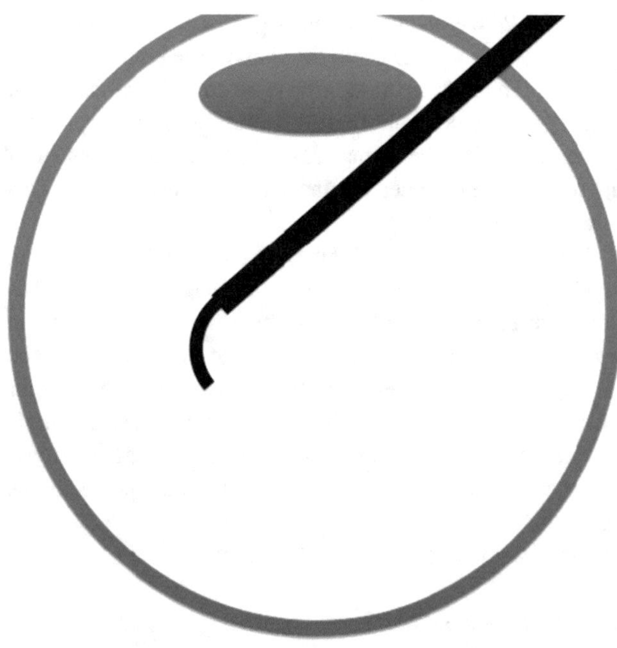

Fig. 2.85 Applying a curve to the fibre optic is useful if applying laser. This allows the surgeon to apply the laser at 90 degrees to the surface to be treated maintaining a focused treatment area

Fig. 2.86 Applying the laser obliquely to the surface creates a diffuse burn, which is elongated and difficult to control

Fig. 2.87 Some fibre optics can be retracted up the sleeve of the instrument to vary the curvature

Yag Laser

Nd: YAG (neodymium-doped yttrium aluminium garnet; Nd:$Y_3Al_5O_{12}$).

Nd: YAG lasers are examples of solid-state lasers because they use laser diode to pump a solid crystal (Nd: YAG crystal), which produces an emission wavelength of 1064 nm (infrared). The wavelength can be frequency doubled to provide a "green" laser for photocoagulation.

Fig. 2.88 The curve aids reaching the whole internal surface, important as the entry point of the fibre optic is fixed

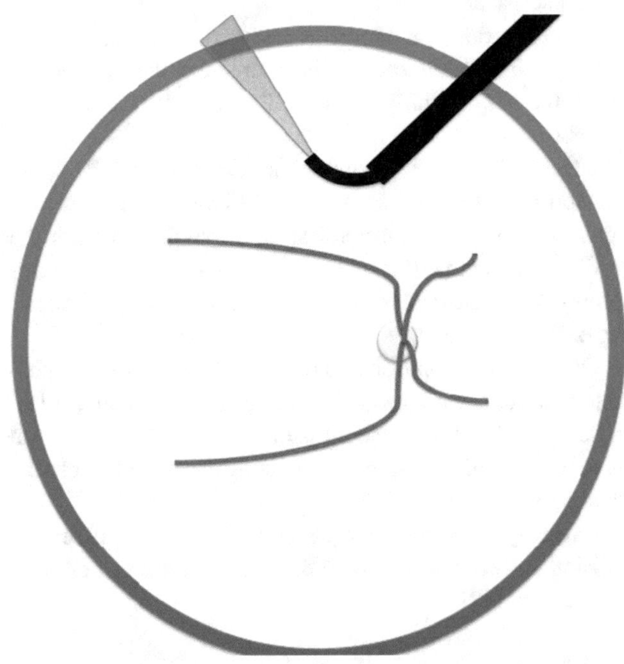

Fig. 2.89 The curve allows the application of laser in different directions whilst maintaining 90 degrees

In ophthalmology, the laser can be operated in Q-switch mode. In this modality, the usual return of light into the medium is prevented during activation of the medium by the diode laser. When maximal energy is reached in the medium, the light can return, causing a short (nanoseconds) and extremely high, the release of energy (kilowatts). The high energy causes ionisation of atoms and plasma formation, i.e.

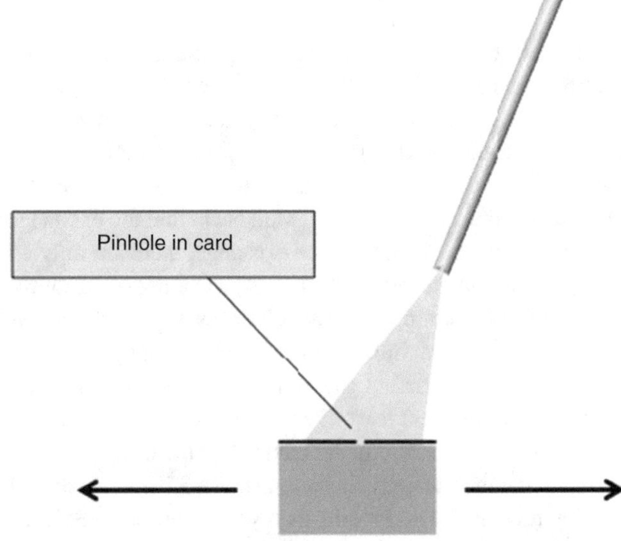

Fig. 2.90 The light intensity increases as the light is closer to the tissue and in the centre of the beam

atoms stripped of electrodes, with a surrounding area of high pressure (creating a destructive shock wave) when applied to the tissue.

These lasers are used to disrupt tissues, which can be reached through optically clear media without the need for the tissue to absorb the wavelength of the laser. They are used on relatively transparent tissues such as a posterior capsule in lens implants or the cornea (intralase). They may be used on tissues where a thermal burn would be undesirable such as peripheral iris.

Using a Contact Lens

For certain moves which require good depth perception and high magnification, and are not restricted by a reduced visual field of view, a contact lens (e.g. Machemer lens) to negate the refraction to the cornea can be used [16]. Disposable lenses are available which can be placed on the cornea with some methylcellulose to provide adherence. For certain difficult macular procedures such as the commencement of internal limiting membrane peel, these can be useful as the membrane can be discriminated from the nerve fibre layer more easily. The field of view is much reduced, and the view is no longer inverted. Be careful when inserting the instruments, it is a long time before they come into view compared with the IVS. If you are using angled instruments take care that you know where the heel of the instrument is in the eye. It is possible to touch the retina with it whilst watching the tips of the forceps. In addition, there is a tendency to have the light pipe closer to the retina risking light toxicity.

Closing

Always close the superior sclerotomies first, and the inferior infusion sclerotomy last as this controls the IOP. Remove both the superior trochars and check they are sealed, then use a 27-gauge needle inserted into the pars plana to vent. This has the advantage that the superior sclerotomies can be check for leaks whilst the air pump is still available before the exchange of gas. If you wait until after the exchange, there are only 15 mls of gas left in the syringe to sort out a leaking sclerotomy.

Keep the air pump on and attach the syringe with the gas to the three-way cannula, close off the air pump and then exchange the long-acting gas by injecting through the infusion cannula. Inject at least 35 mls of the gas to flush out the air in eyes with 25 mm or less axial length. In eyes bigger than this the theoretical volume to achieve 97% saturation of the gas mix in the syringe in the eye is more than 35 mls, therefore, two syringes should be used.

Axial length (mm)	21.5	23.5	25	26.5	28.5	30	31.5
Pseudophakic vitreous cavity volume (ml)	4.06	5.44	6.64	8.02	10.13	11.93	13.94
Flush to 97% saturation (ml)	25	31	36	44	64	68	77

The volume of gas required to flush the vitreous cavity to achieve 97% according to the axial length of the eye [17].

Remove the needle. Keep some gas in a syringe (15 mls) to allow a top-up of gas if some gas leaks during the disconnection of the infusion at the end of the operation.

Note: Take care with the use of the three-way tap. Do not turn the tap so that the air and the gas syringe are in connection because air will enter the syringe and dilute your injection of gas.

Check the intraocular pressure with your fingertip (using the finger's Pacinian corpuscles to assess the pressure!), aiming for 20 mmHg (your fingertip is a better pressure sensor in my view than pressing the eye with an instrument). Alternatively use a Barraquer Terry Scale tonometer contact lens to check the pressure.

Always remove the infusion last. If the globe is soft check for leaks from the sclerotomies, suture if necessary, with 8/0 or 10/0 Vicryl. To elevate the IOP, add BSS to the anterior chamber via a paracentesis or if gas filled inject gas through the pars plana using a 30-gauge needle. Check the pressure again.

Leaks will show as gas bubbles subconjunctivally. This is to be avoided if possible, as finding the sclerotomy becomes more difficult with the conjunctiva elevated.

Subconjunctival gas can be removed by piercing the bubble with a needle.

Liquid leaks are more difficult to see but are suspected if there is a gradual reduction in the IOP. Close the sclerotomies and turn the infusion off. The IOP should be maintained over time but if it drops you have a leak somewhere. Recheck your sclerotomies and try to massage closed once more (apply pressure so the sclera goes blue on the upper surface of the sclerotomy tunnel).

Full concentration fluorescein dropped onto the conjunctiva will indicate a fluid leak (the leaking fluid dilutes the fluorescein changing its colour from orange to green).

Surgical Pearl

Intrascleral Hydration for 23-Gauge Pars Plana Vitrectomy Sclerotomy Closure

At the end of a vitrectomy (for macular hole or pucker or whenever you want to leave air or gas tamponade into the vitreous chamber), if the eye pressure is low after trocar removal, it is often necessary to fill up the eye with air or gas. Massage of the sclerotomy usually is sufficient to achieve sclerotomy closure but, in some cases, if the sclerotomy continues to leak (more frequently using 23G vitrectomy rather than 25G), the surgeon may have to suture them because they are not self-sealing.

A useful trick that can be considered both surgical time sparing, and suture sparing is to hydrate the sclerotomy when the air/gas infusion is still active in the vitreous chamber.

Using a 30G needle mounted on a syringe with BSS, the surgeon injects a little amount of BSS close to the sclerotomy, directly into the scleral stroma (passing through the conjunctiva) so that the stromal oedema will close the sclerotomy. Wash the ocular surface with BBS to check the sealing of the sclerotomy.

Once the infusion trocar is removed (final step), it is possible that the eye is hypotonic from gas or air leaking. Also, in this case, hydrate of the infusion sclerotomy. The eye can be easily and safely refilled by injecting gas directly from the pars-plana.

Basically, it is the same concept of the corneal service incision and corneal tunnel hydro-suture at the end of cataract surgery [18].

Prof. Stanislao Rizzo, Alfonso Savastano. Rome, Italy

Advantages and Disadvantages of 23G, 25G, and 27G Systems

Advantages

- Minimal tissue injury.
- No or minimal suturing.
- Increased patient comfort.
- Shortened duration of closure of surgery.

- Ease of inserting of instruments (no searching for the sclerotomy needed).
- Good peroperative pressure control, especially if trochars with valves are used.
- Rapid rehabilitation of the patient in the postoperative period.
- Shorter duration of postoperative drops.

Disadvantages

- With the conjunctiva intact, in patients with shortened fornixes it more difficult to perform indentation of the eye to view the peripheral retina.
- Risk of hypotony.
- Risk of endophthalmitis.
- Instrumentation, e.g. foreign body forceps that cannot be inserted through the trochars.
- The fine gauge of the instruments alters the ability of the surgeon to move the eye around during surgery.
- Increased duration of vitreous extraction with early systems.

Initially, the transconjunctival systems can be used for less complex cases, e.g. vitreous biopsy, vitreous haemorrhage, macular disease, and simple rhegmatogenous retinal detachments. The role of these systems is now almost universal, and I routinely use 25 G for all cases now and create an extra 20 G sclerotomy in the rare instance that it is required.

Combined Cataract Extraction and PPV

Additional Surgical Steps

- Perform a routine small incision (clear corneal) phacoemulsification procedure with foldable lens implantation at the start of the operation before any of the PPV has been performed.
- Changes in technique.
  1. Keep the corneal section long and make sure that the internal orifice is slightly more central in the cornea, this keeps the iris away from the wound and prevents the effects of pressure drop on egress of fluid lifting the iris into the wound. A wound that is too peripheral is close to the iris. Fluid flow from the wound accelerates near the wound (there is a shallower profile peripherally) causing a pressure drop according to Bernoulli's equation (see appendix) dropping the pressure and causing the iris to lift into the wound.
  2. The capsulorhexis should not be too large as gas bubbles can tilt the lens and cause dislocation of the inferior edge of the optic risking trapping the pupil margin.
  3. Some surgeons set up the vitrectomy before the phaco to allow them to reduce the vitreous volume before the phaco. This is not necessary in routine cases.
  4. Hydrate the wound but be aware that if excessive this may obscure the view of the peripheral retina during the PPV (inferior retina if the wound is superior).
- Check the wound, in general, no suture is necessary for injectable IOLs as the wound is small and secure. If larger wounds are used, for example for foldable rather than injectable IOLs, you may need to secure the wound with a single 10/0 absorbable suture.

In many cases, cataract in the affected eye reduces the view of the retina. It is prudent to remove the cataract at the time of surgery to:

- Improve the view.
- Avoid worsening of the cataract during surgery.
- Avoid worsening of the cataract after surgery thereby delaying visual recovery.

Phacoemulsification of the lens and foldable or injectable intraocular lens implantation (IOL) can be performed as a routine procedure at the time of surgery before commencement of the PPV [19]. The wound should be carefully tunnelled with an anterior tilt and internal opening which is slightly further into the centre of the cornea. This is to ensure that the wound is stable during the PPV. Injectable lenses are desirable because of the reduction in the wound size and increased stability of the anterior chamber peroperatively during the PPV. The wounds from injectable implantation can be left unsutured. Foldable lenses may require a 10/0 absorbable suture to avoid opening of the wound during the PPV and resulting in iris prolapse.

Note: Place the subsequent sclerotomies away from the site of the paracentesis or the cataract wound to avoid opening these on inserting instruments.

Avoid removing the posterior capsule early in the operation because condensation may appear on the exposed IOL when gas is used. If this occurs, e.g. in an eye with a capsulectomy, it is easily remedied by wiping the implant with an instrument such as the flute needle, or if the condensation returns, by placing a small drop of viscoelastic on the posterior of the IOL [20].

There is a tendency for the postoperative refraction to be slightly more myopic (−0.36D) in this combined procedure if gas is used than that predicted by preoperative biometry [21, 22] (Figs. 2.91, 2.92, 2.93, 2.94).

Surgical Pearl

Avoiding Hypotony

Perioperative hypotony can result in a potentially disastrous suprachoroidal haemorrhage. The commonest cause of such

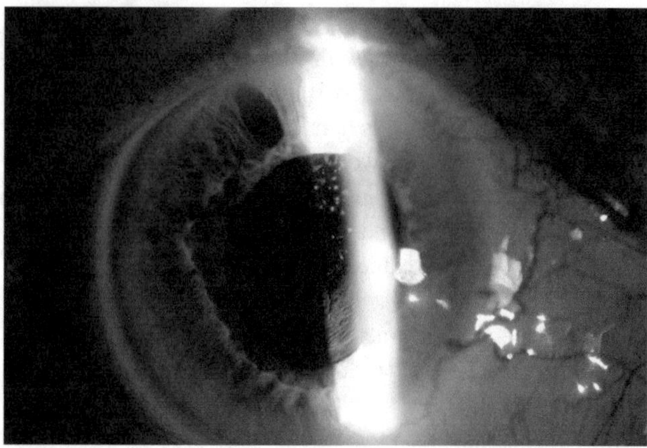

Fig. 2.91 Be careful to avoid iris prolapse during the combined PPV and phaco procedure as this will damage the iris and be visible postoperatively as in this patient. Keeping the phaco wound long and the internal opening more towards the centre of the cornea (when making the incision angle slightly anteriorly) reduces the chance of iris prolapse. Insert a single 10/0 Vicryl suture if the wound is in any way unstable. With injectable lens implants a suture is usually unnecessary

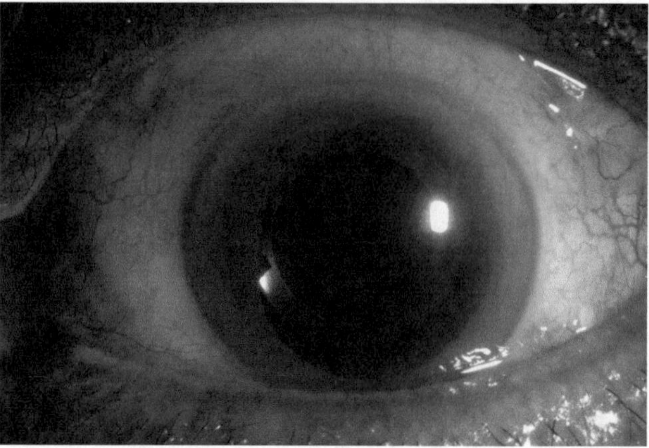

Fig. 2.92 Performing a combined PPV and Phaco and IOL is an effective method for speeding visual recovery but is associated with an increase in posterior synaechiae formation postoperatively

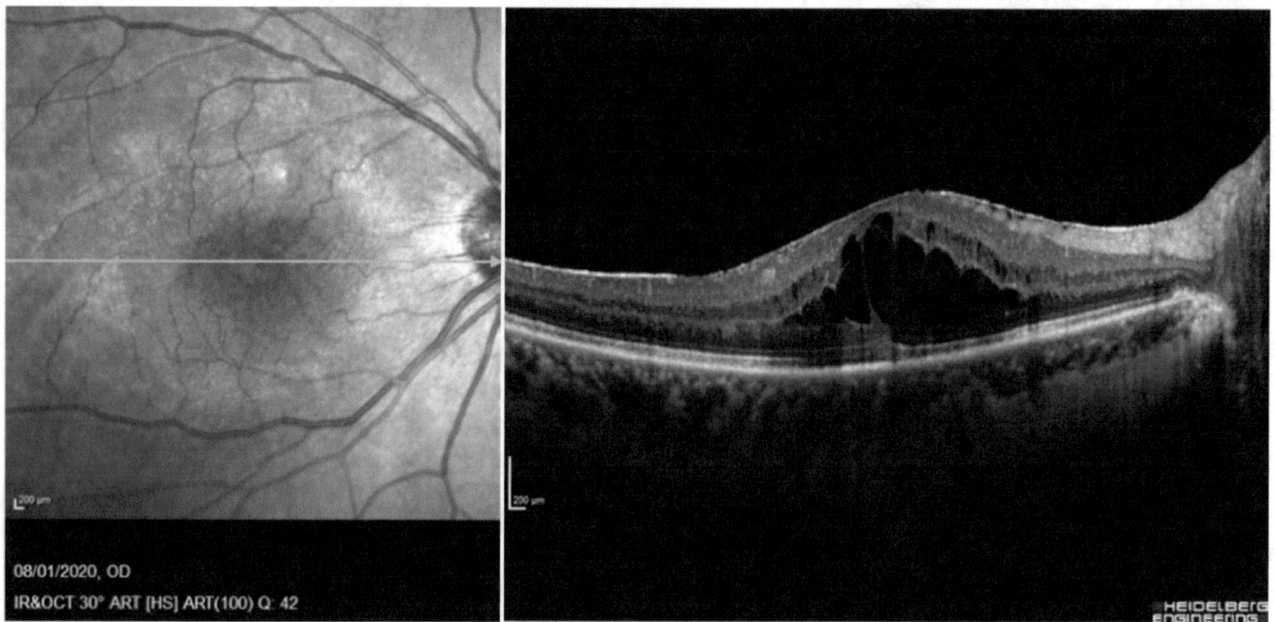

Fig. 2.93 CMO seems to be more common after phacoemulsification and IOL in a vitrectomised eye

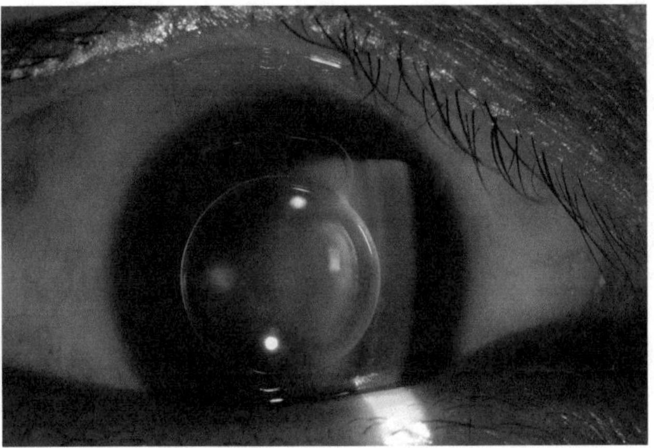

Fig. 2.94 Phakic IOLs in high myopes should be removed in combined PPV and cataract extraction

hypotony is a leaking port or ports. This risk can be reduced with a simple modification of the air–gas exchange procedure: Once the fluid–air exchange has been performed the 2 superior cannulae are removed and checked, one at a time. The IOP is maintained at a safe level throughout by the maintaining the infusion of air (or fluid if not using air). Unhurried closure of each sclerotomy can be ensured using the usual techniques of direct compression or suturing as required. The infusion line can also be temporarily closed as a further check. The air–gas exchange is then performed through a short 25 g needle held on a syringe with the plunger removed, which is inserted until the tip can be seen in mid cavity through the superior pars plana. The infusion cannula is then removed. Pumping the eye up to a high pressure before this is counterproductive, it encourages leaks which are anyway less common from this port. A 27- or 30-gauge needle must always be available to put on the gas syringe to re-inflate the eye if required. One of the sclerotomies can be used for such top-up injections without compromising their closure.

The more usual technique of performing the air–gas exchange before removing the superior cannulae risks a period of uncontrolled hypotony if any of the ports leak. It is all too easy to use up the remaining diluted gas in the syringe while attempting to regain control.

Mr. D Alistair H Laidlaw, St Thomas Hospital, London, UK

How to Decide Whether to Perform Combined Surgery

Perform combined surgery when any cataract is present preoperatively to avoid loss of visualisation of the retina from progression of the cataract during surgery. In eyes with clear lenses perform combined surgery when the risk of developing cataract is high in the postoperative period thereby reducing the number of surgical episodes for the patient.

Combine surgery in patients with:

- Pre-existing cataract
- Macular holes
- Macular puckers
- Elderly RRD

Do not combine surgery

- Diabetic retinopathy
- Young RRD
- Other ischaemic retinopathies

These are not hard and fast rules; take into consideration several other factors. Accommodation.

Unless an accommodative IOL is used the patient loses accommodation after IOL implantation. Accommodation is reported to be retained in crystalline lenses after PPV [23]. Of course, after the age of 50 years, accommodation is lost, and any near focus is from depth of focus only therefore IOL implantation is less detrimental. Fortunately, the loss of accommodation coincides with the age at which the risk of cataract post vitrectomy increases sharply (see complications, cataract earlier in the chapter).

Biometry

There are possible problems obtaining accurate biometry in eyes for PPV, e.g. the retina is anteriorly placed in macula off RRD disrupting axial length measurements. With ERM the retina is thickened and more anterior, thereby causing underestimation of axial length and a myopic postoperative correction. A mean myopic shift of −0.36D has been reported after combined surgery [22, 24]. In addition, the gas bubble may anteriorly displace the IOL causing further myopic shift.

The surgeon may need 3 adjusted A constants:

- Phacoemulsification
- PPV + Phacoemulsification
- PPV + Phacoemulsification and Gas

Other factors

- Astigmatism is changed by PPV making prediction of astigmatism correction during the cataract operation more difficult [22].
- The increased instability of the anterior chamber during surgery can be usually controlled by adjustments to surgical technique and good wound architecture.

- The combined operation has the advantage of improving access to anterior vitreous and peripheral retina removing the risk of crystalline lens touch.
- In the postoperative period combined surgery increases the chance of fibrin and uveitis. This is especially the case in diabetic patients (16%). Posterior synaechiae can occur (6–30%) being increased in diabetics and with gas use. Anterior capsular phimosis and cystoid macular oedema are also seen [25–27]. Ultimately posterior synaechiae can lead to a rare presentation of pupil block glaucoma (Fig. 2.95).

For	Against
Ease of PPV	Loss of crystalline lens too early
Convenience/reduces the number of hospital admissions and anaesthetics	Loss of Accommodation
No period of disability for the patient	Slightly higher postoperative inflammation
Good access to peripheral retina	Posterior synaechiae
Possible increased gas fill	IOL movement
	Inflammation
	Biometry inaccuracy
	Slightly poorer quality cataract surgery

Complications

Capsule rupture rates have been described as 2.2% with this technique [28] and postoperative events as follows: posterior capsular opacification 10.6%, posterior synechiae 4.2%, uveitis 2.1%, angle-closure glaucoma 1.6%, and rhegmatogenous retinal detachment 1.1%.

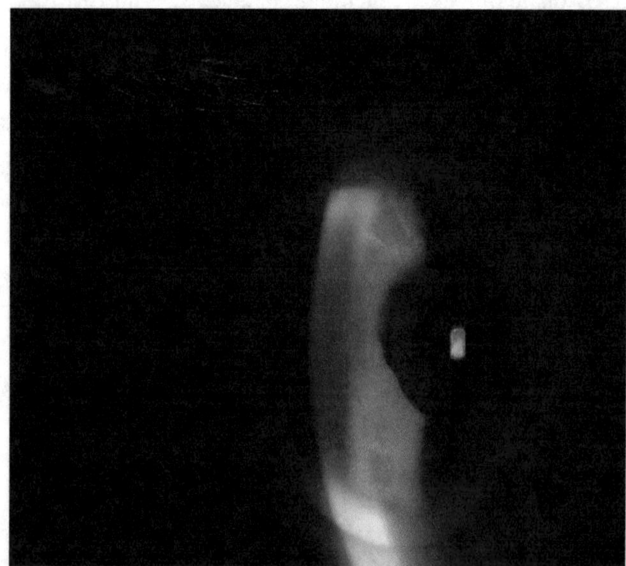

Fig. 2.95 Performing combined cataract extraction and PPV can increase the chance of posterior synaechiae, which in the extreme case can induce 360-degree posterior synaechiae and iris bombe as in this eye, causing pupil block glaucoma

Chandelier Systems and Bimanual Surgery

Using specialised lens systems can allow the illumination of the retina by the microscope lamp [29]. Alternatively, self-retaining chandelier fibre-optic lights can be used, avoid the use of the manual fibre-optic illumination. A high output light source is required, e.g. Xenon to provide adequate illumination. There are various designs of fibre optic (single optic and twin optics), which can be placed in the pars plana at a convenient site that does not interfere with surgery usually 6 or 12 o'clock. The chandelier frees up the second hand to allow the use of two instruments in the eye, e.g. scissors and forceps, or indentation and cutter. This can be useful in complex procedures such as:

- Diabetic tractional retinal detachment.
- Diabetic combined rhegmatogenous and tractional retinal detachment.
- Retinectomy surgery for PVR.
- Trauma.

In 25 gauge surgery chandeliers are often required because poor mobility of the eye requires the surgeon to indent with the second hand to search for retinal breaks or for the application of peripheral laser (Figs. 2.96, 2.97).

Often the illumination is poorer than that obtained by the manual approach because the light cannot be directed to the point of interest. To overcome this, the surgeon can ask an assistant to direct the chandelier illumination during the surgery (Fig. 2.98).

Possible complications:

- Lens touch
- Retinal touch
- Light toxicity

Dyes

Three dyes are used routinely in retinal surgery, Indocyanine green and Brilliant blue for staining of the internal limiting membrane (ILM), and Trypan blue for staining epiretinal membranes (including proliferative vitreoretinopathy) and to a lesser degree the ILM. These will be discussed in Chaps. 11 and 12.

Intracameral Antibiotics

Insertion of 1 mg of intracameral Cefuroxime at the end of surgery is recommended to reduce the risk of postoperative endophthalmitis. At this dose, it will achieve minimal inhibitory concentration (0.13 mg/ml) without reaching toxicity. The concentration for given dose changes with the size of the

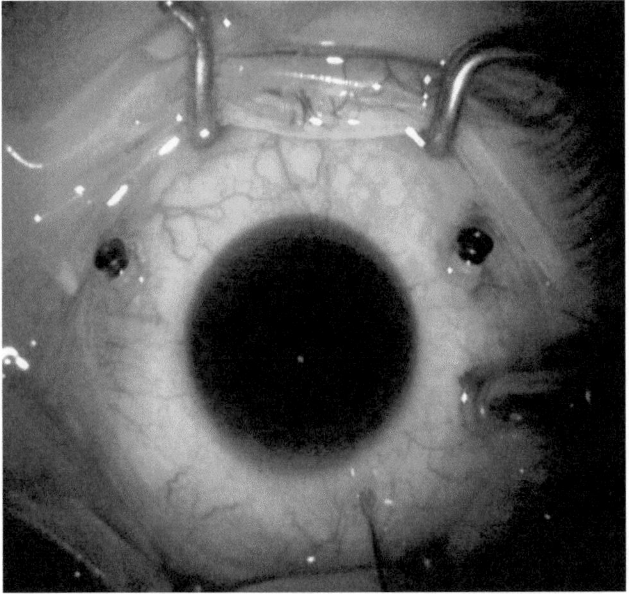

Fig. 2.96 A simple two optic chandelier is inserted by first creating the incisions in the sclera with a needle, be careful not to lose the location of the incisions, therefore remove the needle at the same time as inserting the chandelier tip

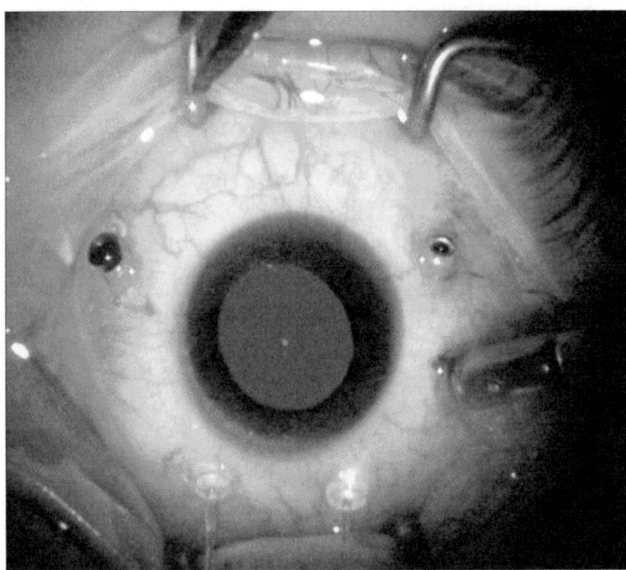

Fig. 2.97 In this case two chandeliers have been inserted in an inferior position

eye and whether a tamponade has been inserted or not (Fig. 2.99).

Intravitreal Injections

Inevitably the vitreoretinal surgeon is going to be involved in burgeoning usage of intravitreal injection, primarily anti-

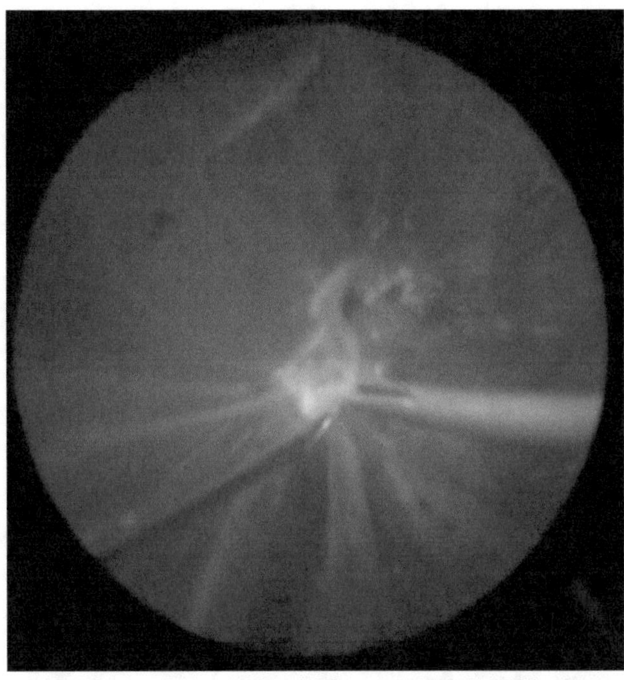

Fig. 2.98 Bimanual surgery being used to dissect membranes in proliferative diabetic retinopathy

mg/ml	4ml	gas	7ml	gas	10ml	gas
cefuroxime 1mg/0.1ml	0.25	1.25	0.14	0.71	0.10	0.50

Fig. 2.99 The concentrations of cefuroxime in the eye after injection of 1 mg/0.1 ml in different sized eyes and with tamponade in situ

VEGF agents but also steroid. Only a basic technique is described.

- Dilate the pupil of the eye for injection.
- Prepare the eye with topical local anaesthesia.
- Once anaesthetised apply topical povidone-iodine (draw some into the minim of anaesthetic and drop onto the conjunctiva).
- Apply a sterile drape to skin and lids.
- Insert a lid speculum.

There are various methods to measure 3.5–4 mm from the limbus for the injection site. The distance can be judged by using a 1-ml syringe and the 0.01 ml markings, make sure you use the same type of syringe each time and have measured 3.5 mm and 4 mm with a caliper at least once on that type of syringe. Otherwise use a disposable measure or caliper.

Using a 30-G needle on a 1-ml syringe, prime the needle (approximately 0.04 mls of dead space) and at 90° to the surface insert the needle tip.

Inject the drug.

Remove the needle and immediately press with a cotton tip to prevent egress of fluid.

Ask the patient if they can see your hand and check the optic nerve perfusion with an indirect ophthalmoscope. If the patient has "blacked out" vision or there is no perfusion of the optic nerve perform a paracentesis to remove some aqueous (use a 1-ml syringe with the plunger removed and a 30-G needle, insert at the limbus and allow aqueous to passively enter the syringe to 0.05 ml). Be aware that in rare circumstances the injection of fluid into the vitreous cavity and removal from the anterior chamber risks aqueous misdirection glaucoma.

Note: If you are injecting a substance into the eye and using tamponade agents, inject the substance when the eye is liquid filled (BSS) just before exchange for the tamponade agent (oil or gas). This ensures the correct concentration of the substance in the remaining aqueous layer.

Injection Medications

AntiVEGF drugs are the commonest injections given and have altered the referral patterns to vitreoretinal surgeons. Other therapies include antimicrobial agents, and intravitreal steroids. These will be discussed in the appropriate chapters.

Indications for antiVEGF injection

- CNV from AMD.
- CNV from other causes.
- Cystoid macular oedema (diabetes, vein occlusion, postoperative).
- Tractional retinal detachment pre-treatment before vitrectomy in diabetic retinopathy.
- Neovascular glaucoma from retinal vein occlusion or diabetic retinopathy.
- Central serous retinopathy.
- Diabetic retinopathy.

Complications

- Endophthalmitis.
  - Bacterial.
  - Sterile.
- Vitreous haemorrhage.
- Lens damage.
- Bubbles of oil in the vitreous cavity from use of silicone syringes.
- Raised IOP.
  - Volumetric.
  - Aqueous misdirection.
- Retinal detachment.
- Central retinal artery occlusion.
- Retinal pigment epithelial rip in CNV.
- Aqueous misdirection (Fig. 2.100).

Slow Release Preparations

Injection capsules and implants have been designed usually to allow slow release of intraocular steroid. These have had variable success being associated with high rates of cataract and glaucoma but some improvement in outcome at 6 months for diabetic retinopathy, retinal vein occlusion, and uveitis [30, 31].

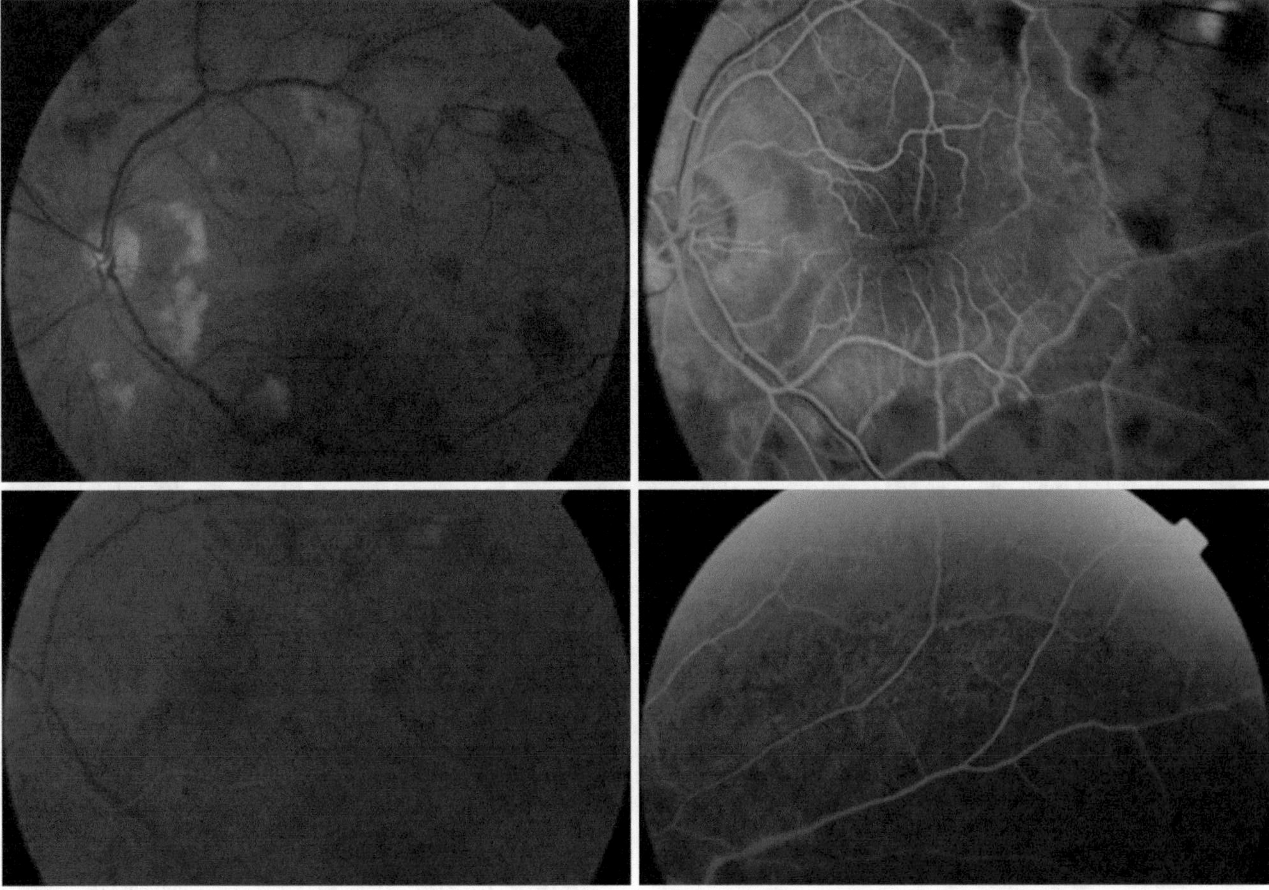

Fig. 2.100 Retinal vascular occlusion from high dose cefuroxime in the eye. This classically occurs with aminoglycosides, but any high dose agent has the potential to be toxic to the retina. Great care must be taken with insertion of intraocular drugs that the agent has a wide margin of safety and is dosaged correctly. Remember additional use of tamponade reduces the aqueous volume in the eye increasing the concentration of a drug by 4–5 times

Summary

The routine procedure is the pars plana vitrectomy which can be adapted to deal with a large variety of retinal conditions. Knowledge of the properties of the various peroperative and postoperative agents that can be employed should be obtained.

Checking small gauge surgery wounds.

References

1. Machemer R, Buettner H, Norton EW, Parel JM. Vitrectomy: a pars plana approach. Trans Am Acad Ophthalmol Otolaryngol. 1971;75(4):813–20.
2. Gupta B, Neffendorf JE, Williamson TH. Trends and emerging patterns of practice in vitreoretinal surgery. Acta Ophthalmol. 2018;96(7):e889–e90. https://doi.org/10.1111/aos.13102.
3. Sugisaka E, Shinoda K, Ishida S, Imamura Y, Ozawa Y, Shinoda H, et al. Patients' descriptions of visual sensations during pars plana vitrectomy under retrobulbar anesthesia. Am J Ophthalmol. 2007;144(2):245–51. S0002-9394(07)00433-3 [pii]. https://doi.org/10.1016/j.ajo.2007.05.001.
4. Desai A, Rubinstein A, Reginald A, Parulekar M, Tanner V. Feasibility of day-case vitreoretinal surgery. Eye. 2008;22(2):169–72. 6702515 [pii]. https://doi.org/10.1038/sj.eye.6702515.
5. Spitznas M. A binocular indirect ophthalmomicroscope (BIOM) for non-contact wide-angle vitreous surgery. Graefes Arch Clin Exp Ophthalmol. 1987;225(1):13–5.
6. Bond LJ, Judd KM, Tucker BJ, Flake M, Boukhny M. Physics of phacoemulsification. United States. Department of Energy; 2003.
7. Fisher RF. Elastic constants of the human lens capsule. J Physiol. 1969;201(1):1–19. https://doi.org/10.1113/jphysiol.1969.sp008739.
8. Weeber HA, Eckert G, Soergel F, Meyer CH, Pechhold W, van der Heijde RG. Dynamic mechanical properties of human lenses. Exp Eye Res. 2005;80(3):425–34.
9. Wallenten KG, Andreasson S, Ghosh F. Retinal function after vitrectomy. Retina. 2008;28(4):558–63. https://doi.org/10.1097/IAE.0b013e31815e9890. 00006982-200804000-00005 [pii]
10. Sato T, Kusaka S, Oshima Y, Fujikado T. Analyses of cutting and aspirating properties of vitreous cutters with high-speed camera. Retina. 2008;28(5):749–54. https://doi.org/10.1097/IAE.0b013e3181631907. 00006982-200805000-00013 [pii]

11. Magalhaes O Jr, Chong L, DeBoer C, Bhadri P, Kerns R, Barnes A, et al. Vitreous dynamics: vitreous flow analysis in 20-, 23-, and 25-gauge cutters. Retina. 2008;28(2):236–41. https://doi.org/10.1097/IAE.0b013e318158e9e0. 00006982-200802000-00006 [pii]
12. Fang SY, DeBoer CM, Humayun MS. Performance analysis of new-generation vitreous cutters. Graefes Arch Clin Exp Ophthalmol. 2008;246(1):61–7. https://doi.org/10.1007/s00417-007-0672-8.
13. DeBoer C, Fang S, Lima LH, McCormick M, Bhadri P, Kerns R, et al. Port geometry and its influence on vitrectomy. Retina. 2008;28(8):1061–7. https://doi.org/10.1097/IAE.0b013e3181840b64. 00006982-200809000-00005 [pii]
14. Peyman GA, Salzano TC, Green JL Jr. Argon endolaser. Arch Ophthalmol. 1981;99(11):2037–8.
15. Folk JC, Sneed SR, Folberg R, Coonan P, Pulido JS. Early retinal adhesion from laser photocoagulation. Ophthalmology. 1989;96(10):1523–5.
16. Machemer R, Parel JM, Norton EW. Vitrectomy: a pars plana approach. Technical improvements and further results. Trans Am Acad Ophthalmol Otolaryngol. 1972;76(2):462–6.
17. Shunmugam M, Shunmugam S, Williamson TH, Laidlaw DA. Air-gas exchange reevaluated: clinically important results of a computer simulation. Invest Ophthalmol Vis Sci. 2011;52(11):8262–5. iovs.11-8258 [pii]. https://doi.org/10.1167/iovs.11-8258.
18. Rizzo S, Pacini B, De Angelis L, Barca F, Savastano A, Giansanti F, et al. Intrascleral hydration for 23-gauge pars plana vitrectomy sclerotomy closure. Retina. 2020; https://doi.org/10.1097/IAE.0000000000002703.
19. Suzuki Y, Sakuraba T, Mizutani H, Matsuhashi H, Nakazawa M. Postoperative complications after simultaneous vitrectomy and cataract surgery. Ophthalmic Surg Lasers. 2001;32(5):391–6.
20. Jaffe GJ. Management of condensation on a foldable acrylic intraocular lens after vitrectomy and fluid-air exchange. Am J Ophthalmol. 1997;124(5):692–3.
21. Falkner-Radler CI, Benesch T, Binder S. Accuracy of preoperative biometry in vitrectomy combined with cataract surgery for patients with epiretinal membranes and macular holes: results of a prospective controlled clinical trial. J Cataract Refract Surg. 2008;34(10):1754–60. S0886-3350(08)00688-3 [pii]. https://doi.org/10.1016/j.jcrs.2008.06.021.
22. Suzuki Y, Sakuraba T, Mizutani H, Matsuhashi H, Nakazawa M. Postoperative refractive error after simultaneous vitrectomy and cataract surgery. Ophthalmic Surg Lasers. 2000;31(4):271–5.
23. Fisher RF. Is the vitreous necessary for accommodation in man? Br J Ophthalmol. 1983;67(3):206.
24. Byrne S, Ng J, Hildreth A, Danjoux JP, Steel DH. Refractive change following pseudophakic vitrectomy. BMC Ophthalmol. 2008;8:19. 1471-2415-8-19 [pii]. https://doi.org/10.1186/1471-2415-8-19.
25. Treumer F, Bunse A, Rudolf M, Roider J. Pars plana vitrectomy, phacoemulsification and intraocular lens implantation. Comparison of clinical complications in a combined versus two-step surgical approach. Graefes Arch Clin Exp Ophthalmol. 2006;244(7):808–15. https://doi.org/10.1007/s00417-005-0146-9.
26. Senn P, Schipper I, Perren B. Combined pars plana vitrectomy, phacoemulsification, and intraocular lens implantation in the capsular bag: a comparison to vitrectomy and subsequent cataract surgery as a two-step procedure. Ophthalmic Surg Lasers. 1995;26(5):420–8.
27. Shinoda K, O'Hira A, Ishida S, Hoshide M, Ogawa LS, Ozawa Y, et al. Posterior synechia of the iris after combined pars plana vitrectomy, phacoemulsification, and intraocular lens implantation. Jpn J Ophthalmol. 2001;45(3):276–80. S0021-5155(01)00319-7 [pii]
28. Fajgenbaum MAP, Neffendorf JE, Wong RS, Laidlaw DAH, Williamson TH. Intraoperative and postoperative complications in phacovitrectomy for epiretinal membrane and macular hole: a clinical audit of 1,000 consecutive eyes. Retina. 2018;38(9):1865–72. https://doi.org/10.1097/IAE.0000000000002034.
29. Horiguchi M, Kojima Y, Shimada Y. New system for fiberoptic-free bimanual vitreous surgery. Arch Ophthalmol. 2002;120(4):491–4.
30. Haller JA, Kuppermann BD, Blumenkranz MS, Williams GA, Weinberg DV, Chou C, et al. Randomized controlled trial of an intravitreous dexamethasone drug delivery system in patients with diabetic macular edema. Arch Ophthalmol. 2010;128(3):289–96. 128/3/289 [pii]. https://doi.org/10.1001/archophthalmol.2010.21.
31. Haller JA, Bandello F, Belfort R Jr, Blumenkranz MS, Gillies M, Heier J, et al. Randomized, sham-controlled trial of dexamethasone intravitreal implant in patients with macular edema due to retinal vein occlusion. Ophthalmology. 2010;117(6):1134–46 e3. S0161-6420(10)00311-8 [pii]. https://doi.org/10.1016/j.ophtha.2010.03.032.

3 Introduction to Vitreoretinal Surgery 2

Contents

T. H. Williamson, *Vitreoretinal Surgery*, https://doi.org/10.1007/978-3-030-68769-4_3

Maintaining a View

Stop and examine all elements in the system.

Microscope

Make sure each portion of the microscope is correctly attached and orientated, e.g. laser filter, stereo inverter, and illumination.

IVS

Inspect the alignment of the IVS and that it is securely attached. Check all the lenses are clean. Condensation can develop on the IVS lens, especially if the drape does not adhere to the skin around the nose. This allows the patient's exhaled air to escape and contact the lens. Replace the drapes if necessary. Cold lenses are more prone to condensation. The complication is more likely to happen when the lens is close to the warm cornea. Move the lens further from the eye until it gradually warms to room temperature. Wiping the lens clears the condensation temporarily.

Cornea

In some patients, the corneal epithelium will become oedematous, especially if the surgery is prolonged and in diabetic patients who have poor epithelial function. Debriding the epithelium with a broad blade restores clarity. Thereafter corneal drying during the surgery will be more rapid. Hydroxymethylcellulose (HPMC) can be used to moisturise the cornea preventing drying. Rarely the corneal stroma will develop a feathery opacity at the commencement of intraocular infusion. This will clear after a few minutes and does not require intervention (Fig. 3.1).

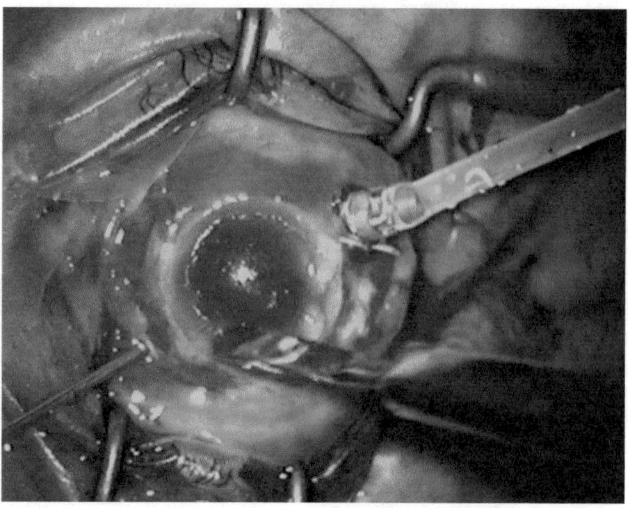

Fig. 3.1 To clear a view from corneal oedema debride the epithelium with a blunt knife

Blood in the Anterior Chamber

If the IOP has dropped during surgery, blood can enter the anterior chamber from the trabecular meshwork. Alternatively, patients with severe vitreous haemorrhage may have a trickle of haemorrhage into the anterior chamber from the vitreous cavity. Perform a paracentesis and wash out the blood with balanced salt solution. If the haemorrhage is recurrent, viscoelastic can be inserted to displace the blood from the pupillary aperture. Remember to remove the viscoelastic later.

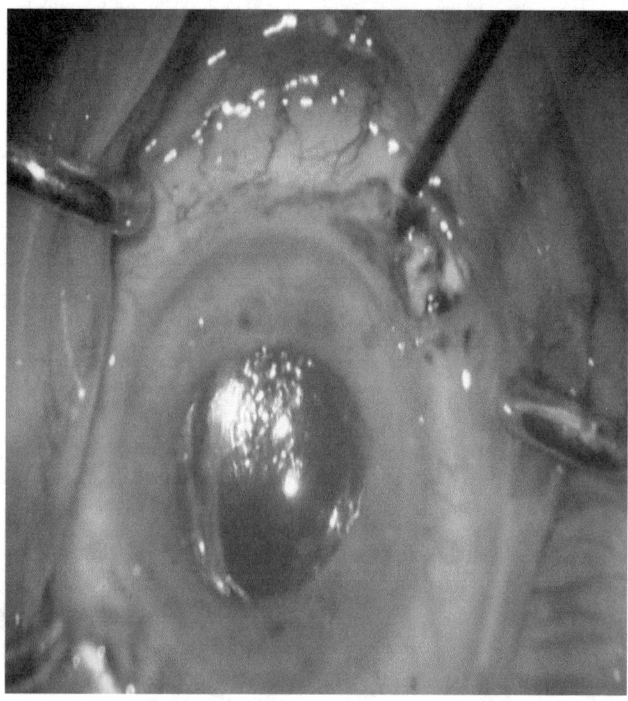

Fig. 3.2 Condensation occurs on lens implants when a posterior capsulotomy has been performed. This can compromise the view during surgery when air is inserted

Condensation on an Intraocular Lens Implant

If the posterior capsule has been removed and gas is in contact with the IOL, condensation may occur on the back of the IOL. First, wipe the back of the lens with a flute needle to add a layer of fluid onto the lens. This is usually enough. If recurrent condensation occurs add a small droplet of viscous fluid HPMC or viscoelastic onto the posterior surface of the IOL and wipe again (Figs. 3.2 and 3.3).

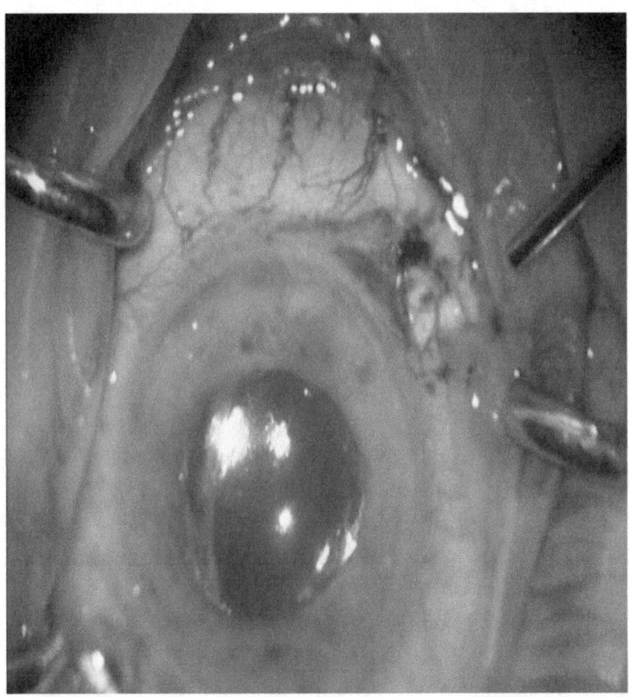

Fig. 3.3 By gently wiping the posterior surface of the lens with the blunt instrument, fluid can be passed over the lens and the view returned. Should the condensation return, some viscoelastic can be placed on the back of the lens and wiped which will retain the view

Cataract Formation

This will only occur peroperatively if the surgery is very prolonged so that the first rule is safe but quick surgery. Preoperatively judge the lens clarity, if there is pre-existing cataract this should be removed by phacoemulsification and lens implantation at the commencement of the surgery. An already cataractous lens is much more at risk of worsening during surgery than a clear lens. In the rare event of a lens clouding, such that the posterior segment is compromised, stabilise the posterior segment (fluid filled), and perform a phacoemulsification cataract extraction and PC IOL insertion and then continue the posterior segment surgery (Fig. 3.4).

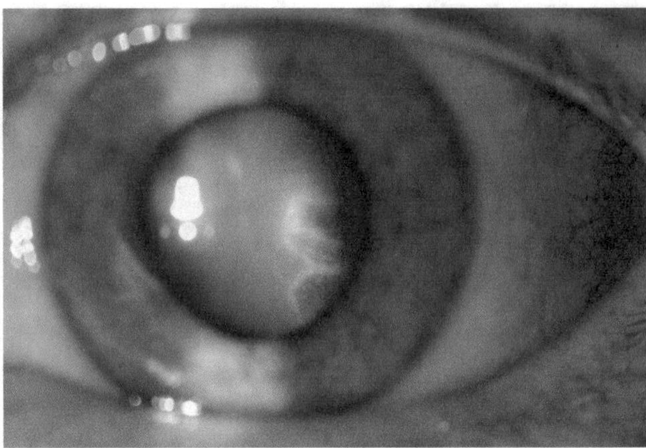

Fig. 3.4 Flow of fluid close to the lens has caused localised lens opacity

Pupillary Dilation

The modern IVS allow visualisation through surprisingly small apertures but if a larger pupil is desired here are some methods:

1. Using a Sub Tenon's LA injection will produce pupillary dilation.
2. Irrigation into the anterior chamber of 0.1 ml of 1% Phenylephrine (1 part of Phenylephrine 10% with 9 parts of balanced salt solution) or 0.1 ml of 2.5% Phenylephrine can be used.
3. Make sure posterior synaechiae have been divided by viscoelastic.
4. If the pupil remains constricted use iris hooks to expand but watch out for a postoperative fibrinous reaction.

Perioperative Complications

Iatrogenic Breaks

These must be identified and treated to avoid postoperative retinal detachment. Apply retinopexy and gas tamponade. Overall, peroperative iatrogenic retinal breaks have been described in 10% of vitrectomy patients [1], 5.5% of patients operated upon for macular hole [2], 20–33% of those with diabetic tractional retinal detachment [3], and 7.3% of those with complex retinal detachment surgery [4]. The complication is commoner in phakic patients and those without posterior vitreous detachment preoperatively [5] and is a risk factor for postoperative retinal detachment in diabetic surgery [6] (Fig. 3.5).

Causes

1. Bites of retina from the cutter produce moderate-sized round breaks. Care must be taken when removing the vitreous in a bullous retinal detachment that the cutter does not bite mobile retina. Remove some SRF to reduce the height of the bulla or splint the retina with some heavy liquid to reduce its mobility.
2. Tears from traction on the retina, e.g. from membrane peel or posterior hyaloid membrane (PHM) peel in macular hole surgery. In epiretinal membrane peel you can only pull on a membrane up to a force equal to the strength of the

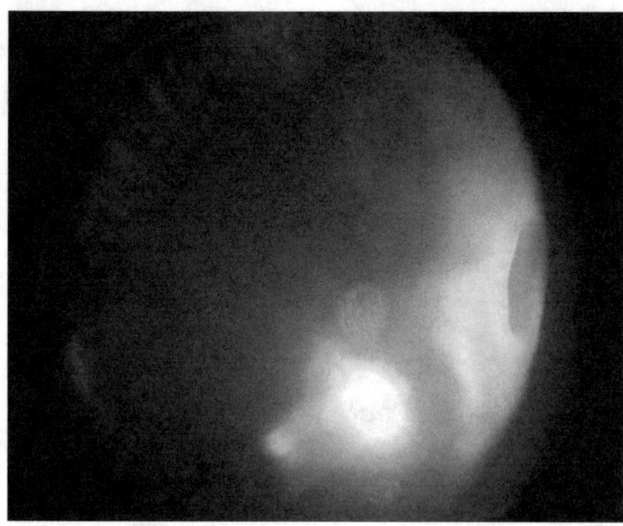

Fig. 3.5 A postoperative detachment has been caused by an entry site break

integrity of the retinal tissue, i.e. the adhesion of the membrane retina must be less than the strength of the retina. Be careful if lattice degeneration is present not to pull the PHM through the lattice lesions as this will tear the retina.

3. Giant retinal tears from traction on the vitreous base. The vitreous base will not separate from the retina. Any force on the vitreous base, e.g. from careless insertion of instruments, will take the retina with it causing a large retinal break.
4. Entry site breaks from vitreous incarceration into the sclerotomies. These may appear after the surgery as the vitreous is slowly drawn into the sclerotomy by postoperative fibrosis thereby producing traction on the retina and retinal tear formation. It is therefore important to remove as much vitreous as possible around trochars and to excise incarcerated vitreous.
5. Scrapes on the retina from contact of instruments onto the retina. You must be aware of the spatial relationships of the inside of the sphere of the eye to avoid scraping the retina whilst moving instruments, e.g. when performing peripheral panretinal photocoagulation. Moving peripherally in the eye requires a compensatory shortening of the length of the shaft of the instrument in the eye, spatial relationships in the eye earlier in the chapter.

Tractional retinal detachment	32.45%
Macular hole	16.13%
Macular pucker	9.38%
Vitreous haemorrhage	8.06%
Trauma	6.84%
Vitritis	4.43%
Others	3.04%
Dropped nucleus	2.83%
Total	10.09%

Rates of iatrogenic retinal breaks according to pathology [5].

Choroidal Haemorrhage

This occurs usually in the suprachoroidal space and is often related to application of a scleral explant (see Chap. 3) [7, 8]. Severe haemorrhage occurs in 0.14–0.17% of PPV [9, 10] but smaller haemorrhages may occur which resolve.

Avoiding SCH at Surgery

1. Be particularly vigilant of patients who may be at risk of SCH (high myopes, patients who have had a previous SCH, arteriopathic status).
2. Maintain constant IOP during surgery and avoiding ocular hypotony.
   1. Self-sealing wounds [11].
   2. Remember basic microsurgical principle of pivoting instruments at the wound, to minimise egress of intraocular fluid.
   3. Surgery systems with IOP control.
3. Minimise inflammation stimulating procedures, such as contact with the iris.
4. Adequate infusion pressures.
   1. Be aware, with systems with passive infusion, if you increase the height of the operating table you must compensate by increasing the height of the infusion bottle.
5. Minimise distortion to the globe and underlying choroidal vasculature.
   1. Take care when pressing on the eye to be smooth and gentle. Think “I don’t want to fracture a blood vessel”.
   2. Tightening sutures over an external ocular device with minimal disturbance to the ocular anatomy and choroidal vasculature.
   3. When suturing onto sclera, be cautious not to pass the suture too deeply.
   4. Insert perfluorocarbon liquids to stabilise the posterior segment in vitrectomised eyes to prevent distortion of the globe during complex anterior segment surgery [12].
6. Check the IOP at the end of the operation.
   1. If there is leakage from the wound.
      1. Fluid filled eye, insert some fluid through a paracentesis into the anterior chamber, watch for posterior movement of the lens iris diaphragm.
      2. Gas filled eye, use a 30G needle on the gas syringe to insert some gas through the pars plana.
   2. Note that the IOP will drop after removal of the lid speculum. The speculum is acting to increase the

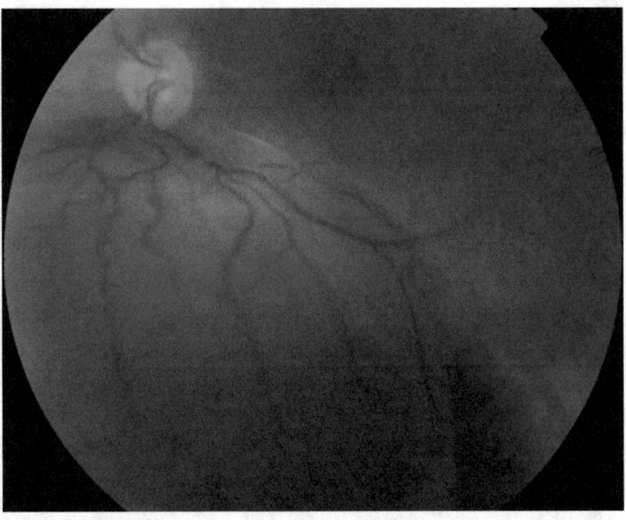

Fig. 3.6 A choroidal haemorrhage from PPV and inferior buckle. The eye has been filled with non-compressible silicone oil to try to limit the spread of the haemorrhage

orbital pressure and therefore the IOP. Therefore, a soft eye before the speculum is removed can become incredibly soft after it is removed. It is safer to have a very firm eye prior to removing the speculum (Fig. 3.6).

What to Do if Choroidal Haemorrhage Occurs?

1. Apply pressure on the superior trochars by squeezing the shafts of the light pipe and your active instrument together, i.e. both towards 12 o'clock. This increases the IOP (changing the shape of the globe from a sphere to an ellipsoid thereby decreases the volume to surface area ratio which increases the pressure, note: a sphere has the minimum surface area for a given volume). With the instruments retained in the eye, leak is prevented from the trochars which would drop the IOP. Do not remove the instruments as this will drop the IOP and allow enlargement of the haemorrhage.
2. Raise the infusion bottle height to 60 cm or pressurised system to 40–50 mmHg.
3. Allow time for a clot to form over the leaking blood vessel before dropping the IOP by removing an instrument, at least 1 minute (count to sixty slowly or watch the clock). Do not be tempted to do anything else until you have given a chance for the clot on the ruptured blood vessel to plug the hole in the vessel wall.
4. If there is only a small haemorrhage at the end of the operation finish the operation and close.
5. It is best to avoid leaving the eye gas filled because gas is compressible and will allow postoperative enlargement of the haemorrhage. If tamponade is required, you should use silicone oil which is non-compressible.
6. If there is a significant haemorrhage ask the assistant to prepare silicone oil for infusion, keep the instruments in the eye and have the assistant attach the oil to the three-way tap on the infusion. Start the oil pump, switch to a flute needle, and fill the eye with oil.

Note: I suspect that choroidal haemorrhages are so catastrophic in anterior segment surgery because the surgeon sees the haemorrhage late, i.e. when the red reflex starts to change. This is not the case in vitreoretinal surgery when the haemorrhage is seen early and can be controlled as above. Therefore, small haemorrhages are seen giving a higher rate of haemorrhage than anterior segment surgery, but these can be kept small and resolve without visual loss.

Haemorrhage from Retinal or Other Blood Vessels

The key is to allow the blood clot to form to plug the hole in the blood vessel.

Sources of Bleeding

Retinal vessels	Severe
Retinal neovascularisation	Variable can be severe
Choroidal neovascularisation	Mild
Choriocapillaris	Moderate (the elasticity of the choroid seems to limit the haemorrhage)

What to do

1. Raise the infusion bottle height and wait.
2. Apply pressure to the bleeding vessel with a blunt instrument, e.g. flute needle tip. This takes skill to apply the instrument without scraping the retina. Keep the instrument in place to allow clotting to occur, at least 1 minute. If you are using the flute needle for this, close the aspiration port throughout, and keep it closed when you take the tip away from the bleeding vessel. Be sure a clot has formed before aspirating with the flute because aspiration drops the IOP and encourages bleeding.
3. Apply endodiathermy. This may be necessary in a few cases that do not stop bleeding with the measures above. The time taken to change over to diathermy often allows further bleeding and obscuration of your view. It is possible to pull the clot off the blood vessel when removing the endo diathermy tip. Therefore, I only use diathermy sparingly.

4. Apply endolaser to burn the tissue without needing or touch the tissue, which prevents pulling the clot off again, as with endodiathermy.

Note: If clearing the clot with a cutter, try to leave a plug of fibrin on the site which has bled, therefore trimming the clot rather than pulling it off. This leaves the hole in the blood vessel "plugged" by a fibrin clot.

Lens Touch

This is seen as a line on the posterior surface of the lens capsule and has been recorded in as much as 9% in complex surgery [4] but should occur in only 2% overall [13]. It is caused by inattention to the position of the posterior surface in relation to the instruments often the light pipe when examining peripheral retina. A bite from the vitrectomy cutter can also occur when removing vitreous from the posterior surface of the capsule; this should be a rare occurrence. Usually, the surgery can be completed with later cataract extraction. Posterior subcapsular cataract forms rapidly in the months after surgery (Figs. 3.7, 3.8, 3.9).

What to do

This is unlikely to compromise the surgery and can be ignored peroperatively but postoperatively there is an increased risk of cataract formation. Routine cataract surgery should be performed and usually without difficulty. In the case of a bite from the capsule, routine phacoemulsification is also possible with the surgeon paying close attention to the hole in the posterior capsule (perhaps because the bite is oval or circular it is a low risk of splitting and spreading).

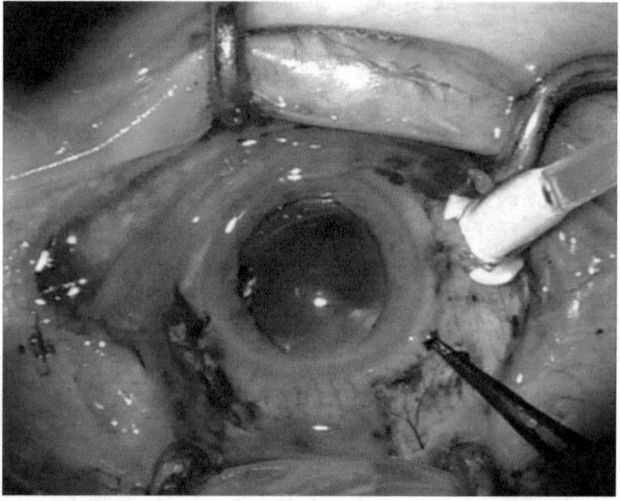

Fig. 3.7 A line can be seen on the posterior lens indicating that the lens has been touched by an instrument

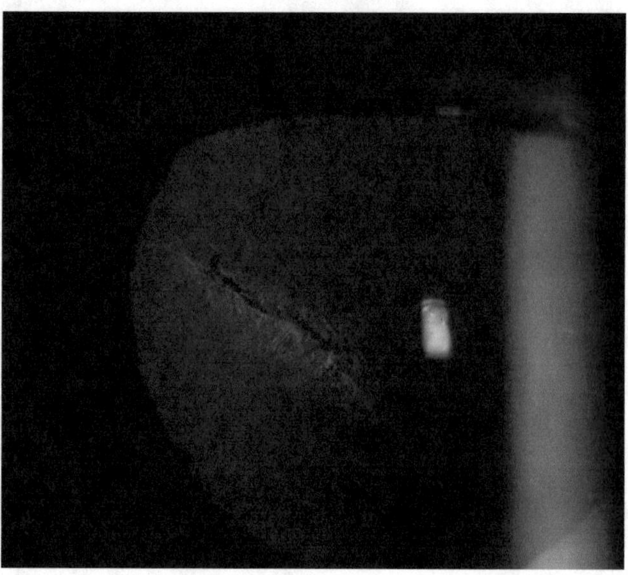

Fig. 3.8 A line can be seen on the posterior capsule indicating a contact of an instrument during the PPV

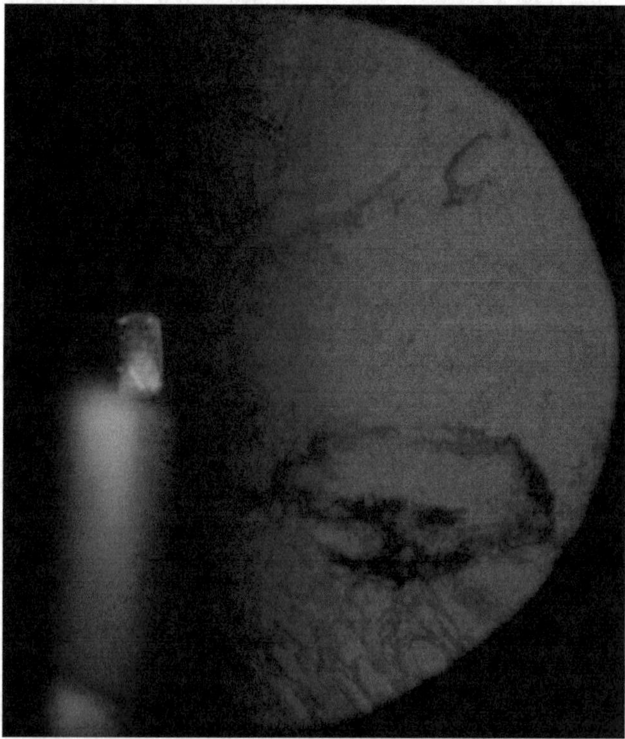

Fig. 3.9 A careless surgeon has taken a bite from the posterior capsule with the vitrectomy cutter. This causes early posterior subcapsular cataract but is easily operated upon by routine phacoemulsification surgery with care taken to avoid enlargement of the capsular defect

If the lens goes white in the post-vitrectomy period before you have a chance to remove it there is a risk that it will swell enough to split the capsule causing a preoperative dropped nucleus.

Hypotony

If you lose IOP during the operation you must restore it as quickly as possible to avoid choroidal haemorrhage. The commonest site causing loss of pressure is the infusion cannula. Check that it has not rotated during a moment of hypotony and resulted in incarceration into vitreous or choroid. Squeeze the tubing to release any incarcerated tissue then use the cutter to remove vitreous or choroidal tissue. If you have inserted heavy liquid up to the ora this can enter the cannula and block it. Again, squeeze the tubing to release then reduce the size of the heavy bubble. If the cannula is satisfactory and the IOP remains low check the infusion line at the three-way tap and at the vitrectomy machine cassette which may be malfunctioning. You may need to re-inflate the eye through a trochar if you are unable to quickly remedy the hypotony. Once the eye is stable (secure trochars and a closed three-way tap) then check for flow of fluid in each junction by disconnecting the tubing of the infusion line to find the blockage. During silicone oil insertion the syringe may disconnect from the three-way tap (a common problem as silicone oil is often supplied in glass syringes that have flimsy connection systems), see silicone oil Chap. 3.

Causes of peroperative hypotony:

1. Blocked infusion cannula.
2. Heavy liquid in the cannula.
3. Faulty cassette.
4. Faulty or wet air filter during air infusion.
5. Water in the air line from incorrect rotation of the three-way tap.
6. Faulty three-way tap.
7. Leaking trochars.
8. Disconnection of an oil infusion syringe.
9. Trochars over draining (Table 3.1, Fig. 3.10).

Table 3.1 Peroperative complications from vitrectomy

Perioperative complications		Avoidance
Trochars	Vitreous incarceration	Good peripheral vitreous gel clearance
	Retinal incarceration	Use of self-sealing trochars with mobile detached retina Early drainage of SRF Use long trochars
Infusion cannula	Non-penetration of choroid or retina	Deep insertion of trochar stents
	Choroidal effusion	Check tip of infusion cannula for full penetration if not incise to allow insertion
	Vitreous and retinal incarceration	Good peripheral vitreous gel clearance
	Lens touch	Good fixation of the cannula Avoid movement of the infusion line off the perpendicular, tape at 6 o'clock so that movement is circumferential rather than radial to the corneoscleral limbus
Intraocular	Iatrogenic retinal breaks / retinal detachment	Avoid traction on the retina High-speed cut rate when near detached retina
	Entry site breaks	Good peripheral vitreous gel clearance Insert forceps and scissors in the closed position Avoid snagging vitreous base during instrument insertion
	Choroidal haemorrhage	Avoid peroperative hypotony Minimise use of scleral buckling during vitrectomy
	Lens touch	Do not reach across to anterior retina in opposite quadrant with instrument or light pipe Be aware of the light pipe during manoeuvres Change hands for access to inferior peripheral gel or retina

Postoperative Complications

Cataract

Cataract formation occurs in almost all patients over the age of 50 years, often within a year but is less rapid in onset under this age. Ischaemic eyes develop cataract more slowly, e.g. diabetic patients with retinopathy and central retinal vein occlusion. Cataract progression in the first 6 months after surgery is likely if there is pre-existing cataract. In patients over 50 years of age, a typical yellow nuclear sclerotic opacity like age-related cataract appears. In those under 50 years, the nuclear sclerosis is white. Risk of postoperative cataract:

Delayed development if the patient is less than 50 years old.

Approximately 30%, when no gas is used:

1. 17–37% when the patient is diabetic [14]. Increased pO2 in the vitreous cavity has been implicated in cataract formation post PPV [15], lower pO2 in diabetes may explain the reduced risk of cataract after PPV in diabetes [16].
2. 80% if the patient is more than 50 years old or gas or silicone oil is used.
3. 70% of PPV for RRD get cataract
4. 83% of macular holes at 3 years have had IOL implantation.

The mean time to phacoemulsification operation after PPV in a Californian practice was 20 months [17]. In one

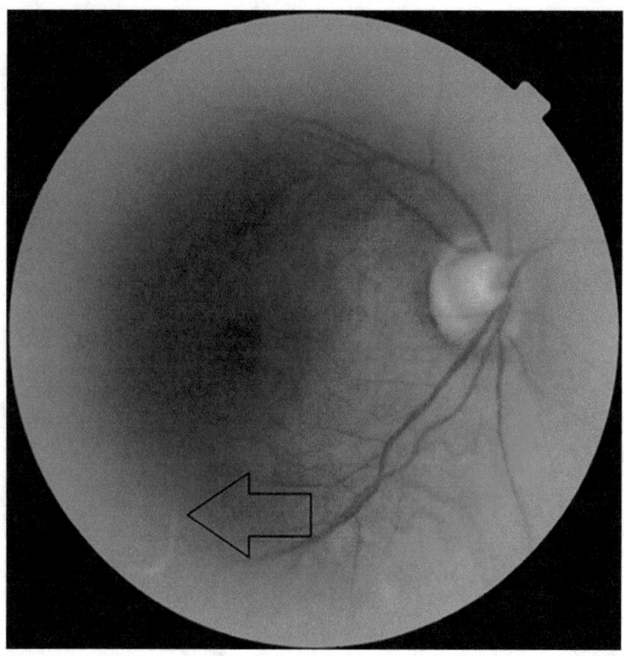

Fig. 3.10 This patient had a floater after a PPV for RRD. There was a filament from a gauze swab in the vitreous cavity which was washed out by repeat PPV. It is important that materials which can produce filaments are not used near vitrectomy surgery in case filaments enter the eye as in this case

study of 301 eyes using 4 grades of cataract, these were the progression rates [18]:

< 50 years	0.13 grades/year
>50 years	0.7 to 0.9 grades/year
Intraocular gas	0.8 grades/year
No gas bubbles	0.5 grades/year

Gas cataracts are feathery posterior subcapsular lens opacities, which are present in some patients when the gas bubble is present. Although these spontaneously resolve once the gas absorbs, they are associated with early onset of nuclear cataract.

Posterior subcapsular cataract occurs if the lens has been touched during surgery.

Post-Vitrectomy Phacoemulsification

The surgery should be performed as a routine phaco operation. The anterior chamber is, however, less stable and prone to reverse pupil block where the AC deepens because of posterior shift of the pupil margin. I place one iris hook inferotemporally to splint the pupil margin. This is enough to prevent this complication and stabilise the AC. Surgery for postoperative cataract has been associated with similar posterior capsular rupture rates to routine cataract but increased zonular dehiscence and dropped nuclear fragments [19].

Endophthalmitis

Endophthalmitis is reported as low as 0.011–0.07% [20–22] in single centre studies but is increased when Medicare insurance forms are examined 0.3–0.4% [23] and appears to involve the usual organisms (see Chap. 12). Early reports of small gauge surgery reported an increased risk of endophthalmitis, but this has not been seen in later studies.

Corneal Changes

Corneal changes are reported in 27% of eyes with tamponade of either oil or gas in PVR eyes [24] in older studies. If fluid can flow freely during vitrectomy corneal changes like gutatta can be seen months after the surgery (Fig. 3.11).

Choroidal Haemorrhage

Choroidal haemorrhage occurs in up to 1% overall but is usually limited in area and associated with other manoeuvres such as external plombage [25]. Two types may be seen, those noticed peroperatively and those only seen postoperatively on the first day. Retrospective studies report lower incidences at 0.1–0.17% but maybe underreporting small bleeds [8–10] and Medicare forms show 0.5% [23]. Identified risk factors are myopia, pseudophakia or aphakia, rhegmatogenous retinal detachment, application of a buckle, previous surgery, and cryotherapy (Fig. 3.12). So far Warfarin therapy had not been associated with haemorrhagic complications from PPV and can be continued [26, 27]. Cases of haemorrhage have been reported with combined antiplatelet

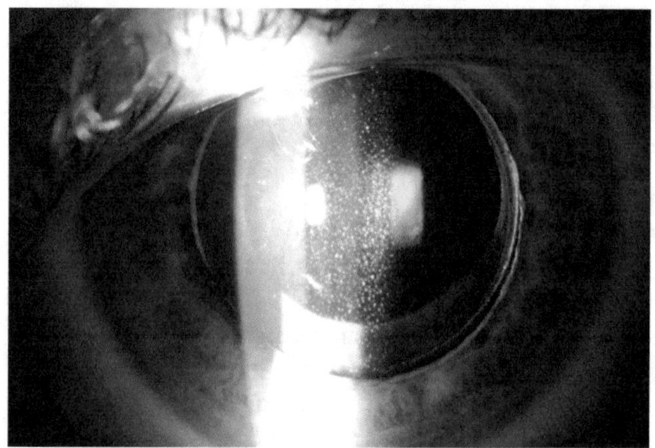

Fig. 3.11 Corneal endothelial changes can be seen after PPV. These appear to be more common if high flow rates of the infusion are used in PPV. Now that flow rates are less because of self-sealing wounds or small gauge vitrectomy corneal changes are less common

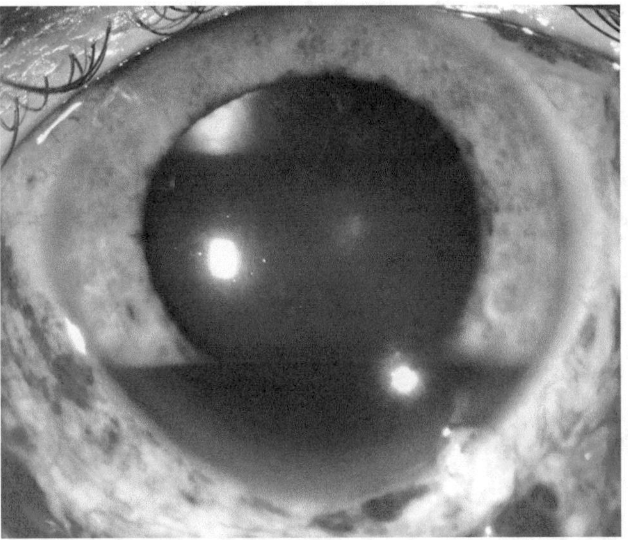

Fig. 3.12 The presence of hyphaema on day one postoperatively suggests a severe posterior segment bleed either intravitreal or suprachoroidal. The patient must be monitored carefully in the postoperative period for elevation of the IOP and repeated ultrasounds performed to detect any RRD. Intervene early if RRD occurs as there is a high chance of PVR

agents, e.g. Clopidogrel [28], but a cohort study has not shown increased risk with these agents [29].

Severe haemorrhage occurs in 0.14–0.17% of pars plana vitrectomy (PPV) but smaller haemorrhages may occur which resolve [7, 8, 10, 23, 27, 30–32]. In vitreoretinal surgery, SCH is associated with the application of a scleral explant [7, 8] or as a result of intraocular hypotony. The former distorts blood vessels risking fracture and bleeds. The latter may be due to a mismatch between intraocular vacuum and infusion pressures. This may be less common with small gauge systems, and vitrectomy systems which attempt to match infusion and vacuum. Tilting eyes during surgery may kink infusion lines and result in sudden reduction in infusion pressure. Finally, as infusion lines in small gauge PPV are not sutured, they can become misplaced. This may result in detachment of the infusion from the trochar giving hypotony. Misdirection of the trochar in the eye may lead to suprachoroidal infusion and secondary rupture of choroidal vessels (Fig. 3.13).

SCH during PPV tends to be more localised partly due to earlier recognition and better intraocular pressure control than in anterior segment surgery (Fig. 3.14).

Finite Element Analysis of Choroidal Haemorrhage

Mahmut Dogramaci

Histopathology

Some SCH may result from rupture of ciliary arteries as they enter the suprachoroidal space. Long posterior ciliary arteries pierce the posterior part of the sclera at some distance from the optic nerve, and run forward between the sclera and choroid, to the ciliary muscle, where they divide into two branches therefore choroidal haemorrhages are observed at or anterior to the equator. Ciliary artery rupture initially leads to extravasation of blood from the artery into the choroid (a tissue which is non expandable), subsequently into the suprachoroidal space which is a space that has the potential to expand [33].

Dynamics of choroidal haemorrhage

To understand the dynamics of choroidal rupture it is worth explaining the process in 2 phases. Phase 1 covers the factors that lead to ciliary artery rupture and phase 2 cover the factors the govern dissemination of blood in extravascular space.

Phase 1: Ciliary Artery Rupture

Ciliary arteries like any other tubular structure could be exposed to two different forms of strain, the first is inflation related strain and the second is elongation related strain. Inflation related strain is when the intra-tubular pressure exceeds the extra-tubular pressure, while elongation related strain is when the tubular structure is stretched in one direction. In both cases, the strains lead to increased levels of stress at the wall of the tubular structure leading to failure and extravasation at its weakest location. One analogy is a hose attached to a tap, an increase in stress levels in the hose can result in its detachment from the tap. Stress levels in the hose can rise if the hose is over inflated because of a blockage in the line and also when it is pulled away from the tap (Fig. 3.15).

Finite element analysis shows that a 30% increment in the pressure at the arteriolar end of a capillary, or reducing the intraocular pressure to zero, both independently increase the shear stress in the capillary blood vessels by 1–2 folds. This mechanically stretches the capillaries by 4% resulting in 43-fold increase in shear stress in the capillary wall. This emphasises the role of globe distortion during surgery in developing choroidal haemorrhage (Fig. 3.16).

It is useful to think about the eye as a fragile tissue that can break or tear if handled carelessly during the operation. Therefore, do not distort the globe and take care when indenting and tightening sutures over an external buckle. Also, it is important to maintain intraocular pressure during the entire length of surgery.

Phase 2 Dissemination of Blood into the Extravascular Space

Rupture of ciliary artery leads to extravasation of blood from the artery into the choroid. Within the choroid, resistance to the expansion is generated from surrounding intact choroidal vasculature, from the outer layers of the eye wall mainly the sclera, from the inner layers of the eye wall mainly Bruch's

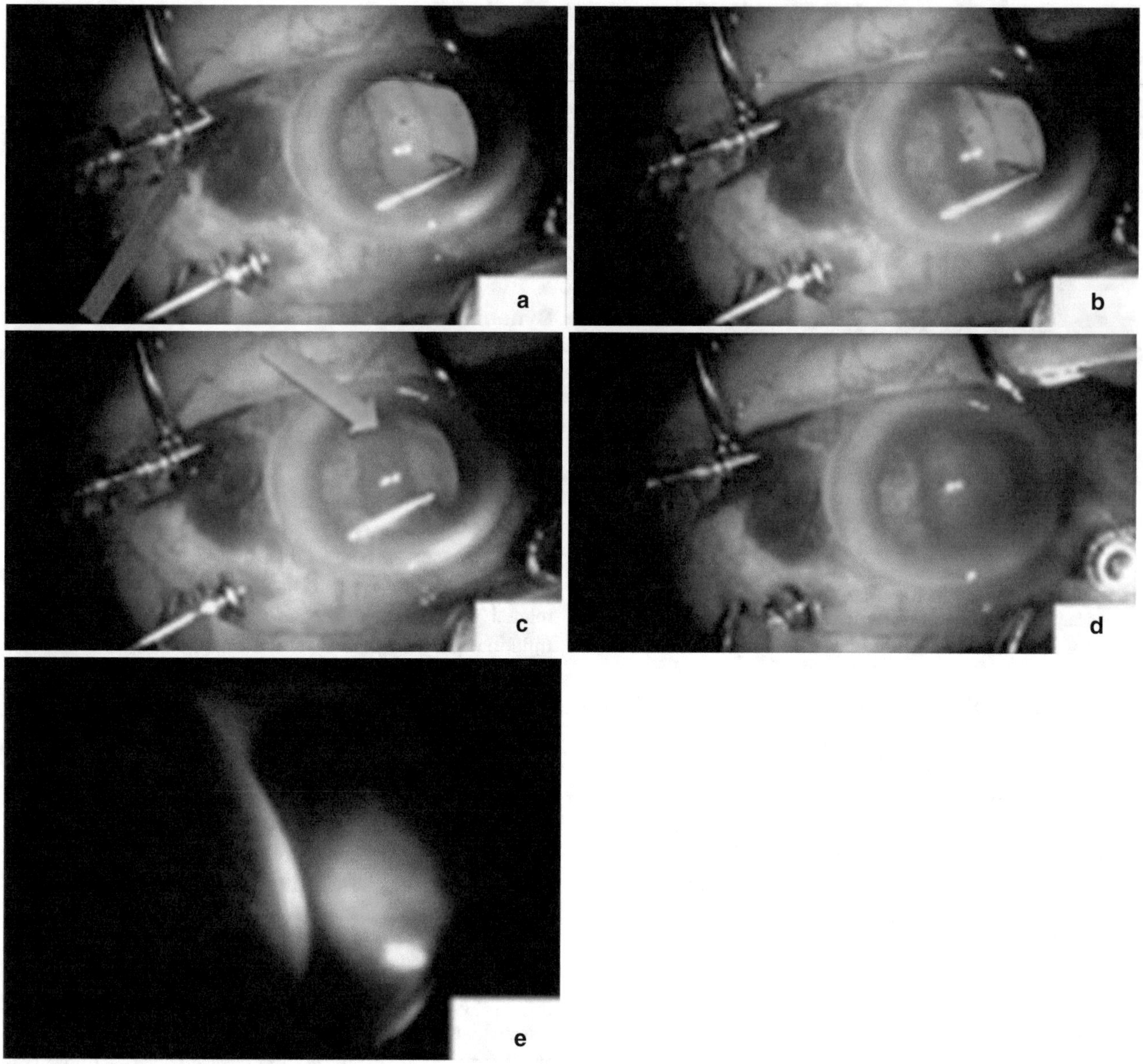

Fig. 3.13 SUPRACHOROIDAL INFUSION (**a**) Note displaced infusion line (red arrow), (**b-c**) Suprachoroidal infusion developing over 3 seconds (blue arrow), (**d**) Loss of red reflex, and (**e**) Posterior segment view (massive suprachoroidal infusion)

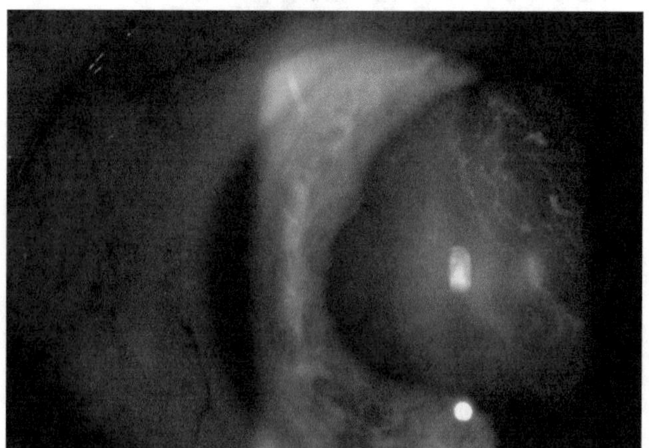

Fig. 3.14 This choroidal haemorrhage is so severe that it has pushed the choroid and retina up behind the lens

membrane and from scattered focal and linear adhesions between the different layers of the eye wall.

Bruch's Membrane and Sclera

Both Bruch's membrane and the sclera have a high stiffness compared to other layers of the eye wall; therefore, they resist deformation. In fact, Bruch's membrane may be up to 3 times stiffer than the sclera itself. Young's modulus for sclera is 5.5 MPa and for Bruch's membrane, the Young's modulus could be as high as 18.8 MPa in elderly patients [11, 34]. However, higher stiffness of a tissue does not necessarily mean better protection against expansion, because the thickness of the tissue is also important. The sclera is many

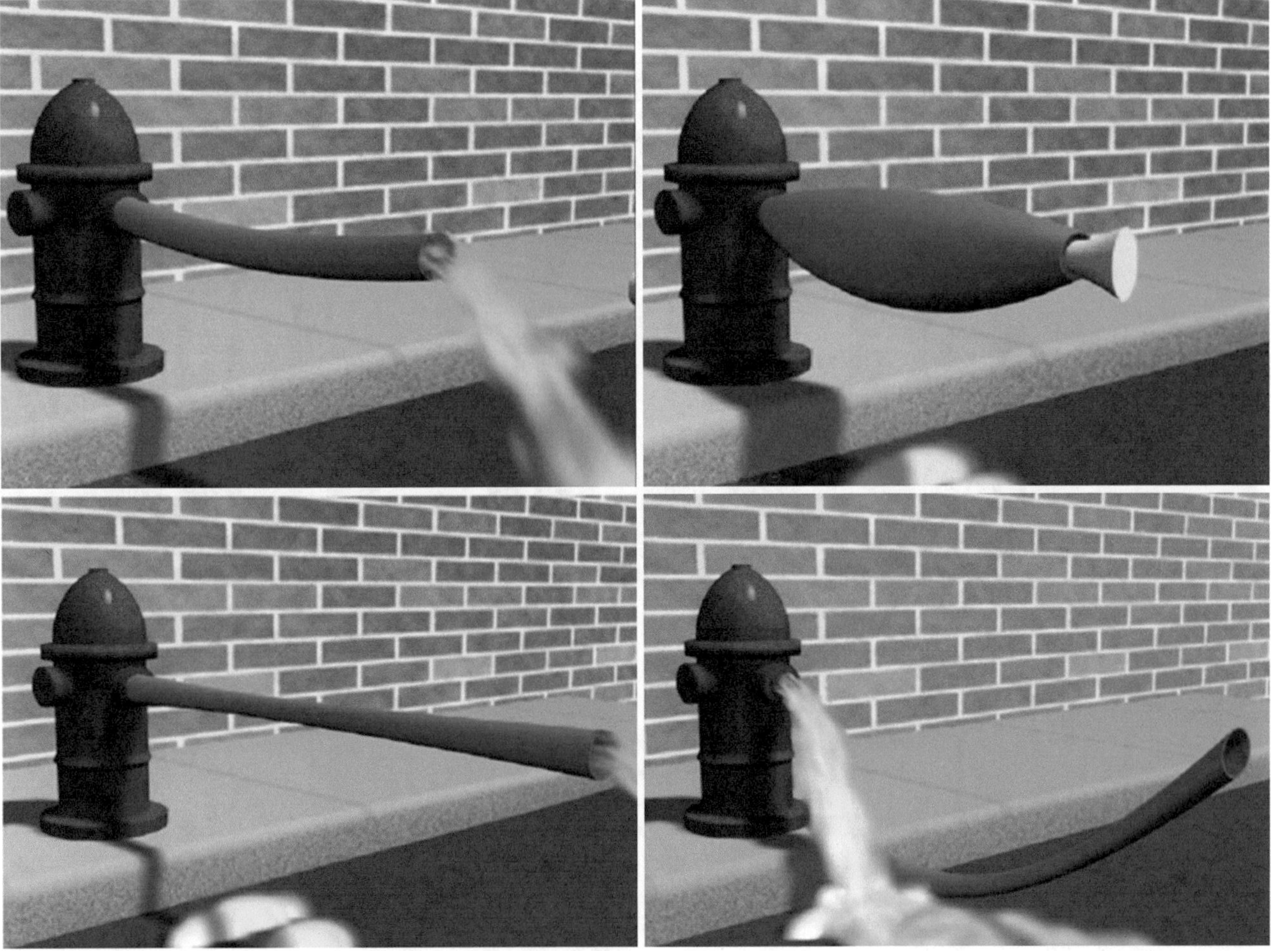

Fig. 3.15 A hose attached to a tap represents a good analogy to ciliary arteries, an increase in stress levels in the hose can result in its' detachment from the tap. Stress levels in the hose can rise if the hose is over inflated because of a blockage in the line and when it is pulled away from the tap. In both cases, the stress generated in the hose lead to the separation of the hose from the tap which is usually its' weakest location

hundreds of times thicker than Bruch's membrane, with an average scleral thickness at the equator of 420 μ, compared to the thickness of Bruch's membrane which is only 2–4 μ [35, 36]. Because of this difference in thickness, when a choroidal haemorrhage puts equal amount of pressure both on the sclera and on the Bruch's membrane, the stress level in Bruch's membrane increases by approximately 15,000 times more than that in the sclera and therefore it deforms more than the sclera. When the stress levels in Bruch's membrane exceeds its yield stress threshold, it ruptures leading to the extravasation of blood into the suprachoroidal space (Figs. 3.17 and 3.18).

In exceptional circumstances, when the sclera is too thin as in myopic patients, some deformation could also happen in the sclera early on during the process, this may allow more space for the expansion of the haemorrhage and minimising the deformation and stress in Bruch's membrane (Fig. 3.19).

Scattered Focal Adhesions Between Eyewall Layers

Focal adhesion between the layers of the eye wall at the ampulla of the veins and arteries as they enter the eye, tends to anchor the layers to each other leading to a cushioned upholstery effect on the surface of the choroidal haemorrhage. Although this kind of adhesion provides protection against free expansion of choroidal haemorrhages into the vitreous cavity, it can also redirect the expansion, leading to circumferential spread of the haemorrhage. This could be missed by an unwary surgeon, who might underestimate the size of the haemorrhage (Fig. 3.20). It is therefore important to carefully check all quadrants for circumferential expansion once a localised choroidal haemorrhage is detected.

Linear Adhesions at Ora Serrata

Linear adhesions at the ora serrata tend to barricade the haemorrhage stopping the expansion of the choroidal swell-

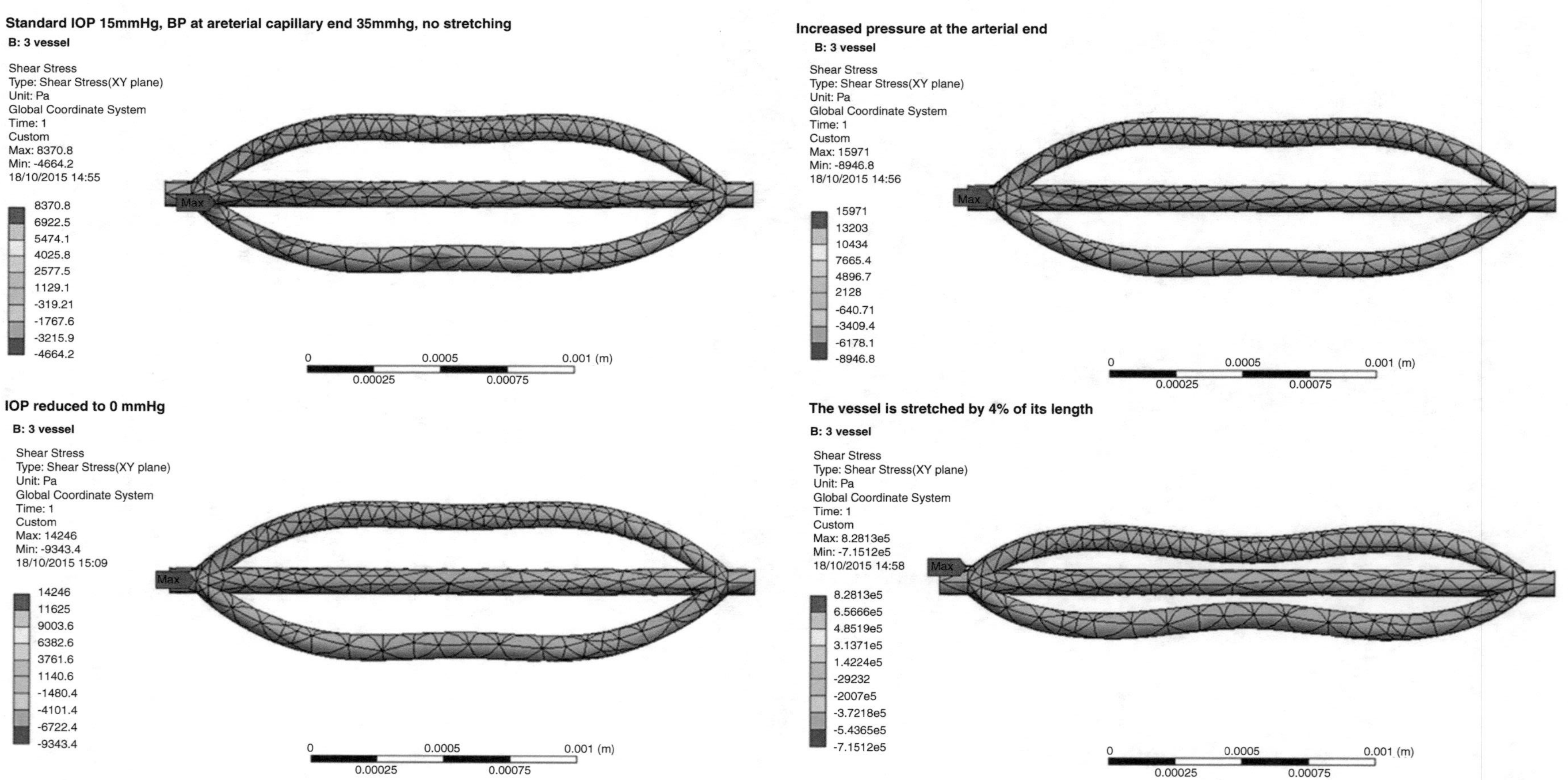

Fig. 3.16 Finite element analysis shows that while a 30% increase in the pressure at arteriolar end of capillary or reducing the intraocular pressure to zero both independently increase the shear stress in the capillary blood vessels by 1–twofold, mechanically stretching the capillaries by 4% will result in 43-fold increase in shear stress in the capillary wall. Upper left shows shear stress at the capillary vessels with intraluminal pressure of 35 mmHg and intraocular pressure of 15 mmHg. Upper right shows shear stress at the capillary vessels with intraluminal pressure of 46 mmHg and intraocular pressure of 15 mmHg. Lower left shows shear stress at the capillary vessels with intraluminal pressure of 35 mmHg and intraocular pressure of zero. Lower right shows shear stress at the capillary vessels with intraluminal pressure of 35 mmHg and intraocular pressure of 15 mmHg being stretched by 4% of its horizontal length

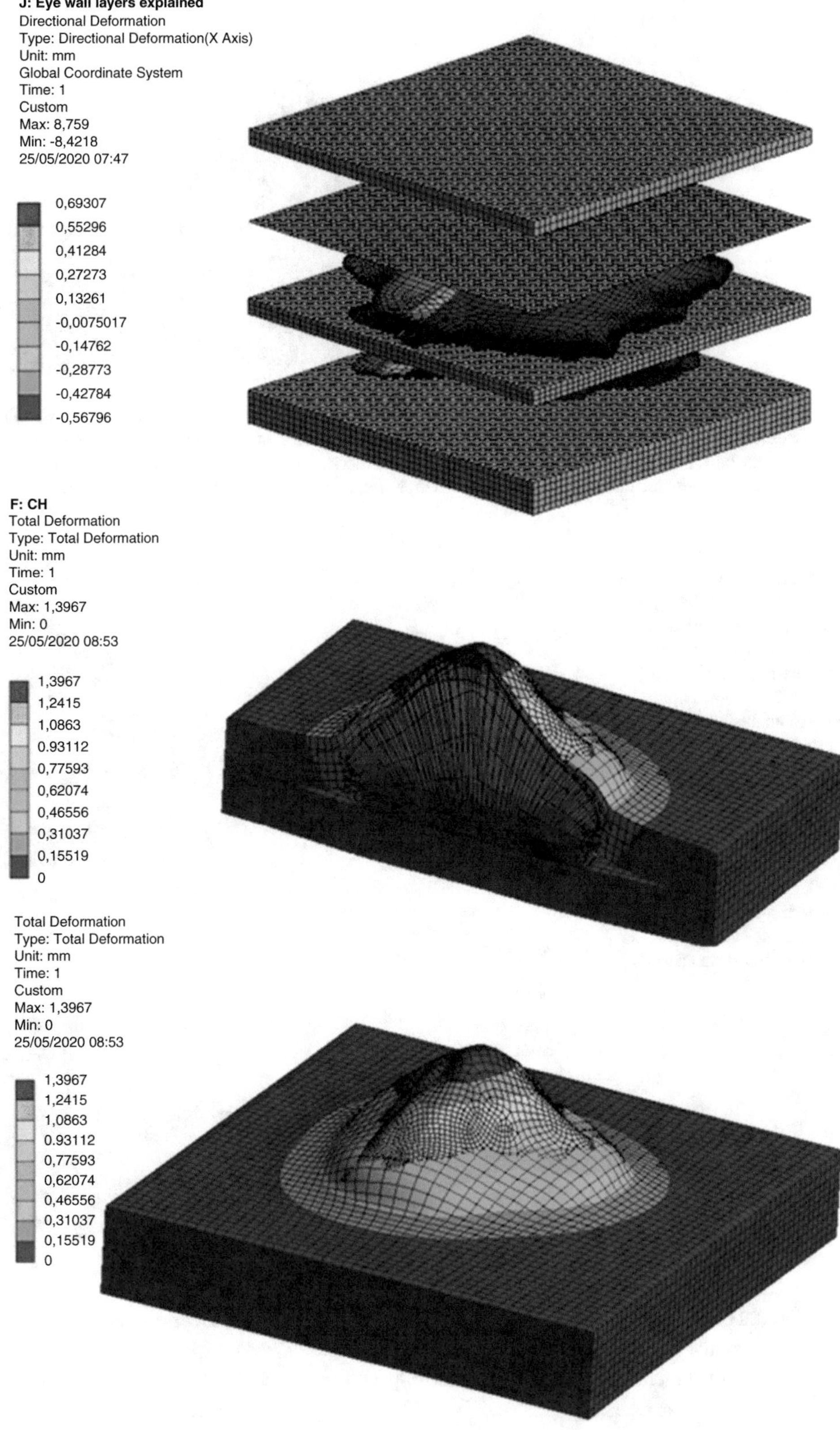

Fig. 3.17 Finite element analysis shows that while a 30% increase in the pressure at arteriolar end of capillary or reducing the intraocular pressure to zero both independently increase the shear stress in the capillary blood vessels by 1–twofold, mechanically stretching the capillaries by 4% will result in 43fold increase in shear stress in the capillary wall. Upper left shows shear stress at the capillary vessels with intraluminal pressure of 35 mmHg and intraocular pressure of 15 mmHg. Upper right shows shear stress at the capillary vessels with intraluminal pressure of 46 mmHg and intraocular pressure of 15 mmHg. Lower left shows shear stress at the capillary vessels with intraluminal pressure of 35 mmHg and intraocular pressure of zero. Lower right shows shear stress at the capillary vessels with intraluminal pressure of 35 mmHg and intraocular pressure of 15 mmHg being stretched by 4% of its horizontal length

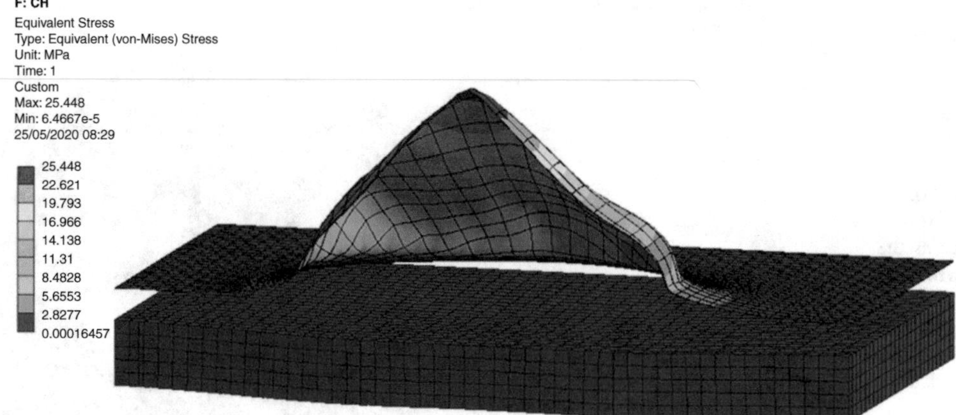

Fig. 3.18 Because of the difference in thickness of Bruch's membrane and the sclera, when a choroidal haemorrhage puts equal amount of pressure both on the sclera and on the Bruch's membrane, the stress level in Bruch's membrane increases by 15,000 times more than that in the sclera and therefore Bruch's membrane deforms more than the sclera does and when the stress levels in Bruch's membrane exceeds its yield stress threshold it ruptures leading to the extravasation of blood into the subretinal space

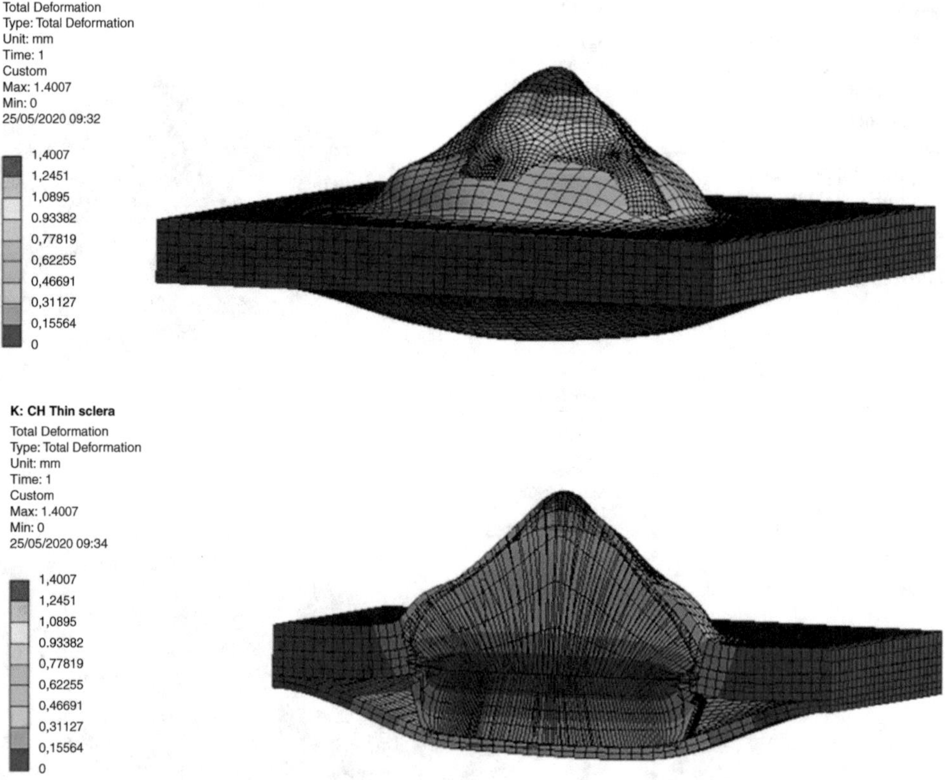

Fig. 3.19 In exceptional circumstances, when the sclera is too thin as in myopic patients, some deformation could also happen in the sclera early on during the process. Top: shows finite element analysis of choroidal haemorrhage with 50% thinner sclera, scleral bulge is visible inferiorly, such a bulge is likely to reduce the stress in Bruch's membrane and result in less deformation and smaller height of choroidal haemorrhage within vitreous cavity. Bottom: A cross-section of the same analysis above

ing (Fig. 3.21). Although this kind of adhesion also provides protection against further expansion, it could lead to increase in the height of the choroidal swelling posteriorly and may result in kissing choroidals.

Important considerations when choroidal haemorrhage arises:

1. Stop leakage and maintain intraocular pressure.
2. Raise the pressure in the globe.
3. Allow time for a clot to form.
4. Finish the operation and close.
5. If a fill of the eye is required liquid is better than gas as the former is non-compressible.

Subsequent Management of SCH

- Observation
- Monitor IOP

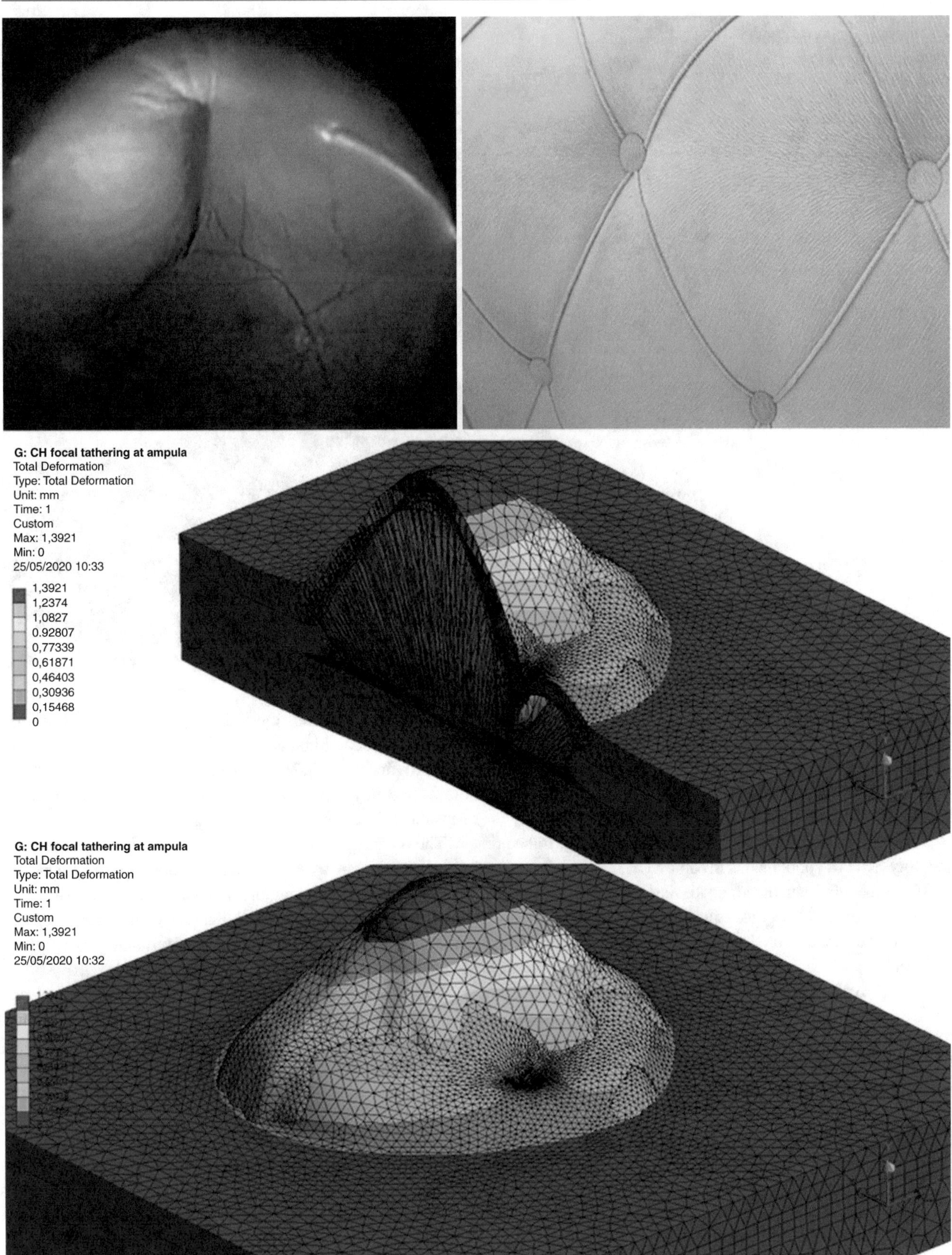

Fig. 3.20 Focal adhesion between the layers of the eye wall at the ampulla tends to anchor the layers of the eye wall to each other leading to tufted upholstery effect on the surface of the choroidal haemorrhage. Although this kind of adhesion provide protection against free expansion of choroidal haemorrhages into vitreous cavity, it can also redirect the expansion leading to circumferential spread

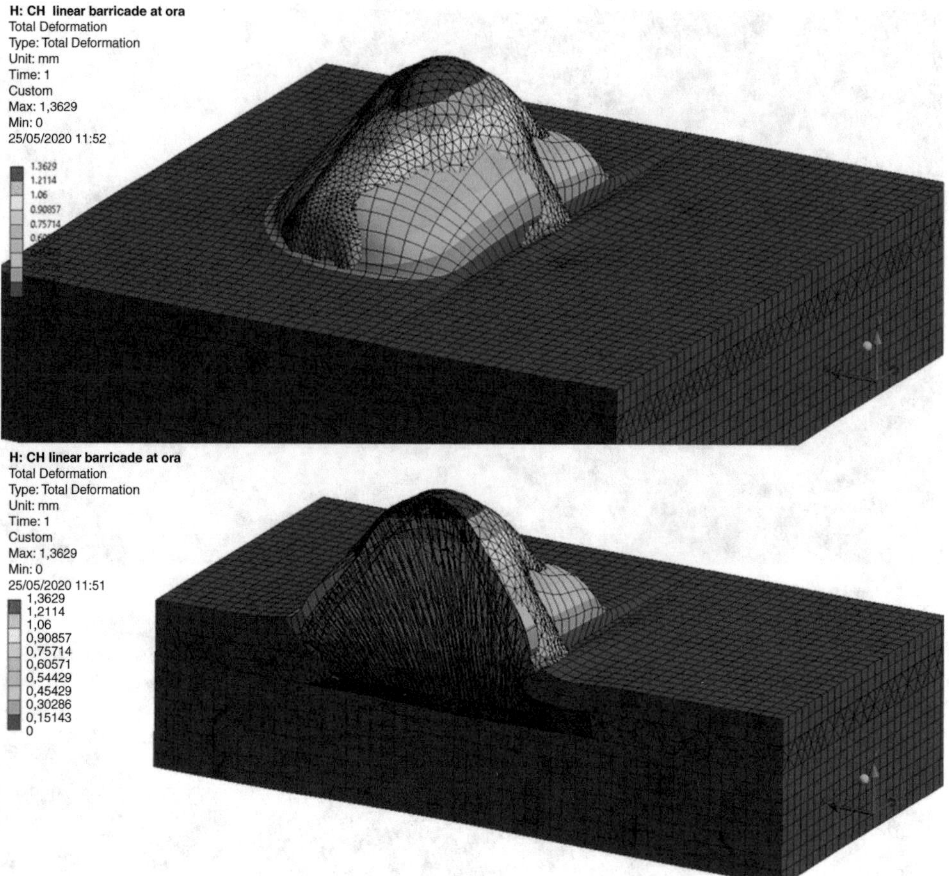

Fig. 3.21 Linear adhesions at ora serrata tend to barricade the haemorrhage stopping the expansion of the choroidal swelling. Although this kind of adhesion also provides protection against further expansion, it could lead to increased height of the choroidal swelling

- Watch for RRD and PVR
- Surgical drainage methods

Small SCH may be observed, particularly if the macula is unaffected. Slow resolution is likely to occur, particularly in SCH which may have a serous element (just as post trabeculectomy SCH or spontaneous myopic SCH).

If the macula is involved, or kissing choroidals are present, intervention is likely to reduce visual morbidity.

In these cases, an initial period of observation is a prudent approach.

This is to allow thrombolysis of the SCH and closure of the rupture in the blood vessel wall by healing. Thrombolysis of whole blood takes up to 20 hours. Larger bleeds can be much slower [37]. Animal models of liquefaction of thrombi in the suprachoroidal space suggest that one to two weeks are necessary for this to occur [38]. The dilemma posed is that evacuating too early may result in a repeat rupture of the blood vessel rupture. Too long a wait, may lead to fibrotic organisation and solidification of the SCH.

Therefore, although small series of earlier interventions are reported [39], most reports suggest a short delay [40, 41].

To aid liquefaction, there are reports of suprachoroidal injection of recombinant tissue plasminogen activator (rTPA) prior to drainage [42]. An example of its use allowing drainage 3 days after massive SCH post complicated extracapsular extraction, is shown in Fig. 3.14.

The technique recommended for SCH drainage involves placement of an anterior chamber infusion (in phakic or pseudophakic eyes). An incision is then made posteriorly, to enter the SCH, but avoiding the vortex veins. Increasing the intraocular pressure with digital pressure and manoeuvring of the eye may allow further expulsion of SCH.

When combined with pars plana vitrectomy, there are techniques suggesting the use of valve-less trocars inserted transsclerally and into the suprachoroidal space to aid drainage [43]. It is recommendable to use non-compressible tamponades such as saline or silicone oil, rather than intraocular gas. Only use the last, if confident that the SCH is unlikely to extend. Finally, short-term perfluorocarbon liquid may be left in situ to aid continued drainage. Sclerotomy sites do not need to be sutured.

When operating on an eye with previous resolved SCH use extra methods to control IOP and choroidal stability. For example, perfluorocarbon liquids can be inserted into the vitreous cavity of vitrectomised eyes to prevent rupture of choroidal vessels during anterior segment surgery [12].

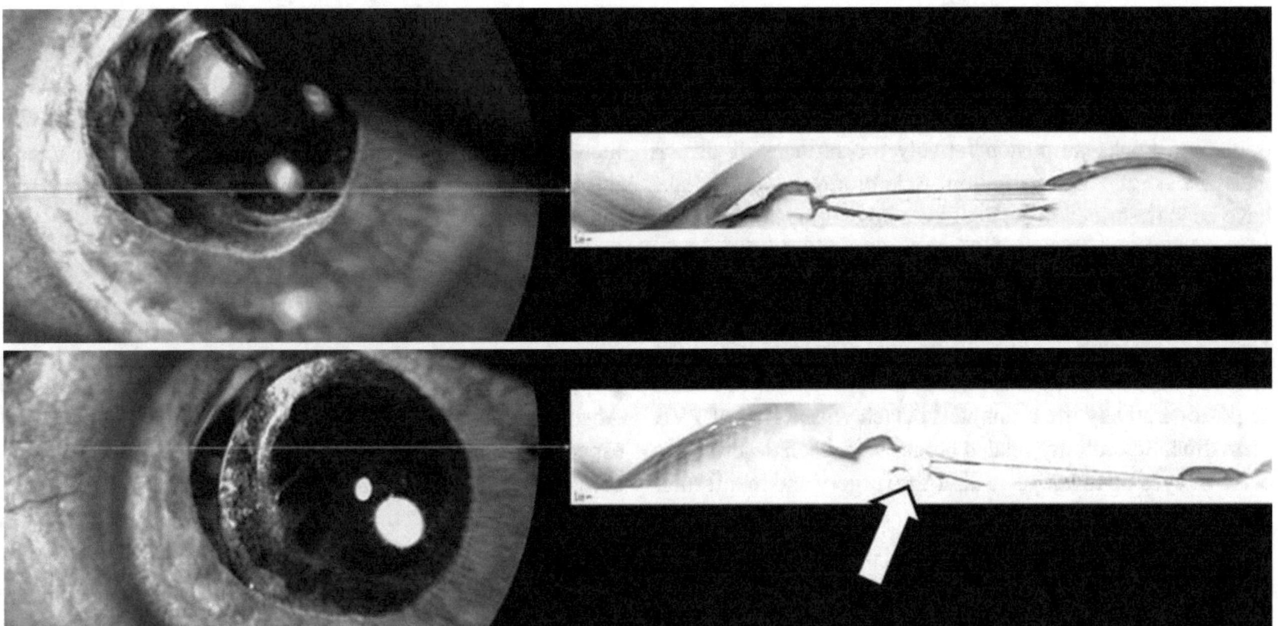

Fig. 3.22 This traumatised eye developed aqueous misdirection and raised IOP with shallowing of the anterior chamber after vitrectomy. A capsulotomy at the edge of the IOL (arrow) allowed the aqueous to flow into the anterior chamber with a drop in the IOP and deepening of the anterior chamber

Raised Intraocular Pressure

Raised IOP is relatively common in the first few weeks after PPV (approximately 25% of patients) occurring from a steroid response to postoperative drops, from intraocular gas expansion and rarely from malignant glaucoma. Most IOP rises to recover very rapidly with medical intervention (within 24 h) suggesting a structural reason for the increase such as temporary collapse of Schlemm's canal. IOP rises are most common in the first two weeks after surgery and therefore many are missed if the patient is not seen until 2 weeks postoperatively.

- 20–30 mmHg treat with prostaglandin analogue but be aware of the possibility for production of cystoid macular oedema.
- IOP over 30 mmHg treats with topical medication with Iopidine as a good first-line therapy.
- IOP over 40 mmHg, add acetazolamide orally.
- Check the IOP in the next two days, often it corrects very quickly.
- Consider moving less IOP-sensitive steroid or even NSAID drops.

More persistent IOP rises to occur with steroid response and will require removal of the topical steroid as quickly as possible.

In the treatment of the aqueous misdirection make sure that there is an open channel between the posterior segment and the anterior segment to allow fluid flow. This requires removal of anterior vitreous and any other tissue (iris or lens capsule), which might occlude flow of aqueous. It is usual to render the eye pseudophakic and to remove the capsule and anterior vitreous behind a peripheral iridectomy.

Often patients with underlying ocular hypertension are discovered at vitrectomy. Long-term increase in IOP because of vitrectomy is uncertain [44] (Fig. 3.22).

A danger is raised IOP from the wrong gas mix which can cause central retinal artery occlusion.

Retinal Breaks and RRD

Inadequate clearance of vitreous from around trochars and careless insertion of instruments can result in retinal breaks just posterior to the trochars, known as entry site breaks. These may develop in the postoperative period as the vitreous contracts into the sclerotomy pulling the retina and causing break formation. Entry site breaks have been described in approximately 3% with aetiology of penetrating trauma increasing the incidence [45]. Inadequate clearance of vitreous from around trochars and careless insertion of instruments can result in retinal breaks just posterior to the trochars, known as entry site breaks. These may develop in the postoperative period as the vitreous contracts into the sclerotomy pulling the retina and causing break formation. Entry site breaks have been described in approximately 3% with aetiology of penetrating trauma increasing the incidence [45].

Other iatrogenic retinal breaks can appear from direct trauma from instruments scraping the retina, the cutter incising retina, peeling of the posterior hyaloid membrane, or traction on the vitreous base. It is important not to miss peroperative breaks as postoperatively the retina will detach with a risk of PVR formation. Sclerotomy-related breaks have been described in 3.1% of eyes up to ten years after the surgery and in a further 2.9% thereafter [45]. Other iatrogenic retinal breaks can appear from direct trauma from instruments scraping the retina, the cutter incising retina, peeling of the posterior hyaloid membrane, or traction on the vitreous base. It is important not to miss peroperative breaks as postoperatively the retina will detach with a risk of PVR formation. Sclerotomy-related breaks have been described in 3.1% of eyes up to ten years after the surgery and in a further 2.9% thereafter [45].

Some surgeons advocate the use of 360° laser to reduce postoperative RRD (from 13% to 3% in one study although these would appear to be high rates of postoperative RRD in routine PPV) [46]. This is not routinely recommended, and it is better to identify breaks and treat these only. Some surgeons advocate the use of 360° laser to reduce postoperative RRD (from 13% to 3% in one study although these would appear to be high rates of postoperative RRD in routine PPV) [46]. This is not routinely recommended, and it is better to identify breaks and treat these only (Fig. 3.23).

Hypotony

Hypotony can occur from leaking trochars. This is unusual with sutured wounds 0.3% [23] but is more common with self-sealing or small gauge surgery. Also, check any cataract extraction wounds. Postoperative hypotony can vary from mild reduction in IOP to choroidal effusions to collapse of the sclera. Mild cases can be monitored and the IOP will increase over a week or two. Severe cases, e.g. with scleral infolding require closure of the leaking wound and re-inflation of the eye.

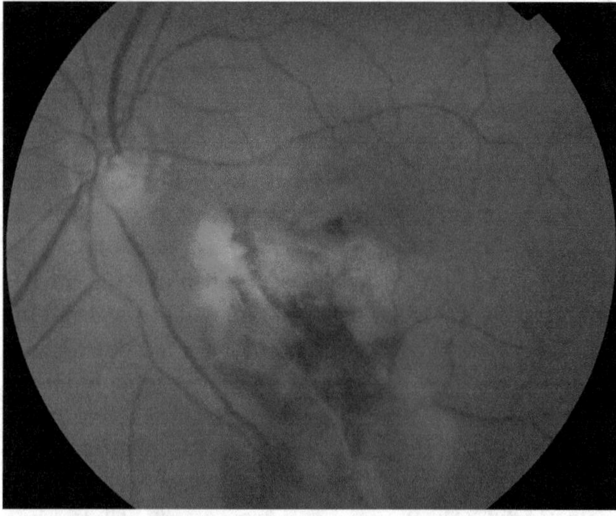

Fig. 3.23 Hitting the retina with an instrument can lead to a severe localised injury to the retina as in this patient where a moment's inattention by the surgeon has allowed an instrument to drift posteriorly and scrape the retina. Always be aware of the position of your instruments in the vitreous cavity if you are distracted during surgery pull the instruments' tips anteriorly towards the sclerotomy sites

Scleritis

Be wary of any inflammation around sclerotomy sites. Absorbable sutures can create an inflammatory reaction especially if they are protruding or on the surface of the conjunctiva. If there is a scleritis response it is worth considering using systemic antibiotics in case, there is an infection as the cause. Infectious scleritis has been described with *Pseudomonas aeruginosa* and methicillin-resistant *Staphylococcus aureus* [47]. An occasional patient may be seen with scleromalacia, the only patients I have seen like this have been lost to follow up and returned at 6 months with the complication. I have presumed that non-compliance with postoperative medication has caused inflammation and scleritis resulting in the scleromalacia. Surgically induced necrotising scleritis (STNS) has been described [48]. This is associated with systemic autoimmune disease. Indeed, necrotising scleritis has been described years after surgery at the sites of surgical wounds in patients with systemic autoimmune disease. Scleritis of this sort will require systemic immunosuppressive therapy. Surgically induced necrotising scleritis (STNS) has been described [48]. This is associated with systemic autoimmune disease. Indeed, necrotising scleritis has been described years after surgery at the sites of surgical wounds in patients with systemic autoimmune disease. Scleritis of this sort will require systemic immunosuppressive therapy.

Scleritis can also occur in relation to scleral buckles.

Sympathetic Uveitis

This is a rare occurrence after vitrectomy. The risk has been described as high as 1 in 500 after PPV in a surveillance survey in the United Kingdom [49, 50]. However, I have not seen a case in 10,000 vitrectomies, and I doubt this high prevalence. The condition is characterised by a panuveitis see Chap. 15 (Figs. 3.24, 3.25, 3.26, 3.27, 3.28, 3.29, 3.30, Table 3.2).

Undo the bow and release the suture from around the flanges of the infusion cannula. Pull the suture tight without pushing down on the globe which will cause egress of fluid or gas when the infusion is removed. Ask the assistant to remove the infusion whilst you close the sclerotomy.

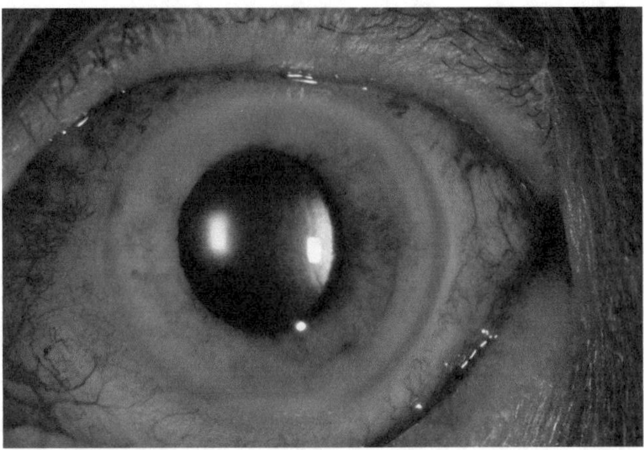

Fig. 3.24 If a patient develops hypopyon and inflammation on the first day postoperatively this may indicate toxic anterior segment syndrome as in this eye with combined PPV and Phaco. This may occur from contamination of the intraocular lens, other instruments, and equipment. You may need to treat as infective with vitreous biopsy and intravitreal antibiotics, but the condition will clear in a week with topical steroids. Unfortunately if severe, complications such as cystoid macular oedema may reduce vision

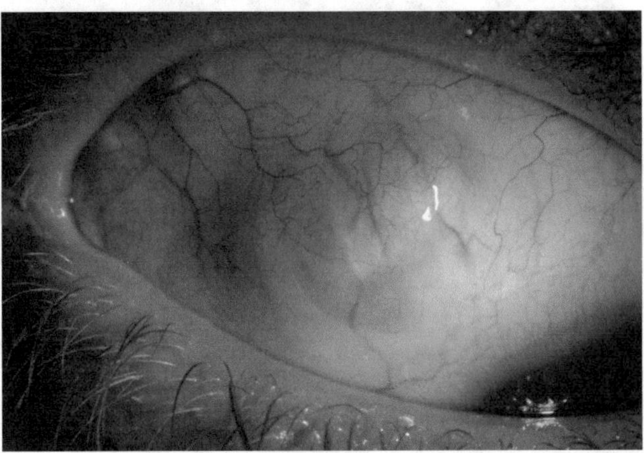

Fig. 3.25 Patients must attend for review in the postoperative period in case of complications. This patient was not seen for 6 months after surgery and reattended with scleromalacia of his sclerotomy sites and corneal scarring. Presumably, he has scleritis (perhaps infectious scleritis) of his sclerotomies which went undetected and untreated and resulted in these unusual complications

Adjustments for Small Gauge Vitrectomy

Steps

1. Measure 3.5– 4 mm from limbus.
2. Insert the inferior stent and trochar transconjunctivally.
3. Remove the stent.
4. Insert the infusion cannula.
5. Tape the infusion line to the margin of the orbit.
6. Check infusion penetrated the vitreous cavity.
7. Measure position and insert superior trochars.
8. Perform the vitrectomy.

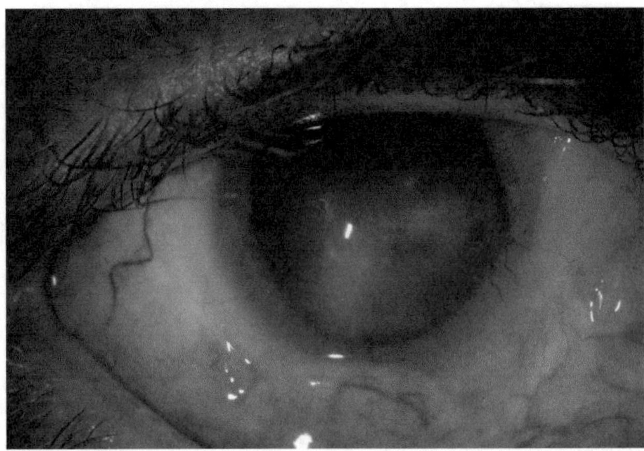

Fig. 3.26 Scleromalacia after the scleritis

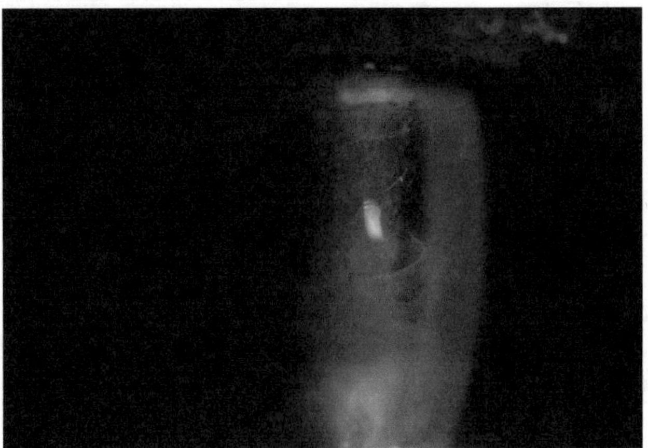

Fig. 3.27 Fibrin can be seen in the anterior chamber after the use of iris hooks to enlarge the pupil. This will clear over two weeks

9. Remove superior trochars and massage wound with squint hook tip.
10. Check IOP and for leaks.
11. Remove infusion sclerotomy and massage wound.
12. Check IOP and for leaks (Figs. 3.31, 3.32, 3.33, 3.34, 3.35, 3.36, 3.37).

Instrumentation

Systems are available which use small bore instrumentation to allow closure of sclerotomies without suturing with comparable complication rates to 20 gauge PPV [51]. These involve specially designed micro instruments such as cutters, scissors, and forceps. The smaller gauge instrumentation provides less illumination and requires higher intensity light sources, e.g. Xenon to provide adequate visualisation. With 25 G illumination additional chandelier fibre-optic illumination is often necessary.

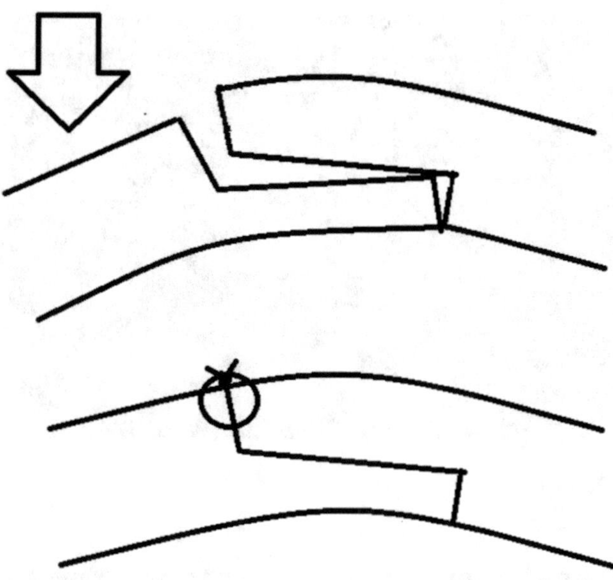

Fig. 3.28 Pressure on one end of a self-sealing wound causes it to leak, only a partial thickness suture is required to stabilise the wound

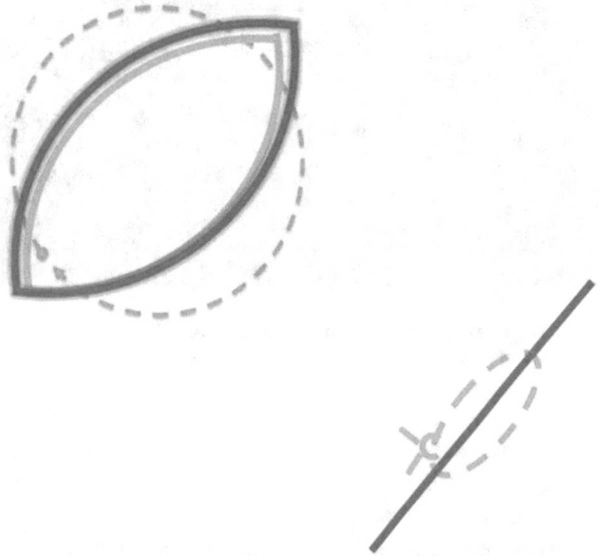

Fig. 3.29 It is possible to bring together a conjunctival wound by passing a suture through the Tenon's (grey line) just under the conjunctiva (blue line) in a circular fashion as shown. Once pulled tight the conjunctival wound is brought together and the suture is covered by the conjunctiva

These systems rely on trochar cannulae inserted into the sclerotomies because the transconjunctival wounds without trochars cause chemosis of the conjunctiva from fluid leak subconjunctivally when instruments are removed. This makes it exceedingly difficult to find the sclerotomy to reinsert instruments without a trochar to indicate the position of the sclerotomy.

There are two systems:

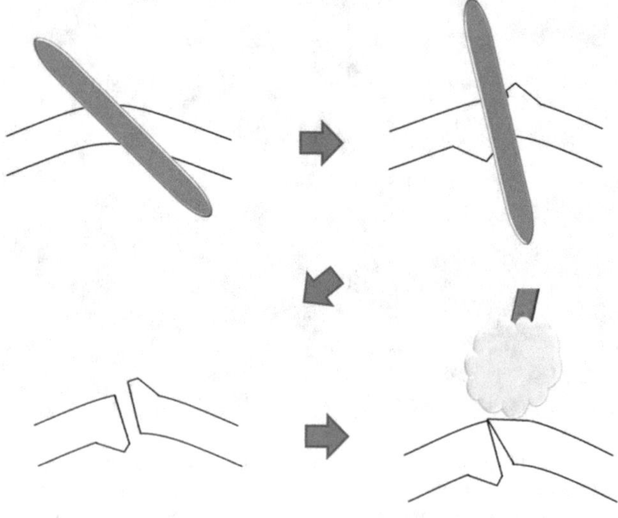

Fig. 3.30 With an angled wound the profile is distorted by the instruments or trochar, only the outer portion of the wound can be corrected by external massage

Table 3.2 The potential complications from pars plana vitrectomy

Postoperative complications of vitrectomy	
Anterior segment	Cataract Glaucoma Conjunctival scarring Subconjunctival haemorrhage Scleritis Corneal endothelial loss Corneal epithelial erosion Sclerotomy leakage Sclerotomy inflammation Sclerotomy infection Uveitis Toxic anterior segment syndrome
Posterior segment	Endophthalmitis Choroidal haemorrhage Retinal detachment Epiretinal membrane Proliferative vitreoretinopathy
Other	Diplopia Surgically induced scleritis Sympathetic ophthalmitis Phthisis bulbi

1. One step: The trochar is loaded on a stent to allow creation of the sclerotomy by direct insertion with removal of the stent after insertion. The angulation of the wound can be less accurate than with a blade (as in the two-step procedure), however, this is the preferred method. Insertion is rapid and there is no risk of losing the sclerotomy site before insertion of the trochar (Fig. 3.38).
2. Two steps: Using a guide on the conjunctiva, a scleral blade is used to create the hole in the sclera and then the

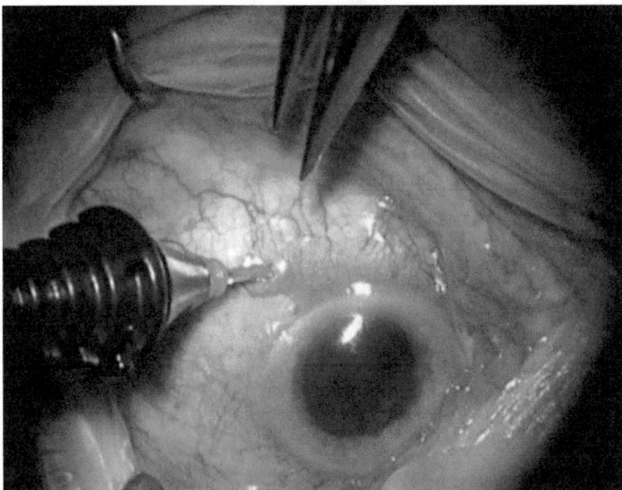

Fig. 3.31 Inserting a 23G trochar mounted on a stent, notice the angle of insertion to create a self-sealing tunnel in the sclera for 2–3 mm before angling directly into the eye

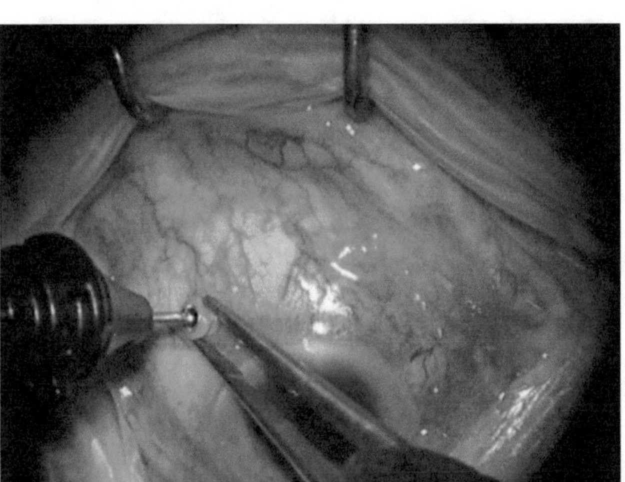

Fig. 3.32 Hold the trochar and remove the stent

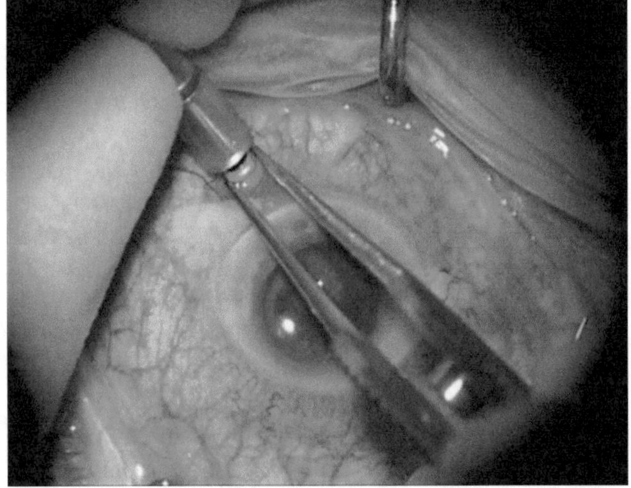

Fig. 3.33 Insert the infusion into the trochar

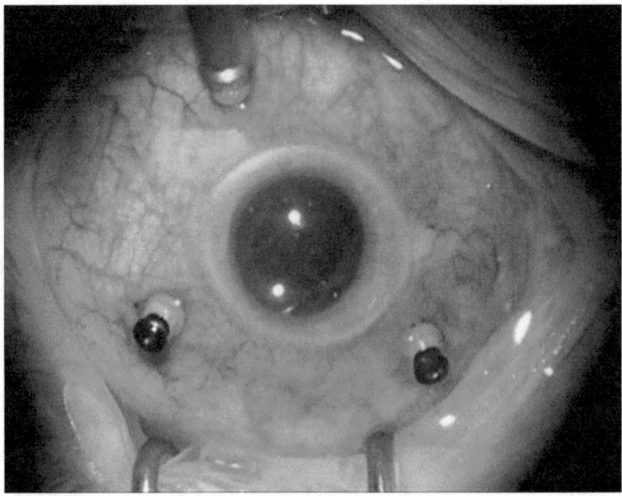

Fig. 3.34 Twenty-three grams set up with plugs in place

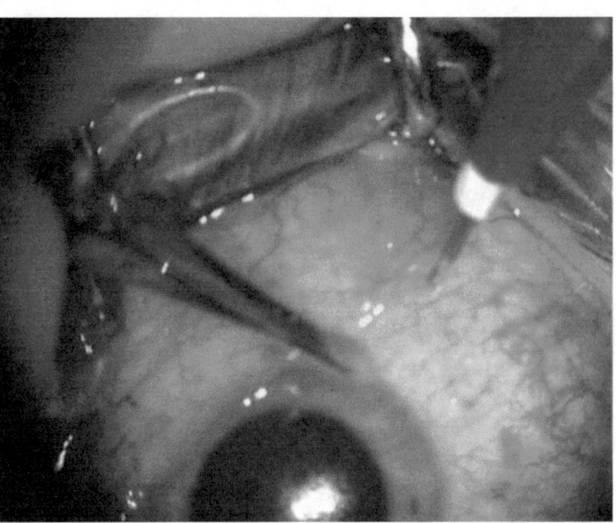

Fig. 3.35 This figure shows the insertion of a stent. The conjunctiva is dragged forward so that when the stent is removed this will release back and the defect in the conjunctiva will be posterior to the hole in the sclera

trochar is inserted through the hole. There is a risk that the conjunctiva will move after creation of the hole causing the surgeon difficulty in locating the hole (Figs. 3.39 and 3.40).

The trochars have various designs from flat to rounder profiles which vary in ease of insertion and wound stability. Some trochars are open to free flow of fluid and require the insertion of plugs to control fluid flow when not in use. Others have simple valve systems to control fluid flow. I prefer a one-step flat blade on the trochar and a valve system for 23-gauge instrumentation. Currently, surgical time saved on closing the sclerotomies is negated by increased time during the intraocular portion of the operation [52, 53]. The patient

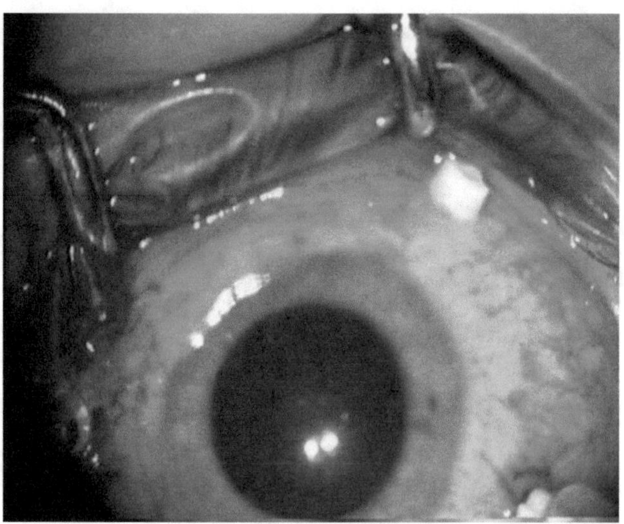

Fig. 3.36 Twenty-five-gauge instrumentation can be inserted via trans-conjunctival and scleral stents which are placed at the beginning of the operation

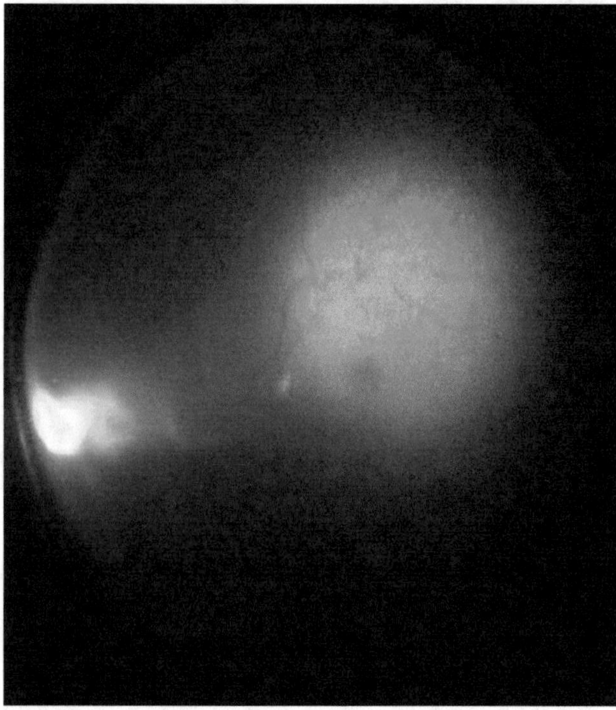

Fig. 3.37 The view of the retina with 25-gauge illumination. Illumination from the 25-gauge system tends to be focused on one area

has much improved postoperative comfort if the wounds remain unsutured.

Surgical Technique

Measure 3.5–4 mm from the corneo-scleral limbus.

1. Method 1. Pull the conjunctiva from 6 mm from the limbus over the site for insertion of the trochar and towards the cornea. This keeps the conjunctival puncture away from the scleral wound when the trochar is removed at the end of surgery. This runs the risk that if the sclerotomy leaks at the end of the operation chemosis will occur and the conjunctiva will need to be incised to find the wound and close it.
2. Method 2. Do not displace the conjunctiva and insert the stent and trochar directly through all layers. Allows easy access to the scleral wound should it leak and without creation of chemosis. Use this technique when learning the method until your sclerotomies reliably seal.

Insert the trochar through the conjunctiva, Tenon's layer, and sclera and circumferentially to the corneo-scleral limbus. Once in the sclera pass the stent parallel to the surface of the sclera for at least 2 mm before angling perpendicular to the surface and inserting it into the vitreous cavity. Hold the flange on the trochar with forceps whilst disconnecting the trochar applicator. Start with the trochar for the infusion infero temporally and attach the infusion line. Check the penetration of the trochar and turn on the infusion. Insert the other two stents and trochars supero nasally and supero temporally in the same fashion. Insert the light pipe and adjust the focus of the IVS and commence the vitrectomy. Illumination will require high output light sources, often Xenon with filters to reduce exposure to retinotoxic light at the extremes of the blue and red spectra.

Use a chandelier fibre optic if the illumination is not adequate, often necessary with 25G but not with 23G. There are various types of chandelier. A double fibre optic with a bent end and flange is adequate.

Note: Two fibre optics are necessary because you are unable to direct the light during bimanual surgery to avoid poorly illuminated areas and shadows.

This can be inserted in a variety of locations but usually 6 or 12 o'clock is convenient. At the end of surgery remove the trochars (infusion last), use the tip of a squint hook to press in the scleral wound immediately after removal to prevent egress of fluid and vitreous. Alternatively, pinch the external portion of the wound together with forceps.

Note: Some surgeons insert a light pipe into the trochar during removal to try to reduce the chance of a vitreous wick being drawn into the wound because a hollow non-valved trochar with fluid flow may engage some vitreous during removal, the vitreous is then drawn into the wound.

It is particularly important to check the wounds for leakage as hypotony is common after these methods and has been blamed for a high rate of endophthalmitis in some series. This may be because a leaking sclerotomy allows conjunctival fluids from the surface to enter the eye (with entry of

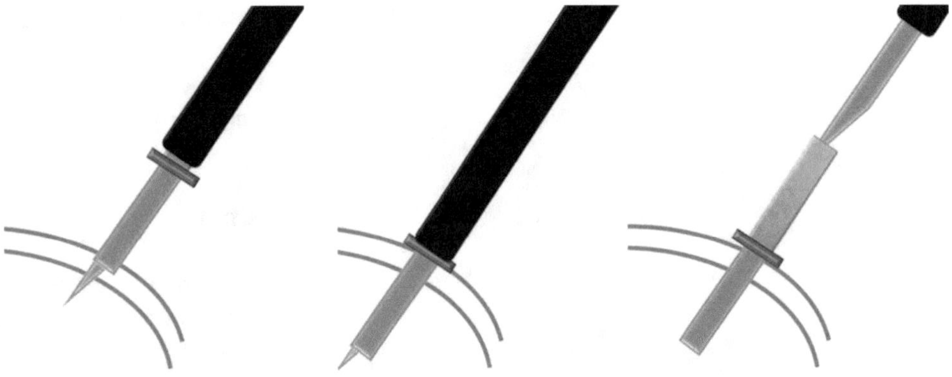

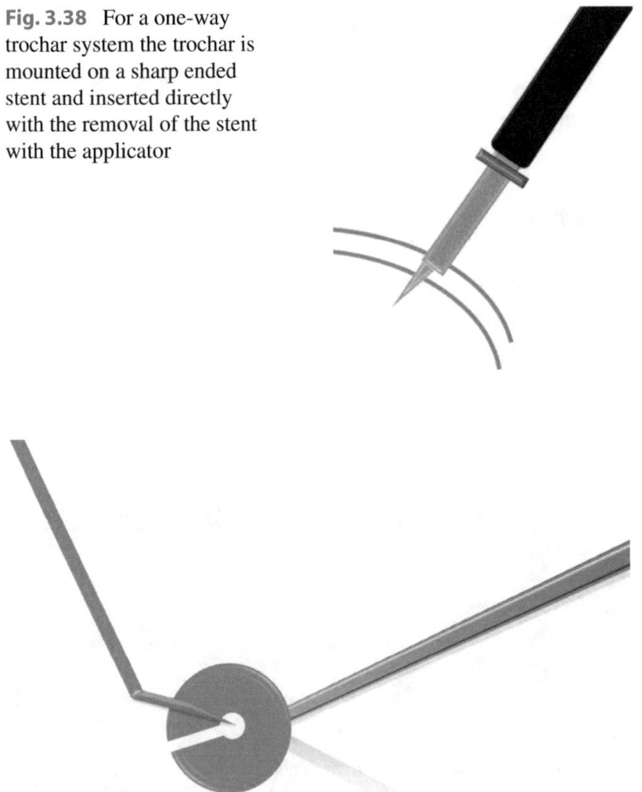

Fig. 3.38 For a one-way trochar system the trochar is mounted on a sharp ended stent and inserted directly with the removal of the stent with the applicator

Fig. 3.39 A two-step procedure for 23G. The guide is used to pull the fornix conjunctiva over the site to be incised. The hole is made in the conjunctiva, Tenon's, and sclera with a blade whilst the conjunctiva is held in place by the serrated under surface of plate of the guide. The blade is removed and the trochar (which has a blunt stent in situ) is inserted

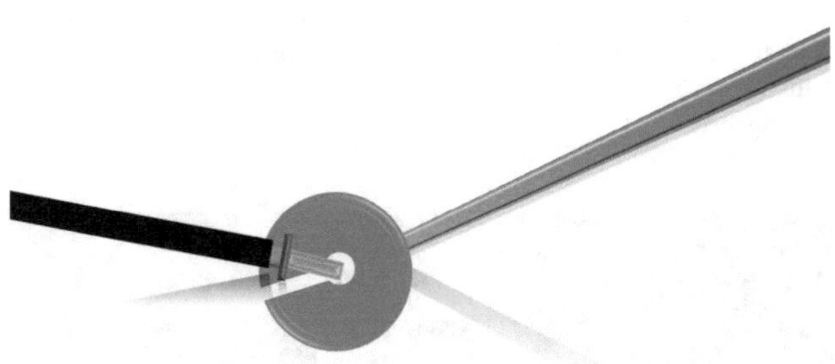

Fig. 3.40 The plate identifies the location of the sclerotomy

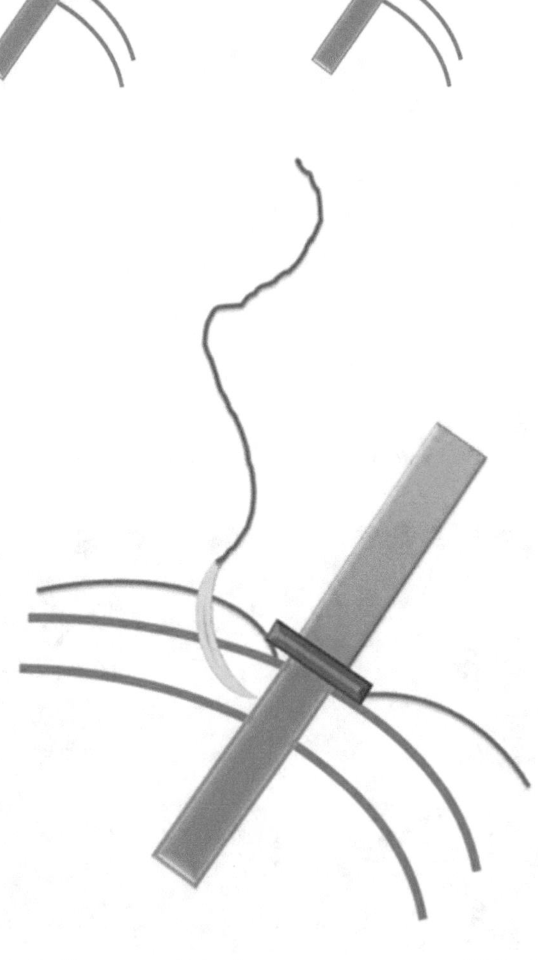

Fig. 3.41 If you are going to insert a suture to secure a 23 G sclerotomy place the needle through the conjunctiva and one side of the wound, then as you remove the stent the location of the sclerotomy is not lost. The needle also holds the conjunctiva preventing chemosis from egress of intraocular fluid

conjunctival floral bacteria). Massage the wound in the opposite direction to the insertion route of the stent (i.e. from the internal hole in the wound to the external hole).

Note: The efficiency of different systems in wound closure varies and therefore wound architecture becomes especially important. When using small gauge some systems can be unstable without suturing, e.g. bevelled 23G, in which case do not pull the conjunctiva as described above, method 1 (it will be impossible to find the sclerotomy at the end of the operation, especially if wound leak has caused chemosis), instead use method 2. If the wounds leak at the end of surgery, sew through the conjunctiva, Tenon's, and the sclera with a single absorbable 10/0 suture. This makes sure you are at the site of the sclerotomy for any suture, but unfortunately it is difficult to bury these knots (Figs. 3.41, 3.42, 3.43, 3.44).

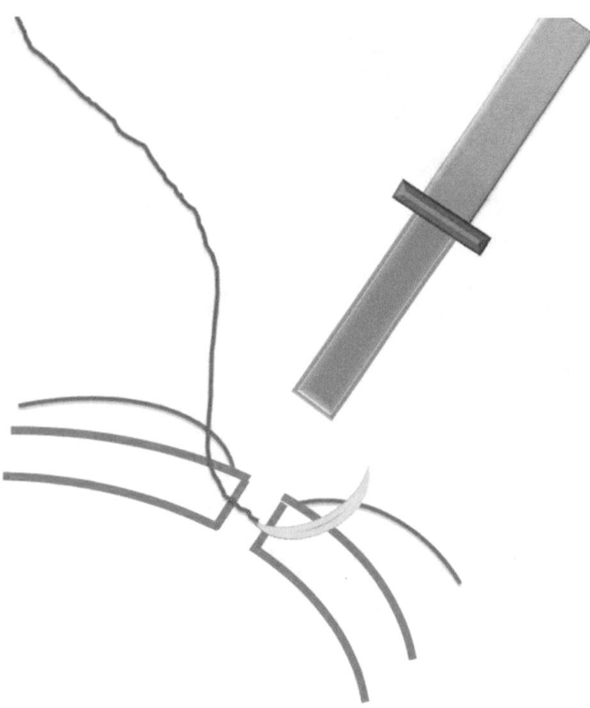

Fig. 3.42 The suture can be inserted as the trochar is removed

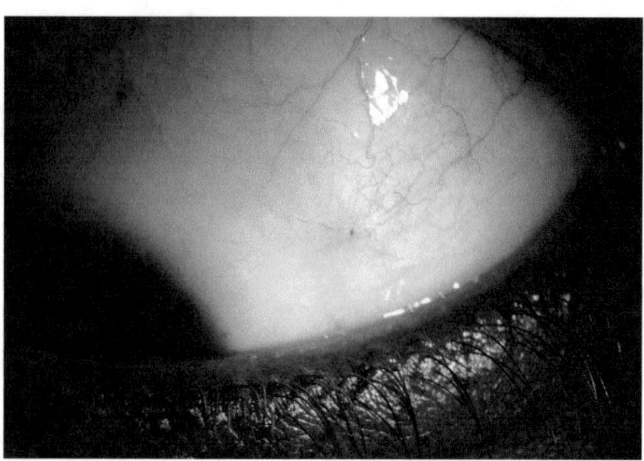

Fig. 3.43 A 10/0 suture to close a 23-gauge sclerotomy and conjunctiva

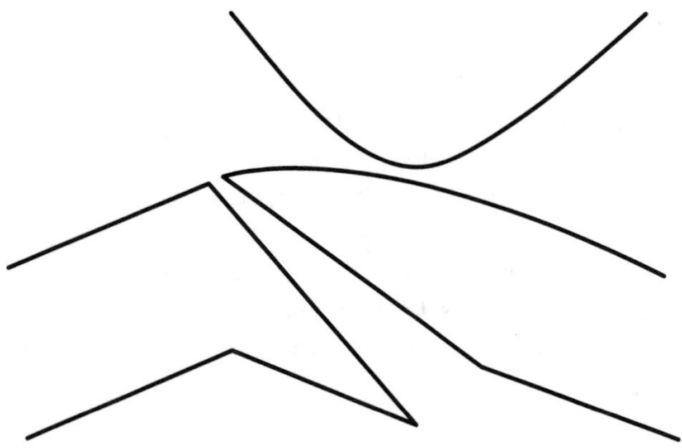

Fig. 3.44 Rubbing the outside of a 45-degree wound (as used in 23 gauge) may close to outer part of the wound but does not affect the inside of the wound

Vitrectomy Technique

The use of a small gauge requires some subtle changes in technique (Figs. 3.45, 3.46, 3.47).

Flexibility

The flexibility of the instruments, especially 25G prevents movement of the eye with pressure on the shaft of the instrument transmitted to the sclerotomy. Some surgeons move the sclerotomies lower in the eye to just above the horizontal so that they can get access to superior retina. If very flexible

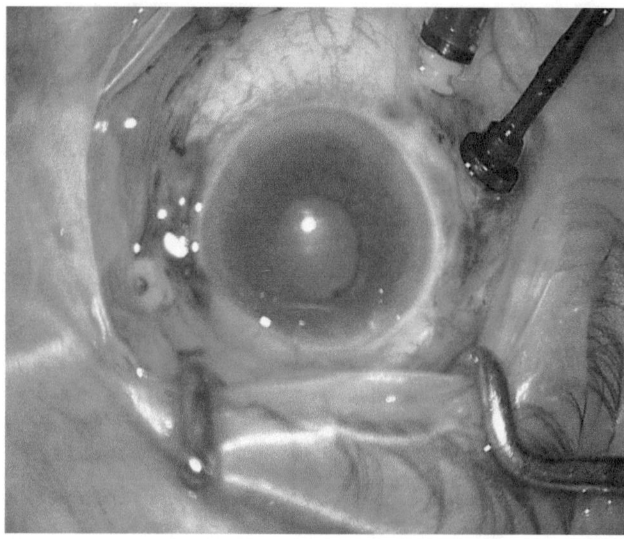

Fig. 3.45 A set up is shown for a 25-gauge sutureless vitrectomy, scleral stents are placed in situ for the infusion and for the instruments, and a chandelier light pipe is inserted to increase the intraocular illumination

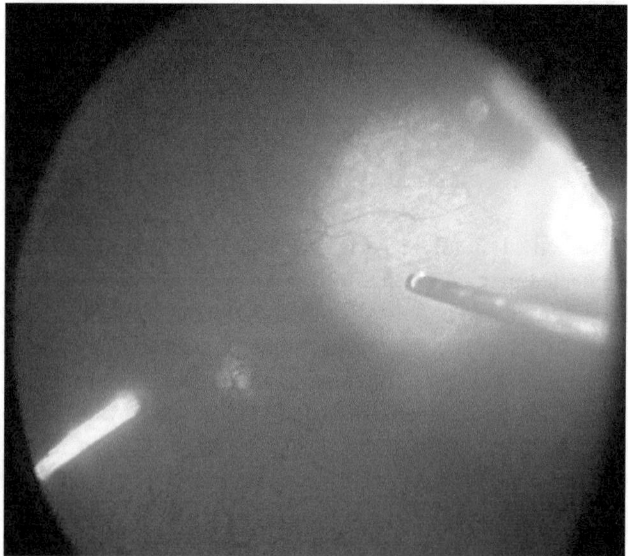

Fig. 3.46 Insertion of a chandelier light pipe improves the overall illumination

instruments are used a chandelier will be needed for illumination leaving both hands available to perform indentation with one hand and use of instruments, e.g. cutter, endolaser, with the other.

Indentation

The intact conjunctiva makes indentation of equatorial retina more difficult, especially on the nasal side which has a shorter fornix. Instead of using the flat edge of a squint hook use the end of the tip or employ a *Williamson* scleral depressor (Vitreq instruments) specially designed for intact conjunctiva. The smaller surface area allows more movement of the conjunctiva and a more posterior indent. Alternatively, make a small incision in the superonasal conjunctiva and Tenon's to allow access of a squint hook to the sub Tenon's space on the nasal side (Fig. 3.48).

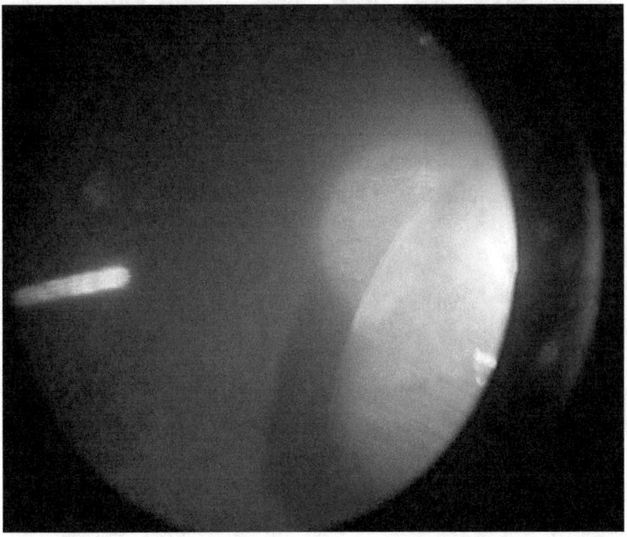

Fig. 3.47 Internal search is compromised in 25 gauge because the conjunctiva is not open. In those patients with short fornixes, internal search and indentation can be reduced

Flow Rates

Flow rates are currently less for small gauge surgery, for example the passive removal of SRF from a retinal break is slower than 20G with a flute needle. Therefore, the surgeon needs to be patient whilst removing vitreous and aspirating fluid. The reduced flow changes the dynamics of the surgery which requires a readjustment of the surgeon to the newer methodology. If you are aspirating fluid and the flow has stopped check that neither of the superior sclerotomies is leaking thereby providing a lower pressure exit for fluid or gas from the vitreous cavity than the shaft of the flute needle. Also, check that the cannula has not become blocked which happens more commonly with small gauge instruments.

Trochar Internal Protrusion

The trochars extend into the vitreous cavity by a few millimetres. This has the effect of reducing your access to the vitreous around the trochar on the same side as the instrument. It may limit your access to anterior retinal tears near the trochar (you will need to access from the other side). In addition, the light pipe illumination will reduce if the light pipe is drawn back too far into the trochar, e.g. when trying to avoid glare in an air-filled eye.

Silicone Oil

Insertion of silicone oil is much slower with a small gauge. Often the infusion cannulae are not strongly enough attached to the infusion needle and they can become detached when the oil pressure is applied therefore only low pressure can be applied slowing the insertion of the oil, e.g. 30 mmHg compared to 50 mmHg when using 20G systems. Removal of silicone oil is surprisingly effective using the oil injector syringe (on extract at 500 mmHg pressure) but use a short 4 mm 23 metal needle to reduce the resistance in the system.

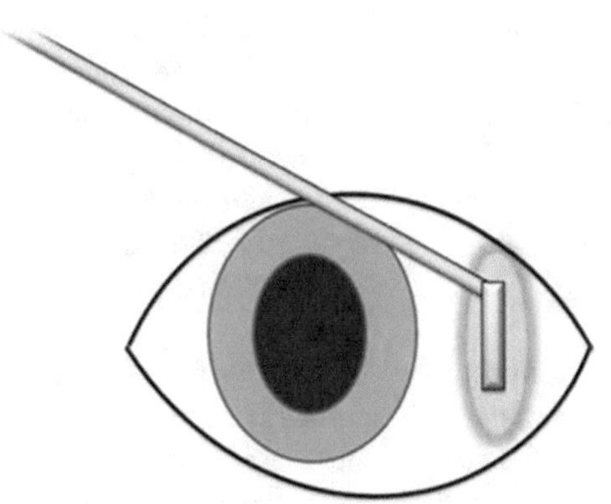

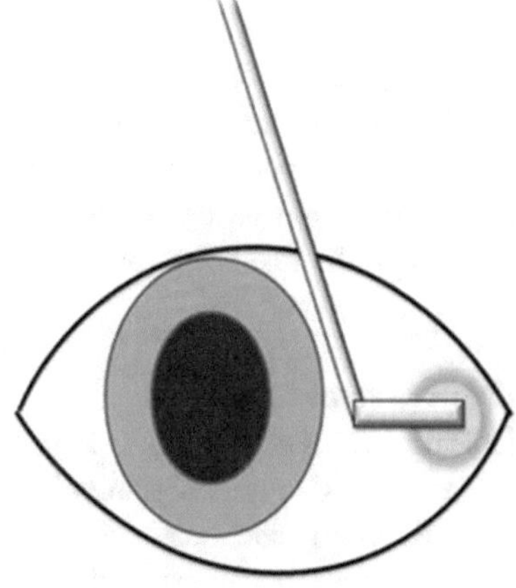

Fig. 3.48 Using the long axis of the end of a squint hook to indent the sclera may not allow posterior indentation transconjunctivally during 23G PPV. Using the tip of the squint hook allows more posterior indentation because the redundant conjunctiva can stretch more readily into the fornix if a smaller point area is indented. For the same reason, the tip of the cryoprobe will reach more posteriorly than the flat edge of the squint hook

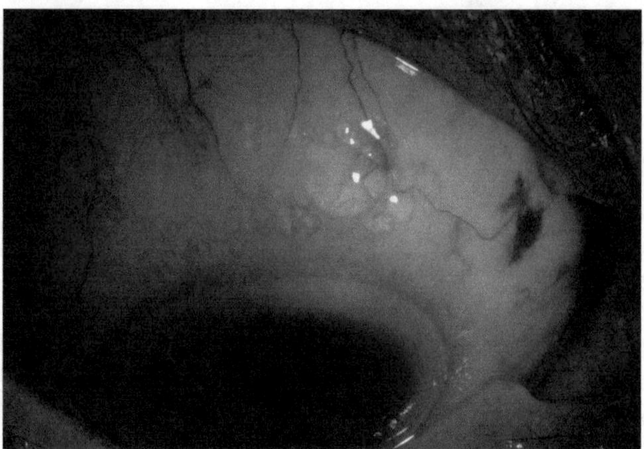

Fig. 3.49 Silicone oil has leaked from a 23G wound and presented into the subconjunctival space. Presumably, a rise in IOP has overcome the interfacial tension of the oil to allow it to exit the small wound

Without the short needle, you will not be able to extract the oil and if the needle is collapsible the negative pressure will close the lumen, and an additional 20G sclerotomy will need to be made (Fig. 3.49).

Complications

Perioperative.

Extrusion of the Trochar on Removal of Instrumentation

In general, the more difficult the trochar is to insert the more stable it is peroperatively. Some trochars are easy to insert but also are more likely to slip out when you remove an instrument. If this happens the conjunctiva will become chemotic and it will be difficult to reinsert the trochar through the original sclerotomy because this will be difficult to find.

If you notice the trochar coming out before the instrument has been removed completely from the eye simply push the trochar down the shaft of the instrument until it has reinserted into the hole. If the instrument has been removed sheath the trochar back onto an instrument insert the instrument into the sclerotomy and repeat the manoeuvre above. If this is not possible you may need to cut down on the conjunctiva and Tenon's to view the sclera and find the sclerotomy before reinserting the trochar. Alternatively, squeeze down onto the lost sclerotomy to close it and make another one (Fig. 3.50).

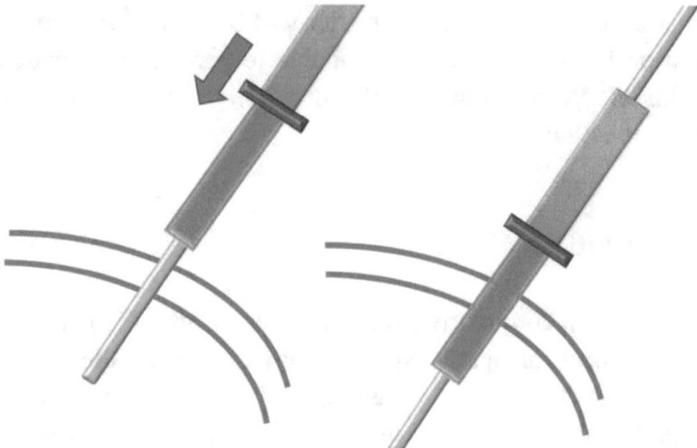

Fig. 3.50 If a stent comes out during removal of an instrument keep the instrument in place (or reinsert the instrument) and push the stent back down the shaft to reinsert

Conjunctival Chemosis

Unfortunately, wound leaks cause conjunctival chemosis so that the sclerotomy is obscured by the swollen conjunctiva. The sclerotomy cannot be found to perform remedial suturing. Therefore, if you are suturing the sclerotomy insert the suture at the same time as removal of the trochar to allow insertion of the suture through the sclerotomy whilst its position is known and to keep the conjunctival (held on the needle) from separating from the sclerotomy. A 10/0 suture can be used to close the sclerotomy and conjunctiva in one. If chemosis has occurred and you wish to suture the sclera use a small radial incision of the conjunctiva and Tenon's to expose the sclera to find the sclerotomy.

Hypotony

Various strategies have been used to try to reduce hypotony including:

1. Trochar blade design, a bevelled and flat blade tip rather than a circular or cutting tip provides a better wound profile for self-sealing.
2. Angled insertion of the trochars.
3. Suturing of the orifices with 10/0 absorbable suture.
4. Massage of the holes.
5. Inserting air into the vitreous cavity.
6. Injecting subconjunctival antibiotic over the sclerotomy sites (beware of the use of aminoglycosides for this, as a case report of Gentamycin induced macular ischaemia has been described from presumed ingress of the antibiotic into the eye postoperatively after subconjunctival injection [54]). Injecting subconjunctival antibiotic over the sclerotomy sites (beware of the use of aminoglycosides for this, as a case report of Gentamycin induced macular ischaemia has been described from presumed ingress of the antibiotic into the eye postoperatively after subconjunctival injection [54]).

Note: When testing the IOP by pressing on the eye do not pressure near the external orifice of the scleral tunnel because the sclerotomy will open. Instead press adjacent to the internal orifice which keeps the tunnel closed.

Endophthalmitis

There has been an increased risk of endophthalmitis in publications, a 12-fold increase in the risk with 25 gauge compared with 20 gauge has been described [55]. Later publications show no difference compared to 20G[25]. There may be a technical reason for the increased risk in the earlier papers. Much has been made of the risk of leakage of these wounds allowing fluid from the ocular surface to enter the eye during a phase of hypotony in the postoperative period.

Postoperative Retinal Break Formation

Iatrogenic break formation has been reported despite the use of smaller gauge instrumentation [56] and appears disappointingly to be similar to 20G. However, entry site breaks may be less frequent because instruments are not pushed through the vitreous base on insertion. Iatrogenic break formation has been reported despite the use of smaller gauge instrumentation [56] and appears disappointingly to be similar to 20G. However, entry site breaks may be less frequent because instruments are not pushed through the vitreous base on insertion.

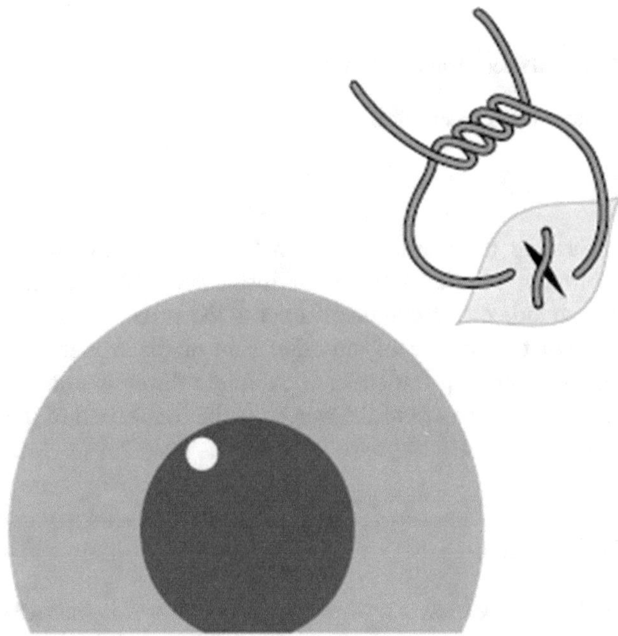

Fig. 3.51 Suture the sclerotomies with 7/0 or 8/0 absorbable sutures then sew the conjunctiva separately

20 Gauge Self-Sealing Sclerotomies

You may wish occasionally to use self-sealing 20G sclerotomies. Some systems do only have Fragmatome available in 20G. These can be made easily by inserting the MVR blade into the sclera circumferentially to the corneo-scleral limbus and advancing just under the sclera parallel to the surface for 2–3 mm before angling the MVR perpendicular to the surface for the final insertion through the inner sclera and choroid. A long tunnel is required for these to be effective postoperatively. These sclerotomies are particularly useful perioperatively where minimal fluid leakage helps to control the IOP and reduces the risk of vitreous and retinal incarceration. If the sclerotomy is self-sealing at the end of the operation (clear any vitreous from the orifice, flatten the outer scleral surface and check for fluid leakage) you may leave it unsutured. In the early stages, suture them on most occasions, therefore, avoiding the risk of postoperative hypotony or gas bubble leakage. As your confidence grows and technique improves you can leave the unsutured (Figs. 3.51, 3.52, 3.53).

For non-sealing sclerotomies, use an 8/0 or 10/0 absorbable suture (e.g. Vicryl), take two bites in a cross-stitch for each sclerotomy perpendicular to the direction of the incision. For self-sealing sclerotomies massage the outer wound to ensure its closure, check carefully for leaks and oversew if necessary.

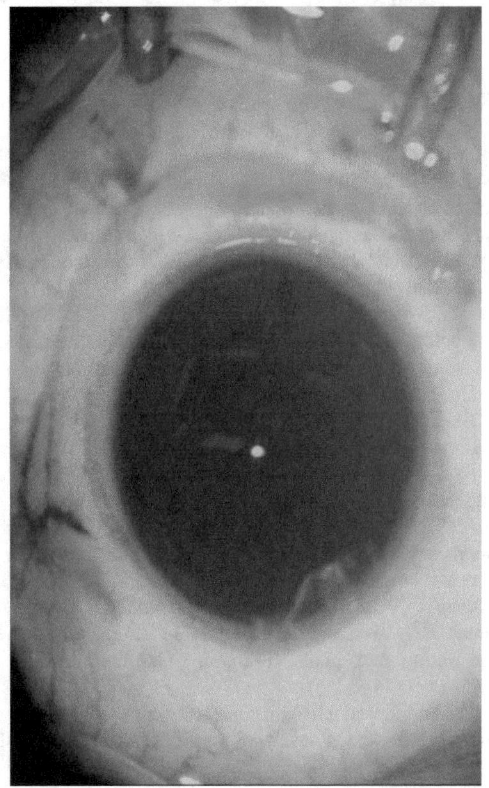

Fig. 3.52 An ideal conjunctiva wound, postoperatively, showing no protruding sutures and minimal disruption to the conjunctiva. Note that the light from the microscope has been blocked centrally to avoid any macular toxicity during closure of the conjunctiva in this patient

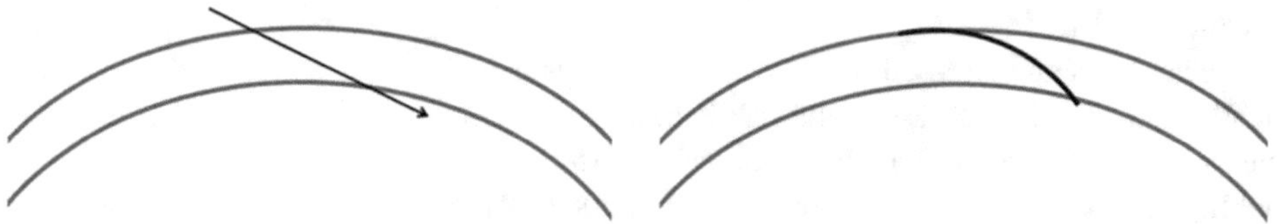

Fig. 3.53 An attempt to create a shelved incision in the curved scleral will often create a curve incision because of movement tissue by the blade

Sew up the conjunctiva with 8/0 or 10/0 absorbable sutures in a buried fashion, i.e. insert the needle through the cut side of the conjunctiva out to the surface and then through the surface of the other side of the wound and then out through the cut side. A single throw is enough usually placed a 1/3 of the way from the limbal end of the wound.

References

1. Carter JB, Michels RG, Glaser BM, de Bustros S. Iatrogenic retinal breaks complicating pars plana vitrectomy. Ophthalmology. 1990;97(7):848–53.
2. Sjaarda RN, Glaser BM, Thompson JT, Murphy RP, Hanham A. Distribution of iatrogenic retinal breaks in macular hole surgery. Ophthalmology. 1995;102(9):1387–92.
3. Han DP, Murphy ML, Mieler WF. A modified en bloc excision technique during vitrectomy for diabetic traction retinal detachment. Results Complicat Ophthalmol. 1994;101(5):803–8.
4. Afrashi F, Erakgun T, Akkin C, Kaskaloglu M, Mentes J. Conventional buckling surgery or primary vitrectomy with silicone oil tamponade in rhegmatogenous retinal detachment with multiple breaks. Graefes Arch Clin Exp Ophthalmol. 2004;242(4):295–300.
5. Dogramaci M, Lee EJ, Williamson TH. The incidence and the risk factors for iatrogenic retinal breaks during pars plana vitrectomy. Eye (Lond). 2012. eye201218 [pii] https://doi.org/10.1038/eye.2012.18.
6. Gupta B, Wong R, Sivaprasad S, Williamson TH. Surgical and visual outcome following 20-gauge vitrectomy in proliferative diabetic retinopathy over a 10-year period, evidence for change in practice. Eye (Lond). 2012. eye2011348 [pii]; https://doi.org/10.1038/eye.2011.348.
7. Lakhanpal V, Schocket SS, Elman MJ, Dogra MR. Intraoperative massive suprachoroidal hemorrhage during pars plana vitrectomy. Ophthalmology. 1990;97(9):1114–9.
8. Tabandeh H, Sullivan PM, Smahliuk P, Flynn HW Jr, Schiffman J. Suprachoroidal hemorrhage during pars plana vitrectomy. Risk factors and outcomes. Ophthalmology. 1999;106(2):236–42.
9. Sharma T, Virdi DS, Parikh S, Gopal L, Badrinath SS, Mukesh BN. A case-control study of suprachoroidal hemorrhage during pars plana vitrectomy. Ophthalmic Surg Lasers. 1997;28(8):640–4.
10. Ghoraba HH, Zayed AI. Suprachoroidal hemorrhage as a complication of vitrectomy. Ophthalmic Surg Lasers. 2001;32(4):281–8.
11. Williamson TH. Intraocular surgery, a basic surgical guide. Springer; 2016.
12. Williamson TH. Vitreoretinal surgery. 2nd ed. Berlin: Springer; 2013.
13. Hoerauf H, Roider J, Herboth T, Hager A, Laqua H. Outcome after vitrectomy in rhegmatogenous retinal detachment and dense vitreous opacities. Klin Monatsbl Augenheilkd. 1997;211(6):369–74.
14. Schachat AP, Oyakawa RT, Michels RG, Rice TA. Complications of vitreous surgery for diabetic retinopathy. II. Postoperative complications. Ophthalmology. 1983;90(5):522–30.
15. Holekamp NM, Shui YB, Beebe DC. Vitrectomy surgery increases oxygen exposure to the lens: a possible mechanism for nuclear cataract formation. Am J Ophthalmol. 2005;139(2):302–10. S0002-9394(04)01147-X [pii]. https://doi.org/10.1016/j.ajo.2004.09.046.
16. Holekamp NM, Shui YB, Beebe D. Lower intraocular oxygen tension in diabetic patients: possible contribution to decreased incidence of nuclear sclerotic cataract. Am J Ophthalmol. 2006;141(6):1027–32.
17. Grusha YO, Masket S, Miller KM. Phacoemulsification and lens implantation after pars plana vitrectomy. Ophthalmology. 1998;105(2):287–94.
18. Thompson JT. The role of patient age and intraocular gas use in cataract progression after vitrectomy for macular holes and epiretinal membranes. Am J Ophthalmol. 2004;137(2):250–7. https://doi.org/10.1016/j.ajo.2003.09.020. S0002939403010948 [pii]
19. Soliman MK, Hardin JS, Jawed F, Uwaydat SH, Faramawi MF, Chu CJ, et al. A database study of visual outcomes and intraoperative complications of postvitrectomy cataract surgery. Ophthalmology. 2018;125(11):1683–91. https://doi.org/10.1016/j.ophtha.2018.05.027.
20. Eifrig CW, Scott IU, Flynn HW Jr, Smiddy WE, Newton J. Endophthalmitis after pars plana vitrectomy: incidence, causative organisms, and visual acuity outcomes. Am J Ophthalmol. 2004;138(5):799–802.
21. Cohen SM, Flynn HW Jr, Murray TG, Smiddy WE. Endophthalmitis after pars plana vitrectomy. Postvitrect Endophthal Study Group Ophthalmol. 1995;102(5):705–12.
22. Wykoff CC, Parrott MB, Flynn HW Jr, Shi W, Miller D, Alfonso EC. Nosocomial acute-onset postoperative endophthalmitis at a university teaching hospital (2002–2009). Am J Ophthalmol. 2010;150(3):392–8 e2. S0002-9394(10)00266-7 [pii]. https://doi.org/10.1016/j.ajo.2010.04.010.
23. Stein JD, Zacks DN, Grossman D, Grabe H, Johnson MW, Sloan FA. Adverse events after pars plana vitrectomy among medicare beneficiaries. Arch Ophthalmol. 2009;127(12):1656–63. 127/12/1656 [pii]. https://doi.org/10.1001/archophthalmol.2009.300.
24. Abrams GW, Azen SP, Barr CC, Lai MY, Hutton WL, Trese MT, et al. The incidence of corneal abnormalities in the Silicone Study. Silicone Study Report 7. Arch Ophthalmol. 1995;113(6):764–9.
25. Narendran N, Williamson TH. The effects of aspirin and warfarin therapy on haemorrhage in vitreoretinal surgery. Acta Ophthalmol Scand. 2003;81(1):38–40.
26. Dayani PN, Grand MG. Maintenance of warfarin anticoagulation for patients undergoing vitreoretinal surgery. Arch Ophthalmol. 2006;124(11):1558–65. 124/11/1558 [pii]. https://doi.org/10.1001/archopht.124.11.1558.
27. Chandra A, Jazayeri F, Williamson TH. Warfarin in vitreoretinal surgery: a case controlled series. Br J Ophthalmol. 2011;95(7):976–8. bjo.2010.187526 [pii]. https://doi.org/10.1136/bjo.2010.187526.
28. Herbert EN, Mokete B, Williamson TH, Laidlaw DA. Haemorrhagic vitreoretinal complications associated with combined antiplatelet agents. Br J Ophthalmol. 2006;90(9):1209–10.
29. Mason JO 3rd, Gupta SR, Compton CJ, Frederick PA, Neimkin MG, Hill ML, et al. Comparison of hemorrhagic complications of warfa-

rin and clopidogrel bisulfate in 25-gauge vitrectomy versus a control group. Ophthalmology. 2010;118(3):543–7. S0161-6420(10)00720-7 [pii]. https://doi.org/10.1016/j.ophtha.2010.07.005.
30. Aras C, Ozdamar A, Karacorlu M. Suprachoroidal hemorrhage during silicone oil removal in Marfan syndrome. Ophthalmic Surg Lasers. 2000;31(4):337–9.
31. Chandra A, Xing W, Kadhim MR, Williamson TH. Suprachoroidal hemorrhage in pars plana vitrectomy: risk factors and outcomes over 10 years. Ophthalmology. 2014;121(1):311–7. https://doi.org/10.1016/j.ophtha.2013.06.021.
32. Tabandeh H, Flynn HW Jr. Suprachoroidal hemorrhage during pars plana vitrectomy. Curr Opin Ophthalmol. 2001;12(3):179–85.
33. Wolter JR. Expulsive hemorrhage: a study of histopathological details. Graefes Arch Clin Exp Ophthalmol. 1982;219(4):155–8.
34. Chan W, Hussain A, Marshall J. Youngs modulus of Bruchs membrane: implications for AMD. Invest Ophthalmol Vis Sci. 2007;48(13):2187.
35. Lee CJ, Vroom JA, Fishman HA, Bent SF. Determination of human lens capsule permeability and its feasibility as a replacement for Bruch's membrane. Biomaterials. 2006;27(8):1670–8.
36. Vurgese S, Panda-Jonas S, Jonas JB. Scleral thickness in human eyes. PloS One. 2012;7(1).
37. Jansen MCWH, Haenen JH, van Asten WN, Thien T. Deep Venous thrombosis: a prospective 3-month follow-up using duplex scanning and strain gauge plethysmography. Clin Sci (Lond). 1998;94:651–66.
38. Lakhanpal V. Experimental and clinical observations on massive suprachoroidal hemorrhage. Trans Am Ophthalmol Soc. 1993;91:545–652.
39. Pakravan M, Yazdani S, Afroozifar M, Kouhestani N, Ghassami M, Shahshahan M. An alternative approach for management of delayed suprachoroidal hemorrhage after glaucoma procedures. J Glaucoma. 2014;23(1):37–40. https://doi.org/10.1097/IJG.0b013e31825afb25.
40. Jin W, Xing Y, Xu Y, Wang W, Yang A. Management of delayed suprachoriodal haemorrhage after intraocular surgery and trauma. Graefes Arch Clin Exp Ophthalmol. 2014;252(8):1189–93. https://doi.org/10.1007/s00417-013-2550-x.
41. Lakhanpal V, Schocket SS, Elman MJ, Nirankari VS. A new modified vitreoretinal surgical approach in the management of massive suprachoroidal hemorrhage. Ophthalmology. 1989;96(6):793–800. https://doi.org/10.1016/s0161-6420(89)32819-3.
42. Fei P, Jin HY, Zhang Q, Li X, Zhao PQ. Tissue plasminogen activator-assisted vitrectomy in the early treatment of acute massive suprachoroidal hemorrhage complicating cataract surgery. Int J Ophthalmol. 2018;11(1):170–1. https://doi.org/10.18240/ijo.2018.01.27.
43. Rezende FA, Kickinger MC, Li G, Prado RF, Regis LG. Transconjunctival drainage of serous and hemorrhagic choroidal detachment. Retina. 2012;32(2):242–9. https://doi.org/10.1097/IAE.0b013e31821c4087.
44. Chang S. LXII Edward Jackson lecture: open angle glaucoma after vitrectomy. Am J Ophthalmol. 2006;141(6):1033–43. S0002-9394(06)00254-6 [pii]. https://doi.org/10.1016/j.ajo.2006.02.014.
45. Al-Harthi E, Abboud EB, Al-Dhibi H, Dhindsa H. Incidence of sclerotomy-related retinal breaks. Retina. 2005;25(3):281–4.
46. Koh HJ, Cheng L, Kosobucki B, Freeman WR. Prophylactic intraoperative 360 degrees laser retinopexy for prevention of retinal detachment. Retina. 2007;27(6):744–9. https://doi.org/10.1097/IAE.0b013e318030ebd7. 00006982-200707000-00012 [pii]
47. Rich RM, Smiddy WE, Davis JL. Infectious scleritis after retinal surgery. Am J Ophthalmol. 2008;145(4):695–9. S0002-9394(07)01008-2 [pii]. https://doi.org/10.1016/j.ajo.2007.11.024.
48. Morley AM, Pavesio C. Surgically induced necrotising scleritis following three-port pars plana vitrectomy without scleral buckling: a series of three cases. Eye (Lond). 2008;22(1):162–4. 6702708 [pii]. https://doi.org/10.1038/sj.eye.6702708.
49. Kilmartin DJ, Dick AD, Forrester JV. Sympathetic ophthalmia risk following vitrectomy: should we counsel patients? Br J Ophthalmol. 2000;84(5):448–9.
50. Kilmartin DJ, Dick AD, Forrester JV. Prospective surveillance of sympathetic ophthalmia in the UK and Republic of Ireland. Br J Ophthalmol. 2000;84(3):259–63.
51. Ibarra MS, Hermel M, Prenner JL, Hassan TS. Longer-term outcomes of transconjunctival sutureless 25-gauge vitrectomy. Am J Ophthalmol. 2005;139(5):831–6.
52. Kellner L, Wimpissinger B, Stolba U, Brannath W, Binder S. 25-gauge vs 20-gauge system for pars plana vitrectomy: a prospective randomised clinical trial. Br J Ophthalmol. 2007;91(7):945–8. bjo.2006.106799 [pii]. https://doi.org/10.1136/bjo.2006.106799.
53. Wimpissinger B, Kellner L, Brannath W, Krepler K, Stolba U, Mihalics C, et al. 23-Gauge versus 20-gauge system for pars plana vitrectomy: a prospective randomised clinical trial. Br J Ophthalmol. 2008;92(11):1483–7. bjo.2008.140509 [pii]. https://doi.org/10.1136/bjo.2008.140509.
54. Kuo HK, Lee JJ. Macular infarction after 23-gauge transconjunctival sutureless vitrectomy and subconjunctival gentamicin for macular pucker: a case report. Can J Ophthalmol. 2009;44(6):720–1. i09-197 [pii]. https://doi.org/10.1139/i09-197.
55. Kunimoto DY, Kaiser RS. Incidence of endophthalmitis after 20- and 25-gauge vitrectomy. Ophthalmology. 2007;114(12):2133–7. S0161-6420(07)00862-7 [pii]. https://doi.org/10.1016/j.ophtha.2007.08.009.
56. Okuda T, Nishimura A, Kobayashi A, Sugiyama K. Postoperative retinal break after 25-gauge transconjunctival sutureless vitrectomy: report of four cases. Graefes Arch Clin Exp Ophthalmol. 2007;245(1):155–7. https://doi.org/10.1007/s00417-006-0354-y.

Principles of Internal Tamponade

4

Contents

Gases

Principles (also see Appendix 1: Useful Formulae and Rules)

It is important to understand Fick's diffusion equation; that is that two gases on either side of a semi-permeable membrane will pass across the semi-permeable membrane until their concentrations are equal on both sides. If one gas travels across the membrane at a slower speed than the other, then this causes a difference in the size of the gas bubbles on either side of the membrane. For example if a large molecule gas like sulpha hexafluoride (SF_6) is placed within the eye, this passes slowly into the bloodstream, to the lungs and out into the atmosphere. However, nitrogen from the atmosphere is highly soluble and passes rapidly through the lungs, blood

T. H. Williamson, *Vitreoretinal Surgery*, https://doi.org/10.1007/978-3-030-68769-4_4

and into the eye, causing the SF_6 gas bubble to enlarge within the eye. For this reason, after a vitrectomy SF_6 and perfluoro propane (C_3F_8) must be mixed with air to prevent a volumetric increase, which would then cause a rise in intraocular pressure.

Additional Surgical Steps

1. Attach the air pump tubing to the three-way tap on the infusion line and switch on the air pump at 30–40 mmHg.
2. With a flat retina, place the tip of a flute cannula close to the optic nerve head to drain the vitreous cavity fluid.
3. Turn the three-way tap to allow insertion of the filtered air.
4. Fill the cavity.
5. Remove the superior trochars and the superior sclerotomies and insert a 26 g needle through the pars plana to allow exhaust of the gases.
6. Prepare the long-acting gas (mixed to the desired concentration with filtered air) by inserting it into a 100 ml syringe (make sure any tubing for drawing up gas is flushed through with the gas before drawing up onto the syringe). Draw up the gas, for the percentage of gas you need. You can usually see how much gas was inserted by holding up the syringe to the light. Look for a condensation line where the syringe stopper was drawn up to with the long-acting gas, e.g. a line at 20 mls. Mistakes can occur with gas mixtures with resultant underfill with too little long-acting gas or severe IOP rise with too much. Therefore, it is worth being careful and observing the processes during gas mixing to ensure the correct dosages are used.
7. Attach the syringe to the three-way tap and flush out the air by inserting over 50 mls. Keep some in case of hypotony during the closure of the surgical wounds.
8. At the end of the operation, the air in the vitreous cavity must be flushed with a volume of gas to achieve the correct gas concentration.

Break closure can be achieved by the use of an internal tamponade such as a gas bubble. This acts in two ways,

1. By "tamponading" the break (The gas is in contact with the edge of the break), so that an accumulation of fluid is not possible through the break. The RPE pumps out the SRF flattening the retina. This is utilised in pneumatic retinopexy where SRF is not drained by the surgeon and the retina can flatten spontaneously after intravitreal gas injection.
2. By forcing the retina flat by displacing the retina outwards. This is primarily reserved for an eye, which has had a vitrectomy, and the retina has already been flattened.

Note: Pneumatic retinopexy, i.e. insertion of gas without vitrectomy, has a success rate of approximately 70% which is lower than conventional or vitrectomy surgery [1–5]. However, it may reduce the need for more extensive surgery if one can accept the relatively low success rates and risk of PVR. In pneumatic retinopexy, rotation of the eye over several hours while the gas bubble is present may also be used to try to flatten the retina.

A gas bubble must have its effect for at least 5 days because the retinopexy requires time to take effect. For this reason, larger molecule gases are used so that the dissipation of the gas bubble from the eye is retarded. The most popular gases are sulpha hexafluoride (SF_6) and perfluoro propane (C_3F_8) [6–9] (Figs. 4.1, 4.2, 4.3, 4.4).

Note: if the retina is completely flat (no SRF) then tamponade is not necessary to close the break, and retinopexy is enough. This is exploited when treating a flat retinal break in the clinic (the retina around the break remains flat despite the need for a few days for the retinopexy to reach full adhesion), presumably because the retinopexy confers some mild adhesion immediately. This has been exploited by Martinez-Vasquez [10], who has described vitrectomy with aqueous tamponade for pseudophakic RRD. This method requires fastidious removal of all of the SRF during the PPV (the SRF is squeezed out by use of heavy liq-

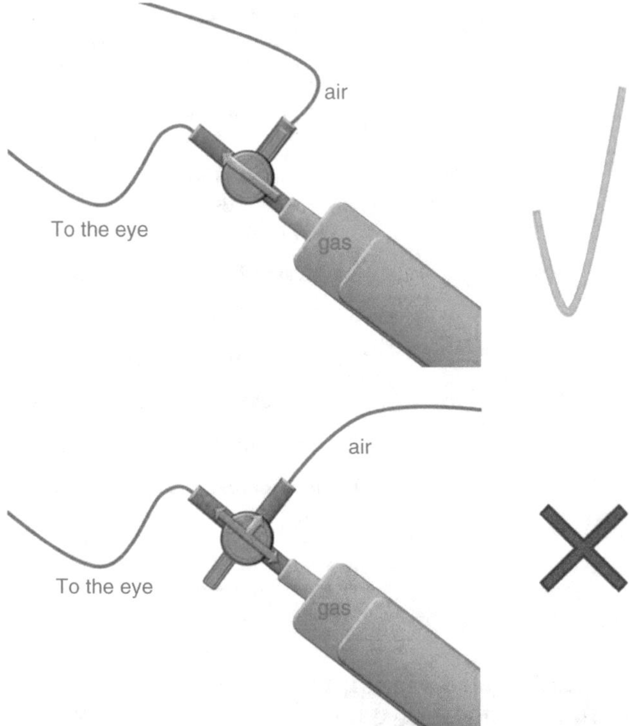

Fig. 4.1 When inserting gas through the three-way tap make sure the tap is closed to the air infusion line otherwise, the gas will enter the air infusion line and you fill not achieve a full flush out of the air

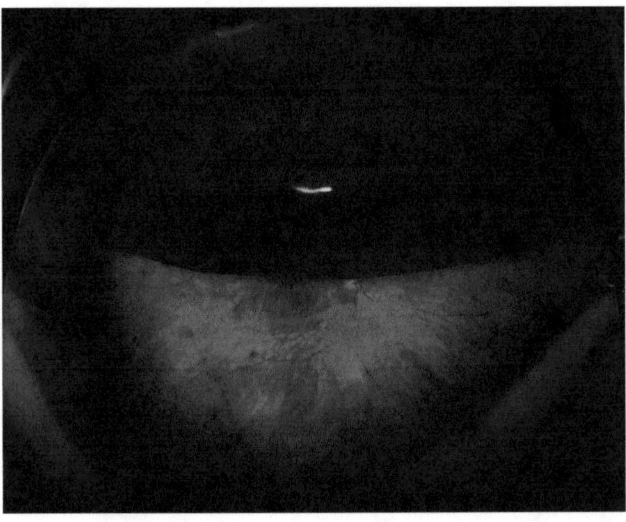

Fig. 4.2 A wide angle view of an intraocular gas bubble notices the flattened inferior surface of the gas bubble. The gravitational effect of the dense vitreous liquid relative to the less dense gas overcomes the surfacel tension (which tries to create a spherical gas bubble), thereby distorting the bubble and flattening the inferior surface

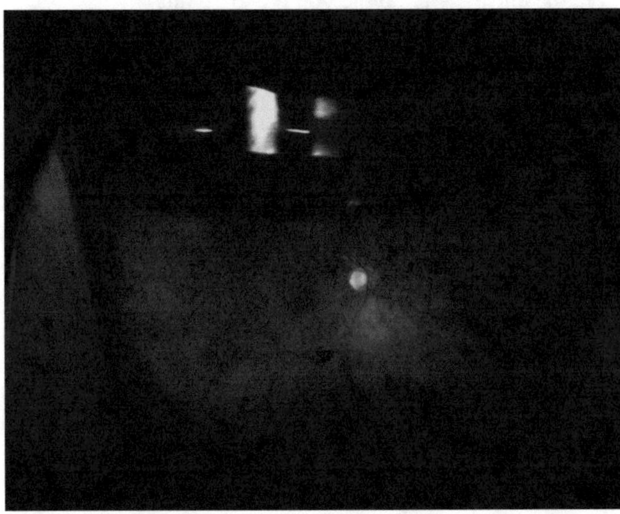

Fig. 4.3 As the gas bubble gets smaller, the inferior surface becomes more curved, when the bubble is very small, it will be spherical

uid posteriorly and air anteriorly, with the air removed again at the end of the operation) and heavy Diode laser retinopexy. As a proof of principle, the method is of interest, but most surgeons would leave the air inside the eye and tamponade as usual. However, the principle is exploited in RRD with inferior holes where a contact of a gas bubble cannot be guaranteed, and the surgeon, with complete removal of SRF, can leave the inferior holes treated with retinopexy and no indentation, see later chapters [11, 12].

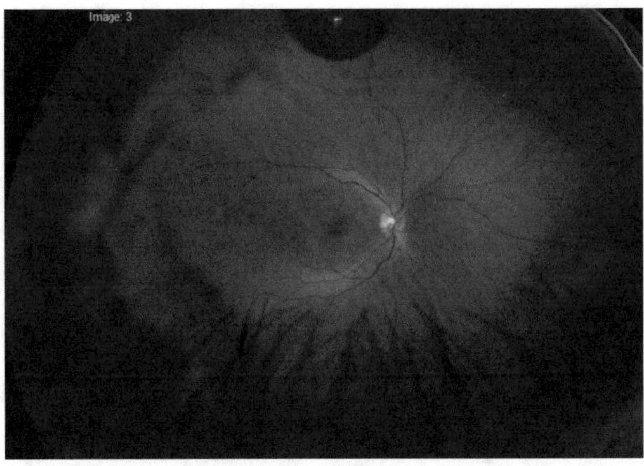

Fig. 4.4 A small residual bubble, notice its spherical configuration

Properties

- Hundred percent SF_6 doubles its volume in 2 days and is present for 2 weeks [13]. Its non-expansible concentration is between 20% and 30% with air.
- C_3F_8 expands four times at 100% concentration, lasts 8 weeks and has a non-expansible concentration with air of 12–16%.

With experience, the concentration most appropriate to the surgeon can be decided upon. 30% SF_6 and 16% C_3F_8 may be suitable to start with.

The gases have a high surface tension of 70 mN/m, i.e. the gas remains as one sphere and does not break up into smaller bubbles. This stops the gas bubble from going through the retinal break allowing contact with the edge of large breaks without the gas entering the subretinal space.

Problems with gas bubbles can be determined from Fick's diffusion equation, for example during surgery with the injection of gas; nitrous dioxide from the anaesthetic will rapidly enter the gas-filled eye. This means that postoperatively the gas bubble will shrink as the lungs exhale this nitrous dioxide. In practice, this may not have a major effect on the size of the gas bubble, but most surgeons prefer to switch off nitrous dioxide when using gases during surgery. A patient with gas in situ should not have a general anaesthetic using nitrous dioxide because this will enter the gas bubble cause expansion and a severe rise in IOP, potentially resulting in central retinal artery occlusion [14] (Figs. 4.5 and 4.6).

The inferior border of a gas bubble has a flattened meniscus. Therefore, it is not possible to know reliably that the gas bubble will tamponade detached inferior breaks. For this reason, surgeons often apply a plombage between the 4 and 8

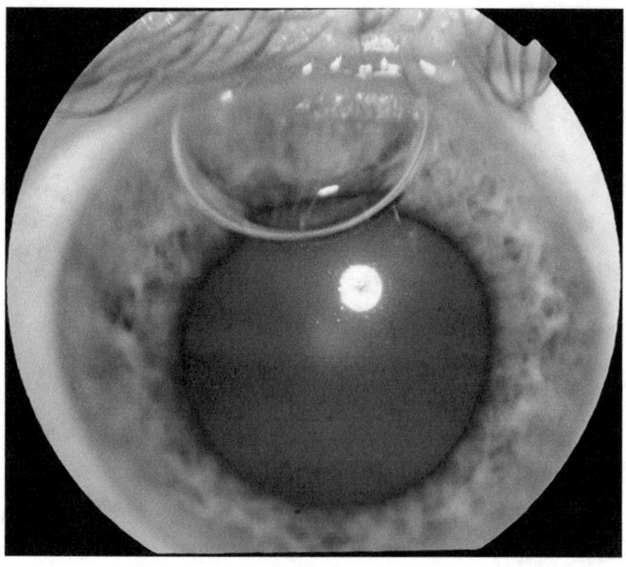

Fig. 4.5 Air can enter the anterior chamber at the end of the operation as in this eye in which there is presumably a defect in the zonule. Attempting to remove the AC gas by aspiration and infusion of fluid can result in a reduced gas fill in the posterior segment because the infusion fluid enters the vitreous cavity (passing with gravity around the lens), and the gas escapes through the sclerotomies. Therefore it is best to have the sclerotomies closed. Any gas leakage must then occur through the anterior segment and can be monitored by the surgeon. If the gas bubble is not removed, the bubble will be present in the postoperative period, usually without any consequences and with gradual absorption

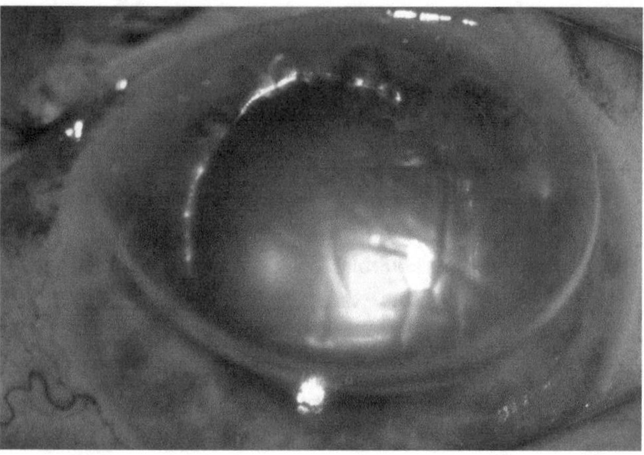

Fig. 4.6 A large air bubble that has leaked into the anterior chamber has caused pupil block

o'clock positions. However, in a vitrectomised situation, this may give a risk of choroidal haemorrhaging because of hypotony, indentation of the choroid and suturing near vortex veins. It is, therefore, sometimes advisable to rely on strict posturing of the patient to tamponade an inferior break. In this circumstance, the patient with an equatorial or pre-equatorial break which is inferiorly placed is postured face up. This may increase the risk of cataract but reliably closes inferior breaks. If an inferior plombage is desired, insert heavy liquids into the eye before placement of the explant. This will limit the size and spread of any haemorrhage should it occur.

A Safe Method for Drawing Up Gas

Most gases are provided in disposable canisters, the assistant fills a 50 ml syringe with the correct percentage of gas and air. Errors can occur, and if the wrong gas is inserted for flushing at the end of surgery, there can be catastrophic visual loss from central retinal artery occlusion. Allowing the assistant to draw up the gas and air has led to 100% gas fills and CRAO from severe IOP rise in the early postoperative period.

Follow this method to minimise the risk of error.

1. The assistant draws the correct amount of gas into the syringe, for example.
   - 8 mls for a 16% gas fill in air
   - 15 mls for a 30% gas fill in air
2. The assistant hands the syringe to the surgeon who draws in the air to make up the volume to 50 mls.

By splitting the responsibility for drawing up the gas by the assistant and the air by the surgeon, it is very difficult to create an error of 100% gas (the surgeon would not have any space to draw up air if the assistant hands over 50 mls of gas). Both must check the type of gas used. The surgeon can double check the correct gas volume has been drawn up by observing a tell-tale condensation mark, e.g. at the 8 ml mark. The only risk of error is that the assistant incorrectly draws up air rather than the long-acting gas. This will lead to the gas bubble duration, which is too short a problem that can be overcome by reoperation or strict posturing. This is preferable to an erroneous 100% long-acting gas and subsequent IOP rise and central retinal artery occlusion. Even better is to use a 100 ml syringe, and then the recalculation from percentage is removed from the process, with 100 ml 20% is 20 mls. I use stickers like Prepdose simple to remind my trainees and myself of the dosage and to mark the syringe on the surgical trolley for best practice (Figs. 4.7, 4.8, 4.9).

Physical Properties

- Contact with the retina
- Expansion
- Effects on IOP
- Duration (Fig. 4.10)

Height (x) and volume (y) in the polar cap, the change in height is very rapid for a small change in volume when the

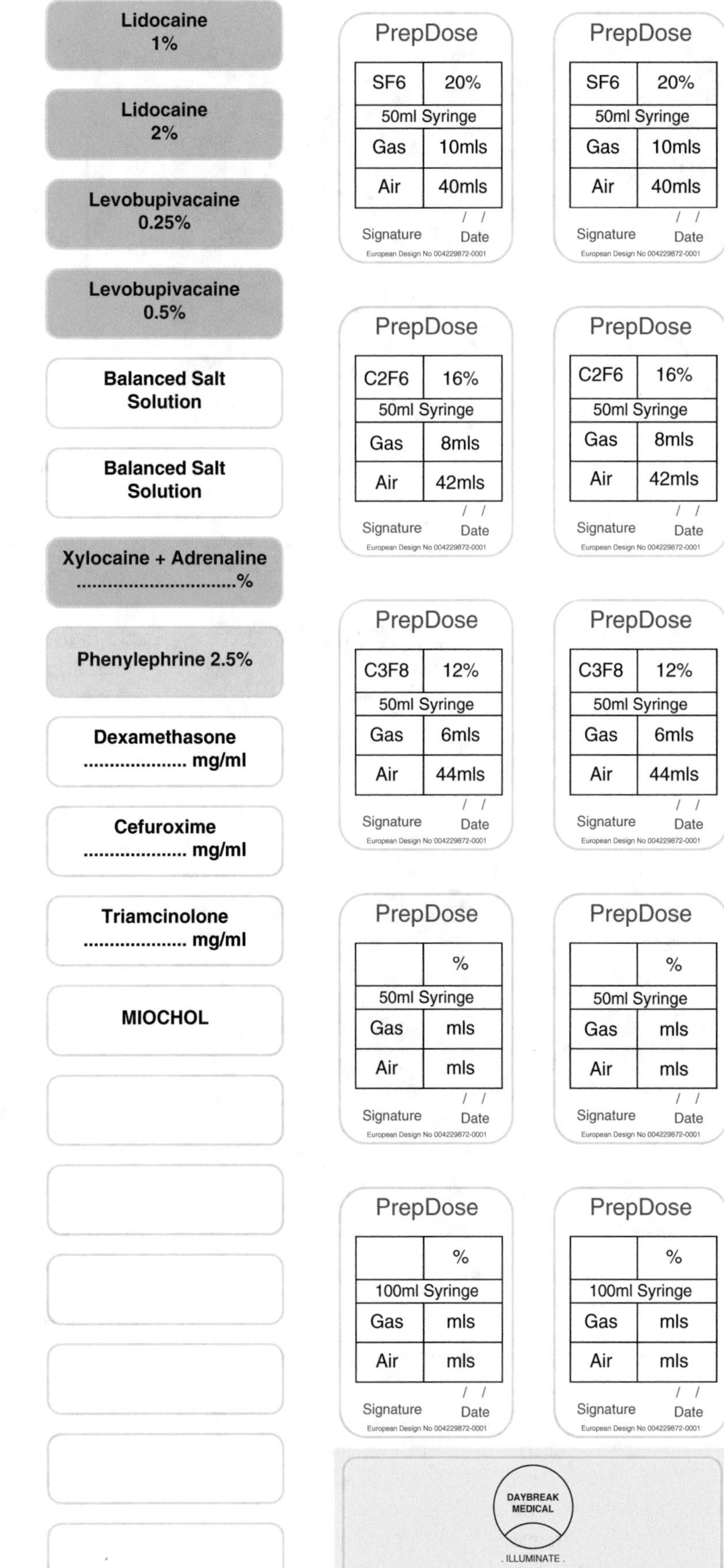

Fig. 4.7 It is recommended to use stickers such as Prepdose to remind yourself of the correct gas concentrations and to record gas usage in the clinical record

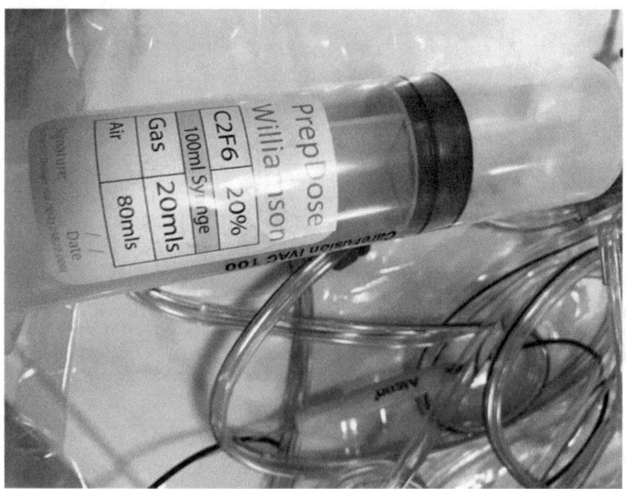

Fig. 4.8 It is important to label any syringes containing drugs on the surgical tray. This is also true for the gas mixture. A label like this can be used to double check the dose mix and increase the safety of the use of gas. Mistakes with gas mixing are under-recognised and often catastrophic for the vision for the patient because of severe IOP elevation

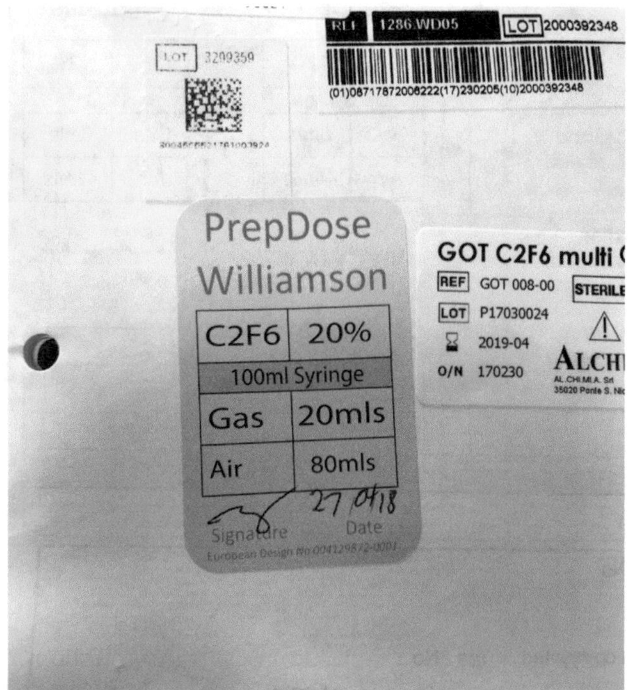

Fig. 4.9 It is recommended to record how you have used the gas mix in the clinical record

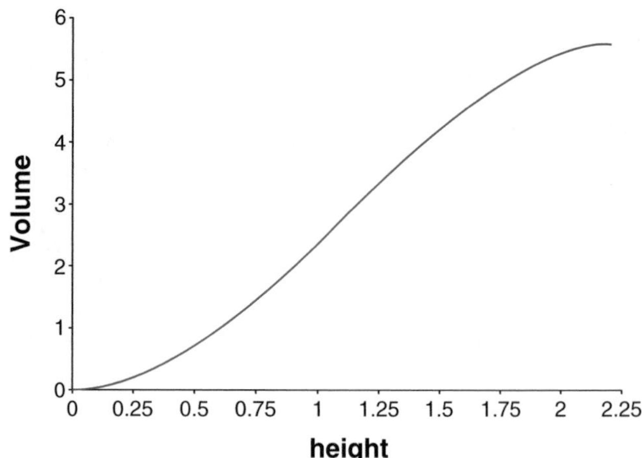

Fig. 4.10 Small changes in volume induce larger changes in the height of the gas bubble at the top and bottom of the sphere than in the middle of the sphere

bubble is at the extremes of the vitreous cavity, i.e. superiorly or inferiorly (Figs. 4.11 and 4.12).

Similarly, the arc of contact will change very rapidly at the inferior and superior extremities of the vitreous cavity because the relative volumes there are less than in the centre of the sphere (Figs. 4.13 and 4.14).

It is important to warn the patient about the visual effects and duration of gas in the eye. The patient will see a horizontal line descend in the eye as the gas bubble gets smaller (inferior edge rising). At just over half of the total duration, the patient will begin to see "over" the gas bubble and be able to use the central vision [15]. When the gas bubble is small, it may break up into a few bubbles. At this point, the gas will disappear in a day or two (Fig. 4.15).

The physical properties of gas in the eye have been calculated and can provide a guide to safe gas concentrations for given fills of the eye at the end of surgery [16]. A complete fill is never achieved. Luckily axial length does not change the concentrations required significantly [17]. However, theoretically if using 100% gas in pneumatic retinopexy, the volume injected should increase with the size of the eye to achieve the same arc of contact on the retina (Figs. 4.16, 4.17, 4.18, 4.19).

Surgical Pearl

An Inexpensive Option for Air–Gas Exchange

Unless the gas comes premixed, in a ready-to-use can, the typically non-expansile concentration is prepared either by diluting the gas externally or intravitreally. The latter results in a somewhat less accurate mixture (which has no relevance in clinical practice) but is very easy to do and is very cost-effective. Here are the steps to be taken:

- Make sure that the label of the gas canister says "undiluted."
- Have the nurse prepare two 2 ml syringes: an empty one and a second with ~2 ml of undiluted gas (for an emmetropic eye; in highly myopic eyes this author uses ~2.5 ml of gas).
- Attach a small (such as 30 g) needle to the empty syringe.

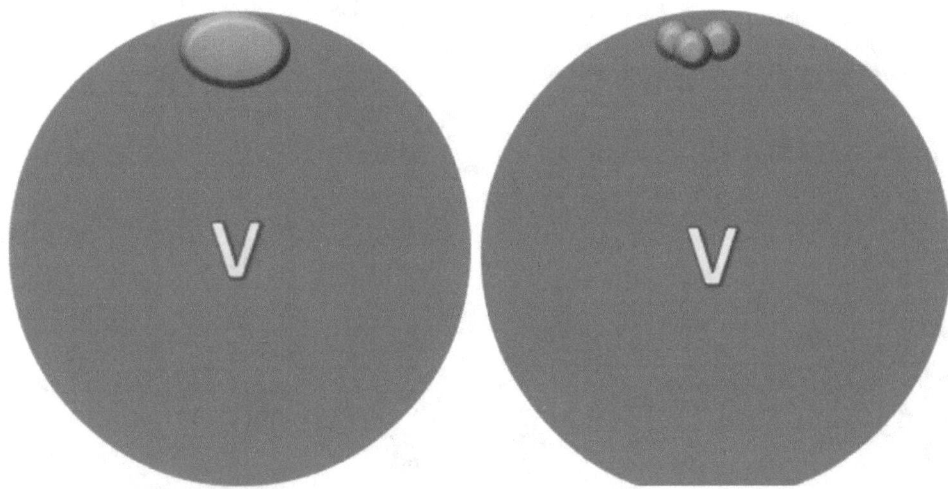

Fig. 4.11 A gas bubb is more spherical when it is small due to increased relative surface tension. This leads to less retinal contact. Alternatively, the bubble might split into smaller bubbles which find it difficult to coalesce. The change in the height of the bubble and surface area contact is faster at the top and bottom of the sphere than the middle

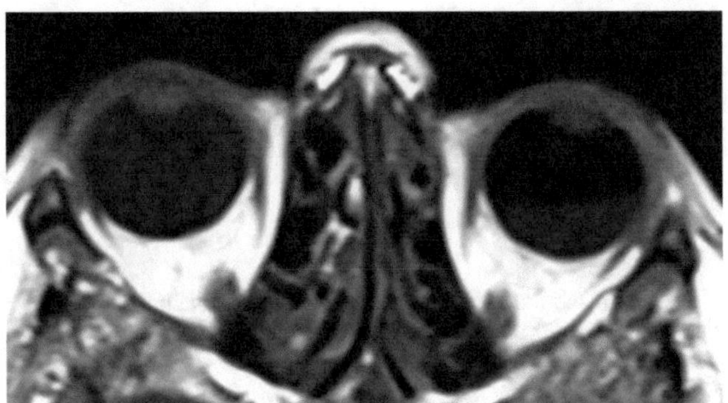

Fig. 4.12 Notice the gas in the vitreous cavity visible on MRI with the patient face up. There is a flattened inferior meniscus

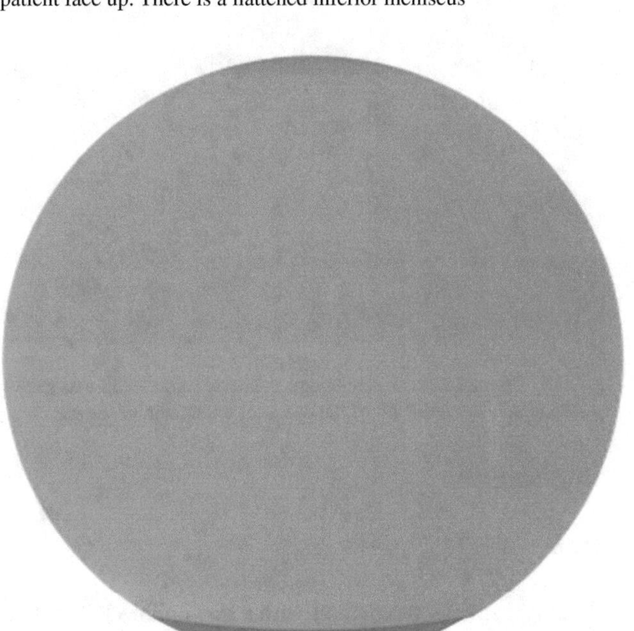

Fig. 4.13 It is rare to see the vitreous cavity fully filled with gas because with the correct concentration of gas, the full fill is only momentary, and the gas bubble recedes rapidly at the bottom of the sphere

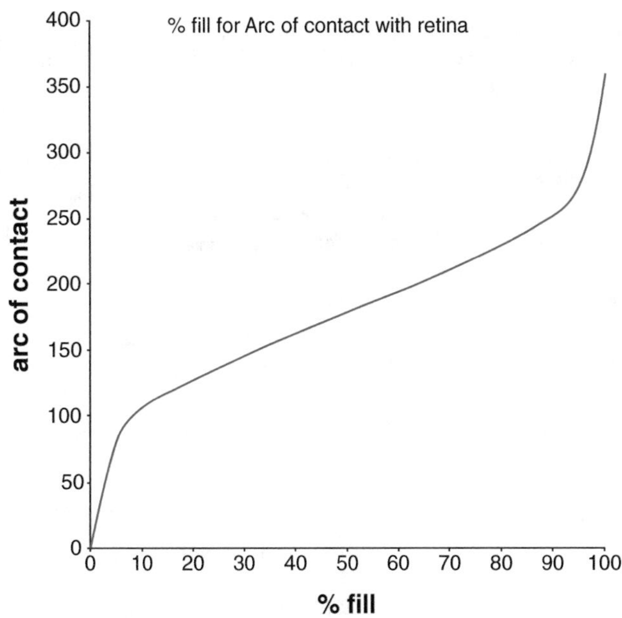

Fig. 4.14 The arc of contact changes rapidly at the extremes, making it difficult to tamponade a 6 o'clock break with gas in the upright position

Duration of gases

gas duration weeks by Temponade	Minimum	Median	Maximum
C2F6	4.0	4.8	6.3
C3F8	8.4	9.4	11.0
SF6	2.0	2.6	3.4

Fig. 4.15 The duration of gas in the eye

% gas in air required for maximum fill after expansion without IOP risk for different fills of gas

Fill (%)	C2F6	C3F8	SF6
10	100	100	100
15	100	100	100
20	100	100	100
25	100	99	100
30	98	78	100
35	79	64	100
40	65	53	100
45	55	44	100
50	46	37	94
55	39	31	78
60	33	27	65
65	27	23	54
70	23	19	45
75	19	16	36
80	15	13	29
85	12	10	22
90	9	8	15
95	5	5	8

Fig. 4.16 Theoretical gas concentrations to use to achieve 100% fill after expansion, depending upon how much of the eye (%) is filled at the end of surgery

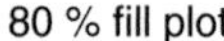

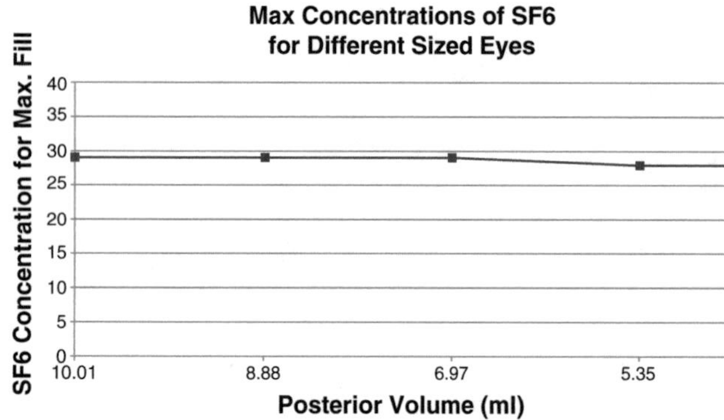

Fig. 4.17 Using mixed gas and filling the eye with gas, and the concentrations are the same for different sized eyes

- Make sure the connection is loose (do not tighten the needle/syringe connection).
- After all scleral wounds have been closed, enter the vitreous cavity with the needle.
- Withdraw ~1.5 ml of air (more if the eye was hard, less if it was soft).
- Keep the needle in the eye in a steady position so as not to damage the retina or the crystalline lens and quickly replace the air-filled syringe with the one containing the gas; this needle/syringe connection must be tight.
- Inject the gas; again, typically the same amount as the withdrawn air (~1.5 ml) but adjusted as necessary by digitally sensing the IOP toward the end of the injection.
- Withdraw the needle while simultaneously pressing on the entry site to prevent gas leakage.

Ferenc Kuhn, Retina Specialists of Alabama, Birmingham, Alabama, USA

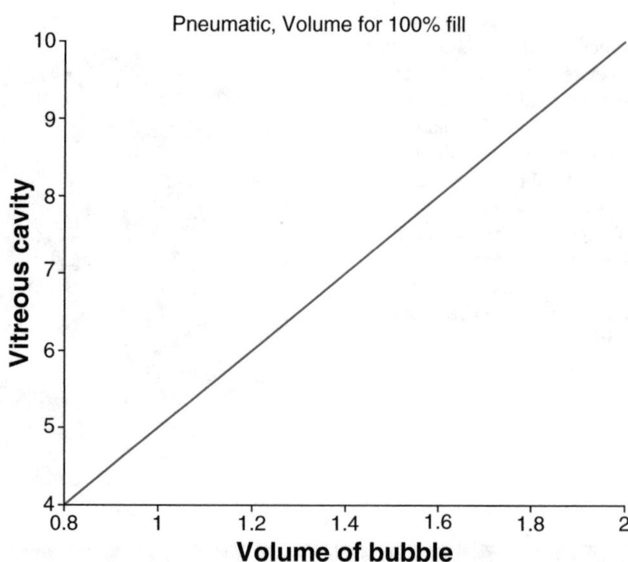

Fig. 4.18 Using gas mixtures and full fill of the vitreous cavity, you do not need to change the gas concentrations. If however, you are putting 100% gas into different sized eyes, you theoretically need to increase the volume injected as the eye increases in volume to achieve the same arc of contact in the eye

% gas in air required for maximum fill after expansion without IOP risk for different fills of gas

Fill (%)	C2F6	C3F8	SF6
10	100	100	100
15	100	100	100
20	100	100	100
25	100	99	100
30	98	78	100
35	79	64	100
40	65	53	100
45	55	44	100
50	46	37	94
55	39	31	78
60	33	27	65
65	27	23	54
70	23	19	45
75	19	16	36
80	15	13	29
85	12	10	22
90	9	8	15
95	5	5	8

Fig. 4.19 The theoretical percentage volumes (with undiluted gases) required to achieve a full fill of the eye after expansion of the gas

Complications

Vision

- Postoperatively, the patient with a gas bubble will notice that they have blurred vision from refractive changes in the eye. As it resolves, a dark line (the inferior edge of the bubble) passes horizontally from superiorly to inferiorly, the bubble gets smaller and more spherical, and gradually multiple small bubbles appear and shortly after complete dissipation of the bubble. Once the bubble edge passes

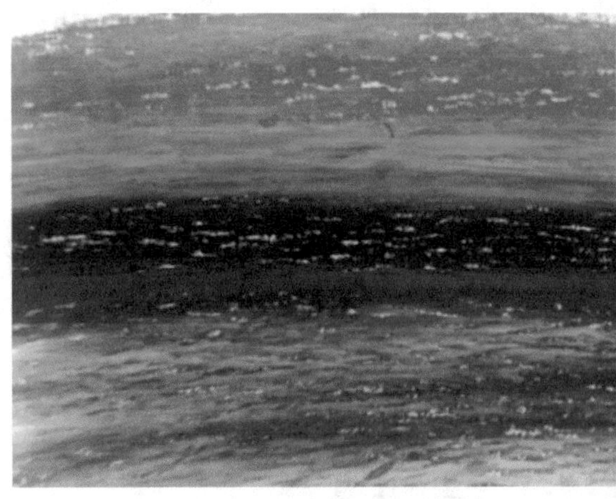

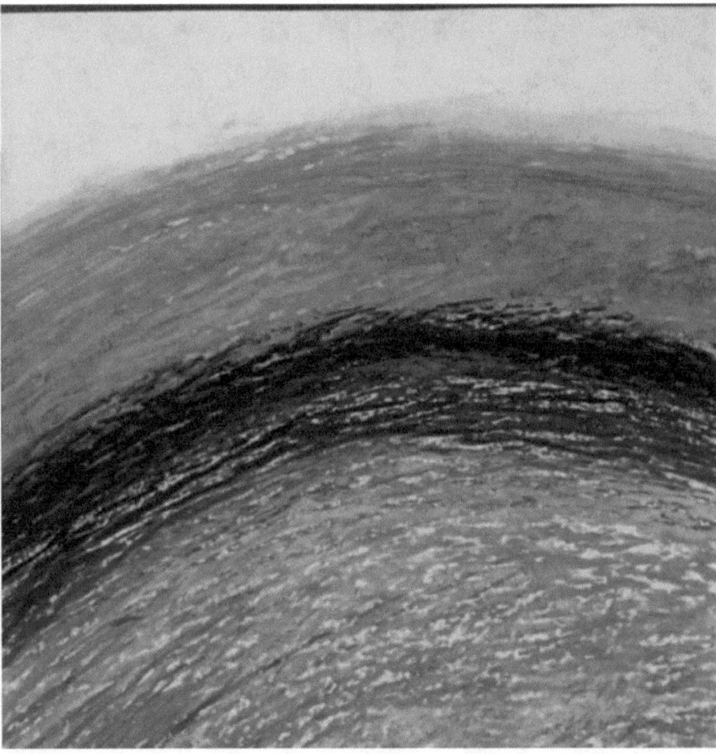

Fig. 4.20 A patient's drawing of visual phenomena around the gas bubble showed diffraction of light and an alteration of colour in the centre of the bubble

above the visual axis (The dark line is now below the patient's central vision), the patient will start to see more clearly (Figs. 4.20 and 4.21).

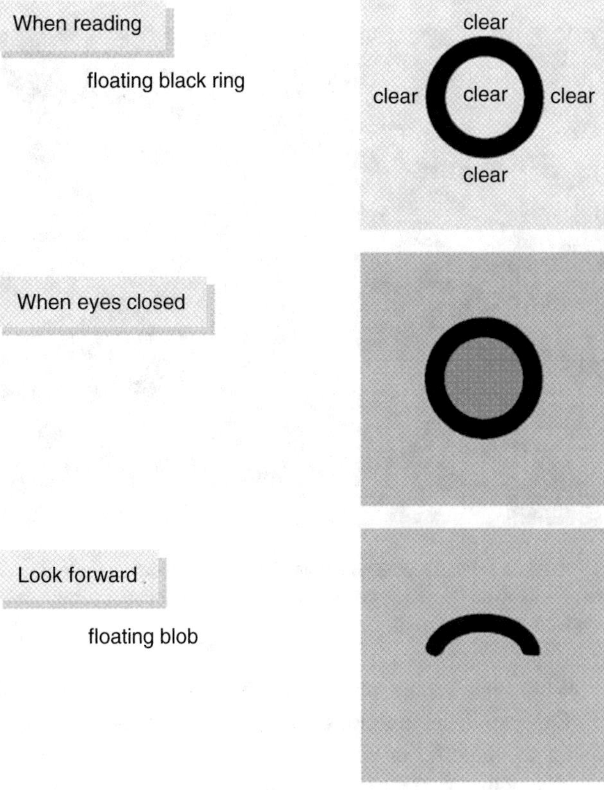

Fig. 4.21 Patients' drawings of their experience of the gas bubble

Refraction

- The phakic or pseudophakic patient is made myopic by the gas bubble and can often see more clearly close to the eye and looking down. The aphakic patient is made even more hypermetropic (Fig. 4.22).

Cataract

- The gas itself may cause a feathery posterior subcapsular cataract or "gas cataract" which is temporary (clears once the gas absorbs) but associated with an increased risk of nuclear sclerotic cataract later (Figs. 4.23, 4.24, 4.25).

IOP

- Raised intraocular pressure may occur after gas expansion in the early stages but can usually be treated medically.
- Severe IOP elevation suggests an error in the composition of the gas during mixing with air at surgery, i.e. the gas is

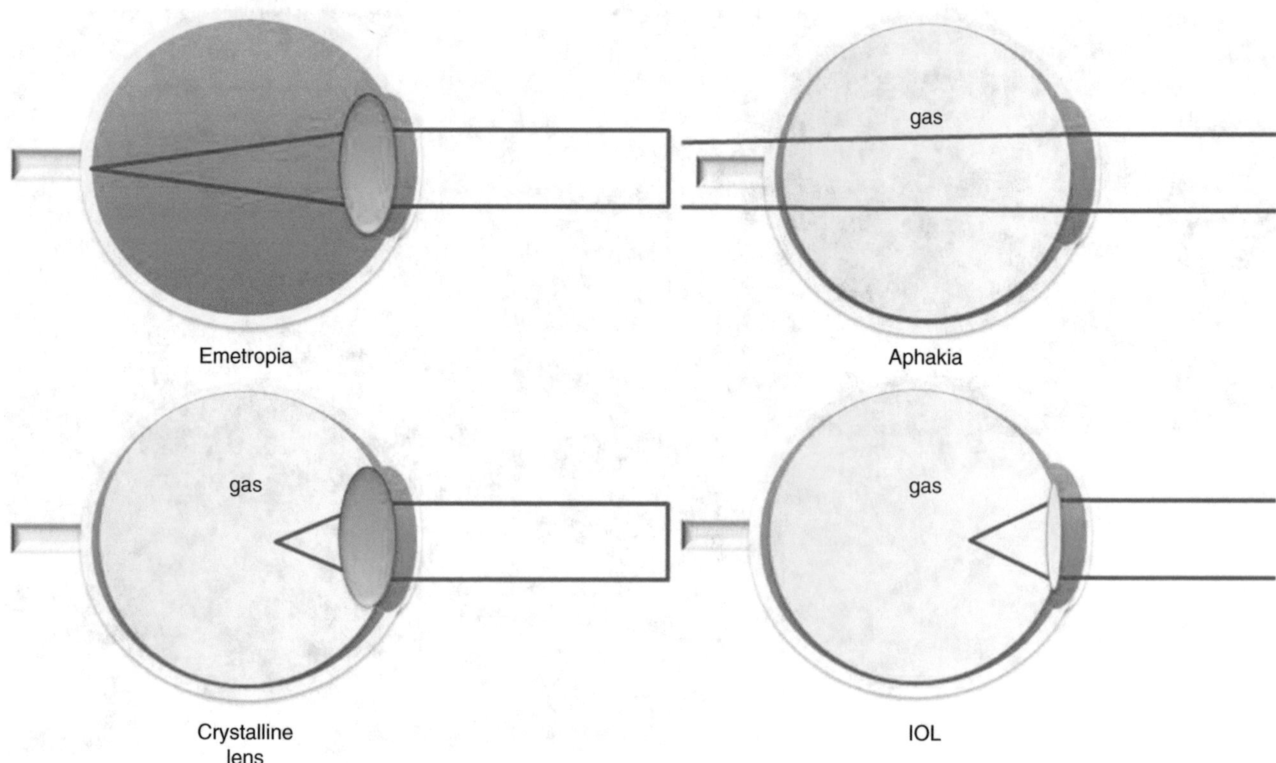

Fig. 4.22 The refraction of the gas-filled phakic or pseudophakic eye is increased because the effective power of the posterior surface of the lens is increased (the difference in the refractive index of air and the lens is greater than the difference between water/vitreous and the lens), causing a large myopic shift. In an aphakic eye, the convexity of the gas bubble in the pupil effectively creates a negative refractive change causing a large hypermetropic shift

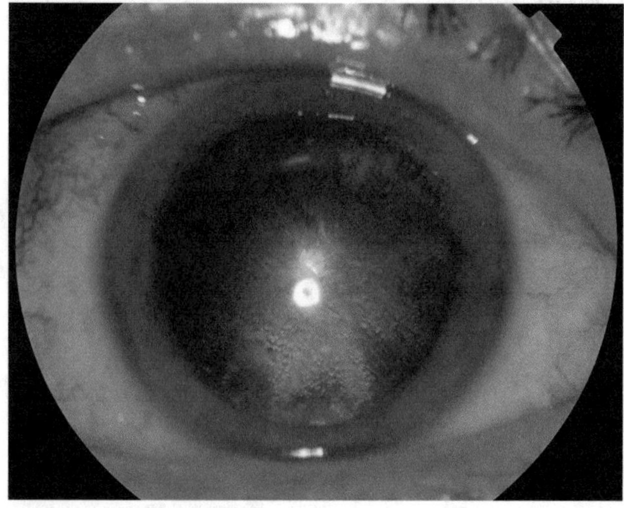

Fig. 4.23 A typical feathery cataract from gas insertion. This will clear but results in an increased chance or early onset nuclear sclerotic cataract formation

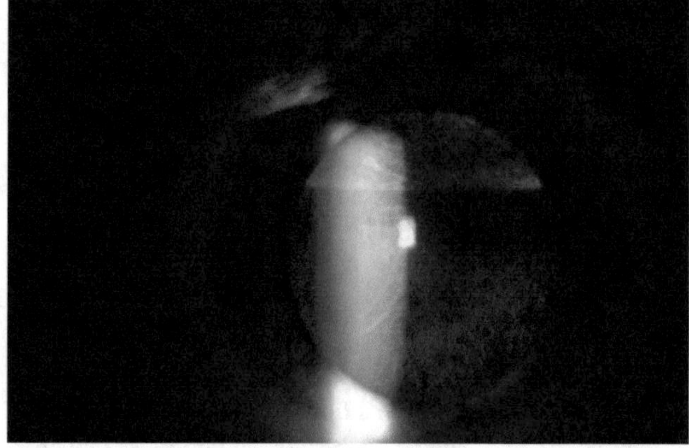

Fig. 4.24 In some patients, gas in the vitreous cavity causes a feathery and bubbly posterior subcapsular cataract in the early postoperative period, e.g. 2 weeks. This clears once the gas absorbs but usually leads to early onset nuclear sclerosis

at too high a concentration and is expanding, causing an IOP rise. If the anterior chamber is shallow and you cannot see the inferior edge of the gas bubble, then a gas mix error is likely. If you have inserted 100% gas in error, it is very unlikely that the eye will recover. If the gas mixture has been inserted at the double the concentration (can occur with 50 ml syringes as the team forgets to halve the percentage value to make the value in mls.

- Some gas may need to be removed, but there is a risk of choroidal haemorrhage during this manoeuvre if the IOP cannot be brought down medically before the gas removal.

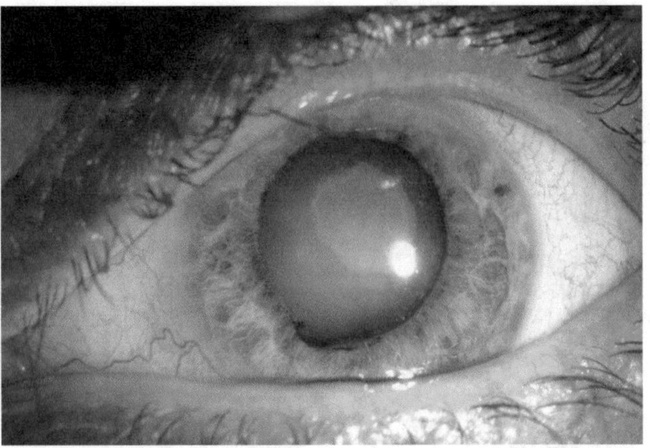

Fig. 4.25 Gas in the anterior chamber postoperatively has led to the formation of an anterior capsular opacity

Removing some gas on its own is not enough as the time to peak expansion increases with increased gas concentration. Therefore, C_3F_8 may take week to reach maximal expansion. It is best to remove all the wrong gas mix and replace the gas with the correct concentration.

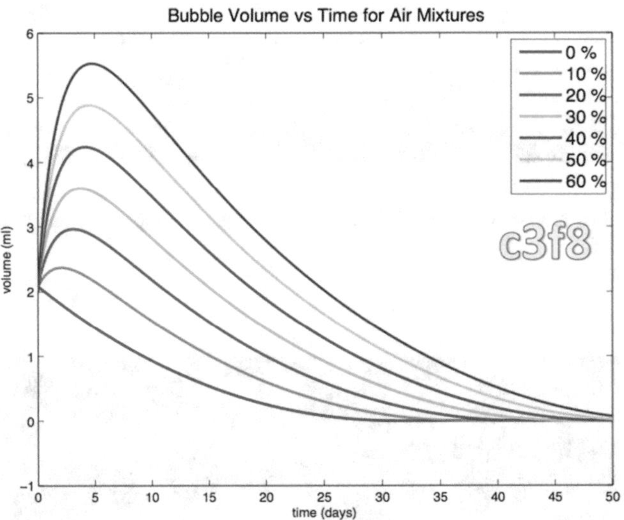

- What to do: Attach a needle to the air pump, increase the pressure to the patient's IOP level and insert the needle into the eye and gradually reduce the air pump pressure to allow a controlled reduction in IOP.
- Then you can proceed to PPV and exchange the gas for the correct concentration. This will require the gas fluid exchange and fluid–air exchange (If you still need the tamponade agent, the pathology may now have resolved, e.g. check if the macular hole is closed), followed by flushing with the correct gas concentration or air if you only need a further week of tamponade as described above (Fig. 4.26).

Loss of the Gas Bubble

- Gas dissipates early, or the bubble size is too small if the concentration inserted has been too low. This risks failure of the surgery because of reduced tamponade area.
  1. What to do: Some of the errors can be compensated for by asking the patient to posture so that the gas bubble contacts the area of pathology, e.g. face down posturing for a macular hole. Occasionally the gas bubble will need to be replaced by repeat operation.
- If the pressure rises significantly, gas may vent through an open sclerotomy leading to underfill.

Gas in the Wrong Place

- If the infusion cannula is unstable during surgery, it may angle forward, risking gas insertion through the zonules of the lens and into the anterior chamber. If the hole in the zonules is large, gas may represent through the hole even after removal of the gas from the AC. This can make visualisation of the retina difficult, in which case the gas can be displaced by viscoelastic. Removal of the viscoelastic may allow the gas back into the AC. In most circumstances gas in the AC postoperatively can be allowed to dissipate without problems (the flattened inferior meniscus allows the aqueous to flow without causing pupil block). Though you may want to keep the pupil dilated. Occasionally pupil block glaucoma will occur, which can be temporarily alleviated by YAG peripheral iridectomy and medication until the gas is absorbed.
- Gas in the suprachoroidal or subretinal spaces is exceedingly rare. Again, movement of the infusion cannula, especially in patients with anterior contraction of the vitreous base (as in PVR) or with detachment into the pars plana, may allow air to infuse under the retina. To leave gas in postoperatively will cause recurrent retinal detachment with PVR.
  1. What to do: The gas can be removed via retinotomy or via a retinal break or choroidectomy. Alternatively, a fine gauge needle can be inserted trans-conjunctivally and through the scleral (while observing the eye internally) to contact the bubble and allow egress (Figs. 4.27 and 4.28) (Tables 4.1 and 4.2).

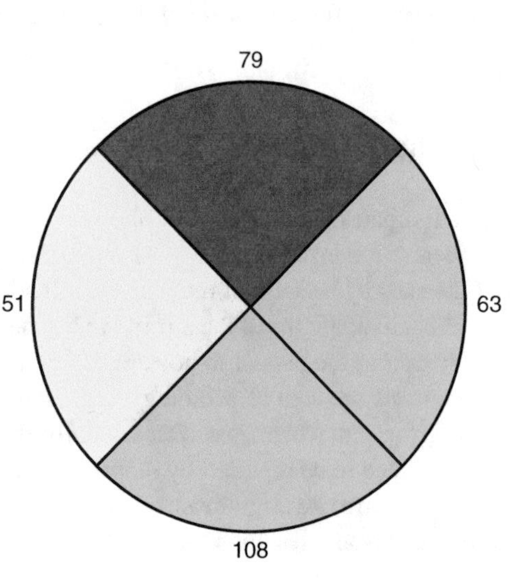

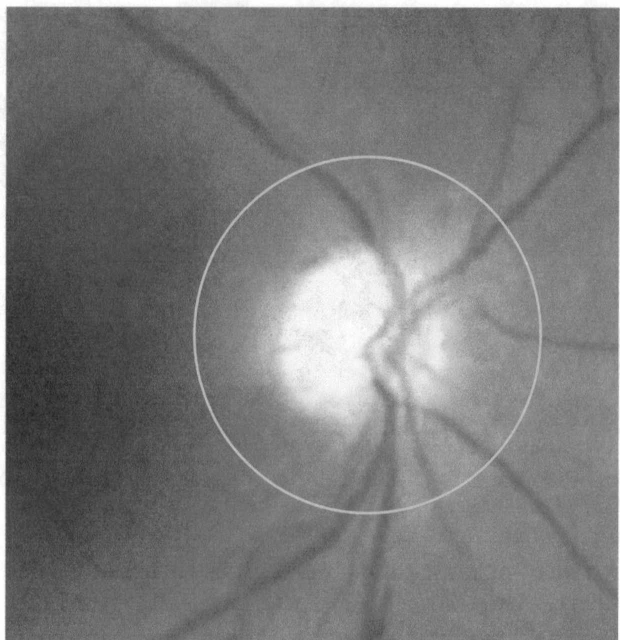

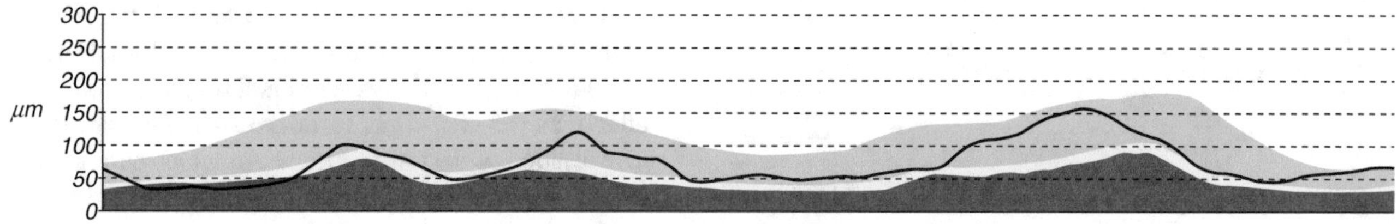

Fig. 4.26 An anterior ischaemic optic neuropathy possibly from IOP rise after PPV showing thinning of the nerve fibre layer superiorly on OCT scan

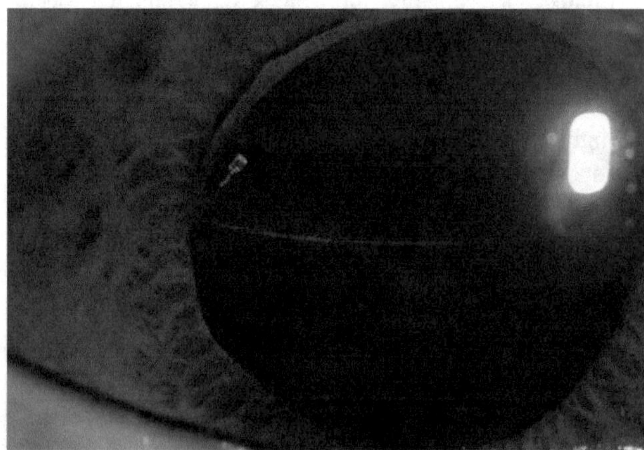

Fig. 4.27 This gas bubble is pushing the IOL forward at the superior edge, which can entrap the edge of the iris. Wait till the gas bubble has gone and then divide the inevitable posterior synechiae from the anterior capsule by passing a cannula between the capsule and the iris, free up the iris margin and relocate the IOL edge behind it

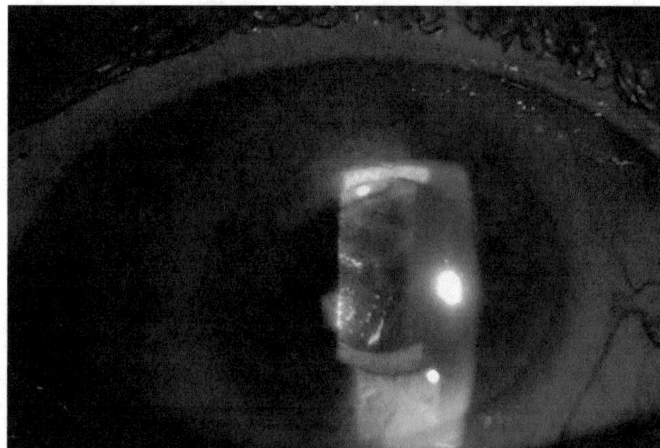

Fig. 4.28 In some patients with combined PPV, gas and cataract extraction, the IOL may be tilted by the gas bubble. The edge of the IOL may move anteriorly to the edge of the pupil causing "capture" of the pupil margin and adhesion of the iris to the lens capsule. This is associated with rapid posterior capsule opacification. Once the gas bubble has re-absorbed, the pupil should be surgically released from the capsule and replaced in its correct position in front of the IOL. A surgical capsulectomy can be performed with a vitrectomy cutter at low cut rate (200 bpm) introduced through pars plana

Table 4.1 Common gases used during pars plana vitrectomy

Gas	Structure	Molecular weight	Expansion of 100% concentration	Duration (days)	Nonexpanding concentration (%)	Uses
Air		29	0	5–7	NA	Flat retinal breaks
Sulpha hexafluoride (SF_6)	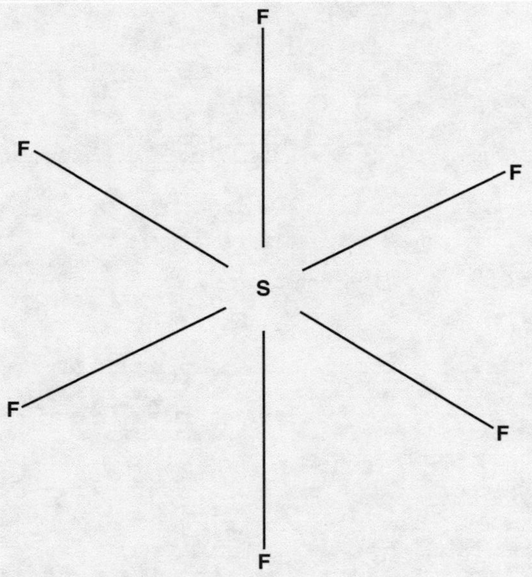 S bonded to six F	146	2	14	20	Superior retinal breaks (above 4–8 o'clock)
Perfluoro ethane (C_2F_6)	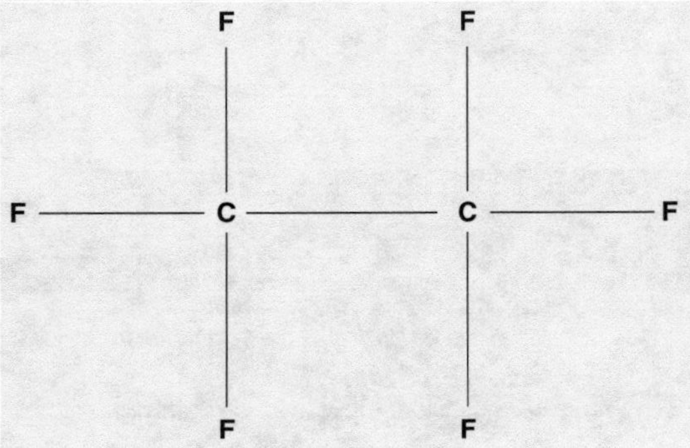 F–C–C–F, each C with F above and below	138	3	30	16	Macular hole surgery

(continued)

Table 4.1 (continued)

Gas	Structure	Molecular weight	Expansion of 100% concentration	Duration (days)	Nonexpanding concentration (%)	Uses
Perfluoro propane (C_3F_8)	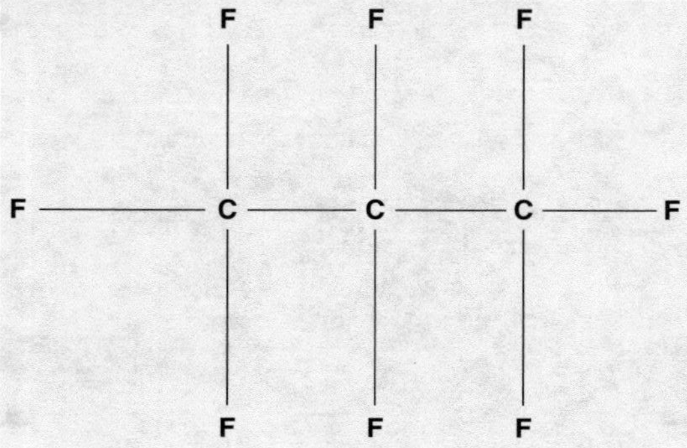	188	4	60	14	Multiple holes Inferior breaks Macular holes Early PVR Diabetic TRD

Table 4.2 Complications from gas insertion

Complications of gas insertion	Abnormality	Frequency
Cataract and lens	Gas cataract Nuclear sclerosis Posterior subcapsular cataract Displacement of an intraocular lens implant (especially sulcus fixated lenses or anterior chamber lenses)	Occasional Common Rare Occasional
Glaucoma	Temporary from gas expansion Angle closure from gas in the anterior chamber Wrong concentration	Common Rare Rare
Gas errors	Wrong gas Wrong concentration Underfill	Rare Rare Rare
Refraction	Myopic shift whilst gas is in situ in phakia and pseudophakia. Hypermetropic shift in aphakia	Always
Gas in the wrong place	Subconjunctival gas from wound leakage Anterior chamber gas from leakage through a zonule dehiscence or capsulotomy	Rare Rare
Visual field loss	Probably from drying of the retinal surface peroperatively, by closing the sclerotomies (valves or plugs), the flow of air over the retina is minimised.	Rare
Dislodgement of lens implant	Superior displacement of the IOL causing pupil capture Displacement of a sulcus IOL risking anterior chamber gas postoperatively	Rare

Important Postoperative Information

Flying or Travel to High Altitude

The patient should avoid flying while the gas bubble is in situ as the drop in cabin pressure causes increased IOP because the bubble tries to expand [18, 19], resulting in pain and a risk of central retinal artery occlusion. Subsequently, after the eye has adjusted to the raised IOP during the descent of the aircraft the eye become hypotonous with a risk of intraocular haemorrhage. Similarly, the patient should not change altitude (e.g. driving across a high mountain pass) because of the variations in atmospheric pressure will increase or decrease the bubble size.

Flying or travelling to high altitude causes a drop in atmospheric pressure which would normally be accompanied by an increase in the volume of the gas bubble [20]. Within the confines of the eye, this expansion cannot occur without loss of aqueous from the eye. If the aqueous volume cannot reduce quickly enough, the IOP elevates, see the table. As aqueous leaves the eye the IOP will gradually fall, some eyes, e.g. glaucomatous eyes with poor aqueous outflow facility, will struggle to reduce their aqueous volume to compensate for the increase in the gas volume required.

The absolute pressure in the eye is atmospheric pressure (760 mmHg) and IOP combined, therefore.

At sea level	776 mmHg (760 mmHg + 16 mmHg)	
At 2400 m altitude	576 mmHg (560 mmHg + 16 mmHg)	
Gas Volume (ml)	IOP rise (mmHg) from a baseline of 16 mmHg	Duration to achieve IOP rise (min)
0.125	26	10
0.25	43	10
0.5	70	10
1.0	105	10
2.0	120	8
4.0	140	8

Table. Pressure changes in a normal sized eye during air travel and cabin depressurisation (sea level to the equivalent pressure of 2400 m altitude). Therefore, any volume around 0.50 ml (one eighth full) or more in a normal sized eye risks producing an IOP, which can occlude ocular circulation.

It is possible to calculate how much the gas bubble must expand to allow the IOP to normalise:

$$\text{Pressure}\,1 \times \text{Volume}\,1 = \text{Pressure}\,2 \times \text{Volume}\,2.$$

$$776 \times V1 = 576 \times V2$$

P1 = 776 mmHg, i.e. atmospheric pressure plus 16 mmHg and P2 = 576 mmHg, atmospheric pressure at 2400 m plus 16 mmHg after the bubble has expanded to allow the IOP to drop to 16 mmHg.

$$\text{Ratio of V1 to V2} = 776/576$$

$$\text{Ratio of V1 to V2} = 1.35$$

Therefore, the bubble must expand to about 1.35 times its initial volume for the pressure to drop back to normal, i.e. the eye will need to lose aqueous to allow the expansion.

How long this will take will depend on the initial gas bubble volume and the rate of aqueous outflow, assuming no wound leak. Larger volumes will prevent the IOP from ever returning to normal, for example a 3.0 ml bubble cannot expand to 1.35 times its initial volume in a 4 ml eye; however, much aqueous escapes.

Note: It is the difference in pressure between atmospheric pressure and absolute eye pressure (measured as IOP) which affects the ocular circulation because measured systemic blood pressure is similarly the difference between atmospheric pressure and the pressure in the blood vessel.

I have calculated the minimal gas volume that would not give a pressure rise and it is 2.5% of the vitreous cavity. This is a gas bubble that is only going to last another few days. Therefore, it is easier to tell patients not to fly with any gas in the eye. Thankfully, the visualisation of the gas bubble is obvious to the patient, and therefore it is easy for the patient to know when the gas has gone.

General Anaesthesia

General anaesthesia should only be performed with the anaesthetist aware of the gas within the eye to allow the avoidance of expansion of the bubble with the anaesthetic gases, particularly nitrous dioxide. Patients have lost all vision from central retinal artery occlusion in this circumstance [14, 21, 22]. Some surgeons provide a wrist band to be worn by the patient, warning about gas in the eye and to alter any general anaesthesia agents used.

Silicone Oil

Additional surgical steps.

Method 1 (has the advantage that the retina can be manipulated during the oil insertion)

1. Attach a silicone oil filled syringe linked to the silicone oil pump set to 50 psi to the three-way tap. Reduce the pressure to 30 psi with 23 gauges to avoid separation of tubing from the infusion trochar.
2. Insert a flute needle and drain intraocular fluids (SRF, then vitreous cavity fluids and then heavy liquids) while actively inserting the oil.
3. Drain fluid off the disc.
4. Leave the IOP at approximately 10 mmHg.

Method 2 (has the advantage of inserting the oil onto the macula first allowing egress of SRF through anterior retinal breaks and may reduce the risk of subretinal oil)

1. Fill the eye with air.
2. Insert the oil through a trochar allowing the air to egress from another trochar.
3. Leave the IOP approximately at 10 mmHg.

Silicone oil is used when more permanent tamponade is required, e.g. for retinal breaks with residual traction from proliferative vitreoretinopathy (PVR) or in trauma. It has a Si-O-Si polymer structure. Two types are in use 1000–1300 mPas and 5000–5900 mPas. There are theoretical advantages for the use of the latter for permanent tamponade or to avoid emulsification of the oil, e.g. in young patients; however the former is easier to handle surgically because of its lower viscosity. 1000–1300 mPas is recommended in most circumstances. In my experience, there appears to be little advantage in using 5000 mPas oil [23].

Properties

1. Viscosity, 1000–1300 mPas or 5000–5900 mPas
2. Molecular weight 25,000 or 50,000
3. Refractive index 1.4
4. Density 0.97 g/cm^3
5. Surface tension 21.3 mN/m
6. Interfacial tension in water 40 mN/m

Silicone oil is clear, inert and floats in aqueous and is highly stable in the eye [24]. It has a flotation force, but its density is only slightly less than water, so the bubble is dominated by its interfacial tension. Therefore, it has a spherical configuration within the eye. Using the principle of "a sphere within a sphere," its contact with the retina is less extensive than a gas bubble (see appendix).

Oil may sometimes be used in complex retinal detachments without PVR when there are multiple breaks requiring multiple retinopexy applications or large breaks such as giant retinal tears. The risk of missing a small break in such a situation, e.g. when ten or twelve breaks are present, means that using gas could result in the early return of the retinal detachment and the onset of PVR. The latter occurs because of the recent operation and the release of cytokines and growth factors from the increased use of retinopexy. A tamponade of silicone oil will prevent retinal redetachment until removal of the oil, thereby allowing the inflammatory mediators in the postoperative period to subside. Thereafter oil removal may reveal a return of the retinal detachment, but this will be hopefully detected early (or even during the oil out operation see ROSO plus) and localised to the area of the retinal break and will not have other influences increasing the risk of PVR. Of course, in this situation, there is a risk that the complications of silicone oil may ensue. However, its short-term use in this situation should avoid most of these (Figs. 4.29, 4.30, 4.31, 4.32).

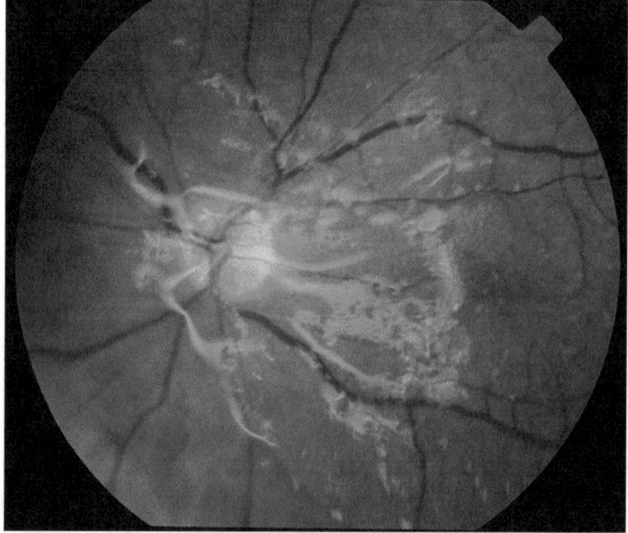

Fig. 4.29 The light reflex from the oil in contact with the retina is visible in an eye with adequate oil fill

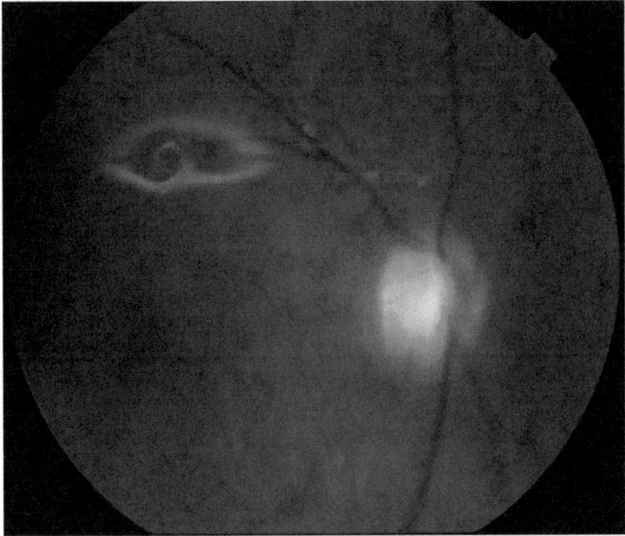

Fig. 4.30 The oil reflex in this patient is on the superior arcade indicating an underfill of oil as the contact area of the silicone oil bubble is superior within the eye

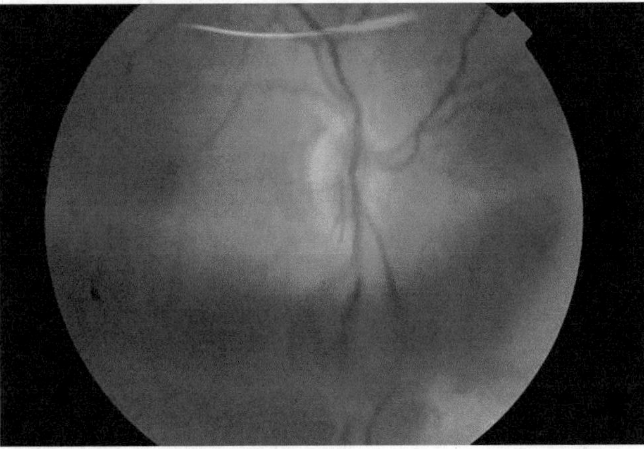

Fig. 4.31 A severe underfill of silicone oil. Note that the oil reflex is above the macula, and the diffraction at the edge of the bubble can be seen. Underfills can occur in eyes with choroidal haemorrhage, as the haemorrhage resolves, the space occupied by the haemorrhage is taken up by aqueous, the oil is suspended in the aqueous with minimal contact with the retina. The vision is reduced from the refractive effects of the edge of the bubble

Silicone Oil in the Anterior Chamber During Surgery

Silicone oil has a higher refractive index than BSS, which can influence the view during surgery. In the aphake the oil bulges through the pupil providing a + lens effect. It is better to flute the aqueous out of the anterior chamber allowing the oil to fill the chamber. The optical properties are then improved for posterior segment visualisation. A sudden change in the view during the surgery in a pseudophakic or phakic patient might indicate oil in the anterior chamber. Inspect the anterior chamber look at the iris if there are reflections of light in the crypts you have oil in the AC. If the view is satisfactory, continue with the operation; if it is reduced, use viscoelastic to displace the oil from the visual axis.

It is important to remove the oil from the AC at the end of the operation, to avoid postoperative pupil block. Close the two superior sclerotomies so that there can be no loss of oil from them. The infusion remains so that the correct pressure can be obtained once the anterior chamber has been closed at the end of the procedure.

You are now able to perform manipulations in the anterior chamber to remove the oil, knowing that the only oil lost from the eye must come through the anterior chamber. You will be able to see any oil that is lost, able to judge whether you are losing too much, and determine whether you will need to refill the posterior chamber (extremely unlikely).

1. Create two paracentesis incisions, one inferiorly and one superiorly. Insert some BSS (balanced salt solution) into the anterior chamber via the inferior paracentesis incision to deepen the AC. You can then remove the oil by engaging it with a wide bore cannula (often supplied with oil injection systems) attached to a 2 ml syringe and using manual aspiration through the superior paracentesis. The infusion of BSS can either be by continuous infusion at moderate pressure (i.e. attached to the BSS infusion line), or by intermittent infusion (insert some BSS with a syringe, remove some oil and repeat until the oil is removed).
2. If the whole of the anterior chamber is filled with oil, you may need to insert a viscoelastic to move the oil to the superior wound (and out of the angle), then aspirate the oil with a wide bore cannula and then insert BSS to allow aspiration of the viscoelastic.

Note you do not want a free flow of infusion fluid into the posterior segment whilst oil is egressing from one of the sclerotomies as eventually you will have an underfill of oil; this is why you must close off the superior sclerotomies. If only the oil in the AC is removed, then you have lost only a maximum of 0.2 mls (volume of the AC) which will not have any effect on the total volume of oil in the eye, which should be 4 mls to 10 ml depending on the eye. Therefore, tamponade is maintained without having to go into the posterior segment to check.

Surgical Tip: The key is pressure; the oil bubble wants to stay as one bubble in the posterior chamber, therefore it requires a pressure differential in the anterior and posterior chambers, i.e. high in the posterior and low in the anterior to allow a bubble of silicone to separate off (breaking its interfacial tension, see appendix) and enter the anterior chamber.

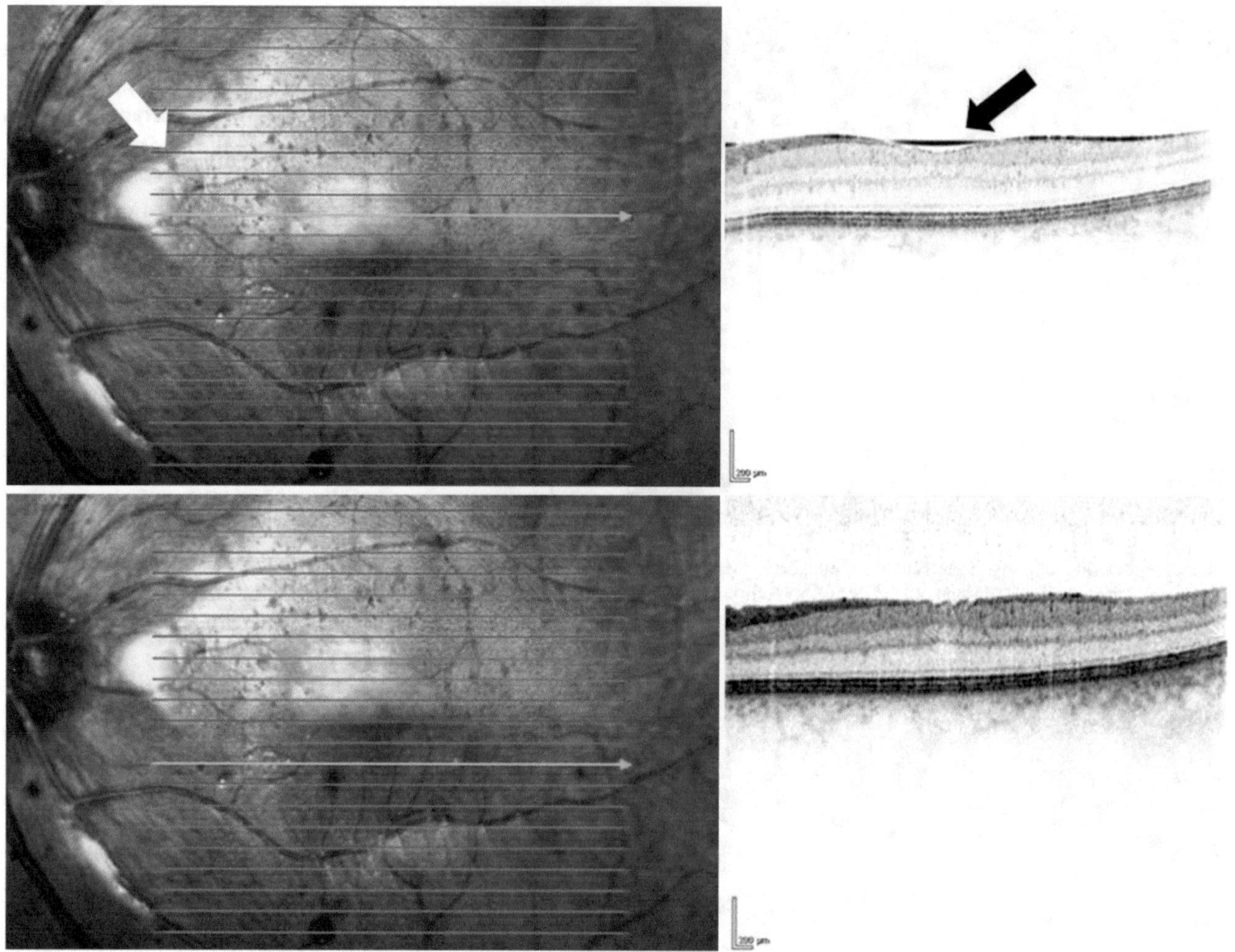

Fig. 4.32 Silicone oil contacts the retina as far inferiorly as the light reflex seen from the retina (white arrow). When the OCT scan is taken through the reflex (indicated by the long green arrow on the upper scan), the oil interface is detected on the oct (black arrow). When the scan is taken below the reflex (green line on the lower scan), the oil interface is no longer seen

Every time you insert an instrument into the anterior chamber, the pressure drops, but if the pressure is already low in the posterior chamber and the pressure is maintained adequately in the AC, there is less chance of separation.

In some eyes, the defect in the zonule allows a bubble of oil to re-enter the eye during these manipulations (seen first as a bulge in the iris and then the bubble floats into the anterior chamber), but this is usually a small bubble that can be removed by repeating step one above. If the lens is dislocated or very unstable (e.g. in a patient with trauma or a complicated cataract extraction) and oil keeps coming through into the anterior chamber, you may need to remove the lens and capsule, leaving the eye aphakic (remember to perform an inferior peripheral iridectomy).

There seems to be a threshold size of the bubble in the AC which can cause pupil block, anything less than 2 mm diameter is safe; however, it is not recommended to leave oil in the AC, therefore by using the techniques above, remove any AC oil at the end of the operation (Figs. 4.33, 4.34, 4.35, 4.36, Table 4.3).

Note: When filling the eye with oil, think "volume rather than pressure." Once the oil is near a maximal fill in the vitreous cavity a tiny increase in volume causes a large increase in IOP because you are inserting a non-compressible liquid into a relatively stiff walled container. To maximise the fill, the key is to remove the residual aqueous layer and SRF. The IOP can be kept at a low level (7 mmHg) without detriment to the fill). The fill is determined by the volumetric removal of the aqueous component and its replacement with a volume of oil and not by increased pressure in the oil bubble (and therefore the aqueous component), which in the rigid container does not increase the volume of the oil.

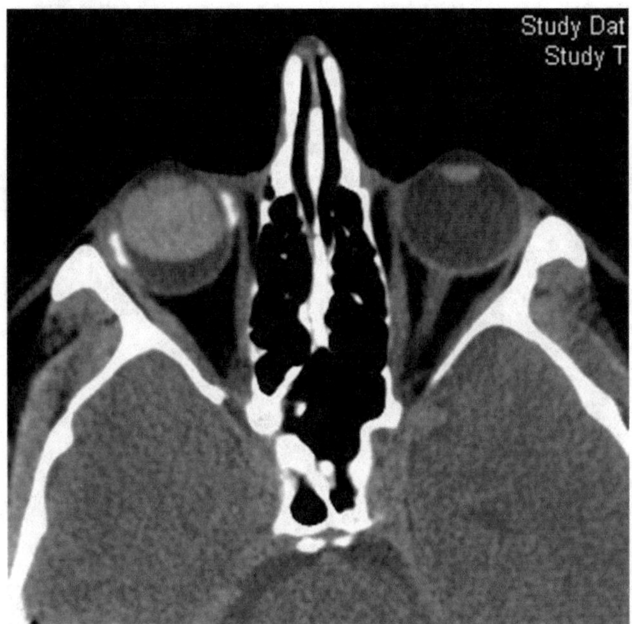

Fig. 4.33 A CT scan of an eye with silicone oil in situ and a silicone encircling band. The curved inferior edge of the oil is apparent, demonstrating the lack of contact with the retina in this case posteriorly (patient is face up)

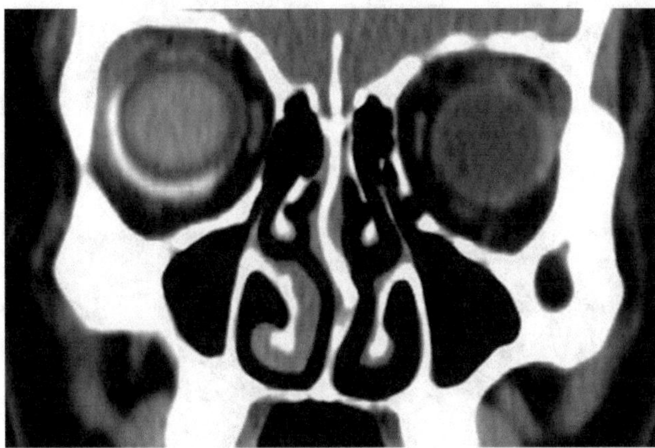

Fig. 4.34 In the face up position the oil can be seen with little contact with the retina in this section

Complications of Silicone Oil

These are numerous.

Refractive Changes

- The oil has a higher refractive index than vitreous or water and therefore induces refractive errors primarily determined on whether the oil surface anteriorly is concave or convex. A concave profile occurs in phakic eyes, the radius of the posterior lens −8.10 mm, effectively reversing the refraction at the posterior lens because the lens and oil have refractive indices of 1.37 for the lens and 1.4 for oil, compared with 1.33 for water/vitreous. This induces a need for a hypermetropic correction of approximately +5D, therefore in a high myope, the myopia is reduced. In pseudophakic eyes, the IOL usually has a flatter profile to the posterior lens surface and has a refractive index as high as 1.55. When oil is inserted, a hypermetropic shift is again induced. In both, the total refraction of the eye is reduced to approximately +50D. In an aphakic eye, the anterior surface is convex inducing a myopic shift in the refraction of approximately +5D, thereby reducing the aphakic correction from +10D to +5D again giving a total refraction of the eye of about +50D.
- Note in a high myope, the hypermetropic shift may reduce the degree of myopia. The opposite occurs in aphakic eyes where the oil bulges through the pupil (reducing the aphakic correction by approximately +5D) (Figs. 4.37 and 4.38).

Cataract

- Silicone is associated with a formation of nuclear sclerotic cataract, which may occur in complex retinal detachments, especially with PVR but is exacerbated by the presence of the oil.

Capsule Opacification

- A posterior capsule in a pseudophake will thicken severely with oil with time (Figs. 4.39 and 4.40).

IOP

- The trabecular meshwork can be filled with silicone oil droplets causing open angle glaucoma in at least 40% [25], which is difficult to treat with 28% remaining refractory to treatment.
- Angle closure glaucoma in aphakic eyes is produced if a peripheral iridectomy closes (seen in up to 33%) and the oil bulges through the pupil [26]. This can be diagnosed in an eye with a deep anterior chamber, with a clear cornea but a raised intraocular pressure. A sheen may be seen in the iris crypts suggesting oil in the anterior chamber, a cross-sectional slit beam reveals that no cells or flare are present in the anterior chamber and there are no visible convection currents suggesting normal aqueous. Reopening of a peripheral iridectomy will re-establish fluid flow pushing the oil back into the posterior chamber reducing the pressure. YAG peripheral iridectomies tend to close over again in a few weeks therefore a surgical iridectomy is preferred. Even the latter may close in 5–33% of eyes with silicone oil [26, 27].

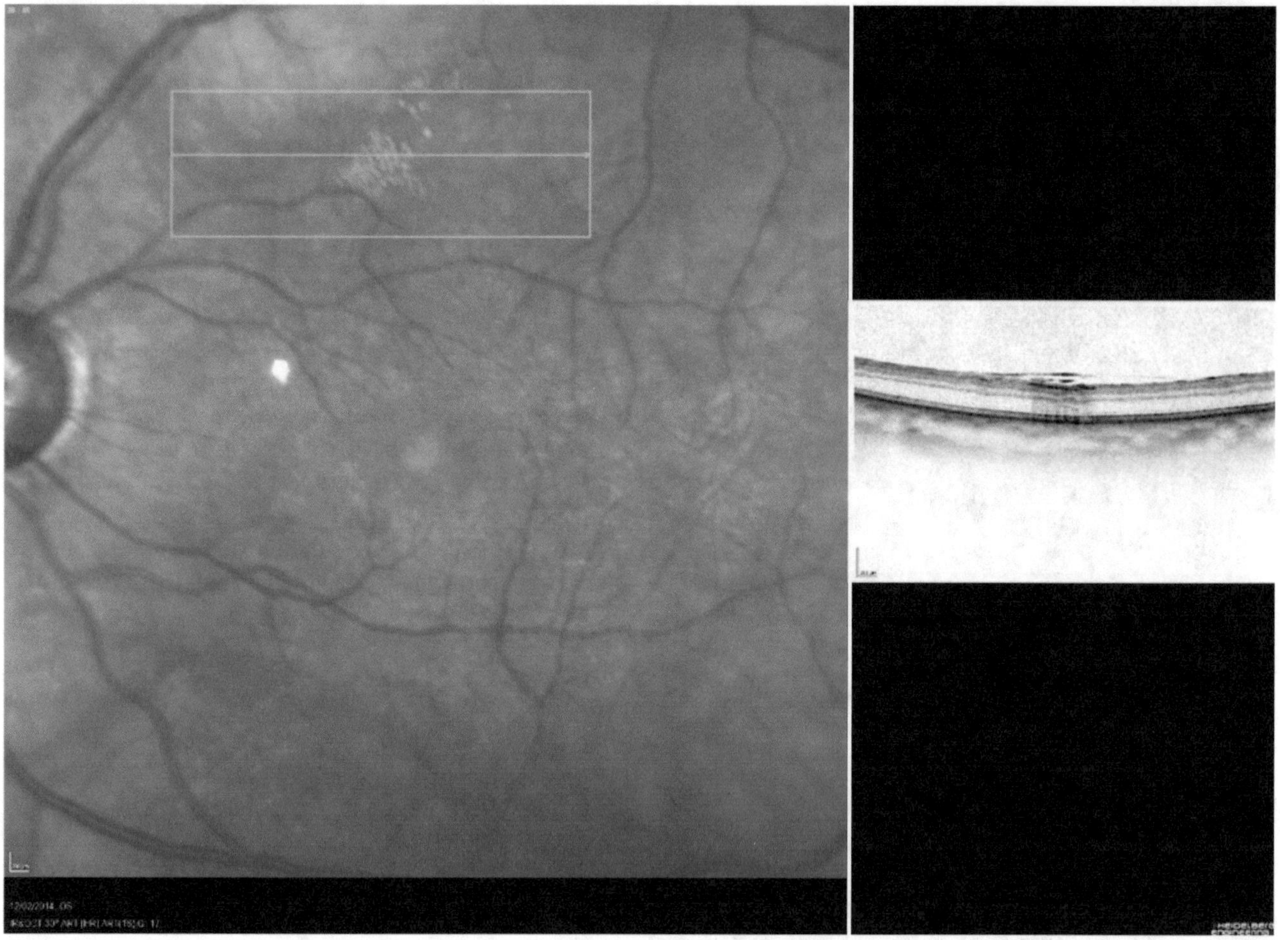

Fig. 4.35 Emulsified oil gets everywhere, here it is under an ERM

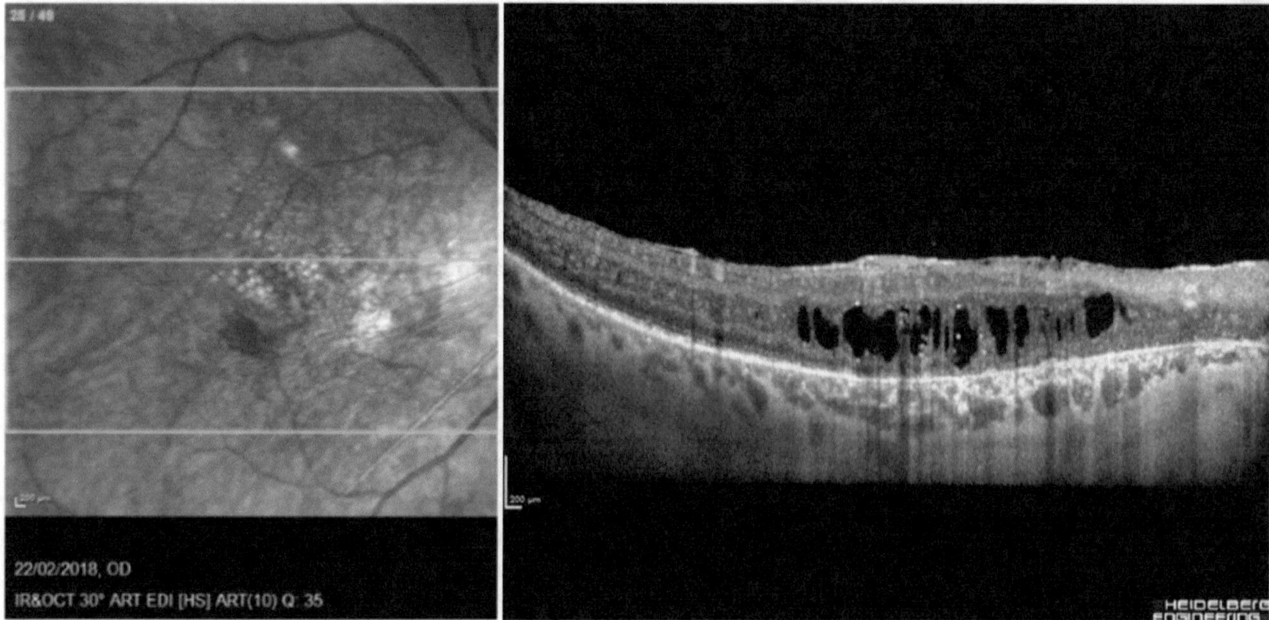

Fig. 4.36 Silicone Oil droplets in the retina

Table 4.3 Silicone oil complications

Silicone oil complications	Duration from surgery			
Complication	0–3 months	3–12 months	1–2 years	2–10 years
Overfill Glaucoma	Yes	No	No	No
Pupil Block Glaucoma in aphakes	Yes	Occasional if peripheral iridectomy closes		
Open angle glaucoma	Unlikely	Occasional	Common	Common
Cataract	Unlikely	Occasional	Common	Common
Oil-induced macular visual loss	Occasional	Occasional	Unlikely	Unlikely
Band Keratopathy	No	No	Unlikely	More Common
Emulsion of Oil	Unlikely	Occasional	Common	Common

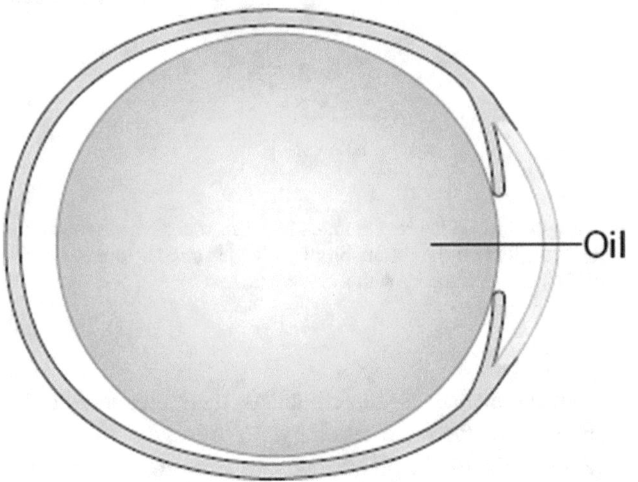

Fig. 4.37 Silicone oil in an aphakic eye produces a convex lens at the point of the pupil, thereby producing a myopic shift. In aphakic eyes, the degree of hypermetropia is reduced by silicone oil insertion

- In phakic or pseudophakic eyes, oil that has dislocated into the anterior chamber, usually peroperatively, can cause an unusual pupil block glaucoma in which the lens is pushed backwards, and the iris is pushed anteriorly [28]. This causes intermittent angle closure glaucoma, which can be difficult to diagnose in the postoperative period. Peripheral iridectomies are usually only temporally effective, and removal of silicone oil is required. If the oil is required for permanent tamponade, the lens capsule complex may need to be removed and an inferior peripheral iridectomy performed in the aphakic eye thus created. Oil presenting into the anterior chamber peroperatively should be evacuated with viscoelastic (see earlier in the chapter, silicone oil in the anterior chamber).
- In some circumstances, there is a deep anterior chamber and the oil is behind the pupil but there is still raised intraocular pressure. This may indicate an overfill situation. In an aphakic eye oil can be removed via a paracentesis reducing the volume of silicone in the eye. In the phakic eye oil will need to be removed through a sclerotomy. The inexperienced surgeon should avoid the temptation to maximise the fill of oil by leaving the eye "hard" (high IOP) at the end of the operation. In fact, because of the physical properties of a sphere filled with a liquid increasing, the IOP does not make a significant change in the volume of the filling liquid in the cavity see appendix.

Cornea

- The oil is associated with the occurrence in some patients of band keratopathy. Some of these eyes are already extensively damaged. The keratopathy may be partly due to the phthisis of the eye, which has been prevented by the oil rather than by contact of the oil on the cornea itself (Fig. 4.41).

Macular Toxicity

- Toxicity to the retina in its severest form may result in occasional patients suffering the loss of central vision either with the oil in situ or around the time of oil removal [29–35]. For the latter always avoid direct illumination of the macula during oil removal (ROSO) as the macula seems to be prone to light toxicity in oil filled eye [36, 37]. Do this by blocking the light passing through the pupil during ROSO. This has eliminated the loss of vision at ROSO in my practice [36], but I have still encountered patients with loss of vision with the oil in the eye. Despite this specific reason for loss of vision with the use of oil in a meta-analysis of comparing gas and oil, visual outcomes were similar overall [38].
- Unfortunately, the loss of vision is permanent often down to 20/200. There is associated relative central scotoma and reduction in colour sensation in the scotoma. The aetiology of the complication is uncertain. OCT images have shown inner retinal cystic changes and loss of the retinal nerve fibre layer, which appear over a period of years postoperatively [39] (Fig. 4.42). These suggest loss of the ganglion cells over time. Electrophysiology has been inconclusive, showing defects in retinal and optic nerve function.
- The rate of the complication at ROSO is uncertain, overall with rates of 0%, 3.3% [12], 4.4% [8], 5.9% [13], 10.9% [14], but subgroup analyses of macula on retinal detachments are as high as 50%. A retrospective paper has shown a very high rate of "unexplained vision loss" in macula on retinal detachment [15] however, the diagnosis of silicone oil-related vision loss was not made in a pro-

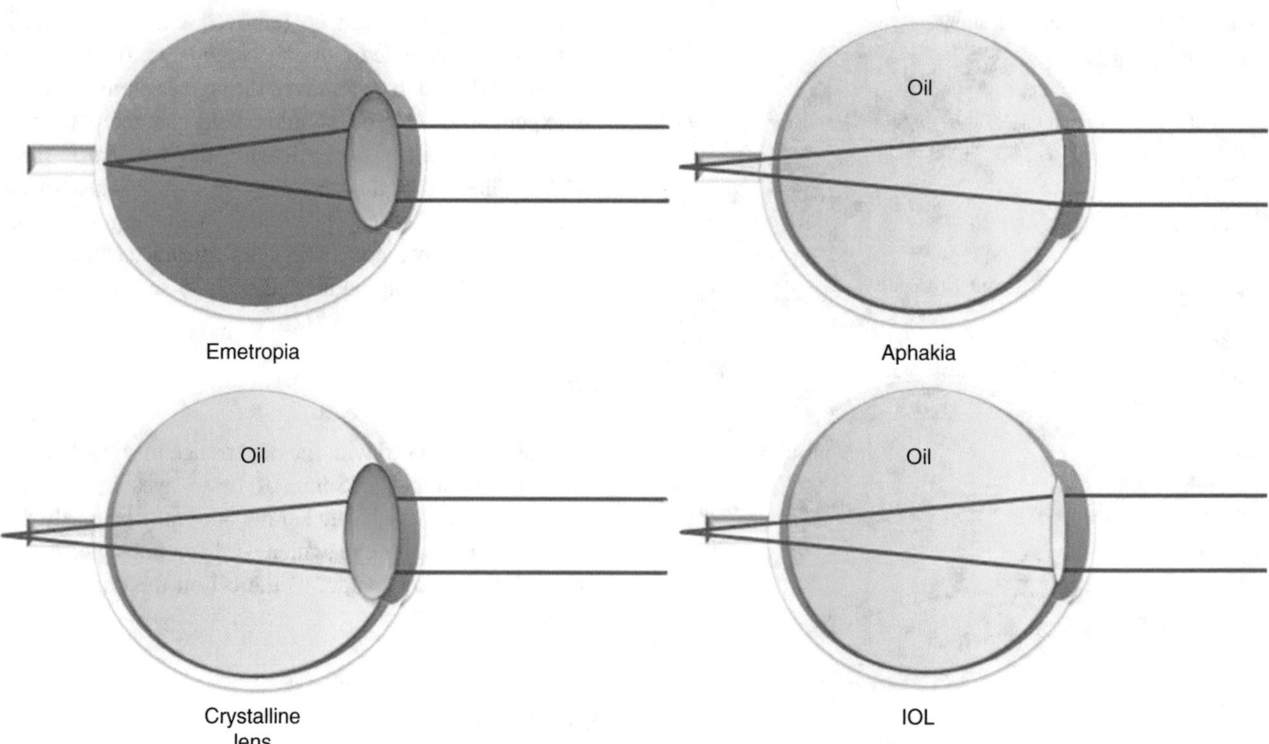

Fig. 4.38 The whole refractive power of the eye is reduced when oil is inserted, therefore the patient needs a + D spectacle lens to compensate. This is because the refractive power of the posterior surface of the crystalline lens is neutralised by the oil, i.e. the difference in refractive index between the oil and the lens is much less than water (vitreous) and the lens. The effect on the refraction of the eye is similar in an eye with aphakia, pseudophakia or with a crystalline lens

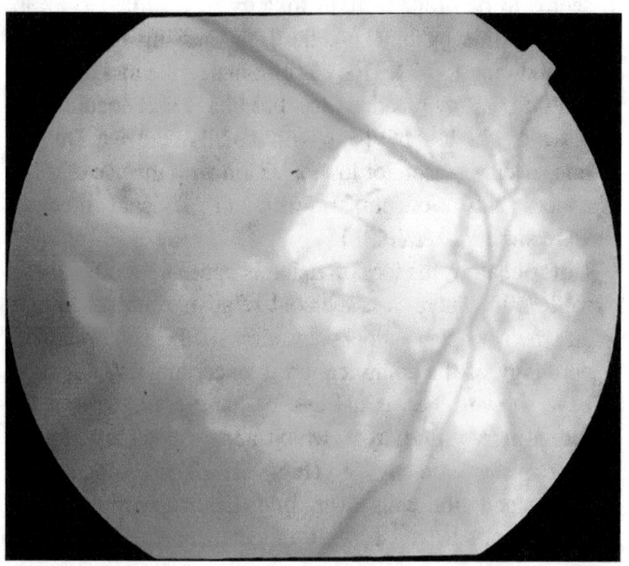

Fig. 4.39 A patient has oil in situ and has low tension glaucoma. This has exacerbated the glaucoma and caused a severe optic disc cup from additional silicone oil and disc glaucoma

spective manner by the clinicians; therefore, some cases may not be the same aetiology.

- Pathologically the oil impregnates all the areas of the eye with characteristic foamy macrophages. Therefore, it has some mild effect on reducing visual acuity through effects on the retina (Figs. 4.43, 4.44, 4.45, 4.46, 4.47, 4.48, 4.49).

Oil in the Wrong Place

- There are complications from oil in the wrong place, such as subretinal, suprachoroidal or subconjunctival (Figs. 4.50, 4.51, 4.52, 4.53).
- Subretinal oil is likely to be associated with a total retinal detachment. This may happen if the infusion cannula tip moves into the subretinal space during infusion of the oil. If the eye goes hypotonous during surgery, the tip may angle under the retina, especially if the anterior retina is elevated because of anterior contraction in proliferative

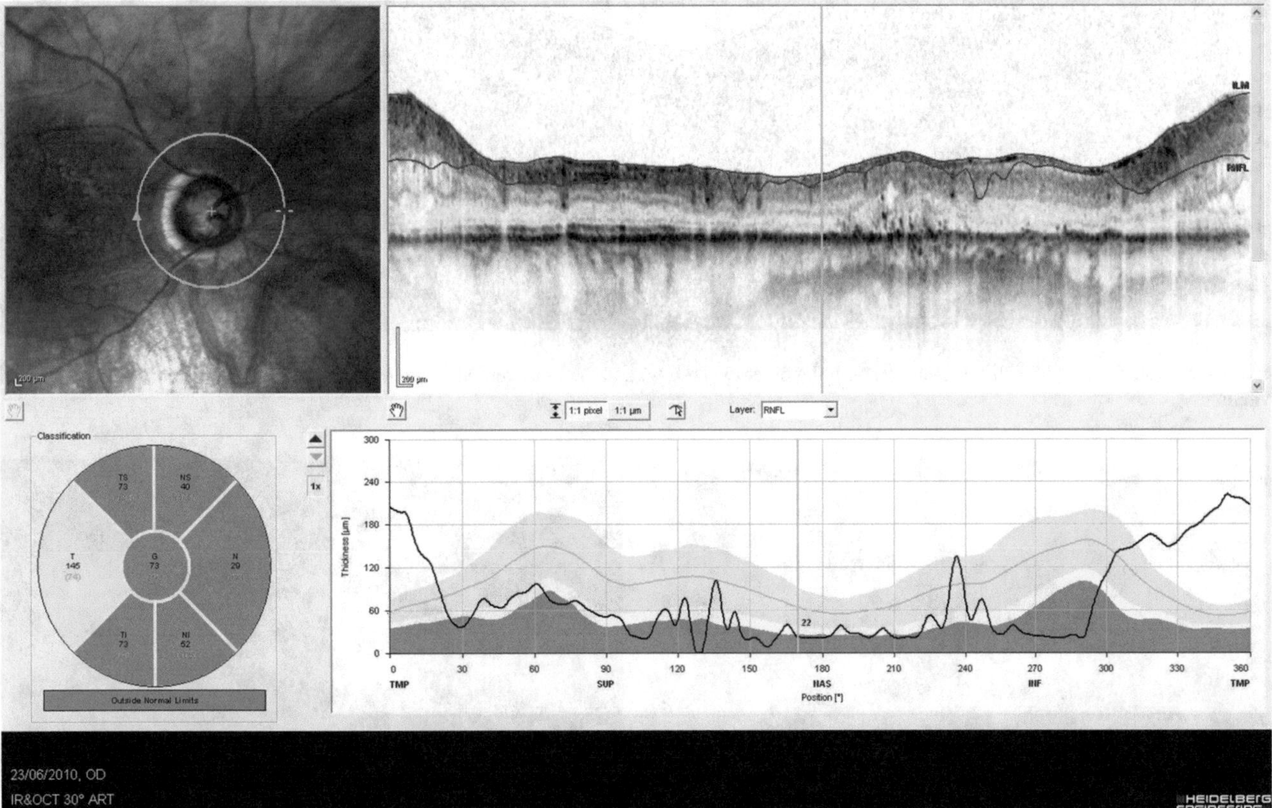

Fig. 4.40 This patient has thinning of the retinal nerve fibre layer from oil-induced glaucoma

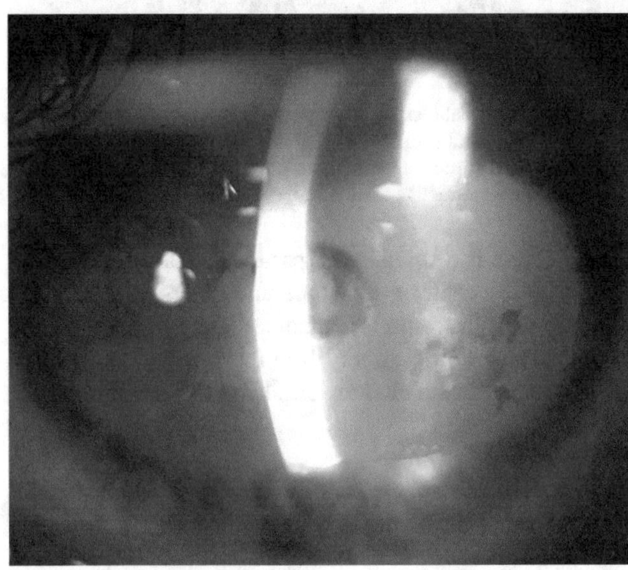

Fig. 4.41 Band keratopathy

vitreoretinopathy or because of retinal detachment into the ciliary body in preoperative hypotony. Once noticed the oil should be evacuated but this will usually require a retinectomy. The retinectomy should be large enough to allow the oil to pass through the hole (at least 2 clock hours), overcoming its surface tension. Postoperative movement of oil into the subretinal space is seen in the presence of large retinal breaks (or breaks that have become larger postoperatively because of traction) with continued contraction of epiretinal membranes usually PVR, e.g. severe tractional and rhegmatogenous retinal detachment in diabetes.

- Suprachoroidal oil is an exceedingly rare occurrence and is again caused by problems with the infusion cannula moving as above but into the suprachoroidal space. A retinectomy and choroidectomy will be needed to evacuate the oil. The incisions should be anterior to allow the oil to float out.

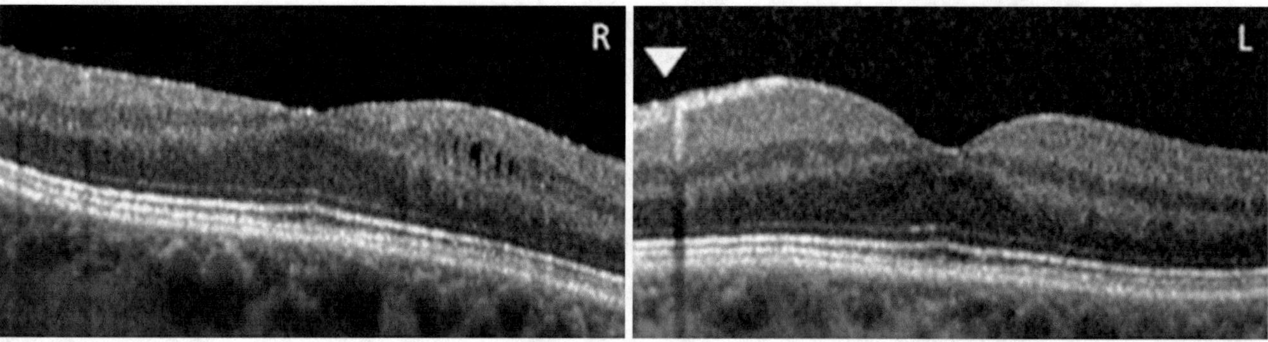

Fig. 4.42 Note the loss of RNFL (compared with the other eye, arrow) and the inner retinal cysts in the right eye of this patient with oil-related vision loss

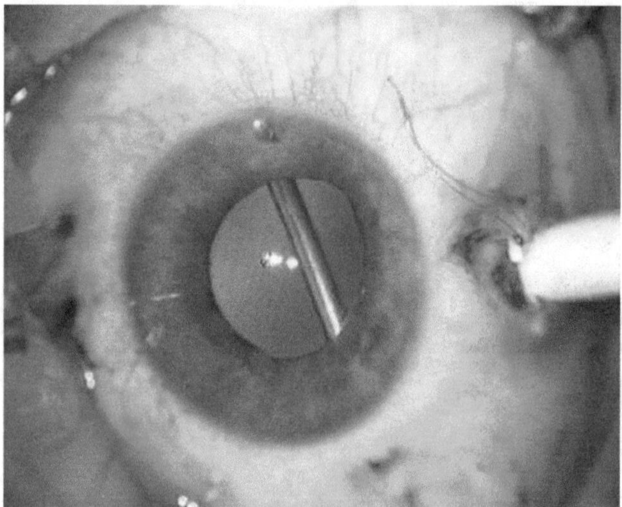

Fig. 4.43 To create an inferior peripheral iridectomy (PI) in an aphake with oil in situ use the cutter on "aspirate only" to engage the iris, then on low cut rate (200 cuts/minute), remove a portion of the peripheral iris. Make sure there is no lens capsule or vitreous behind the PI

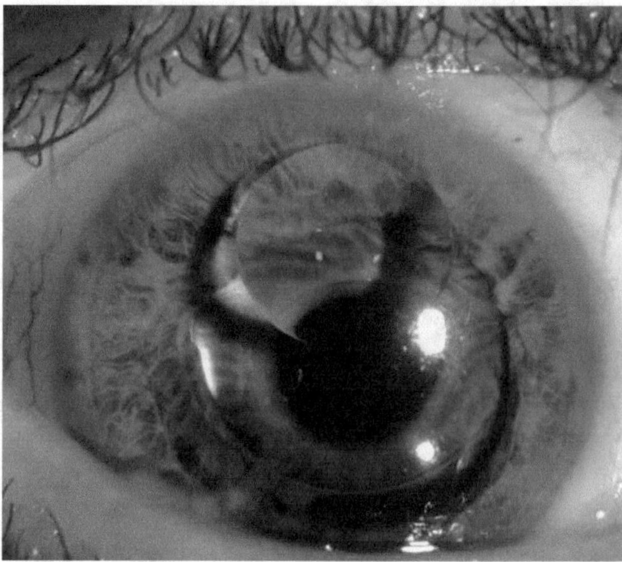

Fig. 4.44 Small bubbles of oil in the AC do not usually cause pupil block. The spherical shape of the bubble minimises the area of oil in contact with the corneal endothelium. Corneal decompensation is rare. The oil can have refractive effects on the vision

- Subconjunctival oil is extremely difficult to remove because it infiltrates the Tenon's layer with multiple small bubbles causing inflammation. It is caused by poor closure of a sclerotomy and possibly raised IOP. This should be seen very rarely. Some surgeons routinely suture the sclerotomies even in small gauge surgery to try to avoid this oil egress.

Surgical Pearl

How to Reduce the Chance of Silicon Oil Coming into Anterior Chamber (AC) at the End of Surgery in an Eye with Zonular Dehiscence

In some complicated cases of PVR or re-surgeries in pseudophakic eyes, there is a chance of silicon oil coming into the anterior chamber at the end of surgery. This is indeed more likely if there is a complicated pseudophakia with disturbed iris or IOL decentring or if one encounters an air bubble coming into the anterior chamber during the air fluid exchange step of the surgery. The following steps could be taken to prevent the chances of silicon oil coming into the AC in such situations

1. In case of complicated pseudophakia, one must make sure, at the beginning of surgery, that vitreous tracking into the anterior chamber or touching the IOL is removed meticulously. Any peaking of the pupil should be corrected by mechanically removing any membrane, lens matter or vitreous. If the IOL is slightly decentred, then care must be taken to try to re-centre it through limbal ports, if possible. This is especially useful in cases where the posterior capsule is compromised along with decentred IOL. This allows an easy path for the oil to come in AC at the end of surgery.

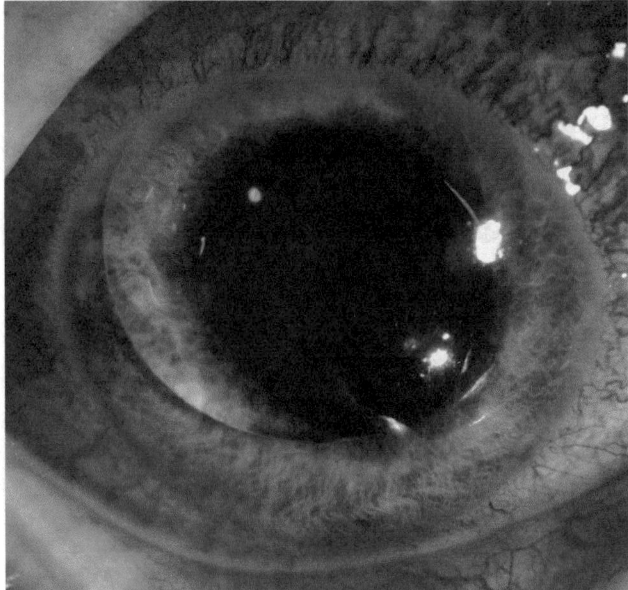

Fig. 4.45 A large bubble of oil in the AC may cause pupil block, which is only temporarily relieved by peripheral iridectomy and usually requires oil removal from the AC and, if possible, from the posterior segment

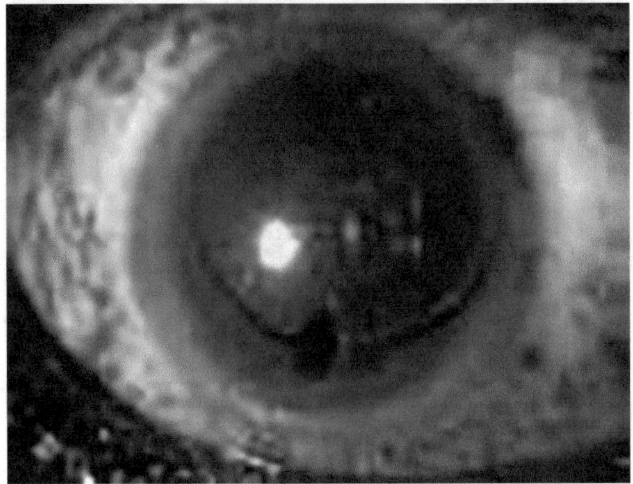

Fig. 4.46 Oil has entered the anterior chamber despite a patent peripheral iridectomy because this eye has become hypotonous and is no longer producing enough aqueous to keep the anterior chamber filled

2. During surgery, if air seeps into the anterior chamber, it usually spoils the view for the surgeon. At this stage, the best solution is to inject viscoelastic into the anterior chamber to replace the air bubble so that the view is well maintained to proceed with the surgery.
3. At the end of the surgery, when the silicon oil is being injected one must make sure that the intraocular pressure does not go up especially at the end of the injection. That can push the oil forcibly through the compromised chamber. Hence gradual injection should be done with careful venting of the residual air.

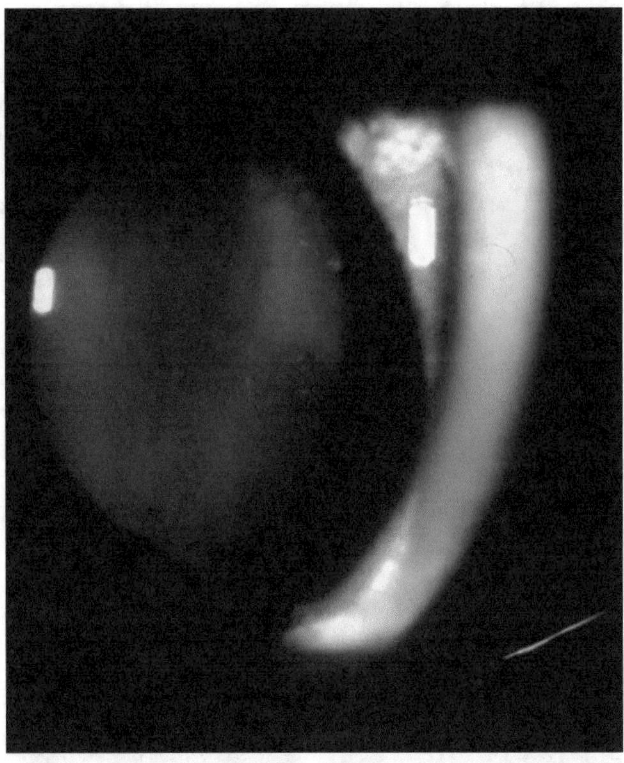

Fig. 4.47 Oil has entered the eye through the zonules of this phakic eye and has pushed the iris forward and created pupil block glaucoma with a deep anterior chamber

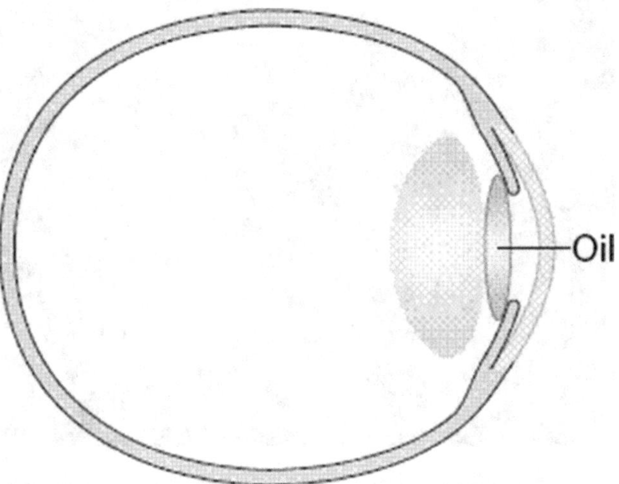

Fig. 4.48 Silicone oil trapped in the anterior chamber can cause forward projection of the pupil and iris and back projection of the intraocular lens, causing pupil block glaucoma

4. At this stage, I would also recommend injecting diluted intraocular carpinol (pilocarpine) injection in the anterior chamber. This allows the pupil to constrict and maintain a good barricade and compartmentalise the oil

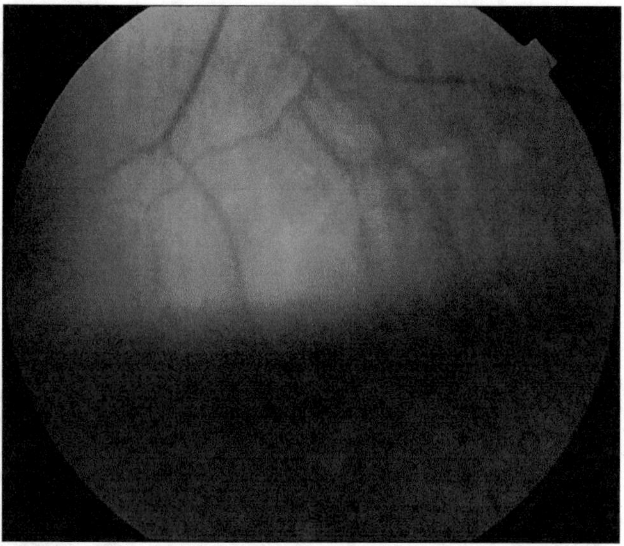

Fig. 4.49 The inferior edge of a silicone oil bubble produces refractive changes, which if the bubble is underfilled can be problematic to the patient with changes in refraction on head movements

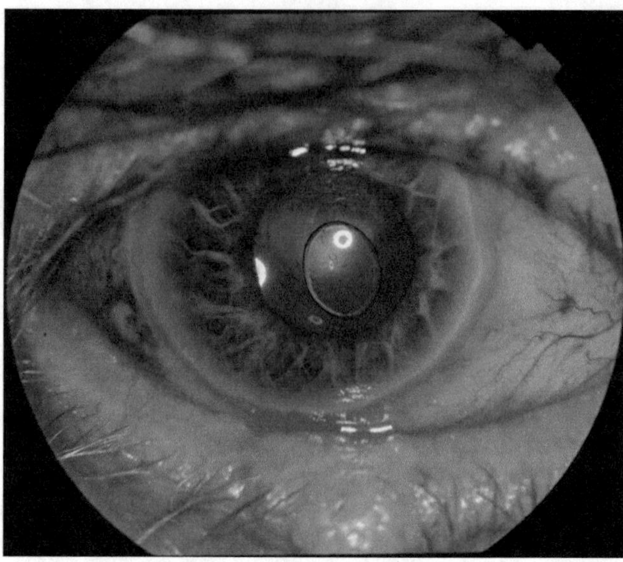

Fig. 4.51 Oil trapped between the IOL and capsule and in the visual axis

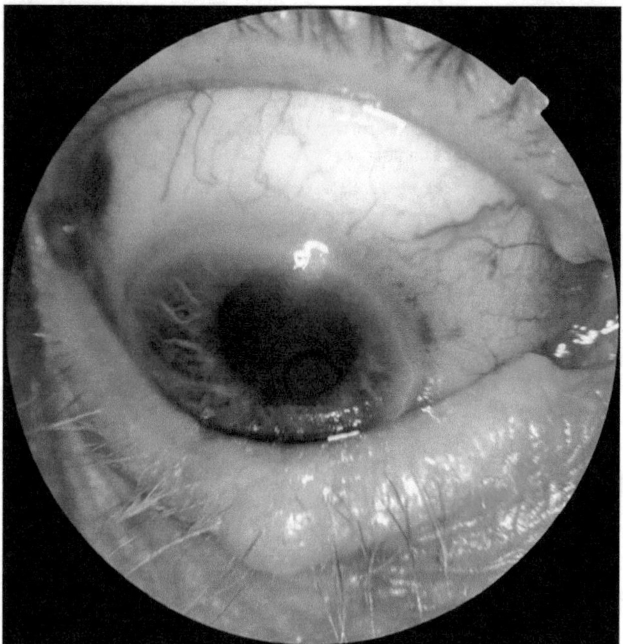

Fig. 4.50 In the first-week post op an oil droplet was noticed inferiorly between the IOL and the posterior capsule, at week two this had risen into the visual axis. A Yag capsulotomy allowed the oil droplet to contact the oil in the posterior chamber into which it was absorbed

behind. At this stage, the final fill of the oil can be achieved, once again keeping in mind that the intraocular pressure of the eye should not go up and a normal tone of the eye, which can be digitally confirmed, should be kept.

Dr. Manish Nagpal, Retina Foundation, Ahmedabad, India

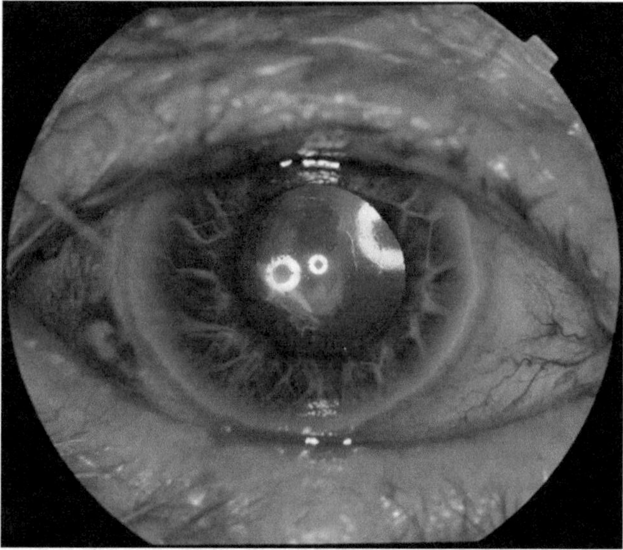

Fig. 4.52 Yag capsulotomy has allowed the oil droplet to move into the oil bubble in the vitreous cavity

Emulsion

- Emulsified oil may reduce visual clarity and cause a white superior opacity in the anterior chamber with droplets producing a superior fluid level. Small residual droplets of oil are common even after oil removal and must not be confused with white cells and inflammation. The patient may experience floating objects in the vision seen especially on looking down at the ground when the oil droplets float up to the macula. In this position, the droplets are next to the retina and are therefore are seen in focus as circles with a dark perimeter (Figs. 4.54 and 4.55).

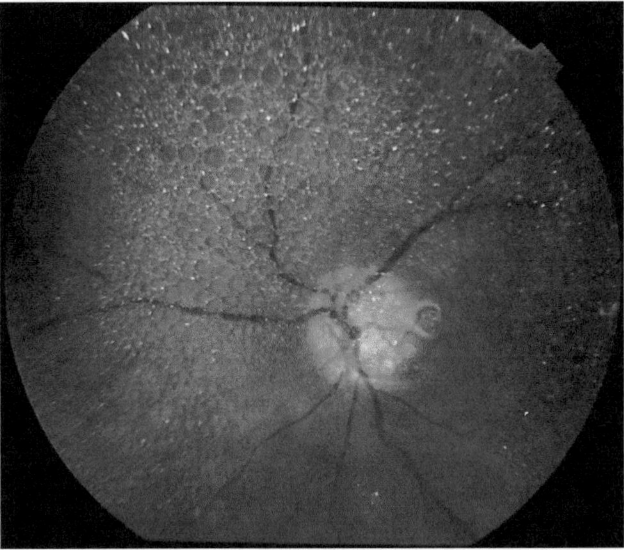

Fig. 4.53 Emulsified droplets of oil are seen on the retina

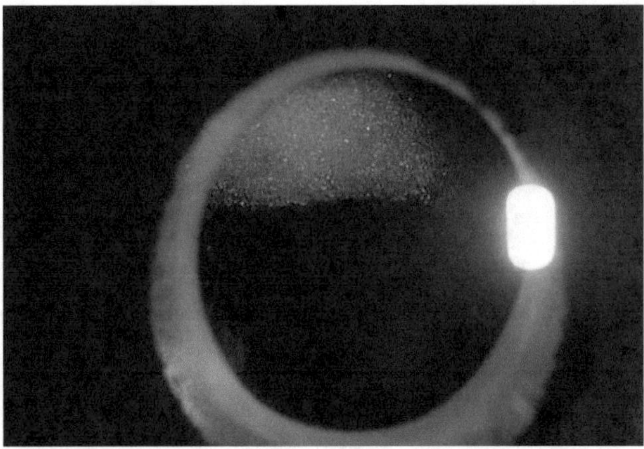

Fig. 4.54 Emulsion of oil between residual anterior vitreous and an IOL in Berger's space

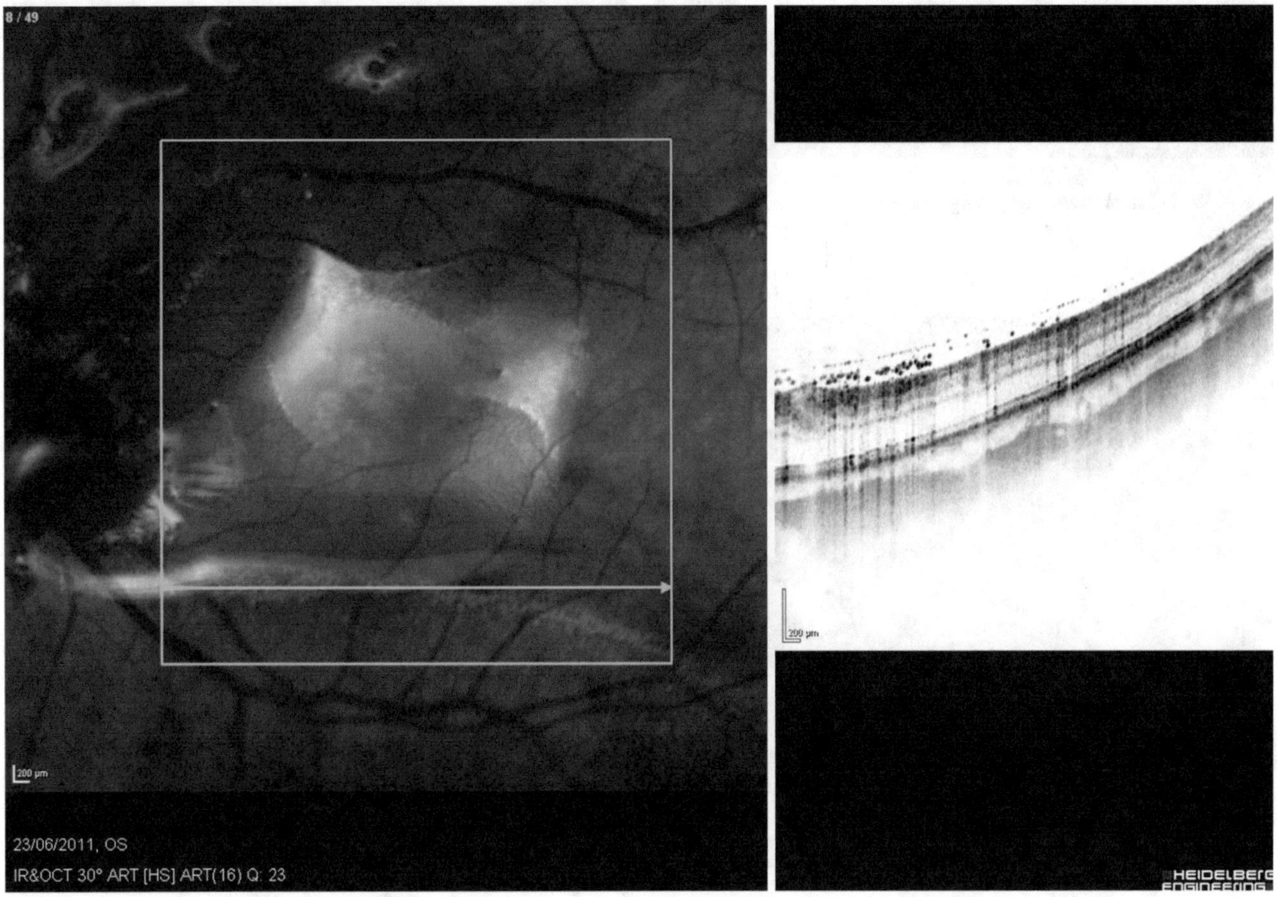

Fig. 4.55 Emulsified oil (small black dots) is seen just inferior to the line of contact of the main oil bubble with the retina (green arrow indicates the line of scan)

Intraocular Lenses

- Oil may adhere to intraocular lenses, especially those made of silicone. Wiping the lens with HPMC can help to remove the oil, occasionally the lens must be exchanged (Figs. 4.56, 4.57, 4.58, 4.59, 4.60, 4.61, 4.62, 4.63, 4.64, Table 4.4).

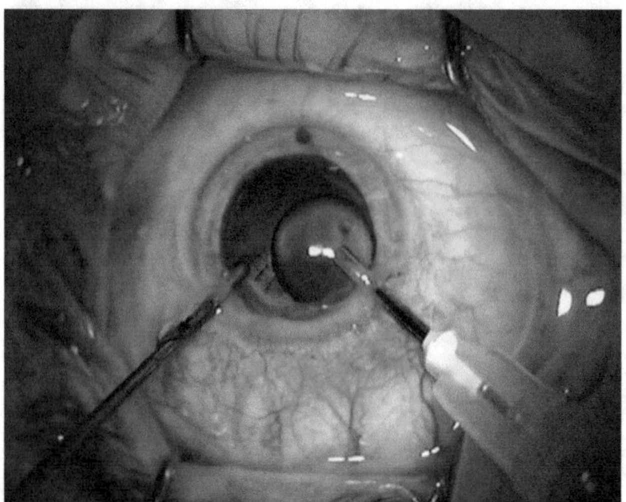

Fig. 4.56 Oil can be removed through the anterior chamber in an aphakic patient

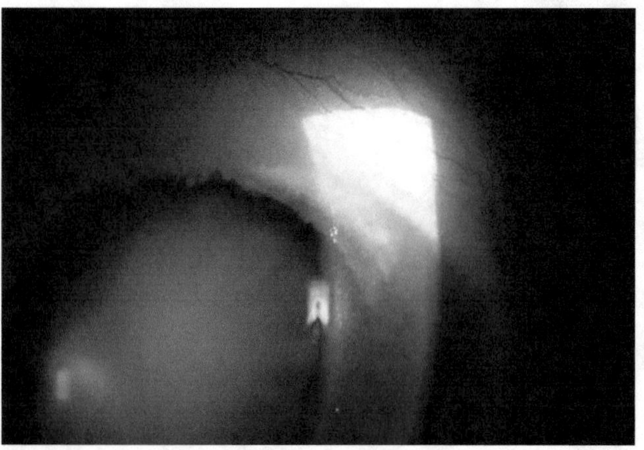

Fig. 4.57 Silicone oil can emulsify in the eye, the droplets float in the anterior chamber producing a "fluid" level in the superior angle

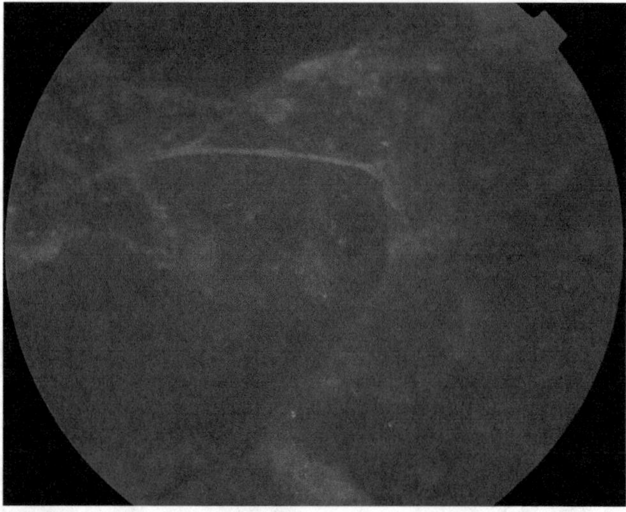

Fig. 4.58 Emulsified silicone oil gets everywhere including attached to epiretinal membranes

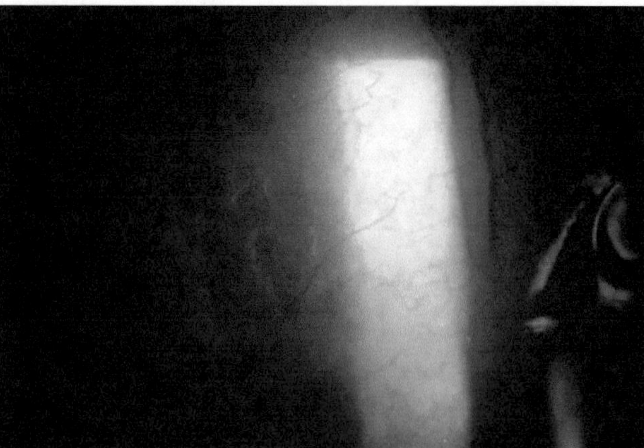

Fig. 4.59 It is not easy for oil to leak through a sclerotomy because of its small size. If leakage occurs, multiple bubbles of oil appear in the Tenon's layer sometimes causing inflammation. Their multiplicity makes removal surgically difficult because the bubbles are loculated within the connective tissue

Surgical Pearl

Silicone Oil and Inflammation

Silicone Oil (SOs) belong to the group of synthetic organosilicon compounds, made of the repetition of –[R2Si–O]– group, characterised by low energy surface and chemical inertness [40]. The stability of SO refers to the capability of the compound to resist changes in its properties over time.

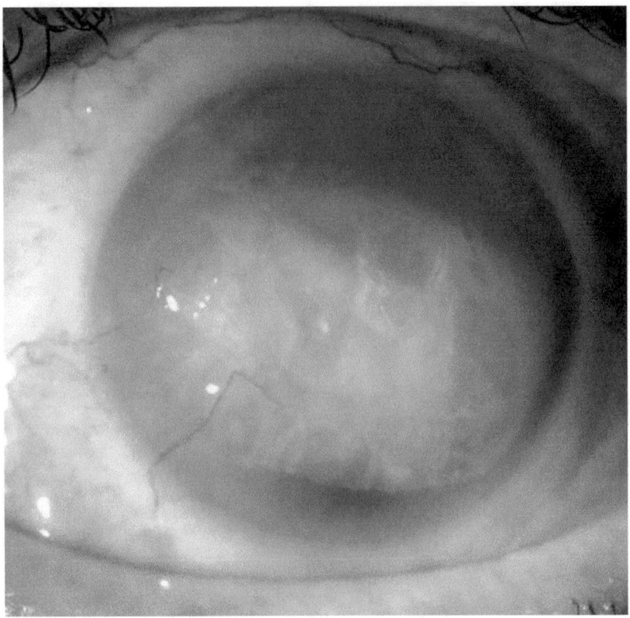

Fig. 4.60 A corneal scar from decompensation of the cornea in an eye with long-term silicone oil in situ

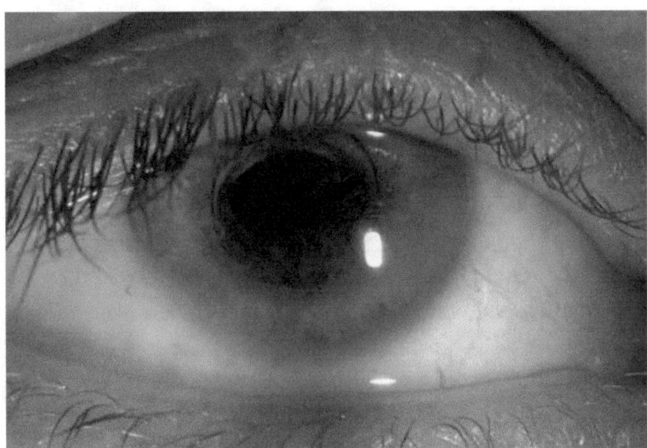

Fig. 4.61 Band keratopathy is a late complication of silicone oil tamponade

Inside the vitreous cavity, the SO bubble tends to remain rounded because the interfacial energy produces an inwards attraction. At the same time, the retina, being hydrophilic, prefers to be in contact with water rather than with SO; therefore, the SO-water-retina forms a meniscus. The interfacial tension (IT) is a cohesion force of a liquid aiming to minimise in a spherical shape the contact area and to increase the "wall tensions." The IT is, thus, responsible for the shape and stability of SOs. The intermediate interfacial tension of SO against water is 40 mN/m. The SO bubble is not able to resist to external forces higher than the IT. In the presence of saccadic eye movements, the system generates the shear stress potentially able to overcome the interfacial tension (IT), which stimulates the breakdown of the originally inert bubble of SO into smaller droplets of SO, defined as emulsion. Emulsion is a mixture of two or more immiscible liquids containing both a dispersed and a continuous phase with the boundary between the phases called the "interface." The formation of SO emulsion inside the eye mainly depends on the balance between the changes in IT induced by surfac-

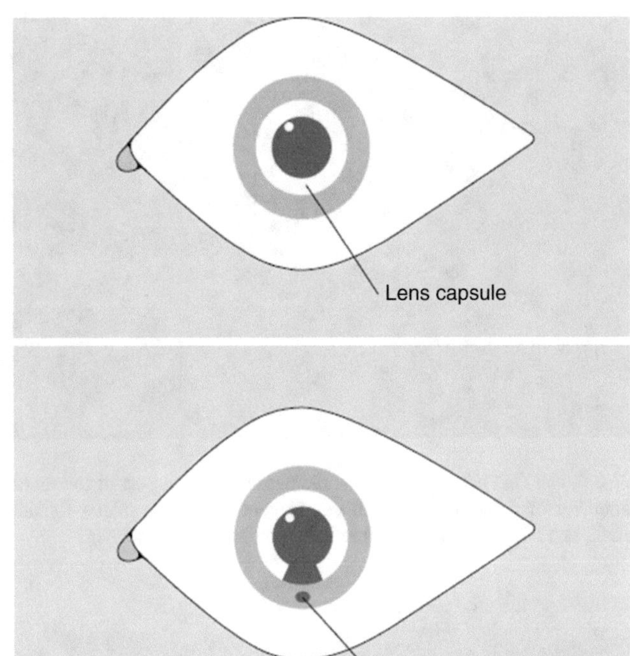

Fig. 4.62 Sometimes, it is necessary to remove the lens of an eye that is about to receive silicone oil. Conventionally the lens was removed in its entirety with the capsule also removed, leaving no structure for subsequent lens implantation. It is possible to preserve some capsule, either anterior or posterior; however, leaving a ring of the capsule will produce posterior synechiae and glaucoma. This can be avoided by excising a small wedge of the capsule at the 6 o'clock position behind a peripheral iridectomy, thereby allowing aqueous to travel into the anterior chamber, avoiding pupil block glaucoma and maintaining capsule for later sulcus fixated lens implantation

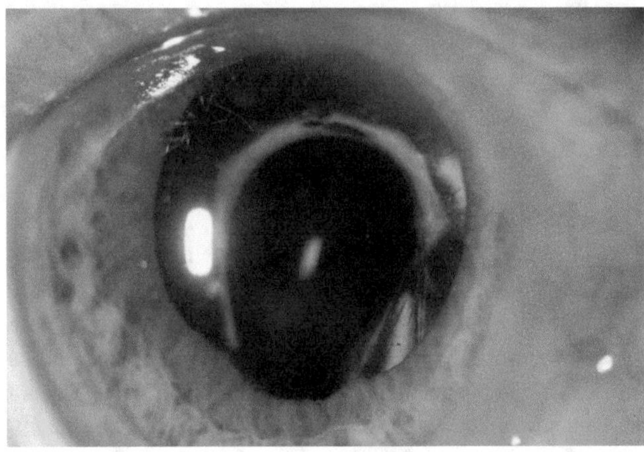

Fig. 4.63 An example of a keyhole capsulectomy postoperatively

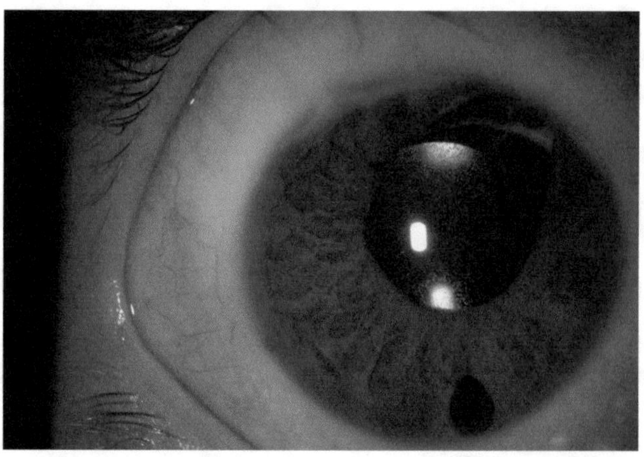

Fig. 4.64 This patient had a keyhole capsulotomy as part of the management of a traumatic retinal detachment with later sulcus fixated IOL. The IOL is stable as seen in this photograph 6 years later

Table 4.4 Silicone oil complications

Complications of Silicone oil	
Cataract	Nuclear sclerotic
Glaucoma	Open angle Pupil block Oil overfill
Refraction	Reduced hypermetropia in aphakes Hypermetropic shift in phakic and pseudophake
Emulsion	
Retinal toxicity	
Oil in the wrong place	Suprachoroidal Subretinal Subconjunctival
Band keratopathy	
Adherence to intraocular lens implant	

tants, heat, changes in pH level and mechanical energy (induced by viscosity and the eye movements) (Fig. 4.65).

The Surfactants

The surfactants are the main compounds able to lower the ST. The surfactants are amphiphilic compounds that contain both hydrophobic and hydrophilic groups, extending in both oil and water with two different tails. The surfactants can be biosurfactants produced by the eye itself or impurity present as low-molecular weight-component (LMWC) in the manufacturing process of SO. Biosurfactants are surface-active substances, such as HDL-apolipoproteins, plasma lipoproteins, red blood cell membranes, growth factors and cytokines, which are mainly released by the RPE cells or by the damaged blood-retinal barrier [41, 42]. In an experimental model, we found that the presence of albumin (at concentration of 70 g/L, corresponding to the physiological serum content) affects remarkably the interfacial properties with an IT reduction of 50% from the baseline. Besides the endogenous emulsifier, the LMWCs present in the SO act as "exogenous surfactants," responsible for lowering the IT. The SO synthesis process generates a mixture of chains with the same structural unit (monomer) but different lengths, defined "impurities," in the form of linear or cyclic siloxanes of different molecular weight. LMWC with M < 1000 g/mol are considered significant chemical impurities of SO. The main role seems to be played by the D4 (octamethylcyclotetrasiloxane). The purification and ultra-purification of SO from short-chained siloxanes significantly decrease the amount of LMWC. The aim is to provide a compound with a concentration of LMWC <1 mg/kg. The latest ultra-purification process consisting in multiple step cleaning with control of purity done by Gas chromatography and mass spectroscopy can provide a concentration of LMWC between 0.2–0.5 mg/kg. We evaluated chemical composition, and molecular and rheological properties in 10 commercially available silicone oils (SilOils), focusing on LMWC. The samples differed significantly in terms of molecular weight distribution and relative LMWC fractions, potentially inducing ocular inflammation and toxicity [43]. The cytotoxic effect of LMWC in conventional 1000 cSt SO with different degrees of purification has also recently been assessed, using in vitro direct contact cytotoxicity tests performed in BALB 3T3 and ARPE-19 according to the ISO 10993-5 (2009) standards evaluation. Although the cellular viability was significantly higher in purified SO, no reduction in cell viability was detected in the tested samples when concentrate of LMWC was added. A direct cytotoxic effect is not likely to be involved in the potential complications

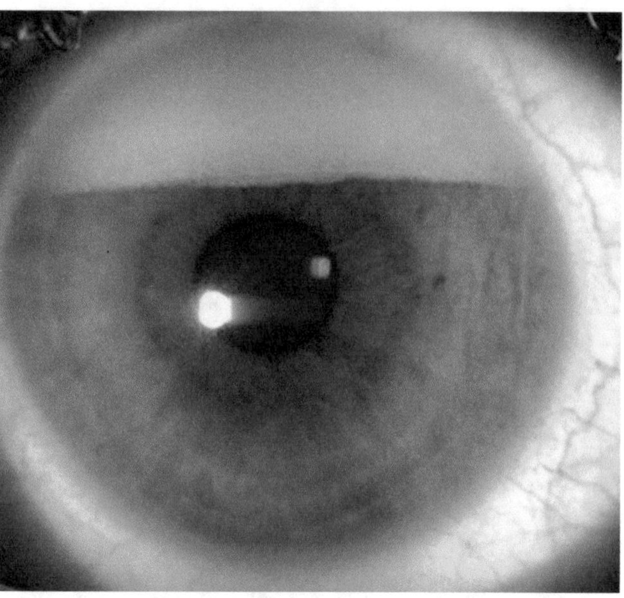

Fig. 4.65 Creaming of silicone oil (SO) in anterior chamber. Migration of the dispersed phase of SO emulsion under the influence of buoyancy. The particles float upwards or sink, and for as long as the particles remain separated, the process is called creaming

related to SO and LMWC. The potential long-term adverse effects of LMWC are not known. However, this mechanism can be related only to the acute cytotoxicity, whereas, with regard to the intraocular use, the capacity of some LMWC to diffuse into surrounding tissues has been already reported [44]. In a real-life scenario, LMWC facilitates the denaturation and aggregation of human serum albumin and, supposedly, other human blood proteins that can be present within the vitreous cavity during surgery as endogenous surfactants. Again, this effect does not determine intraocular cytotoxicity, but it is part of a more complex pathogenetic process leading to SO-related complications. Finally, even small quantitates of detergents or cleaning substances from the sterilisation processes of reusable equipment can increase the risk of emulsification in SO-filled eyes [45].

Inflammation

The SO emulsion is responsible for several complications including retinal toxicity and inflammation. It is almost impossible to distinguish between inflammation caused by the tamponade and the inflammatory reaction that is associated with the underlying retinal pathology. However, focal phenomena of retinal toxicity and necrosis have been described and seem to be related to the direct toxicity and immunogenicity of the impurities or the instability of the agents that modify the IT. The emulsified SO droplets induce a macrophagic foreign body reaction with phagocytosis of SO emulsion by retinal pigment epithelium cells. Such granulomatous reactions with epithelioid cells are responsible for the cascade of inflammation that circumscribed at the interfaces by the presence of SO can lead to retinal necrosis (Fig. 4.66).

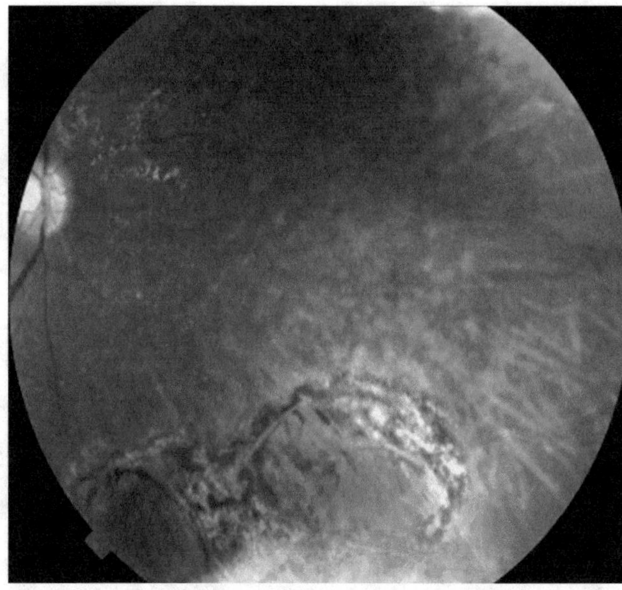

Fig. 4.66 The retina showed signs of extensive inflammation combined with areas of retinal atrophy after use of heavy silicone oil for retinal detachment. An extraordinary fragile retina that broke into two big retinal holes during fluid/air exchange were observed

The Mechanical Energy

The system composed of SO-water-retina is gravitationally unstable because of the eye movements are faster than the re-adaptation of the fluids in the eye. It is not possible to separate viscosity-induced from gravity-induced instability. With the head/eye movements, the mechanical energy increases, and therefore the tendency of SO to emulsify. To decrease the mechanical energy, we can only increase the viscosity by reducing the velocity between the retina and the oil (shear rate). The energy available for dispersion of SO would also be diminished. Viscosity is the measure of the resistance, better defined as the relationship between the shear stress (forces applied) and the shear rate (deformation obtained). In the surgical application of SO, we can distinguish the extensional viscosity from the shear viscosity. Extensional viscosity is measured as the resistance of the SO from the extension and break up into SO droplet. The shear viscosity is measured as the resistance to flow due to the friction induced by a coplanar stress between parcels moving at different speeds. The easiest way to decrease emulsification is to increase extensional viscosity, therefore the length of the molecular chain of the compound, but at the same time we have an increase also of share viscosity (resistance in injection and removal of SO). Williams et al. suggested to add 5–10% high molecular weight SO (423 kDa) to 1000 cSt SO. The resulting SO has the same chemical proprieties of those used in clinical practices but is more resistant to emulsification and is relatively easy to inject and remove [46].

Perfluorocarbon Liquid Toxicity and Interactions

The perfluorocarbon liquids (PFCLs) are synthetic liquid fluorinated carbon-containing compounds, characterised by specific gravity greater than water (ranging from 1.7–2.03 g/cm^3); moderate interfacial tension (approximately 50 mN/m against water); and low viscosity, transparency and immiscibility with water. PFCLs have an intermediate interfacial tension against water at 50 mN/m and a dynamic viscosity of 5.10 mPas [47]. Among all PFCLs, perfluoro-n-octane (PFO) has an high vapour pressure, which allows, in an open system, a more complete PFO removal during fluid–air exchange. Unfortunately, the PFO has also a high spreading coefficient that induces the PFO to dissolve into SO in small amounts. Despite an accurate removal of PFCL under air, small amounts of PFCL are still present in the vitreous cavity and can be responsible for inflammation and changes in SO rheological proprieties [41] (Fig. 4.67). Recently, Pastor et al. reported 117 cases of acute retinal toxicity with severe visual loss, which is mostly characterised by retinal necrosis and vascular occlusion after intraoperative use of perfluoro-n-octane (PFO) Ala-Octa (Alamedics, Dornstadt, Germany)

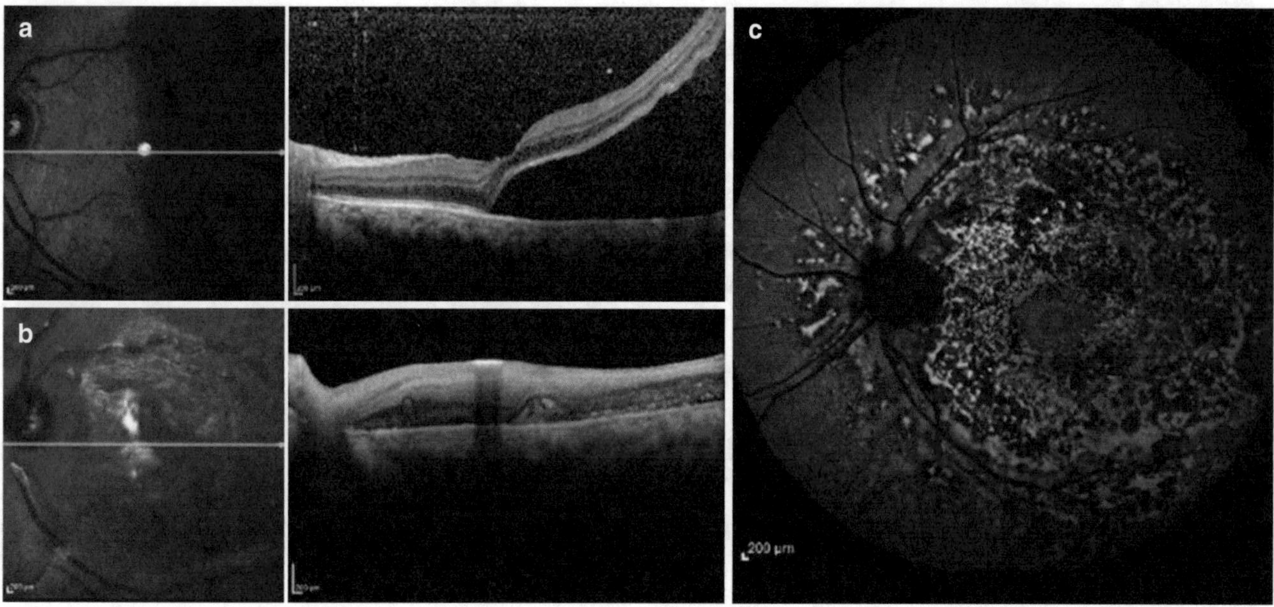

Fig. 4.67 Patient treated for a macula-off retinal detachment (**a**) with vitrectomy, intra-op perfluoro decaline removed by the end of the surgery, endolaser and 1000cSt silicone oil. Seven days after the surgery, is visible accumulation of inflammatory material between the retina and retinal pigment epithelium (RPE) (**b**) and damage of RPE at blue fundus autofluorescence (**c**) (courtesy of Dr. R. Orsi, Dr. V. Battaglino)

[48]. Such severe adverse events raised an animated discussion within the scientific and medical community about the safety of PFCL medical devices, particularly on the validity of the methods used for their safety assessment (ISO 10993-5 and ISO 16672), and emphasised the necessity to review the standardised in vitro cytotoxicity test and the development of chemical analytical methods able to detect the presence of potentially cytotoxic compounds. It has been shown that the direct contact cytotoxicity test according to ISO 10993-5 is a suitable method to detect the cytotoxicity of PFCLs and was validated using quantitative and qualitative approaches in ARPE-19 and BALB/3T3 cells [49]. Alamedics chose these test methods: The Ala-Octa PFO extract was tested with "extract test" that was unsuitable for immiscible and volatile samples, like PFCL. Moreover, the so-called H-value, defined as the ppm content of partially hydrogenated perfluoro alkanes, has been introduced as another PFCL safety criterion, with less than 10 ppm as the safety threshold. We assessed the H-content using a ^{1}H NMR quantitative assay implemented with the electronic reference, and we failed to demonstrate a correlation between the H-content and in vitro cytotoxicity test. Therefore, the H-content alone cannot be predictive of perfluorocarbon ocular endotamponade cytotoxicity in vitro [50].

Interaction Between Heavy Liquid and Silicone Oil Can Lead the Sticky Oil Formation

The first series of sticky oil formation has been described by Veckeneer et al. in 28 eyes tamponaded with SO. The authors reported that 1000 cSt SO and PFCL were used in the previous surgery, and in all cases, the surgeons proceeded with direct PFCL and SO exchange [51]. The proof of the presence of PFCL in the SO bubble has been reported using gas chromatography–mass spectroscopy analysis in samples of sticky SO. Furthermore, Friberg et al., using electron impact ionisation mass spectrometry, described that small amount of PFCL dissolves into solution over time [52]. Sticky oil is defined as SO-like material that remains glued to the retinal surface during SO removal. The stickiness of the compound is related to a reduction in IT of the surrounding aqueous material contaminated with PFCL. We believe that the defined sticky oil is not only "sticky," but it is also a "hyper-viscous" compound produced by interaction between PFCL-SO. Sticky oil formation has been described in eyes previously treated with PFCL and light SO and more frequently with PFCL and HSO. HSO is a mixed compound obtained by adding a semifluorurate (alkane or ether) to SO. The saturation point of HSO is the highest concentration of semifluorurate that dissolves in SO. HSO is a partially fluorinated and saturated compound and, therefore, more unstable than SO. The presence of PFCL induces changes in saturation points. Solubility equilibrium is also temperature-dependent, therefore also changes in temperature modify the saturation of HSO by PFCL. In the absence of PFCL, hyper-viscous solutions have not been formed [53]. In surgical practice, the direct exchange of PFCL with HSO, and probably also the use of PFO, is not recommended during retinal surgery because of the direct contact between the two compounds at the oil interface and because of the high spreading coefficient.

Mario R Romano, Department of Biomedical Sciences, Humanitas University, Rozzano—Milano, Italy

Silicone Oil Removal (Table 4.5)

Additional steps small

1. Prepare for the vitrectomy as before.
2. Use a 4 mm long small gauge cannula attached to an oil injector pump set on extract inserted through one of the trochars (if not available create a 20G sclerotomy).
3. Actively extrude the oil (block the microscope light from entering through the pupil).
4. Perform an internal search.

Whenever silicone oil has been inserted, the aim must be to remove the oil later to maximise vision and reduce the chance of complications. In the Silicone Oil Study, oil was removed from 45% of the eyes in which it was used [54]; however, it is better to aim for a much higher removal rate, perhaps 80%. Different methods are possible. The greatest risk is redetachment of the retina in the early postoperative period. For this reason, it is prudent to re-examine the retina at the time of oil removal and to deal with any redetachment there and then, ROSO plus operation [34].

Insert an infusion line into the pars plana (Take care that the infusion cannula can be more difficult to see because of the refractive properties of the edge of the silicone oil) and set up sclerotomies as for a PPV. Block the central illumination of the microscope light to avoid retinal light toxicity (The macula of the silicone filled eye may be prone to damage). For SG use an attached to a 10 ml syringe which is attached to the oil extraction system (the same one used for oil injection but on extract rather than inject). Insert the cannula into one of the trochars. Aspirate the oil with vacuum of 300 psi and wait for the oil to enter the 10 ml syringe. Keep the tip of the cannula in the oil because if you enter the aqueous layer (which has much less viscosity) the high vacuum can cause a sudden drop in IOP risking choroidal haemorrhage. Be especially careful when the bubble is small. Keep the tip in the oil with the cannula perpendicular to the oil surface. Try to stay in the bubble the whole time; this keeps the bubble on the cannula rather than allowing it to float away. When the bubble is small, it will be hidden behind the iris, aspirate gradually drawing the tip of the cannula to the sclerotomy and slowly out of the eye, the oil bubble should be drawn to the sclerotomy and start to exit through the sclerotomy (keep the sclerotomy at the highest point). Do not aspirate too vigorously just inside the sclerotomy in case you engage the remaining vitreous base and cause traction on the retina.

Table 4.5 Difficulty rating of silicone oil removal

Difficulty Rating	Low
Success Rates	Moderate
Complication Rates	Low
When to Use in Training	Early

Surgical Algorithm

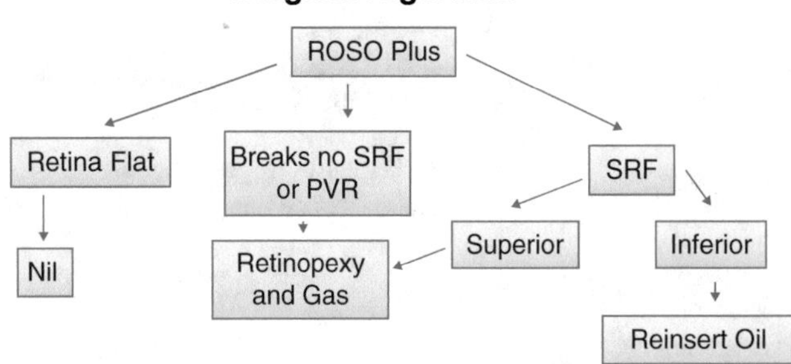

Fig. 4.68 During ROSO plus operation use the algorithm as a guide to manage the retina to minimise postoperative redetachment and reoperation rates

If a short cannula is not available and the eye is phakic or pseudophakic the oil can be removed through an enlarged 2 mm sclerotomy rather than by active suction. If using a 2 mm sclerotomy, the elasticity of the choroid often leads to a small hole in the choroid through which the oil will not pass therefore, it is important to check this and enlarge the hole separately from the scleral incision. Sew up the sclerotomy hole after use and before the internal search; instrumentation will still pass into the eye despite the suture. Create the other sclerotomy and internally search the eye.

Perform the routine PPV approach and internally search the retina for SRF, traction, open breaks or leaking retinectomy edges. The risk of retinal redetachment is extremely high if SRF is found in the inferior retina (Six times more likely than if SRF is found superiorly), and reinsertion of the oil is recommended [34]. If breaks are found without SRF or SRF is found superiorly, these can be treated with retinopexy and gas tamponade (Fig. 4.68).

Alternative Methods

If performing a cataract extraction at the same time, it is possible to perform a posterior capsulotomy to allow the oil to enter the anterior chamber and exit through the cataract excision, in which case insert the IOL after the oil has been removed. If the eye is aphakic a 2 mm corneal incision can be used to allow egress of the oil. These methods do not facilitate re-examination of the retina (ROSO plus).

Retinal Redetachment Rates After Oil Removal

These are high at 15–25% because surgeons tend to use oil in patients with complex vitreoretinal pathologies such as severe trauma, failed tractional retinal detachment surgery or proliferative vitreoretinopathy [55–57]. In addition, there is a

Table 4.6 Properties of various liquids

	Molecular weight	Viscosity mPas	Refractive index	Density g/cm^3
Silicone oil	25,000 or 50,000	1000–1300 or 5000–5900	1.4	0.97
Densiron 68 (heavy oil)	NA	1400	1.39	1.06
Oxane HD (heavy oil)	NA	3300	1.4	1.02
Perfluoro decalin (heavy liquid)	462	2.7	1.3	1.8–2.0
Perfluoro octane (heavy liquid)	438	0.8	1.27	1.76

risk of long-term hypotony of approximately 16% [58]. Some have tried to reduce retinal redetachment rates by applying 360° laser retinopexy to the peripheral retina before the ROSO operation claiming reduced posterior retinal detachment rates from 21% to 11% [59, 60] (Table 4.6).

Heavy Silicone Oils

Silicone oil cannot be relied upon to provide inferior tamponade therefore oils that are denser than water have been developed.

Densiron 68 (fluoron) is a heavy silicone oil made up of polydimethylsiloxane $(CH_3)_3SiO\text{-}9(Si\ (CH_3)_2O)$ n-Si $(CH_3)_3$ and perfluorohexyl octane F6H8.

1. Density 1.06 g/cm^3
2. Viscosity 1400 mPas
3. Refractive index 1.39
4. Interfacial tension in water at 25 °C is 40.82 mN/m

Oxane HD is a combination of silicone oil and partly fluorinated olefin

1. Density 1.02 g/cm^3
2. Viscosity 3300 mPa
3. Refractive index 1.40
4. Interfacial tension in water 40 mN/m

These can be inserted in the same way as silicone oil. Removal is more difficult than with silicone oil because the heavy oils do not float out of the eye; active suction is required with an 18-gauge cannula inserted through a sclerotomy. Metal tip cannulae are best to avoid sticking of the oil to the tip in the final stages of removal. The oils may adhere to the retina but can usually be separated off with care. Some of these oils will separate into their two components, heavy and light which must be considered during removal.

Many surgeons have found uses for heavy oils, for example inferior PVR or giant retinal tears but results may not be improved over the use of conventional silicone oil [61]. My experience is that the heavy oils are not dense enough to reliably deal with inferior PVR and can produce postoperative PVR superiorly. Superior PVR is more difficult to deal with by retinectomy, so that I prefer the predictability of conventional silicone oils (Fig. 4.69).

Heavy Liquids

Additional Surgical Steps [62]

1. Use a heavy liquid-filled syringe and a two-way cannula with the tip close to the fovea.
2. Expand the bubble of heavy liquid with the distal orifice within the bubble and the proximal orifice in the vitreous cavity fluid.
3. For removal use a flute needle in the bubble and try to remove it in one smooth action to avoid losing the bubble when it is small (Fig. 4.70).

Available heavy liquid agents include the perfluorocarbon Liquids (PFCLs) such as decalin, octane or phenanthrene, in which all carbon atoms of the carbon backbone are completely fluorinated. These agents may cause emulsification, vascular changes and structural alterations of the retina and are therefore usually removed at the end of surgery. They are biologically inert, with a specific gravity higher than water, immiscibility with water or blood, and with a high gas binding capacity (Figs. 4.71 and 4.72).

Perfluoro decalin a fluorinated perfluorocarbon has the following properties:

1. $C_{10}F_{18}$
2. Molecular weight 462
3. Densities of 1.8 to 2.0 g/cm^3
4. Refractive index 1.313
5. Boiling point 142 °C
6. Vapour pressure (37 °C) 12.5 mmHg
7. Surface tension (25 °C) 19 mN/m
8. Interface tension in water (20 °C) 57.8 mN/m
9. Viscosity (25 °C) 2.7 mPas

Perfluoro-n-Octane has a high vapour pressure which theoretically allows small droplets at the end of surgery to vaporise into the air or gas bubble, reducing the chance of retained droplets.

1. C_8F_{18}
2. Molecular weight 438
3. Densities of 1.8 g/cm^3

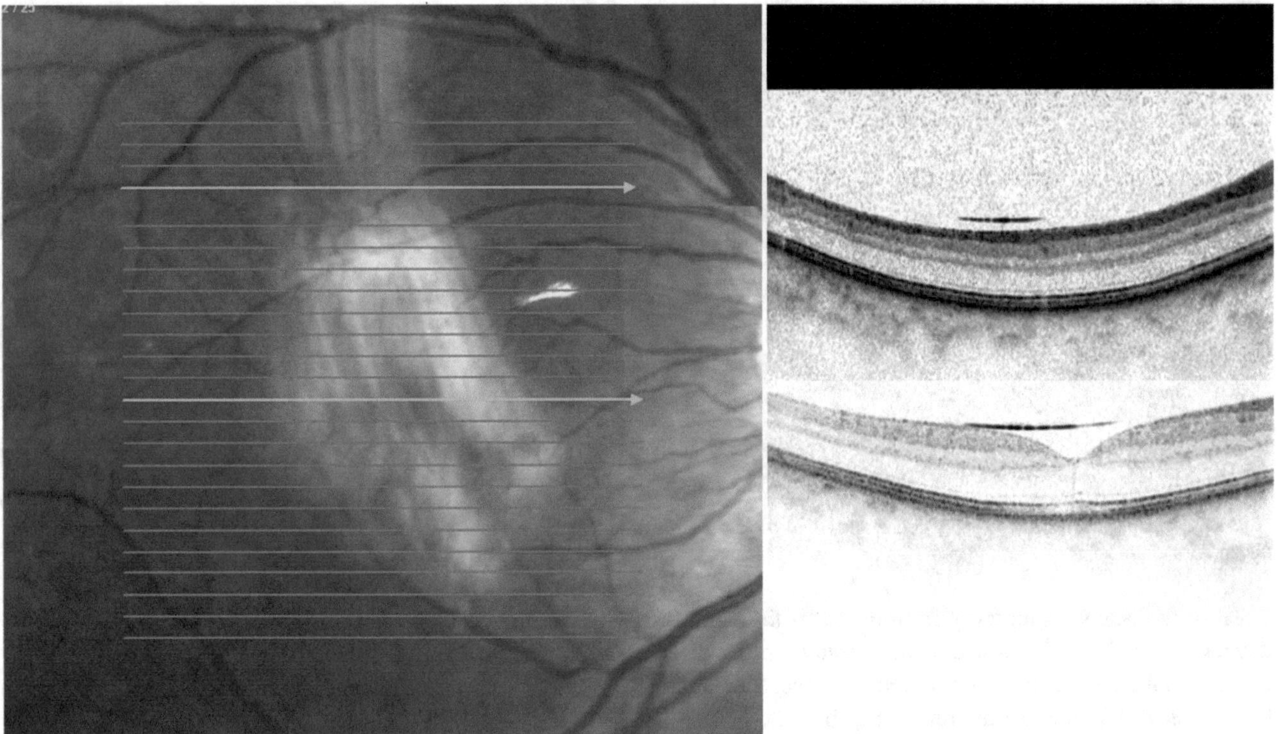

Fig. 4.69 Heavy oil in contact with the retina in the light reflex but not above it

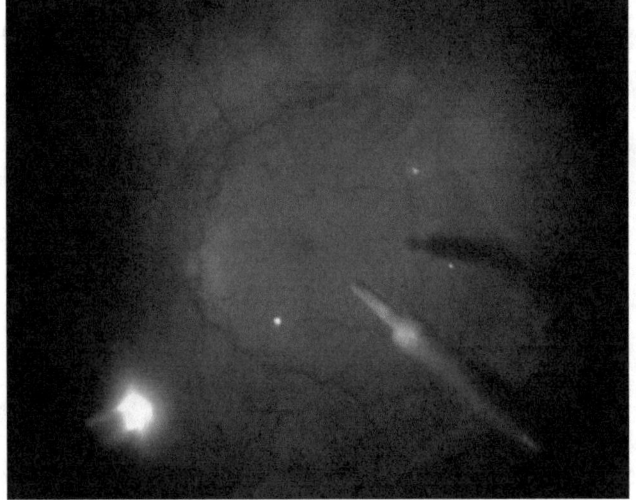

Fig. 4.70 A two-way cannula is used to insert heavy liquids into the eye, the heavies are infused through the distal orifice whilst the vitreous cavity fluid exits through proximal hole on the shaft of the instrument

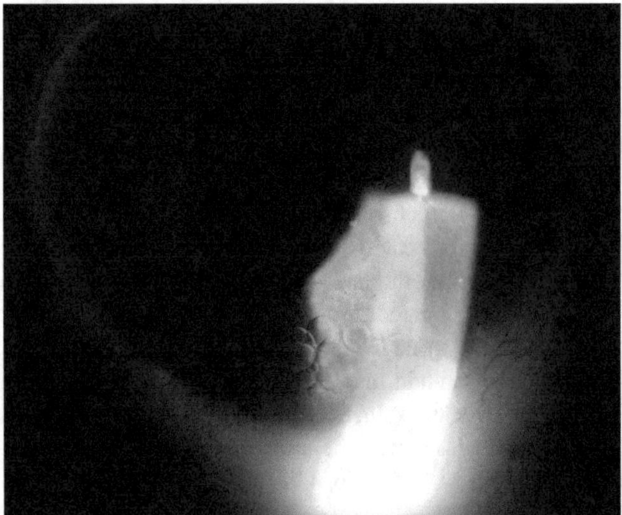

Fig. 4.71 Droplets of heavy liquid are present in the inferior angle of this patient. These can be easily aspirated by using a fine gauge needle and as a paracentesis

4. Refractive index 1.27
5. Boiling point 103 °C
6. Vapour pressure (37 °C) 52 mmHg
7. Surface tension (25 °C) 15 mN/m
8. Interface tension in water (20 °C) >40 mN/m
9. Viscosity (25 °C) 1.4 mPas

These agents are especially useful peroperative tools for:

1. Retinal detachment
2. Giant tears
3. Ocular trauma
4. Assisting laser application
5. Lifting subluxated lenses
6. Peroperative stabilisation of the retina

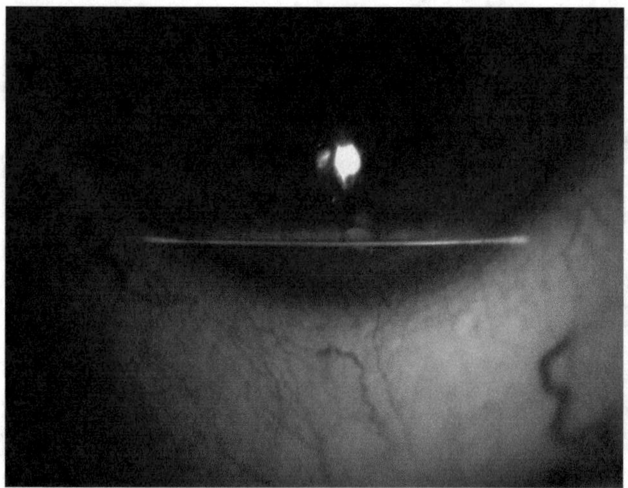

Fig. 4.72 Droplets of retained heavy liquid often find their way into the anterior chamber

Keep the heavy liquid away from breaks if these are on tension (e.g. in PVR) because the liquid easily separates into different bubbles and enters the subretinal space. Small bubbles of heavy liquid under the retina may become immobilised and cause no damage, and larger bubbles are able to move around in the subretinal space causing inferior RPE damage and persistent RD.

Subretinal heavy liquid can migrate to the fovea, use OCT to show an echo lucent bubble. They are very toxic to the retina and the receptors die rapidly (Figs. 4.73 and 4.74).

Subfoveal liquid should be removed; you will need to detach the retina by infusing balanced salt fluid under the retina using a 40 gauge cannula attached to the oil injection pump. Once a bleb of subretinal fluid has been raised, insert air into the vitreous cavity to push the fluid towards the macula. This mobilises the heavy bubble away from the fovea and it can be aspirated through a retinotomy or left to sit inferiorly in the retina if small. Another method described is to insert heavy liquid into the vitreous cavity and create a retinotomy over the subretinal heavy liquid. The subretinal liquid may coalesce with the intravitreal bubble facilitating its removal (Figs. 4.75, 4.76, 4.77, 4.78, 4.79).

"Light" Heavy Liquids

Semi fluorinated alkanes, R(F)R(H), have a perfluorocarbon and a hydrocarbon segment in the molecule. They are physiologically inert, colourless, laser stable liquids with low densities of between 1.1 and 1.7 g/cm^3 and extremely low surface and interface tensions.

They are soluble in perfluorocarbon liquids (PFCL), hydrocarbons and silicone oils.

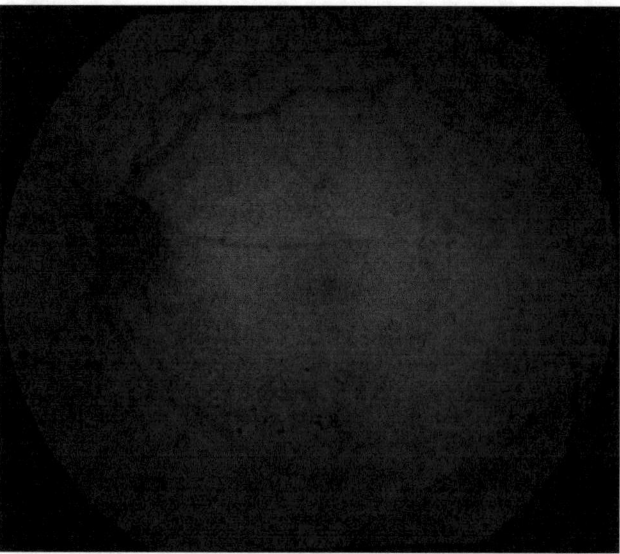

Fig. 4.73 Multiple droplets of subretinal heavy liquid are seen in this patient on fundus autofluorescence

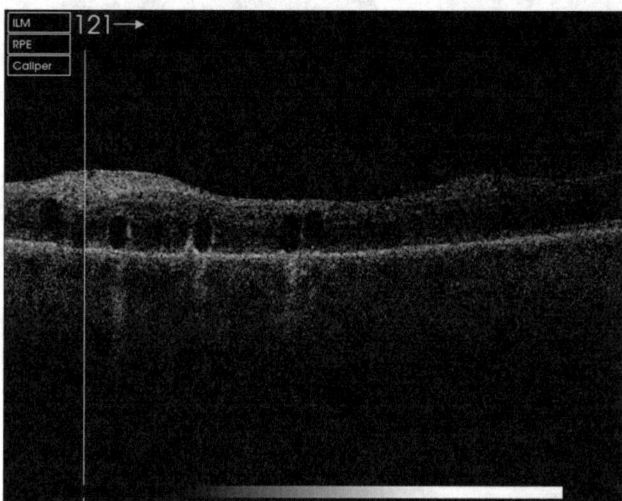

Fig. 4.74 An OCT of the same patient showing the droplets of heavy liquid

Removal of Emulsified Silicone Oil

F6H8, a fluorocarbon liquid that has a density of 1.35 g/cm^3 and can be used for the removal of emulsified silicone oil which it solubilises easing the removal of oil droplets. Fill the vitreous cavity with the light heavy liquid, which advantageously displaces the emulsion, physically aiding its removal, in addition to solubilising residual oil (Fig. 4.80). Alternatively, perform a fluid–air exchange to concentrate the emulsion into a thin fluid layer, then refill with BSS. This can be repeated to maximise the removal of the emulsion.

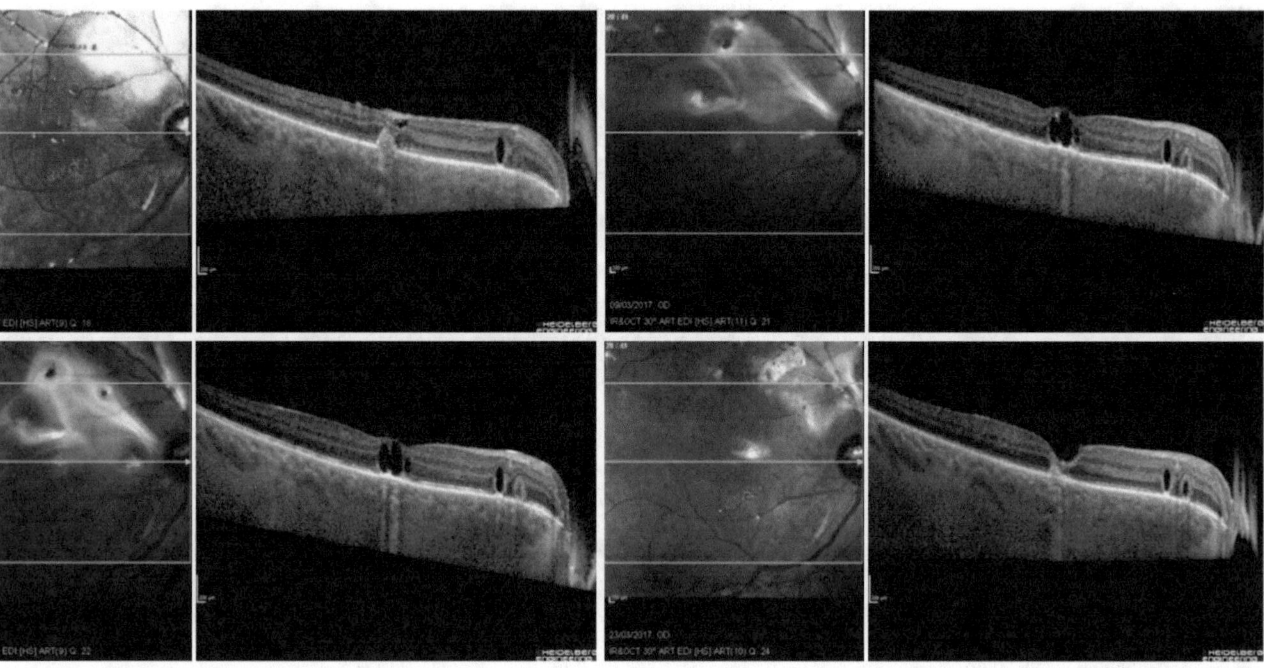

Fig. 4.75 Subretinal heavy liquid which migrated to the fovea and then was removed by redetachment of the macula and upright posture. The heavy liquid is very detrimental to the receptors, and only a thin fovea with poor vision remains

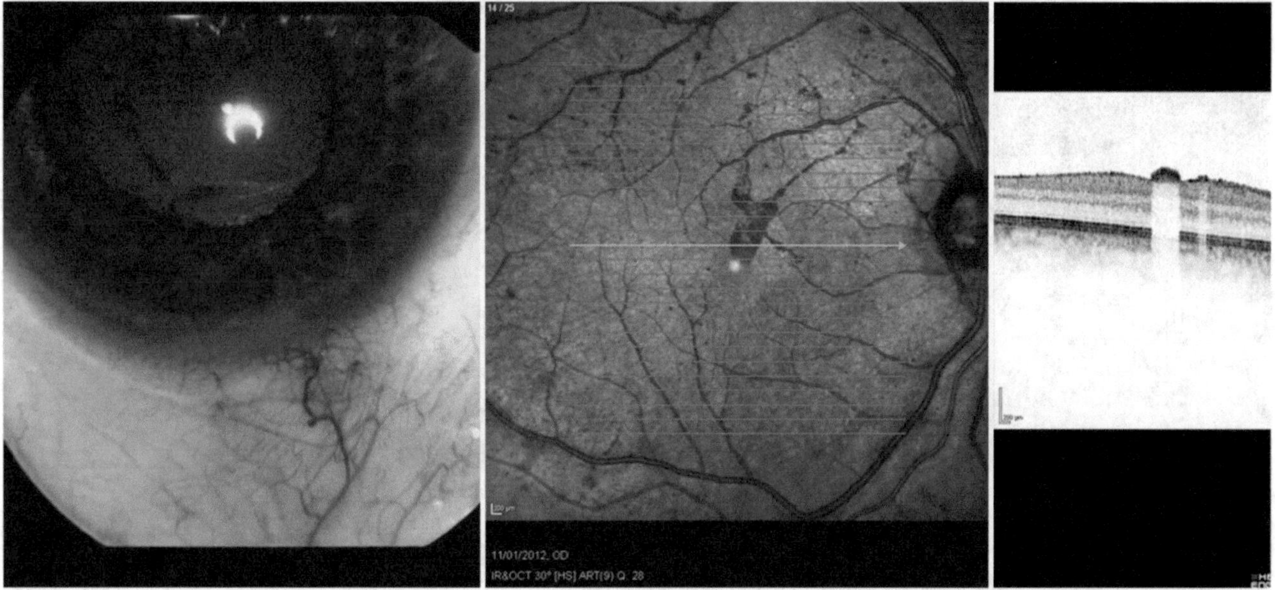

Fig. 4.76 Macrophages will try to remove retained heavy liquids causing chronic inflammation

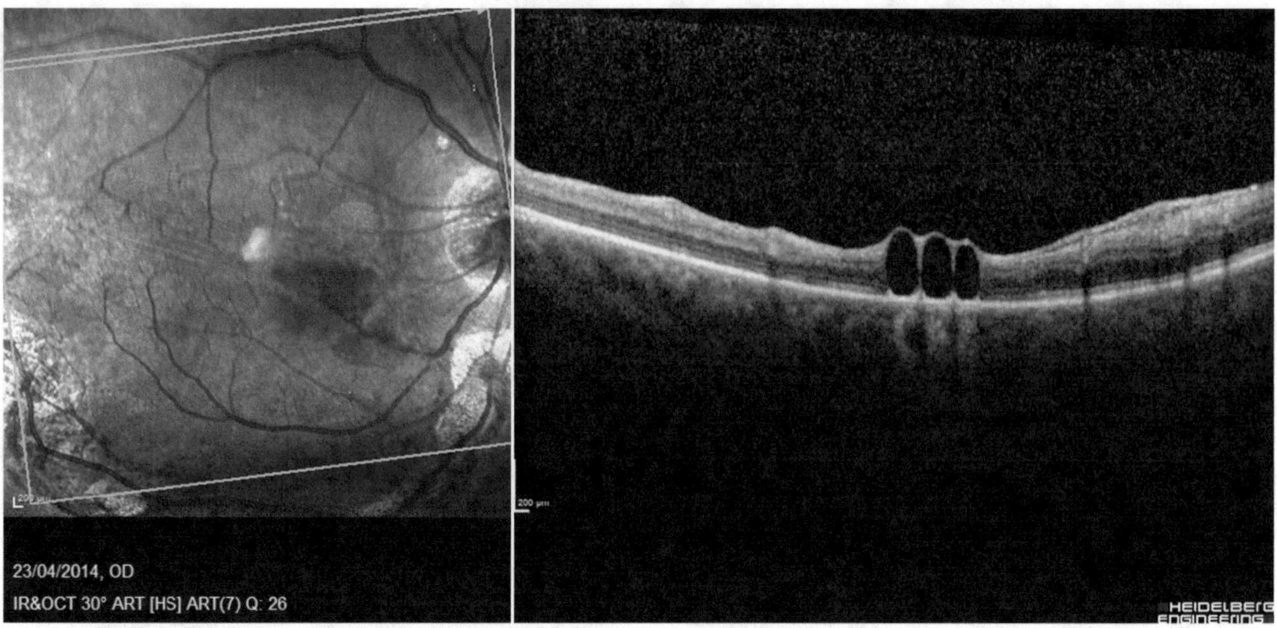

Fig. 4.77 Subretinal heavy liquid

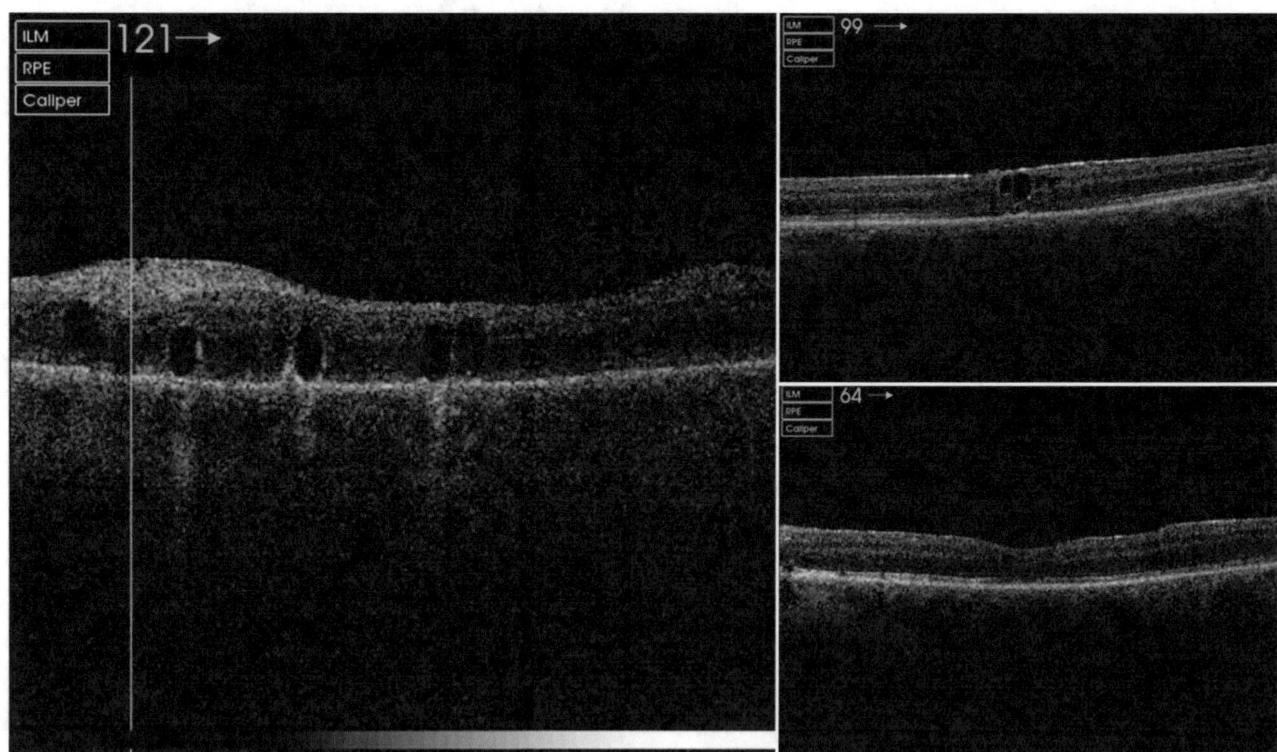

Fig. 4.78 Subretinal heavies have been removed from the fovea, but the receptors are poor centrally postoperatively

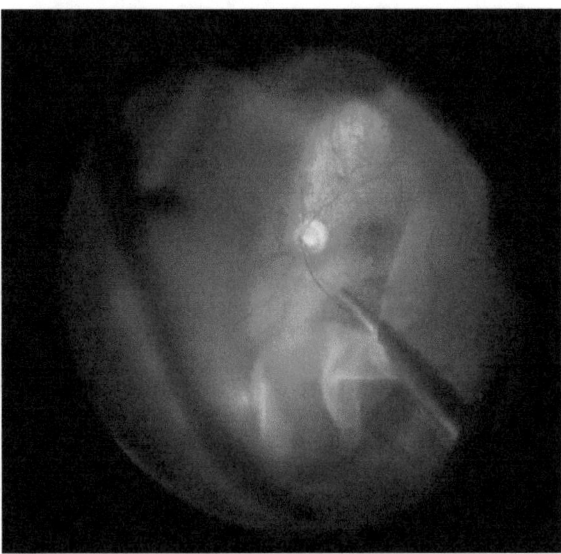

Fig. 4.79 The retina has been incarcerated into the outflow channel of a heavy liquid cannula, this is a risk with mobile retina as in 360 macular translocation or giant retinal tear as in this eye. If you consider this likely to happen, use a single channel flute needle and allow the vitreous cavity fluid to egress through a sclerotomy

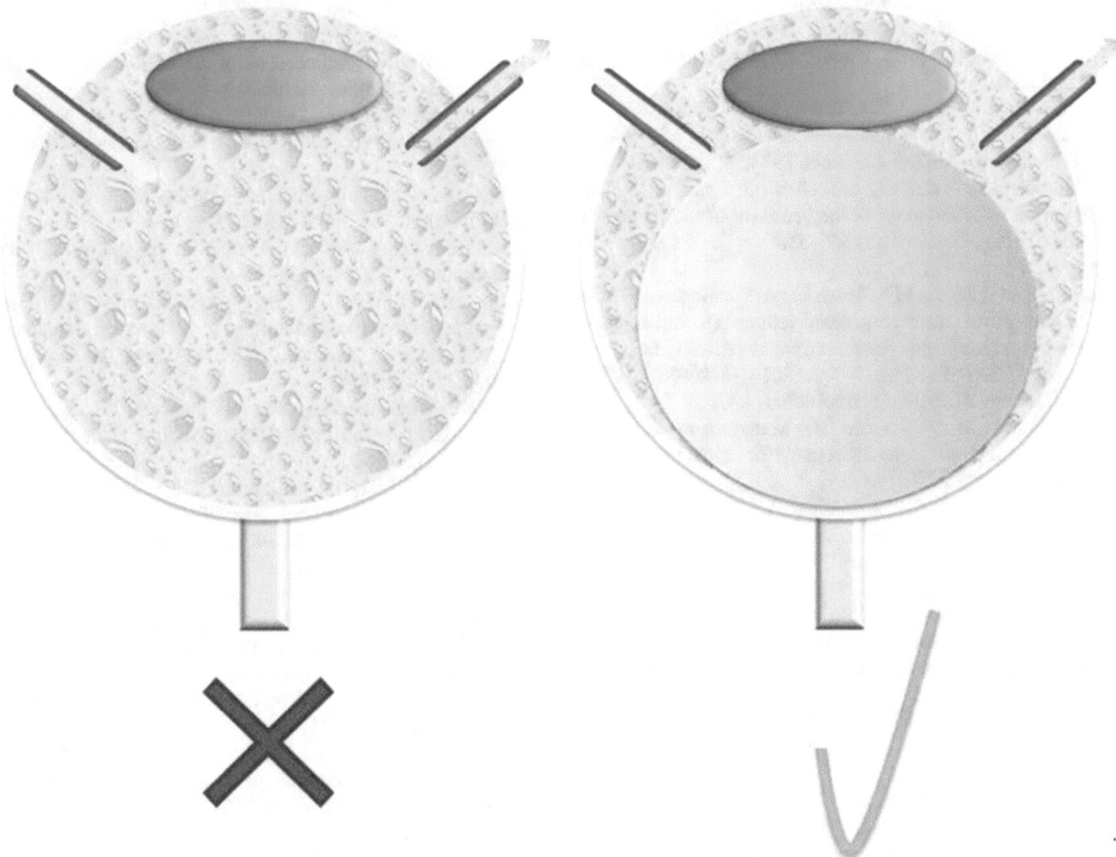

Fig. 4.80 Trying to remove emulsified oil by flushing the vitreous cavity with BSS is ineffective because the oil droplets can enter the BSS and only slowly become less concentrated in the vitreous cavity, with only a few emulsified droplets removed for unit of time (left graphic). Displacing the fluid containing the emulsion with a fluid (gas or F6H8) into which the emulsion cannot dissolve allows the emulsion containing liquid to be extracted rapidly (right graphic). F6H8 also has the advantage that the surface of the F6H8 will absorb some of the oil droplets, which will be removed when the F6H8 is removed

Summary

There are a wide variety of surgical tools available to the vitreoretinal surgeon. Their use depends on personal experience, and each has its own set of additional complications.

References

1. Zaidi AA, Alvarado R, Irvine A. Pneumatic retinopexy: success rate and complications. Br J Ophthalmol. 2006;90(4):427–8. https://doi.org/10.1136/bjo.2005.075515.
2. Yanyali A, Horozoglu F, Bayrak YI, Celik E, Nohutcu AF. Steamroller versus basic technique in pneumatic retinopexy for primary rhegmatogenous retinal detachment. Retina. 2007;27(1):74–82. https://doi.org/10.1097/01.iae.0000256664.02359.c1. 00006982-200701000-00013 [pii]
3. Lowe MA, McDonald HR, Campo RV, Boyer DS, Schatz H. Pneumatic retinopexy. Surgical results. Arch Ophthalmol. 1988;106(12):1672–6.
4. Kulkarni KM, Roth DB, Prenner JL. Current visual and anatomic outcomes of pneumatic retinopexy. Retina. 2007;27(8):1065–70. https://doi.org/10.1097/IAE.0b013e3180546928. 00006982-200710000-00012 [pii]
5. Hilton GF, Kelly NE, Salzano TC, Tornambe PE, Wells JW, Wendel RT. Pneumatic retinopexy. A collaborative report of the first 100 cases. Ophthalmology. 1987;94(4):307–14.
6. Chang S, Lincoff HA, Coleman DJ, Fuchs W, Farber ME. Perfluorocarbon gases in vitreous surgery. Ophthalmology. 1985;92(5):651–6.
7. Chang S, Coleman DJ, Lincoff H, Wilcox LM Jr, Braunstein RA, Maisel JM. Perfluoropropane gas in the management of proliferative vitreoretinopathy. Am J Ophthalmol. 1984;98(2):180–8.
8. Lincoff H, Coleman J, Kreissig I, Richard G, Chang S, Wilcox LM. The perfluorocarbon gases in the treatment of retinal detachment. Ophthalmology. 1983;90(5):546–51.
9. optomap gas.
10. Martinez-Castillo V, Zapata MA, Boixadera A, Fonollosa A, Garcia-Arumi J. Pars plana vitrectomy, laser retinopexy, and aqueous tamponade for pseudophakic rhegmatogenous retinal detachment. Ophthalmology. 2007;114(2):297–302. S0161-6420(06)01058-X [pii]. https://doi.org/10.1016/j.ophtha.2006.07.037.
11. Tanner V, Minihan M, Williamson TH. Management of inferior retinal breaks during pars plana vitrectomy for retinal detachment. Br J Ophthalmol. 2001;85(4):480–2.
12. Martinez-Castillo V, Boixadera A, Verdugo A, Garcia-Arumi J. Pars plana vitrectomy alone for the management of inferior breaks in pseudophakic retinal detachment without facedown position. Ophthalmology. 2005;112(7):1222–6. S0161-6420(05)00306-4 [pii]. https://doi.org/10.1016/j.ophtha.2004.12.046.
13. Lincoff H, Maisel JM, Lincoff A. Intravitreal disappearance rates of four perfluorocarbon gases. Arch Ophthalmol. 1984;102(6):928–9.
14. Hart RH, Vote BJ, Borthwick JH, McGeorge AJ, Worsley DR. Loss of vision caused by expansion of intraocular perfluoropropane (C(3)F(8)) gas during nitrous oxide anesthesia. Am J Ophthalmol. 2002;134(5):761–3.
15. Kontos A, Tee J, Stuart A, Shalchi Z, Williamson TH. Duration of intraocular gases following vitreoretinal surgery. Graefes Arch Clin Exp Ophthalmol. 2017;255(2):231–6. https://doi.org/10.1007/s00417-016-3438-3.
16. Hall SK, Williamson TH, Guillemaut J-Y, Goddard T, Baumann AP, Hutter JC. Modeling the dynamics of tamponade multi-component gases during retina reattachment surgery. AIChe J. 2017;63:3651–62.
17. Williamson TH, Guillemaut JY, Hall SK, Hutter JC, Goddard T. Theoretical gas concentrations achieving 100% fill of the vitreous cavity in the postoperative period: a gas eye model study. Retina. 2018;38(Suppl 1):S60–S4. https://doi.org/10.1097/IAE.0000000000001963.
18. Lincoff H, Weinberger D, Reppucci V, Lincoff A. Air travel with intraocular gas. I. The mechanisms for compensation. Arch Ophthalmol. 1989;107(6):902–6.
19. Lincoff H, Weinberger D, Stergiu P. Air travel with intraocular gas. II. Clinical considerations. Arch Ophthalmol. 1989;107(6):907–10.
20. Aronowitz JD, Brubaker RF. Effect of intraocular gas on intraocular pressure. Arch Ophthalmol. 1976;94(7):1191–6.
21. Fu AD, McDonald HR, Eliott D, Fuller DG, Halperin LS, Ramsay RC, et al. Complications of general anesthesia using nitrous oxide in eyes with preexisting gas bubbles. Retina. 2002;22(5):569–74.
22. Mostafa SM, Wong SH, Snowdon SL, Ansons AM, Kelly JM, McGalliard JN. Nitrous oxide and internal tamponade during vitrectomy. Br J Ophthalmol. 1991;75(12):726–8.
23. Scott IU, Flynn HW Jr, Murray TG, Smiddy WE, Davis JL, Feuer WJ. Outcomes of complex retinal detachment repair using 1000- vs 5000-centistoke silicone oil. Arch Ophthalmol. 2005;123(4):473–8.
24. Lakits A, Nennadal T, Scholda C, Knaus S, Gruber H. Chemical stability of silicone oil in the human eye after prolonged clinical use. Ophthalmology. 1999;106(6):1091–100.
25. Honavar SG, Goyal M, Majji AB, Sen PK, Naduvilath T, Dandona L. Glaucoma after pars plana vitrectomy and silicone oil injection for complicated retinal detachments. Ophthalmology. 1999;106(1):169–76.
26. Madreperla SA, McCuen BW. Inferior peripheral iridectomy in patients receiving silicone oil. Rates of postoperative closure and effect on oil position. Retina. 1995;15(2):87–90.
27. Elliott AJ, Bacon AS, Scott JD. The superior peripheral iridectomy: prevention of pupil block due to silicone oil. Eye. 1990;4(Pt 1):226–9.
28. Jackson TL, Thiagarajan M, Murthy R, Snead MP, Wong D, Williamson TH. Pupil block glaucoma in phakic and pseudophakic patients after vitrectomy with silicone oil injection. Am J Ophthalmol. 2001;132(3):414–6.
29. Herbert EN, Habib M, Steel D, Williamson TH. Central scotoma associated with intraocular silicone oil tamponade develops before oil removal. Graefes Arch Clin Exp Ophthalmol. 2006;244(2):248–52.
30. Herbert EN, Laidlaw DA, Williamson TH, Habib M, Steel D. Loss of vision once silicone oil has been removed. Retina. 2005;25(6):808–9.
31. Herbert EN, Liew SH, Williamson TH. Visual loss after silicone oil removal. Br J Ophthalmol. 2005;89(12):1667–8.
32. Newsom RS, Johnston R, Sullivan P, Aylward B, Holder G, Gregor Z. Visual loss following silicone oil removal. Br J Ophthalmol. 2005;89(12):1668.
33. Wong R, De Luca M, Shunmugam M, Williamson T, Laidlaw A, Vaccaro V. Visual outcome after removal of silicone oil in patients undergoing retinectomy for complex retinal detachment. Int J Ophthalmol. 2016;9(1):108–10. https://doi.org/10.18240/ijo.2016.01.18.
34. Herbert EN, Williamson TH. Combined removal of silicone oil plus internal search (ROSO-plus) following retinal detachment surgery. Eye. 2007;21(7):925–9. 6702341 [pii]. https://doi.org/10.1038/sj.eye.6702341.
35. Herbert EN, Habib M, Steel D, Williamson TH. Central scotoma associated with intraocular silicone oil tamponade develops before oil removal. Graefes Arch Clin Exp Ophthalmol. 2006;244(2):248–52. https://doi.org/10.1007/s00417-005-0076-6.

36. Dogramaci M, Williams K, Lee E, Williamson TH. Foveal light exposure is increased at the time of removal of silicone oil with the potential for phototoxicity. Graefes Arch Clin Exp Ophthalmol. 2013;251(1):35–9. https://doi.org/10.1007/s00417-012-2033-5.
37. Yamada K, Kaneko H, Tsunekawa T, Shimizu H, Suzumura A, Namba R, et al. Silicone oil-associated retinal light exposure under a surgical microscope. Acta Ophthalmol. 2019;97(5):e742–e6. https://doi.org/10.1111/aos.14038.
38. Feng X, Li C, Zheng Q, Qian XG, Shao W, Li Y, et al. Risk of silicone oil as vitreous tamponade in pars plana vitrectomy: a systematic review and meta-analysis. Retina. 2017;37(11):1989–2000. https://doi.org/10.1097/iae.0000000000001553.
39. Shalchi Z, Mahroo OA, Shunmugam M, Mohamed M, Sullivan PM, Williamson TH. Spectral domain optical coherence tomography findings in long-term silicone oil-related visual loss. Retina. 2015;35(3):555–63. https://doi.org/10.1097/IAE.0000000000000325.
40. Mojsiewicz-Pienkowska K, Jamrogiewicz M, Szymkowska K, Krenczkowska D. Direct human contact with siloxanes (silicones) – safety or risk part 1. Characteristics of siloxanes (silicones). Front Pharmacol. 2016;7:132. https://doi.org/10.3389/fphar.2016.00132.
41. Morescalchi F, Costagliola C, Duse S, Gambicorti E, Parolini B, Arcidiacono B, et al. Heavy silicone oil and intraocular inflammation. Biomed Res Int. 2014;2014:574825. https://doi.org/10.1155/2014/574825.
42. Savion N, Alhalel A, Treister G, Bartov E. Role of blood components in ocular silicone oil emulsification. Studies on an in vitro model. Invest Ophthalmol Vis Sci. 1996;37(13):2694–9.
43. Mendichi R, Schieroni AG, Piovani D, Allegrini D, Ferrara M, Romano MR. Comparative study of chemical composition, molecular and rheological properties of silicone oil medical devices. Transl Vis Sci Technol. 2019;8(5):9. https://doi.org/10.1167/tvst.8.5.9.
44. Romano MR, Ferrara M, Gatto C, Giurgola L, Zanoni M, Angi M, et al. Safety of silicone oils as intraocular medical device: an in vitro cytotoxicity study. Exp Eye Res. 2020;194:108018. https://doi.org/10.1016/j.exer.2020.108018.
45. Dresp JH, Menz DH. Preparation and processing of vitreoretinal instrumentation and equipment as a risk factor for silicone oil emulsification. Retina. 2004;24(1):110–5. https://doi.org/10.1097/00006982-200402000-00015.
46. Williams RL, Day M, Garvey MJ, English R, Wong D. Increasing the extensional viscosity of silicone oil reduces the tendency for emulsification. Retina. 2010;30(2):300–4. https://doi.org/10.1097/IAE.0b013e3181babe0c.
47. Peyman GA, Schulman JA, Sullivan B. Perfluorocarbon liquids in ophthalmology. Surv Ophthalmol. 1995;39(5):375–95.
48. Pastor JC, Coco RM, Fernandez-Bueno I, Alonso-Alonso ML, Medina J, Sanz-Arranz A, et al. Acute retinal damage after using a toxic perfluoro-octane for vitreo-retinal surgery. Retina. 2017;37(6):1140–51. https://doi.org/10.1097/IAE.0000000000001680.
49. Romano MR, Ferrara M, Gatto C, Ferrari B, Giurgola L, D'Amato Tothova J. Evaluation of cytotoxicity of perfluorocarbons for intraocular use by cytotoxicity test in vitro in cell lines and human donor retina ex vivo. Transl Vis Sci Technol. 2019;8(5):24. https://doi.org/10.1167/tvst.8.5.24.
50. Ruzza P, Gatto C, Ragazzi E, Romano MR, Honisch C, Tothova JD. H-content is not predictive of perfluorocarbon ocular endotamponade cytotoxicity in vitro. ACS Omega. 2019;4(8):13481–7. https://doi.org/10.1021/acsomega.9b01793.
51. Veckeneer MA, de Voogd S, Lindstedt EW, Menz DH, van Meurs JC. An epidemic of sticky silicone oil at the Rotterdam Eye Hospital. Patient review and chemical analyses. Graefes Arch Clin Exp Ophthalmol. 2008;246(6):917–22. https://doi.org/10.1007/s00417-008-0768-9.
52. Friberg TR, Siska PE, Somayajula K, Williams J, Eller AW. Interactions of perfluorocarbon liquids and silicone oil as characterized by mass spectrometry. Graefes Arch Clin Exp Ophthalmol. 2003;241(10):809–15. https://doi.org/10.1007/s00417-003-0698-5.
53. Romano MR, Vallejo-Garcia JL, Parmeggiani F, Romano V, Vinciguerra P. Interaction between perfluorcarbon liquid and heavy silicone oil: risk factor for "sticky oil" formation. Curr Eye Res. 2012;37(7):563–6. https://doi.org/10.3109/02713683.2012.669511 .
54. Hutton WL, Azen SP, Blumenkranz MS, Lai MY, McCuen BW, Han DP, et al. The effects of silicone oil removal. Silicone Study Report 6. Arch Ophthalmol. 1994;112(6):778–85.
55. Lam RF, Cheung BT, Yuen CY, Wong D, Lam DS, Lai WW. Retinal redetachment after silicone oil removal in proliferative vitreoretinopathy: a prognostic factor analysis. Am J Ophthalmol. 2008;145(3):527–33. S0002-9394(07)00922-1 [pii]. https://doi.org/10.1016/j.ajo.2007.10.015.
56. Falkner CI, Binder S, Kruger A. Outcome after silicone oil removal. Br J Ophthalmol. 2001;85(11):1324–7.
57. Jonas JB, Knorr HL, Rank RM, Budde WM. Retinal redetachment after removal of intraocular silicone oil tamponade. Br J Ophthalmol. 2001;85(10):1203–7.
58. Casswell AG, Gregor ZJ. Silicone oil removal. II. Operative and postoperative complications. Br J Ophthalmol. 1987;71(12):898–902.
59. Laidlaw DA, Karia N, Bunce C, Aylward GW, Gregor ZJ. Is prophylactic 360-degree laser retinopexy protective? Risk factors for retinal redetachment after removal of silicone oil. Ophthalmology. 2002;109(1):153–8.
60. Avitabile T, Longo A, Lentini G, Reibaldi A. Retinal detachment after silicone oil removal is prevented by 360 degrees laser treatment. Br J Ophthalmol. 2008;92(11):1479–82. bjo.2008.140087 [pii]. https://doi.org/10.1136/bjo.2008.140087.
61. Wickham L, Tranos P, Hiscott P, Charteris D. The use of silicone oil-RMN3 (Oxane HD) as heavier-than-water internal tamponade in complicated inferior retinal detachment surgery. Graefes Arch Clin Exp Ophthalmol. 2010;248(9):1225–31. https://doi.org/10.1007/s00417-010-1358-1.
62. Chang S. Perfluorocarbon liquids in vitreoretinal surgery. Int Ophthalmol Clin. 1992;32(2):153–63.

Posterior Vitreous Detachment

5

Contents

Introduction

Posterior vitreous detachment is the commonest and most important event that occurs in the vitreous. As the vitreous ages, the normal architectural features apparent in childhood gradually disappear as degeneration causes syneresis, lacuna (cavity) formation and collapse of the vitreous gel. The collagen fibrils disintegrate and aggregate giving rise to symptomatic floaters [1, 2]. There is a loss of sodium hyaluronate [3] and an increase in vitreous mobility with age [4].

Most individuals will develop posterior vitreous detachment (separation of the posterior hyaloid membrane from the internal limiting membrane), without symptoms or pathological sequelae, usually between the ages of 40–80 years. 27% of patients in their seventh decade and 63% in their eighth decade have PVD [5]. This may occur at a younger age (less than 40 years old) in myopia, diabetes, retinal vascular disorders, trauma and retinitis pigmentosa [6–11]. Presentation with symptomatic PVD (flashes and floaters) may be more common in females than males and in myopia [12].

The detached posterior hyaloid membrane becomes wrinkled and usually separates completely from the retina up to the posterior border of the vitreous base (or up to the posterior aspect of any other vitreoretinal adhesions, which may be present). Acute ischaemic events such as retinal vein occlusion may induce PVD with an increased prevalence of PVD 1 year after the onset of the vein occlusion [13]. No racial differences in the rates of PVD have been found between whites and oriental peoples with disagreement whether black races have less PVD [14–16]. The fellow eye has evidence of PVD in 90% in 3 years [17] with 11% developing symptomatic PVD in the other eye in 2 years often demonstrating similar problems to the first eye such as tears or vitreous haemorrhage [18]. It is thought that the posterior hyaloid membrane is part of the internal limiting membrane, which has separated [19].

PVD is the primary process in the development of most rhegmatogenous retinal detachments because of its role in retinal tear formation. It is also implicated in common macular disorders, such as macular pucker and macular hole formation. Separation of the gel may also tear blood vessels in the retina or in neovascular complexes causing haemorrhaging into the vitreous cavity. The importance of PVD has led many investigators to try methods for the artificial inducement of PVD [20–27], such as plasmin injection as a proteolytic acting on the vitreoretinal interface (Figs. 5.1, 5.2, 5.3).

1. The posterior hyaloid membrane consists of type IV collagen [28].

T. H. Williamson, *Vitreoretinal Surgery*, https://doi.org/10.1007/978-3-030-68769-4_5

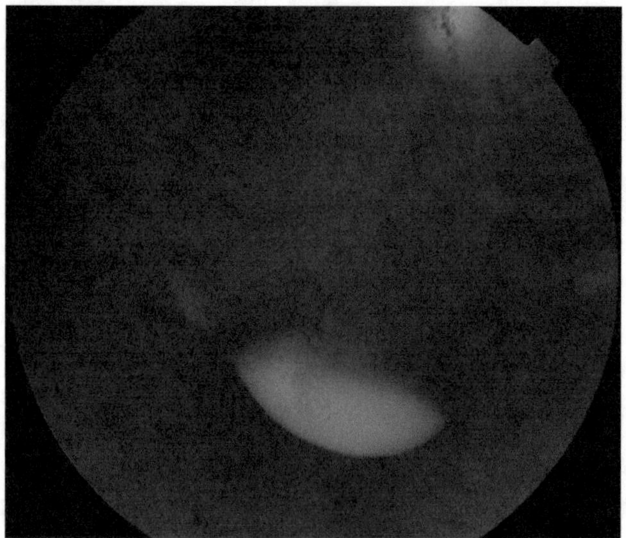

Fig. 5.1 Syneresis of the vitreous causes lacuna formation, in this figure, the presence of a lacuna is demonstrated by the fluid level of old altered blood which is trapped inside a lacuna cavity

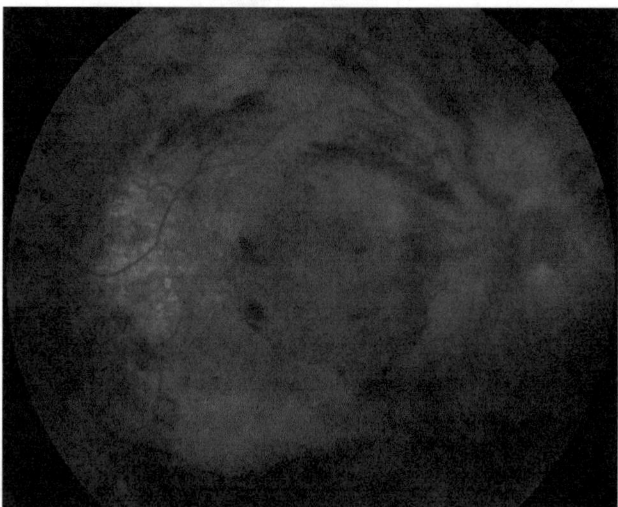

Fig. 5.2 A 13-year-old girl with CRVO in whom the onset was associated with a bout of diarrhoea on ski trip and a short-haul plane journey. She had a familial cholesterolaemia

2. The vitreoretinal adhesions at the vitreous base move gradually posteriorly as the eye ages [29].
3. Epipapillary glial tissue can become avulsed from the disc margin during vitreous detachment and may be seen in ophthalmoscopy as a small ring of tissue in front of the optic disc (Weiss ring). The ring is often incomplete and is absent in 13% of PVDs [30, 31] (Fig. 5.4).

Patients often notice a floater in their vision, describing it as a "cobweb," or "spider" or "fly" which moves with eye movements. OCT has revealed that many adults have an

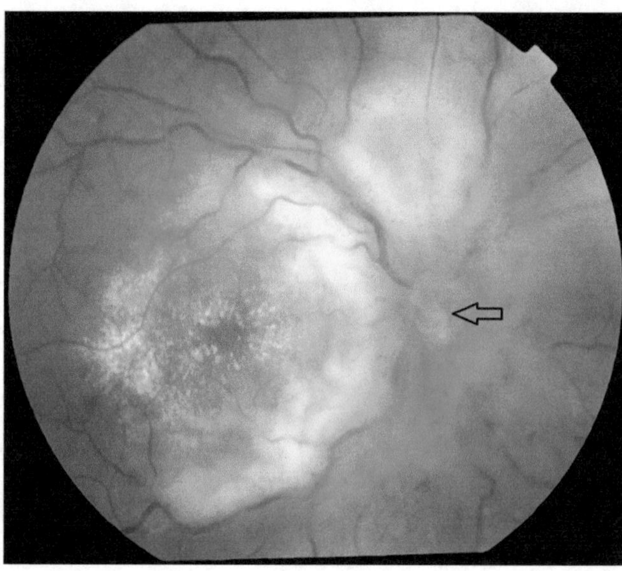

Fig. 5.3 At 2.5 months there is a Weiss ring visible in front of the disc demonstrating induction of a PVD by the CRVO

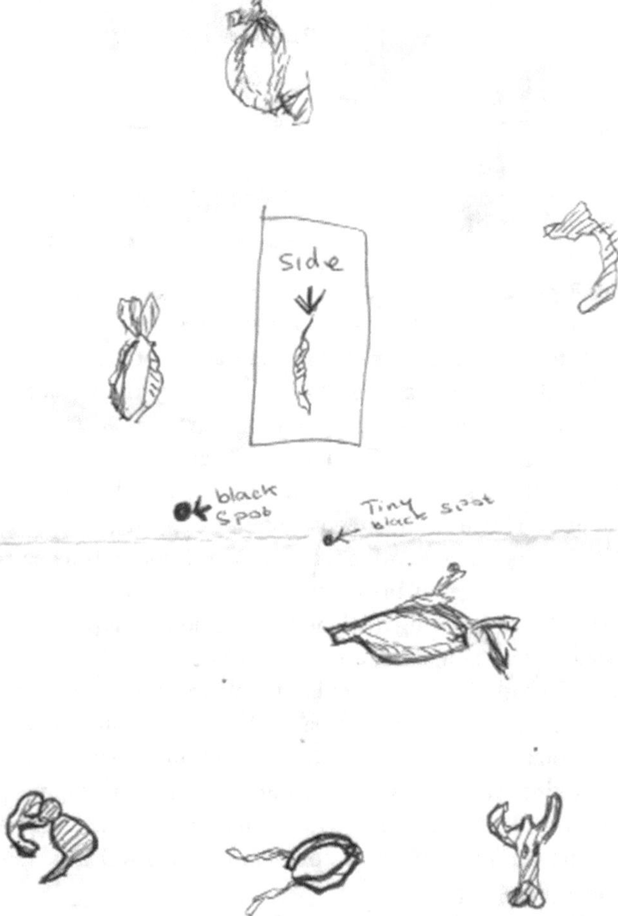

Fig. 5.4 One patient's drawing of his floaters from posterior vitreous detachment showing the Weiss ring moving around in the eye

Table 5.1 Vitreoretinal conditions and the vitreous

Vitreoretinal conditions and the vitreous	
Caused by age-related posterior vitreous detachment	Retinal breaks Rhegmatogenous retinal detachment Macular epiretinal membrane and Vitreomacular traction syndrome Macular hole Vitreous haemorrhage
Associated with pathological vitreous separation	Diabetic tractional retinal detachment Complications of posterior uveitis Trauma

incomplete PVD not visible on biomicroscopy but with separation of the posterior hyaloid membrane from the retina with residual attachments at the optic disc or the fovea [32] (Table 5.1).

Symptoms

Floaters

Floaters must be discriminated from paracentral scotomata. Ask the patient to describe the floater, which should have momentum as the eye moves, i.e. the floater will move with the eye but will continue to move when the eye stops before finally returning to its original position and resting there. In contrast, a scotoma remains in the same position (relative to fixation) in all positions of gaze. The patient may also describe the floater as something in front of the vision or "in the way" of the vision. Scotomata are commonly negative, that is, there is vision missing in the area, but the patient is not aware of the loss until tested (the physiological blind spot, glaucomatous loss). Positive scotomata that the patient is aware of occurs in migraine and retinal inflammation.

Floaters can be described as a cobweb, veils, a ring, spot or multiple spots. These come from the thickened posterior hyaloid membrane, Weiss ring or cells that have been dispersed into the vitreous. Floaters that occur before the age of forty years and are chronic in the presentation are most often due to vitreous degeneration without posterior vitreous detachment. However, it may only take a single floater of recent onset to indicate the development of a posterior vitreous detachment.

Small dark round floaters are usually cells in the vitreous. These may be red blood cells which will usually clear rapidly. Other cells like white cells may indicate inflammation from other conditions and will not clear so rapidly. Post vitrectomy patients may see small dark round floaters, which are inflammatory cells that will disappear eventually.

It is worth remembering, in case a vitrectomy has been performed on floaters, that long-term, post vitrectomy eyes may have an occasional cell like this, pass through the eye.

The patient is often more bothered by a vague smear in the vision rather than floaters. The condensed vitreous fibrils and mobile posterior hyaloid membrane may be the source of this visual phenomenon. The eye with PVD may have subtly reduced vision, with PVD associated with reduced contrast sensitivity. Patients who have vitrectomy and can then look through water rather than old vitreous often not a considerable functional improvement (Figs. 5.5, 5.6, 5.7, 5.8).

Flashes

Introduction

Photopsia is the experience of light from non-photic stimulation. The first description in the modern era was from

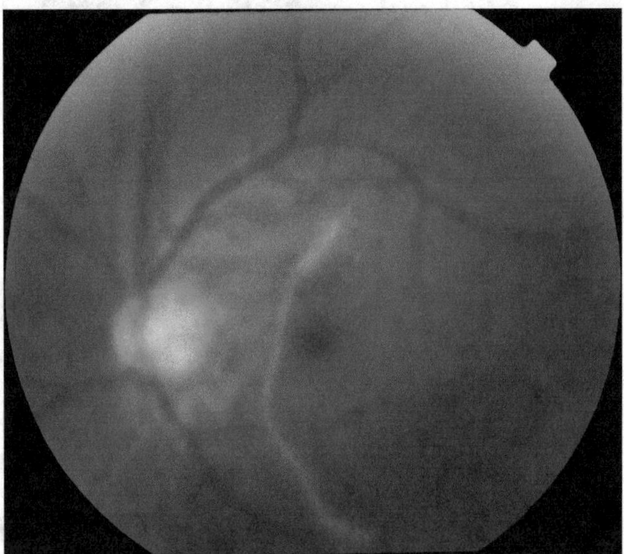

Fig. 5.5 Large "pipe-cleaner" shaped vitreous opacities can be seen in moderate or highly myopic eyes without the presence of PVD. If you operate to remove these for symptomatic reduction of floaters, be aware that a vitreoschisis must be looked for and removed, otherwise the posterior hyaloid may separate later and cause RRD, see Chap. 7

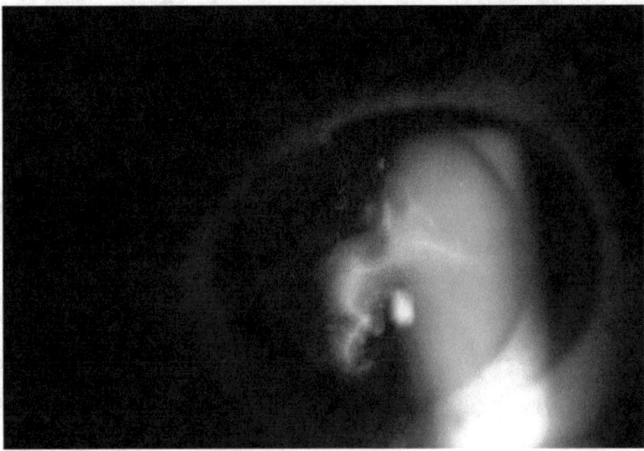

Fig. 5.6 If vitreous opacities are very symptomatic, these can be removed by vitrectomy. Beware of the high myope with apparent PVD who in fact has a vitreoschisis (see Chap. 6)

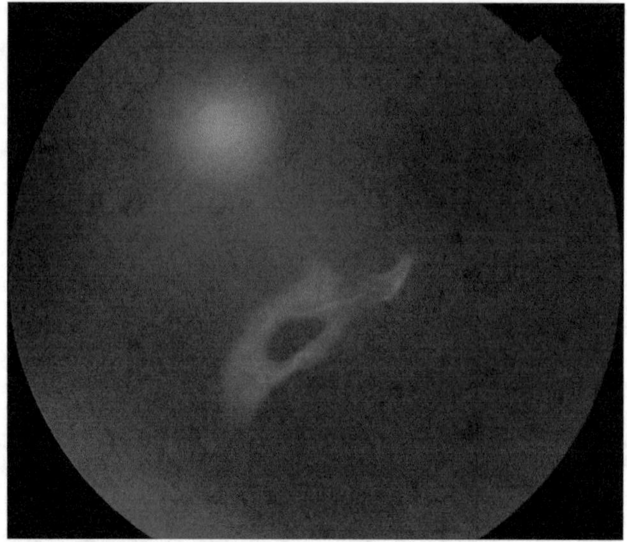

Fig. 5.7 A Weiss ring is apparent in this picture. A Weiss ring may take various forms in different eyes, and as the Weiss ring moves more anteriorly in the eye, it becomes less in focus and less noticeable by the patient

Purkinje in 1819 [33], who attributed it to traction. In 1935. 1940 Moore described "lightning streaks" [34] with a "flash-like appearance of the lights; their position, sometimes slanting but usually vertical, and almost always to the outer side of the eyes, persisting for periods of up to three months; and their association with the sudden development of muscae volitantes, or the presence of visible vitreous opacities."

In 1940 he added more cases using the term lightning flashes [35] and developed streaks in his own eye in 1947 [36]. He initially thought the phenomenon to be wholly benign, although he commented that.

"I used systematically to dilate the pupils and to take the visual fields in fear lest they might indicate some early organic retinal lesion, such as a commencing detachment, vascular disease, or perhaps an early neoplasm" [34].

The flashes were attributed to posterior vitreous detachment (PVD) by Verhoeff [37] in 1941 and the risk of retinal detachment associated with lightning flashes noted by Berens et al. [38] in 1954. In 2008 "black flashes" or negative flashes

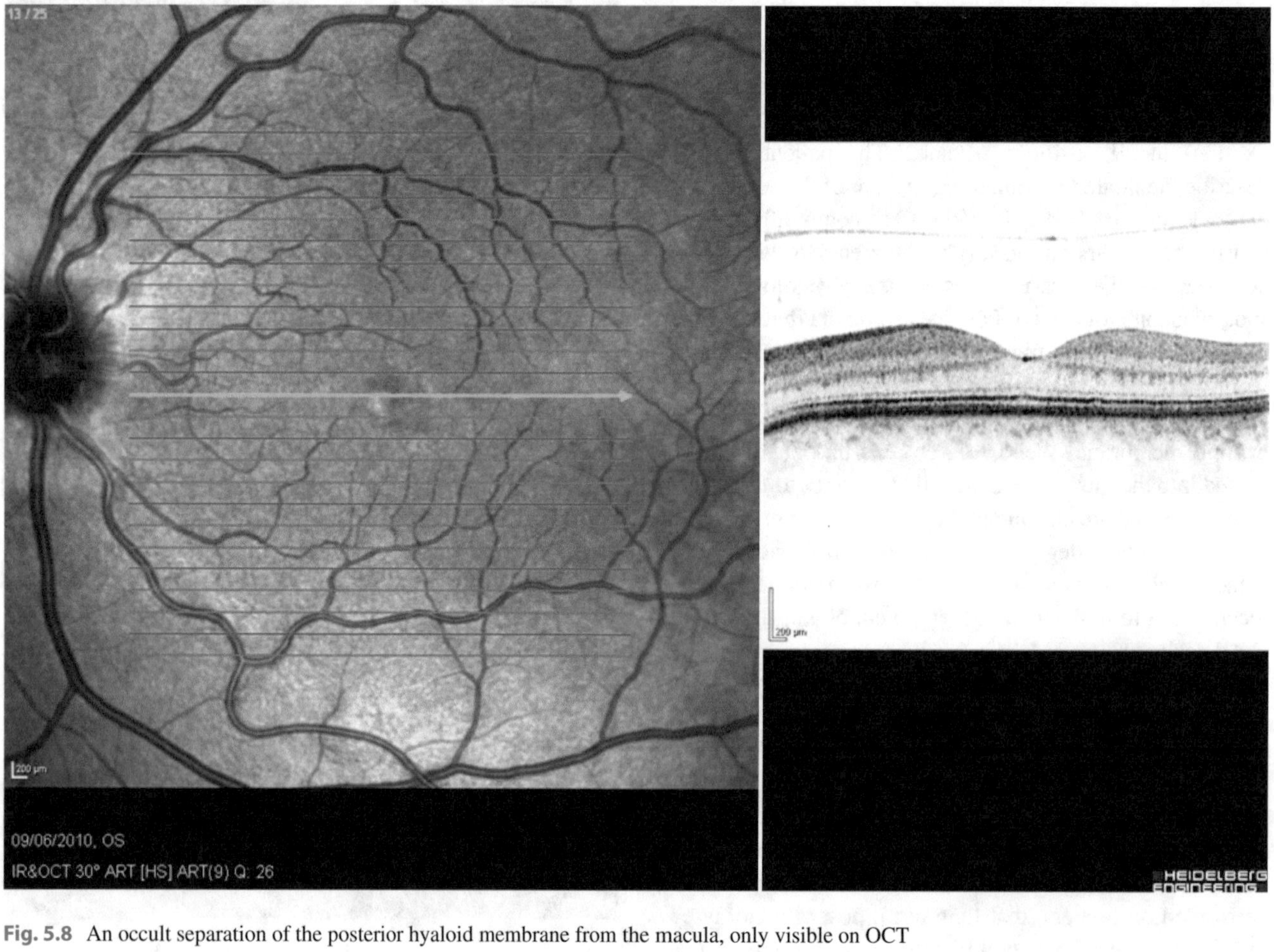

Fig. 5.8 An occult separation of the posterior hyaloid membrane from the macula, only visible on OCT

were described at the commencement of the PVD [39], which have been attributed to traction of the vitreous on the optic nerve head, see below.

Clinical Characteristics

Patients experience "lightning flashes" in the temporal periphery of their visual field that typically lasts a second at a time. Their exact pathogenesis is obscure but may be due to depolarisation of the receptors from tugging of the vitreous base on the retina or by the mobile vitreous impacting the retina on eye movements. If the patient produces repeated eye movements over a short time, the flashes gradually reduce in severity. This may be because the retina loses the ability to respond due to repeated depolarisation of the receptors. Sometimes they are better seen at night.

In some patients, black temporal flashes are seen for a few hours before the lightning flashes and floaters occur [39]. These are thought to be produced by the Weiss ring pulling on the optic nerve head before it separates. The forces applied in this way to the surface of the nerve head block axoplasmic flow in the superficial nerve fibres, thereby inducing a negative peripheral visual phenomenon. As soon as the Weiss ring separates, the symptoms change to floaters and lightning flashes.

Typically, the lightning flashes of PVD are vertical, temporally placed, and instantaneous flashes. If the flashes in a patient with PVD are oblique or horizontally orientated, not in the temporal visual field or not typical instantaneous flashes, the patient is more likely to have a PVD with a retinal tear or rhegmatogenous retinal detachment [40].

These visual phenomena should be discriminated from the flashes that occur with other disorders, such as the zigzag lights of migraine, flickering stars associated with occipital ischemia and the rare coloured lights of the acute zonal outer occult retinopathy (AZOOR) syndromes. Mostly these photopsia are centrally placed in the visual field and therefore can be easily discriminated.

Slower more mid-peripheral flashes are produced by the leading edge of some retinal detachments often shaped like a comet's tail.

Patients who experience symptoms during posterior vitreous separation have a 10% risk of developing a retinal tear [41–43].

Flashes from PVD usually subside in a few months whilst floaters get less but may not disappear entirely [44]. The floaters lessen as the opacities on the posterior surface of the vitreous sink lower in the eye but also because they move anteriorly and are less in focus than when they were nearer the inner surface of the retina. Severe floaters can be bothersome and, in a few patients, PPV is required to clear the vision.

Rarely flashes will persist for years, more often associated with vitreous attached young myope RRD (i.e. flashes associated with RRD rather than PVD) and rarely after PVD. Occasionally patients will have flashes after PPV (Figs. 5.9, 5.10, Table 5.2).

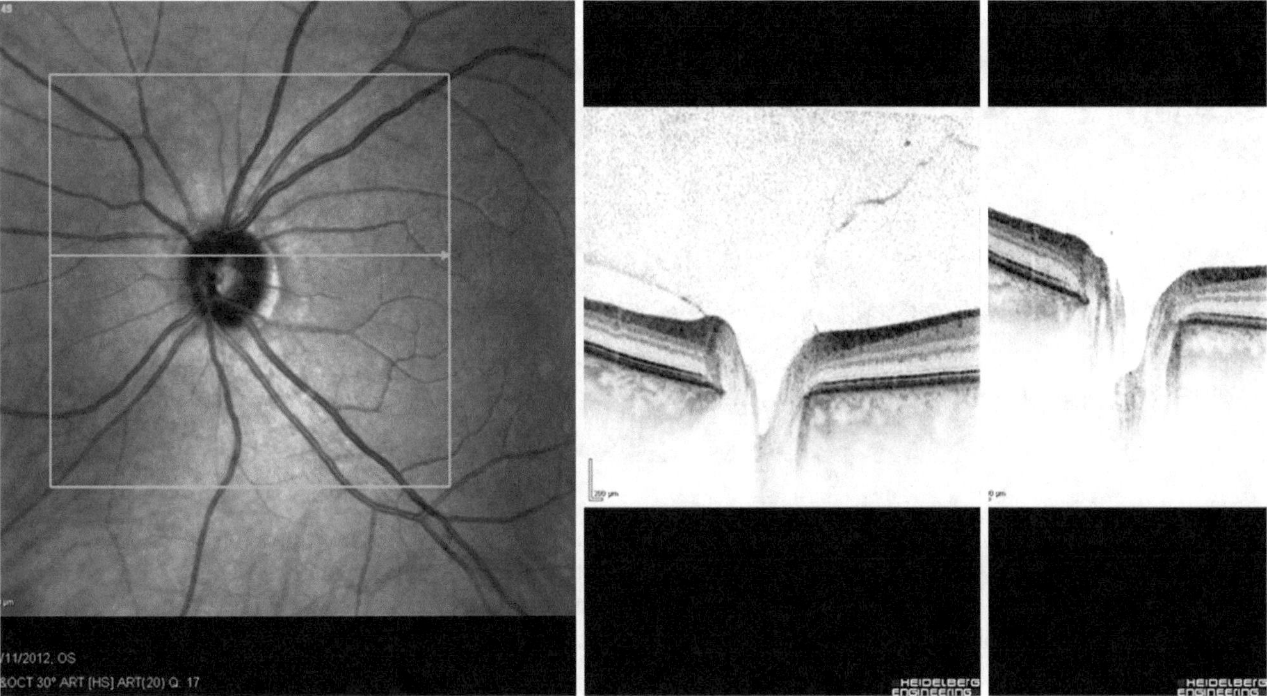

Fig. 5.9 This patient had black flashes from their PVD until the vitreous separated from the optic nerve head

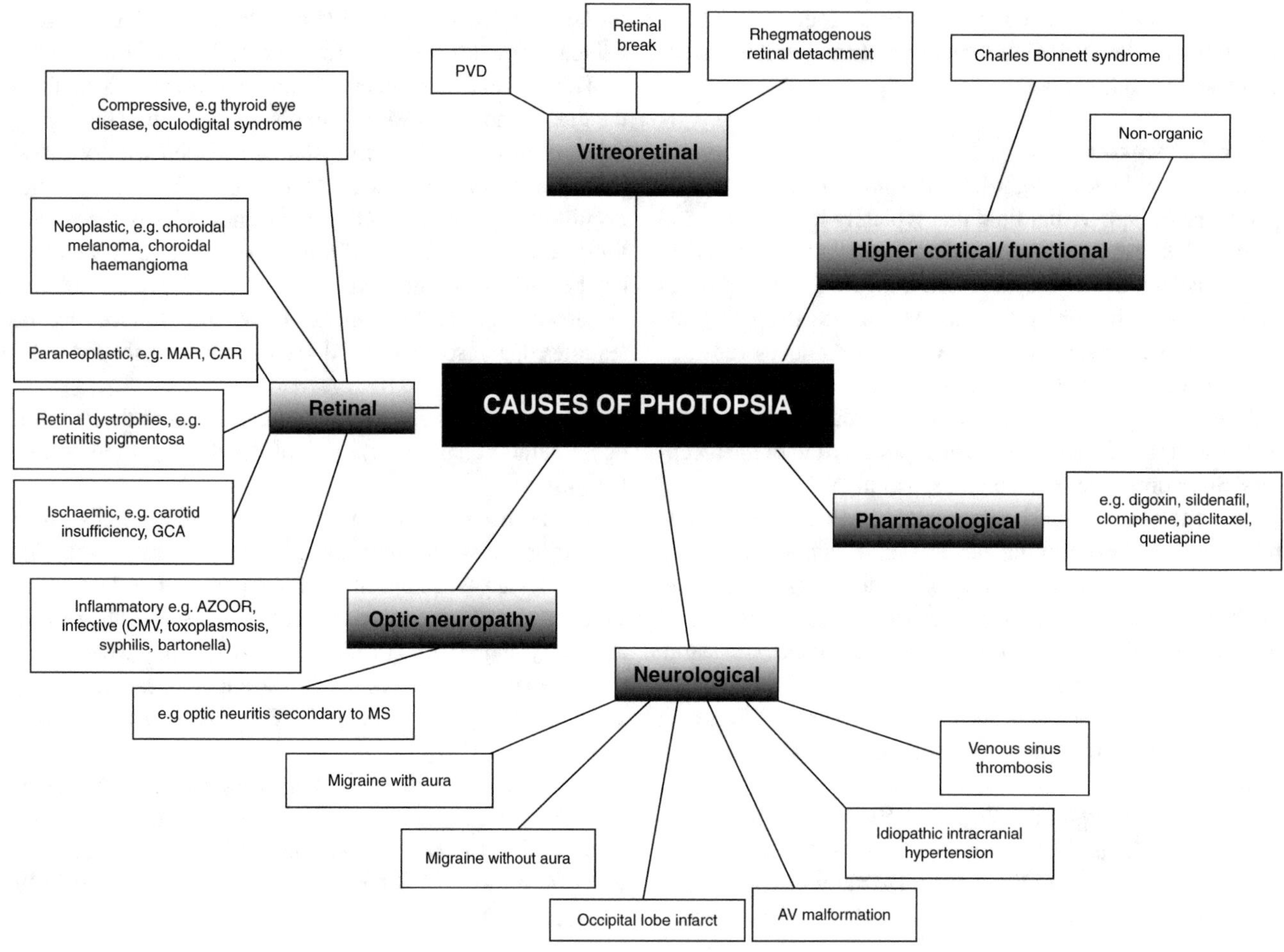

Fig. 5.10 There are multiple causes of photopsia

Table 5.2 Different presentations of flashes

Flashes							
Diagnosis	Duration	Colour	Location	Shape	Stimulus	Other symptoms	Flickering
PVD	Seconds or less	White	Temporal Periphery	Crescentic vertical	Eye Movements	Floaters	No
Migraine	20–30 minutes	Not typically	Paracentral	Arcuate Zigzag	Stress, Food	Scotoma Headache Nausea	Yes
Occipital Ischemia	Minutes	Nil	Central	Petaloid	Neck Movements Exertion		Yes
Cystoid Macular Oedema	Constant	Variable	Central	Pinpricks	Nil	Poor Vision	Yes
Outer retinal or RPE abnormality	Minutes	Blue Purple	Paracentral	Blobs Spirals	Nil	Scotoma	No
Retinal Detachment	Seconds	Golden	Central/ Paracentral	Comet oblique horizontal	Eye Movements	Visual Field Loss	No

Signs

Detection of PVD

A posterior vitreous detachment can be diagnosed by examining the eye with a 90-dioptre lens. Definitively if a Weiss ring is present, then a PVD has occurred. Sometimes this is not obvious, but it is possible to see the posterior hyaloid membrane. This is more subjective, but it can be reassuring to observe the space behind the membrane, if this is optically clear, it suggests that there is no vitreous gel at this location (Figs. 5.11 and 5.12).

A partial posterior vitreous detachment is a diagnosis that should be made only with care. It can be extremely difficult to determine whether there are remaining vitreous attach-

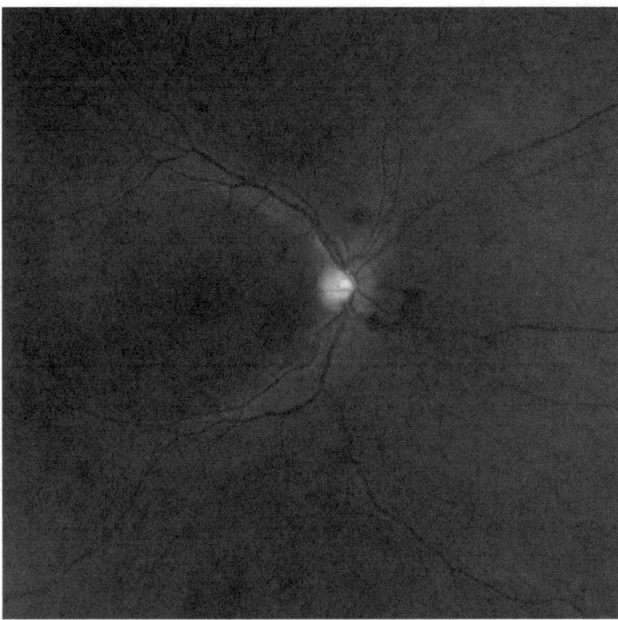

Fig. 5.11 A Weis ring on optomap wide image

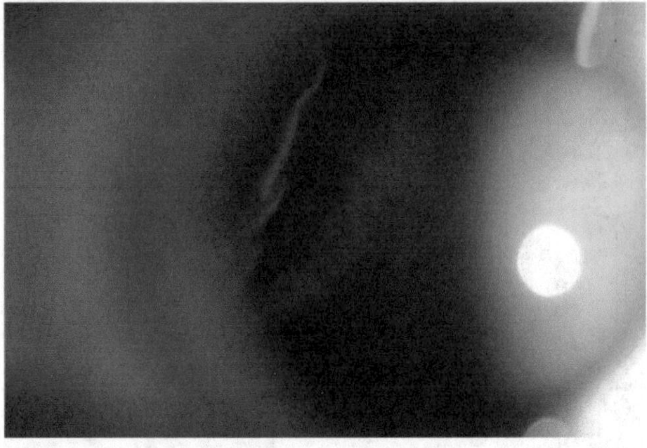

Fig. 5.12 In an eye with forward displacement of a PVD, the posterior hyaloid membrane can be seen in the anterior vitreous cavity

ments. Likely residual attachments are at the optic disc, chorioretinal scars and epiretinal membranes at the macula and neovascular tissue.

Usually a posterior vitreous detachment occurs completely, soon after the onset of symptoms, probably in a few hours. There remain a few patients in whom the posterior vitreous detachment progresses over a few weeks, as evidenced by the formation of new retinal breaks in the first 6 weeks after onset of symptoms in 1.8–3.4% [45].

Shafer's Sign

In most patients with tears, retinal pigment epithelial cells, released through the tear, will be visible in the anterior vitreous (Shafer's sign). This is highly predictive of a retinal tear (approximately 90%) [42, 46–49] (Figs. 5.13 and 5.14).

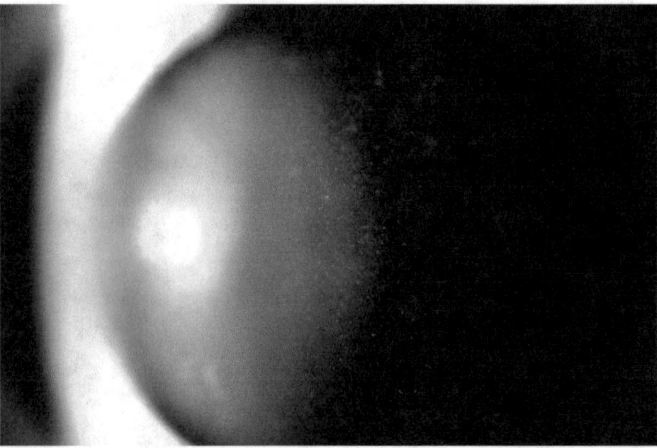

Fig. 5.13 Pigment granules in the vitreous are good indicators of the presence of a retinal tear from PVD

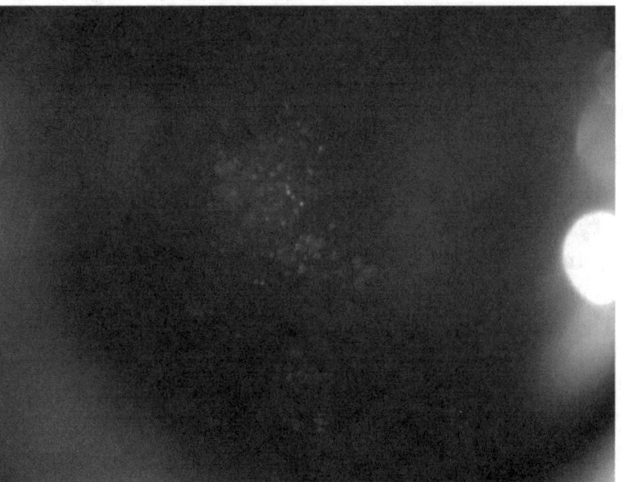

Fig. 5.14 Pigment granules in Shafer's sign

In symptomatic PVD, 10% of patients will develop retinal tears. Most tears are present when the patient presents; however, 10% of tears are be detected at six weeks from the onset of symptoms (constituting theoretically 1% of all cases with symptomatic PVD) [47, 50]. Breaks found in asymptomatic eyes are less likely to lead to retinal detachment [51].

The pigment granules in Shafer's sign are relatively large (diameter of 30–50 μm), pigmented and are seen in the anterior vitreous especially often inferiorly. The patient, therefore, should be examined during eye movements allowing the inferior vitreous to present itself for examination in the pupil. Only one granule is required to make the diagnosis of Shafer's sign and indicate the risk of a retinal tear.

Vitreous Haemorrhage

Red blood cells (RBCs), which are small 6–8 μm, may also be seen and should also raise suspicion of pathology, although this is less indicative than pigment granules with 50% of patients with RBCs in vitreous having retinal tears.

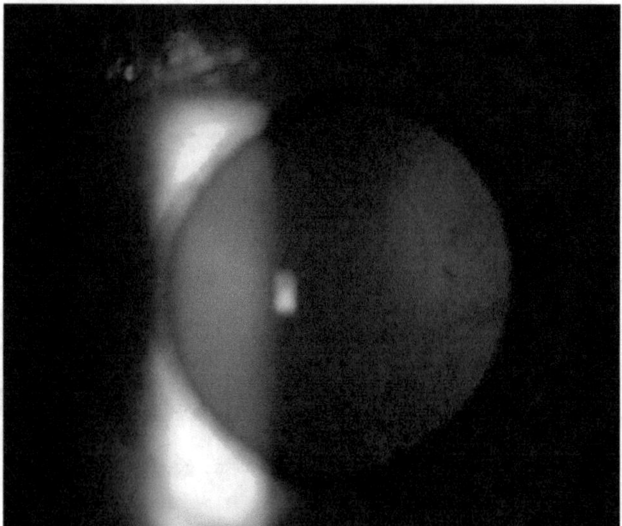

Fig. 5.15 Erythrocytes in the vitreous indicate a 50% of finding and retinal break in an acute PVD

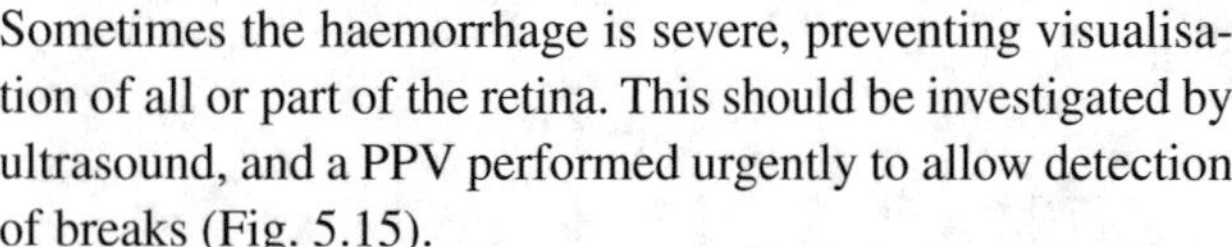

Sometimes the haemorrhage is severe, preventing visualisation of all or part of the retina. This should be investigated by ultrasound, and a PPV performed urgently to allow detection of breaks (Fig. 5.15).

In some patients, a superior break might be seen, but the inferior retina be obscured by inferior vitreous haemorrhage. The surgeon may be tempted to laser the superior break and observe. However, because of the chance of multiple breaks (approximately 50–60%) and the suspected increased risk of PVR, in the presence of haemorrhage it is safer to proceed to PPV, allowing examination of the inferior retina (also see Chap. 5).

Ophthalmoscopy

Note The patient requires 360° examination of the retina with indirect ophthalmoscopy and indentation of the far periphery.

This aids identification of breaks both by introducing the peripheral retina into the view but also allowing a dynamic observation of a break. The break can be opened and more clearly seen by the movement of the retina. Moving the choroid under the break changes the colour of the choroid seen through the orifice of the break, discriminating a break from retinal haemorrhage or pigmentation, which remains the same colour despite indentation.

If a patient presents early with PVD, it is worth re-examining the retina at 6 weeks after symptoms occur because 1.8% to 3.4% will have tears seen at the second examination that were not seen at the first [52]. If patients have a vitreous haemorrhage, retinal haemorrhage or develop new symptoms, they may be more likely to have breaks seen at the second examination (Figs. 5.16 and 5.17).

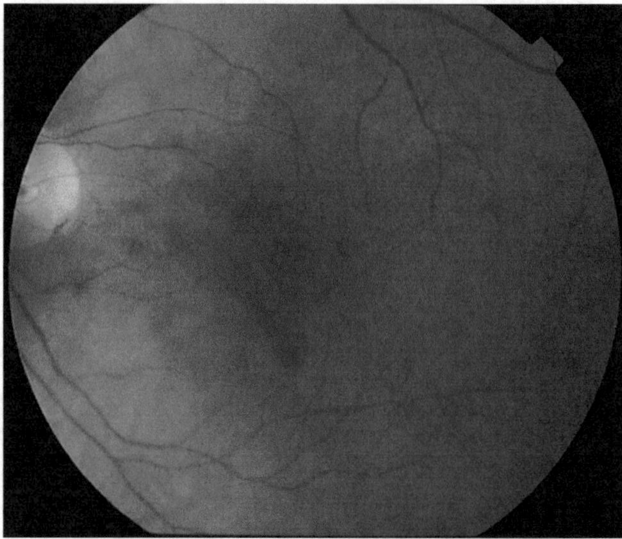

Fig. 5.16 Posterior vitreous detachment can cause a macular haemorrhage from traction on the retina as it detaches, rupturing small blood vessels on the surface

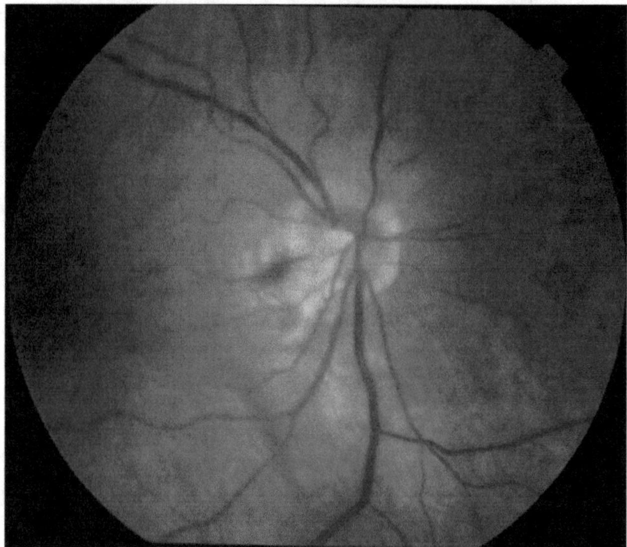

Fig. 5.17 A haemorrhage has occurred at the optic disc in a patient with posterior vitreous detachment

Note if a patient presents early with PVD symptoms of a few days another examination at 1–2 weeks is useful.

	Odds ratio for detection of a retinal break [45]	95% Confidence interval
Subjective vision reduction	5.0	3.1–8.1
Vitreous haemorrhage	10	5.1–20
Absence of vitreous pigmentation	0.23	0.12–0.43

Other signs

PVD may induce optic disc haemorrhages (causing subtle visual field loss) [53, 54], or retinal haemorrhages in the periphery or in the macula [55, 56] (Figs. 5.18, 5.19, 5.20).

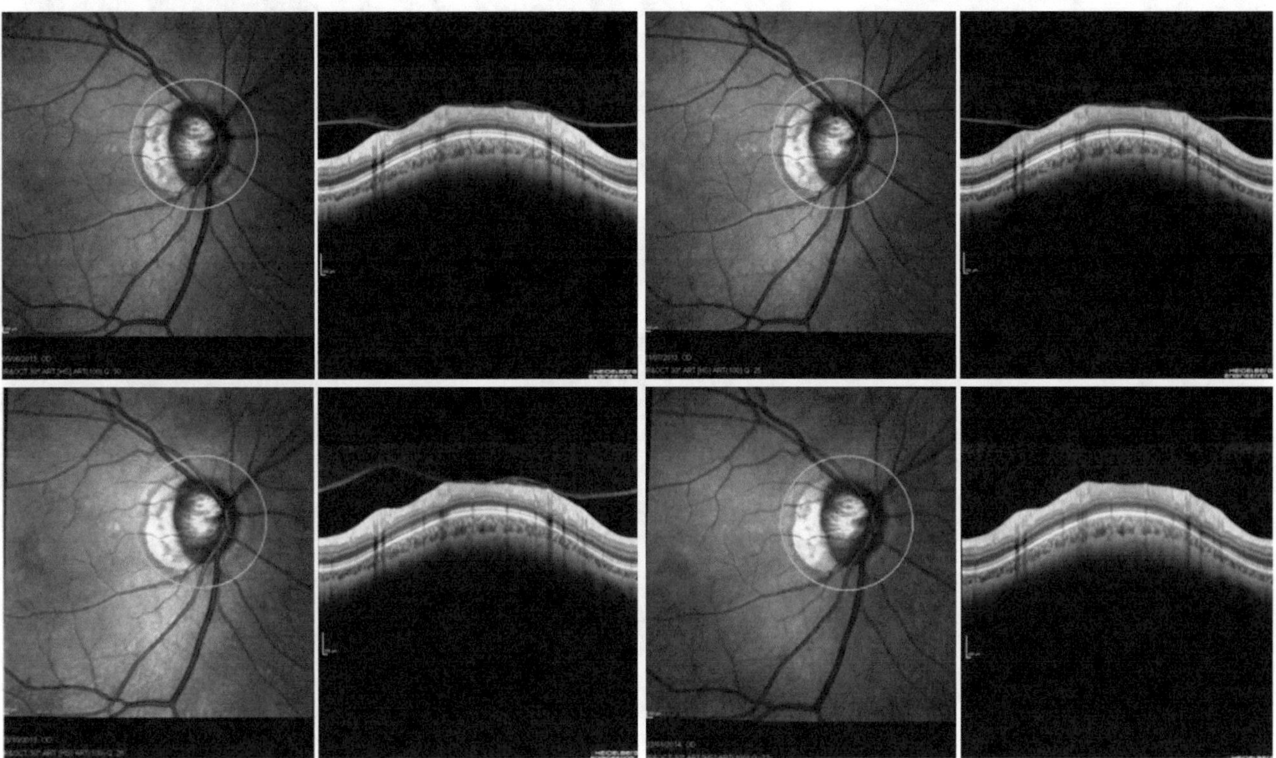

Fig. 5.18 Progressive separation of the vitreous from the disc confirming PVD

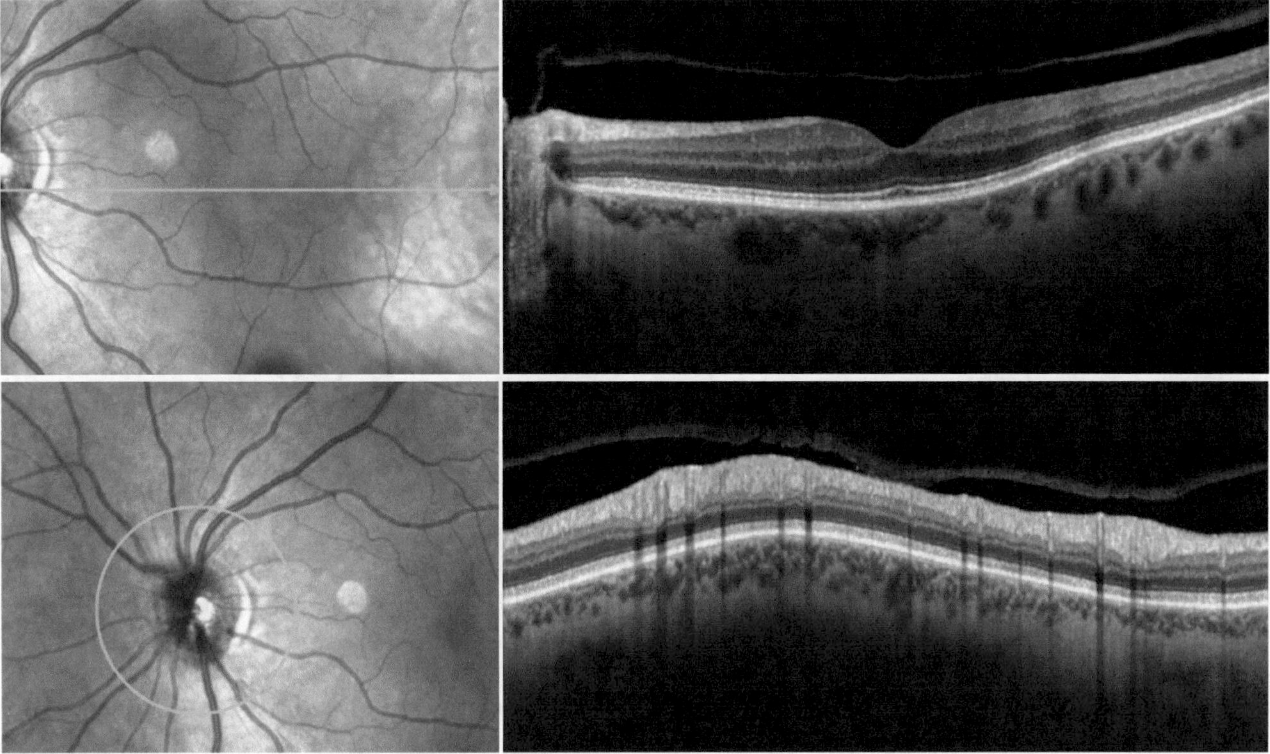

Fig. 5.19 Vitreous almost separated from the posterior pole

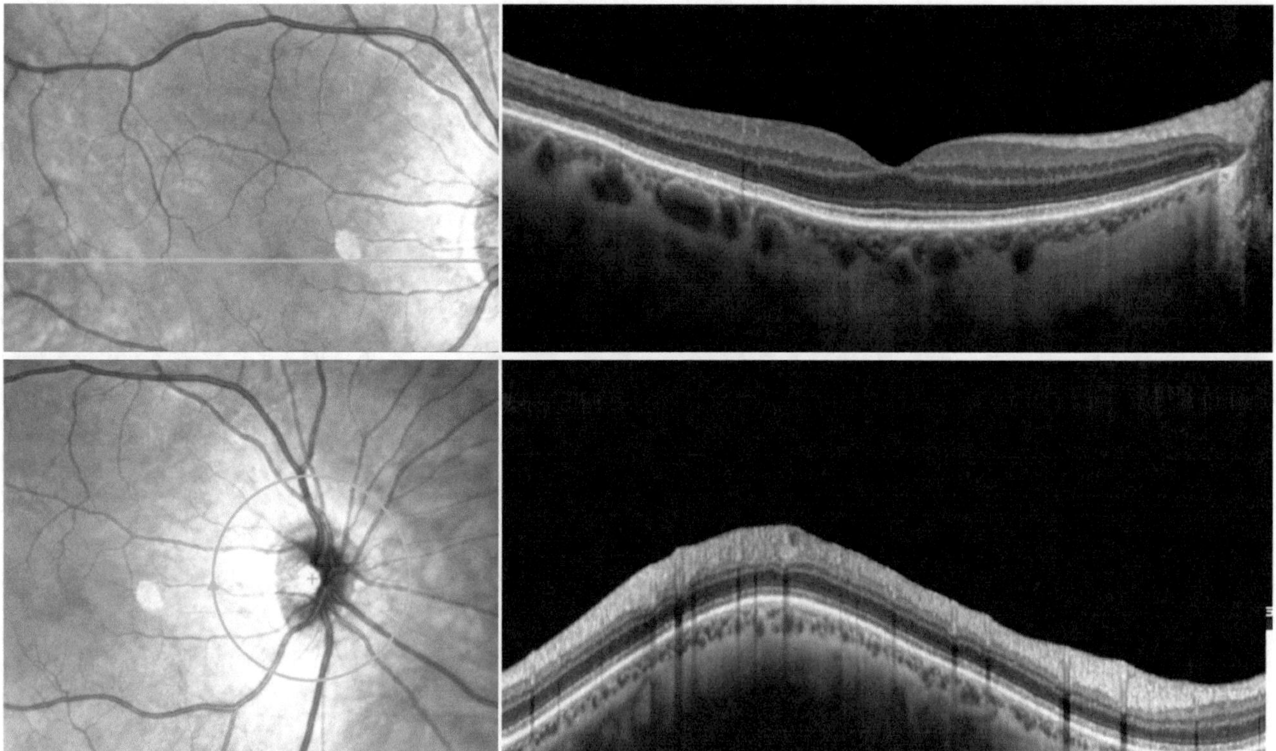

Fig. 5.20 Absence of vitreous confirms posterior vitreous detachment

Retinal Breaks

U Tears

All U tears (or breaks caused by PVD) require treatment by retinopexy, either by laser or cryotherapy. These present with the base of their flaps anteriorly in the direction of the traction of the vitreous. Any retinopexy must surround the whole tear. Tears close to the ora serrata can be treated by retinopexy around the tear and up to the ora serrata. Retinopexy should be performed soon after the diagnosis has been made, e.g. the same day, and subsequent reviews are merely to determine that the retinopexy is adequately encompassing the defect. Retinopexy should be secure after 2 weeks (Fig. 5.21).

Posteriorly placed holes can be treated easily with laser therapy employing a contact lens or a super field lens. More anterior tears require indirect laser ophthalmoscopy and indentation. Alternatively, cryotherapy retinopexy can be applied with a subconjunctival or localised peribulbar local anaesthetic injection in the region of the eye to be treated (Figs. 5.22, 5.23, 5.24).

Note Retinal tears are often multiple (50–60% of eyes), and therefore the surgeon must not be distracted, by finding one tear from examining the rest of the retina for any more tears (Figs. 5.25 and 5.26).

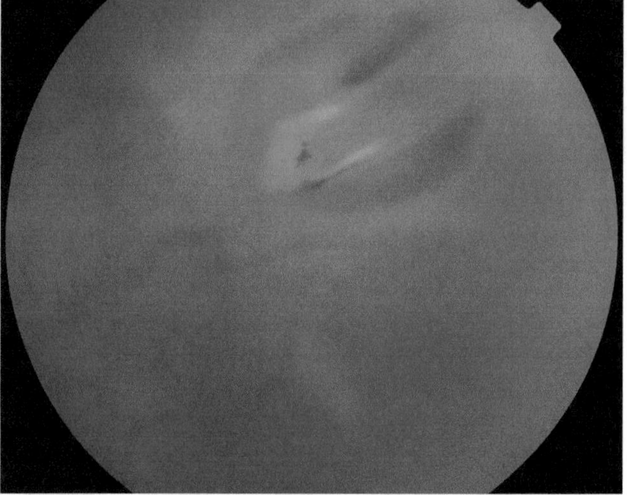

Fig. 5.21 A U tear with a prominent flap

Atrophic Round Holes

Round holes are often seen in asymptomatic eyes associated with snail track or lattice degeneration. These are not associated with posterior vitreous detachment. The work of Norman Byers suggests that these holes do not need to be treated because any retinal detachment associated with these in an asymptomatic eye is unlikely to be progressive with an approximate risk of 1:200 [57, 58].

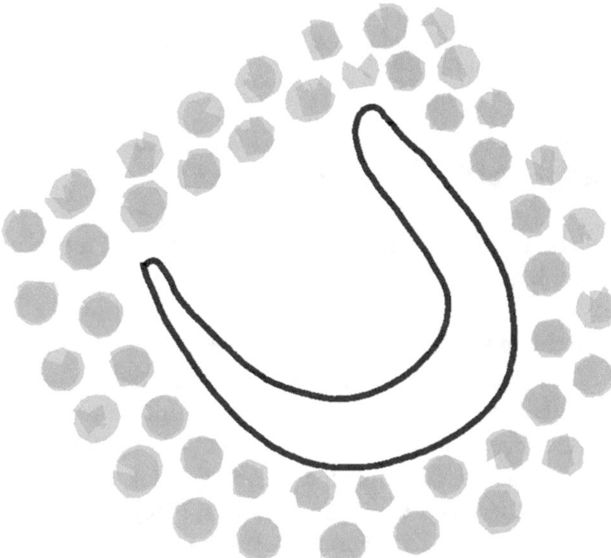

Fig. 5.22 Laser should be placed in two rows around a retinal tear as shown, laser the flat retina close to the edge of the tear

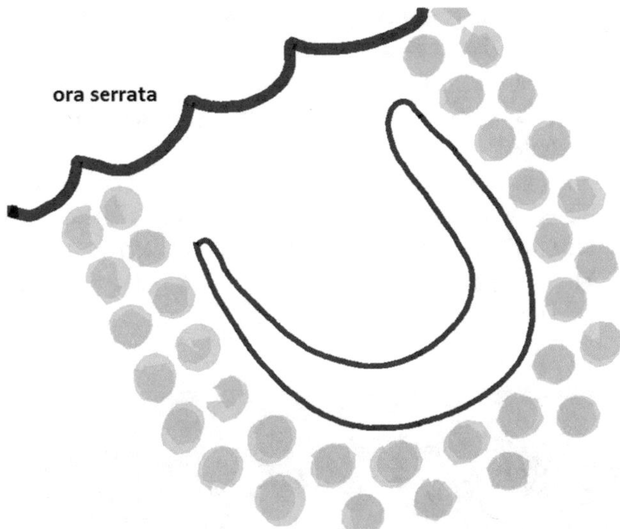

Fig. 5.23 If the retinal tear is close to the ora serrata, laser up to the ora serrata if you are unable to laser around the anterior edge of the tear

However, retinal detachment surgeons will have seen many patients who have presented asymptomatically with macular off retinal detachments from such holes [59]. Therefore, there is a subset of patients that will progress to cause symptomatic retinal detachment. The patient should be made aware of the small risk and symptomatology of retinal detachment.

- Flat round holes do not need treatment.
- Round holes with subretinal fluid may be treated; see Other Retinal Detachments (Fig. 5.27).

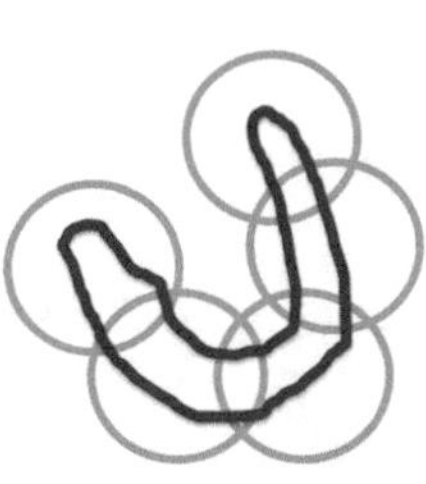

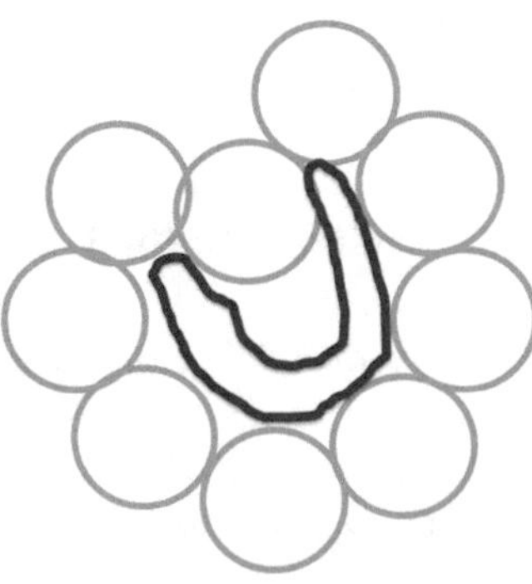

Fig. 5.24 Apply cryotherapy to a large tear as shown on the left, although this applies cryotherapy to the bare RPE in the tear, this is preferable to the increased number of burns required if the retina around the tear is treated as shown on the right

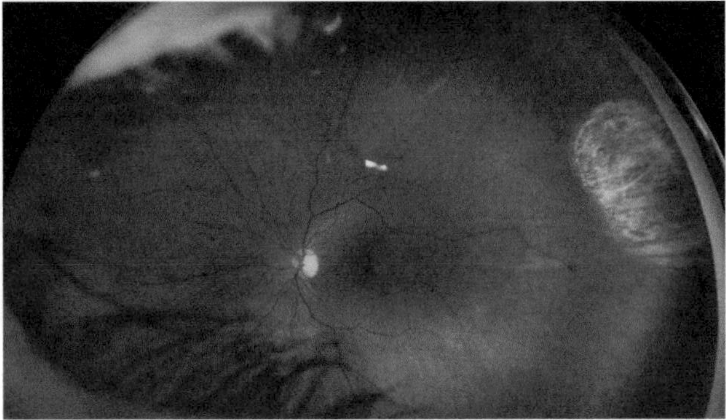

Fig. 5.25 A cryotherapy scar

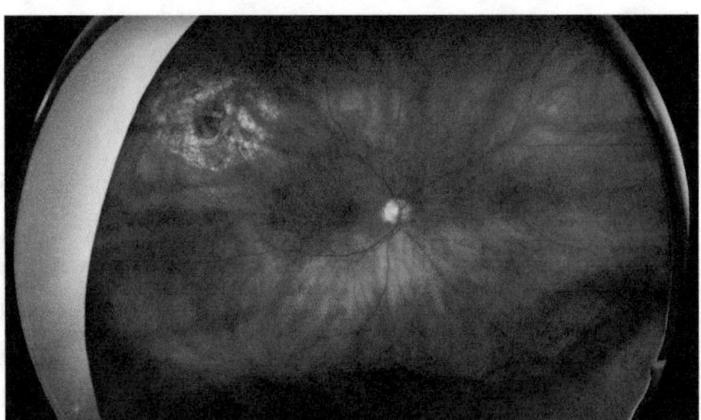

Fig. 5.26 Cryotherapy to a retinal break

Other Breaks

Para vascular tears can occur, often associated with para vascular lattice degeneration (seen in Stickler syndrome). These tears will produce retinal detachment and should be treated immediately.

Other breaks such as dialysis and giant retinal tears usually present with retinal detachment and therefore are not commonly amenable to prophylaxis and will be discussed later (Figs. 5.28 and 5.29).

Progression to Retinal Detachment

Any subretinal fluid around the hole indicates that there is a retinal detachment present. A surgical retinal detachment procedure is usually required. If the SRF is very minimal, cryotherapy can sometimes be successful on its own, probably because the tissue swelling induced by the "burn" causes the hole to close. This, however, should only be tried rarely, and the retina closely monitored for the failure of the procedure.

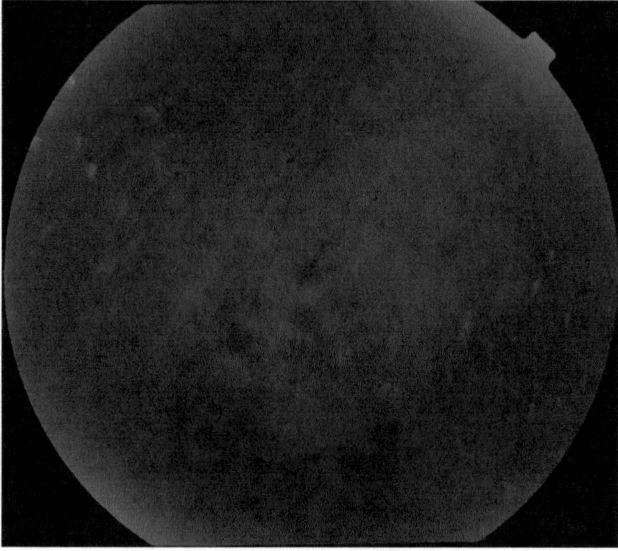

Fig. 5.27 A round hole can be seen in lattice degeneration

Peripheral Retinal Degenerations

Several peripheral degenerations will be seen in the retina (Figs. 5.30, 5.31, 5.32, 5.33).

Associated with Retinal Break Formation

1. Lattice degeneration is usually an equatorial circumferential hyalinisation of the retinal blood vessels with associated pigmentation, giving a crossed pattern. It is often associated with round retinal holes and can be associated with U-shaped tears with PVD. It is present in 5% of eyes but more frequently in moderate myopia [60, 61]. Long-term studies suggest that the chance of tractional tears is 2.9% in 10 years but with very few cases of clinically significant retinal detachment [62]. Routine treatment of lattice is inappropriate because many holes that occur with retinal detachment appear out-with the areas of lattice [63]. Radial lattice in a paravascular orientation may indicate risk of slit-like paravascular tears. In this case, Stickler syndrome should be excluded.
2. Snail track degeneration has no pigmentation and is associated with round tears and retinal detachment with attached vitreous gel. This may be more often seen in the black population and is probably a variant of lattice degeneration [64] (Fig. 5.34).

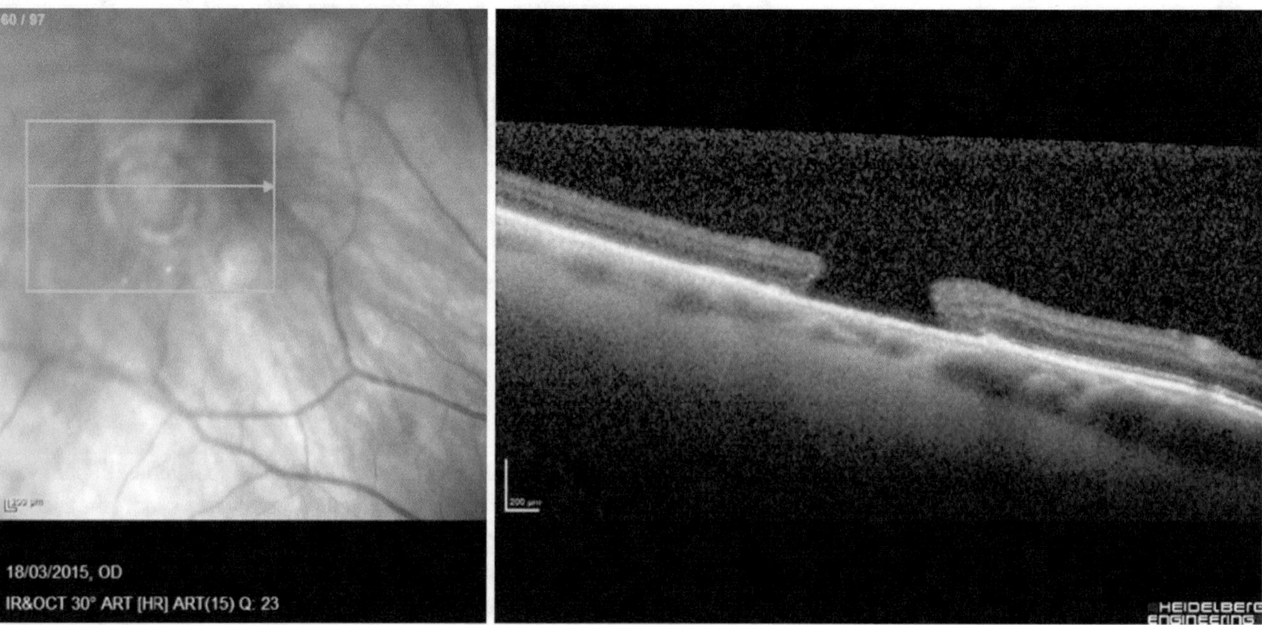

Fig. 5.28 OCT of a peripheral operculated retinal break

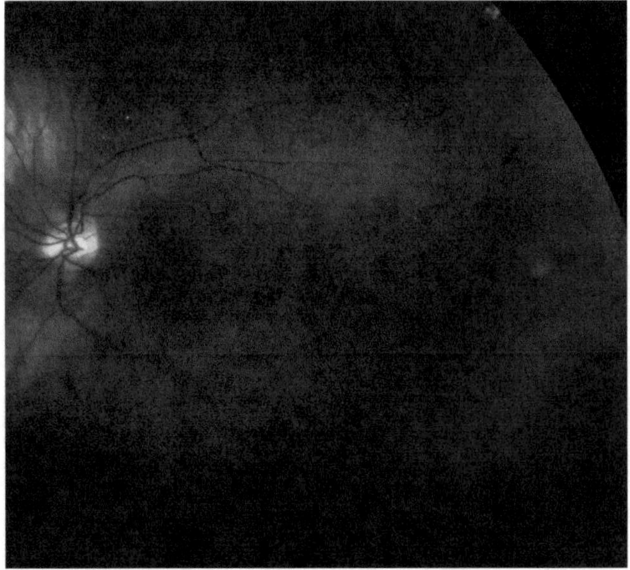

Fig. 5.29 An operculated peripheral retinal break. There is little evidence on how to treat these. Many will not treat these unless there is a bridging blood vessel. Often it is easier to treat the break so that there is no concern about progression to RRD

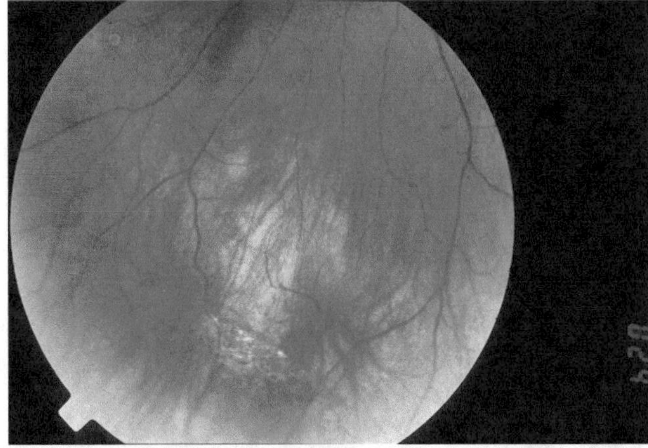

Fig. 5.30 Lattice degeneration is associated with posterior vitreous detachment, U tears and with round hole retinal detachments with vitreous attached. During vitrectomy, should you encounter large areas of lattice, examine the lattice for any holes within it. It is, however, often safe to leave lattice untreated if you are confident that there are no breaks hidden within it. Partial thickness breaks are commonly seen and require no treatment

Associated with Other Retinal Conditions

3. Reticular degeneration is a honeycombed pigmentary change occurring in the aged population and is insignificant apart from an association with age-related macular degeneration [65, 66] (Fig. 5.35).
4. Cystoid changes may be yellow flecks, and this can be associated with retinoschisis.

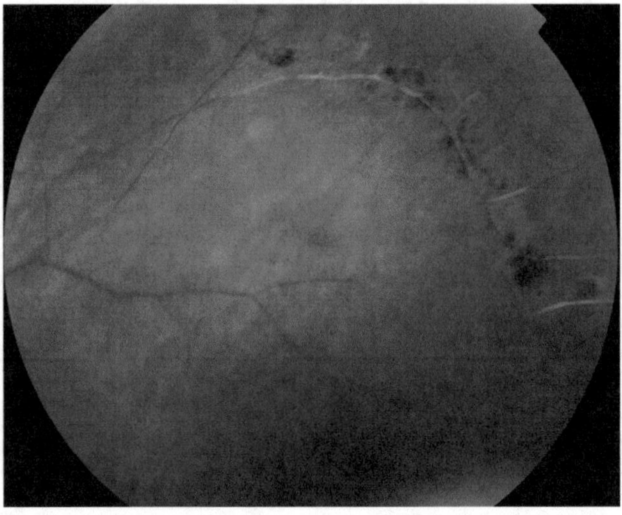

Fig. 5.31 Lattice degeneration

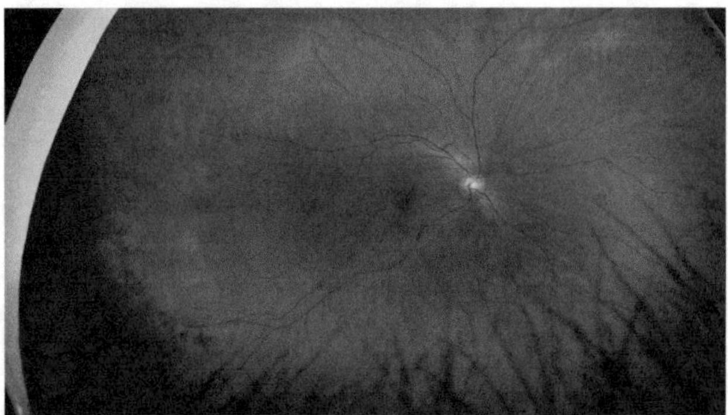

Fig. 5.32 Lattice degeneration

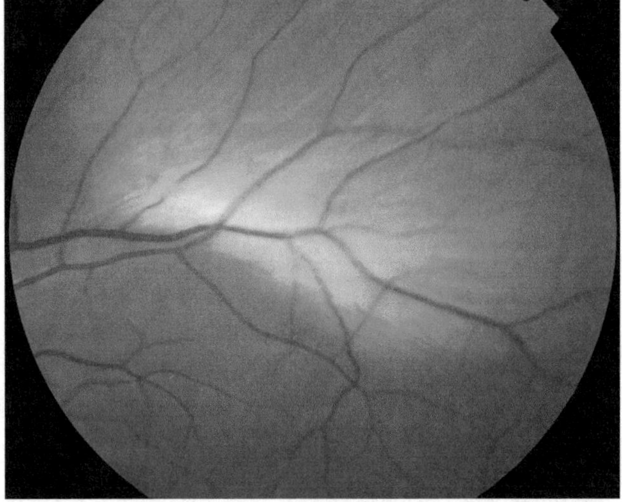

Fig. 5.33 Myelinated nerve fibres will separate with the posterior hyaloid membrane during peel of the membrane, for example during macular hole surgery

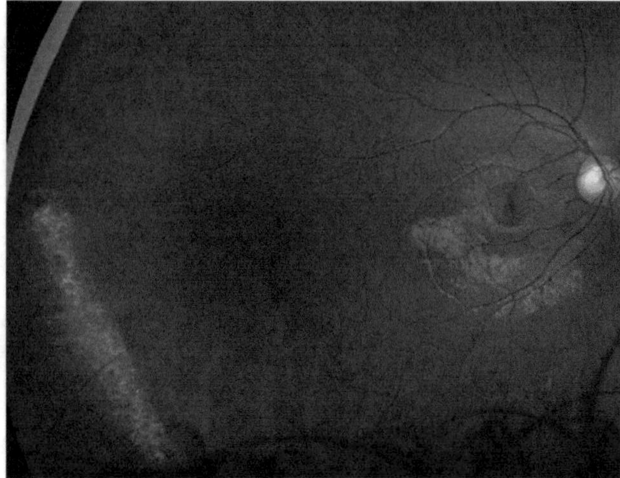

Fig. 5.34 Snail track degeneration is seen in more pigmented fundi and is probably a variant of lattice degeneration

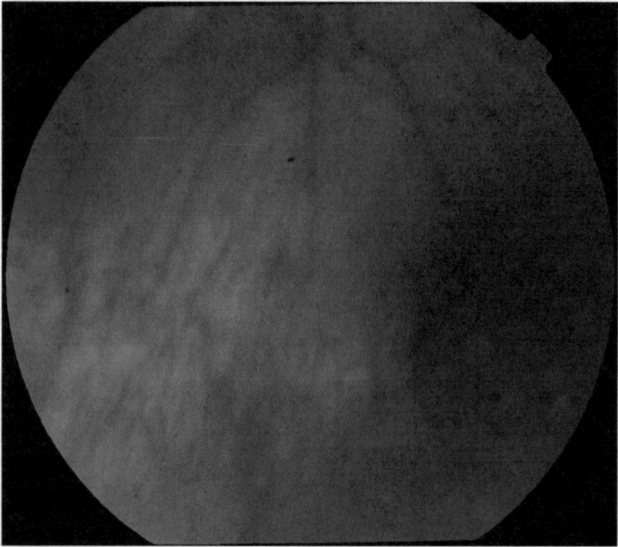

Fig. 5.35 Peripheral reticular degeneration may be associated with age-related macular degeneration

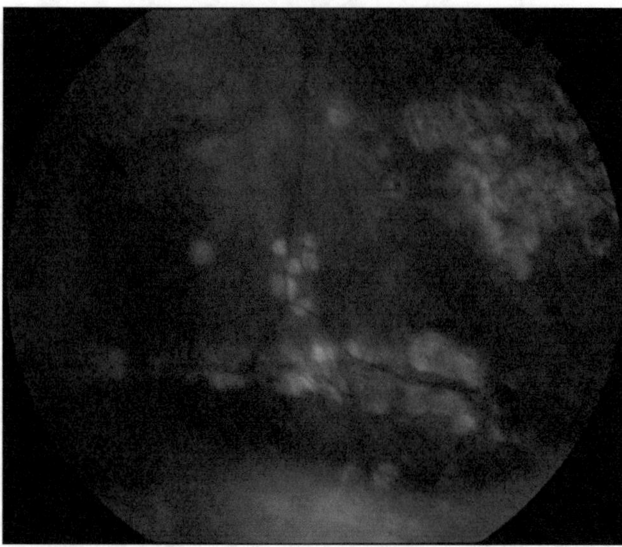

Fig. 5.36 Cobblestone degeneration is commonly encountered by a vitrectomy surgeon and is generally insignificant. Occasionally the degeneration may cause an adhesion of the retina to the choroid, thereby altering the direction of travel of SRF in retinal detachment. On other occasions, however, it can be split by the retinal detachment, leaving atrophic areas of the retina within the retinal detachment itself, which should not be mistaken for retinal holes

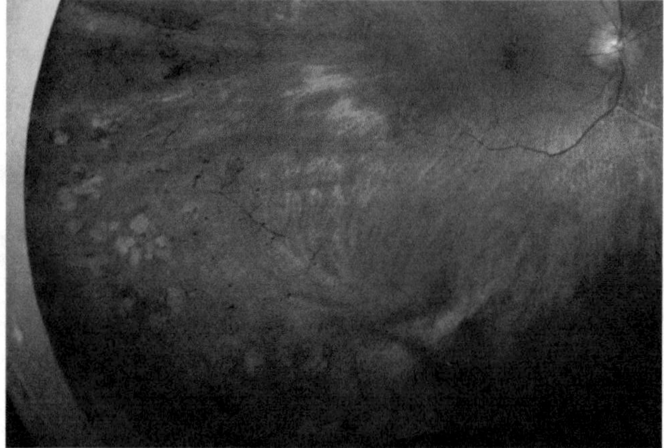

Fig. 5.37 Cobblestone degeneration

Others

5. Cobblestone degeneration is characterised by punched out atrophic areas of depigmentation of the choroid and retina. It is significant in retinal detachment because it may hold back any subretinal fluid, changing the configuration of the retinal detachment (Figs. 5.36 and 5.37).
6. White without pressure shows a crenated edge and pallor of the retina but is not significant in retinal pathology and is often more obvious in highly pigmented fundi. There is a vague association with giant retinal tear formation (Figs. 5.38, 5.39, 5.40).
7. Ora Serrata changes such as oral cysts, bays and meridional complexes may also be seen.

Unfortunately, studies on prophylaxis in retinal detachment do not meet the standards of statistical scrutiny [64], and therefore there is uncertainty about the correct management of many retinal degenerations. However, in most circumstances, retinopexy of these lesions is not required.

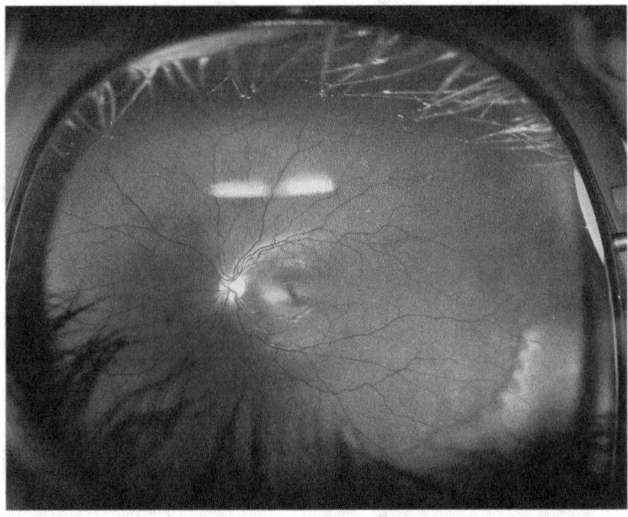

Fig. 5.38 White without pressure is visible in the infero temporal peripheral retina

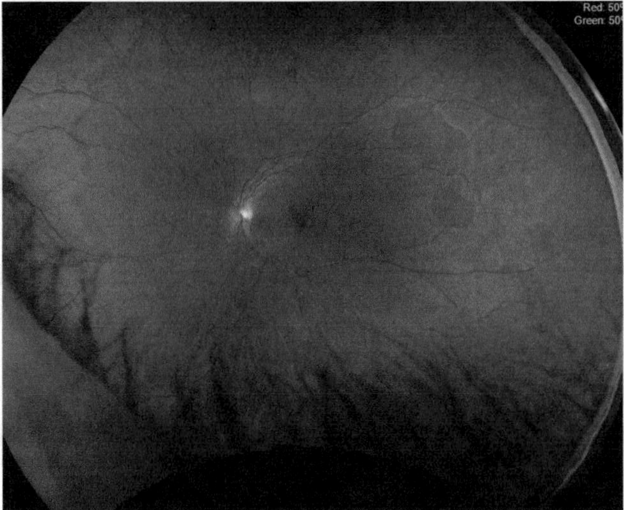

Fig. 5.39 White without pressure

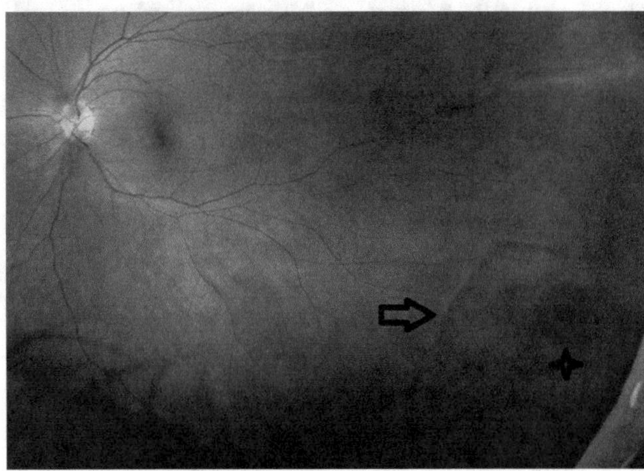

Fig. 5.40 White without pressure and a round hole

Summary

Posterior vitreous detachment is a common accompaniment to the ageing of the eye. The process is implicated in the causation of a large proportion of vitreoretinal disorders.

References

1. Bishop PN, Holmes DF, Kadler KE, McLeod D, Bos KJ. Age-related changes on the surface of vitreous collagen fibrils. Invest Ophthalmol Vis Sci. 2004;45(4):1041–6.
2. Akiba J, Ueno N, Chakrabarti B. Molecular mechanisms of posterior vitreous detachment. Graefes Arch Clin Exp Ophthalmol. 1993;231(7):408–12.
3. Larsson L, Osterlin S. Posterior vitreous detachment. A combined clinical and physiochemical study. Graefes Arch Clin Exp Ophthalmol. 1985;223(2):92–5.
4. Walton KA, Meyer CH, Harkrider CJ, Cox TA, Toth CA. Age-related changes in vitreous mobility as measured by video B scan ultrasound. Exp Eye Res. 2002;74(2):173–80.
5. Foos RY, Wheeler NC. Vitreoretinal juncture. Synchysis senilis and posterior vitreous detachment. Ophthalmology. 1982;89(12):1502–12.
6. Hikichi T, Takahashi M, Trempe CL, Schepens CL. Relationship between premacular cortical vitreous defects and idiopathic premacular fibrosis. Retina. 1995;15(5):413–6.
7. Hikichi T, Trempe CL, Schepens CL. Posterior vitreous detachment as a risk factor for retinal detachment. Ophthalmology. 1995;102(4):527–8.
8. Sebag J. Abnormalities of human vitreous structure in diabetes. Graefes Arch Clin Exp Ophthalmol. 1993;231(5):257–60.
9. Morita H, Funata M, Tokoro T. A clinical study of the development of posterior vitreous detachment in high myopia. Retina. 1995;15(2):117–24.
10. Yonemoto J, Ideta H, Sasaki K, Tanaka S, Hirose A, Oka C. The age of onset of posterior vitreous detachment. Graefes Arch Clin Exp Ophthalmol. 1994;232(2):67–70.
11. Akiba J. Prevalence of posterior vitreous detachment in high myopia. Ophthalmology. 1993;100(9):1384–8.
12. Chuo JY, Lee TY, Hollands H, Morris AH, Reyes RC, Rossiter JD, et al. Risk factors for posterior vitreous detachment: a case-control study. Am J Ophthalmol. 2006;142(6):931–7. S0002-9394(06)00913-5 [pii]. https://doi.org/10.1016/j.ajo.2006.08.002.
13. Kado M, Jalkh AE, Yoshida A, Takahashi M, Wazen N, Trempe CL, et al. Vitreous changes and macular edema in central retinal vein occlusion. Ophthalmic Surg. 1990;21(8):544–9.
14. Hikichi T, Hirokawa H, Kado M, Akiba J, Kakehashi A, Yoshida A, et al. Comparison of the prevalence of posterior vitreous detachment in whites and Japanese. Ophthalmic Surg. 1995;26(1):39–43.
15. Weiss H, Tasman WS. Rhegmatogenous retinal detachments in blacks. Ann Ophthalmol. 1978;10(6):799–806.
16. Foos RY, Simons KB, Wheeler NC. Comparison of lesions predisposing to rhegmatogenous retinal detachment by race of subjects. Am J Ophthalmol. 1983;96(5):644–9.
17. Hikichi T, Yoshida A. Time course of development of posterior vitreous detachment in the fellow eye after development in the first eye. Ophthalmology. 2004;111(9):1705–7.
18. Novak MA, Welch RB. Complications of acute symptomatic posterior vitreous detachment. Am J Ophthalmol. 1984;97(3):308–14.
19. Fincham GS, James S, Spickett C, Hollingshead M, Thrasivoulou C, Poulson AV, et al. Posterior vitreous detachment and the pos-

terior hyaloid membrane. Ophthalmology. 2018;125(2):227–36. https://doi.org/10.1016/j.ophtha.2017.08.001.
20. Unal M, Peyman GA. The efficacy of plasminogen-urokinase combination in inducing posterior vitreous detachment. Retina. 2000;20(1):69–75.
21. Hesse L, Nebeling B, Schroeder B, Heller G, Kroll P. Induction of posterior vitreous detachment in rabbits by intravitreal injection of tissue plasminogen activator following cryopexy. Exp Eye Res. 2000;70(1):31–9.
22. Kakehashi A, Ueno N, Chakrabarti B. Molecular mechanisms of photochemically induced posterior vitreous detachment. Ophthalmic Res. 1994;26(1):51–9.
23. Hikichi T, Yanagiya N, Kado M, Akiba J, Yoshida A. Posterior vitreous detachment induced by injection of plasmin and sulfur hexafluoride in the rabbit vitreous. Retina. 1999;19(1):55–8.
24. Verstraeten TC, Chapman C, Hartzer M, Winkler BS, Trese MT, Williams GA. Pharmacologic induction of posterior vitreous detachment in the rabbit. Arch Ophthalmol. 1993;111(6):849–54.
25. Harooni M, McMillan T, Refojo M. Efficacy and safety of enzymatic posterior vitreous detachment by intravitreal injection of hyaluronidase. Retina. 1998;18(1):16–22.
26. Tezel TH, Del Priore LV, Kaplan HJ. Posterior vitreous detachment with dispase. Retina. 1998;18(1):7–15.
27. Kang SW, Hyung SM, Choi MY, Lee J. Induction of vitreolysis and vitreous detachment with hyaluronidase and perfluoropropane gas. Korean J Ophthalmol. 1995;9(2):69–78.
28. Snead MP, Snead DR, Richards AJ, Harrison JB, Poulson AV, Morris AH, et al. Clinical, histological and ultrastructural studies of the posterior hyaloid membrane. Eye. 2002;16(4):447–53.
29. Wang J, McLeod D, Henson DB, Bishop PN. Age-dependent changes in the basal retinovitreous adhesion. Invest Ophthalmol Vis Sci. 2003;44(5):1793–800.
30. Akiba J, Ishiko S, Yoshida A. Variations of Weiss's ring. Retina. 2001;21(3):243–6.
31. Kakehashi A, Inoda S, Shimizu Y, Makino S, Shimizu H. Predictive value of floaters in the diagnosis of posterior vitreous detachment. Am J Ophthalmol. 1998;125(1):113–5.
32. Uchino E, Uemura A, Ohba N. Initial stages of posterior vitreous detachment in healthy eyes of older persons evaluated by optical coherence tomography. Arch Ophthalmol. 2001;119(10):1475–9.
33. Purkinje JE. Beiträge zur Kenntniss des Sehens in subjectiver Hinsicht (Contributions to the Knowledge of Vision in its Subjective Aspect) Prague J.G. Calve; 1819.
34. Moore RF. Subjective "lightning streaks". Br J Ophthalmol. 1935;19:545–7.
35. Moore RF. Subjective "lightning flashes". Am J Ophthalmol. 1940;23:1255–60.
36. Moore RF. Subjective "lightning streaks". Br J Ophthalmol. 1947;31:46–50.
37. Verhoeff FH. Moore's subjective "lightning streaks". Trans Am Acad Ophthalmol Soc. 1941;39:220–6.
38. Berens C, Cholst M, Emmerich R, McGrath H. Moore's lightning streaks: a discussion of their innocuousness. Trans Am Acad Ophthalmol Soc. 1954;52:35–58.
39. Williamson TH, Watt L, Mokete B. Black or negative flashes in posterior vitreous detachment a transient symptom before lightning flashes commence. Eye. 2008;23:1477. eye2008209 [pii]. https://doi.org/10.1038/eye.2008.209.
40. Goodfellow JF, Mokete B, Williamson TH. Discriminate characteristics of photopsia in posterior vitreous detachment, retinal tears and retinal detachment. Ophthalmic Physiol Opt. 2010;30:20–3. OPO685 [pii]. https://doi.org/10.1111/j.1475-1313.2009.00685.x.
41. van Overdam KA, Bettink-Remeijer MW, Mulder PG, van Meurs JC. Symptoms predictive for the later development of retinal breaks. Arch Ophthalmol. 2001;119(10):1483–6.
42. Sharma S, Walker R, Brown GC, Cruess AF. The importance of qualitative vitreous examination in patients with acute posterior vitreous detachment. Arch Ophthalmol. 1999;117(3):343–6.
43. Hikichi T, Trempe CL. Relationship between floaters, light flashes, or both, and complications of posterior vitreous detachment. Am J Ophthalmol. 1994;117(5):593–8.
44. Serpetopoulos C. Optical explanation of the gradual disappearance of flying dots in posterior vitreous detachment. Surv Ophthalmol. 1997;42(1):92–4.
45. Hollands H, Johnson D, Brox AC, Almeida D, Simel DL, Sharma S. Acute-onset floaters and flashes: is this patient at risk for retinal detachment? JAMA. 2009;302(20):2243–9. 302/20/2243 [pii]. https://doi.org/10.1001/jama.2009.1714.
46. Tanner V, Harle D, Tan J, Foote B, Williamson TH, Chignell AH. Acute posterior vitreous detachment: the predictive value of vitreous pigment and symptomatology. Br J Ophthalmol. 2000;84(11):1264–8.
47. Dayan MR, Jayamanne DG, Andrews RM, Griffiths PG. Flashes and floaters as predictors of vitreoretinal pathology: is follow-up necessary for posterior vitreous detachment? Eye. 1996;10(Pt 4):456–8.
48. Byer NE. Natural history of posterior vitreous detachment with early management as the premier line of defense against retinal detachment. Ophthalmology. 1994;101(9):1503–13.
49. Brod RD, Lightman DA, Packer AJ, Saras HP. Correlation between vitreous pigment granules and retinal breaks in eyes with acute posterior vitreous detachment. Ophthalmology. 1991;98(9):1366–9.
50. Richardson PS, Benson MT, Kirkby GR. The posterior vitreous detachment clinic: do new retinal breaks develop in the six weeks following an isolated symptomatic posterior vitreous detachment? Eye. 1999;13(Pt 2):237–40.
51. Byer NE. What happens to untreated asymptomatic retinal breaks, and are they affected by posterior vitreous detachment? Ophthalmology. 1998;105(6):1045–9.
52. Coffee RE, Westfall AC, Davis GH, Mieler WF, Holz ER. Symptomatic posterior vitreous detachment and the incidence of delayed retinal breaks: case series and meta-analysis. Am J Ophthalmol. 2007;144(3):409–13. S0002-9394(07)00434-5 [pii]. https://doi.org/10.1016/j.ajo.2007.05.002.
53. Katz B, Hoyt WF. Intrapapillary and peripapillary hemorrhage in young patients with incomplete posterior vitreous detachment. Signs of vitreopapillary traction. Ophthalmology. 1995;102(2):349–54.
54. Roberts TV, Gregory-Roberts JC. Optic disc haemorrhages in posterior vitreous detachment. Aust NZ J Ophthalmol. 1991;19(1):61–3.
55. Cibis GW, Watzke RC, Chua J. Retinal hemorrhages in posterior vitreous detachment. Am J Ophthalmol. 1975;80(6):1043–6.
56. Schachat AP, Sommer A. Macular hemorrhages associated with posterior vitreous detachment. Am J Ophthalmol. 1986;102(5):647–9.
57. Byer NE. Subclinical retinal detachment resulting from asymptomatic retinal breaks: prognosis for progression and regression. Ophthalmology. 2001;108(8):1499–503.
58. Byer NE. The natural history of asymptomatic retinal breaks. Ophthalmology. 1982;89(9):1033–9.
59. Murakami-Nagasako F, Ohba N. Phakic retinal detachment associated with atrophic hole of lattice degeneration of the retina. Graefes Arch Clin Exp Ophthalmol. 1983;220(4):175–8.
60. Semes LP, Holland WC, Likens EG. Prevalence and laterality of lattice retinal degeneration within a primary eye care population. Optometry. 2001;72(4):247–50.
61. Celorio JM, Pruett RC. Prevalence of lattice degeneration and its relation to axial length in severe myopia. Am J Ophthalmol. 1991;111(1):20–3.
62. Byer NE. Long-term natural history of lattice degeneration of the retina. Ophthalmology. 1989;96(9):1396–401.

63. Benson WE, Morse PH, Nantawan P. Late complications following cryotherapy of lattice degeneration. Am J Ophthalmol. 1977;84(4):514–6.
64. Shukla M, Ahuja OP. A possible relationship between lattice and snail track degenerations of the retina. Am J Ophthalmol. 1981;92(4):482–5.
65. Lewis H, Straatsma BR, Foos RY, Lightfoot DO. Reticular degeneration of the pigment epithelium. Ophthalmology. 1985;92(11):1485–95.
66. Humphrey WT, Carlson RE, Valone JA Jr. Senile reticular pigmentary degeneration. Am J Ophthalmol. 1984;98(6):717–22.

6 Vitreous Haemorrhage

Contents

Introduction

Vitreous haemorrhage is a common accompaniment to disorders of the retina and will often profoundly reduce vision. A small amount of haemorrhage can reduce the vision severely. Occasionally a good visual acuity can be recorded because the patient, by moving the eye, is able to momentarily visualise the test chart through a clear section of vitreous before the opacified vitreous obscures the vision again. The haemorrhage may be situated in the gel of the vitreous (intragel) or behind a detached gel (retrohyaloid). There may be haemorrhage in the sub ILM, subretinal or suprachoroidal spaces depending upon the aetiology (Fig. 6.1).

Fig. 6.1 Vitreous haemorrhage may be diffuse in the vitreous gel

Aetiology

- The primary cause of spontaneous vitreous haemorrhage is retinal neovascularisation secondary to retinal ischaemia (commonly diabetic retinopathy or retinal vein occlusion). This usually is associated with PVD, i.e. the mobile vitreous tears the fragile new blood vessels, in which case sub hyaloid haemorrhage is common. VH can be seen with the vitreous attached if the blood vessels burst, either spontaneously or during a period of raised systemic blood pressure (e.g. during isometric exertion).
- VH from retinal tears associated with posterior vitreous detachment requires urgent management.

T. H. Williamson, *Vitreoretinal Surgery*, https://doi.org/10.1007/978-3-030-68769-4_6

- Haemorrhage elsewhere in the eye will often disperse into the vitreous cavity, e.g. suprachoroidal blood in trauma, subretinal blood secondary to choroidal neovascularisation or blood under the internal limiting membrane in Terson's syndrome.
- Other common causes of vitreous cavity haemorrhage are retinal macro-aneurysm (often the vitreous is attached) and posterior vitreous detachment without retinal tear formation.
- In infants, retinopathy of prematurity is possible. In children 73% of cases are due to manifest or occult trauma, other common causes are regressed retinopathy of prematurity [1]. Shaken baby syndrome from non-accidental injury should be considered in bilateral vitreous haemorrhage in children. Rarer causes are juvenile retinoschisis, familial exudative vitreoretinopathy, intermediate uveitis, other uveitis, and tumours.
- Sub ILM bleeds are rare and seen in Terson's syndrome, Valsalva-related haemorrhage, blood dyscrasia, and trauma [2]. Terson's syndrome has been reported in 8–14% of patients with subarachnoid haemorrhage [3] (Fig. 6.2).

Aetiology [4–10]

- Diabetic retinopathy
- Branch retinal vein occlusion
- Retinal tear and rhegmatogenous retinal detachment
- Choroidal neovascular membrane
- Macroaneurysm
- Posterior vitreous detachment
- Trauma
- Sickle cell retinopathy
- Central retinal vein occlusion
- Terson's syndrome
- Retinal vasculitis
- Intermediate uveitis
- Retinoschisis
- Needle-stick injury
- Tumour (vasoproliferative)
- Familial exudative vitreoretinopathy
- Retinal telangiectasia
- Valsalva manoeuvre

Natural History

The blood in the vitreous gel initially forms a localised clot, but subsequent fibrinolysis causes dispersion of the haemorrhage throughout the gel. During haemolysis biconcave erythrocytes lose most of their enclosed haemoglobin and change to spheroidal erythroclasts. Biodegradation of the released haemoglobin produces pigments, which often stain the gel an ochre-yellow or orange colour. Such staining of a detached erythroclast clogged vitreous cortex produces an "ochre membrane" at the posterior hyaloid face.

The mechanisms of spontaneous absorption of vitreous haemorrhage have not been clearly elucidated, through phagocytosis by macrophages, outflow of cells through the trabecular meshwork, and syneretic disintegration of the gel play a part. Cells in the trabecular meshwork can reduce aqueous drainage causing raised intraocular pressure and creating "erythroclastic glaucoma". Another rare consequence of vitreous haemorrhage is "synchisis scintillans", a localised form of cholesterolosis bulbi. It is characterised by the presence of cholesterol crystals in the vitreous cavity, which tend to sediment inferiorly, but may be seen to scatter and shower throughout the vitreous cavity after eye movements (Fig. 6.3).

Erythroclastic Glaucoma

The macrophage-mediated removal of red blood cells clogs up the trabecular meshwork causing a rise in IOP. If a vitreous haemorrhage is left in the eye for weeks or months glaucoma is an occasional risk. If undetected and untreated a cupped optic disc can result. If you plan not to operate on an eye with vitreous haemorrhage and are awaiting spontaneous resolution of the haemorrhage the eye will require periodic IOP checks. If glaucoma occurs the definitive therapy is removal of the blood by PPV.

Investigation

The priority with vitreous haemorrhage is determining the aetiology because some causes require immediate intervention. Many cases can be determined from the history of the patient.

- Diabetic retinopathy.
- Branch retinal vein occlusion with a previous symptomatology.
  - Previous loss of vision 1 year ago/laser.
- Trauma.
  - Traumatic history.
- Central retinal vein occlusion.
  - Loss of vision 2 years ago.
- Terson's syndrome.
  - Headache, neurological signs, and symptoms.
- Needle-stick injury.
  - Careless anaesthesia.
- Sickle cell.
  - Race and blood tests.

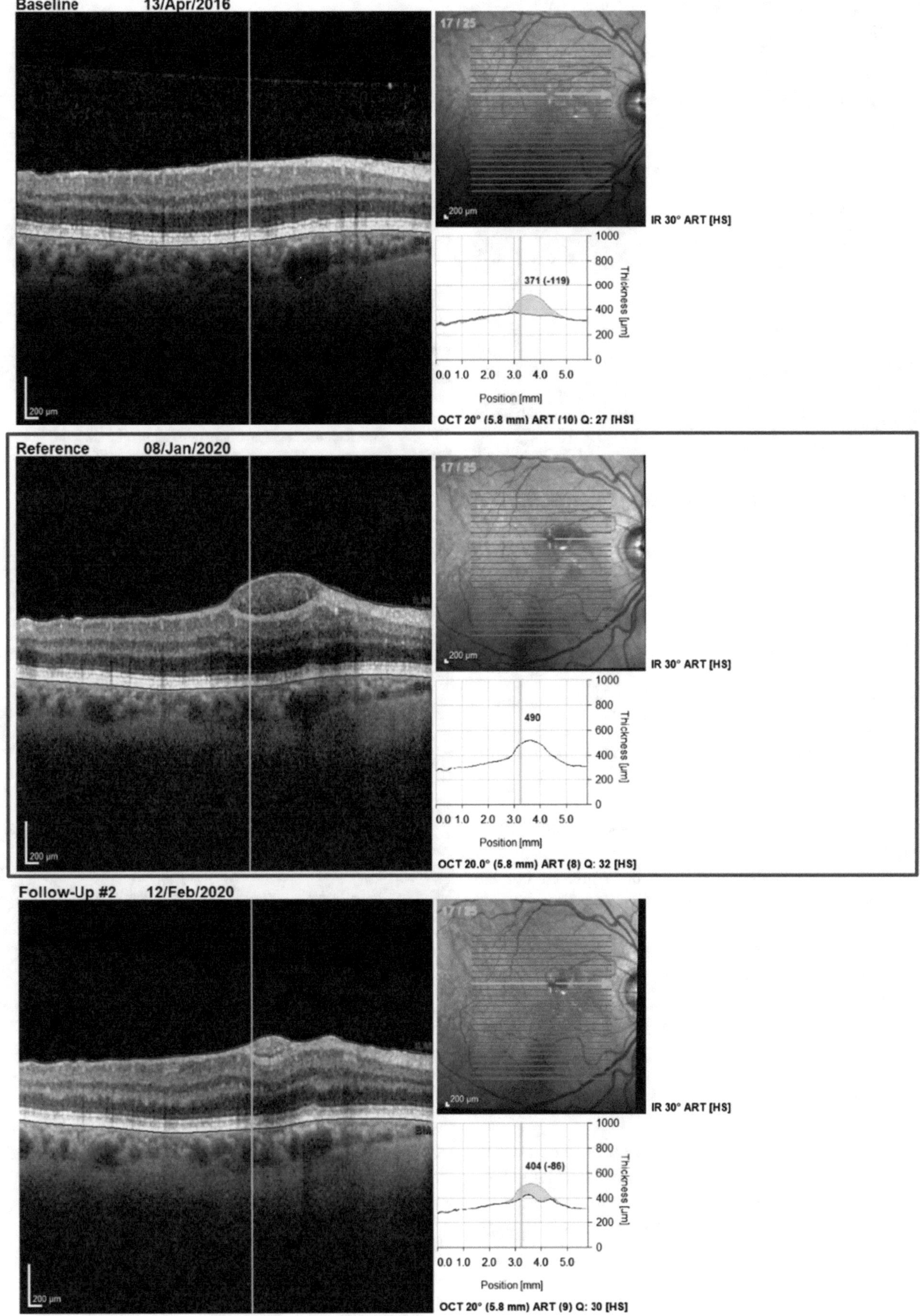

Fig. 6.2 A small preretinal haemorrhage after a coughing fit which spontaneously resolves

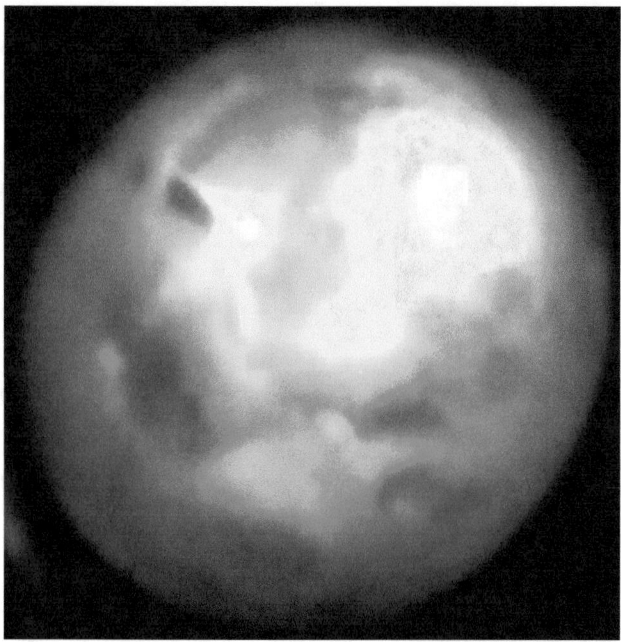

Fig. 6.3 Very thick vitreous haemorrhage has an ochre colour as in this patient with Bechet's disease

- Retinal vasculitis.
  - Previous treatment.

Others are not so obvious:

- Branch retinal vein occlusion previously asymptomatic.
- Choroidal neovascular membrane.
  - Often the presenting complaint in these patients with or without signs of AMD in the other eye.
- Macroaneurysm.
- Posterior vitreous detachment with or without retinal tears.
  - Flashes and floaters may have been present but are inconclusive clinical features.
- Retinal vasculitis.
- Intermediate uveitis.
  - Beware the 20-year-old patient with vitreous haemorrhage, they may have had undiagnosed panuveitis. Ask for a history of floaters prior to the onset of the vitreous haemorrhage.
- Retinoschisis.
- Tumour.

Vitreous haemorrhage may be mild or localised in which case it may be possible to see the cause with slit-lamp biomicroscopy and a 90D lens. However, with the indirect ophthalmoscope more of the retina can be visualised through the haemorrhage. Scleral indentation may be required to exclude retinal tears. If a view is not available ultrasound is the mainstay of investigation (Figs. 6.4, 6.5, 6.6, 6.7, 6.8, 6.9, 6.10, 6.11).

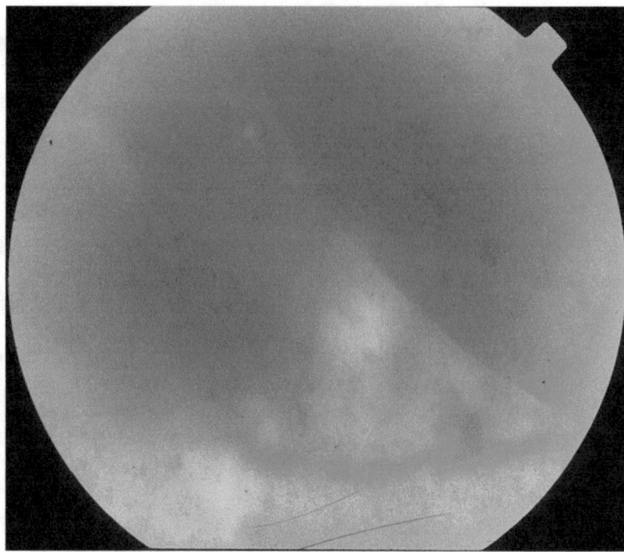

Fig. 6.4 The haemorrhage is often most dense behind the posterior hyaloid membrane and can produce the appearance of bullae of blood, no to be mistaken with bullous retinal detachment

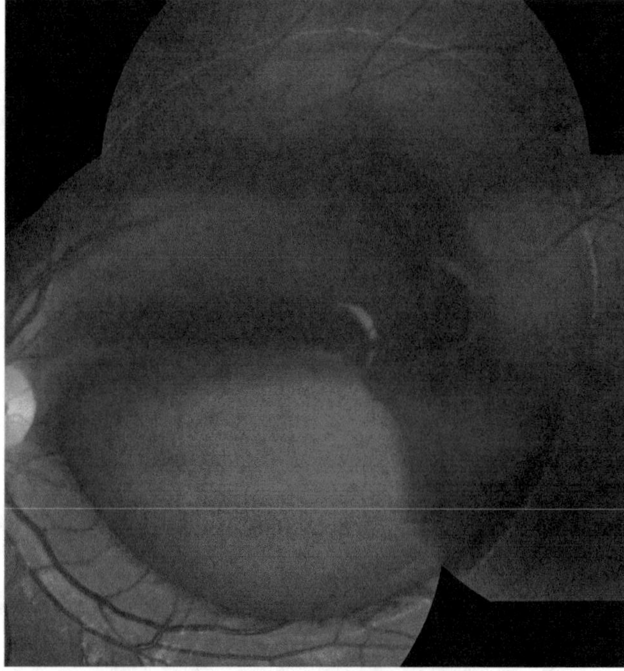

Fig. 6.5 Subhyaloid haemorrhage showing separation of the posterior vitreous face in a dome and a fluid level of erythrocytes

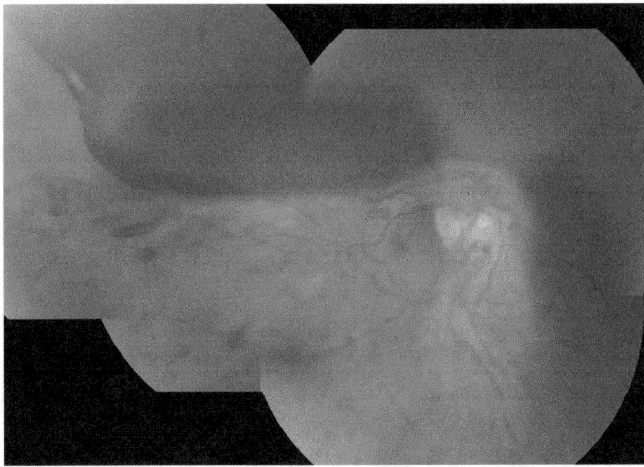

Fig. 6.6 A bulla of subhyaloid haemorrhage is seen demarcated by neovascular membrane

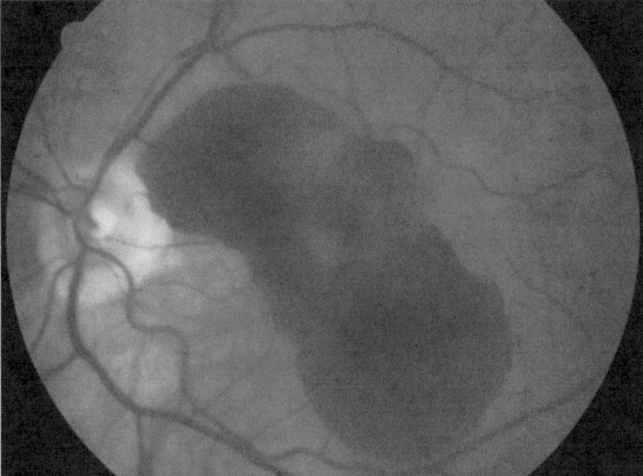

Fig. 6.7 Preretinal haemorrhage is present after breaking through the retina from a bleeding retinal lesion such as choroidal neovascular membrane

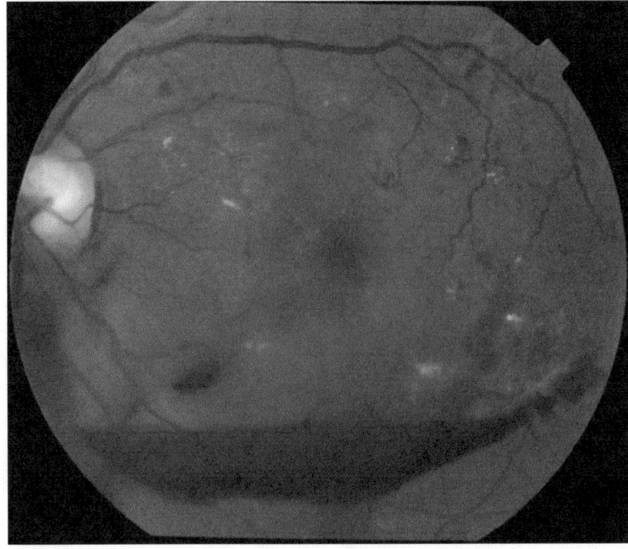

Fig. 6.8 If the vitreous is still attached the haemorrhage is trapped in front of the retina, i.e. described as retrohyaloid or subhyaloid or preretinal

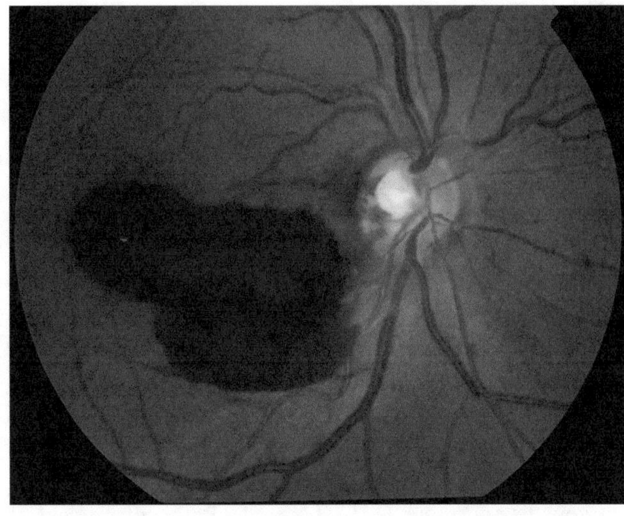

Fig. 6.9 A subretinal haemorrhage from a Valsalva manoeuvre

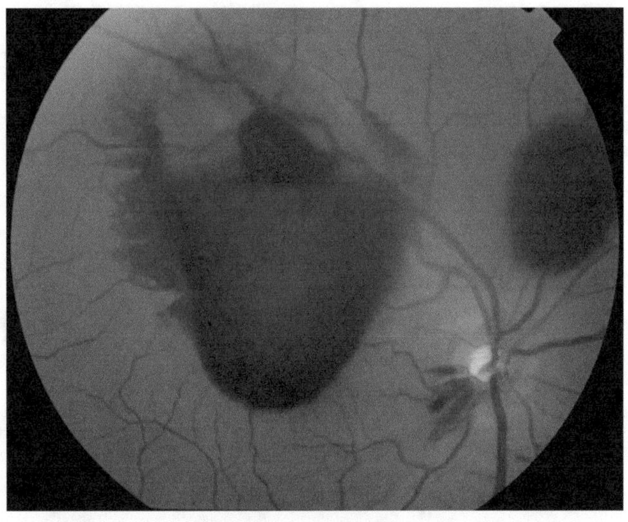

Fig. 6.10 A Valsalva induced pre-retinal haemorrhage

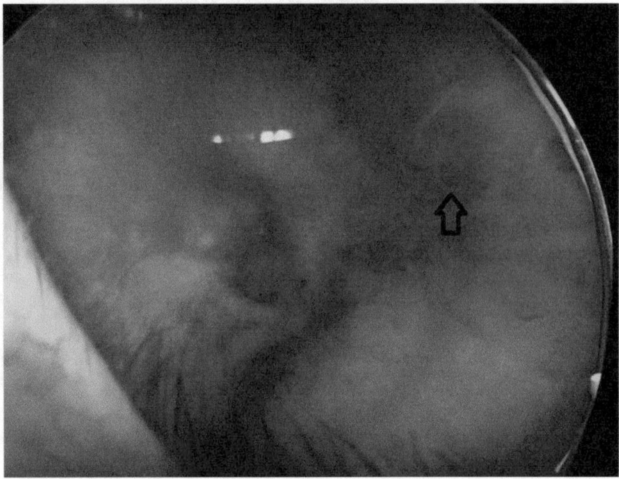

Fig. 6.11 A retinal break and vitreous haemorrhage

Ultrasound

All vitreoretinal clinics should have ultrasonography available. If the surgeon learns this skill, he or she will be able to make rapid assessment and diagnosis of the eye by interpreting information on the dynamics of the vitreous and the retina. In vitreous haemorrhage, first determine whether the retina is flat by taking cross-sections of the whole eye. A sinuous continuous high echo that starts at the ora serrata and ends around the optic nerve head is typical of a detached retina. In contrast, a posterior vitreous detachment will move with a more rapid and flimsy action. If the vitreous is detached watch out for the flap of a retinal tear attached to the peripheral vitreous, a sensitivity of 56% has been estimated for detecting retinal tears on ultrasound in eyes with vitreous haemorrhage [11]. There may be an attachment of the vitreous to the disc if disc new vessels are present in diabetes or with BRVO but most often there is no attachment at the disc. Diffuse increased echo behind the gel indicates retrohyaloid blood. If this is seen behind a high echo membrane, which may appear like retina, it helps identify the membrane as thickened posterior cortical vitreous gel. In comparison, retinal detachments have clear fluid on ultrasound behind their echogenic signal, i.e. SRF in the subretinal space. If the vitreous is still attached this may aid in diagnosis suggesting diabetic retinopathy or an unusual cause such as Terson's syndrome (Chap. 16). The focal attachments of an otherwise detached vitreous can be helpful, e.g. the vitreous attached to new vessels at the disc or elsewhere, tractional retinal detachments or incarceration sites in trauma or needle stick injury.

Other conditions will provide clues of their own. Choroidal neovascular membranes that bleed tend to produce severe subretinal haemorrhage which be a dense immobile craggy mass at the posterior pole. The patient will usually have signs of high-risk age-related macular degeneration in the other eye, e.g. soft drusen or disciform scar. The patient is commonly on an anticoagulant or antiplatelet medication.

Tumours have their own characteristic shapes, e.g. collar stud melanoma. Colour Doppler imaging helps by demonstrating a tumour circulation in elevated, e.g. metastases and malignant melanomas. Vasoproliferative tumours are flatter and more difficult to detect with Doppler.

Retinoschisis provides a thin dome-shaped peripheral elevation. X-linked retinoschisis is particularly associated with vitreous haemorrhage in the young (Figs. 6.12 and 6.13).

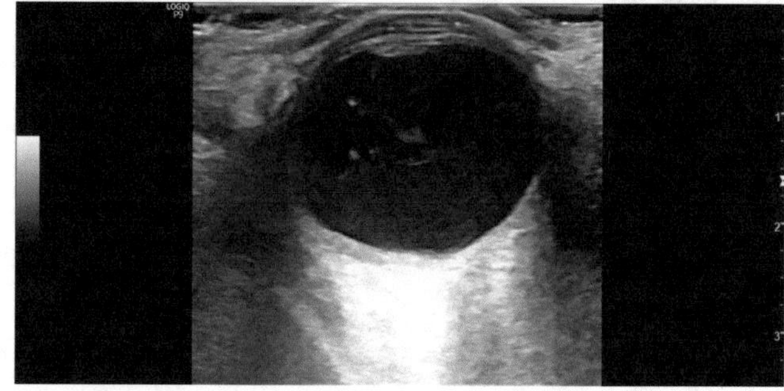

Fig. 6.12 Subhyaloid haemorrhage on US with PVD

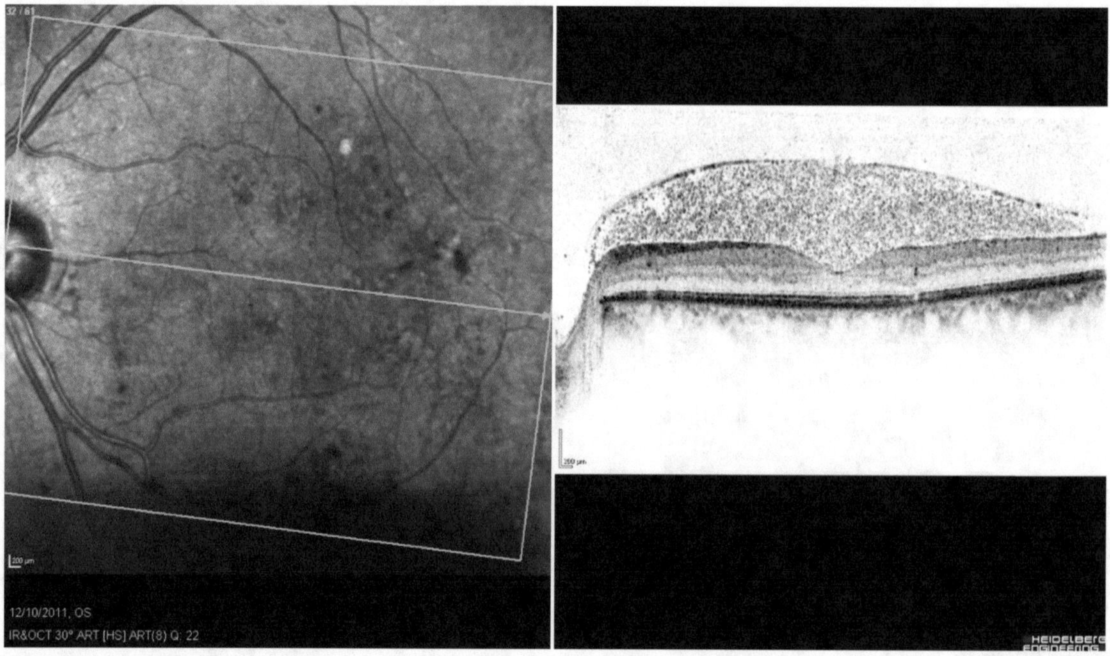

Fig. 6.13 Subhyaloid haemorrhage

Ultrasound features

- Vitreous detached or not.
  - If attached not a retinal tear!
- Evidence of neovascularisation.
  - BVO or CRVO.
  - But beware of the posterior retinal break which can be attached to the gel and look like posterior neovascularisation.
- Subretinal haemorrhage.
  - Large craggy mass under the retina.
  - CNV can be posterior or peripheral.

Management

- Do you have a retinal tear?
  - Can you wait?
  - Do you need to operate soon?
- You cannot afford to miss the threat of a retinal detachment.
  - Risk of retinal tear going on to RRD.
  - Risk of proliferative vitreoretinopathy in RRD with VH.

A patient with fundus obscuring VH should have an ultrasound performed on each visit (Figs. 6.14, 6.15, 6.16).

Surgery

Mild vitreous haemorrhage may clear spontaneously. Depending upon the aetiology recurrences can occur. Monitoring is required to detect retinal detachment or erythroclastic glaucoma. If the surgeon determines that there is a risk of retinal detachment early vitrectomy is advisable to allow inspection of the retina and treatment of any breaks. It is advisable to have a low threshhold for performing PPV when the diagnosis is uncertain because of the significant risk of retinal detachment (Figs. 6.17 and 6.18, Table 6.1).

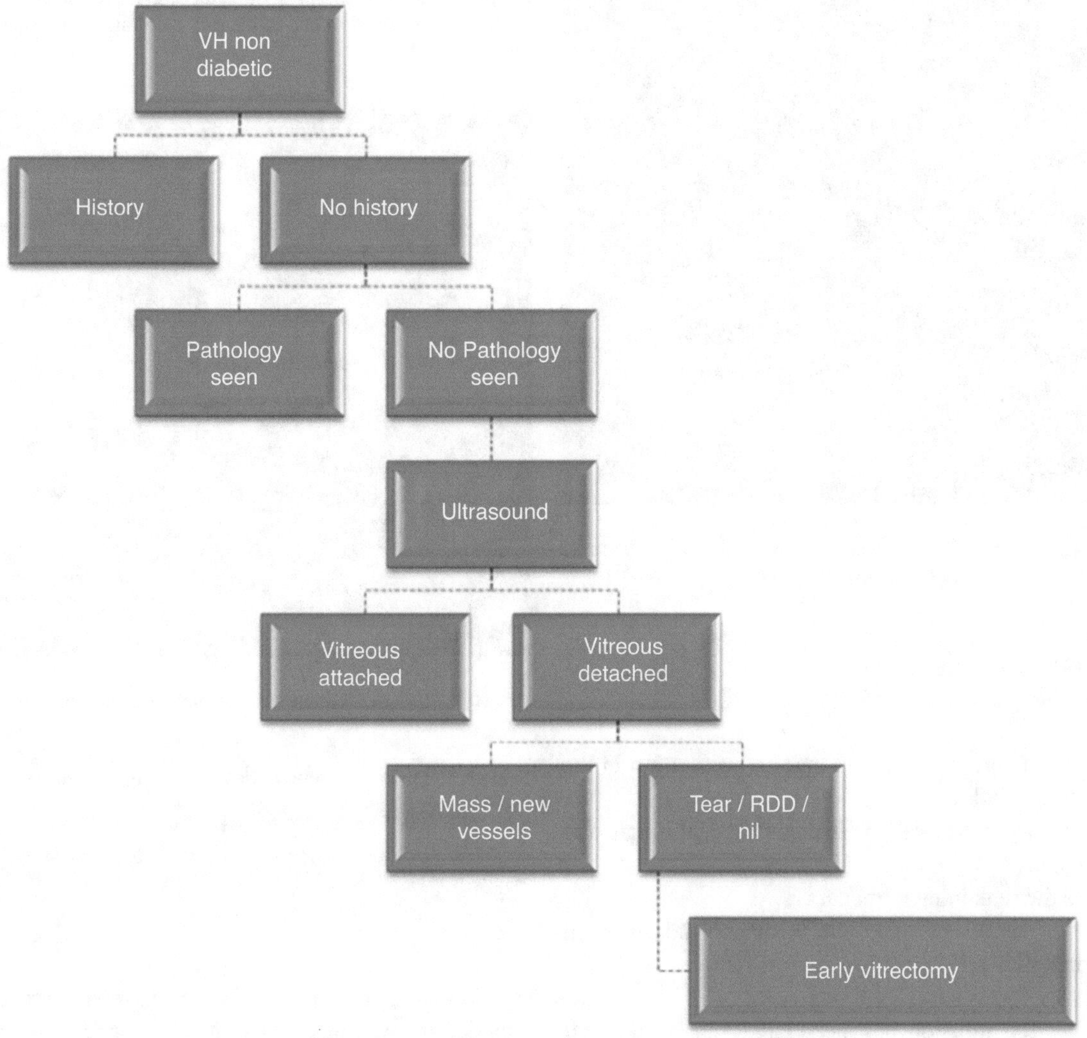

Fig. 6.14 In non-diabetic vitreous haemorrhage there are clues from the history, the examination, and ultrasound which can help you avoid having to do an early vitrectomy (operation performed within a week)

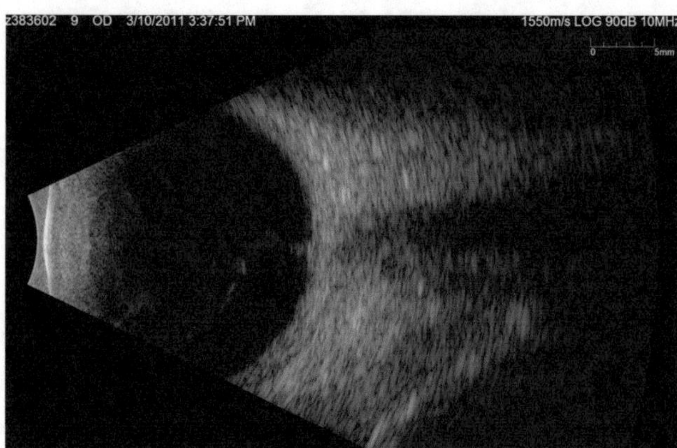

Fig. 6.15 The vitreous is detached but an attachment can be seen at the optic disc, suggesting a neovascular frond from the disc to the vitreous as the cause of the vitreous haemorrhage

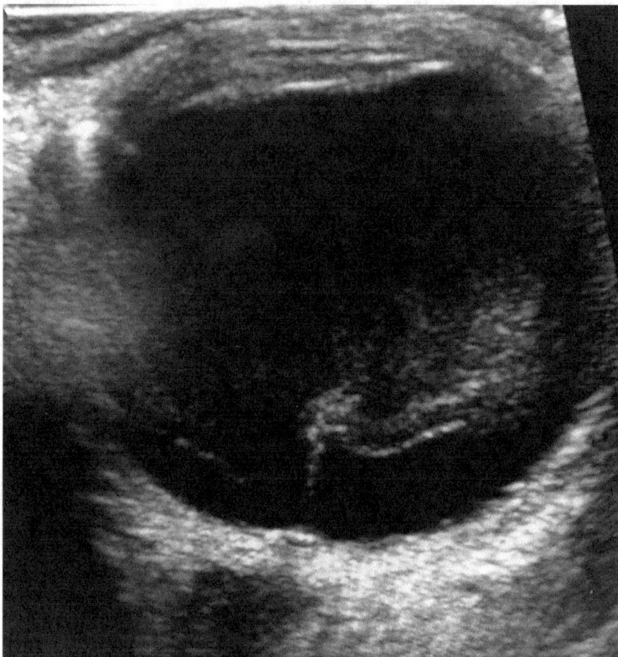

Fig. 6.16 An ultrasound of vitreous haemorrhage with evidence of disc attachment, usually indicating disc new vessels

Vitrectomy

Additional surgical steps:

- Remove the core vitreous and make a perforation in the posterior hyaloid.
- Remove any retrohyaloid haemorrhage through the perforation.
- Remove the remaining vitreous.
- Find the cause of the haemorrhage and treat it appropriately.

Checking the infusion has penetrated can be difficult because of overlying blood. Make sure that you can see the infusion by removing haemorrhagic vitreous around the cannula before switching on the infusion (see clearing the infusion Chap. 2). Start by removing the core vitreous to clear a

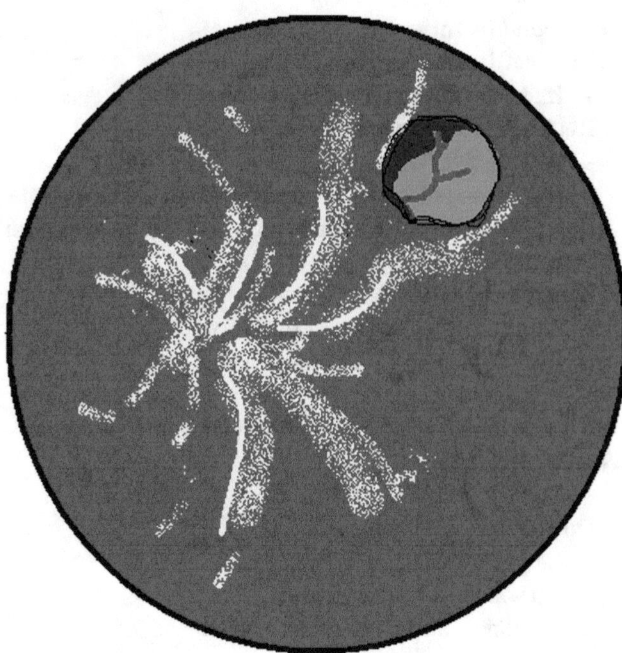

Fig. 6.17 When removing very dense blood during PPV, create a small peripheral hole, in the posterior vitreous, flush out the retrohyaloid blood to clear the view and to identify the retina, before removing the rest of the gel

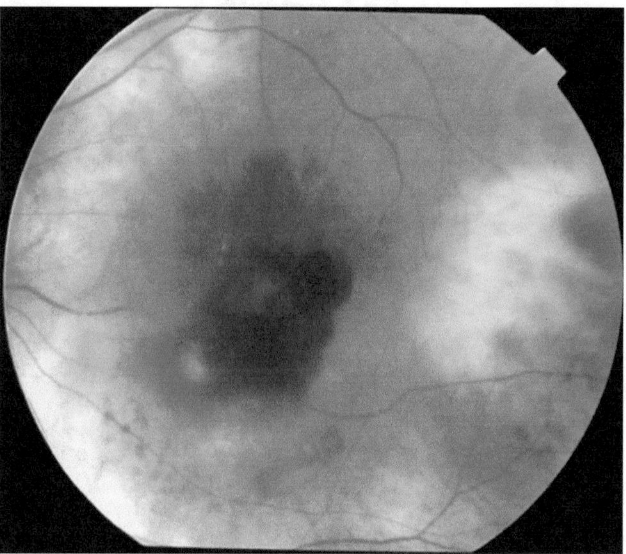

Fig. 6.18 This macroaneurysm has bled into the vitreous cavity

Table 6.1 Difficulty rating of PPV for vitreous haemorrhage

Difficulty rating	Low
Success rates	High
Complication rates	Low
When to use in training	Early

view. If the eye has PVD make a hole in the posterior hyaloid membrane (PHM) and drain out any subhyaloid haemorrhage.

- This allows visualisation of the retina to check that it is attached and not at risk of damage whilst you remove further vitreous.
- Failure to remove the subhyaloid haemorrhage allows the haemorrhage to mix with the infusion fluid causing repeated loss of the view during the remaining vitrectomy.

Once the vitreous has been removed trim the vitreous base to leave as little haemorrhage in the eye as possible. There is usually a clear layer of vitreous in the denser cortical gel next to the retina which gives you a clue when to stop removing gel before hitting the retina. Residual haemorrhage leaks out postoperatively and can cause erythroclastic glaucoma. In addition, good clearance of the vitreous base allows full inspection of the retina. The cause of the haemorrhage should be determined and treated, retinopexy and gas for retinal tear or detachment, or laser therapy for vein occlusion (Figs. 6.19, 6.20, 6.21, 6.22).

Postoperative vitreous cavity haemorrhage is common in some conditions receiving PPV for VH. The haemorrhage will clear more rapidly if the vitreous has been removed. The same rules apply for monitoring the IOP and performing repeated ultrasounds. In general, if you can see the optic disc of blood vessels, the VCH will clear spontaneously within a few weeks. If the haemorrhage is denser, a vitrectomy to washout the haemorrhage is useful for visual rehabilitation and to avoid complications.

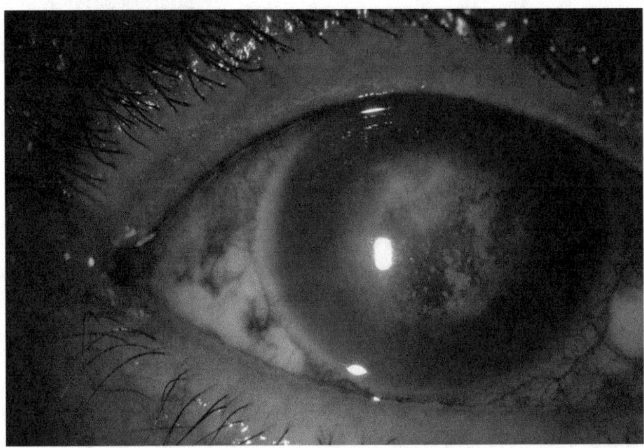

Fig. 6.19 This patient presented from the intensive care unit with suspected bilateral endogenous endophthalmitis, with absent anterior chambers with white infiltration. It was diagnosed later that the patient had probably suffered severe intraocular haemorrhaging from severely reduced platelets, presumably causing choroidal haemorrhage (with anterior chamber shallowing), followed by vitreous and then anterior chamber haemorrhage (old white blood clot). The patient regained 20/20 vision over the course of year after anterior segment reconstruction, vitrectomy, and later penetrating keratoplasty. Images show the right eye preoperatively and postoperatively (anterior segment and fundus) and the untreated left eye

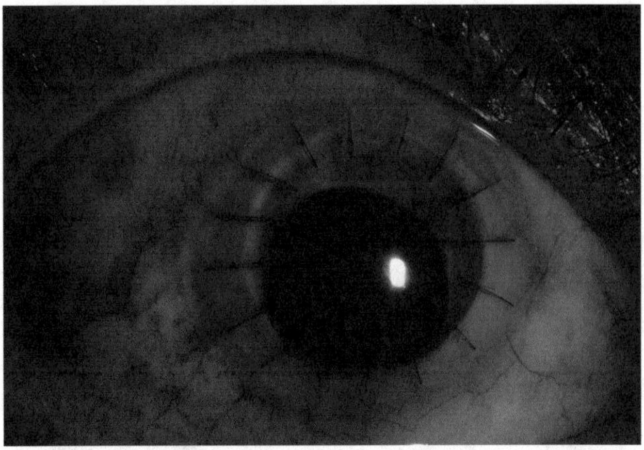

Fig. 6.20 The cornea was grafted

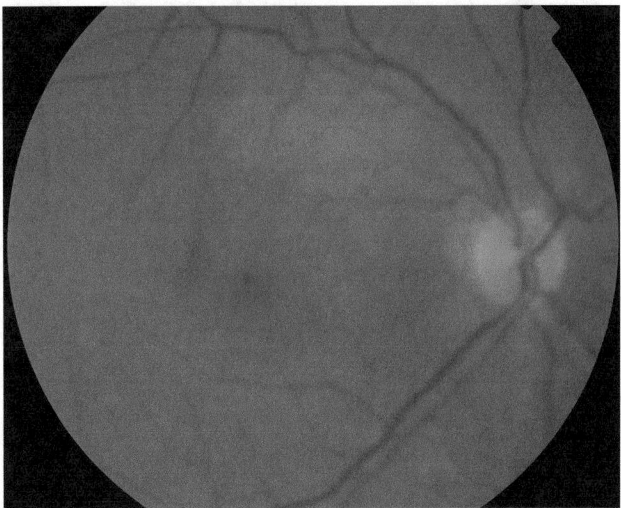

Fig. 6.21 The retina was healthy

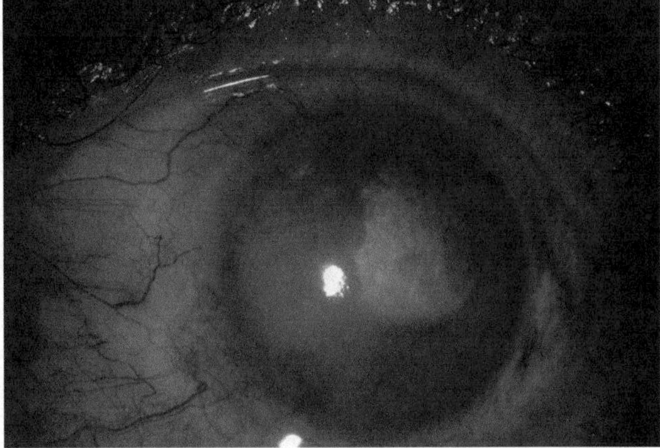

Fig. 6.22 The left eye shows corneal staining

Summary

Vitreous haemorrhage is a common presenting complaint in vitreoretinal clinics. It is easily treated by vitrectomy.

References

1. Spirn MJ, Lynn MJ, Hubbard GB III. Vitreous hemorrhage in children. Ophthalmology. 2006;113(5):848–52.
2. De Maeyer K, Van Ginderdeuren R, Postelmans L, Stalmans P, Van Calster J. Sub-inner limiting membrane haemorrhage: causes and treatment with vitrectomy. Br J Ophthalmol. 2007;91(7):869–72. bjo.2006.109132 [pii]. https://doi.org/10.1136/bjo.2006.109132.
3. Garweg JG, Koerner F. Outcome indicators for vitrectomy in Terson syndrome. Acta Ophthalmol. 2009;87(2):222–6. AOS1200 [pii]. https://doi.org/10.1111/j.1755-3768.2008.01200.x.
4. Lauer AK, Smith JR, Robertson JE, Rosenbaum JT. Vitreous hemorrhage is a common complication of pediatric pars planitis. Ophthalmology. 2002;109(1):95–8.
5. Zhao P, Hayashi H, Oshima K, Nakagawa N, Ohsato M. Vitrectomy for macular hemorrhage associated with retinal arterial macroaneurysm. Ophthalmology. 2000;107(3):613–7.
6. Kuhn F, Morris R, Witherspoon CD, Mester V. Terson syndrome. Results of vitrectomy and the significance of vitreous hemorrhage in patients with subarachnoid hemorrhage. Ophthalmology. 1998;105(3):472–7.
7. Dana MR, Werner MS, Viana MA, Shapiro MJ. Spontaneous and traumatic vitreous hemorrhage. Ophthalmology. 1993;100(9):1377–83.
8. el Bawa F, Jarrett WH, Harbin TS Jr, Fine SL, Michels RG, Schachat AP, et al. Massive hemorrhage complicating age-related macular degeneration. Clinicopathologic correlation and role of anticoagulants. Ophthalmology. 1986;93(12):1581–92.
9. Lean JS, Gregor Z. The acute vitreous haemorrhage. Br J Ophthalmol. 1980;64(7):469–71.
10. Sarrafizadeh R, Hassan TS, Ruby AJ, Williams GA, Garretson BR, Capone A Jr, et al. Incidence of retinal detachment and visual outcome in eyes presenting with posterior vitreous separation and dense fundus-obscuring vitreous hemorrhage. Ophthalmology. 2001;108(12):2273–8.
11. Tan HS, Mura M, Bijl HM. Early vitrectomy for vitreous hemorrhage associated with retinal tears. Am J Ophthalmol. 150(4):529–33. S0002-9394(10)00261-8 [pii]. https://doi.org/10.1016/j.ajo.2010.04.005.

Rhegmatogenous Retinal Detachment 1

7

Contents

Introduction

Strictly speaking, "retinal detachment" is a misnomer. The term denotes the separation of the neuroepithelium from the pigment epithelium (rather than detachment of the retina, which consists of the neuroepithelium and the RPE, from the choroid) and therefore implies re-establishment of the space between the original layers of the embryonic optic cup. The incidence is approximately 10/100,000 [1] and presentation is more common in affluent populations and possibly males. Black races are probably less affected than white [2].

The most common cause of retinal detachment is the formation of a "break" or full-thickness discontinuity in the neuroepithelium with the recruitment of fluid from the vitreous cavity into the subretinal space via the break, creating "rhegmatogenous retinal detachment." Classically, breaks are subdivided into "tears" (secondary to dynamic vitreoretinal traction) and "holes" (secondary to localised retinal disintegration or atrophy).

Natural History

The commonest RRD is associated with PVD and tractional retinal tear formation. This occurs in middle age and slightly commoner in males. Most RRD like this commence in the superotemporal region as a one quadrant RRD and then extend inferiorly picking up inferior breaks and increasing the extent of the RRD and detaching the fovea. Success rates of primary surgery are reduced with the number of quadrants of retinal involvement and whether inferior breaks are elevated by SRF [3]. It is therefore important that RRDs are referred promptly and not just for macula on or off.

The fovea is sensitive to detachment with cones more likely to be damaged or lost if detached than rods. For those patients with short duration of macular off RRD surgery should be performed promptly to restore the cones to their blood supply (the choroid). Early macula off RRD (for 1–3 days) should be regarded as urgent as macula on RRD for the urgency of surgery because patients do worse visually if they are left beyond 3 days from the detachment of the fovea. Even if operations are performed in macula on RRD within 24 h 1% of patients will progress to macula off by the

T. H. Williamson, *Vitreoretinal Surgery*, https://doi.org/10.1007/978-3-030-68769-4_7

time of surgery. This, thankfully, has little effect on their visual outcomes (Figs. 7.1 and 7.2).

Finally, longer duration of RRD leads to loss of receptors and development of PVR, further reducing anatomical and visual success. Risk of surgery to the other eye is 7% at 10 years [4].

Tears with Posterior Vitreous Detachment

Most retinal tears occur in association with posterior vitreous detachment by the operation of "dynamic vitreous traction." This term denotes the transmission of rotational energy (generated by saccadic contraction of the extraocular muscles) to the vitreous gel through the coats of the eye (sclera, choroid and retina). While the vitreous remains attached to the retina, this energy transmission is dispersed throughout the total area of vitreoretinal contact. After posterior vitreous detachment, however, the forces produce considerable movement in the posterior gel. The vitreous base provides the centre of energy while the posterior vitreous responds to the energy by accelerating into a violent movement (Figs. 7.3 and 7.4).

If there is any area of "abnormal" adhesion of the retina to the gel, the movement of the gel exerts considerable dynamic traction on the retina, sometimes producing a U-shaped tear of the retina. The base of the tongue of the retina, which produces the "U," is anteriorly placed because the vitreous separates first posteriorly, tearing the retina at a point of adhesion, and the action of the vitreous extends the tear anteriorly towards the vitreous base. If the flap of the tear separates completely from the retina, the piece of the avulsed neurosensory retina is seen attached to the posterior vitreous membrane as an operculum, and a round tear is produced.

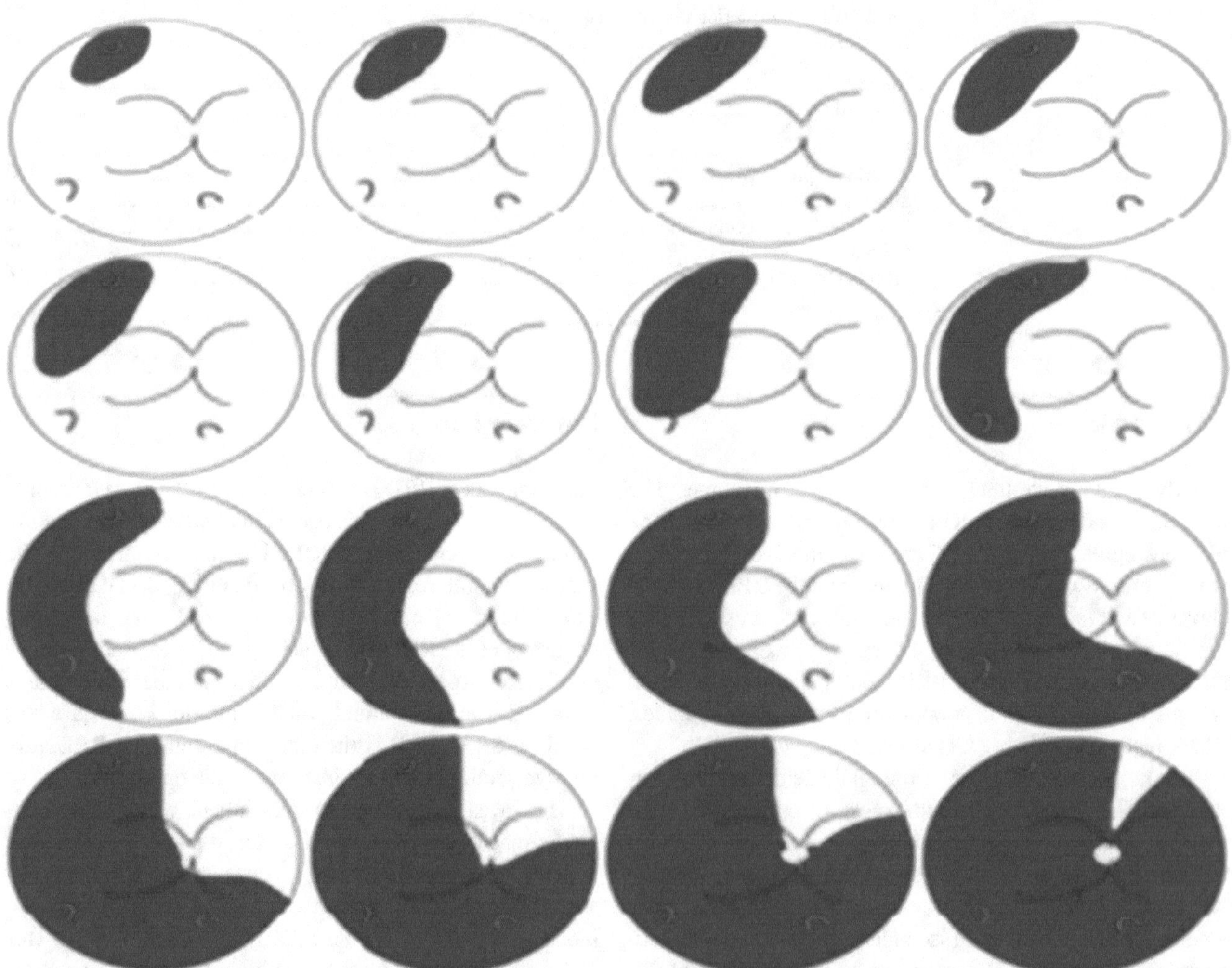

Fig. 7.1 Most PVD-related RRD starts in the superotemporal region and spread around the retina picking any inferior retinal breaks as they go. Detached inferior breaks and increased quadrants of RRD are associated with the poorer primary success of the surgery. Primary success of surgery is associated with visual outcome. It is therefore important to operate when the RRD is limited to the superotemporal region. Rapid referral and prompt treatment are essential for good results, not only relying on whether the fovea has detached or not

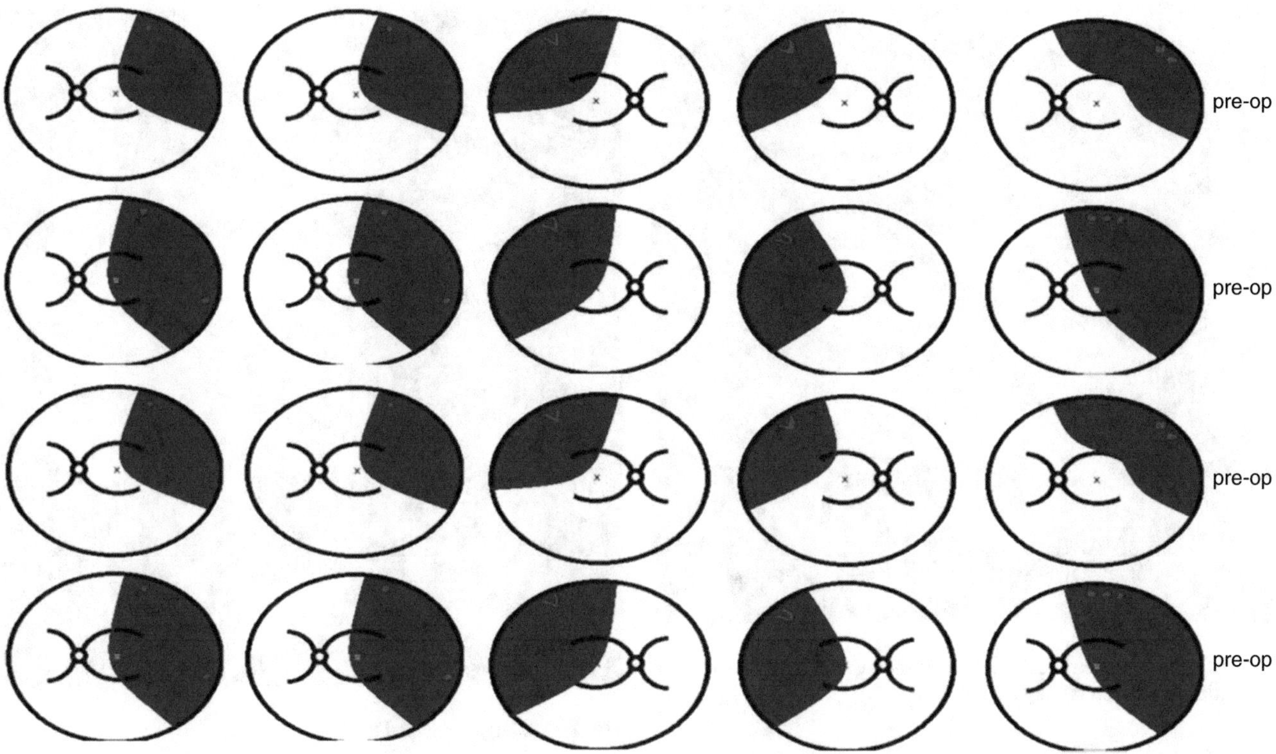

Fig. 7.2 The retinal drawings of 10 patients in whom the fovea detached while waiting for surgery. These were primarily bullous superotemporal RRD near the macula at presentation. The short duration of foveal detachment was associated with high levels of visual recovery

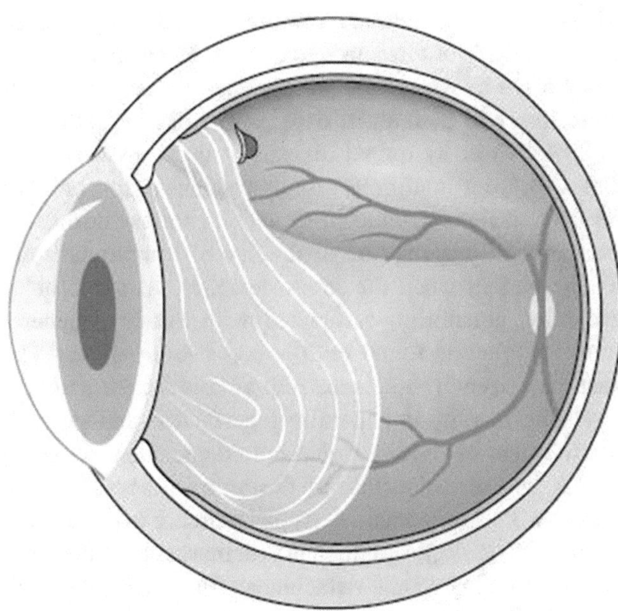

Fig. 7.3 A retinal tear occurs when the vitreous separates from the retina posteriorly. The vitreous produces traction on its attachments to the retina, thereby tearing the retina, producing a retinal break

Ninety percent of tears are present at the initial examination after a symptomatic PVD. Approximately 10% are not seen at the initial presentation or develop later; therefore a follow-up examination is recommended [5].

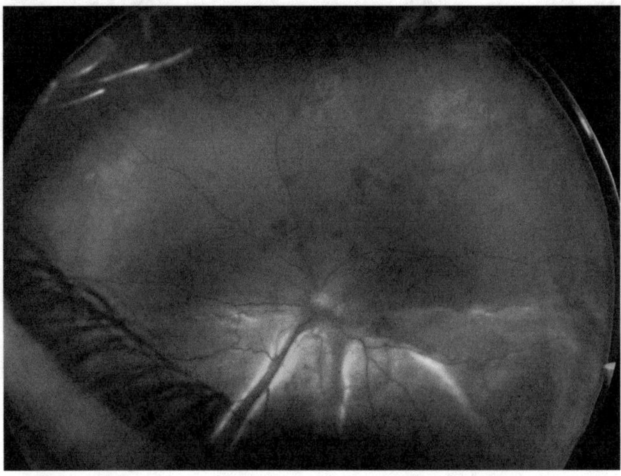

Fig. 7.4 A retinal detachment with 12 o'clock break and mild vitreous haemorrhage

If the symptoms are of a few days' duration review in one week if longer review at 4–6 weeks (Figs. 7.5 and 7.6).

Haemorrhage from rupture of a blood vessel that crosses a U tear may produce a "tadpole" floater or shower of floaters. Floaters may also be seen from the posterior vitreous detachment and photopsia (flashing lights) from traction on the retina.

The vitreous is adherent to the rim of lattice lesions. U tears in lattice, therefore, tear along the posterior border of

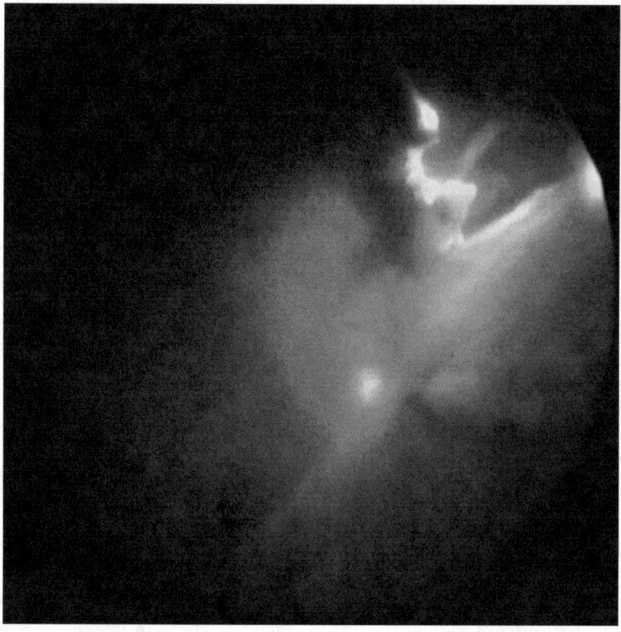

Fig. 7.5 A clot of fibrin can be seen extending from an artery torn by the action of PVD in tearing the retina

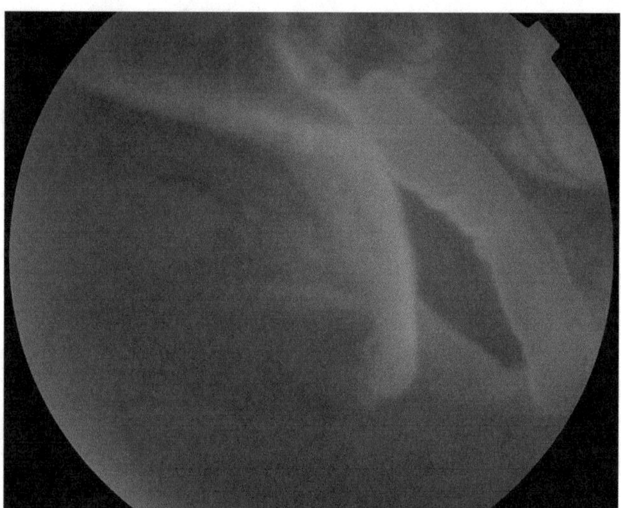

Fig. 7.6 A large retinal tear

the lattice and then extend anteriorly around the edge of the lesion.

Multiple tiny flap breaks at the posterior border of the vitreous base are particularly associated with aphakia or pseudophakia. The reasons for this are not clear, but cataract extraction alters the architecture of the vitreous through loss of the posterior bulge of the crystalline lens into the anterior vitreous (Fig. 7.7).

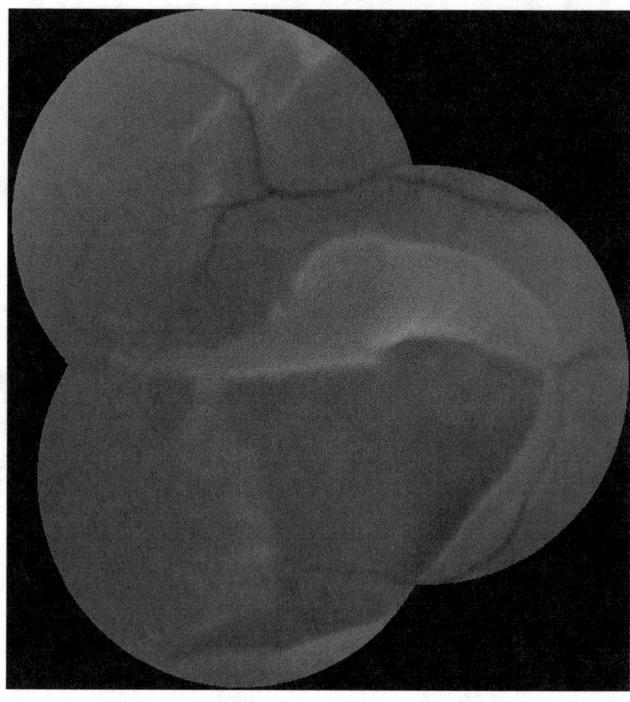

Fig. 7.7 A large U-shaped tear

Breaks without Posterior Vitreous Detachment

Rhegmatogenous retinal detachment may be produced without posterior vitreous detachment by atrophic retinal holes often in young myopic patients (these patients are more likely to be female, 64%, with bilateral pathology in 83% [6]) or by retinal dialysis at the ora serrata (see Chap. 6). Both conditions usually produce a slow onset of retinal detachment, which may only be noticed during the coincidental examination of the eye or symptomatically by the patient when the fovea detaches. Atrophic holes are often equatorial, associated with lattice degeneration, myopia and found in 20–40-year-old patients. The vast majority will not cause retinal detachment and prophylactic therapy is generally regarded as unnecessary. Recruitment of fluid in round hole detachment probably occurs by the connection of the hole to lacunae in the vitreous. This may cause a stepped increase in the detachment with multiple pigmentary demarcation lines in a chronic-looking retinal detachment (Figs. 7.8, 7.9, 7.10, 7.11, 7.12).

Retinal dialyses are ellipsoid separations of the retina at the ora serrata that are usually situated inferotemporally. They differ from U tears because the gel is attached to the posterior rather than the anterior margin of the break, and posterior vitreous detachment is absent.

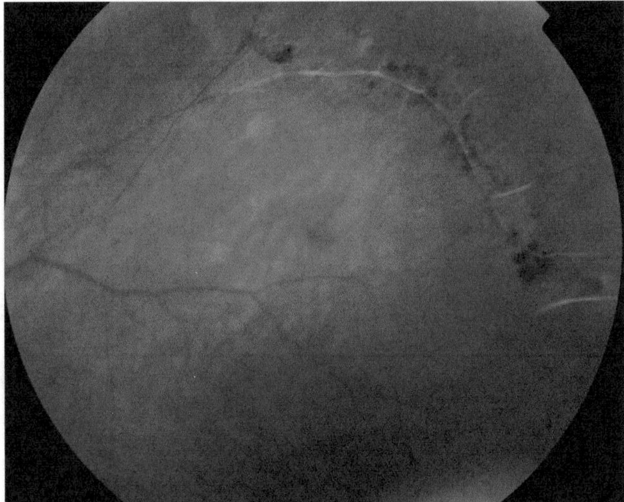

Fig. 7.8 Lattice degeneration

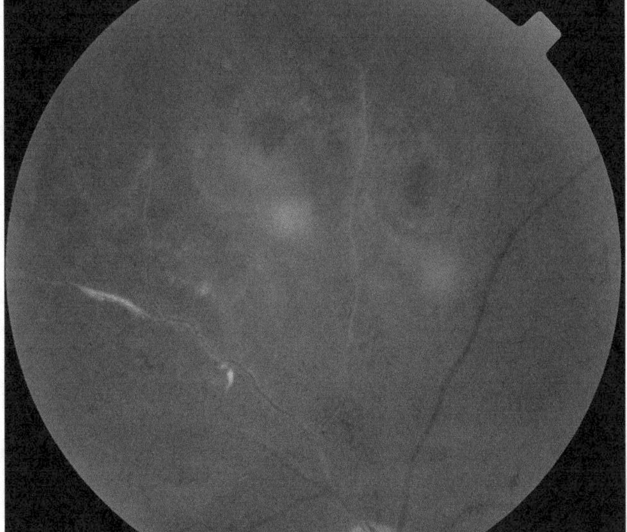

Fig. 7.9 These round breaks have overlying opercula of the retina (seen out of focus), suggesting previous vitreal traction, these breaks are at low risk of causing retinal detachment

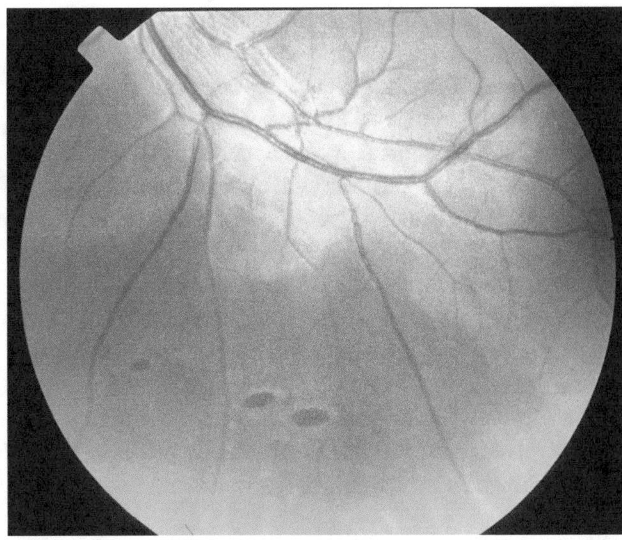

Fig. 7.10 Round holes are present in an inferior retina in this patient. These can be ignored if they are asymptomatic as the chances of their progression to retinal detachment are probably less than 1/200

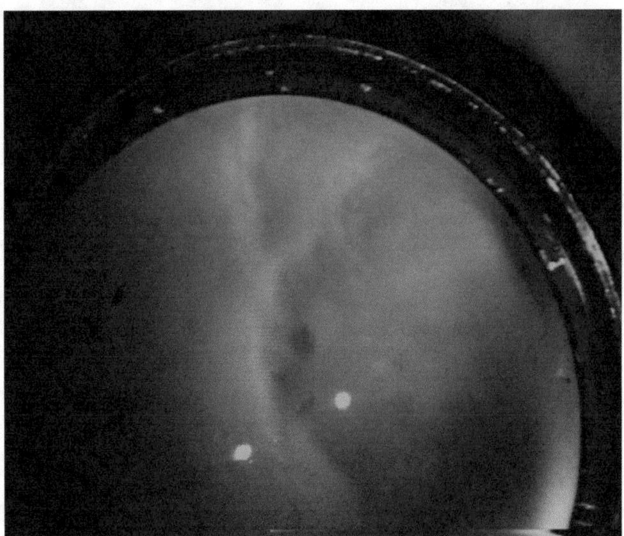

Fig. 7.11 A round hole is visible on the indentation of this eye

Natural History

- Most retinal detachments, if untreated will progress to totality or near totality. The visual loss is profound, and potential recovery of vision by surgery reduces as the weeks go by.
- The accumulation of SRF in the periphery seems to be important for the development of loss of vision as patients with RRD lose more vision in comparison to CSR for the same foveal.
- Initially, the retina is thickened and less transparent than normal.
- If the retina remains detached for many months, it becomes progressively atrophic.
- The longer the retina remains detached, the higher the risk of a scarring response, proliferative vitreoretinopathy (see PVR Chap. 8) (Figs. 7.13, 7.14, 7.15).

Chronic RRD

In a longstanding subtotal retinal detachment, a "high-water mark" or pigment demarcation line of retinal pigment hyperplasia may appear, which sometimes limits the further extension of the detachment. Multiple high-water marks in the detached retina indicate recurrent extension of the detachment and are more often seen in slower onset detachments associated with round holes or dialyses. Other indices of longstanding detachment include retinal cysts (secondary retinoschisis) [7], oxalate crystals on the macula [8] and peripheral neovascularisation (Figs. 7.16, 7.17, 7.18, 7.19, 7.20, 7.21, 7.22, 7.23, 7.24, 7.25, 7.26, 7.27, 7.28).

Very rarely, the retina reattaches spontaneously, sometimes leaving pigmented chorioretinal changes but most often, surgery is required to reattach the retina. After successful surgery, the rods recover their function surprisingly well and any visual field defect disappears. If the fovea has been involved, recovery of function of the cones is good if the detachment is treated quickly (within one week of onset).

Fig. 7.12 A round hole seen on a slit lamp camera

After prolonged detachment of the fovea, central vision may be permanently impaired (Figs. 7.29, 7.30, 7.31, 7.32).

Descriptive statistics for a north European population [9].

Mean age	53 years
Bilateral	10%
Lattice Degeneration	15%
Total Detachment	17%
More than one break	41%
No break found	11%
More dialyses	<20 years old
Tears = atrophic holes	20–40-year olds
Predominantly tears	>40-year-old
Bilateral simultaneous [10]	2.3%

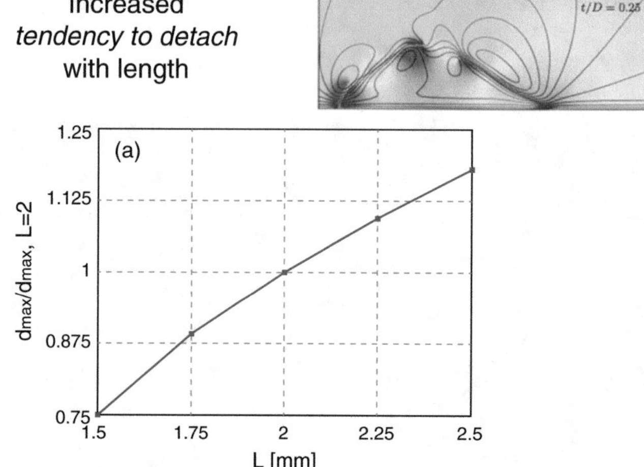

Fig. 7.14 The forces increase as the detachment increases

Fig. 7.13 Forces are applied to the retina from fluid currents passing through a retinal break

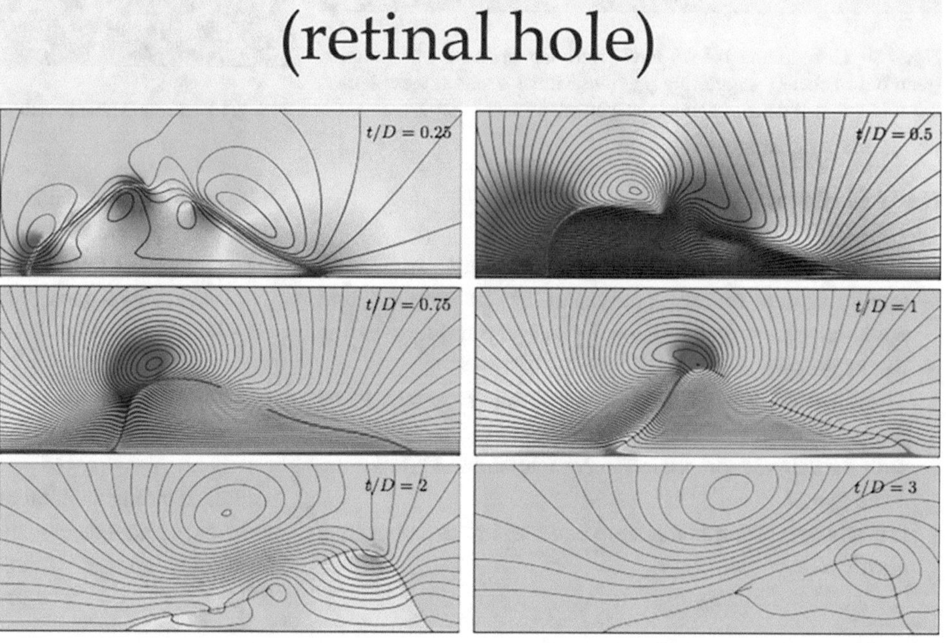

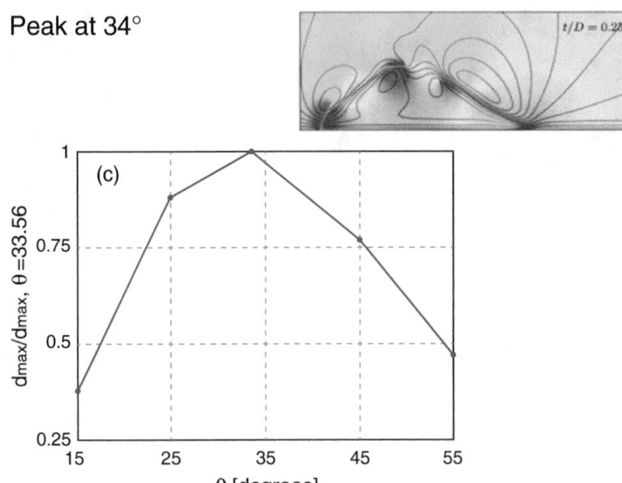

Fig. 7.15 The force on the adhesion of the retina to the RPE is maximal at 34 degrees

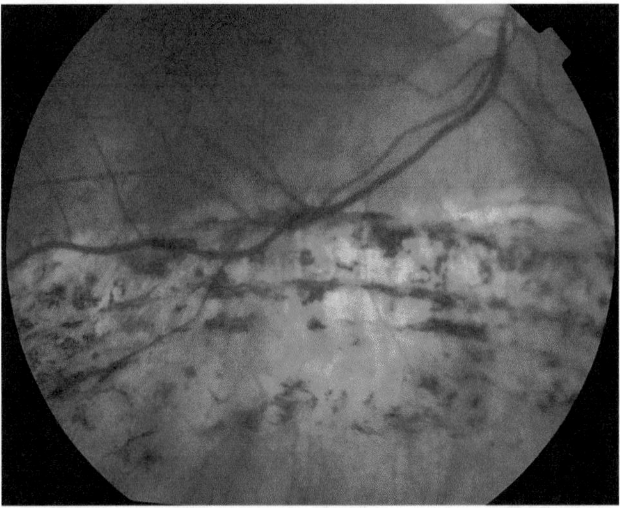

Fig. 7.17 An RRD may spontaneously reattach, leaving RPE hypertrophy and atrophy. The arcs of pigment hyperplasia in this patient suggest that the RRD advanced, stopped and advanced again, a phenomenon is seen in vitreous attached RRD. One theory for this observation is that lacunae of fluid vitreous empty through a retinal hole, providing fluid for the subretinal space and advancement of the RRD edge. The RRD does not move again until other lacunae form and empties through a hole. In the meantime, RPE hyperplasia occurs at the juncture of the detached and attached retina creating arcs of pigmentation. Spontaneous reattachment may occur when vitreous gel plugs the retinal hole, and the RPE is able to clear the SRF

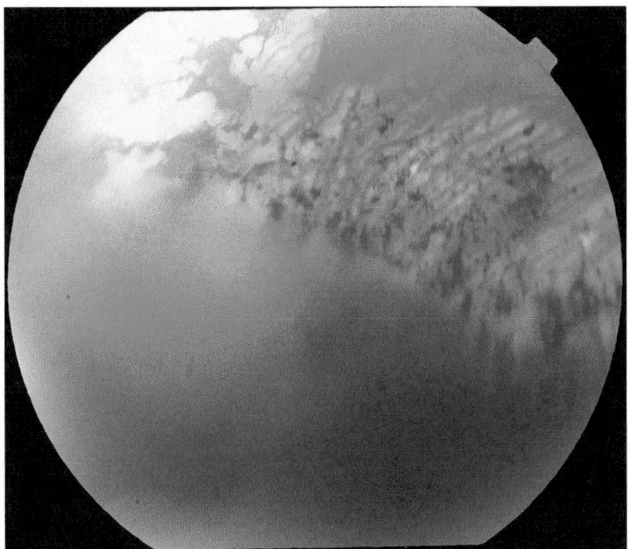

Fig. 7.16 A demarcation line is shown around this retinal detachment which has been chronic in nature. It is unlikely that the retinal detachment will extend through this demarcation, and therefore surgery is not required

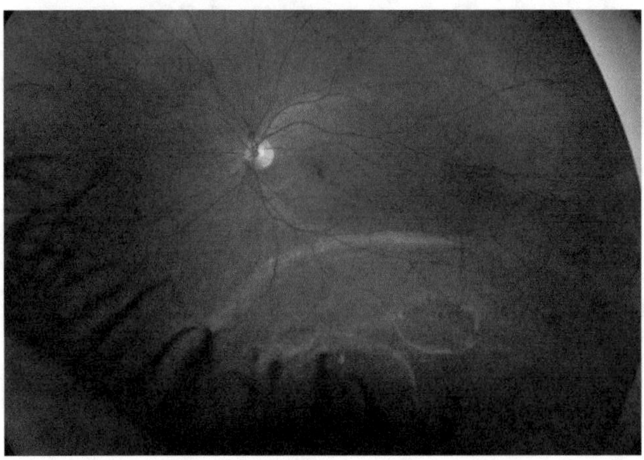

Fig. 7.18 A chronic RRD with retinal cysts

Risk to the Other Eye

Chance of RRD in the fellow eye, later on, is 12% with an 12% chance of requirement for retinopexy to a tear [11].

Clinical Features

The patient may experience symptoms of flashes and floaters (indicating posterior vitreous detachment with or without vitreous haemorrhage) followed by visual field loss. Some slow onset retinal detachments will produce the symptom of a slow flashing light (often moving like a slow comet tail) lasting a few seconds and situated in the visual field appropriate to the leading edge of SRF. When the fovea detaches, there is loss of central vision, with the fovea just off, the visual acuity may vary from 20/40 to 20/200. As the fovea lifts, the patient may experience distortion of vision. When the macula is fully detached, the vision may be 20/200 to hand movements.

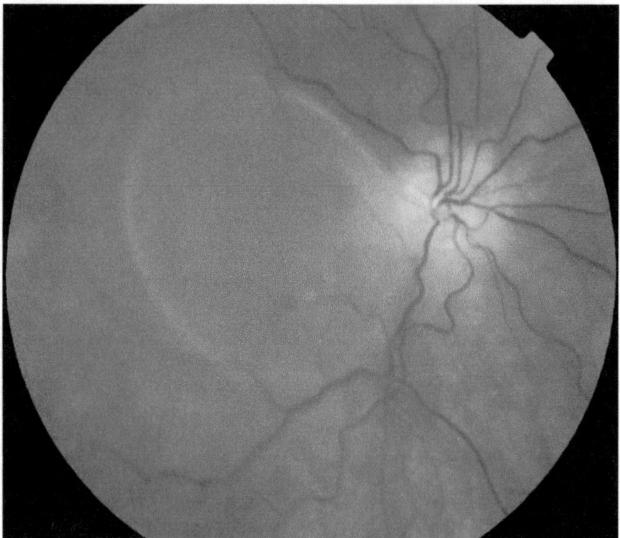

Fig. 7.19 A retinal cyst has formed in the macular area in this patient with chronic RRD

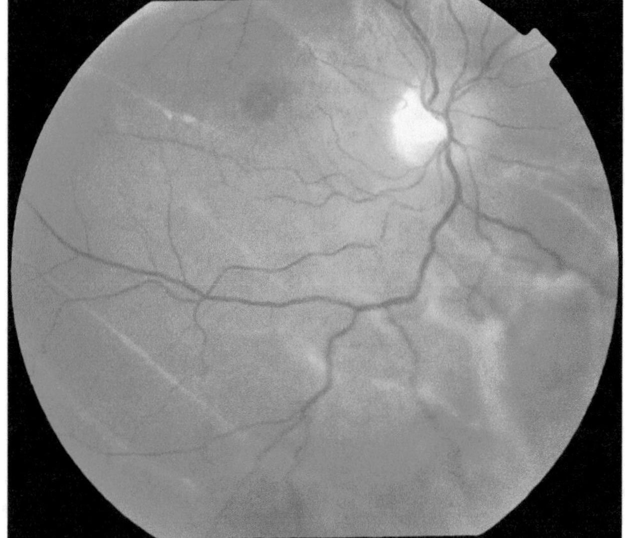

Fig. 7.20 Subretinal bands in a chronic RRD, these are commoner in vitreous attached RRD, e.g. retinal dialysis or round hole (young myope) RRD

Anterior Segment Signs

A few cells and some flare can be seen in the anterior chamber. Rarely a severe anterior uveitis occurs, perhaps indicating a high risk of PVR. IOP is often lower than the fellow eye. Occasionally a high IOP can be produced by blockage of the trabecular meshwork by the remnants of receptor outer segments (Schwartz's syndrome) [12, 13]. Iris neovascularization has been described, which reverses after resolution of the RRD [14].

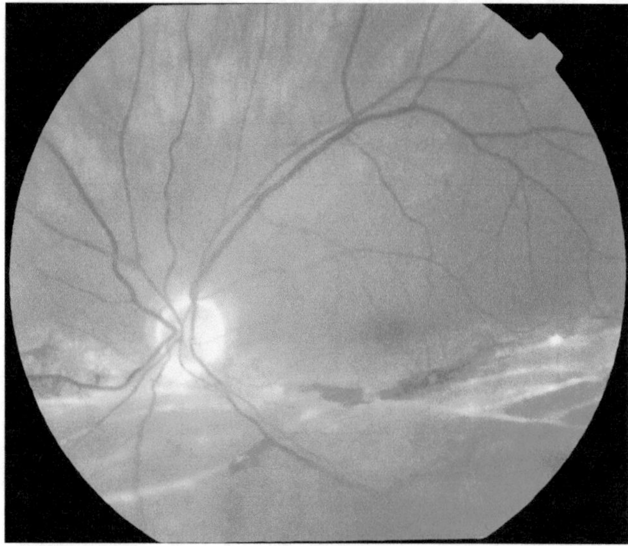

Fig. 7.21 The fovea was in place in this chronic RRD with subretinal bands. The retinal hole appeared to be plugged with vitreous, perhaps preventing further fluid vitreous entry through the break and further spread of the RRD

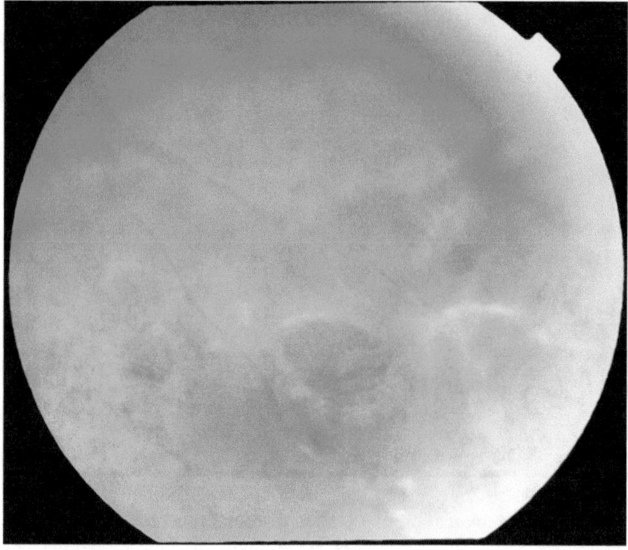

Fig. 7.22 The retinal hole can be seen

Signs in the Vitreous

Retinal tear formation is usually associated with the release of retinal pigment epithelial cells into the vitreous cavity (see Chap. 3). The presence of pigment cells in the retrolental gel (Shafer's sign) [15] in a phakic eye strongly implies the presence of a retinal break. Differentiation of these cells into fibroblast-like cells and synthesis of new collagen within the gel and on the posterior hyaloid interface results in retraction and immobilisation of the gel. An early sign of this process is seen when the cells change from diffuse single cells to

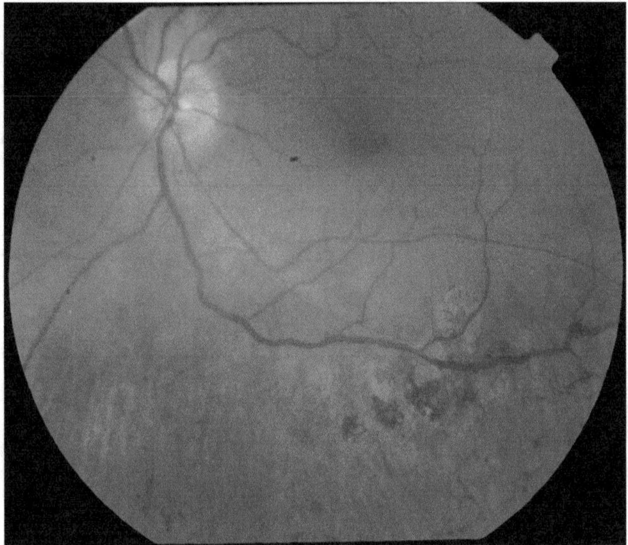

Fig. 7.23 If an RRD spontaneously reattaches retinal pigment, epithelial changes may occur

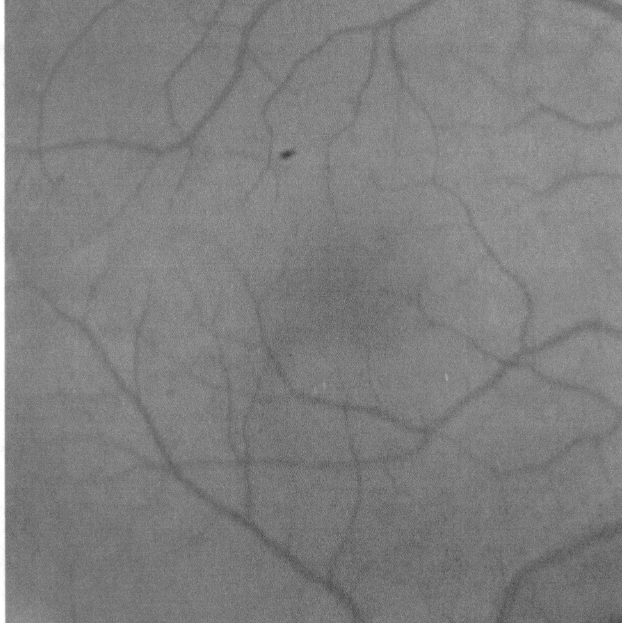

Fig. 7.24 Tiny white flecks can be seen in the fovea in patients with chronic retinal detachment. These are signs of oxalosis, a secondary complication from the chronicity of the retinal detachment

groups or "clumps" of cells in the gel. Such changes are frequently associated with the proliferation and contraction of cellular membranes on the retinal surface in proliferative vitreoretinopathy (PVR). Vitreous haemorrhage may obscure the view of the retina and breaks. Suspect that any patient with vitreous haemorrhage of unknown aetiology has a retinal tear or detachment.

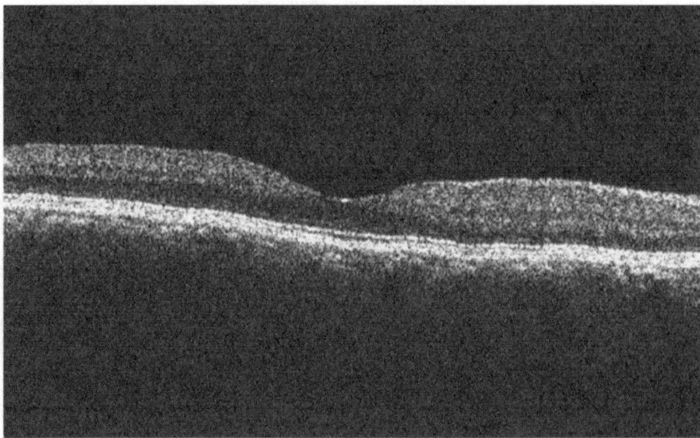

Fig. 7.25 A tiny speck of oxalate can be seen on the foveal surface on OCT (grey scale image)

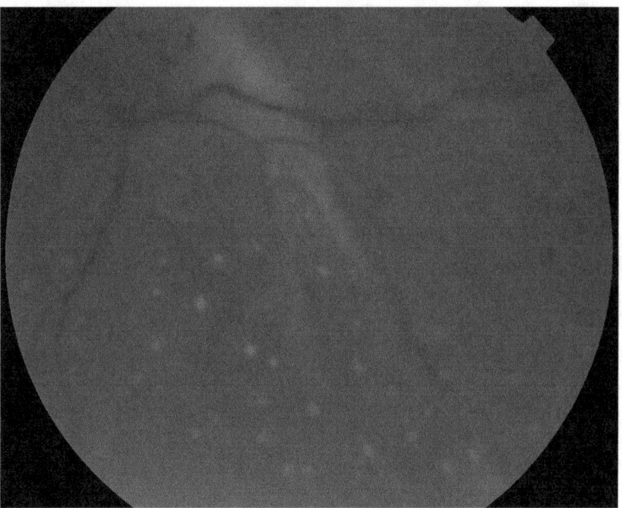

Fig. 7.26 Some longstanding RRDs, e.g. from retinal dialysis, will show white spots on the outer retina. These fade after reattachment of the retina

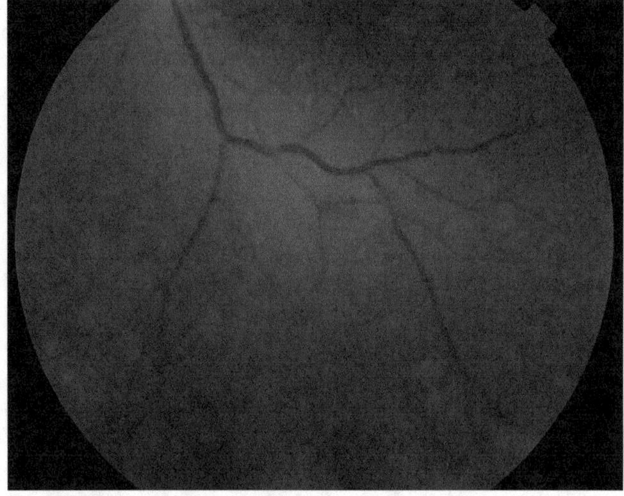

Fig. 7.27 The white spots fade after retinal reattachment

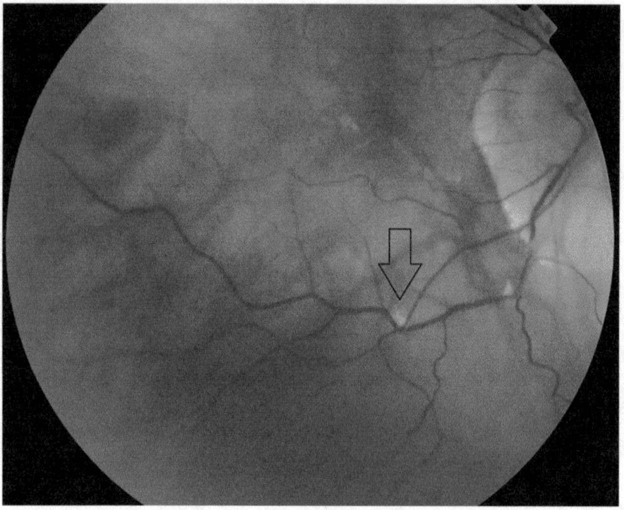

Fig. 7.28 The arrow indicates a point of adhesion that appears to have stopped the progress of a chronic inferior RRD

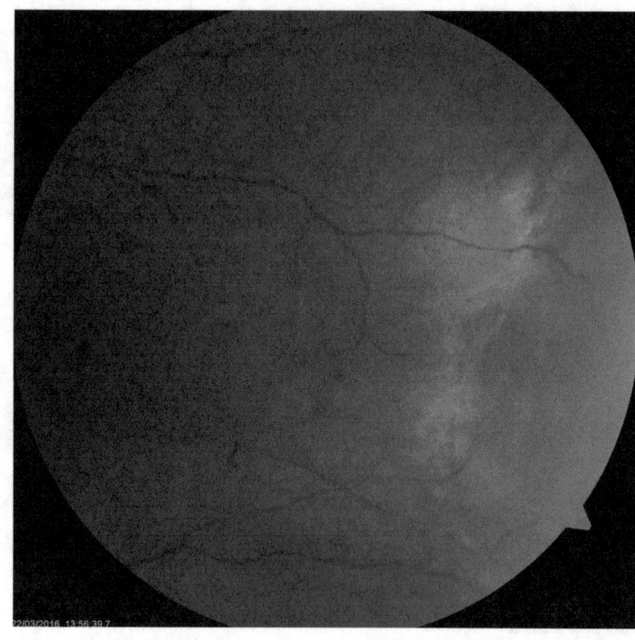

Fig. 7.30 A chronic RRD with a demarcation line

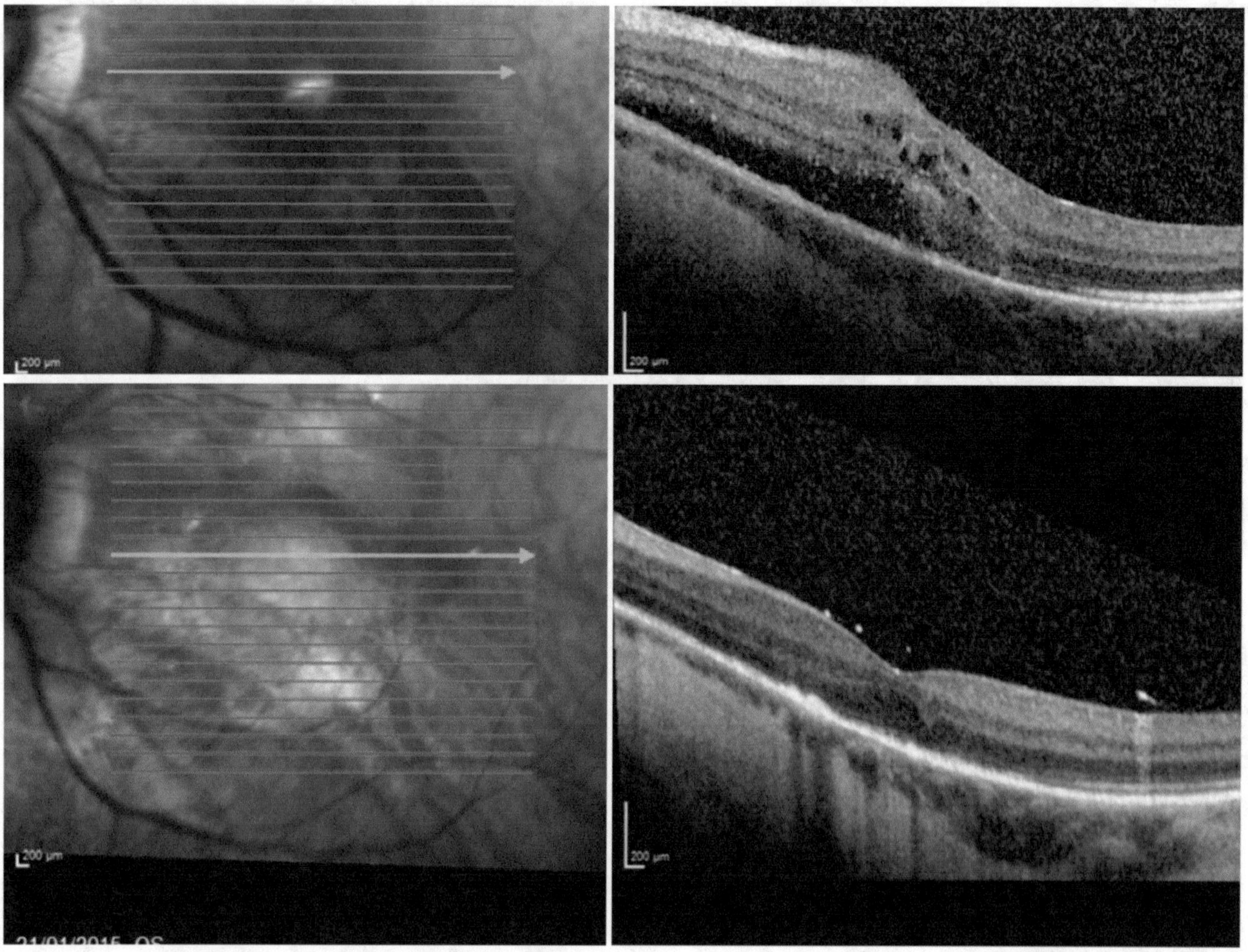

Fig. 7.29 Chronic RRD without recovery of the ellipsoid layer after surgery

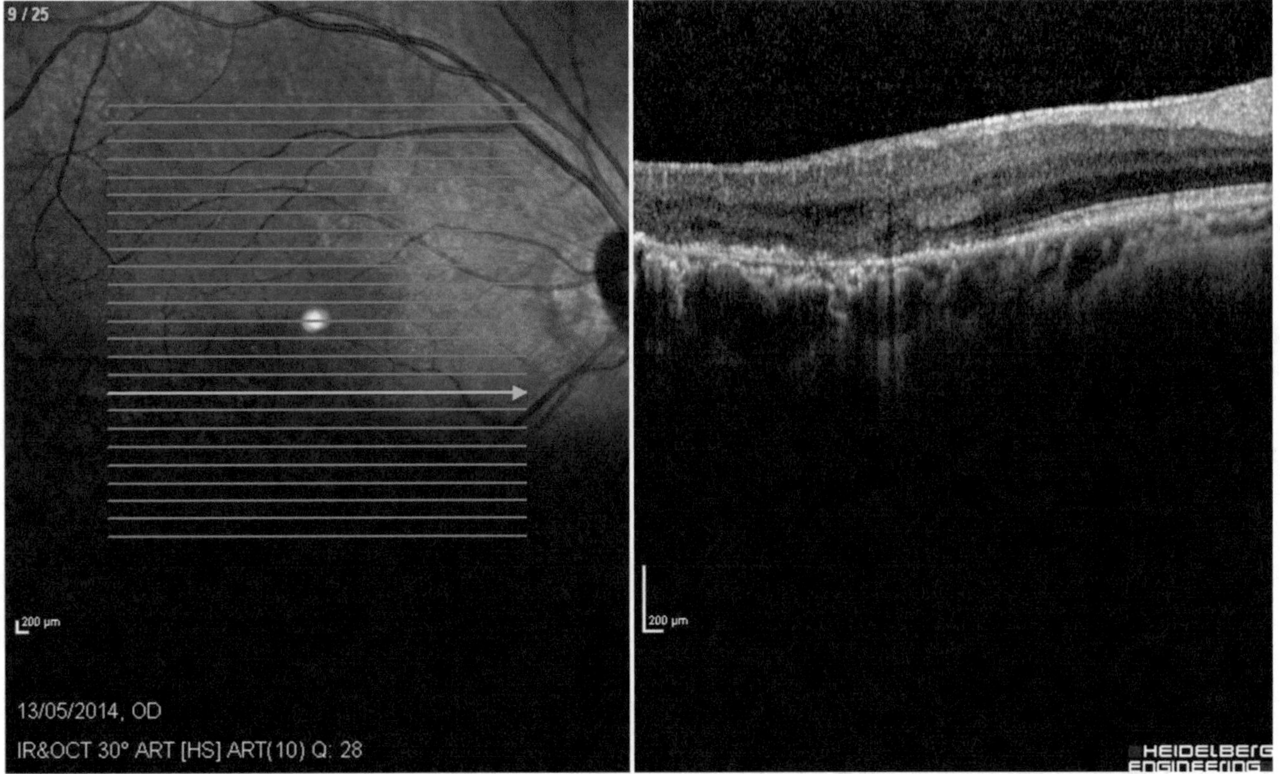

Fig. 7.31 Loss of receptors in the inferior macula from a chronic RRD

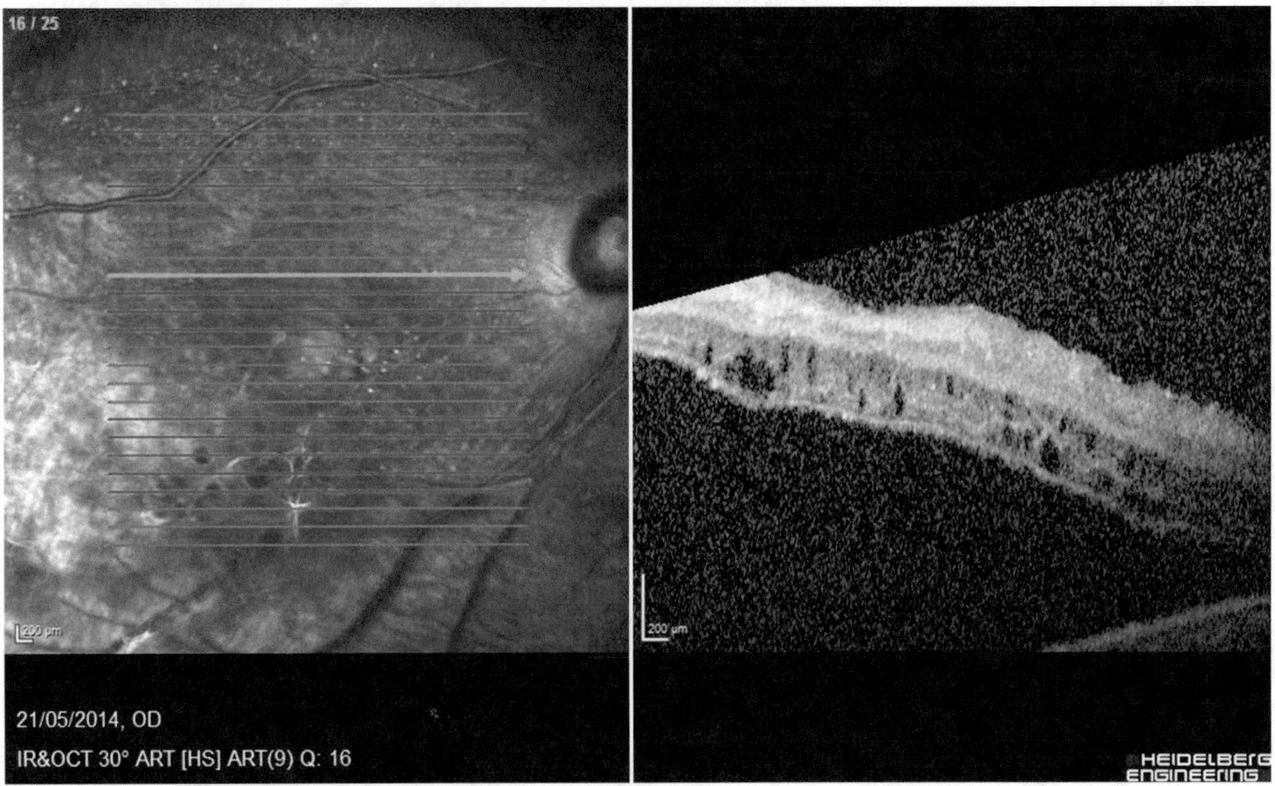

Fig. 7.32 A chronic RRD showing loss of outer retinal architecture

Subretinal Fluid Accumulation

Separation of the neuroepithelium from the pigment epithelium occurs first in the immediate vicinity of the break. Progressively more subretinal fluid is recruited from the vitreous cavity (from the retro hyaloid space or from syneretic gel), increasing the area and elevation of retinal separation. Progression has been estimated at 1.8 disc diameters per day [16] so that fovea on patients can become fovea off by the time of surgery. If the globe is completely immobilised at an early stage, the retina may partially or even completely reattach, suggesting that three mechanisms may be implicated.

Movement of the eye (and the resultant vitreous gel movement) causes extension of the retinal detachment through the action of dynamic vitreoretinal traction (Figs. 7.33, 7.34, 7.35, 7.36, 7.37).

The movement of the gel induces fluid currents in the retrohyaloid space, which forcefully elevates the neurosensory retina [17].

Gravity encourages the spread of the subretinal fluid.

The last mechanism causes a pattern of spread of subretinal fluid first described by Lincoff that may be used by the surgeon to aid localisation of a retinal break [18].

A tear between 11 and 1 o'clock causes a retinal detachment, which becomes total soon after its onset.

Tears above the horizontal meridian (3 o'clock to 9 o'clock) produce subtotal detachments. Fluid is recruited, progressing downwards on the same side as the tear at first and then upwards on the opposite side of the disc (but to a level lower than that on the side of the tear).

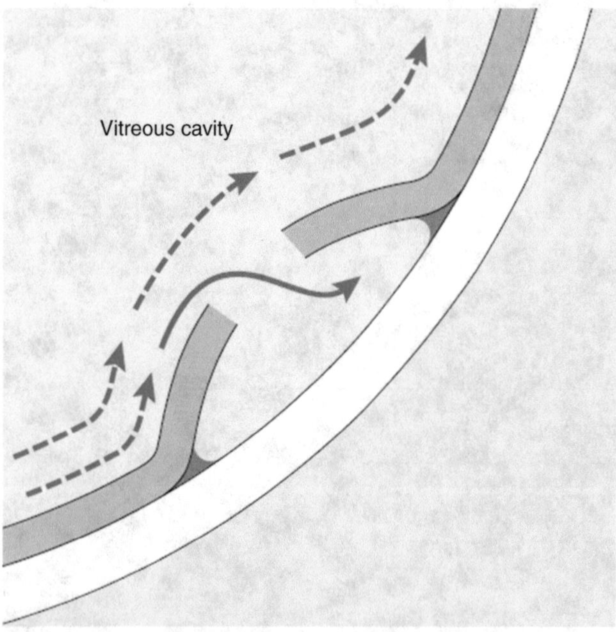

Fig. 7.33 Fluid currents from the vitreous cavity may contribute to the lifting of the retina in rhegmatogenous retinal detachment

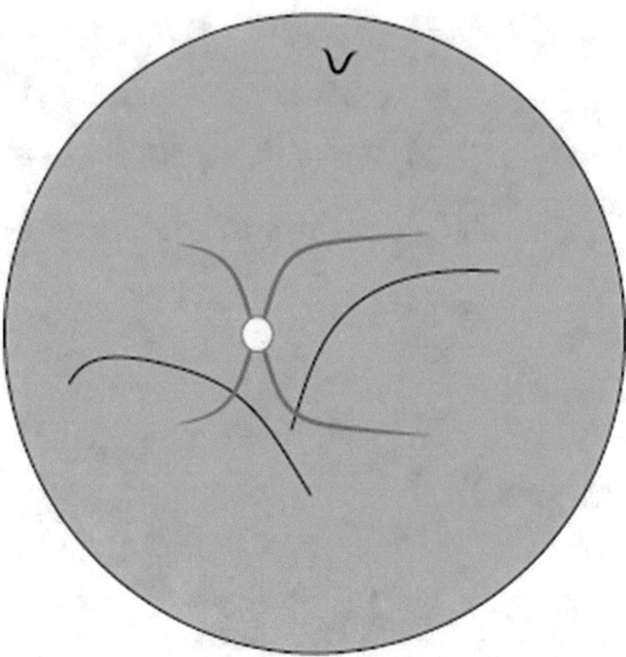

Fig. 7.34 A break at 12 o clock causes a total bullous RRD

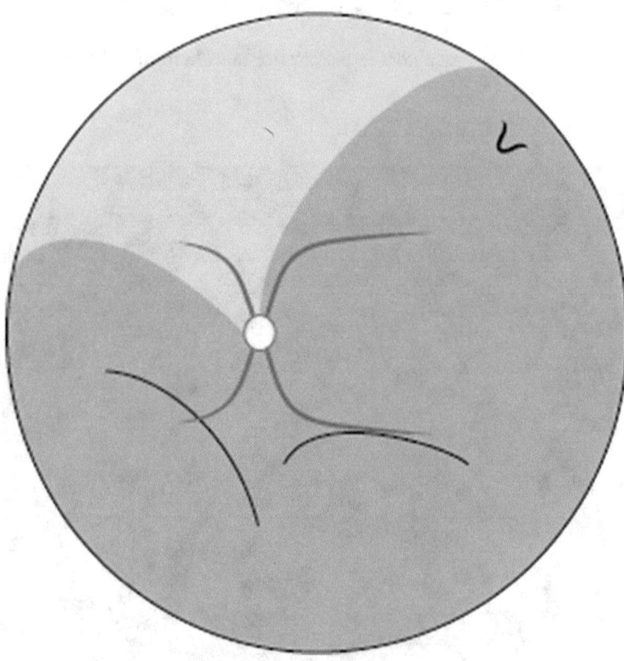

Fig. 7.35 The retinal break in a bullous RRD is usually located 1 to 2 clock hours from the superior edge on the highest side

Inferior subretinal fluid from a superior tear tends to separate partially into two bullae with a cleft or "cleavage" of less elevated retina in the 6 o'clock meridian.

A break located below the horizontal meridian tends to accumulate fluid more slowly compared with that descending from above. The upper limits of the detachment form

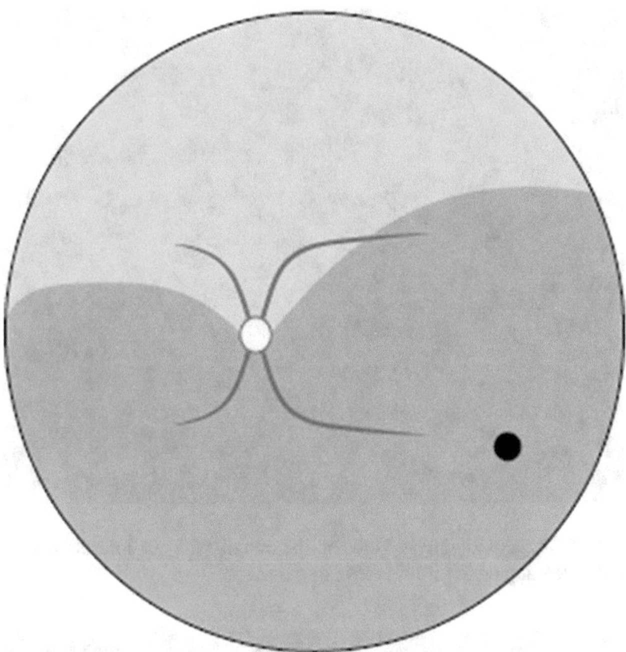

Fig. 7.36 The break in a non-bullous RRD is usually inferior and on the side of the highest retinal detachment upper edge

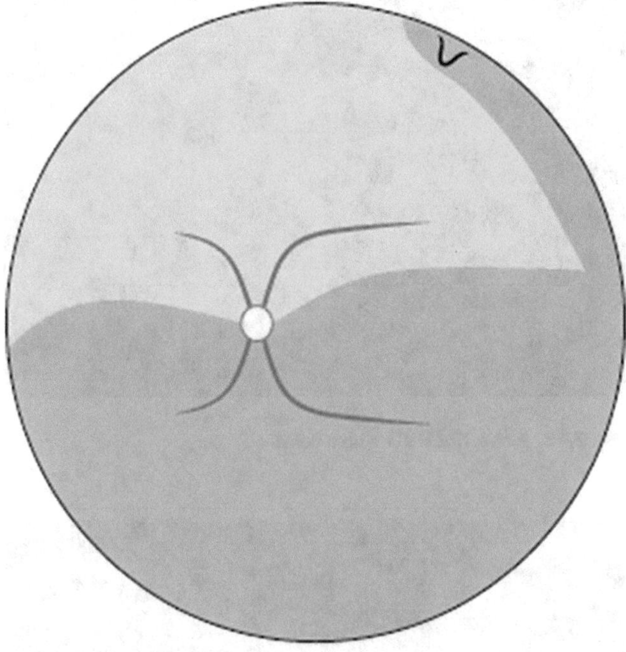

Fig. 7.37 Occasionally, a small anterior break will cause an inferior RRD by tracking SRF down the anterior retina

convex curved edges on each side, the higher edge indicating the side of the break. Bullae are not seen with inferior breaks.

Occasionally a small anterior and superior tear leaks fluid down the post oral retina, causing an inferior retinal detachment. Therefore, inferior retinal detachments can occur from both superior and inferior tears (Figs. 7.38 and 7.39).

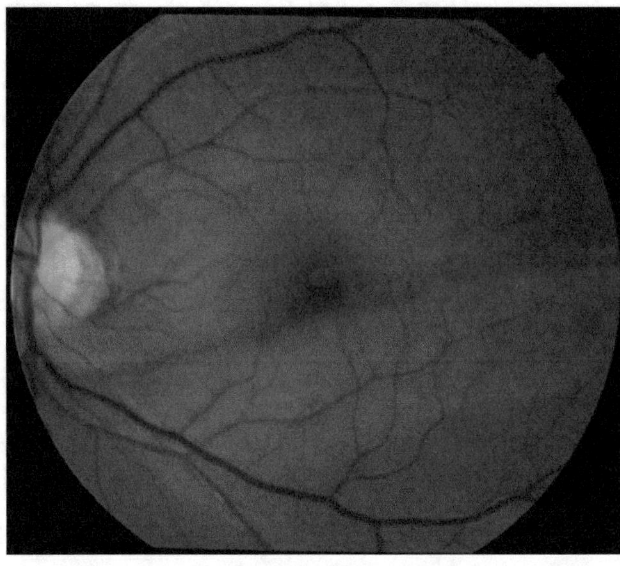

Fig. 7.38 An RRD near the fovea

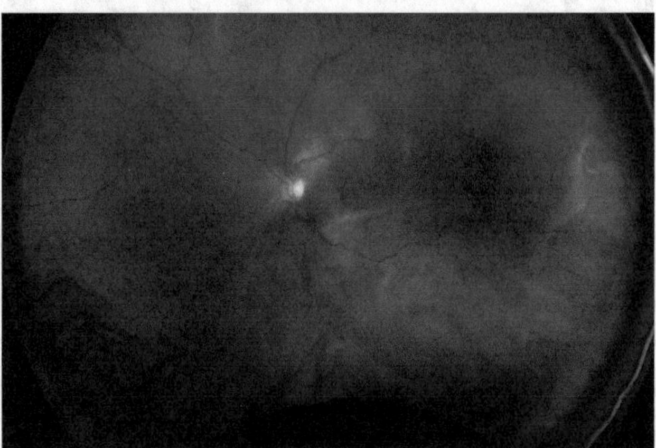

Fig. 7.39 A shallow inferior RRD

Subretinal fluid accumulates more quickly if fluid is recruited from the retrohyaloid space (e.g. via a U tear after posterior vitreous detachment) compared with breaks occurring without posterior vitreous detachment (e.g. atrophic holes and dialyses). In the latter potential recruitment of fluid from syneretic gel may be limited by the size of the lacuna in the gel. As a retinal detachment progresses, the patient notices an increasing field defect corresponding to the detached area. Central vision is distorted and diminished as the fovea detaches (Figs. 7.40 and 7.41).

Retinal Break Patterns in RRD

Breaks are more common temporally and superiorly than nasally or inferiorly in PVD-related RRD. See the next chapter for more details (Figs. 7.42, 7.43, 7.44, 7.45).

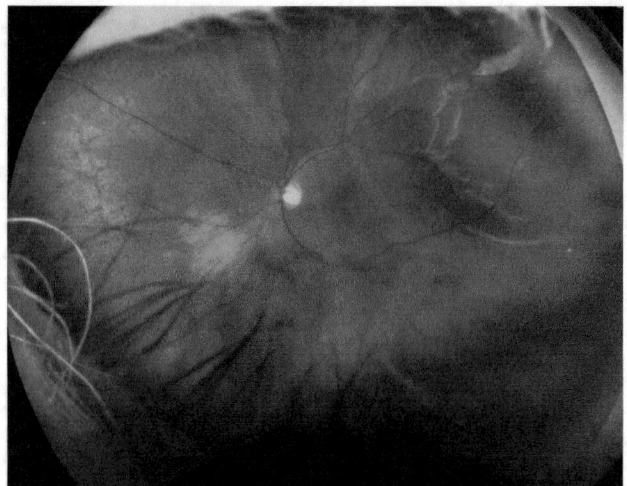

Fig. 7.40 A retinal tear with RRD

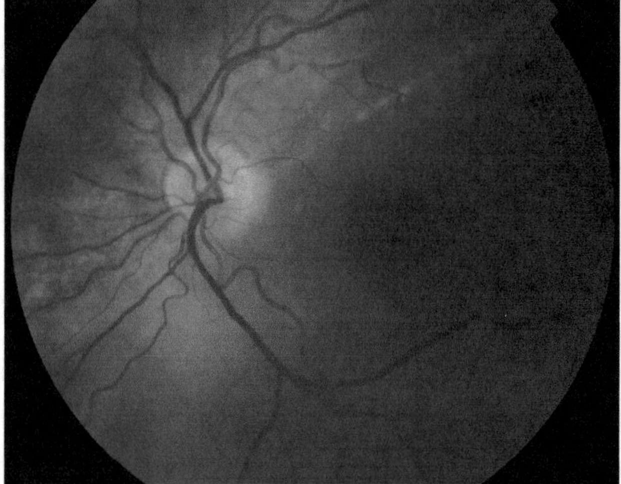

Fig. 7.41 A cystic fovea in RRD should not be confused with a secondary macular hole

Macula Off or On

When the fovea of the macula detaches (usually called macula off) the chances of return of full central vision is reduced. A recent macula off RRD (under 3 days) is as urgent as macula on and should be operated upon as soon as possible (within 24 h) [19]. If the delay is likely, posturing the break to the lowest point in the eye may reduce SRF and restrict the extension of the RRD and further elevation of the fovea [20]. This may require the patient to keep their heads as still as possible to be effective and to avoid interruptions in the posturing regime [21, 22]. Superotemporal retinal detachments already close to the arcades are most at risk of converting from macula on RRD to off while waiting for surgery [23] (Figs. 7.46, 7.47, 7.48, 7.49, 7.50, Table 7.1).

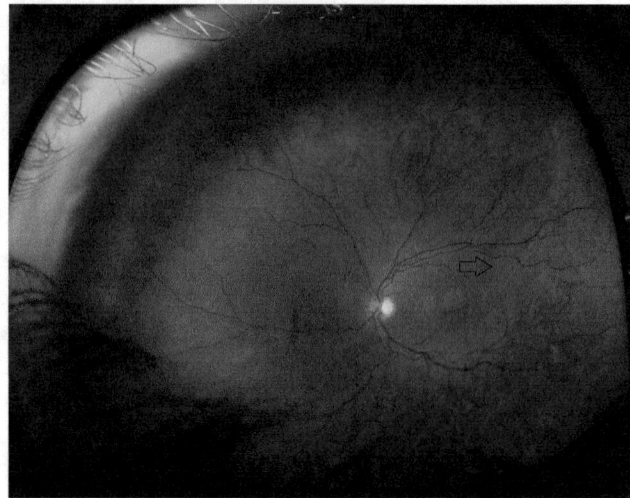

Fig. 7.42 A wide-angle view of the retina with an inferotemporal RRD, leading edge (arrow) close to the fovea

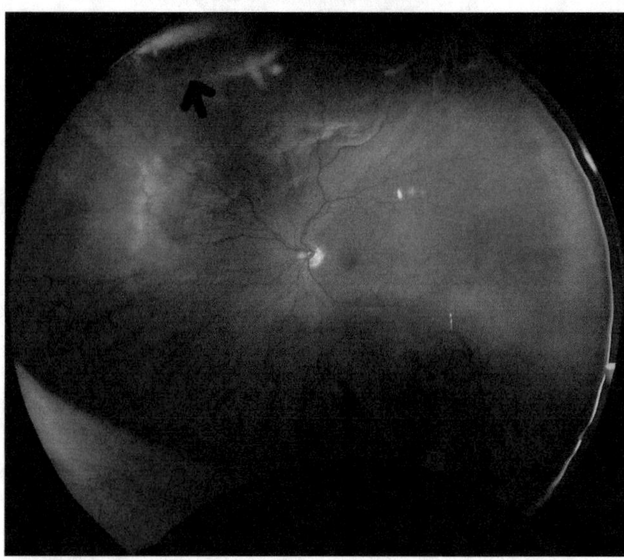

Fig. 7.43 A superior RRD with a break

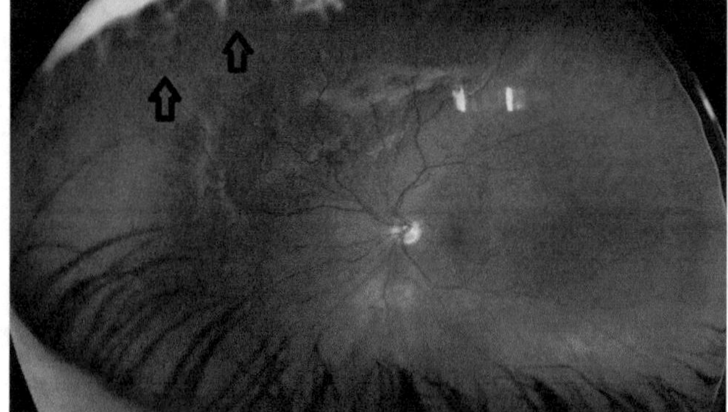

Fig. 7.44 An RRD with superotemporal retinal breaks

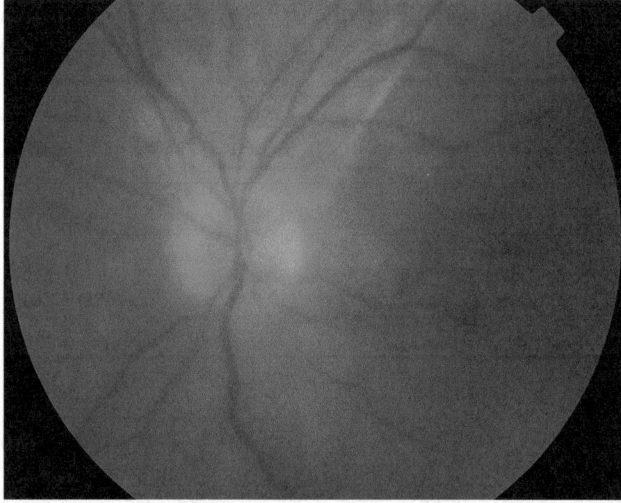

Fig. 7.45 Young chronic RRD

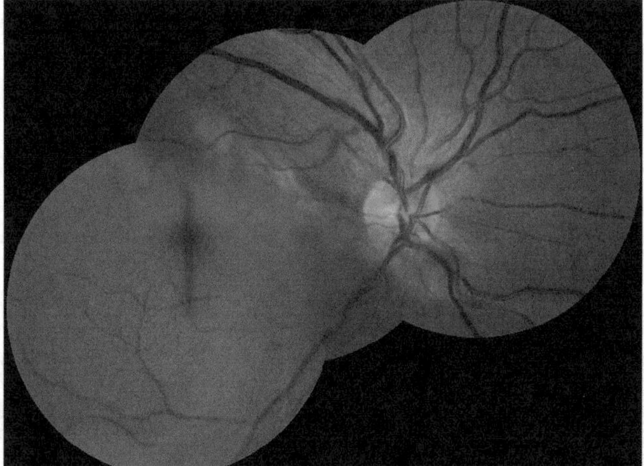

Fig. 7.46 A composite picture shows an RRD passing through the macula

Chance of 20/40 or better after fovea off retinal detachment [24].

10 days or less	71%
11 days to 6 weeks	27%
More than 6 weeks	14%

Macula off retinal detachment is more likely to suffer subtle changes in vision such as distortion postoperatively, therefore it is preferable to avoid the detachment of the fovea by performing surgery on "macula on" retinal detachment promptly, e.g. within 24 h. Chronic retinal detachments (e.g. when the vitreous is attached) in which there is a slow accumulation of subretinal fluid can be left longer before surgery. By posturing a retinal break to the dependant portion of the eye, accumulation of SRF can be reduced or even reversed while the patient is waiting for surgery.

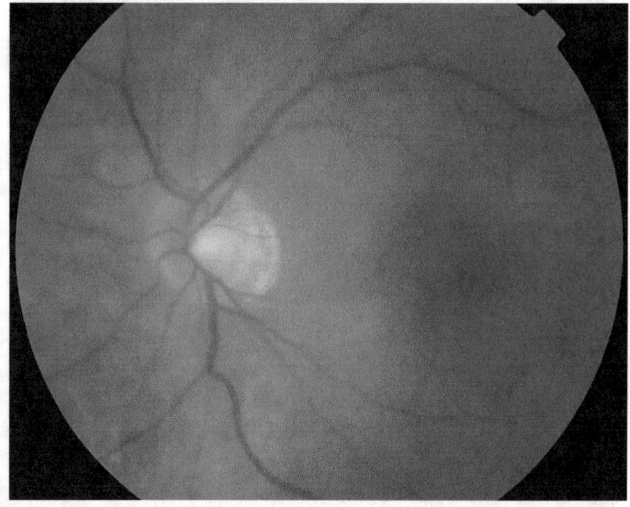

Fig. 7.47 It may not be obvious that the fovea is detached, in which case OCT is useful

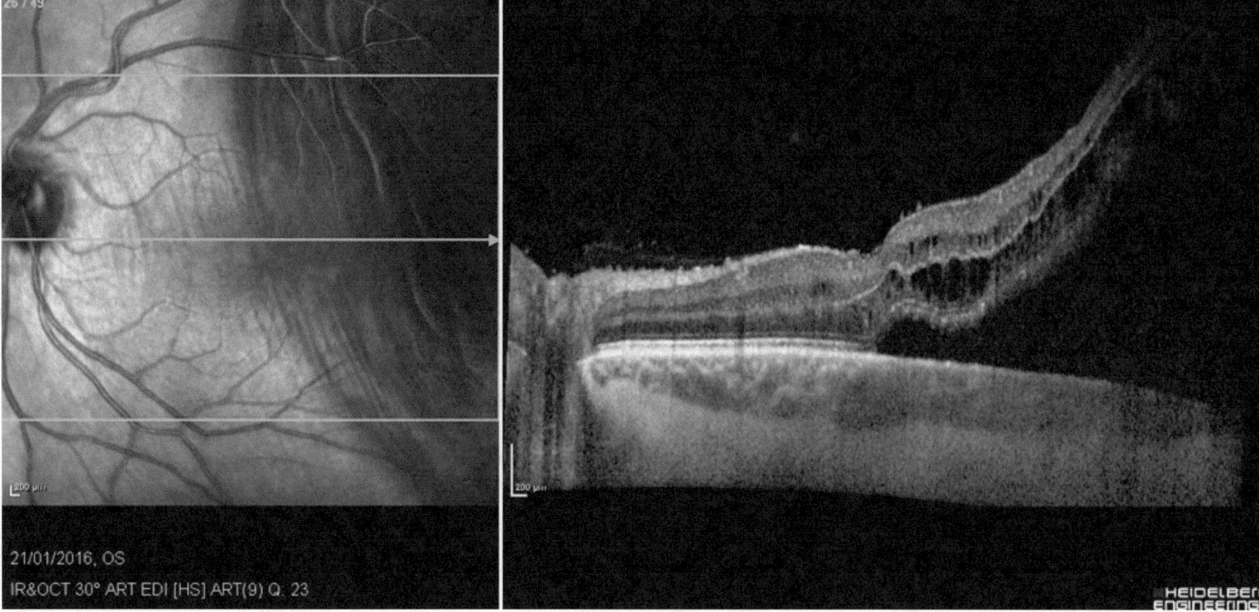

Fig. 7.48 A fovea detached by RRD

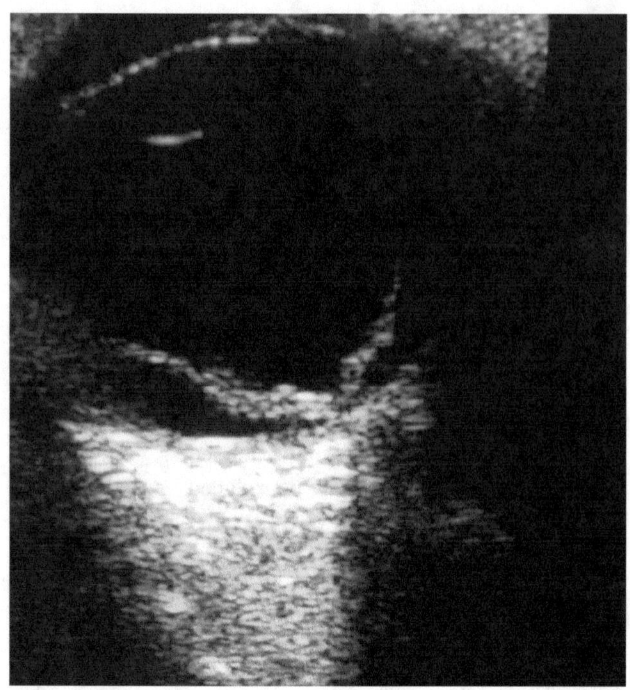

Fig. 7.49 Open RRD on US

For a temporal hole in the left eye or a nasal hole in the right eye, the patient would be asked to lie with their left cheek down to the ground.

For a nasal hole in the left eye or a temporal hole in the right eye, the patient would be asked to lie with their right cheek down to the ground.

For a superior hole, the patient lies supine with no pillows and the foot of the bed raised.

Table 7.1 Referral procedure for RRD

Condition	Characteristics	Referral	Why?
RRD with PVD	Macula on	Immediate	Prevent macula detaching
	Macula off less than 1 week	1–3 days	Macula should recover fully
	Macula off 1–2 weeks	1 week	Macula should recover well
	Macula off 2–6 weeks	1–2 weeks	Macula will show moderate recovery
	Macula off >6 weeks	2–3 weeks	Macula unlikely to recover well
RRD without PVD		1–2 weeks	Slow progression

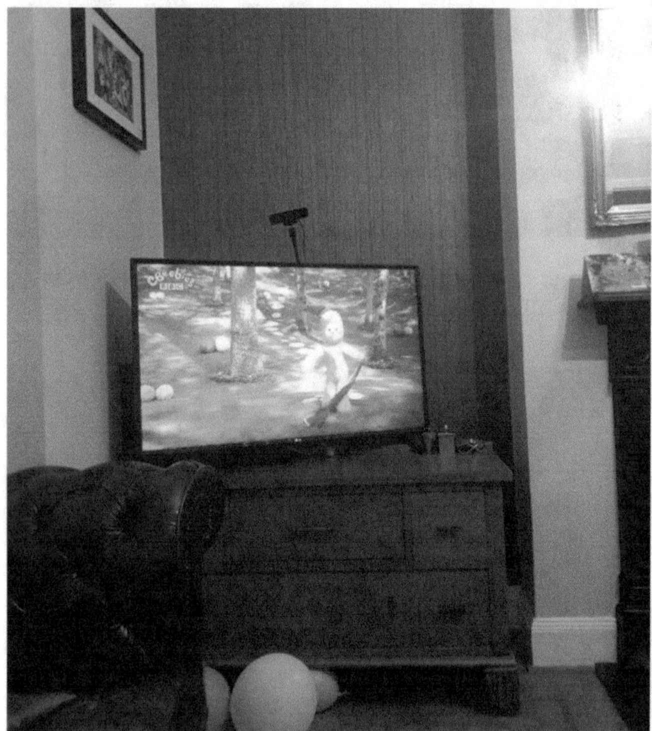

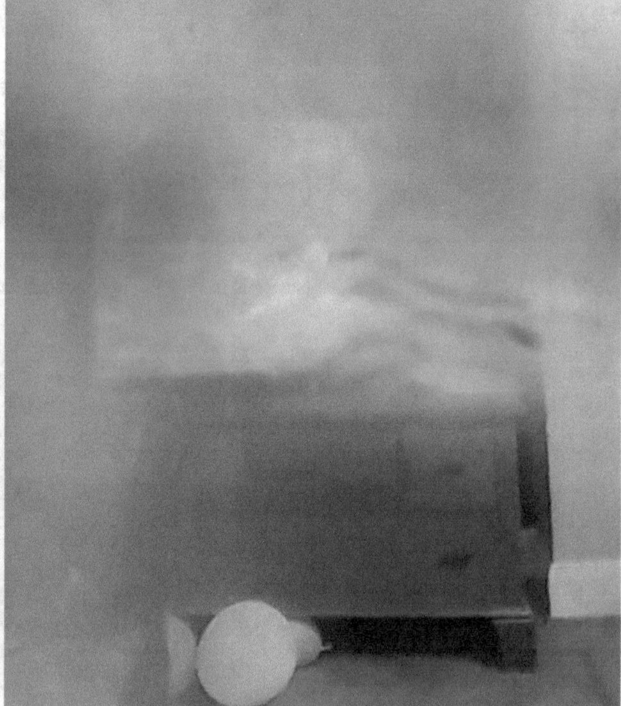

Fig. 7.50 A patient's representation of the loss of their vision when the RD passes through the macula

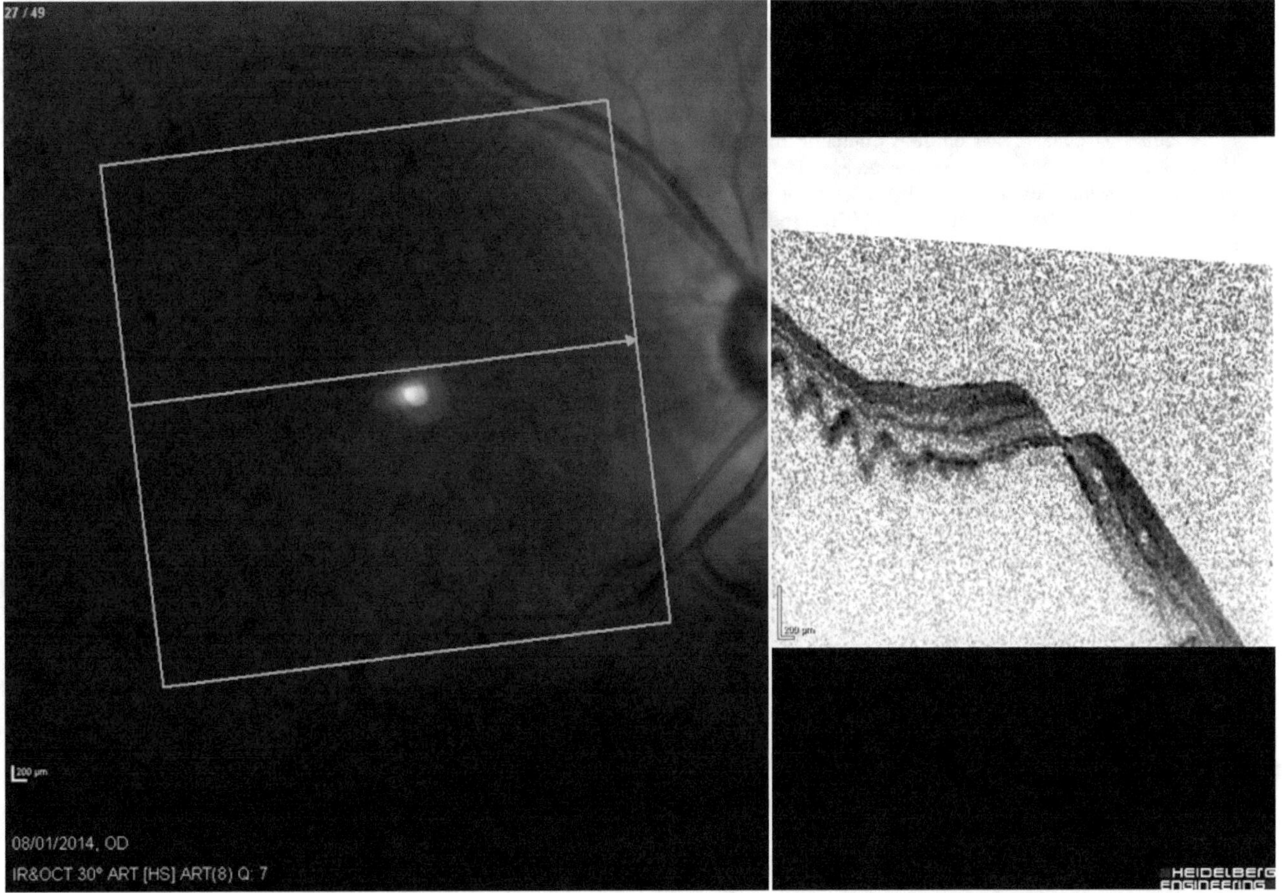

Fig. 7.51 The outer retina has a longer cord length than the inner retina so that when the retina detached the outer retina must fold as shown

For inferior holes sit the patient upright (Fig. 7.51).

References

1. Saidkasimova S, Mitry D, Singh J, Yorston D, Charteris DG. Retinal detachment in Scotland is associated with affluence. Br J Ophthalmol. 2009;93(12):1591–4. bjo.2009.162347 [pii]. https://doi.org/10.1136/bjo.2009.162347.
2. Day S, Grossman DS, Mruthyunjaya P, Sloan FA, Lee PP. One-year outcomes after retinal detachment surgery among medicare beneficiaries. Am J Ophthalmol. 150(3):338–45. S0002-9394(10)00265-5 [pii]. https://doi.org/10.1016/j.ajo.2010.04.009.
3. Williamson TH, Lee EJ, Shunmugam M. Characteristics of rhegmatogenous retinal detachment and their relationship to success rates of surgery. Retina. 2014;34(7):1421–7. https://doi.org/10.1097/IAE.0000000000000094.
4. Fajgenbaum MAP, Wong RS, Laidlaw DAH, Williamson TH. Vitreoretinal surgery on the fellow eye: a retrospective analysis of 18 years of surgical data from a tertiary center in England. Indian J Ophthalmol. 2018;66(5):681–6. https://doi.org/10.4103/ijo.IJO_1176_17.
5. Sharma MC, Regillo CD, Shuler MF, Borrillo JL, Benson WE. Determination of the incidence and clinical characteristics of subsequent retinal tears following treatment of the acute posterior vitreous detachment-related initial retinal tears. Am J Ophthalmol. 2004;138(2):280–4.
6. Ung T, Comer MB, Ang AJ, Sheard R, Lee C, Poulson AV, et al. Clinical features and surgical management of retinal detachment secondary to round retinal holes. Eye. 2004.
7. Marcus DF, Aaberg TM. Intraretinal macrocysts in retinal detachment. Arch Ophthalmol. 1979;97(7):1273–5.
8. Ahmed I, McDonald HR, Schatz H, Johnson RN, Ai E, Cruess AF, et al. Crystalline retinopathy associated with chronic retinal detachment. Arch Ophthalmol. 1998;116(11):1449–53.
9. Laatikainen L, Tolppanen EM. Characteristics of rhegmatogenous retinal detachment. Acta Ophthalmol. 1985;63(2):146–54.
10. Krohn J, Seland JH. Simultaneous, bilateral rhegmatogenous retinal detachment. Acta Ophthalmol Scand. 2000;78(3):354–8.
11. Gonzales CR, Gupta A, Schwartz SD, Kreiger AE. The fellow eye of patients with rhegmatogenous retinal detachment. Ophthalmology. 2004;111(3):518–21.
12. Netland PA, Mukai S, Covington HI. Elevated intraocular pressure secondary to rhegmatogenous retinal detachment. Surv Ophthalmol. 1994;39(3):234–40.
13. Schwartz A. Chronic open-angle glaucoma secondary to rhegmatogenous retinal detachment. Trans Am Ophthalmol Soc. 1972;70:178–89.

14. Tanaka S, Ideta H, Yonemoto J, Sasaki K, Hirose A, Oka C. Neovascularization of the iris in rhegmatogenous retinal detachment. Am J Ophthalmol. 1991;112(6):632–4.
15. Shafer DM, Stratford DP, Schepens CL, Regan CJD. Binocular indirect opthalmoscopy. Controversial aspects of the management of the retinal detachment. London: J&A Churchill; 2005. p. 51.
16. Ho SF, Fitt A, Frimpong-Ansah K, Benson MT. The management of primary rhegmatogenous retinal detachment not involving the fovea. Eye (Lond). 2006;20(9):1049–53. 6702083 [pii]. https://doi.org/10.1038/sj.eye.6702083.
17. Hammer ME, Burch TG, Rinder D. Viscosity of subretinal fluid and its clinical correlations. Retina. 1986;6(4):234–8.
18. Lincoff H, Gieser R. Finding the retinal hole. Arch Ophthalmol. 1971;85(5):565–9.
19. Williamson TH, Shunmugam M, Rodrigues I, Dogramaci M, Lee E. Characteristics of rhegmatogenous retinal detachment and their relationship to visual outcome. Eye (Lond). 2013;27(9):1063–9. https://doi.org/10.1038/eye.2013.136.
20. de Jong JH, Vigueras-Guillen JP, Simon TC, Timman R, Peto T, Vermeer KA, et al. Preoperative posturing of patients with macula-on retinal detachment reduces progression toward the fovea. Ophthalmology. 2017;124(10):1510–22. https://doi.org/10.1016/j.ophtha.2017.04.004.
21. de Jong JH, Vigueras-Guillen JP, Wubbels RJ, Timman R, Vermeer KA, van Meurs JC. The Influence of prolongation of interruptions of preoperative posturing and other clinical factors on the progress of macula-on retinal detachment. Ophthalmol Retina. 2019;3(11):938–46. https://doi.org/10.1016/j.oret.2019.05.004.
22. Vroon J, de Jong JH, Aboulatta A, Eliasy A, van der Helm FCT, van Meurs JC, et al. Numerical study of the effect of head and eye movement on progression of retinal detachment. Biomech Model Mechanobiol. 2018;17(4):975–83. https://doi.org/10.1007/s10237-018-1006-y.
23. Kontos A, Williamson TH. Rate and risk factors for the conversion of fovea-on to fovea-off rhegmatogenous retinal detachment while awaiting surgery. Br J Ophthalmol. 2017;101(8):1011–5. https://doi.org/10.1136/bjophthalmol-2016-309178.
24. Hassan TS, Sarrafizadeh R, Ruby AJ, Garretson BR, Kuczynski B, Williams GA. The effect of duration of macular detachment on results after the scleral buckle repair of primary, macula-off retinal detachments. Ophthalmology. 2002;109(1):146–52.

Rhegmatogenous Retinal Detachment

8

Contents

T. H. Williamson, *Vitreoretinal Surgery*, https://doi.org/10.1007/978-3-030-68769-4_8

Surgery

Flat Retinal Breaks

Retinopexy

If a patient presents with a retinal break which is at high risk of producing a retinal detachment (U tear, paravascular tear, operculated tear, or dialysis) but has no subretinal fluid, then retinopexy is applied to prevent accumulation of fluid underneath the neurosensory retina [1]. This can be applied as laser therapy around the break (usually in two rows around the circumference of the break) or by trans-scleral cryotherapy. Both methods produce damage to the neurosensory retina, to the retinal pigment epithelium, and perhaps to Bruch's layer and the choroid. The resultant reparative scar formation occurs in approximately 5–10 days and seals the layers of the retina together preventing fluid accumulation.

Cryotherapy

Cryotherapy employs the Joule–Thomson effect whereby expansion of certain gases, such as nitrous oxide or carbon dioxide, results in a reduction in temperature. The gas is compressed and then released through a small hole in a cryotherapy instrument tip, causing a rapid expansion of the gas and reduction in the temperature. Cryotherapy has the advantage that it can be applied trans-scleral without discernible damage to the conjunctiva, Tenon's layer, and the sclera if not used excessively whilst creating a freeze and therefore a scar in the retina.

It takes effect and has maximum adhesion in approximately ten days but causes dispersion of retinal pigment epithelial cells into the vitreous giving an increased risk of PVR especially in the presence of U tears with curled edges or tears greater than 180° [2]. Apply cryotherapy sparingly, usually one freeze in the centre of the break. Although this may increase the chance of RPE dispersion through the break, it is preferable to multiple freezes around the tear, which increase the pro-inflammatory effects of the treatment (and the risk of PVR) and the discomfort to the patient. Cryotherapy is especially useful for anterior breaks which are difficult to laser because it allows simultaneous indentation, a single cryotherapy application is often a less traumatic experience for the patient than a difficult laser session.

Cryotherapy in the Clinic Setting

1. Insert topical anaesthesia.
2. Insert a lid speculum if required, sometimes not necessary.
3. Give a localised injection of anaesthesia in the fashion of a peribulbar injection in the quadrant of the orbit with the retinal break. Warn the patient that they may experience some photopsia.
4. Always check that the tip will freeze and unfreeze before applying to the eye (these machines are notoriously unreliable).
5. Apply the cryotherapy tip trans-conjunctivally and use the tip to indent whilst observing with the indirect ophthalmoscope. Make sure you are visualising the tip and not the shaft of the cryotherapy probe when producing the indent otherwise the freeze will be posterior to the site that you are attempting to treat.
6. Once you are under the break, start the freeze commence until the break has been surrounded with ice crystals, do not overdo the freeze it only needs to encompass the break by the equivalent of two rows of laser.
7. Provide topical postoperative antibiotics for a few days (Fig. 8.1).

Complications

- Extraocular muscle injury causing diplopia, wait and the muscles will recover.
- Eyelid injury, loss of pigmentation. Avoid freezing through the lid.
- Subconjunctival haemorrhage or tearing of the conjunctiva.
- An over freeze causing a retinal tear and haemorrhage. You only need to see the retina freeze in the early stages not a severe freeze with massive ice crystal formation.
- Never pull off a frozen tip as this may tear the sclera, be patient before removing the tip, allow it to thaw.

Laser (Fig. 8.2)

Argon, diode, or visible spectrum diode laser induce tissue injury, and therefore scarring from thermal burns on the tissues (photocoagulation). Nonvisible diode can cause a disproportionate injury to the choroid and must be used with care. The laser should extend anteriorly around the tear or if not possible should extend to the ora serrata. Argon laser therapy can be applied either by a contact lens with a slit lamp or by indirect ophthalmoscopy with indentation. Maximum adhesion is approximately five days and requires two rows of burns around a break for maximal adhesion. Trans-scleral diode laser has also been used [3].

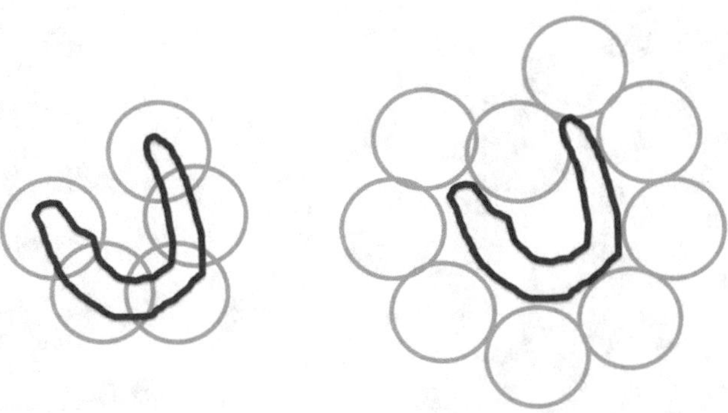

Fig. 8.1 Apply cryotherapy to a large tear as shown on the left although this applies cryotherapy to the bare RPE in the tear, this is preferable to the increased number of burns required if the retina around the tear is treated as shown on the right

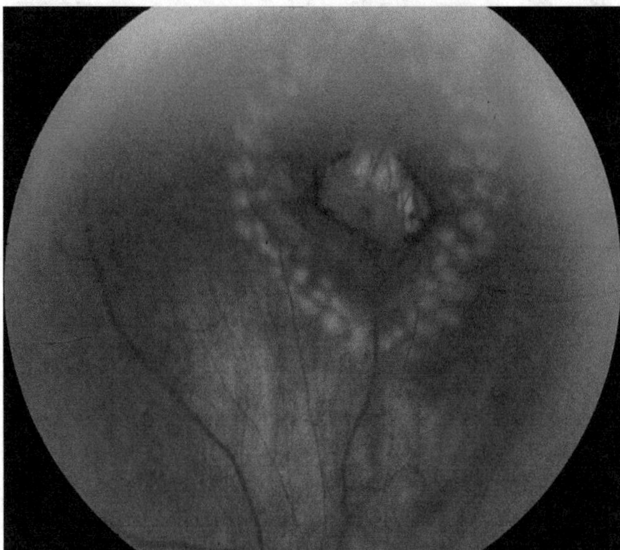

Fig. 8.2 A tear has been treated with laser retinopexy

Typical laser settings for argon green.

- 200–300 mW power
- 0.1–0.2 msec duration
- Spot size 200–500 μm.
- Repeat interval 0.1 sec.

Laser in the Clinic Setting

- Can be applied at the slit lamp using various contact lenses for posterior and equatorial tears (contact lenses have the advantage over non-contact fundus lenses of helping control eye movements during the laser session).
- Can be applied with indirect ophthalmoscopy thereby allowing indentation for anterior breaks.
- Apply laser of adequate power to produce a blanching spot.
- Two rows 360° around the break or for very anterior breaks around the posterior and lateral borders of the break and up to the ora serrata (Figs. 8.3, 8.4, and 8.5).

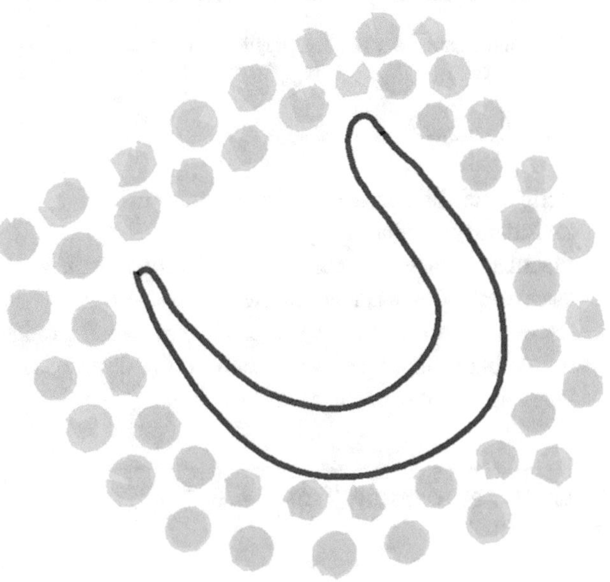

Fig. 8.3 Laser should be placed in two rows around a retinal tear as shown, laser the flat retina close to the edge of the tear

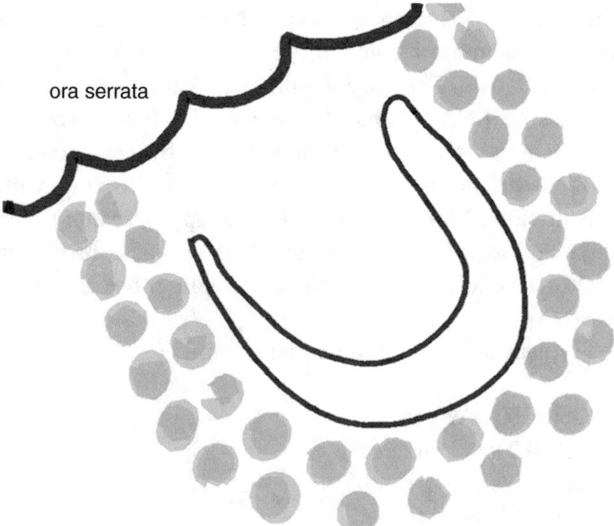

Fig. 8.4 If the retinal tear is close to the ora serrata, laser up to the ora serrata if you are unable to laser around the anterior edge of the tear

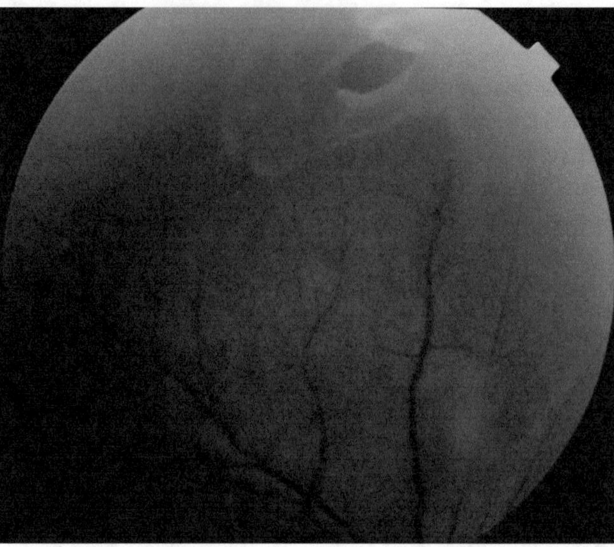

Fig. 8.6 This tear has SRF extending around its edge

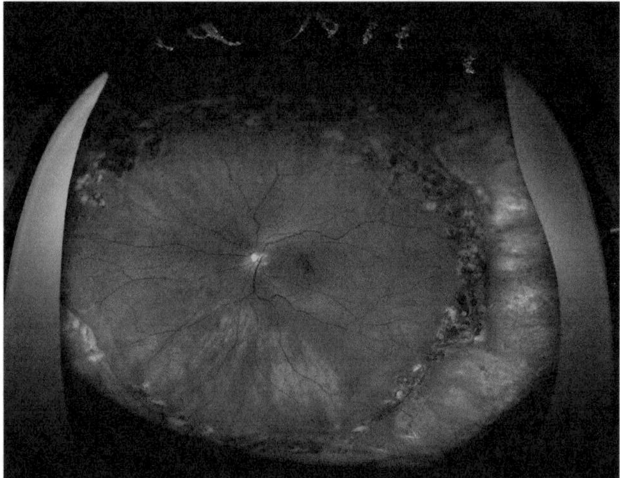

Fig. 8.5 360-degree laser has been applied to this RRD to try to prevent recurrence

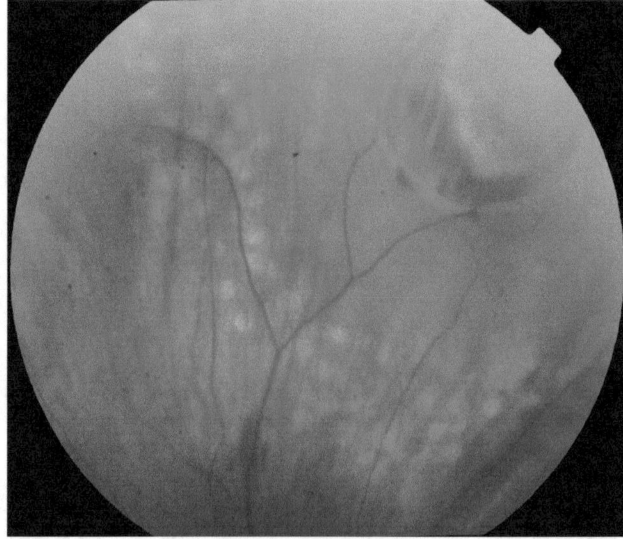

Fig. 8.7 The SRF around this tear is likely to lead to failure of the laser retinopexy

Complications

- Retinal bleeding press on the eye to minimise.
- Lens damage, reduce the power.
- Macular damage, take care with 3 mirror lenses, keep the laser on standby when not in use.
- Excessive burns, only use laser powers which produce retinal blanching, take care when lasering during scleral indentation not to get an excessive burn.

Retinal Detachment (Figs. 8.6, 8.7, 8.8, 8.9, and 8.10)

The definition of rhegmatogenous retinal detachment is a retinal break with subretinal fluid. This may be as little as a small cuff of fluid or as much as total retinal detachment. Once the detachment has occurred, identification and closure of the retinal break or breaks are the primary aim of surgery (Figs. 8.11 and 8.12).

Attachment of a silastic explant to the sclera of the eye to create a dent in the sphere of the eye underneath the break or breaks allows the retina to reattach. This may occur because of relief of traction or because of an alteration in the fluid currents in the eye.

Alternatively, the vitreous can be removed by pars plana vitrectomy and a long-acting gas bubble, such as sulpha hexafluoride or perfluoropropane, inserted into the vitreous cavity. The gas bubble contacts the rim of the break preventing the passage of fluid through the break (tamponade). Thereafter, subretinal fluid will be reabsorbed by the RPE and the retina will flatten.

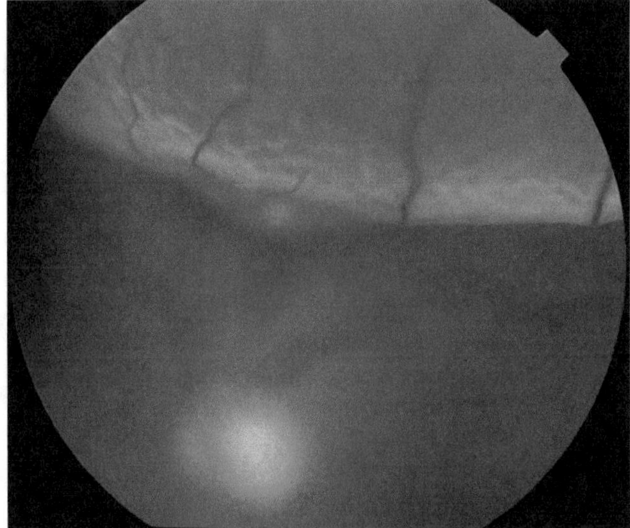

Fig. 8.8 The superior bulla of an RRD

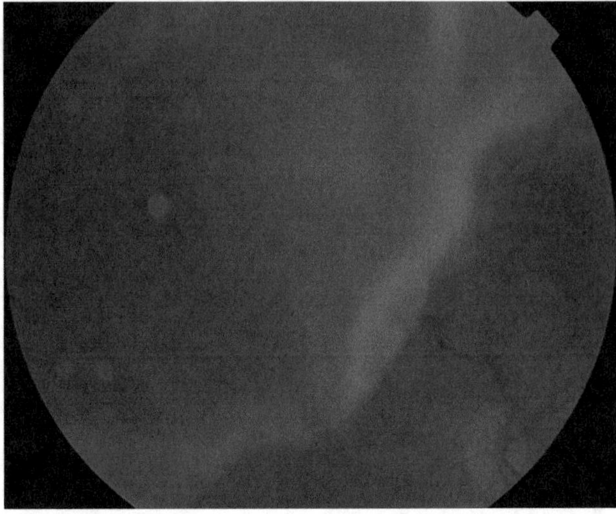

Fig. 8.10 A superior bullous RRD may overhang the macula blocking a view of the fovea. It is therefore difficult to judge whether the fovea is detached. Usually the fovea is found to have this SRF peroperatively

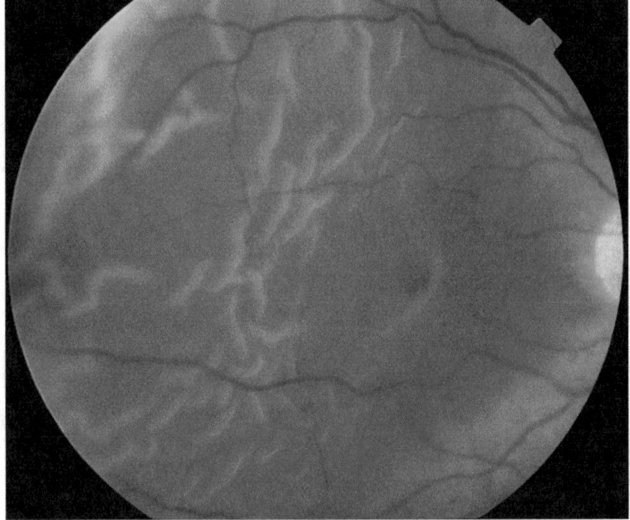

Fig. 8.9 Wrinkling of the retina in RRD

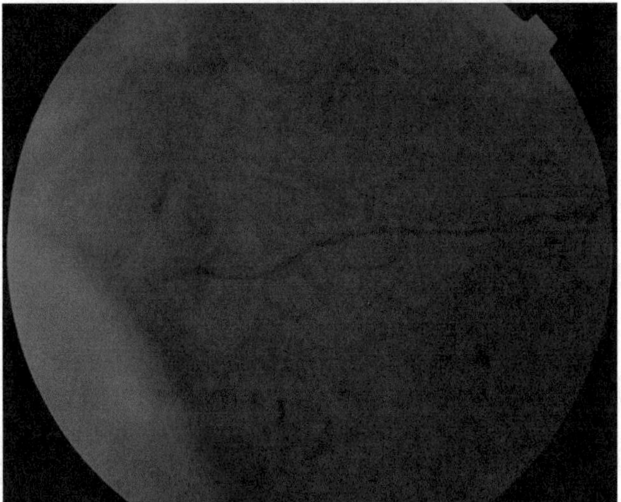

Fig. 8.11 Choroidal effusions should not be confused with retinal detachment, the appearance is of an immobile smooth elevation with a green or brown underlying colour due to the detachment of the RPE

The gas bubble is only temporary and the indentation from an explant may gradually lessen therefore retinopexy is also applied to seal the tear and avoid re-accumulation of the subretinal fluid.

The shortening on the retina produced by proliferative vitreoretinopathy may prevent retinal reattachment unless the fibrous membranes are surgically removed, or the retina cut to fit the inside of the eye (retinectomy). In this circumstance silicone oil may be inserted into the vitreous cavity to provide long-term support to the retina allowing time for the proliferative vitreoretinopathy process to stop. Silicone oil in the vitreous cavity is associated with several complications including cataract, glaucoma, refractive changes, and low-grade retinal toxicity.

This type of surgery requires a preoperative assessment of the patient, particularly determining whether the patient requires conventional surgery or vitrectomy.

Although it is possible to perform most of these operations by vitrectomy alone, this may be inconvenient for the patient in that they will often develop a cataract requiring further surgery later. They may also be required to position their heads for 1–2 weeks and will have delayed visual recovery for 2 to 8 weeks depending on the gas used. A conventional procedure, on the other hand, does not produce cataract and requires no posturing in most circumstances. However, it requires the development of additional surgical

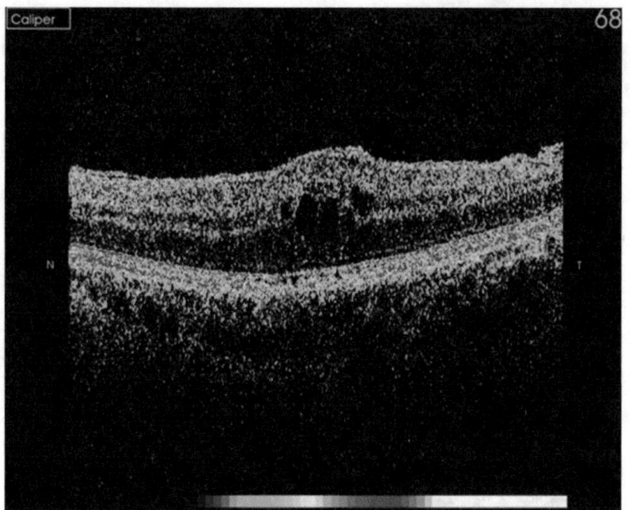

Fig. 8.12 This patient had a persistent inferior retinal detachment postoperatively with CMO present. Some surgeons argue that peripheral RRD has secondary effects on the macular receptors

skills and visualisation of retinal breaks can be more difficult via indirect ophthalmoscopy.

I treat most RRD with PVD with by PPV and those with attached vitreous are operated by non-drain, however there is wide variation in methods worldwide and therefore non-drain, pneumatic retinopexy, and PPV are all described in this text.

Principles

The principles of surgery are break closure, relief of traction, alteration of fluid currents, and retinopexy [4]. Under normal circumstances the retina is held in place by physiological forces such as hydrostatic and osmotic pressure, weak intracellular bonds, and the intracellular matrix. If a break appears in the retina, these forces are not sufficient to prevent the accumulation of subretinal fluid, which usually comes from fluid vitreous behind the posterior hyaloid.

Break Closure

Any treatment of a retinal detachment depends primarily on identification of all the breaks in the patient. A small "pinprick" break will quite easily result in a redetachment if it is missed and remains untreated. Therefore, careful inspection of the retina is of paramount importance. Once identified, the breaks can be closed in several ways. In conventional surgery this is performed by placing an indent underneath the break or breaks [5]. In vitrectomy surgery the break is opposed to the RPE by the action of a gas bubble (or silicone oil) on the retina.

Relief of Traction

The placement of a plombage may also have the effect of relieving traction by shortening the distance to the centre of the eye if vitreous traction is present. However, it is likely that vitreous traction is already relieved by production of the retinal detachment. The traction of the vitreous on the retina is negated by the removal of the vitreous in vitrectomy. Traction becomes important when this is adjacent to a retinal break, for example in PVR, (proliferative vitreoretinopathy) when the break is prevented from closing onto an indent or onto the back of the eye with gas. Traction by scar tissue is removed during membranectomy in PVR surgery.

Alteration of Fluid Currents (Figs. 8.13 and 8.14)

Fluid currents are present in the retina in the presence of PVD, which help lift the retina through their action on a retinal break. The effect of currents can be seen in the non-drain retinal detachment repair where appropriate placement of a plombage will allow resolution of SRF and closure of the break onto the indent, even if at the end of the operation, the break is not flat onto the indent itself. Although it is not necessary to close the break onto the indent at the end of surgery, it is important that the indent is in the correct position to modified fluid currents to produce break closure over the next twenty four to thirty six hours. The indent produces an increase in the velocity of the fluid over the indent because the cross-sectional area through which the flow of fluid can

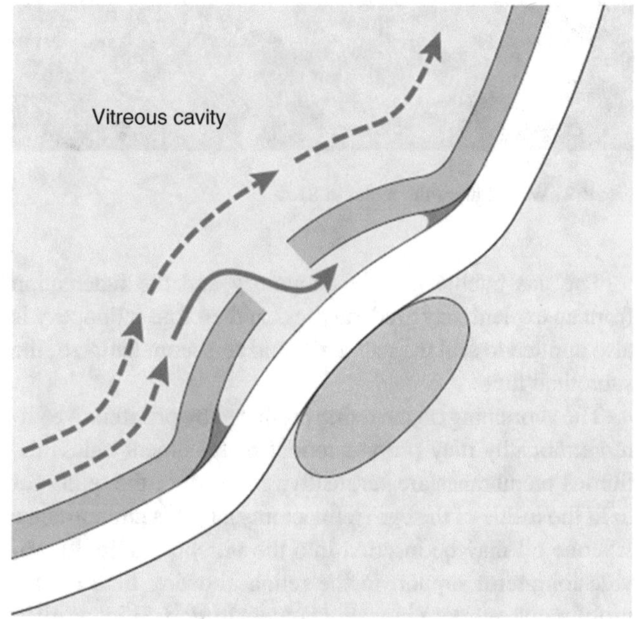

Fig. 8.13 Application of an indent under a tear alters the fluid currents, by increasing the velocity of fluid flow, the pressure is dropped drawing the retina to the sclera (Bernoulli's principle)

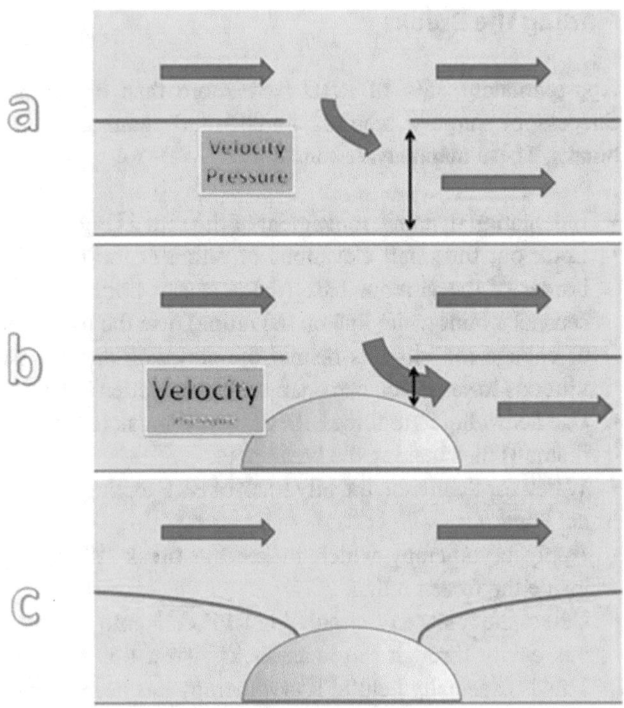

Fig. 8.14 If fluid passes over a membrane with a hole in it, the fluid enters through the hole (**a**). If an indentation is inserted under the hole the space the fluid must go through narrow (double arrow), for the same flow the velocity of the fluid increases (**b**). According to Bernoulli's principle this drops the pressure at this point, causing the membrane to move towards the indent eventually closing the hole on the indent and preventing any other fluid entering (**c**)

pass through the break has been reduced. This in turn induces a pressure drop by Bernoulli's principle (velocity of a fluid increases causing a decrease in pressure in the fluid) causing the retina to move onto the indent. For this reason, it is not necessary to perform drainage of SRF in all patients.

Bernoulli's principle states that as the speed of a moving fluid increases, the pressure within the fluid decreases.

Retinopexy

Retinopexy is important because the means of closing the break is often temporary, such as with absorption of a gas bubble or when a plombage gradually loosens with ageing or becomes adrift from loosening of the sutures. Once retinopexy has taken effect it is entirely appropriate to remove a plombage at ten days. This has been exploited by Lincoff and his balloon indent procedure [6] whereby a balloon is inserted into the orbit to produce an indent of the eye and is later deflated and removed. Similarly, internal tamponade is only necessary until the retinopexy has sealed the break (Table 8.1).

The percentages of operations performed in my team for RRD between 1998 and 2006 showed more conventional surgeries. The team now rarely perform DACE or pneumatic retinopexy, and nondrain is confined to those patients with attached vitreous. Pars plana vitrectomy is used in 90% and non-drain in 10% in 2021.

Table 8.1 Proportion of methods used historically for RRD in my team in 1998–2006

Operations for RRD (n = 1528)	%
PNEUMATIC RETINOPEXY	0.7
NON-DRAIN	22.8
DACE	1.6
PPV	74.9

Table 8.2 Difficulty rating of PPV for RRD

Difficulty Rating	Moderate
Success rates	High
Complication rates	Medium
When to use in training	Early

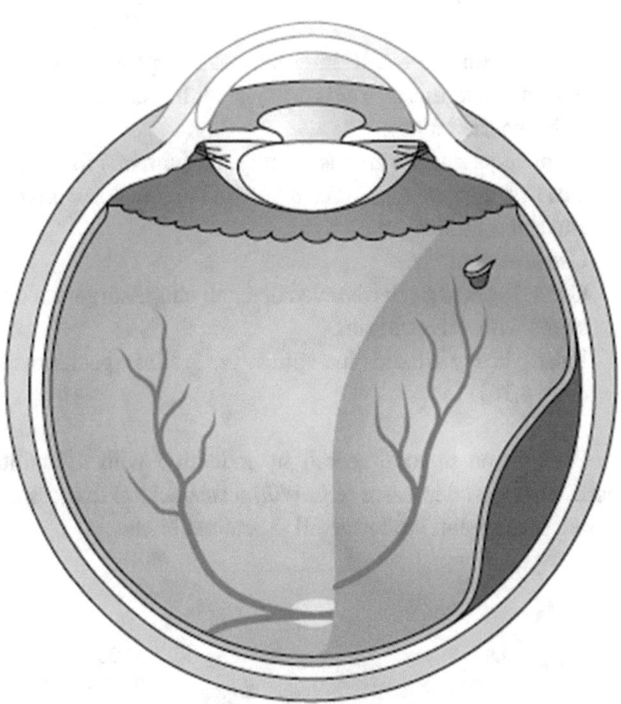

Fig. 8.15 The eye is orientated with the lens superiorly for PPV

Pars Plana Vitrectomy (Table 8.2)

Additional Surgical Steps

1. Search for breaks with deep scleral indentation.
2. Apply cryotherapy.
3. Drain subretinal fluid (SRF).
4. Drain SRF and insert air.
5. Drain residual vitreous cavity fluid off disc.
6. Apply cryotherapy or laser retinopexy as required.
7. Exchange long-acting gas (Fig. 8.15).

Introduction

PPV is becoming more popular for RRD repair because of the ease of application and good visualisation of the retina with wide-angle viewing systems. Examination of Medicare data for fees in the USA shows a 72% increase in the use of PPV for RRD and a 69% reduction in the use of scleral buckles from 1997 to 2007 [7]. In addition, cataract can easily be dealt with peroperatively or postoperatively by phacoemulsification and posterior chamber lens implant. Perform the PPV in the usual way. Take care if operating on a bullous RRD not to encourage incarceration of the retina into the sclerotomies or into the infusion cannula. So far randomised studies support the use of PPV or scleral buckle in RRD surgery [8].

To avoid this:

- Try to drain some SRF internally early in the procedure from a break (this also aids removal of the gel without risk of biting the retina).
- Remove as much vitreous as possible (vitreous incarcerates first then the retina) from around the infusion cannula and sclerotomies.
- Use scleral plugs.
- Use self-sealing sclerotomies or small gauge surgery with stents with valves in situ.
- Insert heavy liquid to splint the retina posteriorly (Fig. 8.16).

Perform an internal search by indenting with a squint hook or scleral depressor (e.g. *Williamson* scleral depressor, Vitreq instruments) to locate all the retinal breaks.

Finding the Breaks

Approximately 55% of RRD have more than one break. Success of surgery requires finding and treating all the breaks. These manoeuvres can help:

- Indentation dynamic movement of the retina (Fig. 8.17).
- Look out for small elevations of retina at the posterior border of the vitreous base (the posterior border can be seen as a faint white line on the retina), use the light pipe to engage the vitreous behind the elevation and lift the vitreous to see if you can open the break hidden behind it.
- Use heavy liquid to force SRF out of the break (especially if small) thus making the break pout.
- Watch for Schlieren, the oily track of SRF exiting the retinal break.
- Apply cryotherapy which makes the break "shine" up inside the frozen retina.
- Detect the release of circulating RPE cells into the vitreous cavity through the hole, looks like a tiny volcano. This is especially helpful if cryotherapy has been applied and confirmation of the presence of a break is required.
- Apply laser retinopexy which will blanch the attached retina around the break but not the bare RPE in the centre of the break.
- Gently aspirate over the suspected break with the flute needle to see if SRF will drain through the suspected break, take care that you do not create a hole by doing this thereby fooling yourself that you have found the break.

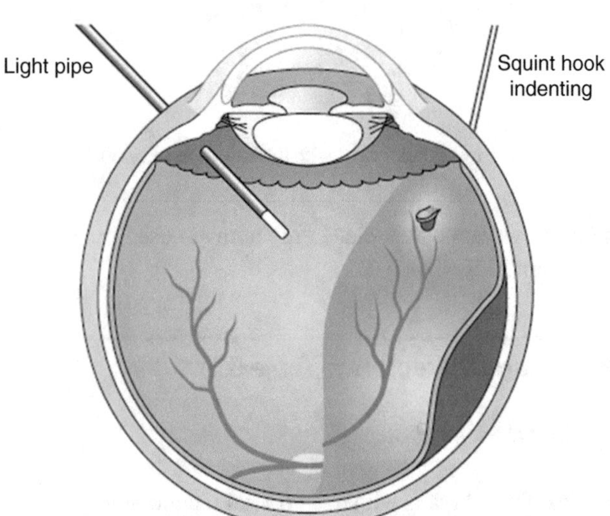

Fig. 8.16 During vitrectomy indentation is required to bring peripheral retina into view and to aid internal search for retinal breaks

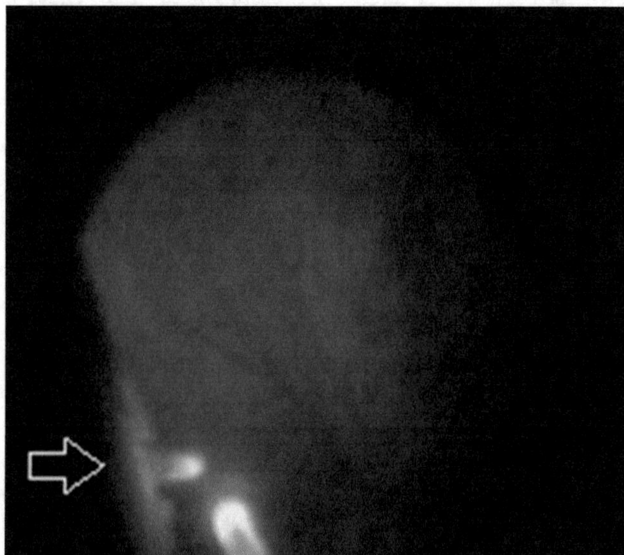

Fig. 8.17 The flap of a U-shaped tear can be seen on indentation during PPV

- If you have tried everything else, use a 40 gauge needle to inject some trypan blue dye into the subretinal space, heavy liquids can be inserted to move the dye towards the periphery and egress of the dye through the break will allow location of the break (dye extrusion, De-Tech, method) [9, 10].

Apply cryotherapy or endolaser to any flat breaks and any which are indentable. Any breaks which are not indentable can be treated with retinopexy after insertion of the air. Laser must be applied to flat retina and therefore is applied after air insertion or with heavy liquid in situ. Laser should be used if there are large breaks or multiple breaks to help prevent overuse of cryotherapy which increases the risk of PVR. Many surgeons like to mark the edge of retinal breaks with a small burn from endodiathermy. This allows visualisation of the burn and therefore the location of the tear after the air insertion (unmarked breaks are difficult to see after air injection) to allow easy retinopexy. Alternatively remember where the break is using anatomical landmarks such as blood vessels to direct you to the break (Fig. 8.18).

Advantages and Disadvantages of Retinopexy under Air

Advantages of retinopexy under air:

- Breaks are flat allowing laser application.
- Cryotherapy application is much quicker under air because of the insulating properties of the air.

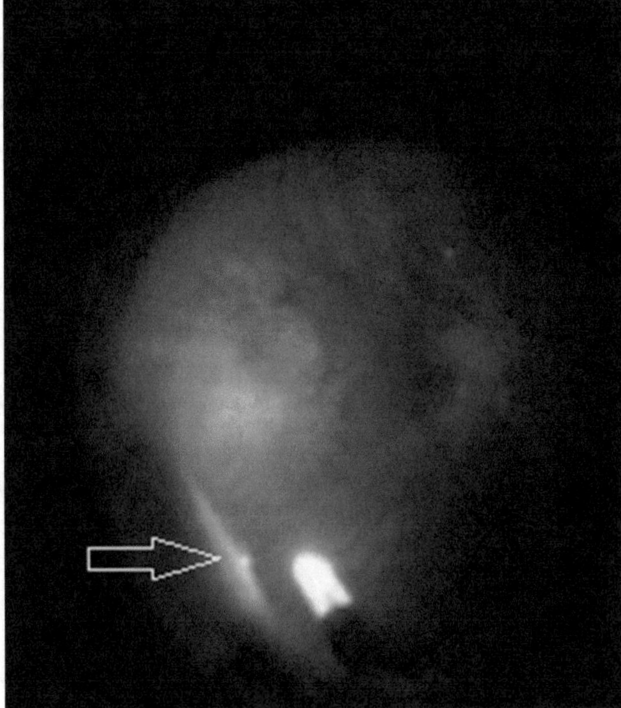

Fig. 8.18 If you see a tiny tag like this, there may be small U tear in its posterior edge. Lift the vitreous frill to expose the break

- Peripheral laser can be easier to apply because the air allows a wider field of view (but with reduced magnification) with the IVS in a phakic patient.

Disadvantages

- Breaks are more difficult to visualise.
- Cryotherapy releases RPE cells which will not be removed (air fluid exchange has already been completed).
- Condensation on the IOL in the presence of a capsulotomy reduces the view.
- Posterior lenticular opacification in a phakic patient reduces the view.
- Glare from the tip of the endo-illumination is increased. If you are using a bullet light pipe, cut off the exposed end to make it flush with the sleeve to reduce glare (Figs. 8.19 and 8.20).

Draining Subretinal Fluid

Drain the SRF internally with a flute needle placed over one of the breaks. It helps to drain as much SRF as possible by fluid/fluid exchange before going to air/fluid. With the retina as flat as possible commence inserting air through the infusion (using the air pump of the vitrectomy machine). There will be a moment when the vitreous cavity is half filled when the view of the needle tip and the break is lost. Keep the needle over the break and advance very slightly into the eye to compensate for the flattening of the retina. Do not stop draining. The moment of poor visualisation will pass, and the view will return and the SRF drainage can be completed.

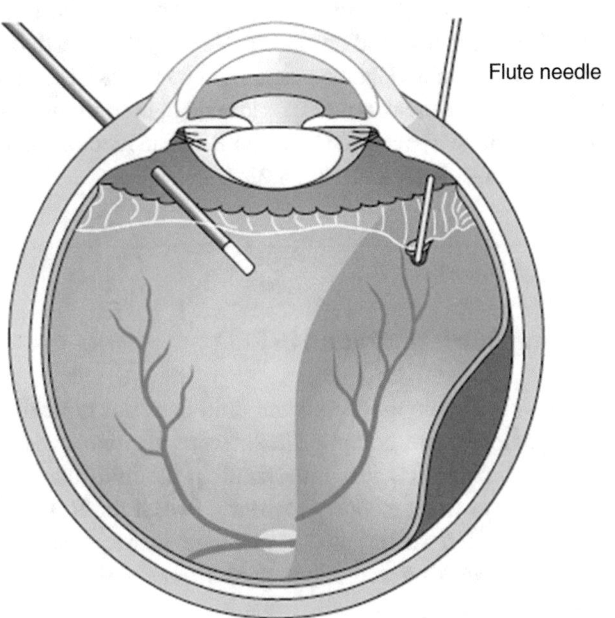

Fig. 8.19 Subretinal fluid can be drained by placing a "flute" instrument just anterior to the posterior edge of the retinal break, thereby avoiding vitreous attached to the anterior edge of the break

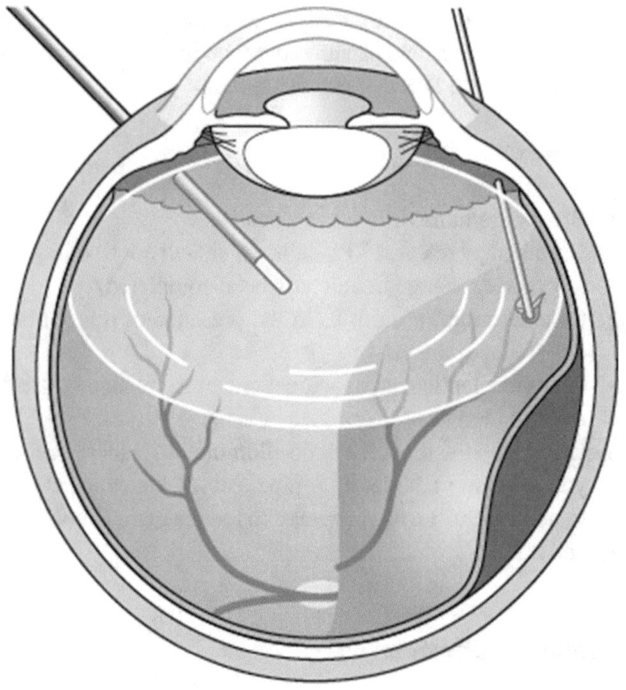

Fig. 8.20 Injecting air during a vitrectomy whilst draining SRF through a retinal break. By flattening the retina extensively before insertion of air complete SRF drainage is facilitated. Keep the flute needle over the break till a maximal air fill and SRF drainage has been achieved before draining any fluid from the back of the eye

When bubbling is heard from the flute needle only air is being removed and the needle tip should be advanced gently towards the break to drain more SRF.

Once the retina is flattened, drain off any vitreous cavity fluid from the optic disc.

Note: When coming away from the break to observe the posterior retina and the remaining SRF do not be tempted to drain vitreous cavity fluid off the disc. If you do, you will be left with a pool of SRF at the macula and no means of draining it because the break is now closed and not in communications with the SRF (refill the eye with BSS and recommence drainage) (Figs. 8.21, 8.22, and 8.23).

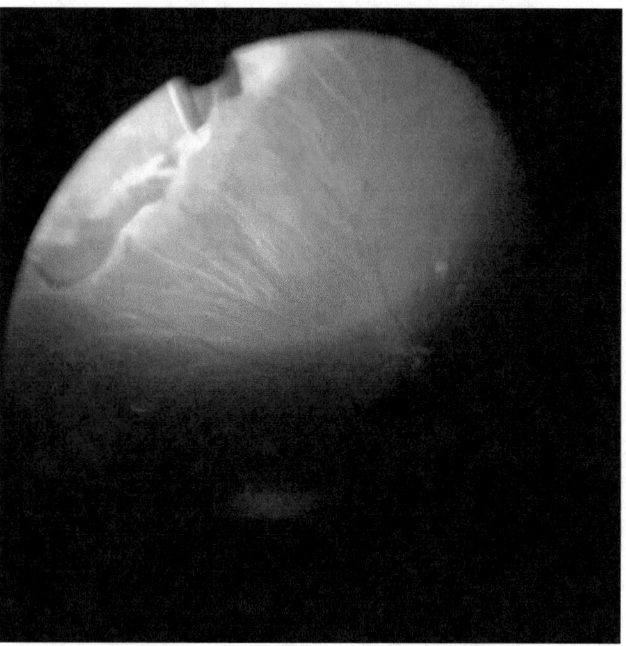

Fig. 8.21 A large retinal break

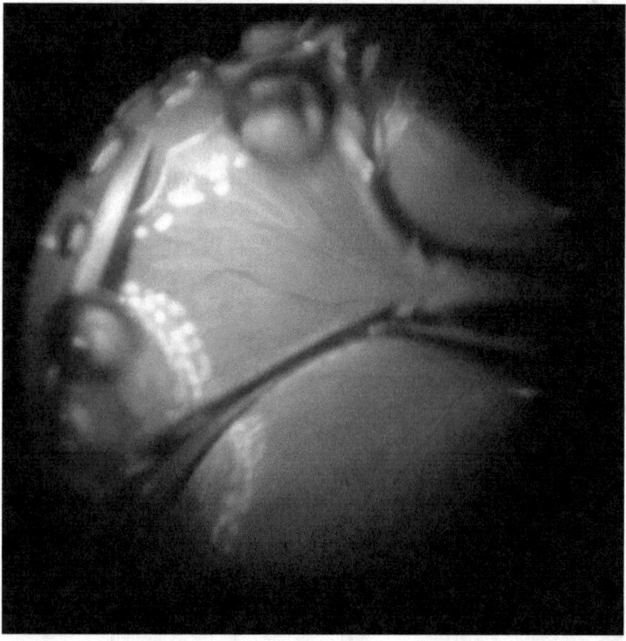

Fig. 8.22 During fluid gas exchange there is a moment when you will lose sight of the break and drainage instrument. Be confident to maintain the instrument over the break and the view will return. Do not be tempted to drain from the back of the eye to regain your view. If you do so, you will move the bubble posteriorly past the break and it will be flattened, and no longer easy to drain from. This will risk trapping SRF posteriorly

Surgical Pearl

Draining Subretinal Fluid in RRD

Whilst a small amount of residual fluid does not typically cause postoperative complications, there are two exceptions. One, if the RD was longstanding, the fluid may be too viscous to spontaneously reabsorb; two, if the RD was fovea-sparing, a steamroller manoeuvre is necessary to prevent the shifting subretinal fluid from detaching the fovea.

To maximise the efficacy of draining the subretinal fluid during vitrectomy for RD, do the following:

- turn the eye so that the break is at the lowest part of the globe,
- (if there are multiple breaks, use the most central one—not the largest of the breaks)
- position the flute needle just over the break,

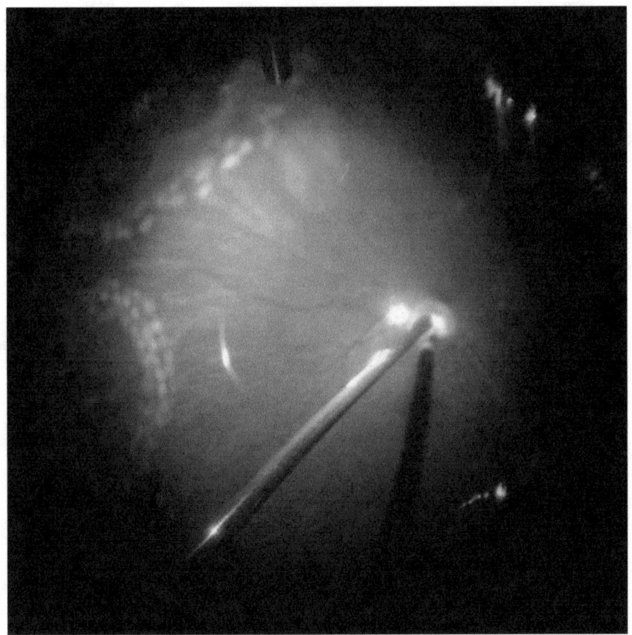

Fig. 8.23 Drain vitreous fluid off the disc to maximise the size of the gas bubble

- (no need to enter the subretinal space with the flute needle unless the RD is bullous and the retina is highly mobile; in such an eye either the flute needle must carefully be advanced just behind the retina or heavy liquid be used to reduce retinal movements)
- switch the infusion from BSS to air,
- do not change the position of either the eye or the flute needle (this is difficult since visibility is initially lost but crucial since otherwise the fluid streaming into the flute needle is interrupted; the retina collapses back and residual subretinal fluid is the consequence).

Ferenc Kuhn, Retina Specialists of Alabama, Birmingham, Alabama, USA

When to Use Heavy Liquids

To avoid retinal incarceration into sclerotomies.

Flute needle or infusion cannula. Some retinae are very bullous and mobile. These can incarcerate into sclerotomies, flute needle or infusion cannula. If the breaks are large drainage of SRF alone may not control the situation because re-accumulation of fluid is very rapid. Insert heavy liquids via a two-way needle onto the optic disc. Keep the tip of the needle just in the heavy liquid bubble to maintain a single bubble. Expand the bubble to force some SRF out through a break. Even a small bubble will help control the situation by stabilising the retina.

Note: If an incarceration of the retina into a sclerotomy or the infusion cannula is encountered, the insertion of heavy liquid into the vitreous cavity will usually free the retina. Search the damaged retina for new breaks and treat appropriately. A small incarceration into the flute can be extracted using a back flush or by removing the light pipe to release some of the intracavity pressure.

To flatten the retina when there is a difficult to reach break.

Heavy liquid can be used to flatten the retina followed by air/heavy exchange. This minimises the need to drain SRF out of a break. If the retina is flat under the heavy liquid, retinopexy can be applied at this stage (useful for giant retinal tears, see Chap. 6).

Take Care. If inserting a large bubble for this purpose, small bubbles can separate off at the vitreous base and be left in the eye. These may enter the anterior chamber postoperatively. How the heavy liquid enters the anterior chamber is uncertain, but it is likely to pass through a small hole in the zonules which may act in the fashion of a lobster pot allowing liquid to enter the AC but not to leave again. Anterior chamber heavy liquid can be removed by paracentesis with a fine gauge needle.

To change the contour of the retina when it is not possible to find the breaks.

In some retinae it is not possible to identify the break. Inserting heavy liquid causes the break (usually an exceedingly small U tear) to pout as the SRF leaves (you may spot the Schlieren, i.e. oily tube of SRF in the vitreous cavity fluid exiting the break). This may be enough to allow detection of the break on re-inspection by indentation.

Removal of Heavy Liquid

Fluid/heavy liquid exchange is straightforward but more often air/heavy liquid exchange is desirable in RRD because this has the advantage that the SRF is pushed anteriorly and peripherally by the heavy liquid during the exchange. Perform the air/SRF exchange and then lastly the air/heavy liquid to maintain a flattened macula. Heavy liquid can be difficult to see under air so make sure that it is taken out in one smooth action so that visualisation of the position of the bubble as it gets smaller is not lost. Stopping and restarting are not recommended because the position of the remaining liquid may be lost.

Choice of Tamponade

A long-acting gas is inserted to support the retina whilst the retinopexy takes effect.

- SF6 can be used for any breaks above the horizontal meridian.
- SF6 can be used for breaks above 4 and 8 clock hours but posture may be needed.

- C3F8 is used if breaks are below 4 and 8 clock hours to ensure that there is a large bubble for longer aiding contact of the bubble to the inferior breaks.

A method of fastidious removal of SRF, heavy diode laser retinopexy, and no gas tamponade has been described with successful retinal reattachment [11]. This method involves inserting air on top of heavy liquid to extract the SRF with subsequent removal of the air again. Most surgeons would leave the air in and exchange with a gas mixture.

Avoiding Retinal Folds (Figs. 8.24 and 8.25)

It is essential that a large bulla of retina is not left at the macula when a gas bubble is in the eye because when the patient changes posture the retina can be folded by the action of the gas. Try to minimise the amount of SRF left in the eye at the end of surgery. If a small bulla remains in the eye do not completely fill the eye with air, i.e. do not drain all of the vitreous cavity fluid off the disc. Immediately after the surgery posture the patient face down for a duration of 2 hours. Roll the patient onto the face down position, do not allow the patient to be upright at any point as this risks folding the retina.

Some surgeons will add in extra steps to try to help avoid folds. The need for these steps depends on the individual surgeon's skills in draining fluid.

- Insertion of heavy liquid to aid drainage of SRF [12, 13].
- Posterior retinotomy to aid SRF aspiration.
- Incomplete gas fill at the end of surgery.
- Insertion of a small bubble of 100% gas.

Retinal folds are problematic because they induce oblique diplopia and distortion which are difficult to remedy postoperatively.

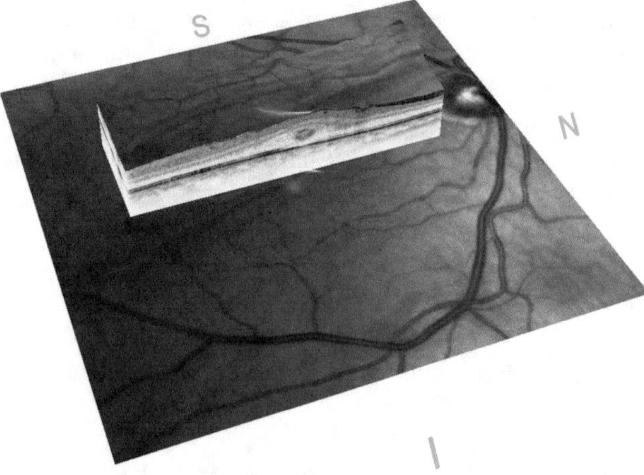

Fig. 8.24 A retinal fold after PPV for RRD in an eye in which the edge of the RRD was transecting the fovea. A fold is seen in the deep layers of the retina

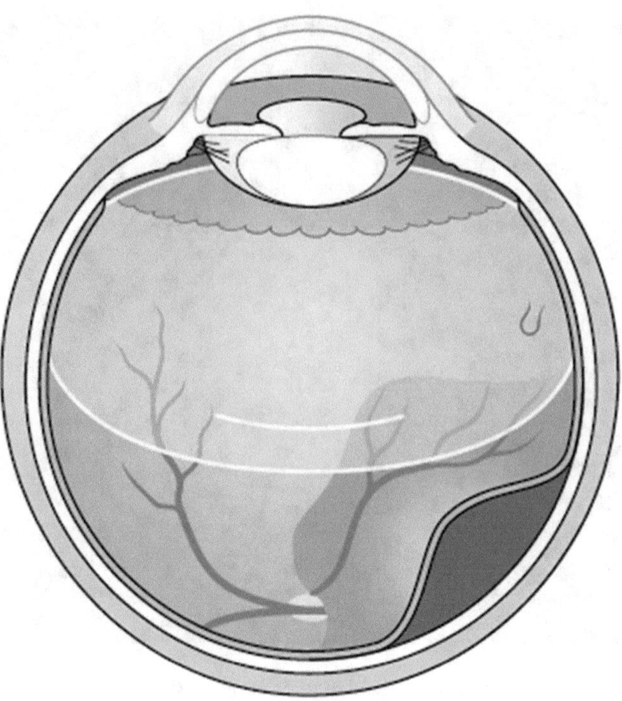

Fig. 8.25 Closure of the hole before drainage of residual SRF means that the SRF will be trapped at the posterior pole and there will be no channel for removing that SRF as the hole is now flattened

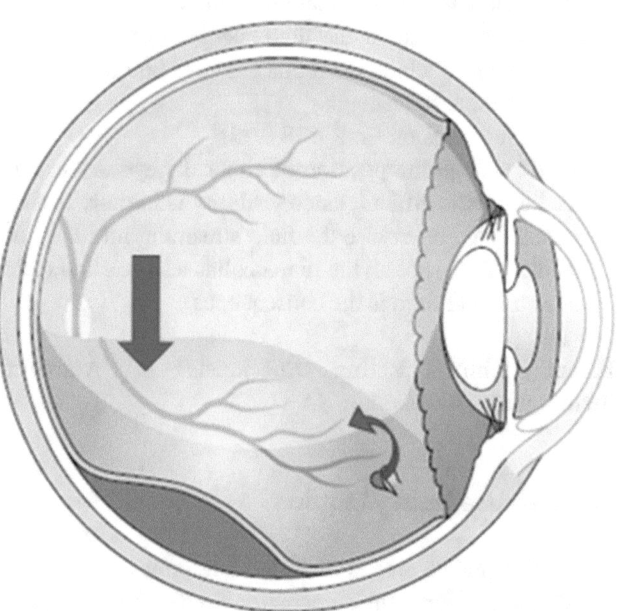

Fig. 8.26 Hanging the retina off the optic nerve (washing line method) allows the SRF to leave a temporal break and should reduce the chance of a retinal fold. Immediate face down posture seems to help avoid macular retinal folds

Once the SRF is drained apply laser or cryotherapy as required to any untreated breaks (it may be prudent to re-treat the break that was drained from if there was any difficulty encountered in case if extension of the tear (Fig. 8.26).

Mathematical Modelling of Retinal Displacement after PPV and Gas Tamponade for Retinal Detachment Repair

Mahmut Dogramaci

It is hypothesised that retinal shifts after PPV for RRD could be caused by a combination of forces generated from SRF gravity and intraocular gas buoyancy [14]. Finite element analysis showed that the density of SRF increases by at least 2.5 folds within the initial 1-2 hours after surgery accompanied by minor reduction in its volume. The increase in density of SRF is possibly due to an increase in total protein, lactic acid, dextrose, and phospholipids concentration as the pigment epithelium actively transports subretinal fluid [15]. Whilst the absence of significant change in SRF volume is possibly due to the guttering effect of postoperative postures leading to the accumulation of subretinal fluid during the same period [16] (Fig. 8.27).

Inferior Breaks (Figs. 8.28 and 8.29)

Controversy exists over the best way to deal with breaks between 4 and 8 clock hours inferiorly [17–20]. High success rates have been described with PPV and gas alone but sometimes with extensive laser application [21]. A solid silicone buckle can be applied but carries a risk of inducing a choroidal haemorrhage [22–25] and adds the potential complications of the explant. If this is used, it is recommended to place the sutures for the explant with closed self-sealing sclerotomies and to have heavy liquid in the eye during placement of the explant. The latter applies a force on the retina because of its increased density and helps limit any spread of any choroidal haemorrhage. PPV without buckle and with face up posturing for the first postoperative week has been used but must only be tried when the risk of PVR is low and a complete gas fill has been obtained [20, 26] (Figs. 8.30, 8.31, 8.32, 8.33, 8.34, and 8.35).

Posterior Breaks

These are easily dealt with as they facilitate SRF drainage and laser retinopexy. Sometimes in myopes the vitreous is still attached to the anterior break edge usually it is not possible to actively detach the vitreous further anteriorly at the break, but it can be detached further anteriorly elsewhere. Leave the vitreous at the break and tamponade as usual. Myopic macular holes are dealt with in Chap. 6 (Fig. 8.36).

Multiple Breaks

Occasionally an excessive amount of retinopexy is required because there are many breaks, or some breaks are exceptionally large. In this situation the judicious use of endolaser reduces the chance of PVR. Even so occasionally the risk of a small missed break or PVR is too high and silicone oil should be inserted (see Chap. 7). If this is done, the pro-inflammatory effects of the operation (and therefore the increased risk of PVR) can be allowed to subside before taking the risk of retinal redetachment (i.e. at oil removal). If long-acting gas is inserted, the patient must be watched more

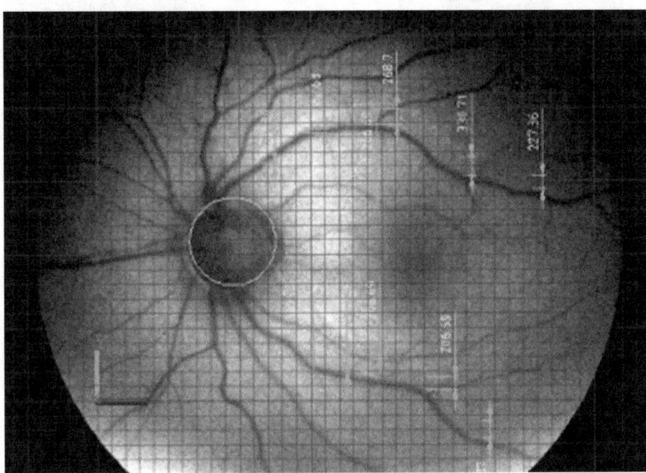

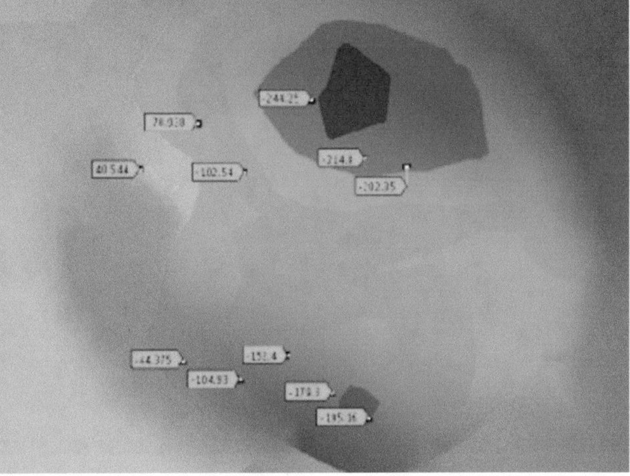

Fig. 8.27 Finite element analysis showing shift values in sample points in AF pictures (left) being compared to their corresponding points in the computer model (right). The retina has shifted downward in this patient as he adopted upright posture immediately after surgery. Finite element analysis for this eye was performed with the eye model being placed in upright orientation in relation to gravity and for the time starting immediately after surgery

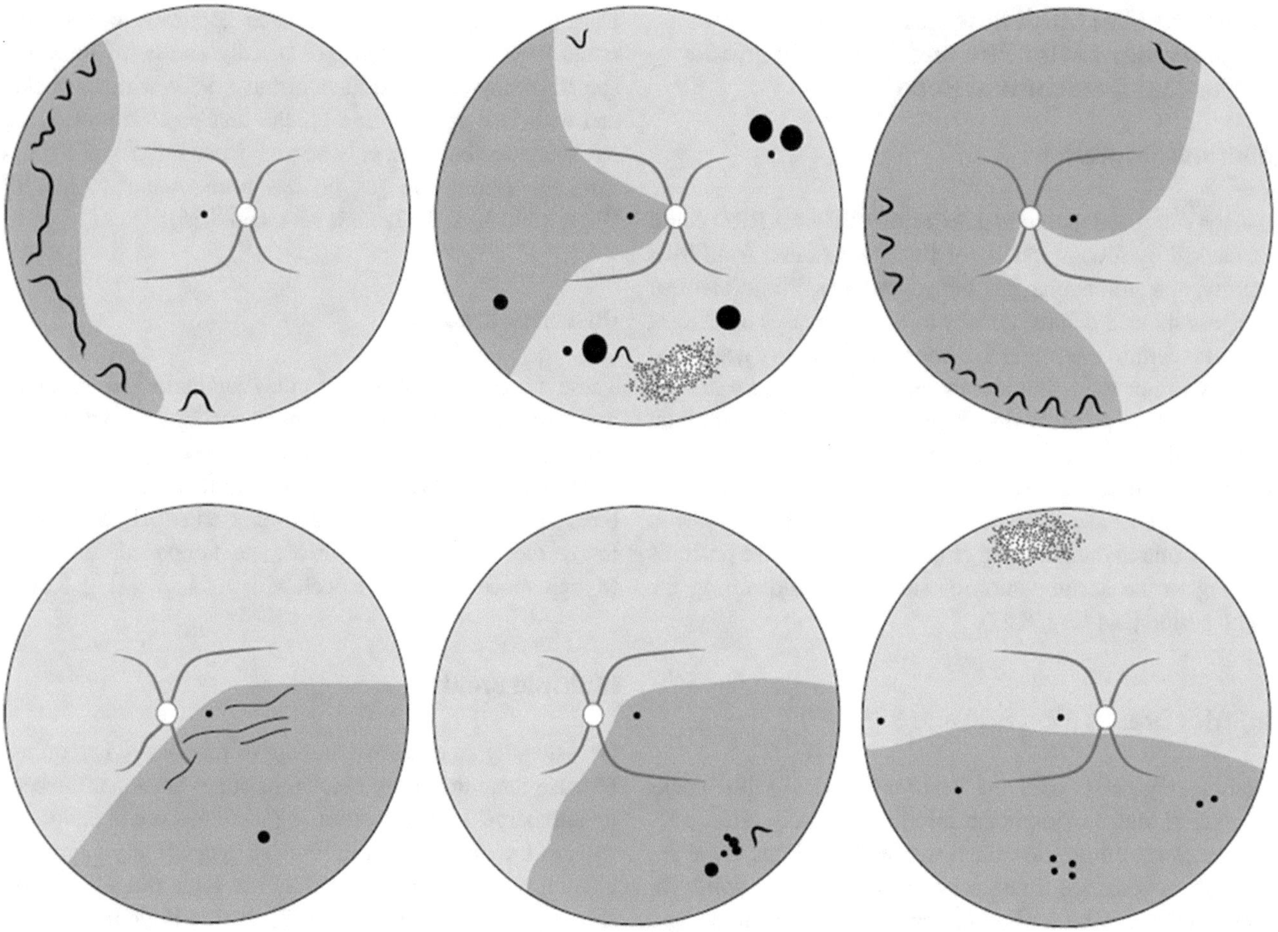

Fig. 8.28 Inferior holes can often be treated by PPV and long-acting gas and posture if there is no risk of inferior proliferative vitreoretinopathy and the patient is willing to posture “face up”. The upper three retinas were treated by PPV and gas and the lower row treated by non-drain repair

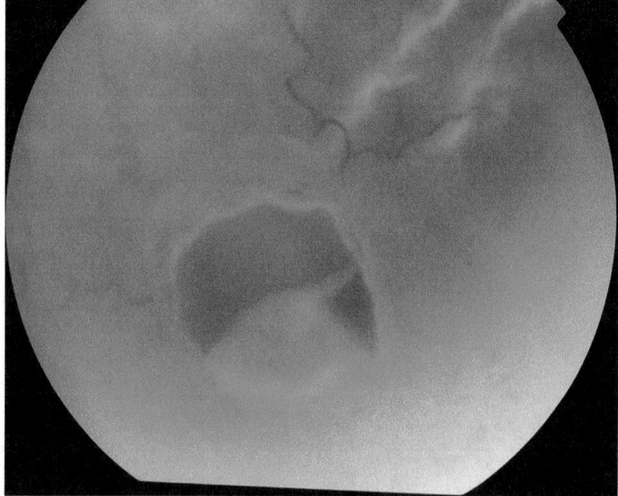

Fig. 8.29 An inferior U tear

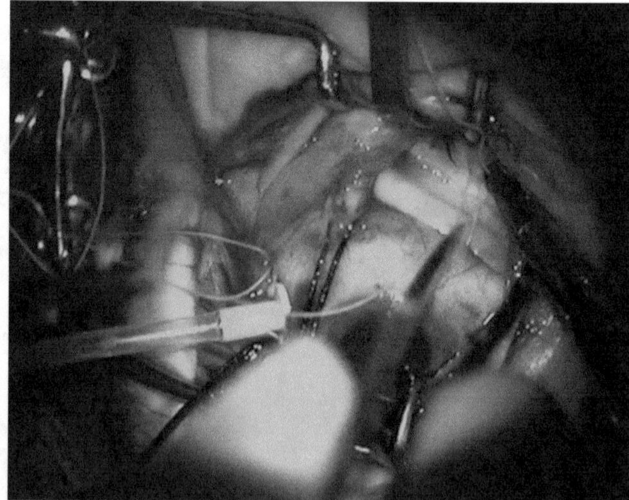

Fig. 8.30 Placing a solid silicone explant onto an eye during PPV is difficult because the eye is soft, and the infusion cannula is in the way. With small gauge systems move the infusion to one of the superior trochars

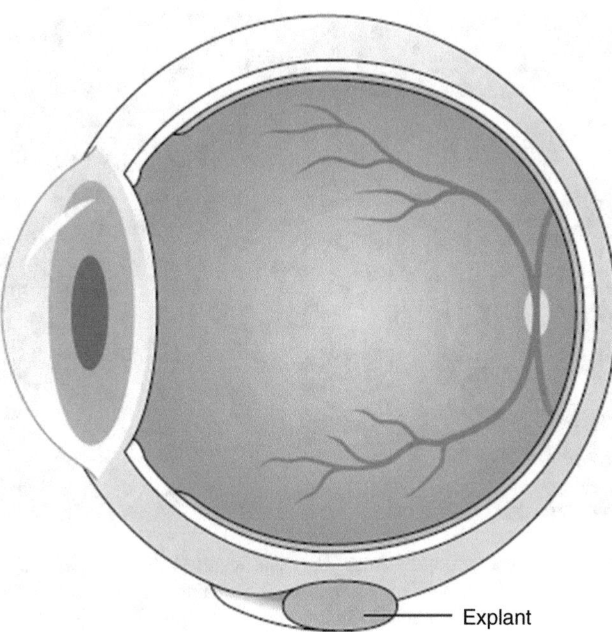

Fig. 8.31 Applying an inferior buckle to a vitrectomised eye runs the risk of inducing a choroidal haemorrhage

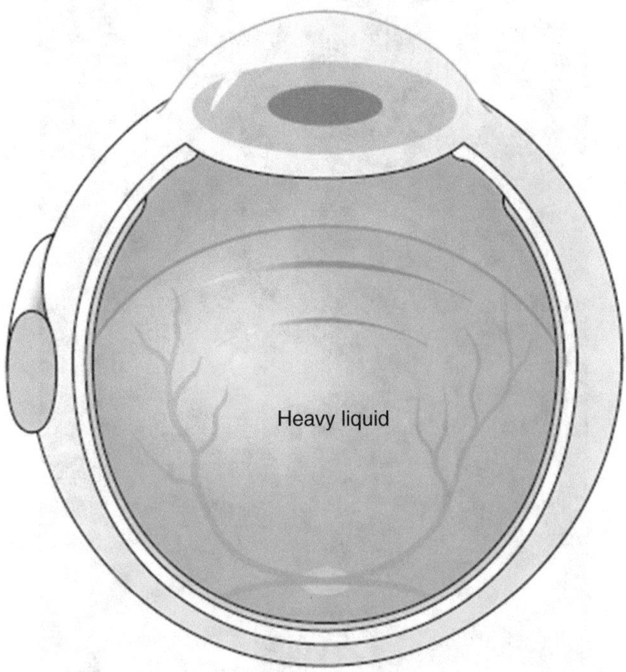

Fig. 8.32 One way to restrict any extension of choroidal haemorrhage is to insert heavy liquids into the eye before the buckle is attached

often in the postoperative period. If the retina detaches, reoperation must be performed immediately before PVR can become established.

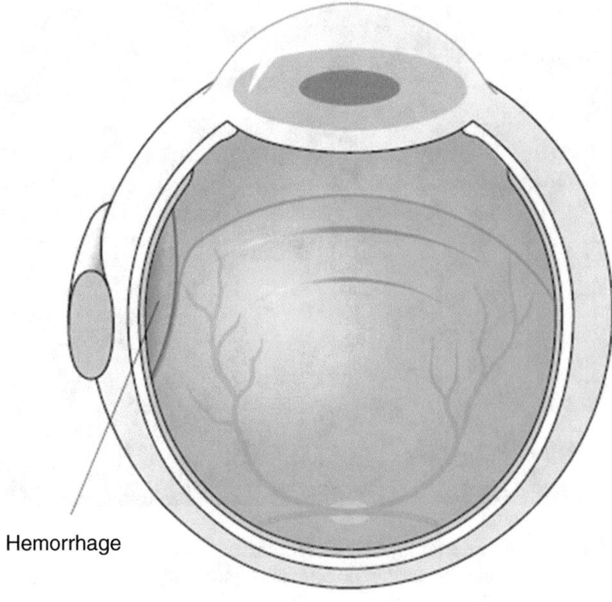

Fig. 8.33 Should a haemorrhage occur it will be restricted to the site of the buckle and not spread to the posterior pole

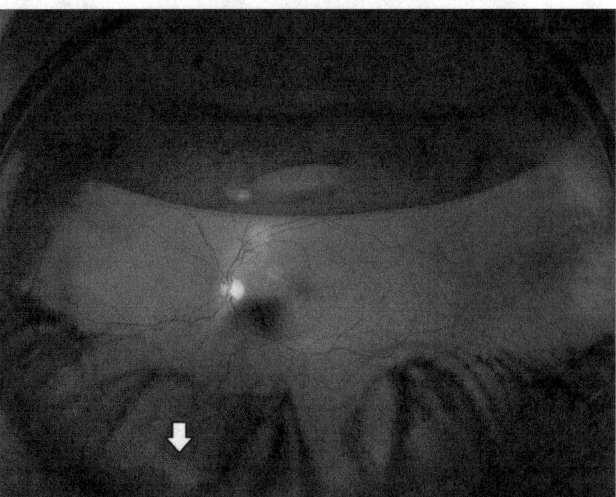

Fig. 8.34 An indentation is shown (arrow) from an inferior buckle. Gas is seen superiorly

Medial Opacities

Cataract and vitreous haemorrhage can be removed during surgery. If the vitreous haemorrhage is severe, care must be taken to identify the position of the RRD behind the haemorrhage to avoid injury to the retina with the cutter. Corneal opacities and small pupils can usually be overcome with use of the wide-angle viewing system which is effective through surprisingly small apertures (Figs. 8.37 and 8.38).

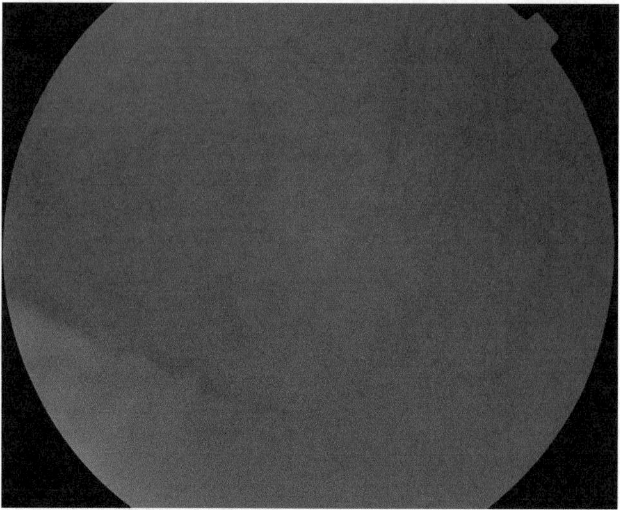

Fig. 8.35 An inferior indentation from a solid silicone explant used to treat inferior breaks during vitrectomy. Minor fold in the retina as in this case will flatten with time

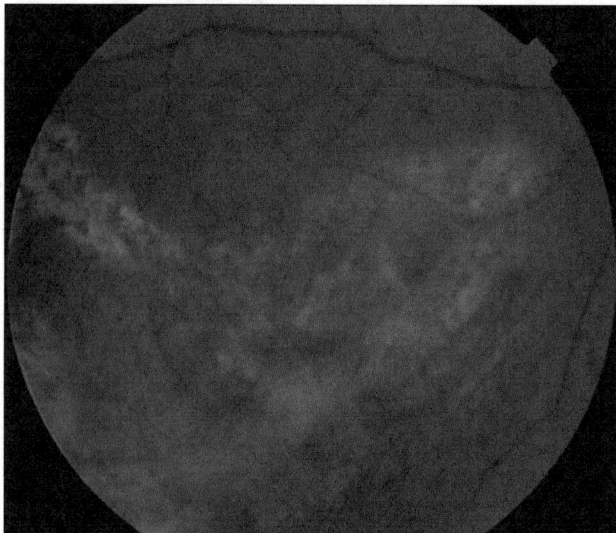

Fig. 8.36 A large tear postoperatively with laser retinopexy

Complications

- Retinal incarceration into sclerotomies or the infusion cannula.
  - Perform good vitreous clearance, early SRF drainage and use of heavy liquids (Figs. 8.39 and 8.40).
- Choroidal haemorrhage.
  - Maintain the IOP throughout surgery.
  - Avoid scleral buckles.

Iatrogenic retinal breaks

- Retinal bites with the cutter, low vacuum near bullous retina, early SRF drainage, use of heavy liquids.

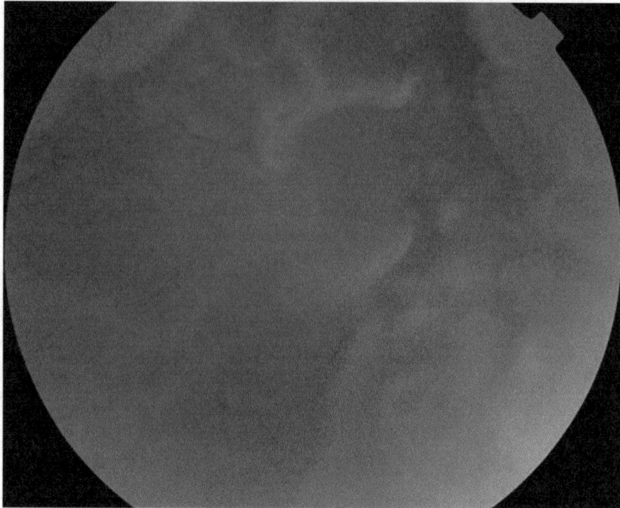

Fig. 8.37 The hypotony from RRD can result in choroidal effusion. Why hypotony occurs in RRD is uncertain but may be due to the detachment spreading anteriorly into the ciliary epithelium

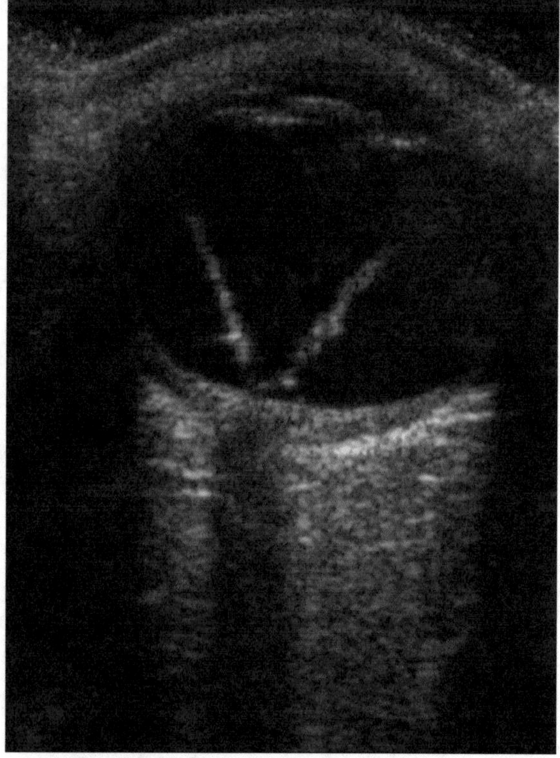

Fig. 8.38 An ultrasound of a hypotonous eye with a total funnel retinal detachment from trauma

  - Take care with mobile bullous RRD.
  - Drain SRF early during vitreous removal.
  - Use heavy liquid if the retina is still very mobile.
  - Use high speed cutters which are more predictable near mobile retina, smaller more frequent bites mean less movement of the retina with each bite.

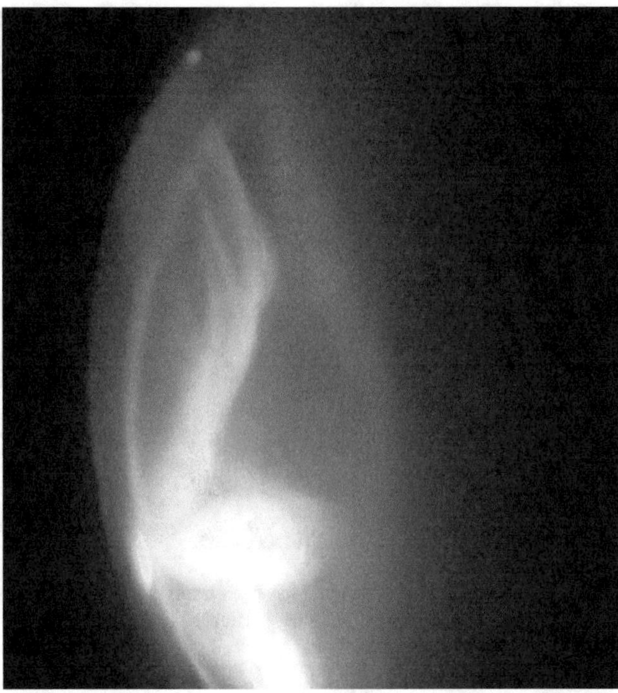

Fig. 8.39 The vitreous and retina are incarcerated into a sclerotomy. The incarceration is reversed by the insertion of heavy liquid

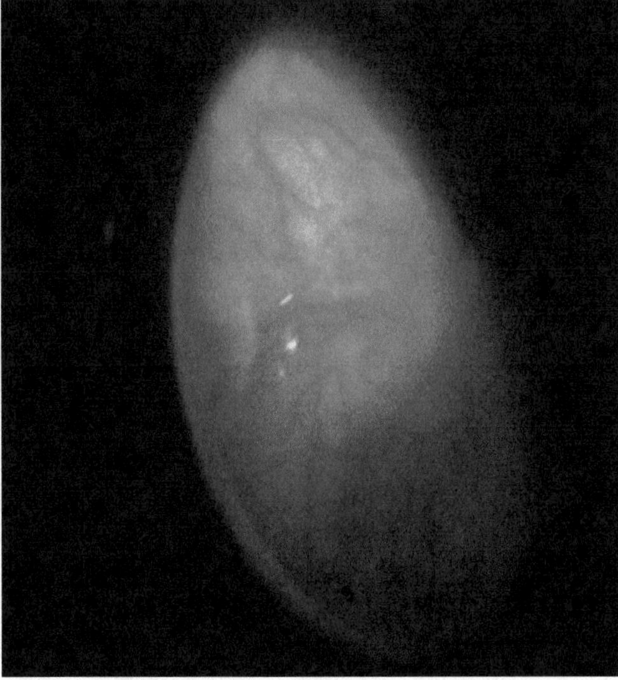

Fig. 8.40 Insertion of heavy liquid resolves the incarceration

- Entry site breaks.
  - Perform a good vitreous clearance especially at the sclerotomies to avoid vitreous and then incarceration of the bullous retina.
  - Close instruments on insertion.

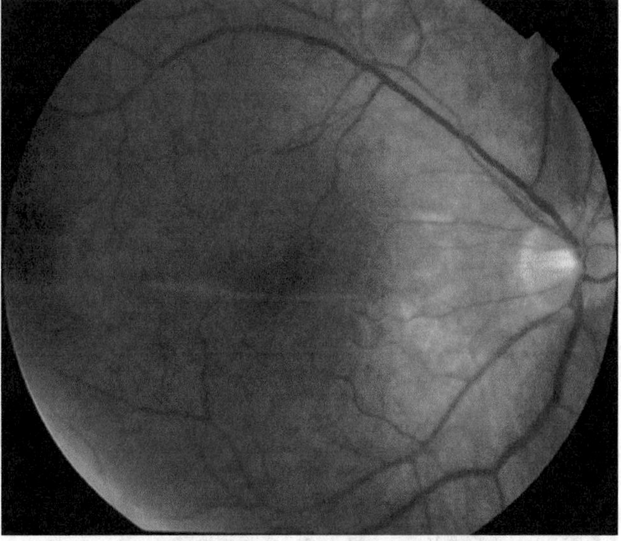

Fig. 8.41 If fluid is left at the posterior pole during vitrectomy and gas tamponade, during postoperative positioning, this can cause a fold in the retinal detachment. If this fold passes through the fovea as in this patient, it can cause considerable problems with distortion and diplopia, which can be difficult to alleviate

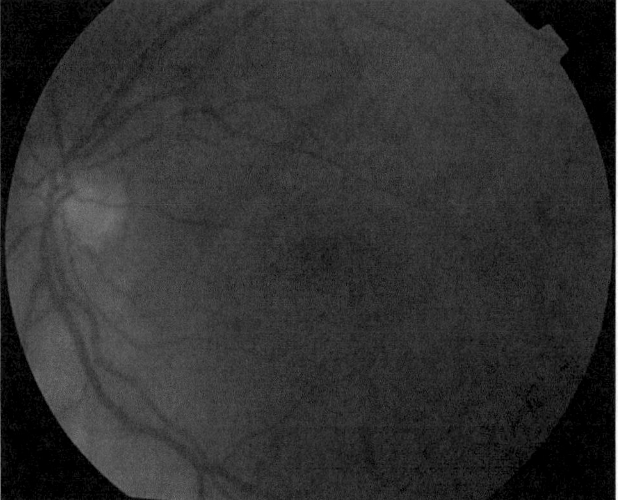

Fig. 8.42 When the macula is just elevated as in this patient there is a risk of retinal folding postoperatively. The surgeon must be careful that SRF at the end of the operation is not trapped in the macula. Depending on access to the retinal break for drainage you may need to insert heavy liquids prior to the air exchange to maximise extrusion of SRF through the break during the air/heavy exchange

  - Make sure that vitreous incarceration into sclerotomies is minimal without vitreous wicks and that sclerotomies are secure at the end of surgery (i.e. no leaks and no vitreous present outside the sclerotomy) (Figs. 8.41, 8.42, 8.43, 8.44, 8.45, 8.46, 8.47, and 8.48).
- Retinal folding.
  - Good SRF drainage, i.e. do not leave SRF in the macula at the end of the operation.

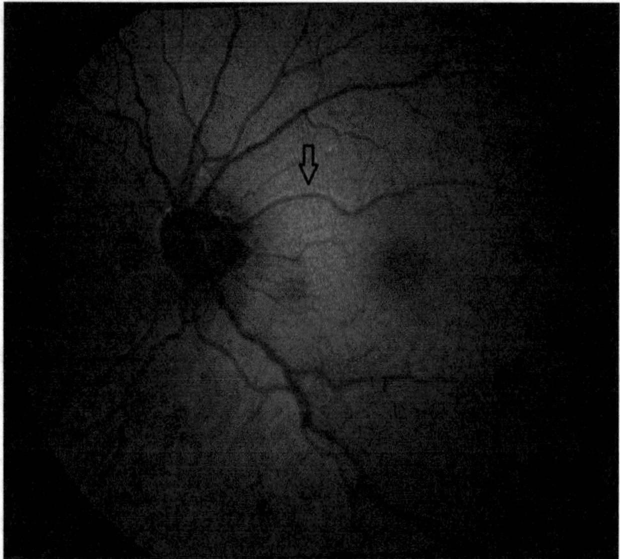

Fig. 8.43 Displacement of the retina after RRD surgery can be demonstrated by the increased fluorescence of the RPE, which previously was posterior to the blood vessels and is now uncovered and shows as a white line adjacent to the blood vessel

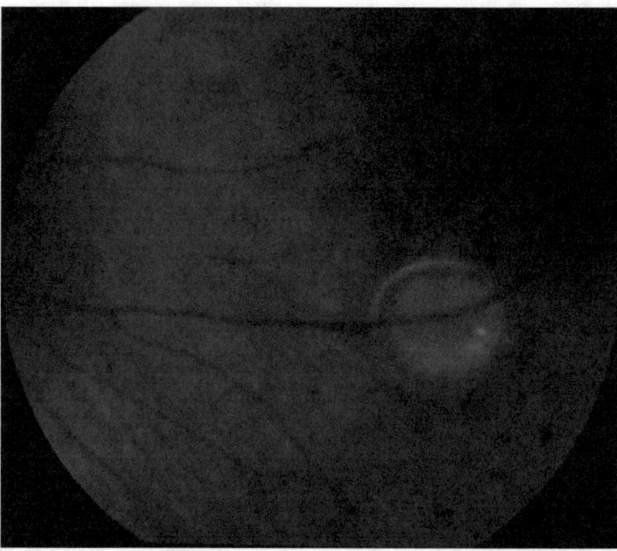

Fig. 8.45 A droplet of heavy liquid has been trapped under the retina. Small bubbles will not move and cause damage. Larger bubbles will move causing diffuse RPE disruption

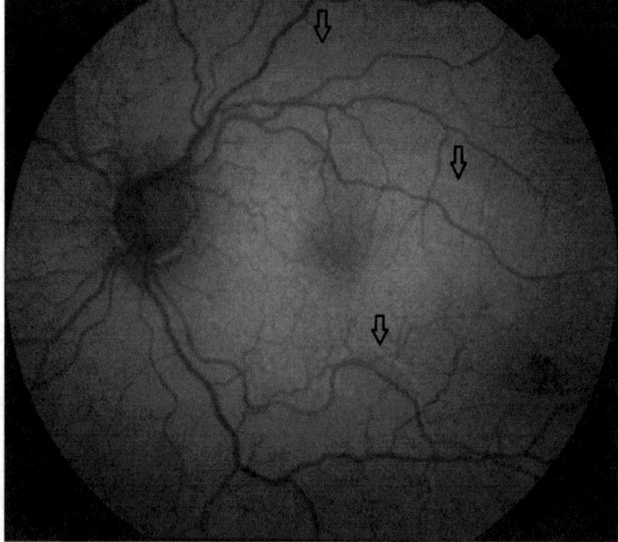

Fig. 8.44 The arrows indicate autofluorescence of RPE cells which were formerly covered by blood vessels and are now exposed after RRD and retinal reattachment. Comparing the blood vessels with the white lines illustrates how far the retina has rotated around the disc and away from its original position even in this eye without retinal folds

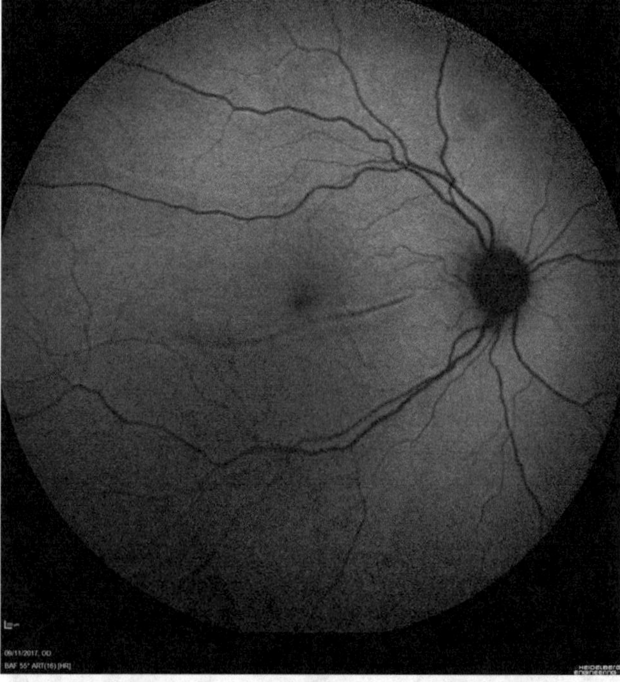

Fig. 8.46 A postoperative retinal fold

  - Face down posturing for first 2 hours postoperatively if there is persistent SRF thereby allowing the RPE to pump out the residual SRF before the gas contacts the macular retina.
  - Underfill with gas, e.g. 80% fill at the end of the operation, to keep the gas away from the macula during face up posture (Fig. 8.49).
- Lens touch.
  - Be aware of the instrument shafts especially when searching for anterior breaks (Figs. 8.50, 8.51, and 8.52)

Surgery for Eyes with no Breaks Found

There are rare eyes in which no retinal break is found despite thorough searching, insertion of heavy liquids, etc. Flatten

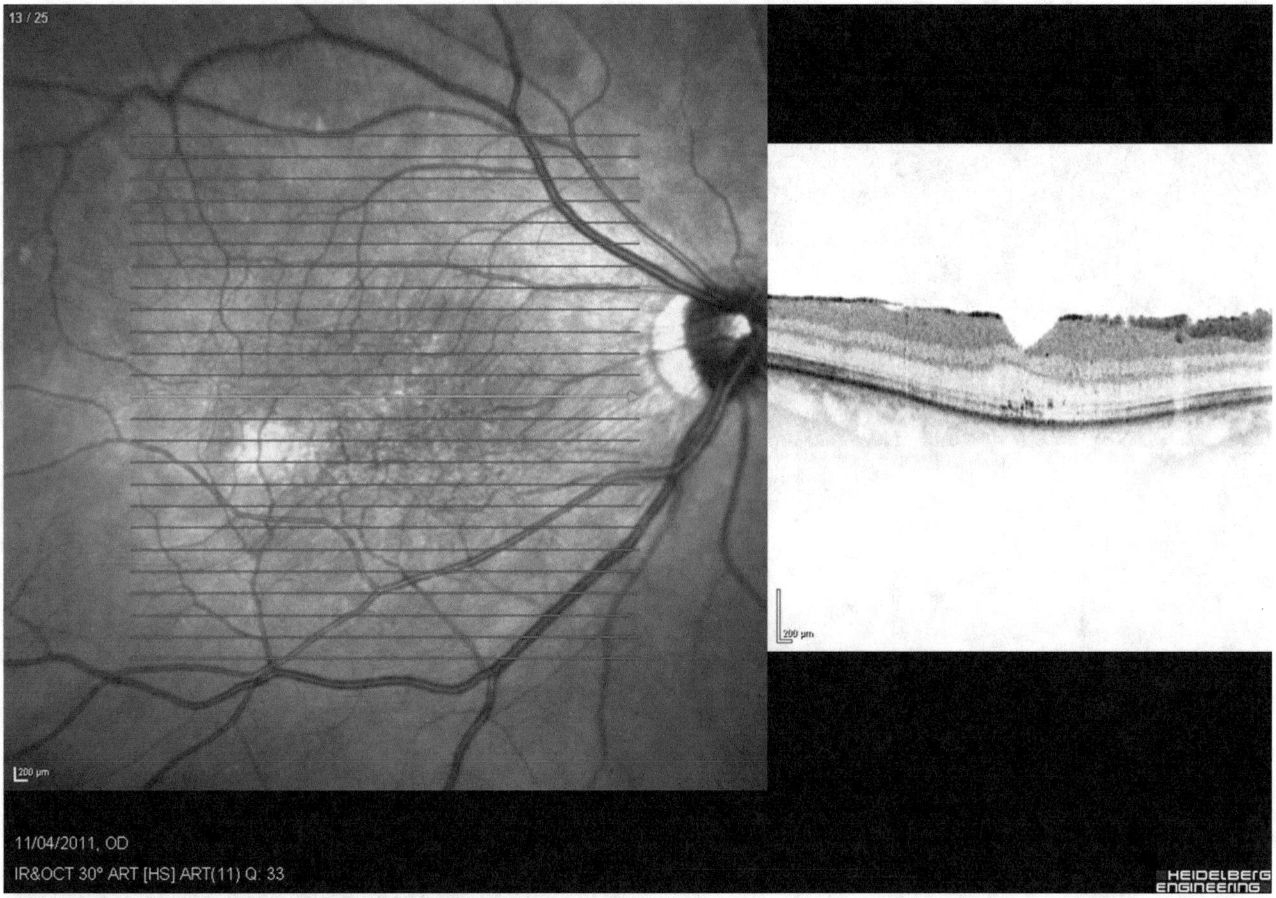

Fig. 8.47 This patient has had a repair of RRD by PPV but has pigment dispersed under the fovea and ERM

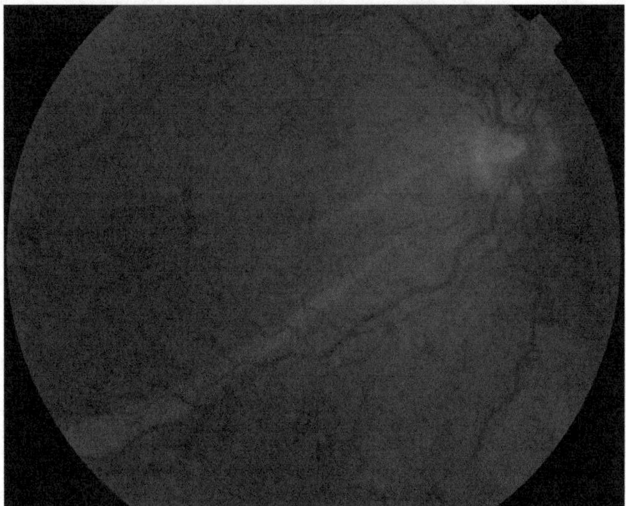

Fig. 8.48 A fold in the retina postoperatively such as this causes postoperative distortion and sometimes diplopia from difficulty fusing the abnormal image with the normal image of the other eye. This can be difficult to remedy, redetachment of the retina can be attempted by reoperation and infusing fluid subretinally via a 40 gauge needle (see macular translocation surgery Chap. 8) but this has risks such as creation of a macular hole during infusion under the fovea

the retina with heavy liquid and internal air tamponade. If the retina cannot be flattened satisfactorily in this way, a posterior retinotomy can be used to allow SRF drainage. Make the retinotomy in detached retina as superiorly and anteriorly as possible. First use endodiathermy to create a weak site on the retina, then aspirate over the weak spot with the flute needle (this creates a smaller hole than a vitrectomy cutter bite). Apply laser around the retinotomy after air insertion. Apply laser also to the quadrant in which the retinal break should be according to Lincoff's rules, 3 rows straddling the posterior border of the vitreous base. If you are unsure where the break should be, apply three rows to straddle the vitreous base in detached retina or 360° if a total RRD. This has a 70% chance of successful outcome [27–29] (Fig. 8.53).

Use of 360° Laser or Routine 360° Encirclage

In modern surgery using the latest retinal viewing systems the chance of not finding any break should be low at 1% therefore direct treatment of RRD pathology is recommended. It should not now be necessary to use 360° laser or encirclage to compensate for the small chance of missing a

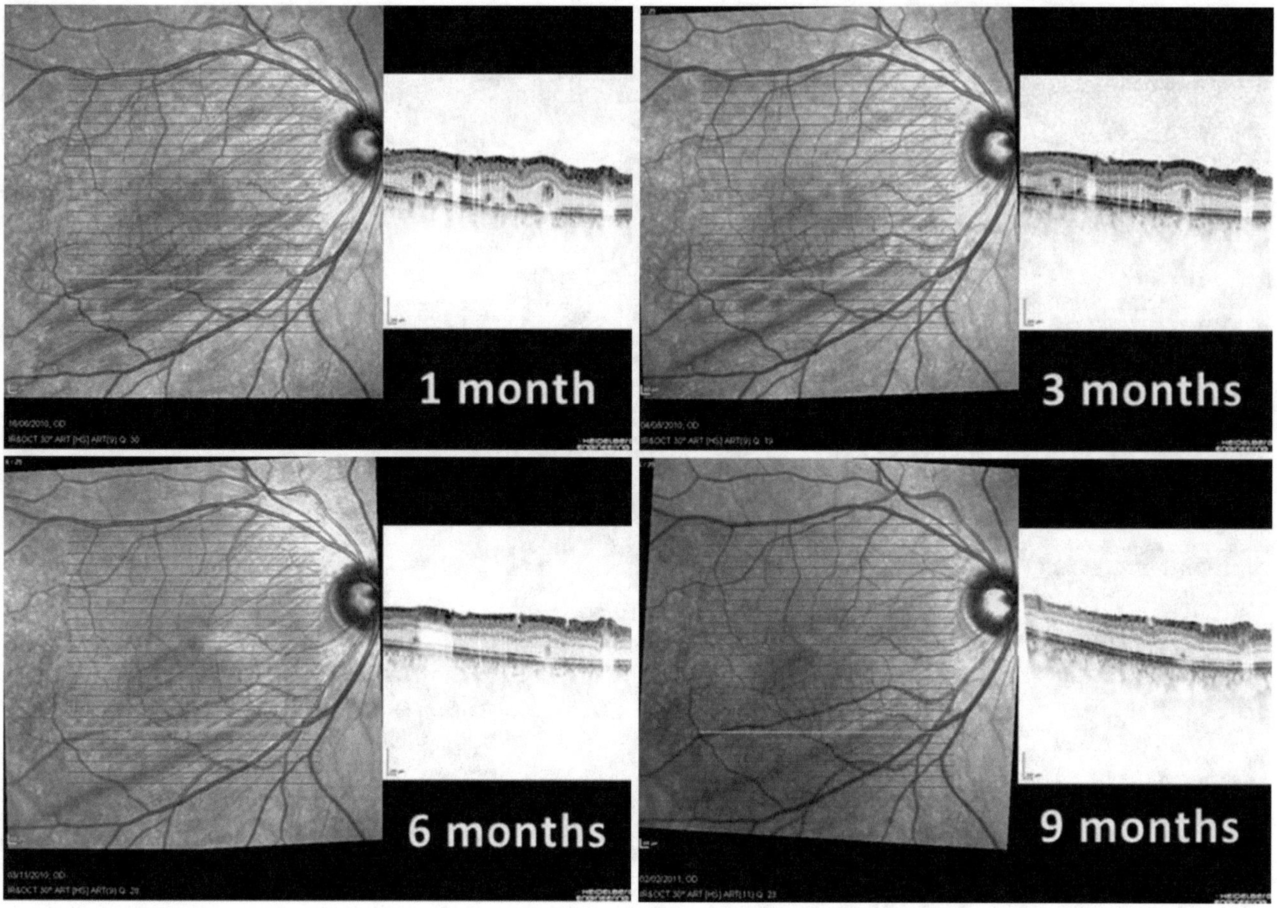

Fig. 8.49 This patient with postoperative folding of the retina after PPV and gas for rhegmatogenous retinal detachment shows gradual reduction of the folding over 9 months

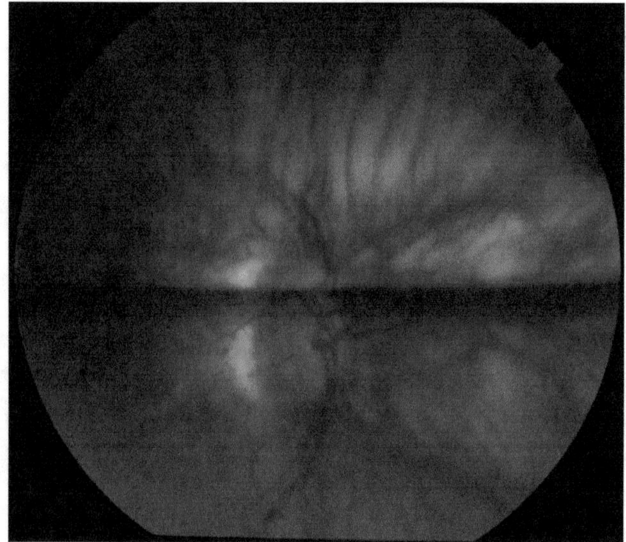

Fig. 8.50 A 50% fill of gas

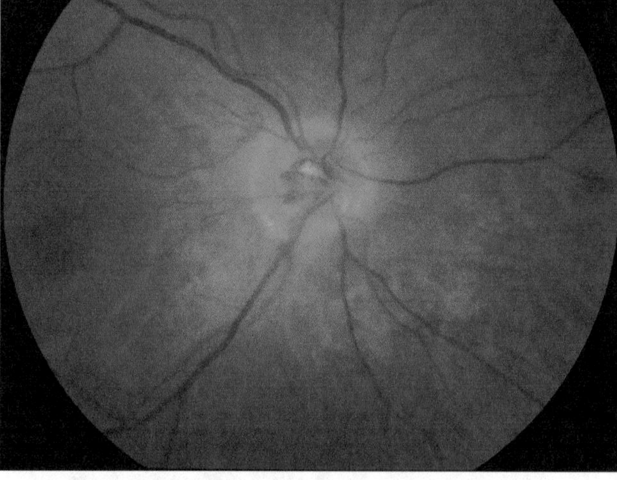

Fig. 8.51 Pigment has settled onto the optic nerve head after cryotherapy, perhaps a sign of overly heavy cryotherapy retinopexy

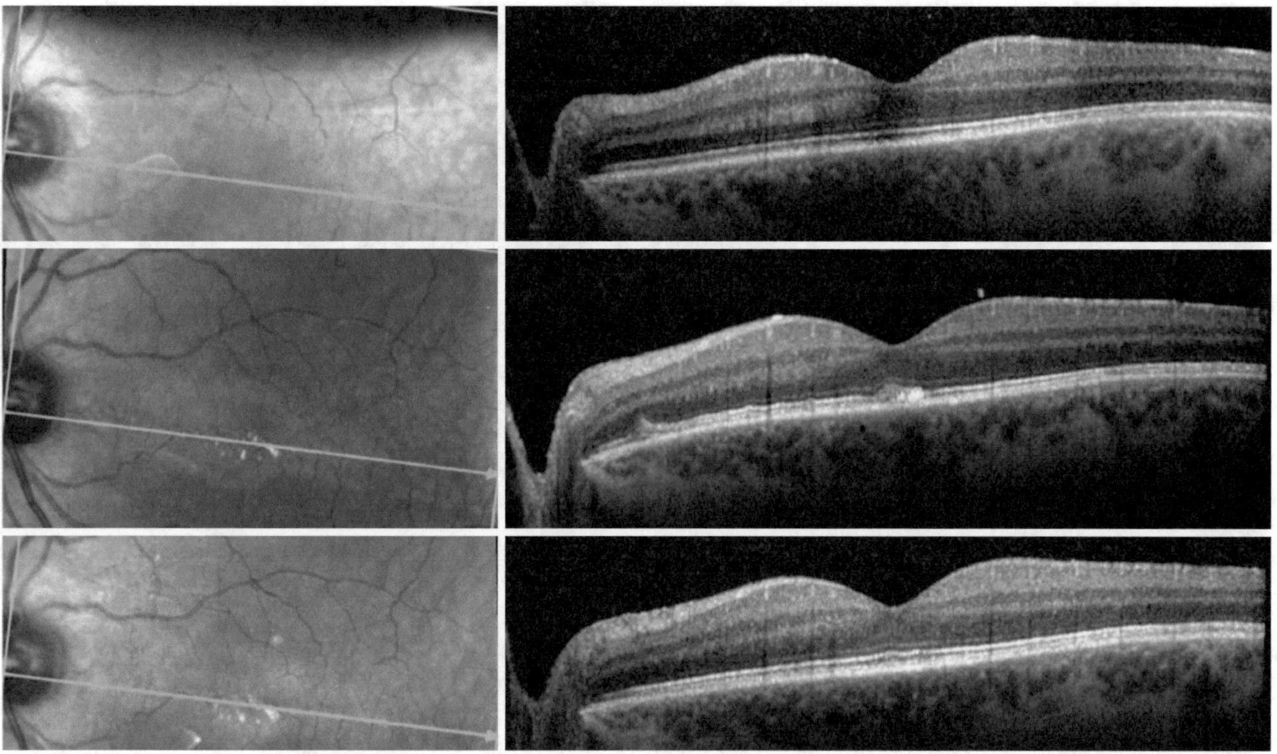

Fig. 8.52 Pigment cells were migrated into the fovea on RRD. The pigment faded with time, top image most recent

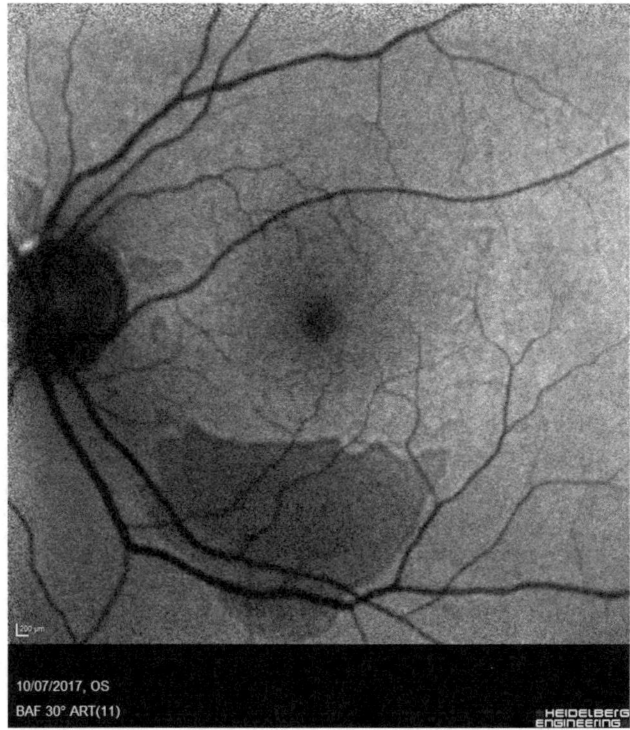

Fig. 8.53 SRF has been pushed through the macula by the gas bubble in a macula on RRD

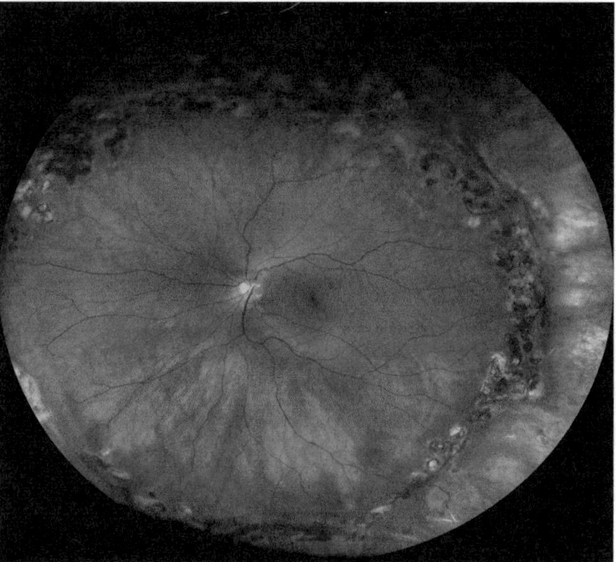

Fig. 8.54 360 laser and encirclage have been used but this is usually unnecessary and instead individual breaks can be treated to minimise the area of retina requiring treatment

break. Older studies reported 8% of patients in whom no break was seen with more chances of missed break resulting in redetachment [30, 31] and therefore prophylactic measures were justifiable. Even so 360° laser or routine 360° encirclage are used by some surgeons for eyes with RRD. There are several problems with this approach. (Figs. 8.54 and 8.55).

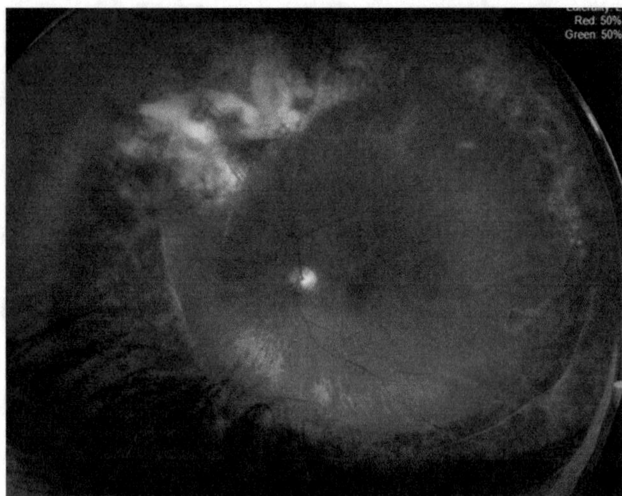

Fig. 8.55 360-degree laser has been applied for this RRD. This method is increasing in popularity for use in all cases as an alternative to treating only the retinal breaks that are detected

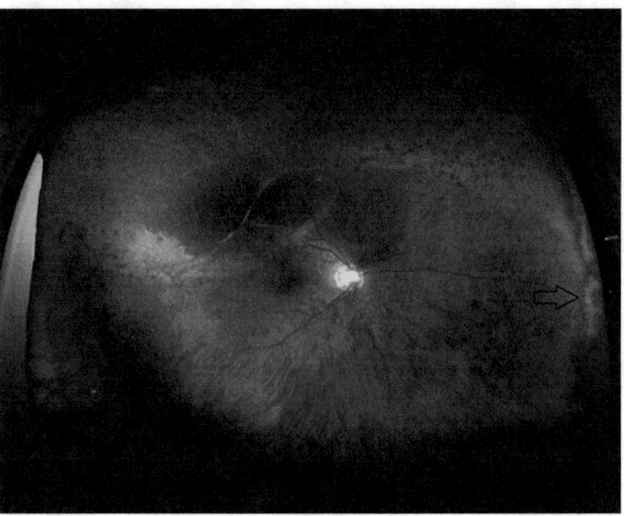

Fig. 8.56 A 360 encirclage has been used but has caused a large myopic shift from -5D to -8D resulting in anisometropia in this patient

- Any extra retinopexy especially cryotherapy increases the chance of PVR.
- Blue light hazard (damage to retinal cones) from laser.
- Some patients are aware of the loss of visual field associated with retinopexy.
- The surgeon is not encouraged to determine the exact pathology present in each case and therefore is at risk of losing the skills to find all breaks and the ability to recognise patterns of RRD pathology.
- Isolated RRD anterior to laser stimulates ischaemia and inflammation which can secondarily cause CMO and ERM in the macula.
- Heavy treatment affects the anterior segment with loss of iris function and flare.
- Encirclage requires opening of the conjunctiva.
- Encirclage has the potential for suture related complications.
- Encirclage may change the refraction of the eye because the eye is elongated by the reduction of the equatorial circumference, in extreme cases resulting in an hourglass shape to the eye (Figs. 8.54 and 8.56).

Posturing

The patient does not need to posture if the breaks are above the horizontal meridian. Use posturing for breaks inferior to 3 and 9 o'clock. They should posture for 50 minutes in the hour for the first 7 days postoperatively.

For a temporal hole in the left eye or a nasal hole in the right eye the patient would be asked to lie with their right cheek down to the ground.

For a nasal hole in the left eye or a temporal hole in the right eye the patient would be asked to lie with their left cheek down to the ground.

For an inferior hole, the patient lies supine (face up) with no pillows and the foot of the bed raised if possible.

Surgical Pearl

Surgery for Rhegmatogenous Retinal Detachment

- You do not need to use PFCL in every case—I use them in cases of very mobile retinas to stabilise and when breaks are very anterior and SRF chronic to maximise SRF drainage. If used inject into the enlarging PFCL bubble to avoid small bubbles and do not fill to anywhere near the infusion line to avoid bubble creation during indentation.
- The Tindall effect using triamcinolone and trans-scleral light pipe indentation is a useful technique in lightly pigmented Caucasian patients and avoids the need for chandeliers in many cases.
- If you cannot find a break, then use subretinal blue assisted searching. I use heavy BBG and a 38 g cannula and then PFCL to express the dye through the break.
- Tilting head to drain SRF can massively increase SRF drainage through breaks without resorting to PFCL or posterior retinotomies. Residual SRF is rarely of importance and resolves in <24 hours in most cases. It is not necessary to drain all fluid unless patient is old, or RRD is chronic, with inferior breaks.
- If you need to do a giant retinotomy to reattach a retina with PVR always do it greater than 200 degrees. Small retinotomies have a high incidence of edge contraction.

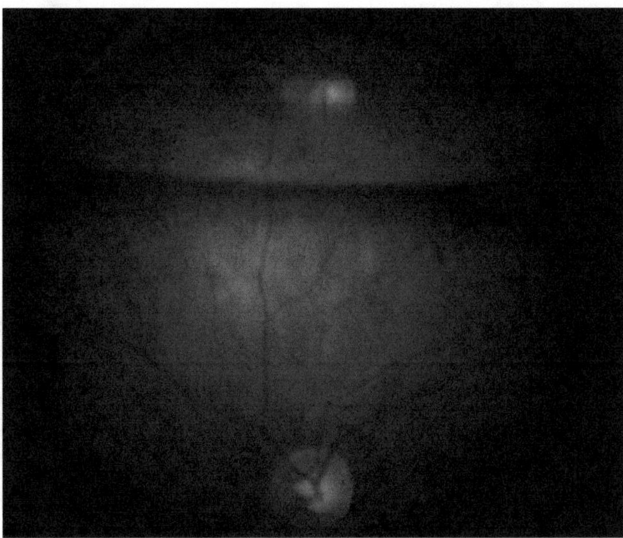

Fig. 8.57 A 20% fill of gas

Professor David Steel, Sunderland Eye Hospital, Sunderland, UK (Figs. 8.57 and 8.58)

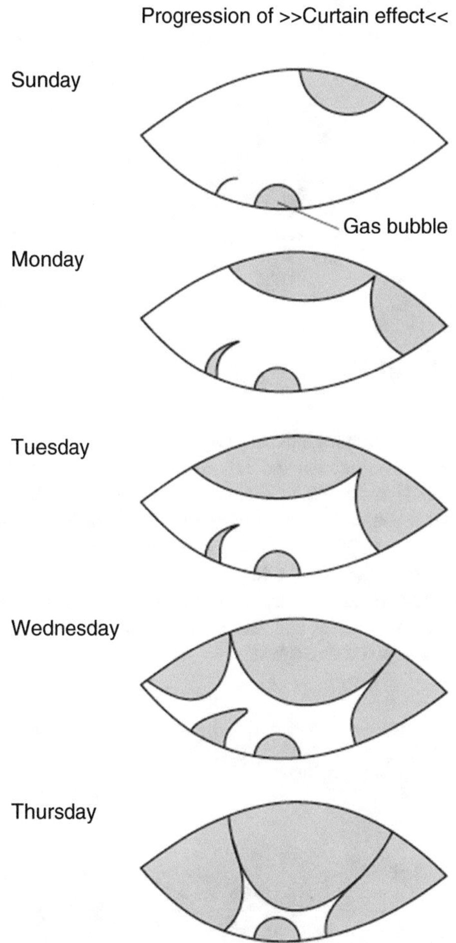

Fig. 8.58 This is the patient's perception of recurrence of his retinal detachment. As the patient's visualisation of events is inverted, he sees the gas bubble at the bottom of the diagram and the retinal detachment returning at the top of his diagram

The Non-Drain Procedure

Surgery for RRD evolved over the twentieth century from surgery with scleral buckling [32] to PPV and gas [33]. The non-drain retinal detachment procedure involves placement of a silicone sponge underneath a retinal tear. Placement of the sponge is crucial to the success of the procedure. A 3, 4, 5, or 7 mm silicone sponge can be used but, in the majority, a 5 mm sponge is appropriate. Some surgeons use a solid silicone explant which provides a broader but shallower indent. Preoperatively the facility for using this operation can be determined by the ability to "indent the tear", i.e. it should be possible to oppose the retinal pigment epithelium to the neurosensory retina indicating that it will be possible to apply cryotherapy retinopexy during surgery without drainage of subretinal fluid (SRF) (Table 8.3).

Table 8.3 Difficulty rating of the non-drain procedure

Difficulty Rating	Moderate
Success rates	High
Complication rates	Low
When to use in training	Early

Operative Stages

- Open the conjunctiva and sling the recti muscles.
- Search for retinal breaks with the indirect ophthalmoscope and scleral indentation.
- Apply cryotherapy to the breaks.
- Mark the site of the breaks on the external sclera.
- Pre-place the scleral sutures.
- Insert the sponge.
- Tie one suture.
- Perform a paracentesis to remove some aqueous.
- Tie the remaining sutures.
- Check the optic nerve perfusion and break position on the indent.
- Close the conjunctiva (Figs. 8.59, 8.60, and 8.61).

When starting with this surgery open the conjunctiva 360° to facilitate isolation of the recti muscles and to ease indentation of the sclera. Later when skills are more honed restrict the conjunctival perimetry if you wish. Start by making a radial cut of 2–3 mm (usually one snip of the scissors) in the conjunctiva and Tenon's layer on one of the oblique meridians (thereby avoiding the extraocular muscle insertions), sweep one of the blades of a blunt ended scissor under the

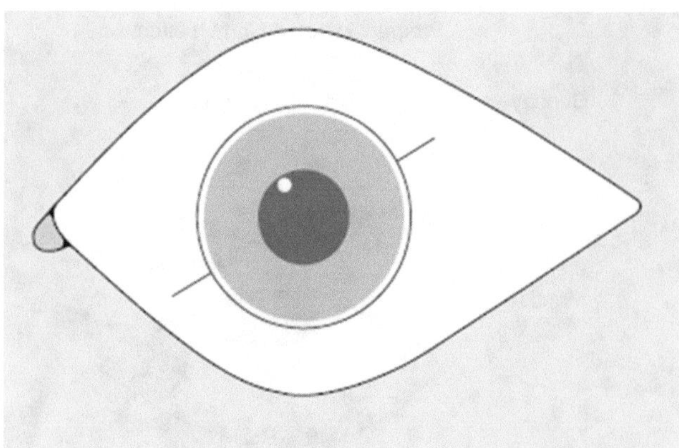

Fig. 8.59 Use a limbal conjunctival perimetry for a non-drain procedure. Incise the conjunctiva and Tenons close to the limbus and sweep the scissor blade under the Tenons and up to the limbus. Keep as close to the limbus as possible by pulling with the scissor blade towards the cornea. Make two small radial slits as shown to allow the conjunctiva to open for access to the sclera otherwise there is a risk of tearing of the conjunctiva later in the surgery. Keep the slits on the oblique axis to avoid extraocular muscles and place them in quadrants where you are not proposing to place an explant

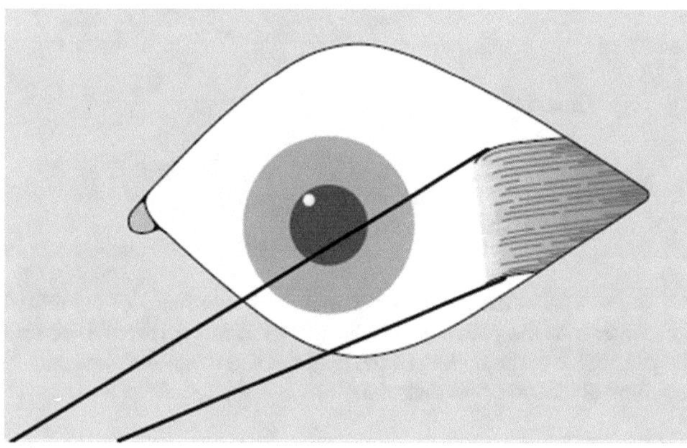

Fig. 8.60 26. Sling the extraocular muscles

Tenons, and anteriorly towards the limbus of the cornea and sclera to leave as little tissue as possible at the limbus. Repeat the sweep and cut all around the limbus. Make a second radial cut 180° from the first.

Note: It is preferable not to make the radial cuts in the quadrant in which the explant is being placed. This keeps intact conjunctiva and Tenons over the explant in the postoperative period. Pass a squint hook instrument behind the rectus insertion to be able to pull the muscle anteriorly. Next take a damp piece of swab in forceps and push the conjunctiva and Tenons posteriorly over one of the longitudinal borders of the rectus muscle and then the other border of the muscle. The aim is to free the muscle from its attachments to Tenons. Do this to all the recti muscles. This should leave clean sclera between the muscle insertions, tendon, and anterior muscle

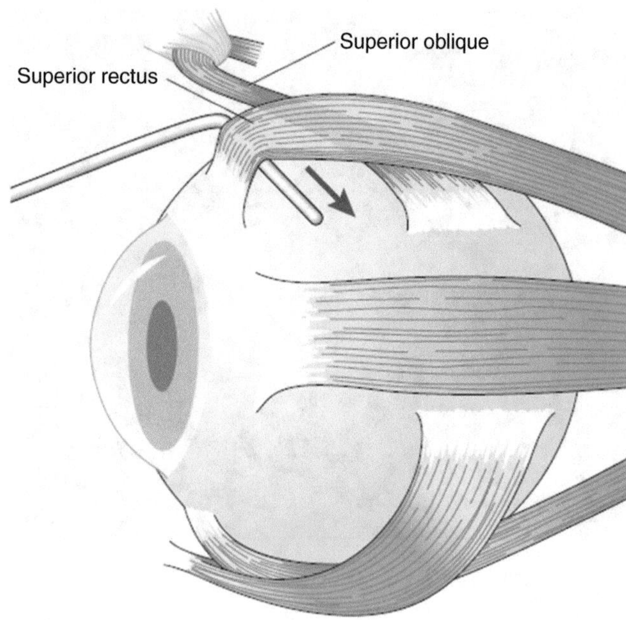

Fig. 8.61 When hooking the superior rectus take care not to hook the superior oblique

belly with no attached Tenons. If any is attached, clear this off now because it will only hamper the surgery later.

Slinging the muscles:

- Whilst holding the position of the muscle with the squint hook.
- Pass a 2/0 braided suture (20 cm long) through the eyelet of an instrument, for example, an aneurysm needle (this is a bent tool with an eyelet at its tip) whilst holding the muscle insertion forward with the squint hook.
- Pass the aneurysm needle under the muscle insertion.
- Remove the squint hook.
- Pull one of the ends of the suture through.
- Hold that end of the suture (press it against the orbital rim with the squint hook).
- Remove the artery needle and disengage it from the suture.
- Tie the ends of the suture with a simple knot and weigh down by clamping the end with an artery clip.

Always sling both horizontal recti with a suture. The horizontal slings will allow movement of the eye in a circumferential manner if, for example, there is difficulty viewing a particular portion of the retina because of the anatomy of the patient, e.g. a large nose, deep socket, or kyphoscoliosis of the patient. With superior breaks also sling the superior rectus if inferior breaks sling the inferior rectus. The slings will be required to move the eye to expose the sclera overlying the break for the application of the explant (Figs. 8.62, 8.63, 8.64, and 8.65).

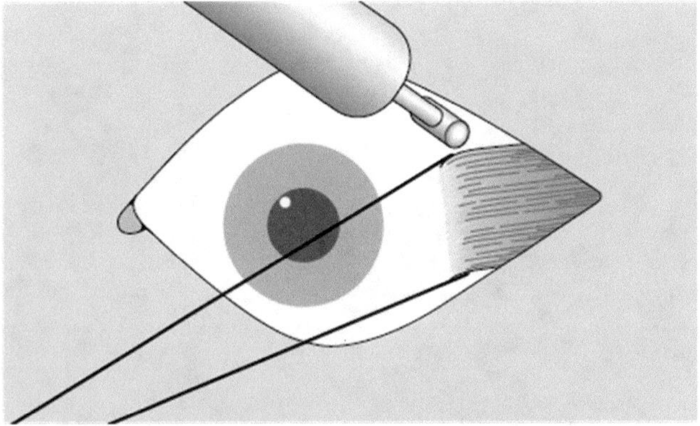

Fig. 8.62 Indent the sclera to view the peripheral retina

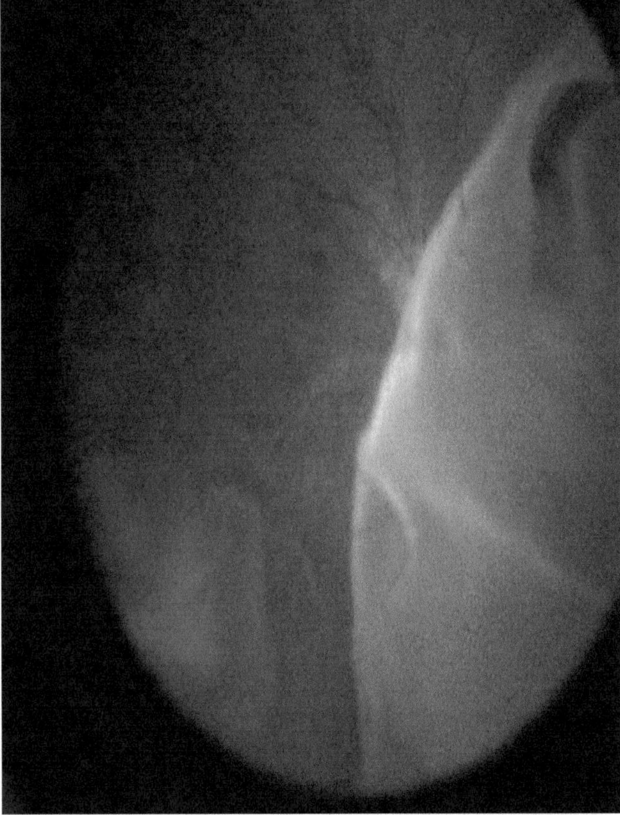

Fig. 8.63 A U tear can be seen on indentation of the sclera to allow visualisation of the peripheral retina

Search the eye with binocular indirect ophthalmoscope (BIO) and 20D lens or equivalent and indentation for 360° (use a thimble with attached prong and T bar on the end or a squint hook). Remember start at one shoulder whilst viewing the 12 o'clock retina and work around the head to the other shoulder and back to the 12 o'clock position. The slings help to manoeuvre the eye during indentation. The weight of the artery clips helps stabilise the eye during this search (reducing rotation and posterior displacement of the globe).

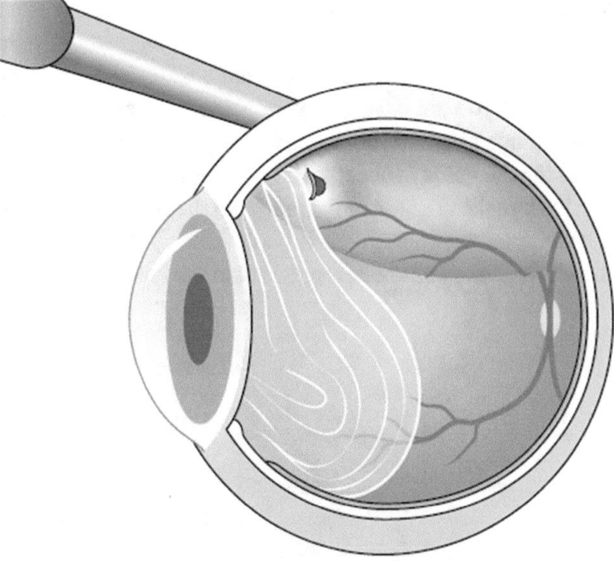

Fig. 8.64 Indent the break with the cryotherapy probe

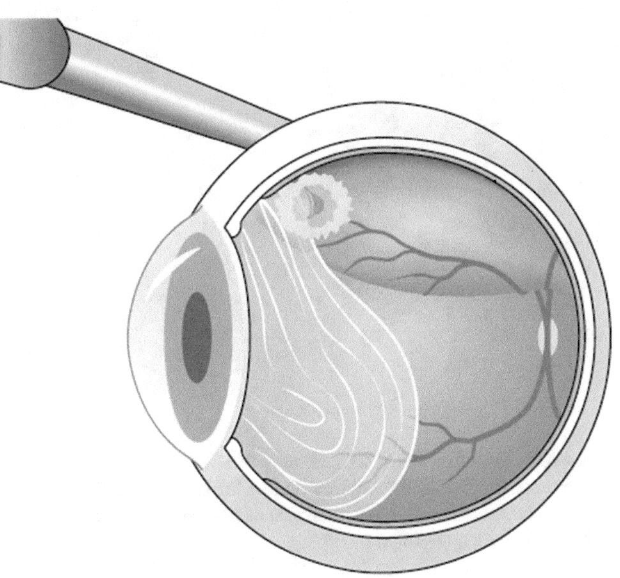

Fig. 8.65 Apply the freeze

Note: To further stabilise the eye place, the fifth finger of the hand holding the lens and press down on to one of the horizontal slings and the orbital rim. This stops the eye moving both circumferentially and posteriorly into the orbit during indentation.

Apply cryotherapy to all the breaks. Usually each break only requires one freeze starting in the middle of the break and extended to the equivalent of two laser rows around the break. Produce a mark on the external sclera, indicating the site of the breaks, using an indenter, e.g. Glass indenter, a thimble shaped instrument with a prong attached with a 1 mm diameter elevated circular rim at its end. After indentation this leaves a circular mark on the sclera. Dry the sclera and mark the spot with ink from a sterile indelible marker pen. Swab again to remove excess ink otherwise it will stain the Tenons (Figs. 8.66, 8.67, 8.68, and 8.69).

Note: If you are unsure of your accuracy grasp the sclera at the mark gently with toothed forceps and indent whilst checking the break is over the indent internally with the BIO.

Observe the position of the marks on the sclera breaks and decide upon the appropriate explant (plomb) that can cover the marks. Much has been argued about the type and orientation of the plomb. A circumferential plomb is easy to apply and successful in most cases. If using a sponge, two factors determine the choice of size.

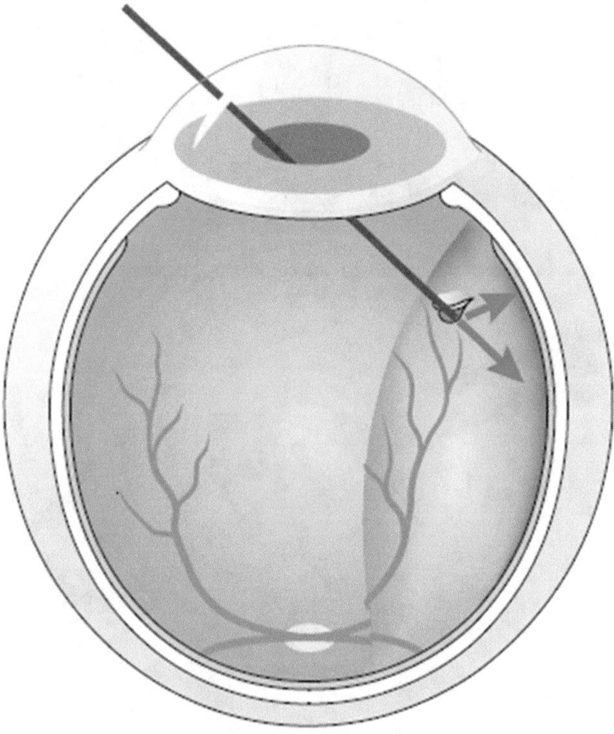

Fig. 8.66 Visualisation of a break in a retinal detachment by indirect ophthalmoscopy gives the impression that the break should settle more posteriorly because of the phenomenon of parallax. Take this into consideration when applying a plombage

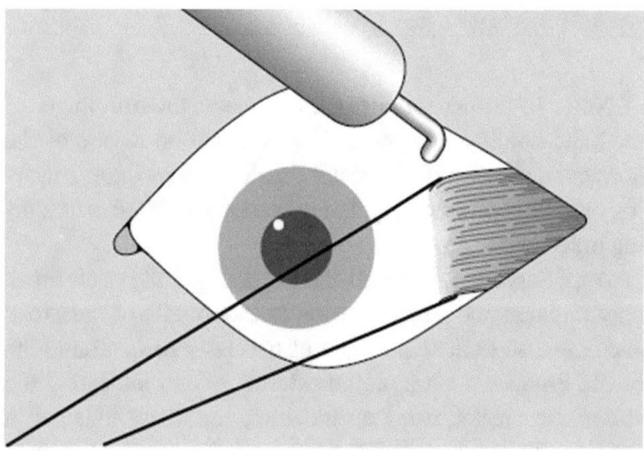

Fig. 8.67 With indentation mark on the external sclera the position of the break or breaks

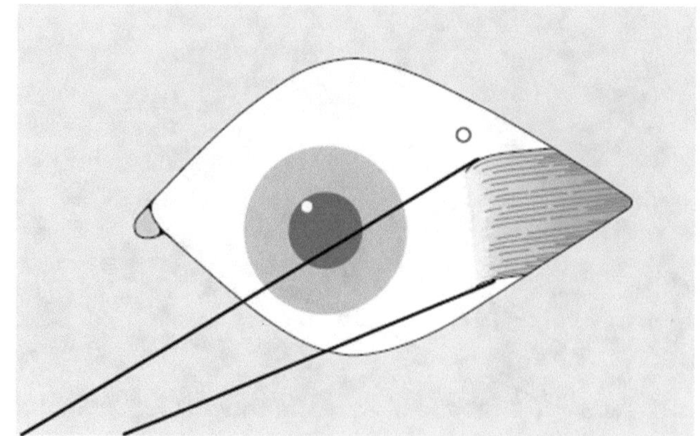

Fig. 8.68 The mark is used to guide the placement of the sutures

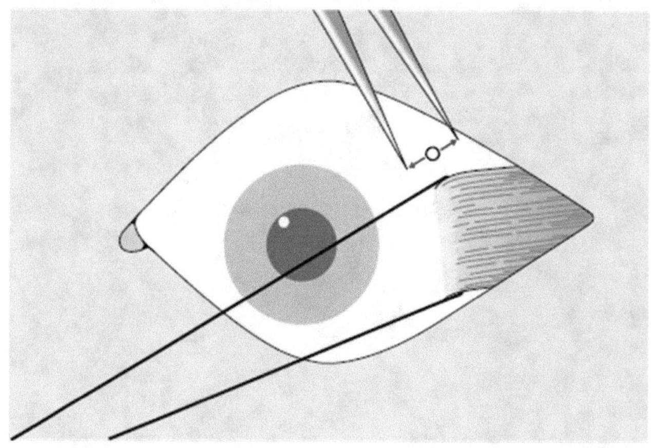

Fig. 8.69 Place the sutures an equal distance from the mark

- The size of the break or breaks, bigger breaks requiring larger indentation surface area.
- The presence of multiple breaks in different circumferential positions, e.g. in a young person's low myope round hole retinal detachment.
- Height of break from the RPE, e.g. in retinal dialysis.

Note: Try to use the smallest explant to achieve placement of the break or breaks on the apical ridge of the indentation. If there are multiple breaks in different circumferential meridians, you will need a larger plombage and not all breaks will be on the apex but try to keep them as close as possible, i.e. on the apical 1/3 of the total area of the indent.

Use 5/0 non-absorbable sutures at a width of 1.5x the diameter of the sponge (approximately, ½ the circumference of the cross-section of the plomb, i.e. 0.5 x 2πr), e.g. 7.5 mm for a 5 mm sponge or 6 mm for a 4 mm sponge. Insert the suture with a spatulated needle into the sclera for 2–3 mm for each insertion and as deep into the sclera without going into the suprachoroidal space. The sclera will allow a plane to open for the suture to pass along.

Note: If you can see the dark of the needle as it passes through the sclera you are too shallow and there is a risk the suture will tear through the sclera during suture tightening. Remove the needle and try again (Figs. 8.70, 8.71, 8.72, 8.73, and 8.74).

Each incision is orientated parallel to the explant.

Signs that the stitch is too deep are as follows:

- Extrusion of SRF (straw coloured viscous fluid).
- Haemorrhage from the suture track.
- A speck of pigment appears at the end of the suture track.

If too deep, inspect the inside of the eye with the BIO. A white spot will be seen in the choroid and some subretinal bleeding may be encountered. In the latter circumstance indent the eye to increase the IOP and to limit the spread of the bleed long enough to allow clotting to occur. Occasionally fluid vitreous will come out of a deep stitch causing progressive collapse of the eye. The vitreous fluid passes through the retinal break and then out through the needle track (also seen rarely with external drain procedures). In this circumstance indent the break if possible, to do so. This prevents further recruitment of fluid vitreous into the subretinal space. Re-inflate the eye with an air bubble, which will also prevent further extrusion of fluid (see DACE procedure).

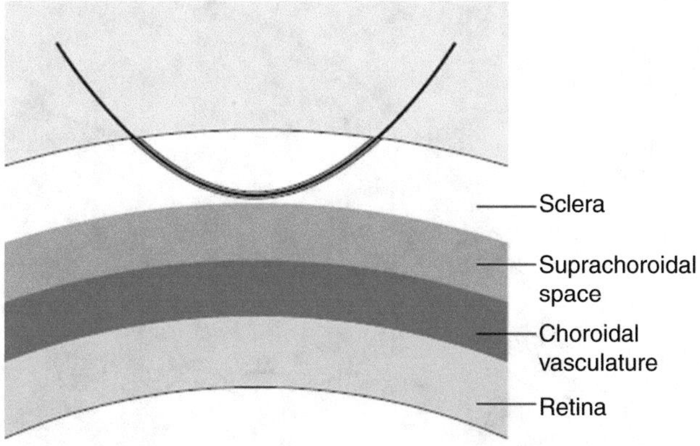

Fig. 8.70 The scleral suture should go deep through the sclera without penetrating it

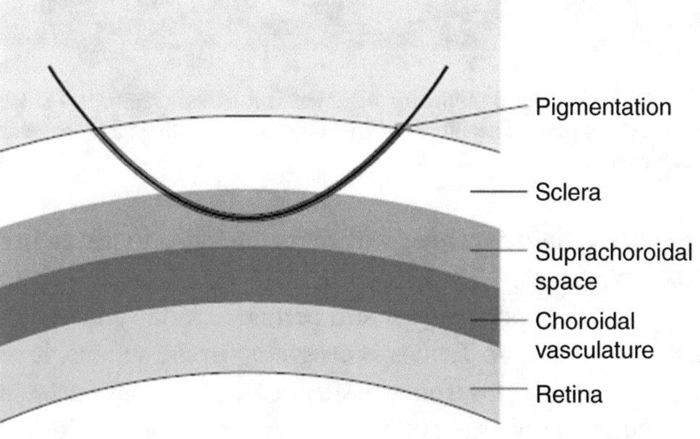

Fig. 8.71 Penetration into the suprachoroidal space is often evidenced by the presence of some pigmentation in the suture track

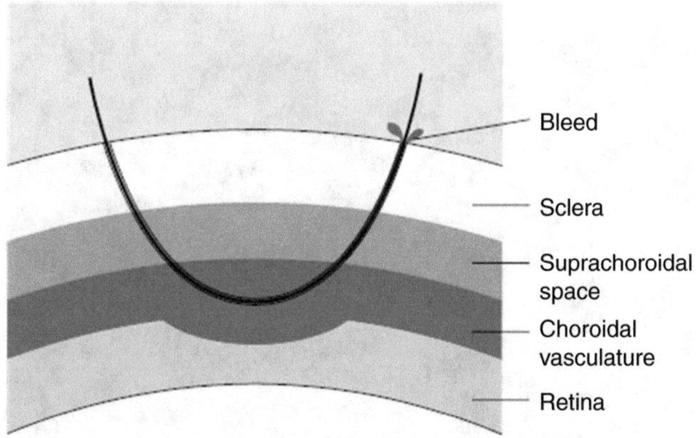

Fig. 8.72 Penetration into the choroid can cause a bleed subretinally or into the choroid. This may be indicated by the presence of bleed at the far end of the needle track

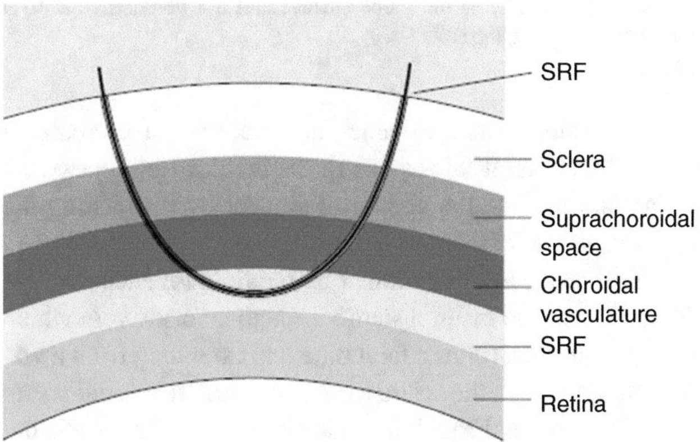

Fig. 8.73 If the stitch is too deep, subretinal fluid can leak through the suture track causing hypotony of the eye

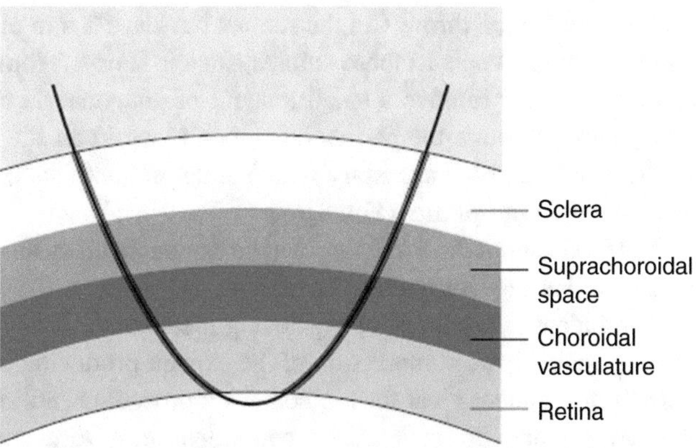

Fig. 8.74 It is possible to produce a retinal perforation if the patient has flat retina at the site of the insertion of a sclera suture

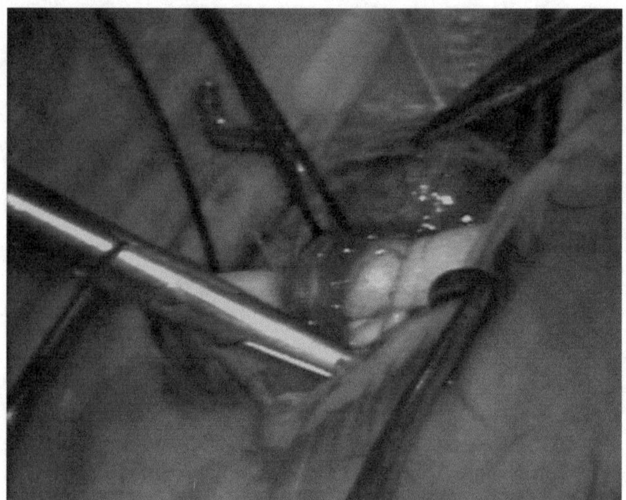

Fig. 8.75 When applying tension to the sutures be careful to apply pressure tangentially to the globe surface and not perpendicular to it which risks tearing the sclera

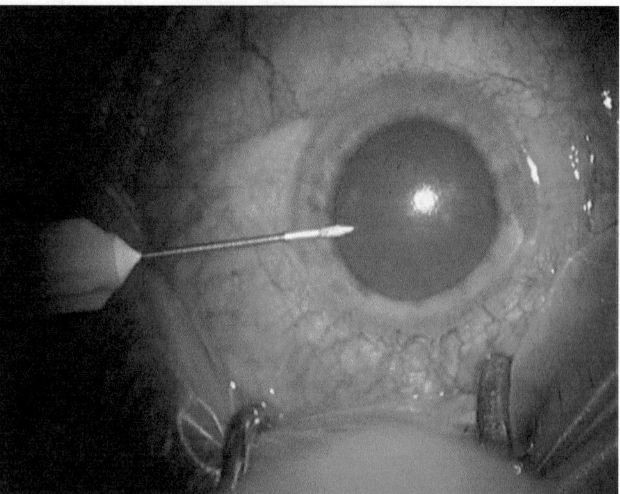

Fig. 8.76 It can be useful to release some aqueous after the first stitch is applied to a plomb in a non-drain procedure to prevent an IOP rise from compromising the blood supply to the optic nerve head. Insert a 30-gauge needle attached to a 1 ml syringe with the plunger removed. The aqueous will exit slowly through the needle and the quantity of aqueous can be monitored as it enters the syringe. Usually removal of 0.1 mls is adequate to maintain a normal IOP

If the retina has been penetrated, i.e. you have created a retinal break, treat this as one of the breaks. Retinopexy the retina and include the site on the indent by readjusting the explant (Fig. 8.75).

Usually two or three sutures are required for each explant. Be careful not to insert a suture through a vortex vein which may pass unseen (or as a faint blue line extending from a visible vein) through the sclera for a 1 or 2 mm. It is usually safe to insert a suture through the insertion of a rectus muscle but make sure to bite into some sclera to avoid tearing the suture out. If this happens, take another bite further away from the edge of the explant.

Insert the explant and tie the first suture with 3 throws then 1 throw and 1 throw. Cut the sutures but leave 2 mm of length from the knots as these sutures can slip. For a 5 mm sponge or larger remove a small amount of aqueous via a paracentesis through the peripheral cornea to avoid an IOP rise (this is usually unnecessary with 3 and 4 mm explants). Tie the remaining sutures (Fig. 8.76).

Note: Never put the stitch through the explant itself as this will make subsequent removal hazardous.

The indent is produced by tightening the sutures. A silicone sponge allows compression of the explant producing a narrow high indent ideal for the non-drain procedure. Solid silicone explants produce a flat broad indent (easy to place under the retinal break) but in my experience too often requiring postoperative gas injection because of lack of resolution of SRF. Check that the breaks are on the apex of the indent. If the breaks are not correctly placed on the indent, reposition the sutures. Move all bites to achieve the appropriate repositioning. Usually you will have to move them further than anticipated at first. The breaks need not be flat on the indent. If the break is close to the surface of the indent, the altered fluid dynamics will cause the retina to flatten in a few hours (Figs. 8.77, 8.78, 8.79, and 8.80).

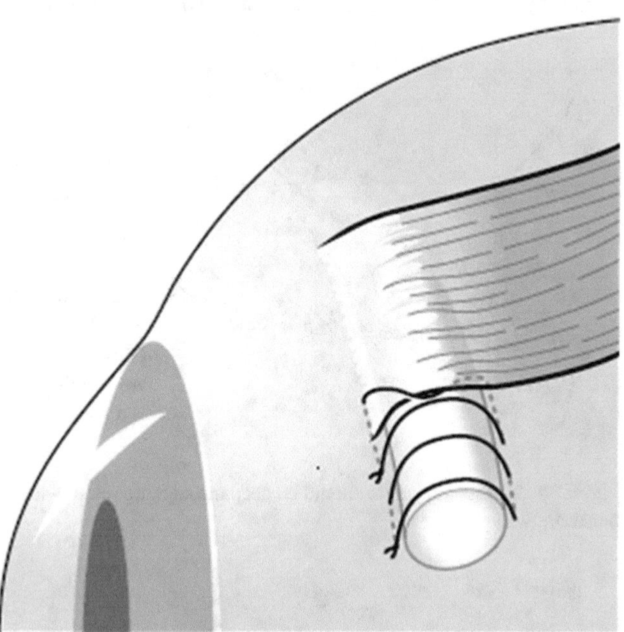

Fig. 8.77 Placing a plombage underneath a muscle requires a stitch which can be passed around the edge of the muscle without any sequelae such as diplopia

Check the optic nerve is still perfused. At the end of surgery make sure no Tenons is caught up in the sutures, if so clear out the Tenons from any site. I suspect Tenons adherent to sutures in this way provides a focal point for scar formation that increases the risk of postoperative diplopia. To aid

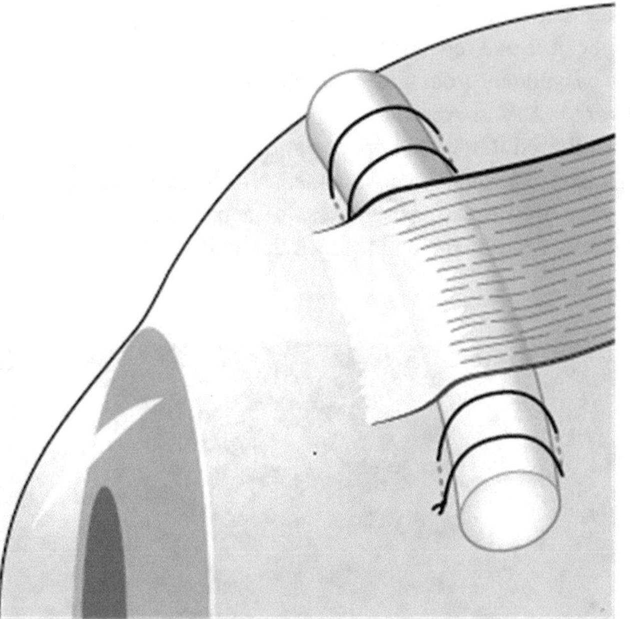

Fig. 8.78 If the plomb passes completely under the muscle to the other side of the muscle, stitches should be placed on either side of the muscle, avoiding suturing through the thin sclera underneath the muscle

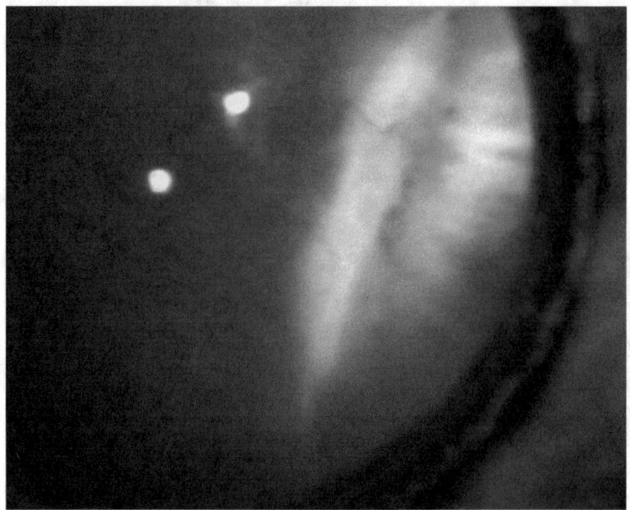

Fig. 8.79 The break should be seen situated over the apex of the indent but does not need to be flat on the plomb at the end of the operation

in the correct apposition of the conjunctiva grasp the horizontal recti insertions with non-toothed forceps and gently push the globe back into the orbit. This causes the conjunctival and Tenon's layers to return to their correct position around the limbus. It is now easy to see where the radial cuts in the conjunctiva are for suturing. Close the conjunctiva with an absorbable 7/0 suture at each of the radial incisions. Insert the suture through the Tenons then conjunctiva on the one side and then the conjunctiva and the Tenons on the other side of the wound with one suture. Bury the knot under the Tenons. Apply subconjunctival antibiotics.

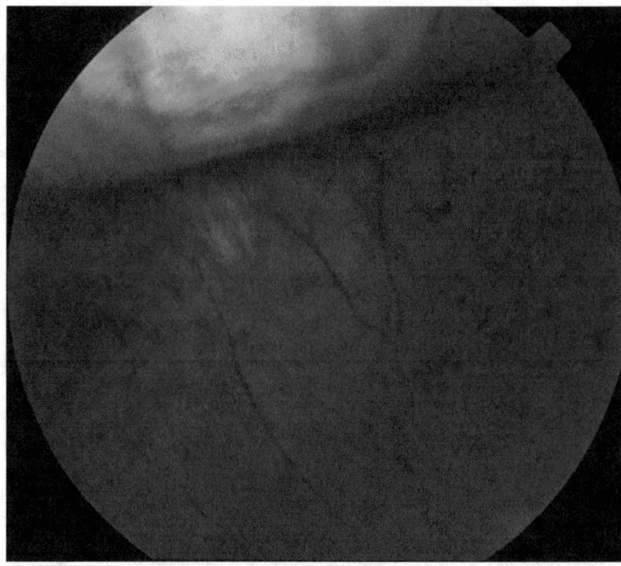

Fig. 8.80 An internal indent is seen with a cryotherapy scar

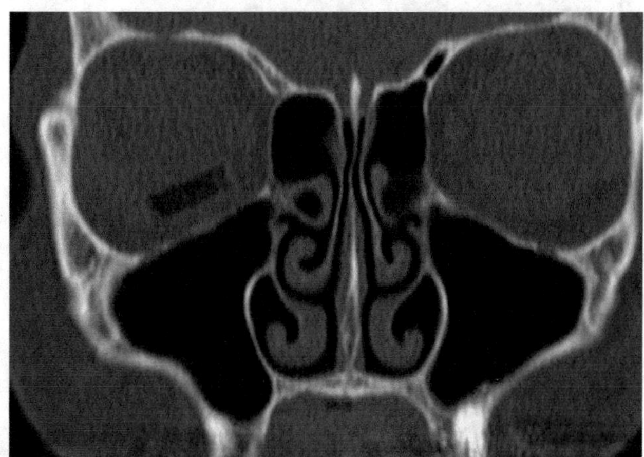

Fig. 8.81 An explant showing on MRI scan

Postoperative Care

The next day postoperatively much of the subretinal fluid will have reabsorbed and in fact the retina is usually flat. A topical steroid, antibiotic and cycloplegic should be used for 1 month. This procedure has a low morbidity depending on the experience of the surgeon (Figs. 8.81, 8.82, and 8.83).

Complications

Peroperative

Explant

Sutures tear out. Replace with a scleral bite further away from the explant avoid by making sure that the stitches are deep and long and taking care when compressing the explant during tightening of the suture. Do not attempt plombage in high myopes with thin sclera perform PPV instead (Figs. 8.83, 8.84, and 8.85).

Deep stitch, remove and check the retina.

Scleral tear [34] can happen rarely when clearing scar tissue from the sclera in a redo operation especially from under the extraocular muscles, it is important to recognise the complication and repair the sclera.

Hypotony from a deep stitch and drainage of SRF insert air see DACE procedure.

Raised IOP causing poor optic nerve blood flow. Perform a paracentesis to remove aqueous or massage the eye with your fingertip to cause egress of aqueous through the trabecular meshwork and recheck the optic nerve.

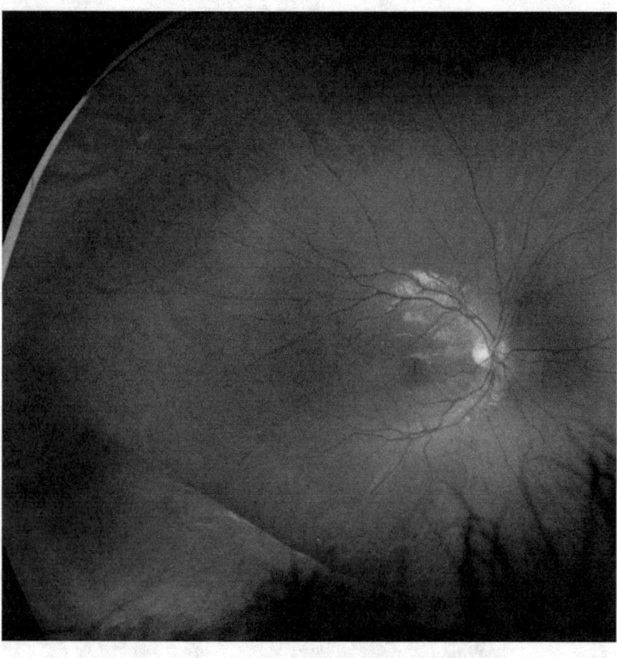

Fig. 8.82 An inferior indentation to treat RRD

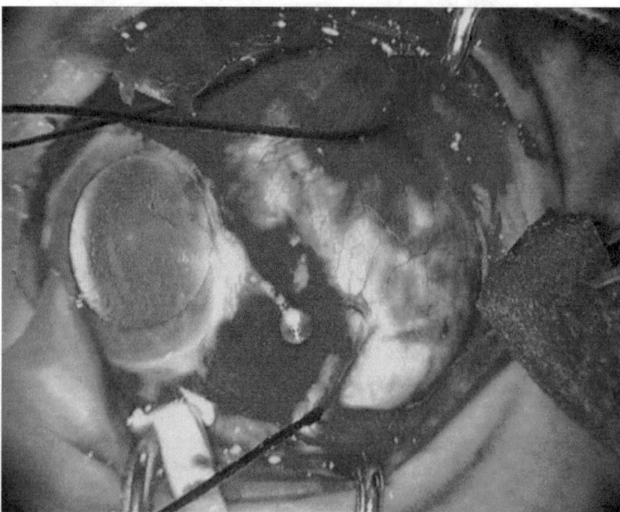

Fig. 8.84 In highly myopic patients, thin sclera may be evident underneath the muscles and elsewhere, as thin blue striae in the sclera. This is a contra-indication to external buckle

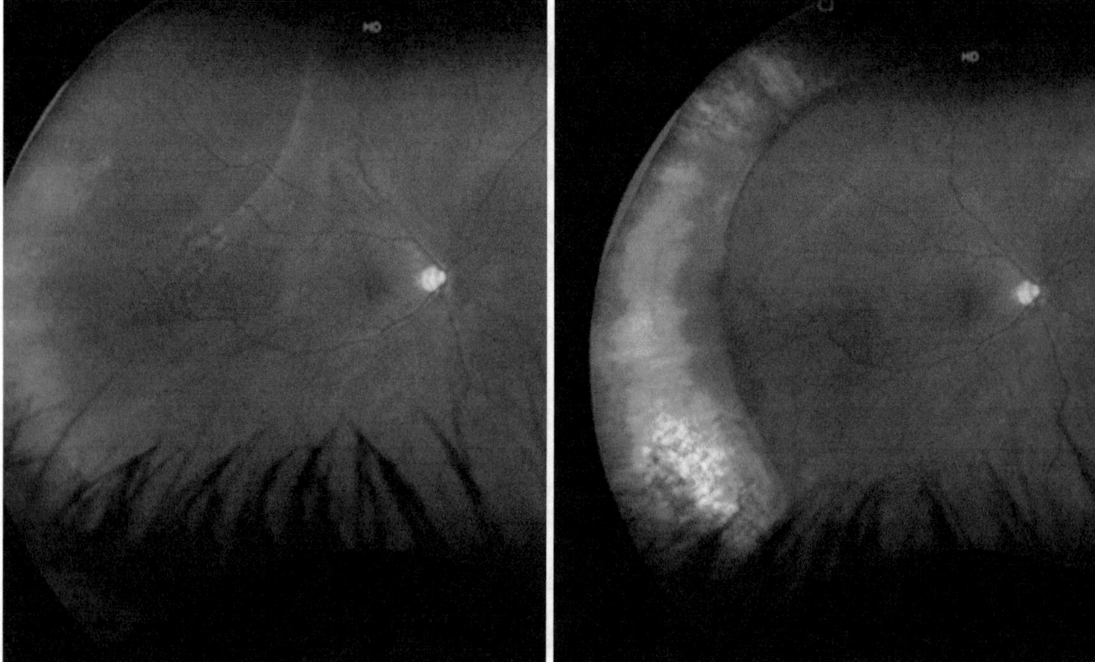

Fig. 8.83 Treatment of RRD by non-drain explant procedure

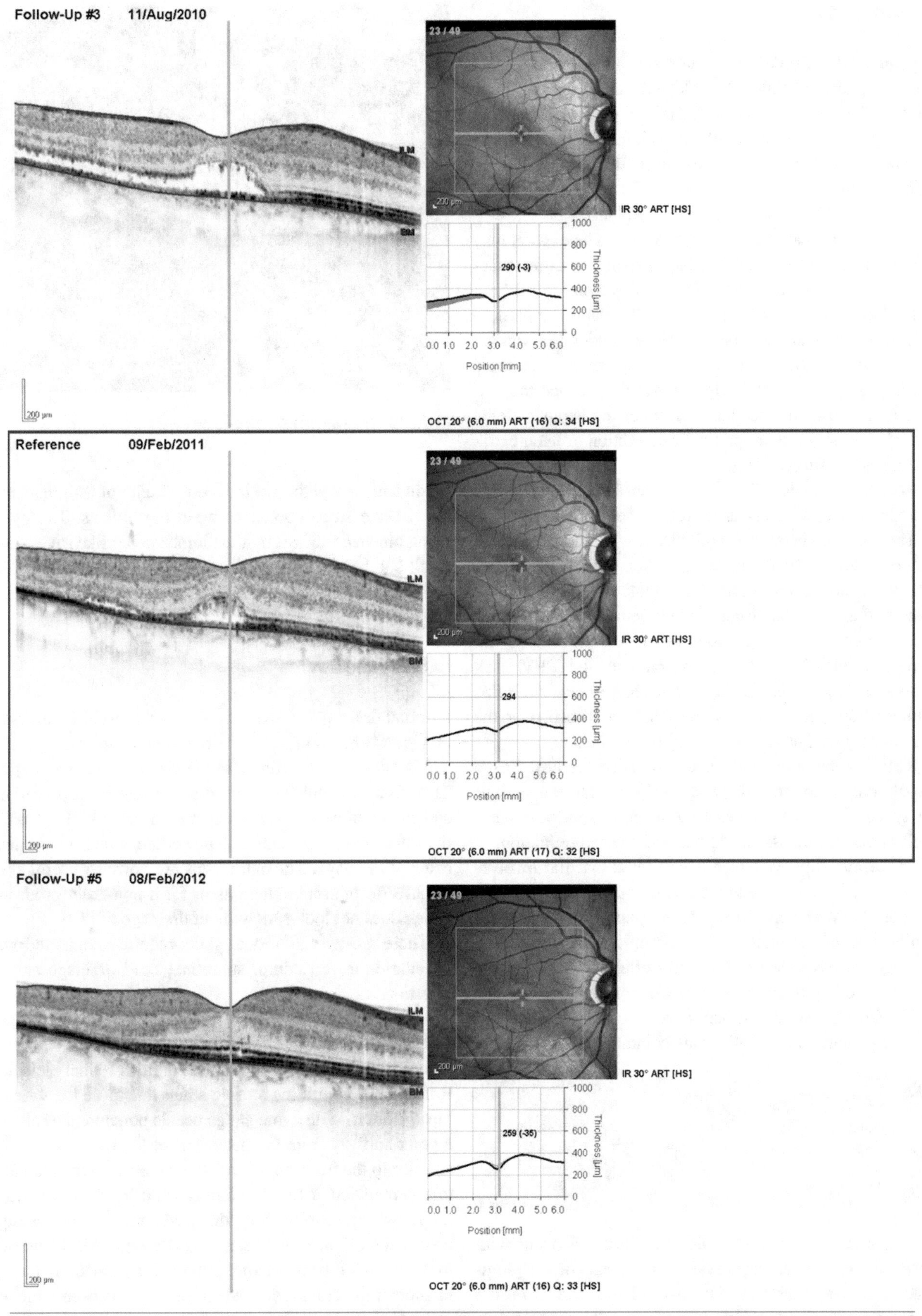

Fig. 8.85 Slow SRF resolution after a non-drain repair often taking 9-12 months

Postoperative

Explant erosion through the conjunctiva, remove the explant in the outpatient setting if the hole in the conjunctiva is large enough. The eye will not heal until the explant is removed.

Explant infection early. Infections immediately after surgery are often seen as a localised scleritis should be treated with systemic antibiotics and will usually settle.

Explant infection late, remove the explant.

Cosmetic problems remove the explant. The explant may be visible if anteriorly placed or large, in some circumstances this is cosmetically unacceptable for the patient.

Diplopia removes the explant early. Explants are particularly likely to cause diplopia if placed under the vertical recti. Scar formation around the explant can be very rapid and is soon established. Early removal will reduce the scar formation and reduce the bulk effects of the explant. Some patients will still require prismatic correction or even extraocular muscle surgery.

Raised IOP is usually due to a steroid response to the postoperative drops and can be treated medically.

The macula vision can be reduced by persistent SRF in the postoperative period under the fovea. This is very common when non-drain is used for macula off chronic round hole or dialysis related detachment [35–37]. The viscous SRF becomes loculated under the fovea preventing full recovery of visual acuity. No convincing method (PPV, laser, intravitreal injections) has been described to deal with this complication. The SRF may eventually reabsorb over the course of a year but visual recovery is variable.

RPE dispersion into the macula from cryotherapy. Heavy use of cryotherapy may disperse RPE cells into the subretinal space which may settle in the macular area postoperatively. This may be associated with mild visual reduction.

Distortion. Any eye which has suffered macular involvement may have a change in the image seen by the patient in the postoperative period [38]. Many patients experience a minification of the image and some mild distortion. Often these symptoms lessen at 6 months after surgery however they may be accompanied with a reduction in stereopsis.

HD-OCT allows assessment of the recovery in the fovea in these patients, abnormalities are common [39]:

Foveal changes	62%
Disruption of the inner/outer segment line	43%
Later restored in	50%
Disruption of the external limiting membrane	39%
ERM	23%
CMO	4%

Astigmatism is rare after plombage but can occur with steepening of the corneal curvature in the axis of the plombage. This case illustrates the effect of the indents on the cornea where inferotemporal and superonasal circumferential indents in a right eye induced −3.25D of astigmatism at 145°, i.e. a steep cornea between the indents. The eye is being pinched inwards by the plombs rather like squeezing a small ball between two fingers (Figs. 8.86, 8.87, 8.88, 8.89, and 8.90).

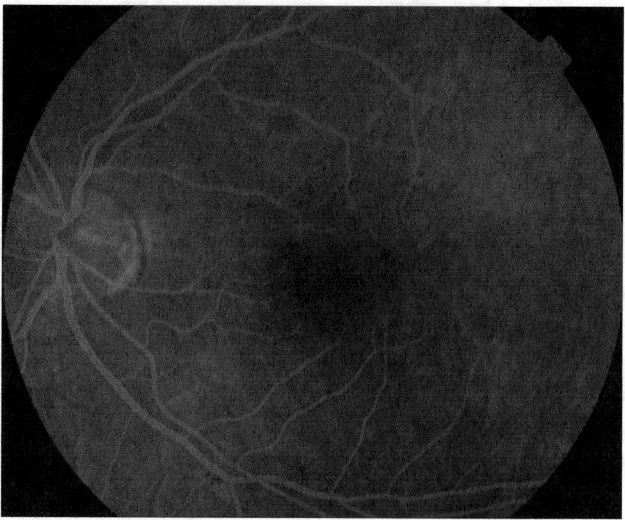

Fig. 8.86 Trapped SRF is not seen on FFA

Extra Manoeuvres

External drainage of SRF has a risk of choroidal, subretinal or vitreous haemorrhage which varies between 3 and 10% and but can be catastrophic to the vision of the patient [40]. Therefore, it is not favoured in all conventional procedures and many surgeons, including me, proceed to PPV rather than perform a conventional procedure which might need external drainage. The extra steps are however useful skills to have for unusual situations or for a non-drain procedure which does not look safe without drainage of SRF.

There are two additional skills required compared with the non-drain procedure, subretinal fluid drainage and air insertion.

Subretinal Fluid (SRF) Drainage

Select a quadrant where there is a bullous retinal elevation. Rotate the eye with the muscle slings to expose the sclera in this quadrant. With a fine gauge needle puncture the sclera at a point halfway from the insertions of the recti muscles but anterior to the insertion of the vortex veins. Make the puncture perpendicular to the sclera (a bend in the needle tip of 2 mm will prevent inserting the needle too far); any oblique hole will close too easily stopping drainage. Allow the SRF to drain out whilst maintaining the IOP by indenting the eye in another quadrant. Once adequate SRF has been removed, insert air into the vitreous cavity.

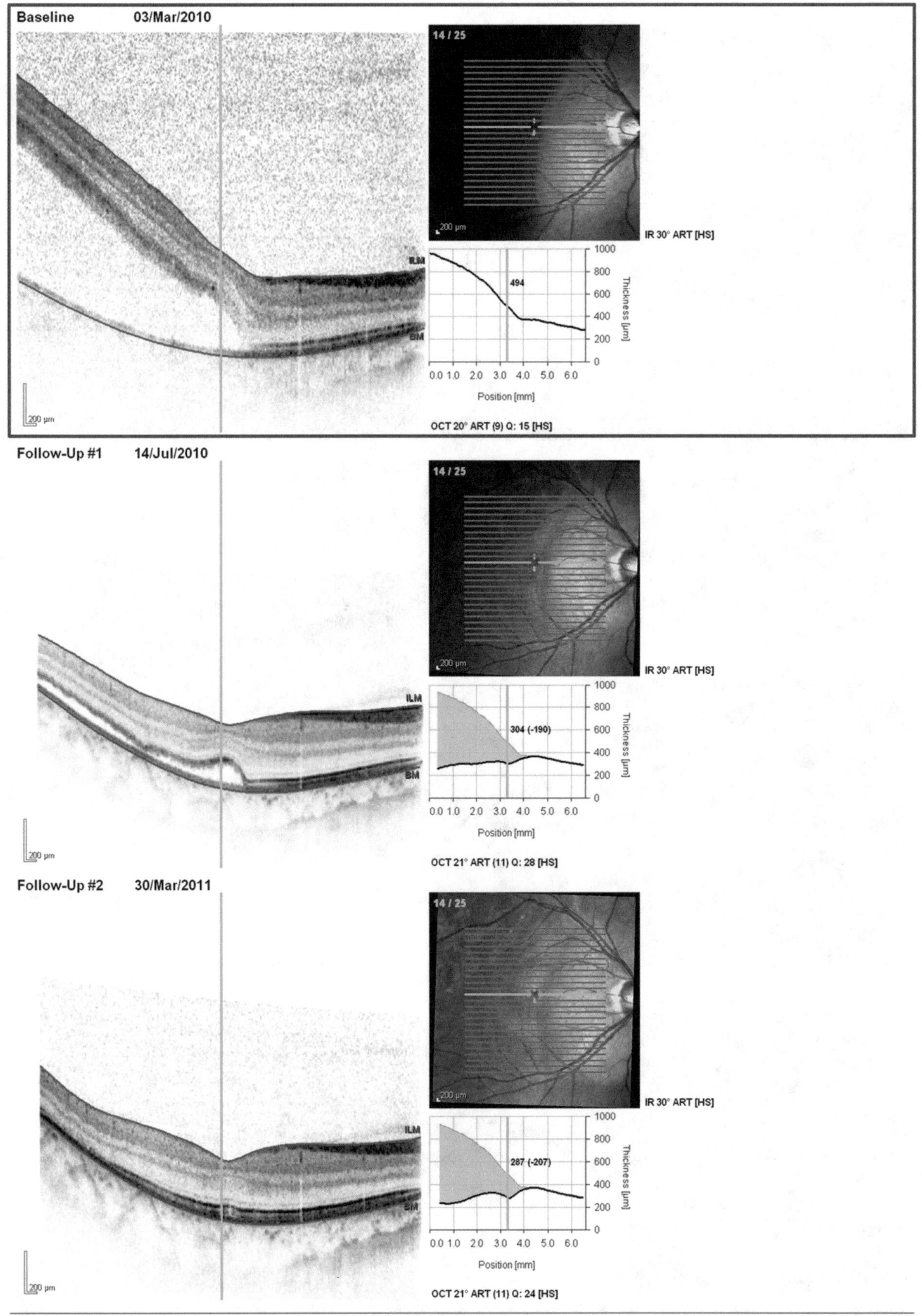

Fig. 8.87 A sequence of OCTs showing the preoperative macula with fovea detached, fovea at 4 months and finally attached at 12 months

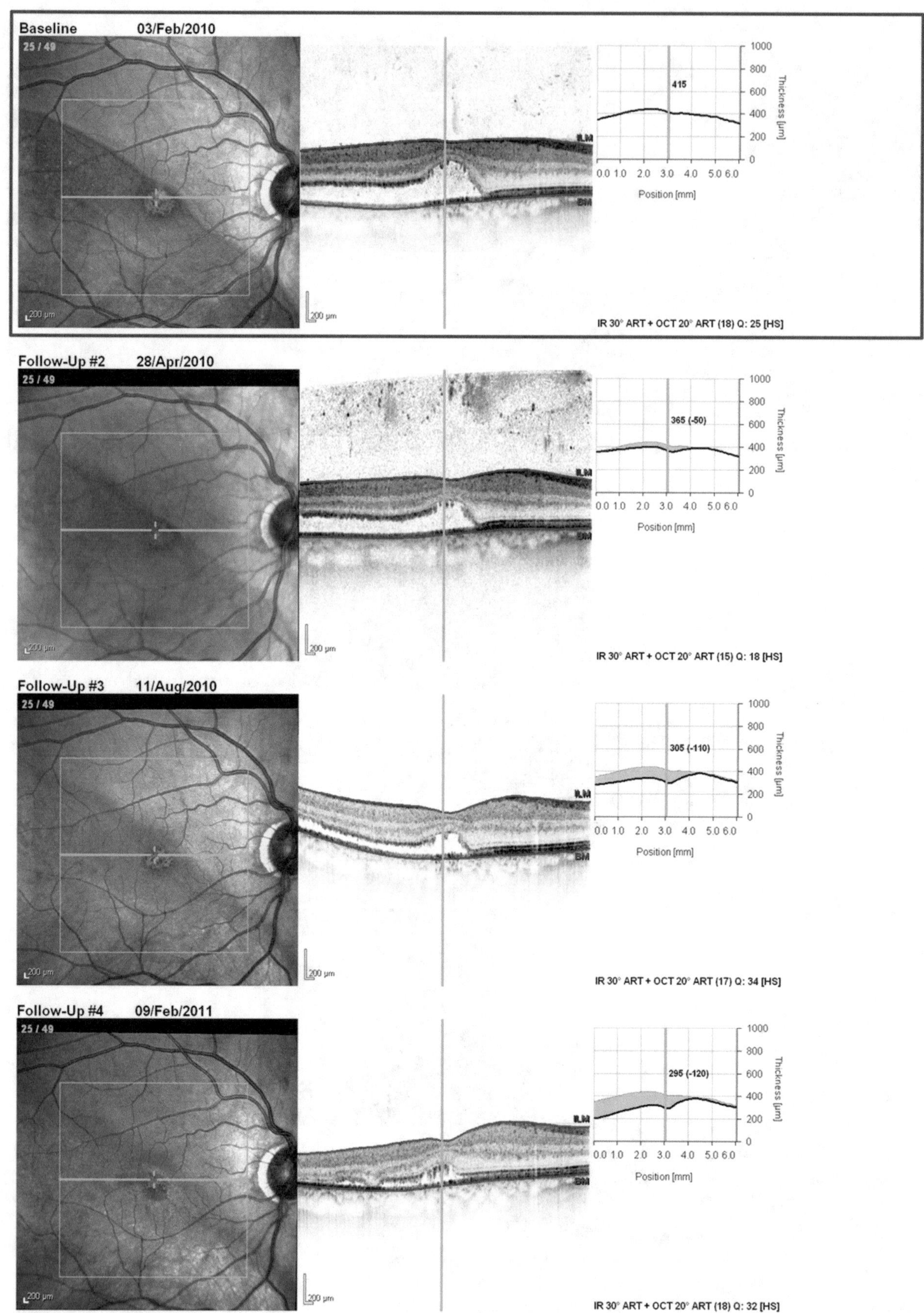

Fig. 8.88 A sequence of OCTs show gradual reduction of persistent SRF under the fovea in patient with atrophic round hole retinal detachment treated with non-drain surgery

Air Insertion (Figs. 8.91, 8.92, 8.93, 8.94, 8.95, and 8.96)

Use a fine gauge needle attached to the air insertion pump of the vitrectomy machine with the pressure set at 70 mmHg. Insert through the pars plana (3.5 to 4 mm from the limbus) rotate the eye to make this insertion at the highest point of the globe. Check that the needle is in the vitreous cavity and perpendicular to the sclera. Take the pressure off the indenting hand (do this quickly but smoothly). Insert the gas at the highest point and quickly. Both actions help to achieve a single

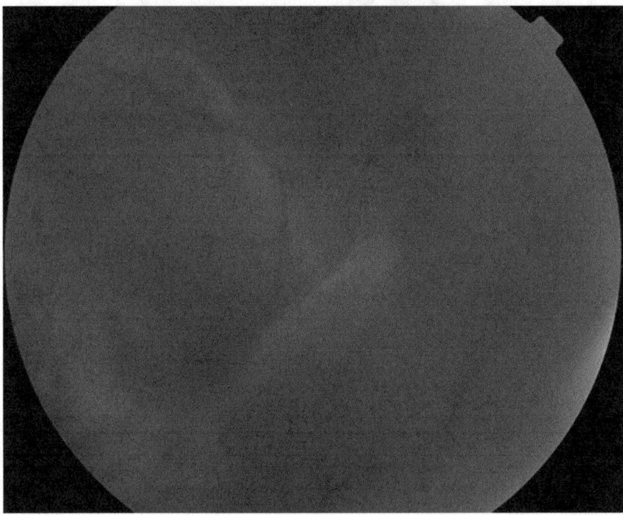

Fig. 8.89 Creating a large indent with an external plombage reduces the internal diameter of the eye wall. This leads to redundancy of the retina, the internal circumference of the eye wall is too small to allow the retina to reattach, and fold in the retina is produced as in this patient in whom a large indent has been applied. The retina will flatten if there is no retinal break in the fold

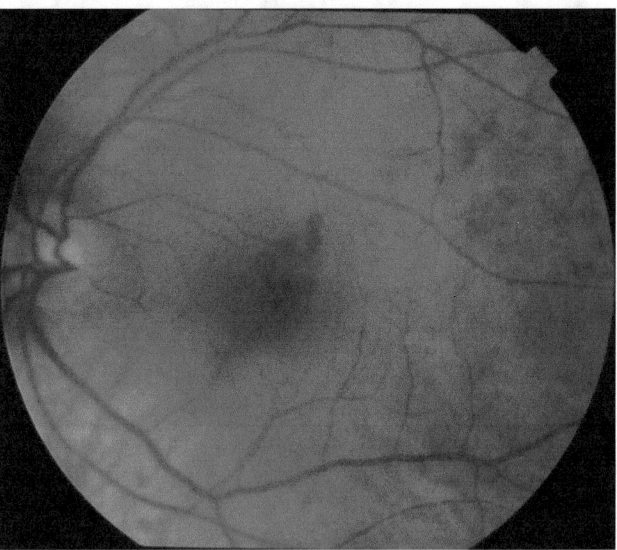

Fig. 8.91 RP cells have been dispersed by heavy use of cryotherapy in this non-drain retinal detachment. These have settled under the fovea and restricted visual recover: there is masking defect on fluorescein angiography

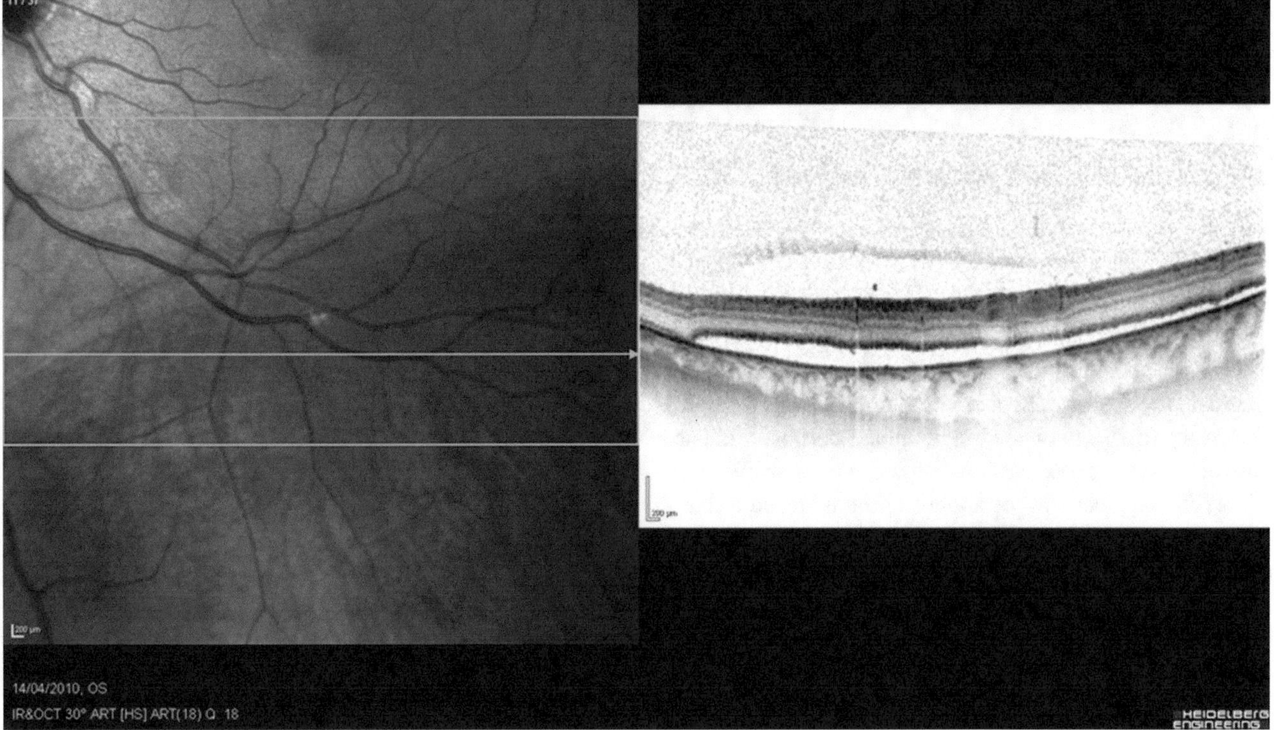

Fig. 8.90 SRF can be trapped peripherally despite reattachment of the retina after non-drain surgery

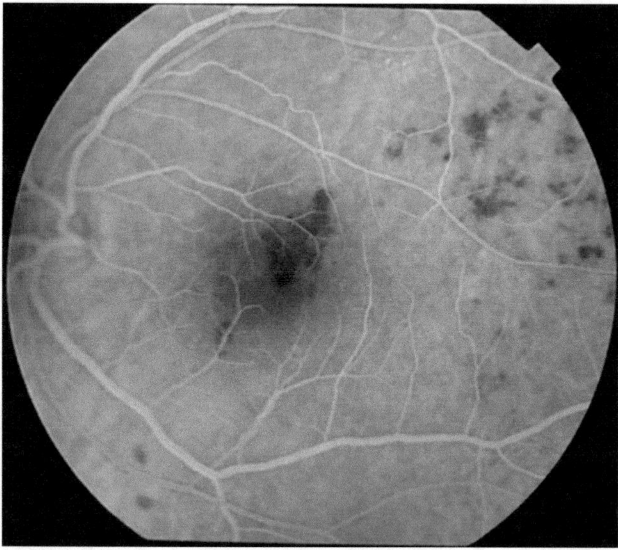

Fig. 8.92 On FFA the RPE cells mask underlying choroidal perfusion

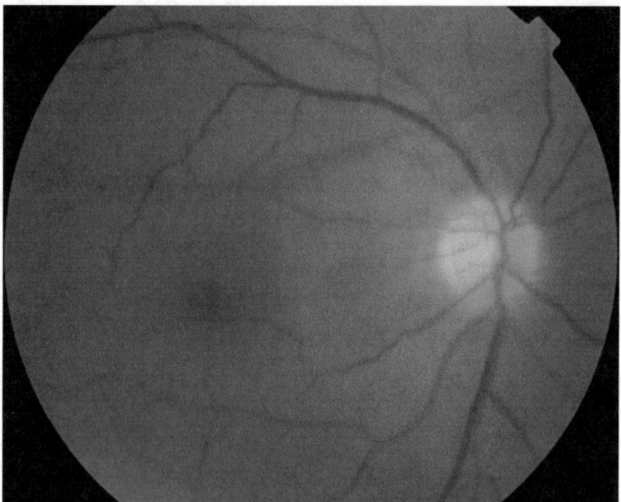

Fig. 8.93 In this postoperative image pigment can be seen which has settled at the leading edge of the flattened retinal detachment

bubble in the eye allowing a good view for the cryotherapy and the placement of the explant. The air is only inserted to re-inflate the eye, any effect on the tamponade of the break is secondary (fluid is not used to re-inflate because fluid will pass through the break causing re-accumulation of SRF).

Cryotherapy can now be applied to the flattened retina. A solid silicone explant is used because there is a gas filled eye (and therefore a compressible vitreous cavity). The solid explant produces less pressure on the sclera and avoids too high and indent.

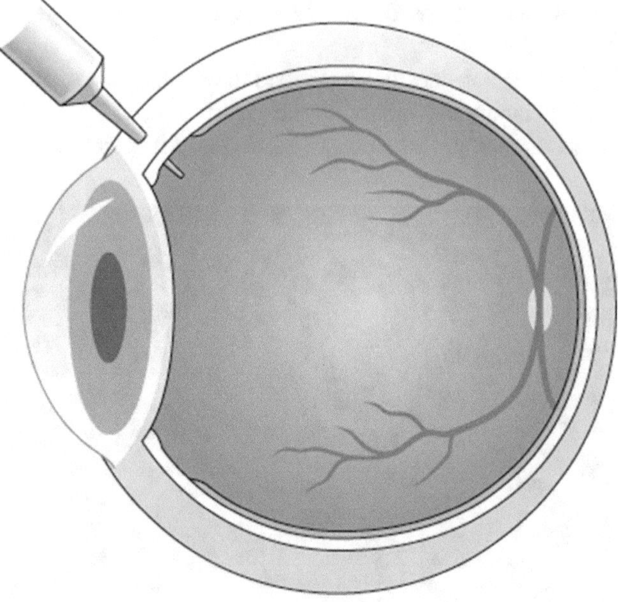

Fig. 8.94 When inserting air, inject into the pars plana

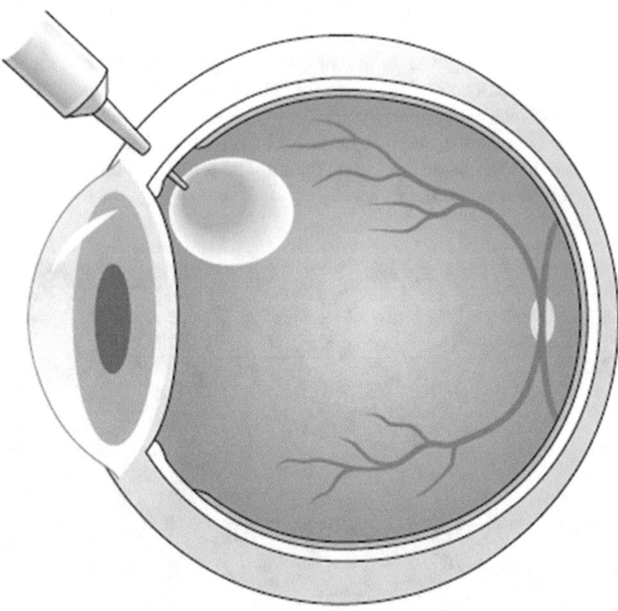

Fig. 8.95 Inject at the highest point

Complications

Drainage

Retinal incarceration, this is rare if the drainage incision is small, e.g. from a fine needle tip, includes the incarceration site on the indent if there is a large incarceration if you can.

Choroidal or subretinal haemorrhage raises the IOP with pressure from your instruments on the globe until the bleeding stops. Consider converting to PPV to remove any sub-macular blood. This is an advanced step and should only be performed if you are confident of your skills at inserting a flute needle through a retinal break and towards the subretinal space. Beware if you perform a PPV in eyes with vitreous attached you will need to detach the vitreous and run a risk of producing retinal tears. Performing a PPV in a patient with dialysis brings you awfully close to the back of the lens to access the break risking damage to the lens. It is however possible to access the macular subretinal space from a peripheral dialysis using a flute needle (Fig. 8.97).

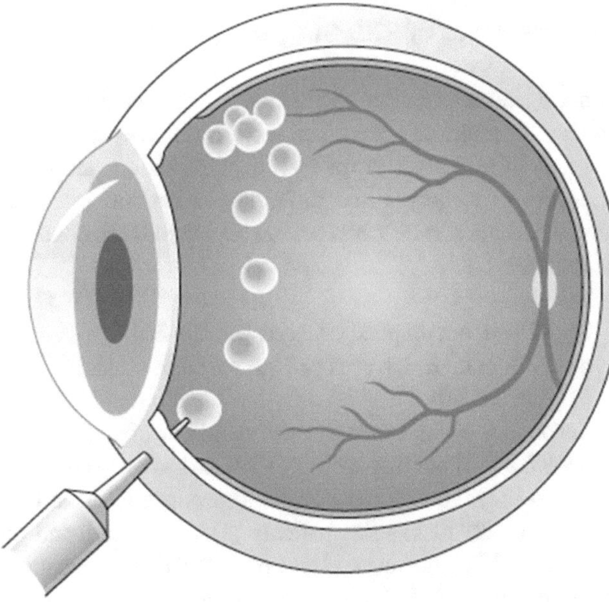

Fig. 8.96 Injecting inferiorly allows separation of the air into separate bubbles

Fluid vitreous loss, close the sclerotomy, inject air into the vitreous cavity.

Retinal tear, include on the indent.

Hypotony, inject air into the vitreous cavity.

Air Injection

Injury to lens, leave for later cataract extraction.

Air in the wrong place

- Anterior chamber, remove if the procedure is not completed, otherwise leave to dissipate postoperatively.
- Anterior to the vitreous producing a doughnut air injection, leave in place.
- Subretinal or suprachoroidal air, exceedingly rare, you may need to convert to a PPV to remove.

Fish egging of the air (multiple separate bubbles of gas), proceed with surgery but with reduce visualisation.

Raised intraocular pressure, perform anterior chamber paracentesis to remove some aqueous.

Pneumatic Retinopexy (Table 8.4)

Successful reattachment of the retina can be achieved by injection of gas and retinopexy without PPV [41] especially with single superior breaks in the presence of a posterior vitreous detachment. However the success rates are lower than other methods approximately 65% reattachment with one

Table 8.4 Difficulty rating of pneumatic retinopexy

Difficulty Rating	Low
Success rates	Moderate
Complication rates	Low
When to use in training	Early

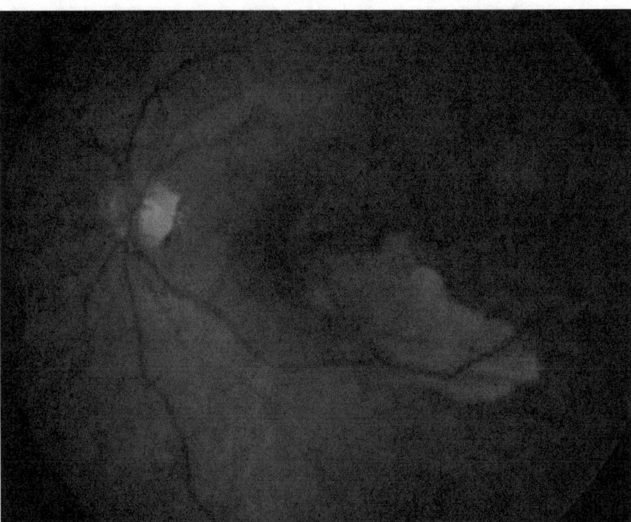

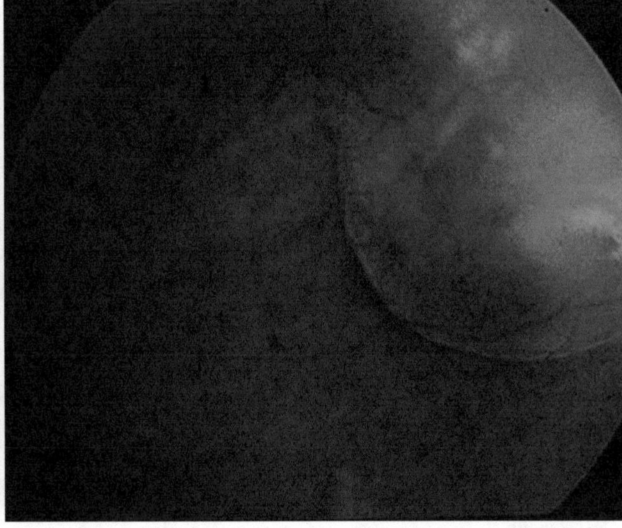

Fig. 8.97 A large buckle placed peripherally has been associated with the formation of a subretinal haemorrhage which is tracked down to the macula. This has severely restricted the visual recovery in this patient

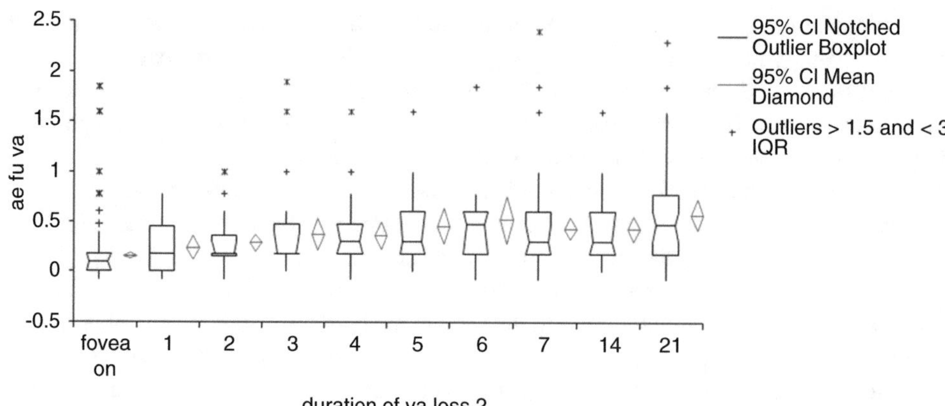

Fig. 8.98 There is small reduction in visual recovery from fovea on RRD to fovea off RRD approximately 6/6 to 6/7.5. Patients with 1-3 days of visual loss do very well. There is a slight drop after 3 days and progressive drop in visual recovery thereafter

procedure [42, 43] and there is the risk of inducing new inferior retinal breaks [44]. Even in the best hands and with selection of easy cases (1-2 breaks) the success rate is 80% [45] probably 10% less than the expected success rate from PPV on the same cases. For these reasons I only use this in special circumstances such as a patient who is unfit to attend more extensive surgery. As an office procedure the method can show improved visual recovery over scleral buckling especially if strict criteria are applied to treat superior RRD with small retinal breaks and no PVR [46, 47]. The PIVOT trial has shown improved visual results with reduced risk of macular folds with pneumatic retinopexy versus PPV [48].

Surgical Steps

- Apply cryotherapy via scleral indentation with the cryotherapy probe to the break.
- Inject 100% SF6 0.5 ml via the pars plana with a 30G needle.
- Remove some aqueous via a paracentesis to equalise the IOP if required.

Apply head posturing by the patient in the first few days so that the gas bubble contacts the break or breaks and monitors the patient daily to ensure retinal reattachment and no IOP rises. Be careful that SRF is not pushed into the fovea in a macula on RRD. If this is a risk, start the patient off with face down posture gradually rotating to upright over a few hours to push SRF through the break before it is closed by the gas.

Complications

- New retinal break formation in the inferior retina causing redetachment.
- Missed or new retinal breaks are the commonest cause (75%) of redetachment.
- IOP rises.

Success Rates of RRD Surgery

Primary (flat retina after one operation) and secondary (flat retina after multiple operations) success rates depend on the case mix of patients, rates of PVR at presentation, and speed of access to surgery. Little difference in success rates has been seen between PPV and scleral buckle [49] (Fig. 8.98).

Primary

- 81–92% in uncomplicated cases [21, 50–56]
- 65–70% in high risk eyes or 75% when no break is found [21, 29, 57–60]
- Secondary or final success rates should be approximately 95–97% [61] but this drops in PVR and when no break is found [27]. You should be able to produce a visual outcome of 20/40 in most patients [21], 83% of fovea on patients [62], however visual outcome if the macula is detached is reduced to a 44% chance of 20/40 or better. Patients may describe metamorphopsia (change in image shape) after macula off retinal detachment and this may be accompanied by a reduction in stereo acuity [38]. There appears to be a very small difference in fovea on RRD and one day fovea off RRD [63]. Those with fovea off for less than 3 days do better and should be operated upon promptly to restore the anatomy and allow the receptors to recover.
- So far no difference in success rates has been found between buckling procedures and PPV [64–66] (Fig. 8.99).

In an analysis of Medicare insurance forms (looking at individual patients rather than eye)s pneumatic retinopexy was twice as likely to be followed by further surgery (40%) than PPV or scleral buckling (20%) despite PPV being used for more complex cases, but with PPV having twice the adverse complication rate (2%) [67] (Figs. 8.100, 8.101, 8.102, 8.103, 8.104, 8.105, 8.106, 8.107,and 8.108).

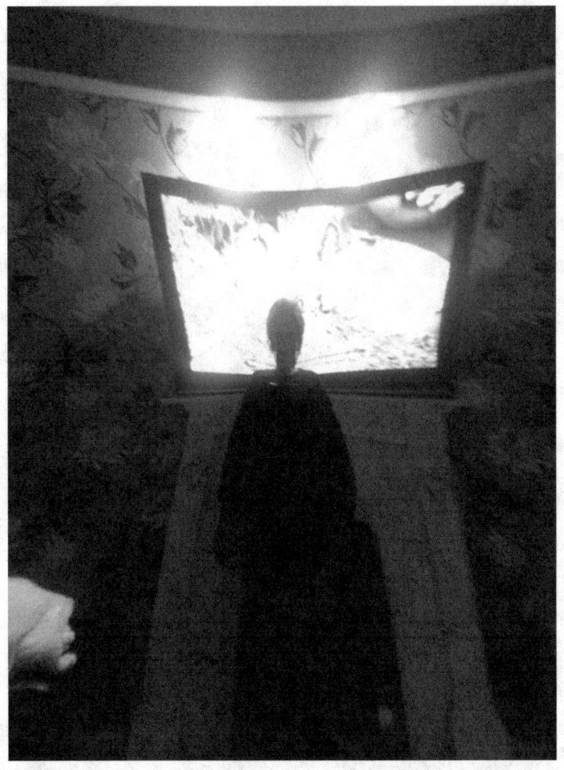

Fig. 8.99 A patient's representation of their central micropsia after retinal detachment. Presumably, the central receptors are more prone to being spread apart by the action the SRF on the fovea. Often patients will describe a small head on top of a body. Some retinal remodelling seems to occur, and the symptom resolves to some degree over 6–9 months

Causes of Failure

Surgical capability will affect the success rate of such technical operations. Missing and therefore failing to treat breaks or new breaks will lead to redetachment in half of failures. PVR is less predictable and controllable causing failure in the remainder [68]. In addition, severe complications of surgery must be added such as endophthalmitis and choroidal haemorrhage. Persistent thin areas of subretinal fluid have been described on OCT, occasionally affecting the macula and thereby reducing visual acuity in buckling procedures [35, 37]. Late macular breaks have been described in rare cases after scleral buckle [69]. Late redetachment over 1 year can occur in approximately 2% [70]. The cause is usually from new break formation although old breaks can reopen (Figs. 8.109, 8.110, and 8.111).

Surgery for Redetachment

Despite the surgeon's greatest efforts redetachment of the retina occurs at rates of 10–15%. The rate of redetachment is linked to the PVR rate at presentation with higher rates with more PVR.

Causes of redetachment are as follows:

- PVR, the surgery stimulates the PVR to progress overcoming the effects of internal tamponade and reopening retinal breaks causing RRD.

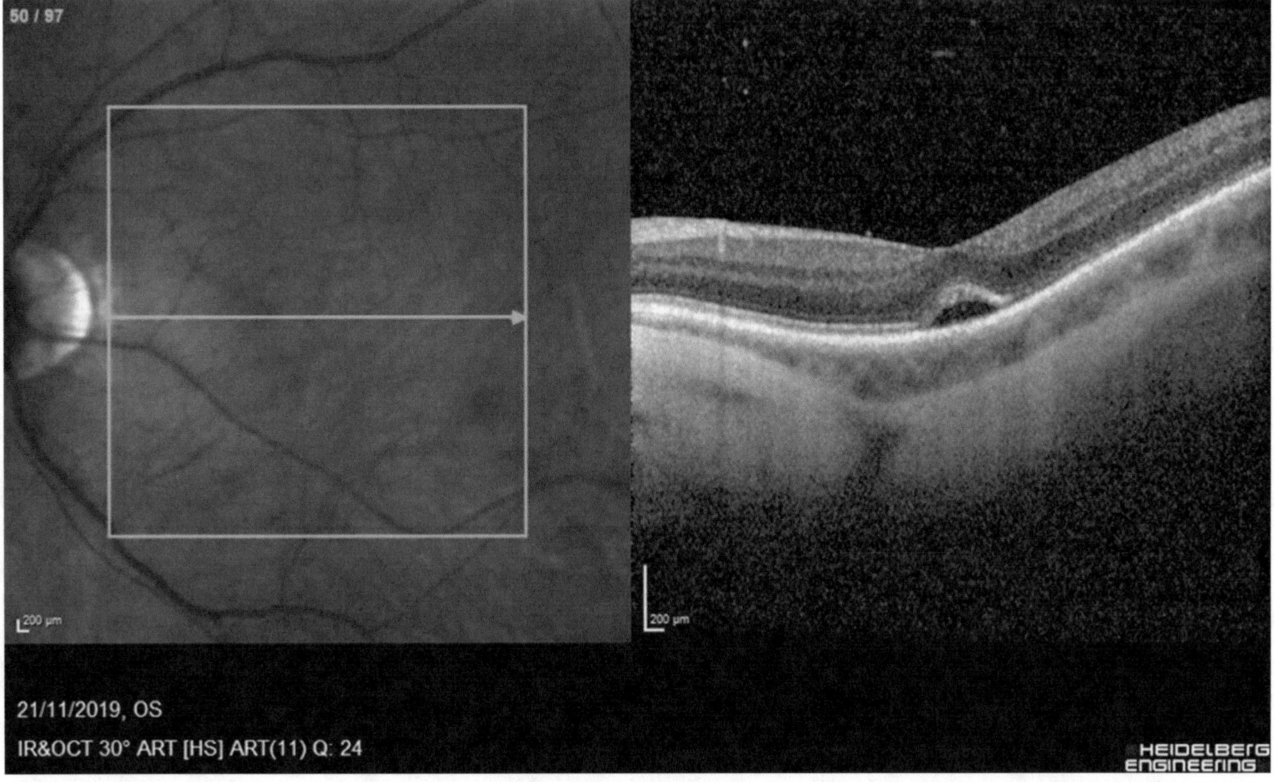

Fig. 8.100 SRF in the fovea postoperatively in a patient with macula on RRD preoperatively

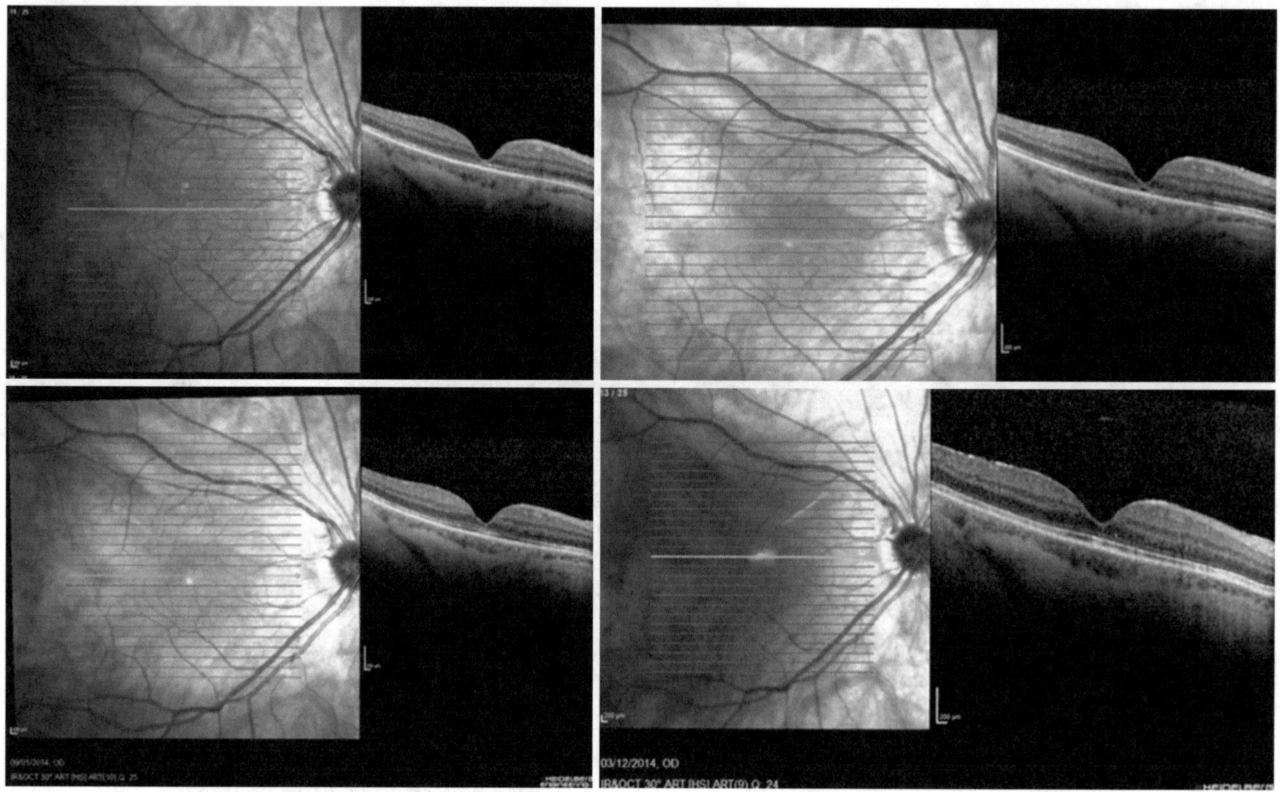

Fig. 8.101 The fovea in this eye was thin after RRD surgery with vision of 6/36/ gradually over time it thickened, and the vision was 6/11 finally

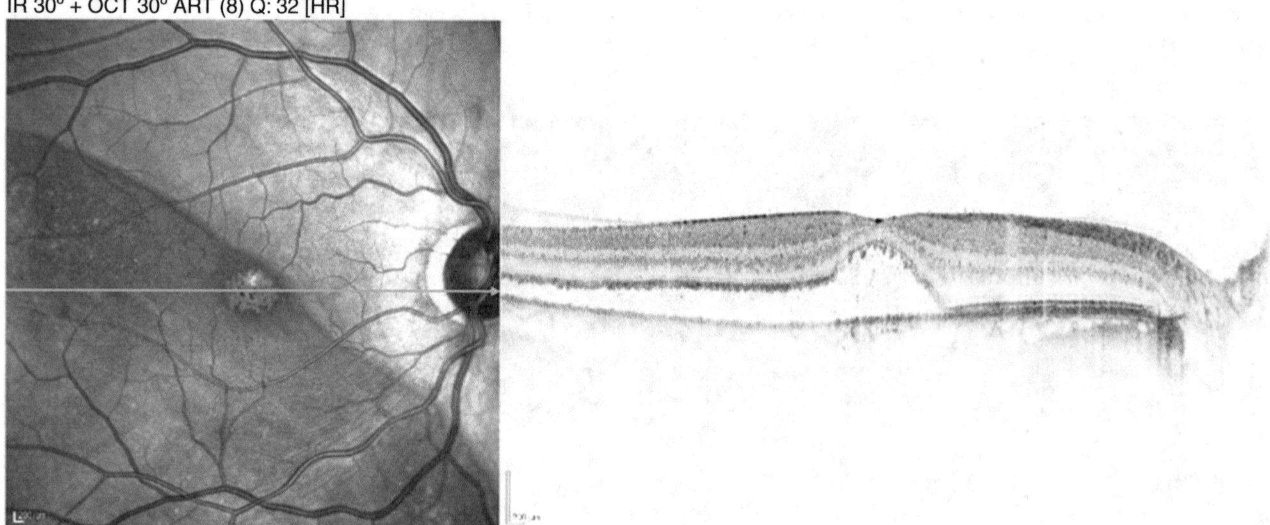

Fig. 8.102 SRF trapped in the fovea after non-drain surgery

  - Be aware of the presence of PVR at presentation, use longer acting gases or silicone oil, restrict the use of cryotherapy.
- Missed retinal breaks, tiny retinal breaks may be missed during the first surgery; usually these are easier to see at the second operation because slight contraction of the remaining vitreous base causes the breaks to open slightly.
- New retinal breaks, occasionally larger breaks appear that are unlikely to be missed from the first operation these may be produced from problems at the sclerotomies (entry site breaks) or secondary to PVR.
- PVR and missed/new breaks, often the two accompany each other and it is not possible to say with certainty which is the cause of the redetachment. However, if a

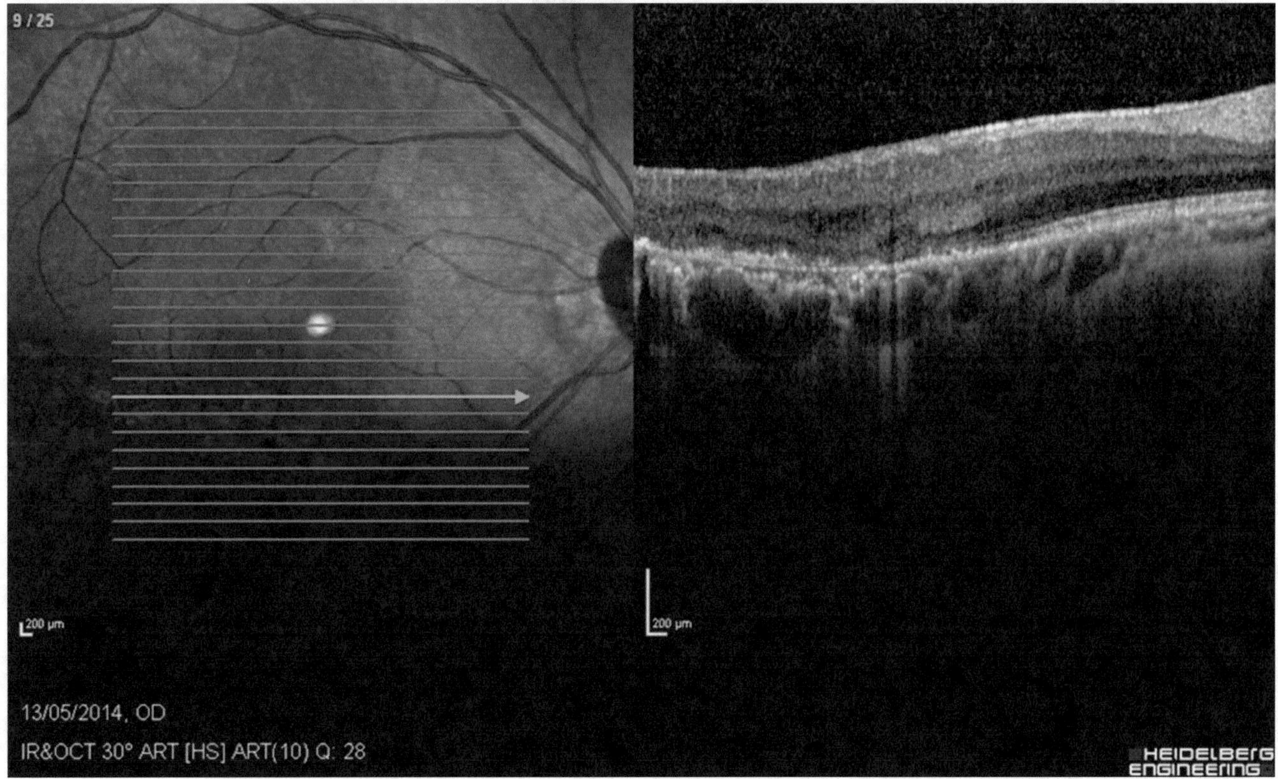

Fig. 8.103 This chronic retinal detachment has been reattached but there is evidence of damage in the retina with loss of the ellipsoid layer

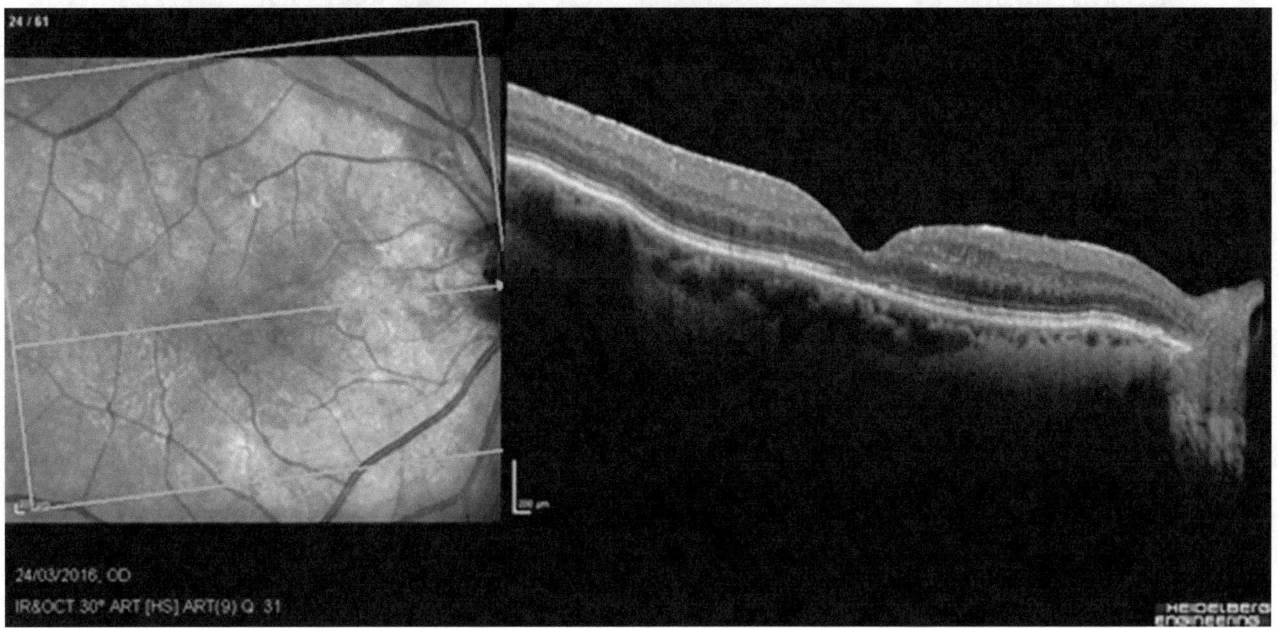

Fig. 8.104 Broken ellipsoid after RRD

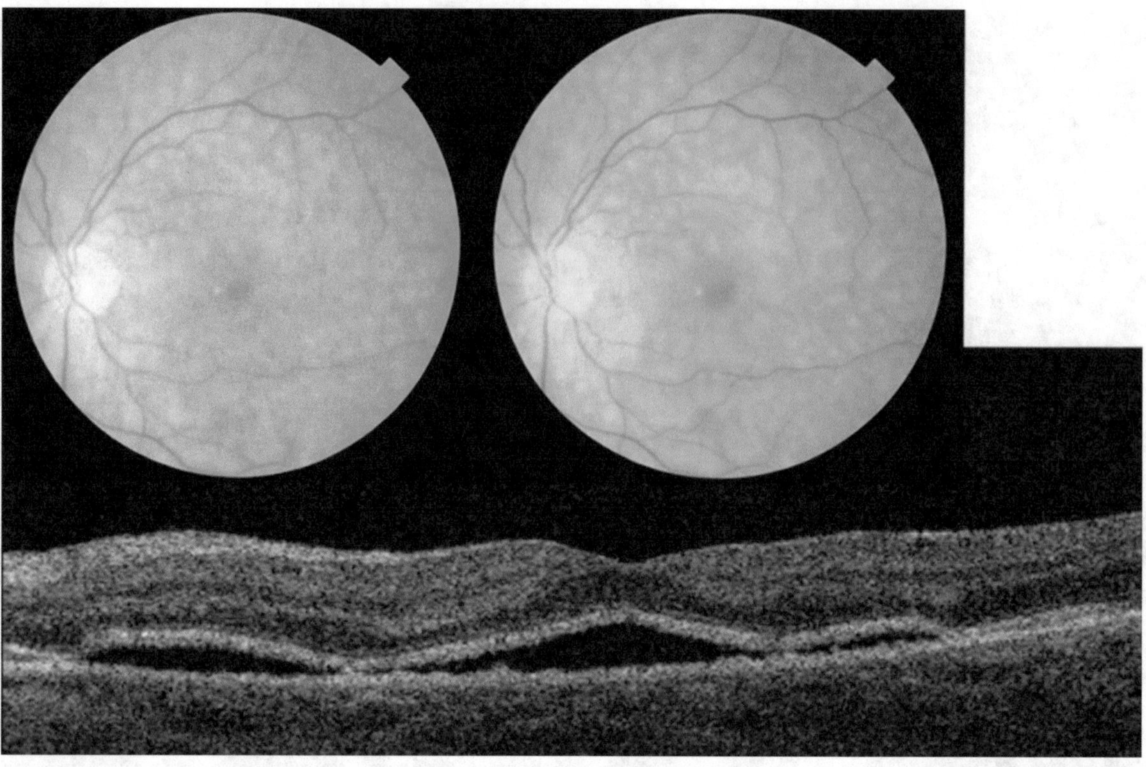

Fig. 8.105 An eye with multiple areas of persistent SRF after RRD surgery. These areas are presumed to have high viscosity fluid which the RPE has difficulty removing. The SRF will usually resolve over a year

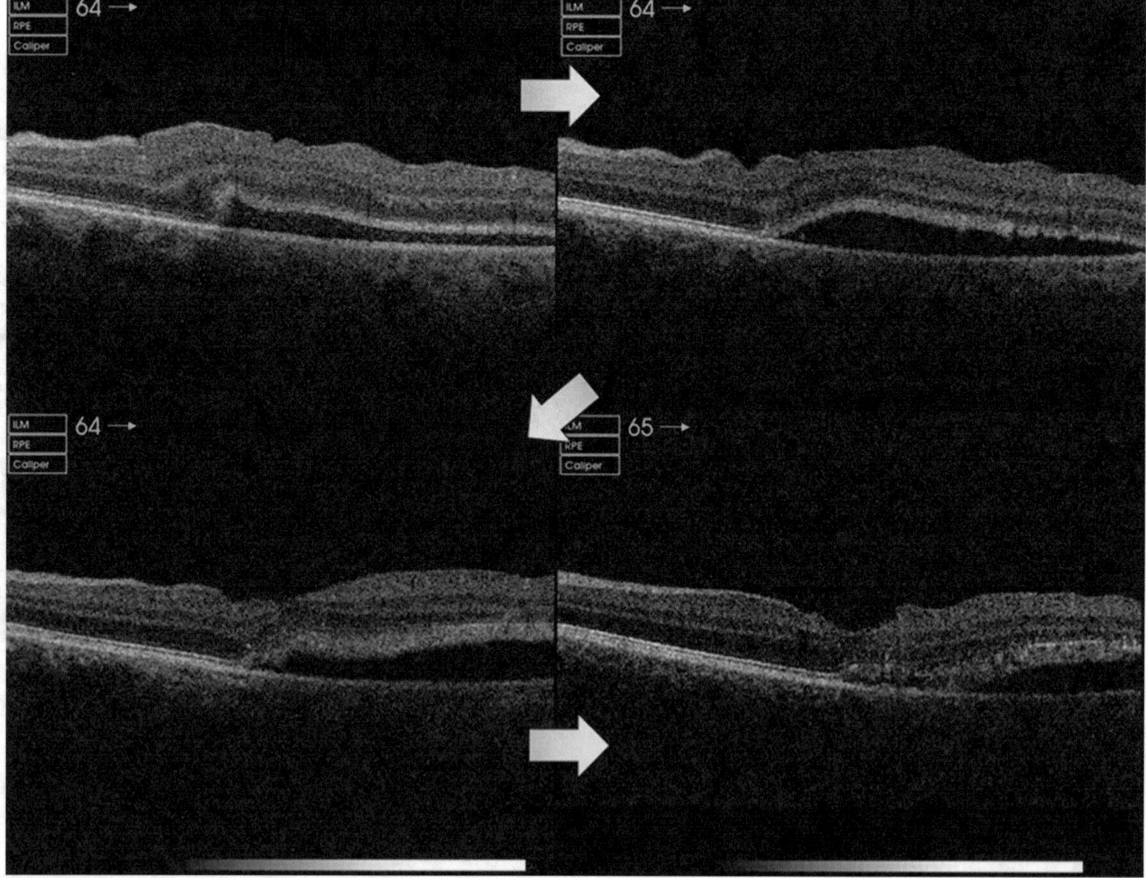

Fig. 8.106 A round hole RRD with slow SRF resolution

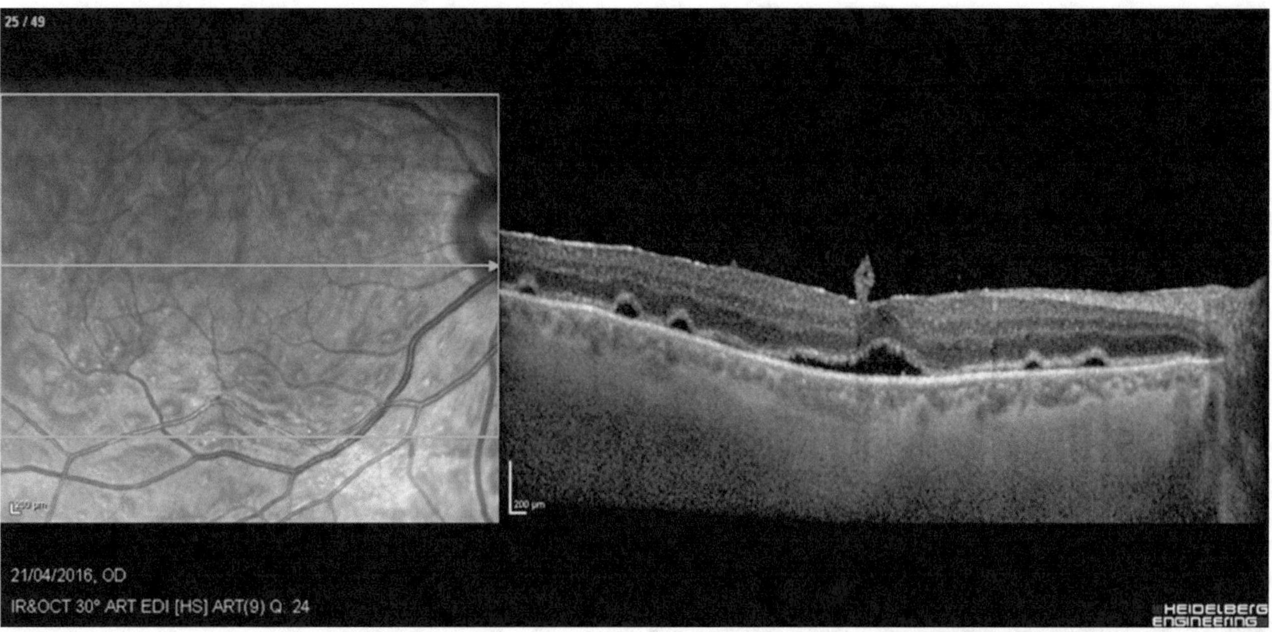

Fig. 8.107 Persistent SRF after RRD

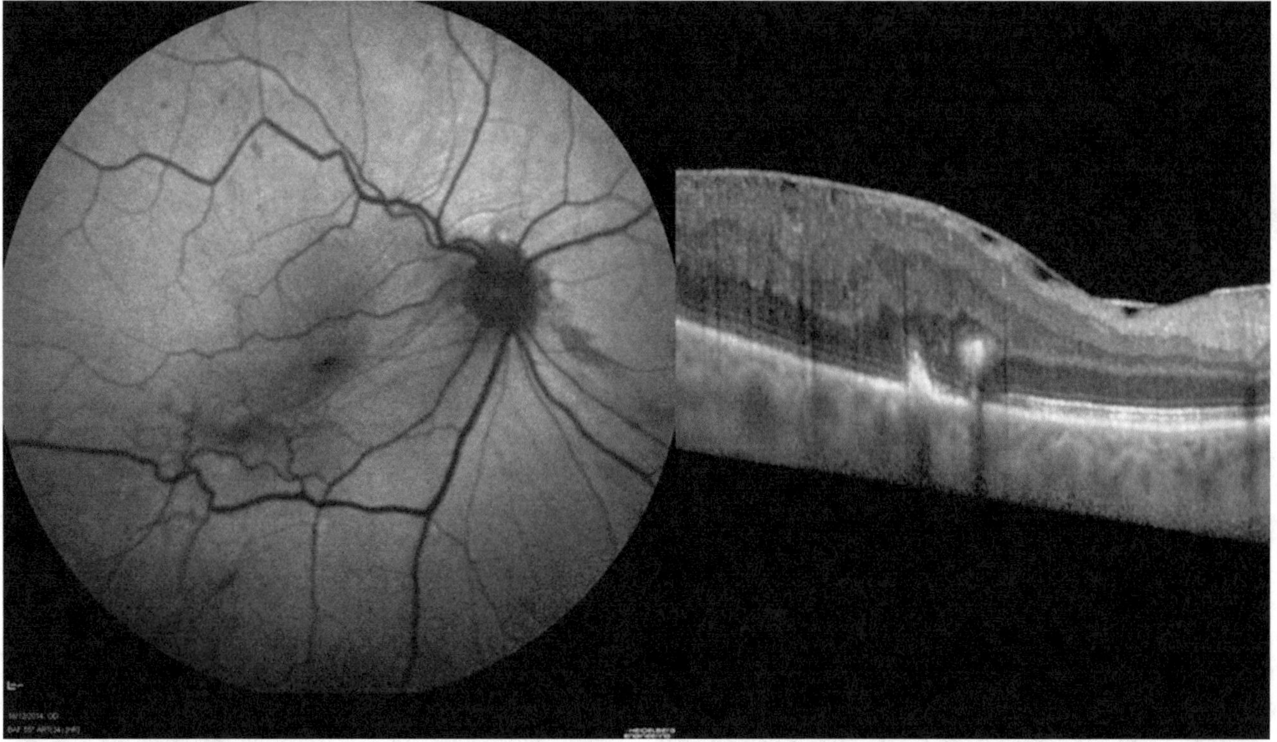

Fig. 8.108 RRD fold and ERM

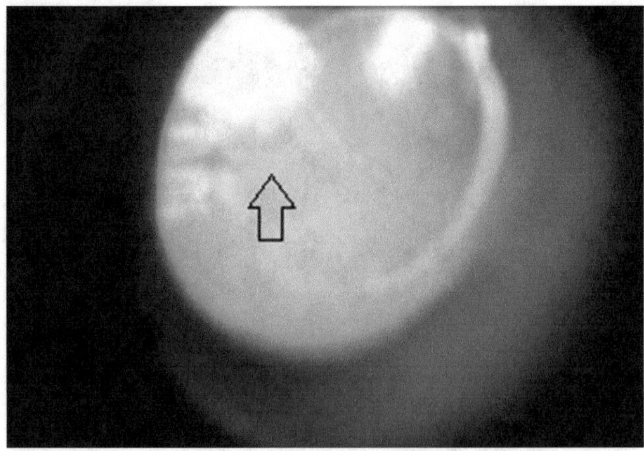

Fig. 8.109 A retina has re-detached from a break on the edge of cryotherapy scar, this is an exceedingly rare occurrence

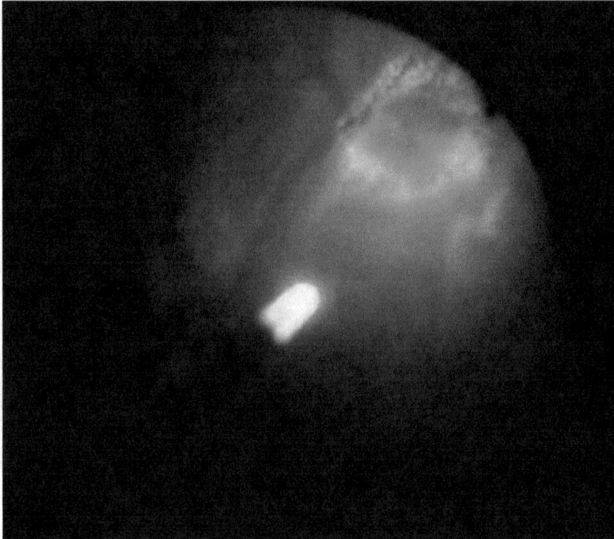

Fig. 8.110 If you see a redetachment through a treated break like this, the commonest cause is another untreated break that was missed during the operation, allowing the SRF to return and elevate the lasered break

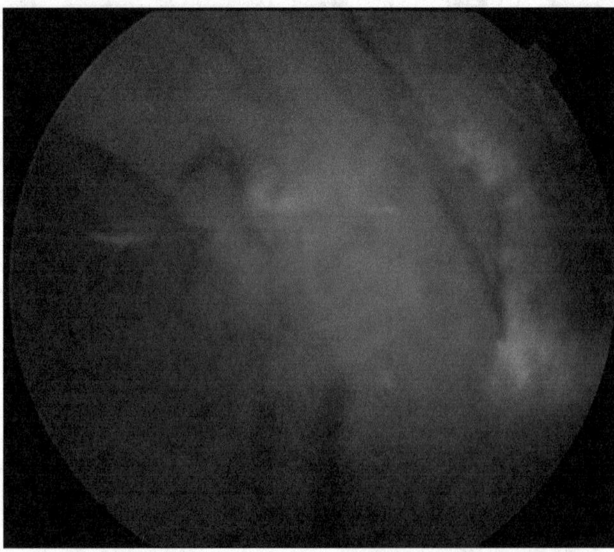

Fig. 8.111 A rolled up retinal detachment which is inoperable

break is found which was not treated at the first operation by retinopexy, it was probably missed or created at the first surgery and is therefore the cause of the redetachment, the PVR is secondary. This emphasises the importance of seeing and treating all pathology at the first operation and therefore the need for a technically competent surgeon.

Again, chose the operation appropriate to the pathology, i.e. non-drain surgery for vitreous attached RRD or PPV for vitreous detached RRD.

Redo Vitreous Attached RRD Surgery

In vitreous attached surgery the RRD will often go concave in shape with resolution of most of the SRF but not all. Often the retina is too stiff to enter the space immediately behind the indentation especially with high indents from the use of sponges. There may be small areas of peripheral concave loculated SRF, unfortunately often also at the macula. These will settle but can take up to one year to do so, they do not require reoperation.

If the RRD is unchanged from preoperatively or there is convex SRF, there is likely to be a break which is still open or pre-existing PVR which is preventing flattening of a break on the indent. In the former find the break and treat with redo non-drain procedure in the latter proceed to PPV and PVR surgery. Usually subretinal PVR bands (which are common with vitreous attached RRD) will only tent up the retina but the RPE pump will allow the rest of the retina to settle, again the residual RRD will be concave.

Redo non-drain, either a round hole has been missed or a dialysis not covered properly. Reopen the conjunctiva, remove the existing explant, the thick fibrous capsule should be excised otherwise it will prevent indention and restrict adequate searching in that area and make sewing on the new explant will be more difficult. Produce an indent under any open detached breaks.

Note the eye will be softer after removal of the indent.

Redo Vitreous Detached RRD

Again, the reason for the recurrent RRD is open breaks which have been missed or are new. If there is no PVR, the eye requires PPV, finds and treats the breaks, and inserts gas. Often a missed break is easier to see in the second operation because slight contraction of the vitreous base opens the breaks by curling the flap anteriorly. If you have detected the recurrent RRD early in the postoperative period, the SRF should be localised near the break. If you are still unable to find the break scatter laser can be applied to the localised area of RRD at the location of the posterior border of the vitreous base, making sure that you laser to the ora serrata at the ends of your treatment area to stop SRF spreading anteri-

Table 8.5 Success rates for patients are reduced for secondary procedures compared to primary operations. Especially if they have presented with PVR, approximately 50% can be fixed with one operation, whereas the others may need multiple operations

		Attached no tamponade		Attached +/− OIL	
		Yes	No	Yes	No
All		88 (66%)	45 (34%)	107 (80%)	26 (20%)
PVR b/c at presentation	Yes	19 (59%)	13 (41%)	22 (69%)	10 (31%)
	No	69 (68%)	32 (32%)	85 (84%)	16 (16%)
Chi-square test		P < 0.001		P < 0.001	

orly past the laser. Do not delay the repeat surgery as PVR is a risk if the retina is not flattened soon. If PVR is the cause of the redetachment, proceed to PVR surgery. Usually postoperative PVR is associated with risk factors such as preoperative PVR, intraocular haemorrhage, multiple breaks, large breaks, complicated surgery, and excessive retinopexy Table 8.5.

Secondary Macular Holes

Macular holes can be found associated with RRD preoperatively and can spontaneously close after surgery without any additional procedures [71]. Holes that develop after surgery can occur in 1% of patients usually after scleral buckle of macular off RRD [69]. Those that do not close spontaneously can be treated by PPV and gas as for idiopathic macular holes. Posterior breaks have been described in the postoperative period around the arcades after PPV which can be treated by laser retinopexy although it is possible that no treatment is required [72].

Detachment with Choroidal Effusions

If the retina detaches into the pars ciliaris hypotony occurs and choroidal effusions may form. These can be drained early in the PPV through the sclerotomies using positive pressure from the infusion (take care when inserting the infusion that the tip has penetrated in to the vitreous cavity) [73, 74]. The fluid is often greenish in colour. Once the suprachoroidal fluid has drained the RRD can be managed by the usual processes although some advocate the use of silicone oil because these patients probably have an increased risk of PVR [75]. Others suggest preoperative systemic steroid therapy [76]. Note very rarely a sequence of events is seen whereby:

1. A break causes RRD.
2. RRD causes hypotony.

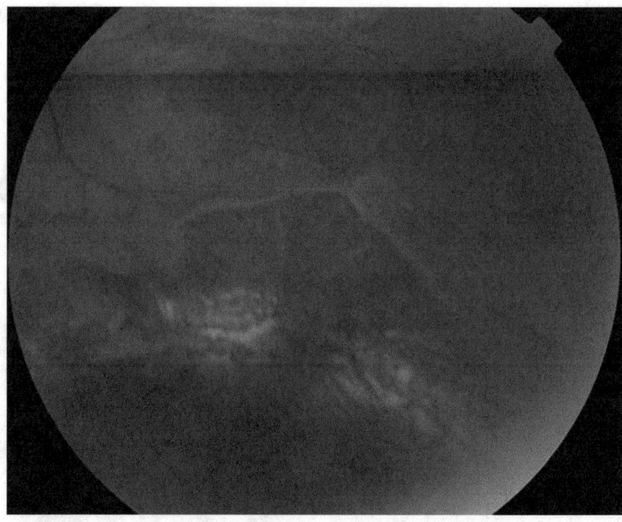

Fig. 8.112 This inferior retinal U tear has lifted through the laser as the gas bubble has absorbed

3. Hypotony causes effusions.
4. Effusions indent onto the retinal break.
5. The RRD subsides.
6. Leaving a flat retinal break on an apparently spontaneous choroidal effusion, laser the break and wait for the effusions to settle (Figs. 8.112 and 8.113).

Removal of Explant

There are occasions when an explant will require removal approximately 1 in 25 explants:

Diplopia

If the explant is placed beneath the extraocular muscles especially the vertical recti (there is a reduced fusion range vertically) diplopia can be induced. Remember that the indent is only required for as long as the retinopexy needs to take effect. Therefore, an explant can be removed at 2 weeks post-op. If diplopia occurs early removal of the plombage will usually resolve the situation. Sometimes diplopia is from unmasked prior phoria, e.g. old fourth nerve palsy.

Erosion through Conjunctiva

With time the end of an explant can erode through the conjunctiva causing pain and discharge in the eye. If the erosion is large enough, the explant should be removed at the slit lamp. The wound will granulate and close spontaneously. The wound cannot be repaired over the explant and it must be removed before orbital infection occurs.

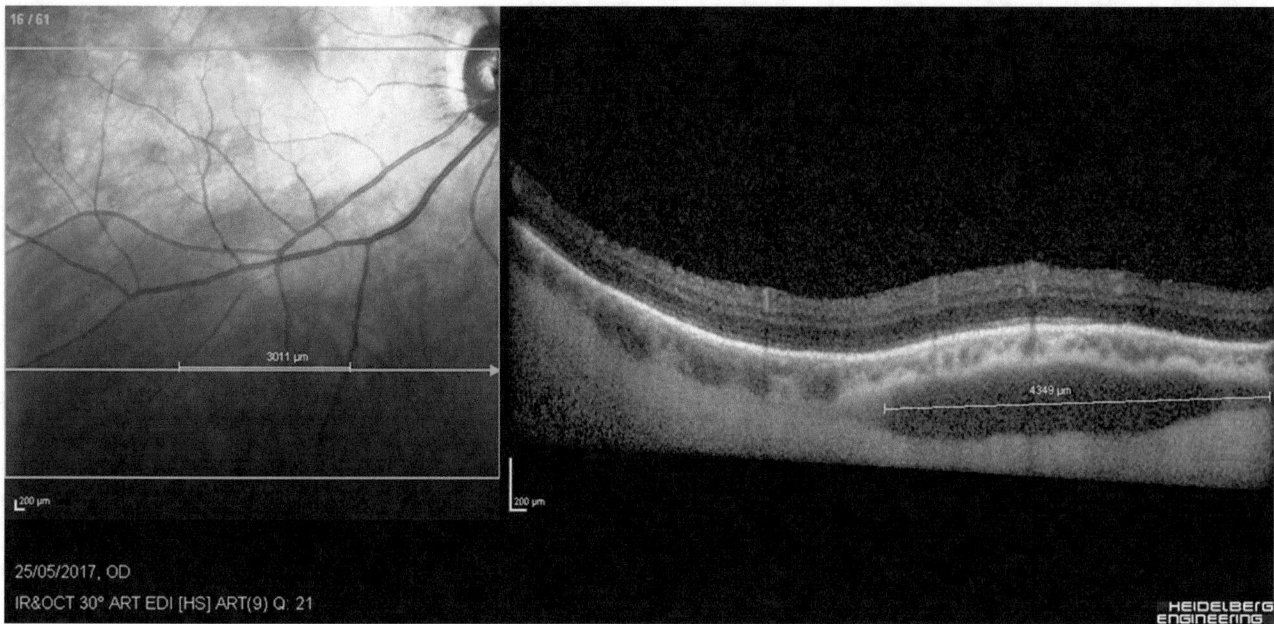

Fig. 8.113 Posterior suprachoroidal fluid after an RRD repair by PPV

Infection

An inflamed explant early in the postoperative period should be assumed to be infected and systemic oral antibiotics prescribed. Usually this will settle the inflammation. Late onset infection is usually associated with erosion through the conjunctiva.

Cosmesis

Plombage is often used in young patients with attached vitreous and therefore the appearance of the eye is important. Patients should be warned that they may feel the explant under the lid, and it may be visible on extreme eye movements but that it can be removed to improve the appearance.

Irritation

If the end of the explant is high, an area of drying can occur in the conjunctiva.

Surgery for Removal of the Explant

Inject some local anaesthetic over the end of the explant that is most accessible. Cut down through the conjunctiva and Tenons onto the end of the explant. The explant is covered very rapidly in the postoperative period by a thick fibrous capsule. Cut down onto the explant through this capsule and make sure the incision is large enough to allow the explant to pull through. The capsule is inelastic therefore the hole needs to be large enough accommodate the circumference of the end of the explant (1/2× $2\pi r$, or approximately 1.5× the diameter of a cylindrical explant). Once the end of the explant is exposed the explant will exit very easily. Remove any sutures near the incision, allow the conjunctiva to close without suturing (Fig. 8.114).

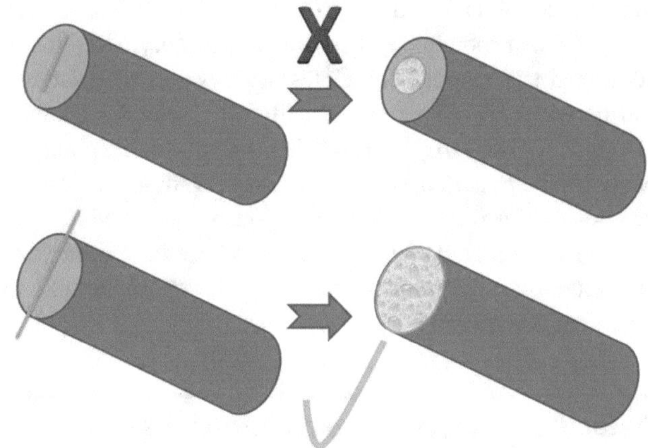

Fig. 8.114 Make sure the incision in the tough capsule at the end of the plomb will be big enough to allow the plomb to come out, approximately 1.5× the diameter of a cylindrical plomb

Summary

RRD can be treated by non-drain retinal detachment repair (vitreous attached RRD) or PPV and gas insertion (vitreous detached RRD). Using only these two surgical procedures almost all RRD without proliferative vitreoretinopathy can be dealt with. The skills of SRF drainage and air injection from the DACE procedure and pneumatic retinopexy are useful in case the surgeon has unexpected problems perioperatively which these methods could remedy. There is a need for new methodology and gluing retinal breaks directly shows initial promise [77].

References

1. Gonin J. The treatment of detached retina by searing the retinal tears. Arch Ophthalmol. 1930;4:621–3.
2. Bonnet M, Fleury J, Guenoun S, Yaniali A, Dumas C, Hajjar C. Cryopexy in primary rhegmatogenous retinal detachment: a risk factor for postoperative proliferative vitreoretinopathy? Graefes Arch Clin Exp Ophthalmol. 1996;234(12):739–43.
3. Haller JA, Blair N, De Juan E, de Bustros S, Goldberg MF, Muldoon T, et al. Multicenter trial of transscleral diode laser retinopexy in retinal detachment surgery. Trans Am Ophthalmol Soc. 1997;95:221–30.
4. Custodis E. Beobachtungen bei der diathermischen Behandlung der Netzhautatablosung und ein Minweis zur Therapie der Operation der Netzhautablosung. Ber Dtsch Opthalmol Ges. 1952;57:227–9.
5. Goldbaum MH, Smithline M, Poole TA, Lincoff HA. Geometric analysis of radial buckling. Am J Ophthalmol. 1975;79(6):958–65.
6. Oge I, Birinci H, Havuz E, Kaman A. Lincoff temporary balloon buckle in retinal detachment surgery. Eur J Ophthalmol. 2001;11(4):372–6.
7. Ramulu PY, Do DV, Corcoran KJ, Corcoran SL, Robin AL. Use of retinal procedures in medicare beneficiaries from 1997 to 2007. Arch Ophthalmol. 128(10):1335–40. https://doi.org/10.1001/archophthalmol.2010.224.
8. Heimann H, Bartz-Schmidt KU, Bornfeld N, Weiss C, Hilgers RD, Foerster MH. Scleral buckling versus primary vitrectomy in rhegmatogenous retinal detachment: a prospective randomized multicenter clinical study. Ophthalmology. 2007;114(12):2142–54. https://doi.org/10.1016/j.ophtha.2007.09.013.
9. Jackson TL, Kwan AS, Laidlaw AH, Aylward W. Identification of retinal breaks using subretinal trypan blue injection. Ophthalmology. 2007;114(3):587–90. https://doi.org/10.1016/j.ophtha.2006.05.079.
10. Wong R, Gupta B, Aylward GW, Laidlaw DA. Dye extrusion technique (DE-TECH): occult retinal break detection with subretinal dye extrusion during vitrectomy for retinal detachment repair. Retina. 2009;29(4):492–6. https://doi.org/10.1097/IAE.0b013e31819bab72.
11. Martinez-Castillo V, Zapata MA, Boixadera A, Fonollosa A, Garcia-Arumi J. Pars plana vitrectomy, laser retinopexy, and aqueous tamponade for pseudophakic rhegmatogenous retinal detachment. Ophthalmology. 2007;114(2):297–302. https://doi.org/10.1016/j.ophtha.2006.07.037.
12. Guber J, Schawkat M, Lang C, Scholl HPN, Valmaggia C. How to prevent retinal shift after Rhegmatogenous retinal detachment repair: a prospective. Randomized Study Ophthalmol Retina. 2019;3(5):417–21. https://doi.org/10.1016/j.oret.2019.01.010.
13. Vidne O, Blum Meirovitch S, Rabina G, Abd Eelkader A, Prat D, Barequet D, et al. Perfluorocarbon liquid vs. subretinal fluid drainage during vitrectomy for the primary repair of Rhegmatogenous retinal detachment: a comparative study. Curr Eye Res. 2018;43(11):1389–94. https://doi.org/10.1080/02713683.2018.1490436.
14. Heimann H, Bopp S. Retinal folds following retinal detachment surgery. Ophthalmologica. 226(Suppl 1):18–26. https://doi.org/10.1159/000328380.
15. Quintyn J-C, Brasseur G. Subretinal fluid in primary rhegmatogenous retinal detachment: physiopathology and composition. Surv Ophthalmol. 2004;49(1):96–108.
16. Hakimbashi M, Amini P, Khatibi A, Goldbaum MH. Retinal detachment from guttering also a problem after vitrectomy. Invest Ophthalmol Vis Sci. 2012;53(14):5796.
17. Martinez-Castillo VJ, Garcia-Arumi J, Boixadera A. Pars Plana vitrectomy alone for the Management of Pseudophakic Rhegmatogenous Retinal Detachment with only inferior breaks. Ophthalmology. 2016;123(7):1563–9. https://doi.org/10.1016/j.ophtha.2016.03.032.
18. Martinez-Castillo V, Boixadera A, Verdugo A, Garcia-Arumi J. Pars plana vitrectomy alone for the management of inferior breaks in pseudophakic retinal detachment without facedown position. Ophthalmology. 2005;112(7):1222–6. https://doi.org/10.1016/j.ophtha.2004.12.046.
19. Martinez-Castillo V, Verdugo A, Boixadera A, Garcia-Arumi J, Corcostegui B. Management of inferior breaks in pseudophakic rhegmatogenous retinal detachment with pars plana vitrectomy and air. Arch Ophthalmol. 2005;123(8):1078–81. https://doi.org/10.1001/archopht.123.8.1078.
20. Sharma A, Grigoropoulos V, Williamson TH. Management of primary rhegmatogenous retinal detachment with inferior breaks. Br J Ophthalmol. 2004;88(11):1372–5.
21. Campo RV, Sipperley JO, Sneed SR, Park DW, Dugel PU, Jacobsen J, et al. Pars plana vitrectomy without scleral buckle for pseudophakic retinal detachments. Ophthalmology. 1999;106(9):1811–5.
22. Sharma T, Virdi DS, Parikh S, Gopal L, Badrinath SS, Mukesh BN. A case-control study of suprachoroidal hemorrhage during pars plana vitrectomy. Ophthalmic Surg Lasers. 1997;28(8):640–4.
23. Piper JG, Han DP, Abrams GW, Mieler WF. Perioperative choroidal hemorrhage at pars plana vitrectomy. A case-control study. Ophthalmology. 1993;100(5):699–704.
24. Tabandeh H, Flynn HW Jr. Suprachoroidal hemorrhage during pars plana vitrectomy. Curr Opin Ophthalmol. 2001;12(3):179–85.
25. Wickham L, Connor M, Aylward GW. Vitrectomy and gas for inferior break retinal detachments: are the results comparable to vitrectomy, gas, and scleral buckle? Br J Ophthalmol. 2004;88(11):1376–9.
26. Tanner V, Minihan M, Williamson TH. Management of inferior retinal breaks during pars plana vitrectomy for retinal detachment. Br J Ophthalmol. 2001;85(4):480–2.
27. Salicone A, Smiddy WE, Venkatraman A, Feuer W. Management of retinal detachment when no break is found. Ophthalmology. 2006;113(3):398–403.
28. Wu WC, Chen MT, Hsu SY, Chang CW. Management of pseudophakic retinal detachment with undetectable retinal breaks. Ophthalmic Surg Lasers. 2002;33(4):314–8.
29. Wong D, Billington BM, Chignell AH. Pars plana vitrectomy for retinal detachment with unseen retinal holes. Graefes Arch Clin Exp Ophthalmol. 1987;225(4):269–71.
30. Phillips CI. Distribution of breaks in Aphakic and "senile" eyes with retinal detachments. Br J Ophthalmol. 1963;47:744–52.
31. Ashrafzadeh MT, Schepens CL, Elzeneiny II, Moura R, Morse P, Kraushar MF. Aphakic and phakic retinal detachment I Preoperative findings. Arch Ophthalmol. 1973;89(6):476–83.
32. Custodis E. Scleral prebuckling with plastic plombage. Bibl Ophthalmol. 1965;65:140–3.
33. Machemer R, Parel JM, Norton EW. Vitrectomy: a pars plana approach. Technical improvements and further results. Trans Am Acad Ophthalmol Otolaryngol. 1972;76(2):462–6.
34. Tabandeh H, Flaxel C, Sullivan PM, Leaver PK, Flynn HW Jr, Schiffman J. Scleral rupture during retinal detachment surgery: risk factors, management options, and outcomes. Ophthalmology. 2000;107(5):848–52.

35. Wolfensberger TJ, Gonvers M. Optical coherence tomography in the evaluation of incomplete visual acuity recovery after macula-off retinal detachments. Graefes Arch Clin Exp Ophthalmol. 2002;240(2):85–9.
36. Wolfensberger TJ. Foveal reattachment after macula-off retinal detachment occurs faster after vitrectomy than after buckle surgery. Ophthalmology. 2004;111(7):1340–3.
37. Baba T, Hirose A, Moriyama M, Mochizuki M. Tomographic image and visual recovery of acute macula-off rhegmatogenous retinal detachment. Graefes Arch Clin Exp Ophthalmol. 2004;242(7):576–81.
38. Ugarte M, Williamson TH. Horizontal and vertical micropsia following macula-off rhegmatogenous retinal-detachment surgical repair. Graefes Arch Clin Exp Ophthalmol. 2006;244(11):1545–8.
39. Wakabayashi T, Oshima Y, Fujimoto H, Murakami Y, Sakaguchi H, Kusaka S, et al. Foveal microstructure and visual acuity after retinal detachment repair: imaging analysis by Fourier-domain optical coherence tomography. Ophthalmology. 2009;116(3):519–28. https://doi.org/10.1016/j.ophtha.2008.10.001.
40. Jaffe GJ, Brownlow R, Hines J. Modified external needle drainage procedure for rhegmatogenous retinal detachment. Retina. 2003;23(1):80–5.
41. Hilton GF, Grizzard WS. Pneumatic retinopexy. A two-step outpatient operation without conjunctival incision. Ophthalmology. 1986;93(5):626–41.
42. McAllister IL, Meyers SM, Zegarra H, Gutman FA, Zakov ZN, Beck GJ. Comparison of pneumatic retinopexy with alternative surgical techniques. Ophthalmology. 1988;95(7):877–83.
43. Han DP, Mohsin NC, Guse CE, Hartz A, Tarkanian CN. Comparison of pneumatic retinopexy and scleral buckling in the management of primary rhegmatogenous retinal detachment. Southern Wisconsin pneumatic Retinopexy study group. Am J Ophthalmol. 1998;126(5):658–68.
44. Poliner LS, Grand MG, Schoch LH, Olk RJ, Johnston GP, Okun E, et al. New retinal detachment after pneumatic retinopexy. Ophthalmology. 1987;94(4):315–8.
45. Mudvari SS, Ravage ZB, Rezaei KA. Retinal detachment after primary pneumatic retinopexy. Retina. 2009;29(10):1474–8. https://doi.org/10.1097/IAE.0b013e3181ae70f3.
46. Tornambe PE, Hilton GF. Pneumatic retinopexy. A multicenter randomized controlled clinical trial comparing pneumatic retinopexy with scleral buckling. The retinal detachment study group. Ophthalmology. 1989;96(6):772–83.
47. Tornambe PE, Hilton GF, Brinton DA, Flood TP, Green S, Grizzard WS, et al. Pneumatic retinopexy. A two-year follow-up study of the multicenter clinical trial comparing pneumatic retinopexy with scleral buckling. Ophthalmology. 1991;98(7):1115–23.
48. Hillier RJ, Felfeli T, Berger AR, Wong DT, Altomare F, Dai D, et al. The pneumatic Retinopexy versus vitrectomy for the Management of Primary Rhegmatogenous Retinal Detachment Outcomes Randomized Trial (PIVOT). Ophthalmology. 2019;126(4):531–9. https://doi.org/10.1016/j.ophtha.2018.11.014.
49. Znaor L, Medic A, Binder S, Vucinovic A, Marin Lovric J, Puljak L. Pars plana vitrectomy versus scleral buckling for repairing simple rhegmatogenous retinal detachments. Cochrane Database Syst Rev. 2019;3:Cd009562. https://doi.org/10.1002/14651858.CD009562.pub2.
50. Ah-Fat FG, Sharma MC, Majid MA, McGalliard JN, Wong D. Trends in vitreoretinal surgery at a tertiary referral Centre: 1987 to 1996. Br J Ophthalmol. 1999;83(4):396–8.
51. Girard P, Karpouzas I. Pseudophakic retinal detachment: anatomic and visual results. Graefes Arch Clin Exp Ophthalmol. 1995;233(6):324–30.
52. La Heij EC, Derhaag PF, Hendrikse F. Results of scleral buckling operations in primary rhegmatogenous retinal detachment. Doc Ophthalmol. 2000;100(1):17–25.
53. Oshima Y, Emi K, Motokura M, Yamanishi S. Survey of surgical indications and results of primary pars plana vitrectomy for rhegmatogenous retinal detachments. Jpn J Ophthalmol. 1999;43(2):120–6.
54. Thompson JA, Snead MP, Billington BM, Barrie T, Thompson JR, Sparrow JM. National audit of the outcome of primary surgery for rhegmatogenous retinal detachment. II. Clinical outcomes. Eye. 2002;16(6):771–7.
55. Minihan M, Tanner V, Williamson TH. Primary rhegmatogenous retinal detachment: 20 years of change. Br J Ophthalmol. 2001;85(5):546–8.
56. Sallam AB, Donachie PHJ, Yorston D, Steel DHW, Williamson TH, Jackson TL, et al. Royal college of ophthalmologists' national database study of vitreoretinal surgery: report 7, Intersurgeon variations in primary Rhegmatogenous retinal detachment failure. Retina. 2018;38(2):334–42. https://doi.org/10.1097/IAE.0000000000001538.
57. Hakin KN, Lavin MJ, Leaver PK. Primary vitrectomy for rhegmatogenous retinal detachment. Graefes Arch Clin Exp Ophthalmol. 1993;231(6):344–6.
58. Heimann H, Bornfeld N, Friedrichs W, Helbig H, Kellner U, Korra A, et al. Primary vitrectomy without scleral buckling for rhegmatogenous retinal detachment. Graefes Arch Clin Exp Ophthalmol. 1996;234(9):561–8.
59. Schmidt JC, Rodrigues EB, Hoerle S, Meyer CH, Kroll P. Primary vitrectomy in complicated rhegmatogenous retinal detachment--a survey of 205 eyes. Ophthalmologica. 2003;217(6):387–92.
60. Tewari HK, Kedar S, Kumar A, Garg SP, Verma LK. Comparison of scleral buckling with combined scleral buckling and pars plana vitrectomy in the management of rhegmatogenous retinal detachment with unseen retinal breaks. Clin Exp Ophthalmol. 2003;31(5):403–7.
61. Doyle E, Herbert EN, Bunce C, Williamson TH, Laidlaw DA. How effective is macula-off retinal detachment surgery. Might good outcome be predicted? Eye. 2006.
62. Ho SF, Fitt A, Frimpong-Ansah K, Benson MT. The management of primary rhegmatogenous retinal detachment not involving the fovea. Eye (Lond). 2006;20(9):1049–53. https://doi.org/10.1038/sj.eye.6702083.
63. Williamson TH, Shunmugam M, Rodrigues I, Dogramaci M, Lee E. Characteristics of rhegmatogenous retinal detachment and their relationship to visual outcome. Eye (Lond). 2013;27(9):1063–9. https://doi.org/10.1038/eye.2013.136.
64. Miki D, Hida T, Hotta K, Shinoda K, Hirakata A. Comparison of scleral buckling and vitrectomy for retinal detachment resulting from flap tears in superior quadrants. Jpn J Ophthalmol. 2001;45(2):187–91.
65. Oshima Y, Yamanishi S, Sawa M, Motokura M, Harino S, Emi K. Two-year follow-up study comparing primary vitrectomy with scleral buckling for macula-off rhegmatogenous retinal detachment. Jpn J Ophthalmol. 2000;44(5):538–49.
66. Ahmadieh H, Moradian S, Faghihi H, Parvaresh MM, Ghanbari H, Mehryar M, et al. Anatomic and visual outcomes of scleral buckling versus primary vitrectomy in pseudophakic and aphakic retinal detachment: six-month follow-up results of a single operation--report no. 1. Ophthalmology. 2005;112(8):1421–9. https://doi.org/10.1016/j.ophtha.2005.02.018.
67. Day S, Grossman DS, Mruthyunjaya P, Sloan FA, Lee PP. One-year outcomes after retinal detachment surgery among medicare beneficiaries. Am J Ophthalmol. 150(3):338–45. https://doi.org/10.1016/j.ajo.2010.04.009.
68. Richardson EC, Verma S, Green WT, Woon H, Chignell AH. Primary vitrectomy for rhegmatogenous retinal detachment: an analysis of failure. Eur J Ophthalmol. 2000;10(2):160–6.
69. Moshfeghi AA, Salam GA, Deramo VA, Shakin EP, Ferrone PJ, Shakin JL, et al. Management of macular holes that develop after retinal detachment repair. Am J Ophthalmol. 2003;136(5):895–9.

70. Foster RE, Meyers SM. Recurrent retinal detachment more than 1 year after reattachment. Ophthalmology. 2002;109(10):1821–7.
71. Riordan-Eva P, Chignell AH. Full thickness macular breaks in rhegmatogenous retinal detachment with peripheral retinal breaks. Br J Ophthalmol. 1992;76(6):346–8.
72. Okada K, Sakata H, Mizote H, Minamoto A, Narai A, Choshi K. Postoperative posterior retinal holes after pars plana vitrectomy for primary retinal detachment. Retina. 1997;17(2):99–104.
73. Ghoraba HH. Primary vitrectomy for the management of rhegmatogenous retinal detachment associated with choroidal detachment. Graefes Arch Clin Exp Ophthalmol. 2001;239(10):733–6.
74. Yang CM. Pars plana vitrectomy in the treatment of combined rhegmatogenous retinal detachment and choroidal detachment in aphakic or pseudophakic patients. Ophthalmic Surg Lasers. 1997;28(4):288–93.
75. Loo A, Fitt AW, Ramchandani M, Kirkby GR. Pars plana vitrectomy with silicone oil in the management of combined rhegmatogenous retinal and choroidal detachment. Eye. 2001;15(Pt 5):612–5.
76. Sharma T, Gopal L, Badrinath SS. Primary vitrectomy for rhegmatogenous retinal detachment associated with choroidal detachment. Ophthalmology. 1998;105(12):2282–5.
77. Tyagi M, Basu S. Glue-assisted retinopexy for rhegmatogenous retinal detachments (GuARD): a novel surgical technique for closing retinal breaks. Indian J Ophthalmol. 2019;67(5):677–80. https://doi.org/10.4103/ijo.IJO_1943_18.

Different Presentations of Rhegmatogenous Retinal Detachments

9

Contents

T. H. Williamson, *Vitreoretinal Surgery*, https://doi.org/10.1007/978-3-030-68769-4_9

Age-Related RRD from PVD

The commonest RRD is caused by an age-related PVD this can be treated using the principles defined in the previous chapter. The clinical characteristics (PVD, U-shaped breaks, usually acute onset retinal detachment) have been used as the basis for the cases described in the previous chapter and are summarised here:

Clinical features in Age-Related RRD from PVD	
Sex	Males > females
Age	>40 years
Refraction	All refractions but more common in myopia
Bilaterality	25% [1]
Fellow eye at presentation	10%
Onset	Rapid
Vitreous	Detached
Retinal break type	U tears, operculated breaks
Retinal break size	Variable
Mean number of breaks	2.5
Multiple breaks >1	56%
Retinal break position	All but temporal>nasal and superior>inferior
Fovea off	55%
PVR	Preretinal A, B, and C
Surgery	PPV and gas
Primary success rate	87%

Most commonly these are now treated by PPV and gas with later phacoemulsification cataract extraction and IOL if necessary. However, scleral buckling procedures can also be applied.

Atrophic Hole RRD with Attached Vitreous

Clinical features in atrophic hole RRD in young myopic patients	
Sex	Females>males
Age	20–40 years
Refraction	Myopia (mean – 5.5D)
Bilaterality	12% with bilateral RRD, retinal holes in the other eye 63%
Fellow eye at presentation	10%
Onset	Slow
Vitreous	Attached
Retinal break type	Atrophic round holes
Retinal break size	Small
Retinal break position	Inferior > superior, temporal > nasal
Mean number of breaks	3.6
Multiple breaks >1	70%
Fovea off	40%
Retinal degeneration	Lattice
PVR	Subretinal bands
Surgery	Non-drain scleral explant
Primary success rate	93%

Young myopic patients in the third and fourth decade of age may present with a chronic RRD usually inferiorly sited. These can be treated by non-drain explant surgery as described in the previous chapter. 64% are female and 83% myopic [2, 3]. Abnormalities in the fellow eyes are common (63%), with bilateral RRD in 12% [4]. These patients can go on to develop PVD with RRD from U tears later in life.

Pseudophakic RRD

Cataract surgery has evolved rapidly in the last fifty years with progression from intracapsular surgery to extracapsular surgery to phacoemulsification, and aphakia to pseudophakia postoperatively. This has led to a reduction in complications and an improvement in the standard of surgery and postoperative outcome from cataract surgery worldwide. The relationship between cataract surgery and rhegmatogenous retinal detachment (RRD) is only partially defined from data from Medicare, other insurance datasets [5–7], and Scandinavian public health records.

[8, 9] and large population based studies such as The Rochester Study [10, 11], there remains an increased risk of retinal detachment associated with cataract operations despite progress in surgical technique. The four year incidence of retinal detachment after all cataract extractions has been described as 1.17%, increasing with vitreous loss to 4.9% but reduced in phacoemulsification to 0.4% [12]. This is regarded as higher than would be expected in the normal population. The connection seems to be with the occurrence of phacoemulsification rather than the presence of cataract. Approximately 10–17% of these eyes have a history of vitreous loss during the cataract surgery [13]. The pattern of retinal tears is like older studies of aphakia with less chance of large breaks, superotemporal breaks, or presentation with vitreous haemorrhage and more inferonasal breaks than phakic RRD. Surgical repair is by PPV in most circumstances (Table 9.1).

Aphakic RRD

Studies have been performed in this area in the 1960s and 1970s when intracapsular cataract surgery and aphakia were common [14–18]. Schepen's group in 1973 showed an increase in nasal breaks in aphakia versus phakia, 65% and 50.6%, respectively [19]. The older studies used a system of counting the number of breaks in each quadrant, providing a total number of breaks in each quadrant over a cohort. Applying statistical analysis using this methodology is more complicated because breaks from the same eye are not independent variables. The use of this method explains the increased percentages described in these studies. Similarly, Phillips in 1963 found increased rates of breaks ante-

Table 9.1 showing a univariate comparison of various features of pseudophakic RRD with aged related PVD induced RRD, patients were older than 50 years

Variable	Pseudophakic eyes	Phakic eyes	Significantly different
Age in years	69	64	Yes
Sex (% female)	31	41	Yes
Presenting visual acuity (mean)	20/180	20/160	
Duration of visual loss in days (mean)	15	31	
Vitreous haemorrhage At presentation (%)	7	17	Yes
Presence of PVR (%)	14	14	
Number of breaks (mean ± S.D.)	2.5	2.7	
Fovea off (%)	64	55	
Small breaks (%)	56	46	Yes
Medium breaks (%)	60	59	
Large breaks (%)	13	27	Yes
Superotemporal break (%)	64	75	Yes
Inferotemporal break (%)	27	32	
Superonasal break (%)	38	38	
Inferonasal break (%)	21	14	Yes
Anterior break (%)	28	21	
Posterior break (%)	13	17	
Flat inferior break (%)	9	13	
Inferior breaks in the RRD	23	16	
Visual acuity at last follow-up (mean)	20/55	20/55	
Any RD at final follow-up (%)	5	4.0	
Oil in at final follow-up (%)	10	5	
Phthisis at final follow-up (%)	1	0	

riorly, nasally, and inferonasally in aphakic retinal detachment compared with phakic retinal detachments [20]. His group attempted to exclude patients with vitreous loss during cataract surgery from analysis.

Retinal Dialysis

Clinical Features

(Figs. 9.1 and 9.2) Retinal dialysis is a dehiscence of the anterior retina at the ora serrata. There is classically no posterior vitreous detachment. This means that the RRD progresses very slowly and often presents by coincidental observation or when the macula finally detaches. In the latter situation because of the slow onset and delay in noticing the foveal detachment, visual recovery is seldom complete even after successful surgery. The chronicity results in subretinal fibrosis and retinal cysts but a low rate of preretinal PVR is described [21, 22]. If PVR is present, subretinal bands are more common than other types of PVR. The dialysis is usually stiff and smooth-edged and the retinal detachment immobile unless of recent onset of a few weeks.

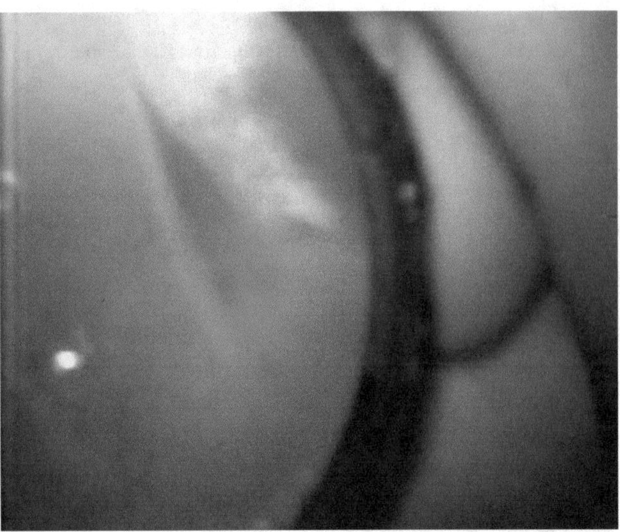

Fig. 9.1 A retinal dialysis is seen by indirect ophthalmoscopy and indentation

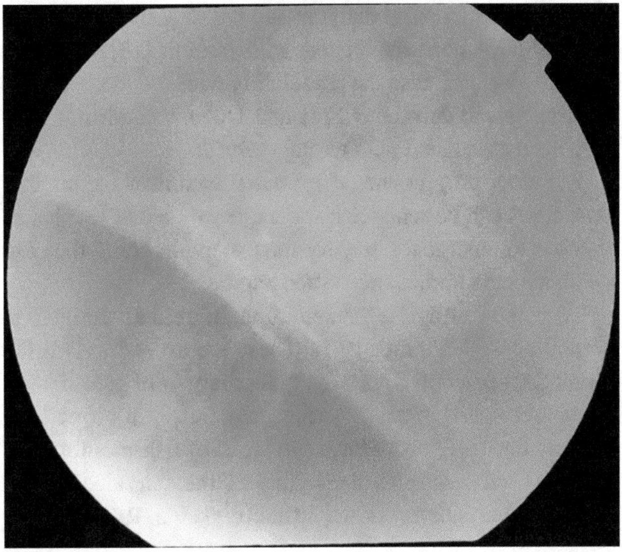

Fig. 9.2 A retinal dialysis

Clinical features in RRD from retinal dialysis	
Sex	Males > females
Age	20–40 years
Refraction	Emmetropia
Fellow eye at presentation	8%
Onset	Slow
Vitreous	Attached
Retinal break type	Retinal dialysis
Retinal break size	Large and medium

Clinical features in RRD from retinal dialysis	
Retinal break quadrant	Inferotemporal (superonasal more likely to be traumatic)
Median number of breaks	1
Multiple breaks >1	30%
Fovea off	40%
PVR	Subretinal bands
Surgery	Non-drain explant procedure
Primary success rate	92%

A separation of the vitreous base is sometimes seen as a "bucket handle" in the inner surface of the dialysis especially in traumatic cases. Blunt trauma has been associated with dialysis formation but a history of trauma is not always present and some are thought to be spontaneous [23]. In the latter a familial basis has been sought but remains uncertain [24, 25]. On rare occasions a retinal dialysis is seen a few days after a severe contusion injury in which case the dialysis and retina are mobile.

The commonest sites are inferotemporal and superonasal. 56% of inferotemporal dialyses and the 87% of superonasal dialyses have been associated with trauma [26]. 14% are bilateral in which case the association with trauma is said to be less. Atopic dermatitis [27] and Down's syndrome [28] have been associated with retinal dialysis.

The slow progression of retinal detachment means that most cases can be scheduled for surgery on a daytime list as opposed to emergency surgery the exception being the case which appears immediately after trauma.

Occasionally a late presentation of retinal dialysis is associated with C grade PVR. These are exceedingly difficult to fix, see PVR. Similarly, giant dialysis of greater than 90 degrees may occur. These may require vitrectomy because buckling procedures will lead to fish-mouthing of the break secondary to shortening of the scleral diameter leading to redundancy of the retina.(Figs. 9.3, 9.4, and 9.5).

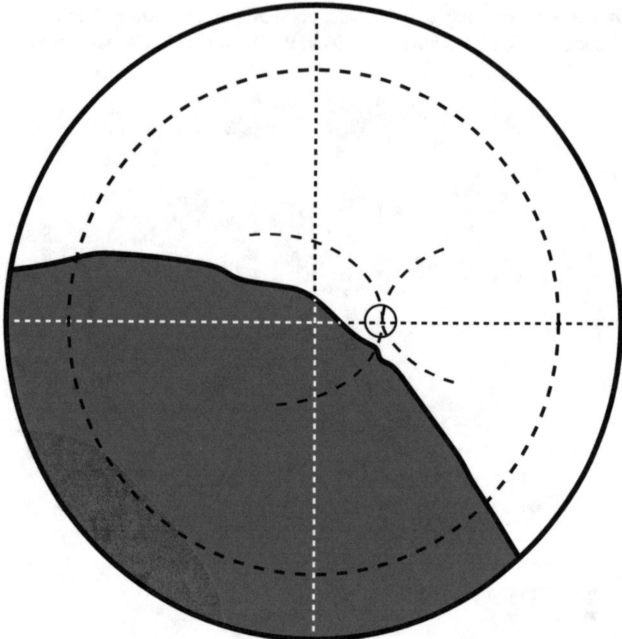

Fig. 9.3 A drawing of an inferotemporal retinal dialysis

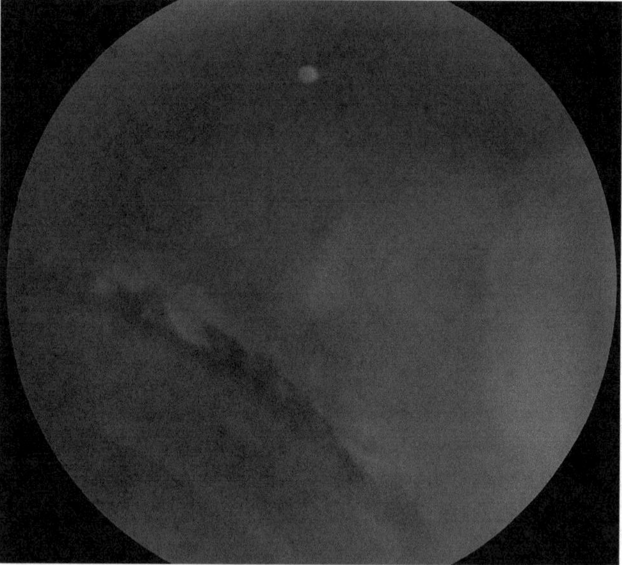

Fig. 9.4 A dialysis with a pigment demarcation line indicating stability

Surgery for Retinal Dialysis (Table 9.2)

The approach is the same as the non-drain procedure, but a few adaptations are required to cope with the characteristics of the dialysis. The operation can be technically demanding but the results are potentially particularly good.

Search

Particular attention should be paid to the ora serrata over 360° because this is the position of any likely pathology. The indentation is very anterior as you are indenting the ora and therefore requires good control of the movement of the eye, use the muscle slings to fix the position of the eye (rest your fifth finger on the sling to stabilise the eye) during indentation. Carefully examine the ends of the dialysis for small extra dialyses. Very shallow dialysis will close when indented and can be missed. Move your indent in a circumferential direction around the ora so that the dialysis is partially opened on the edge of the indent to overcome this problem. I have seen U tears (surprisingly) accompanying the dialysis on rare occasion; therefore, the whole retina needs to be searched.

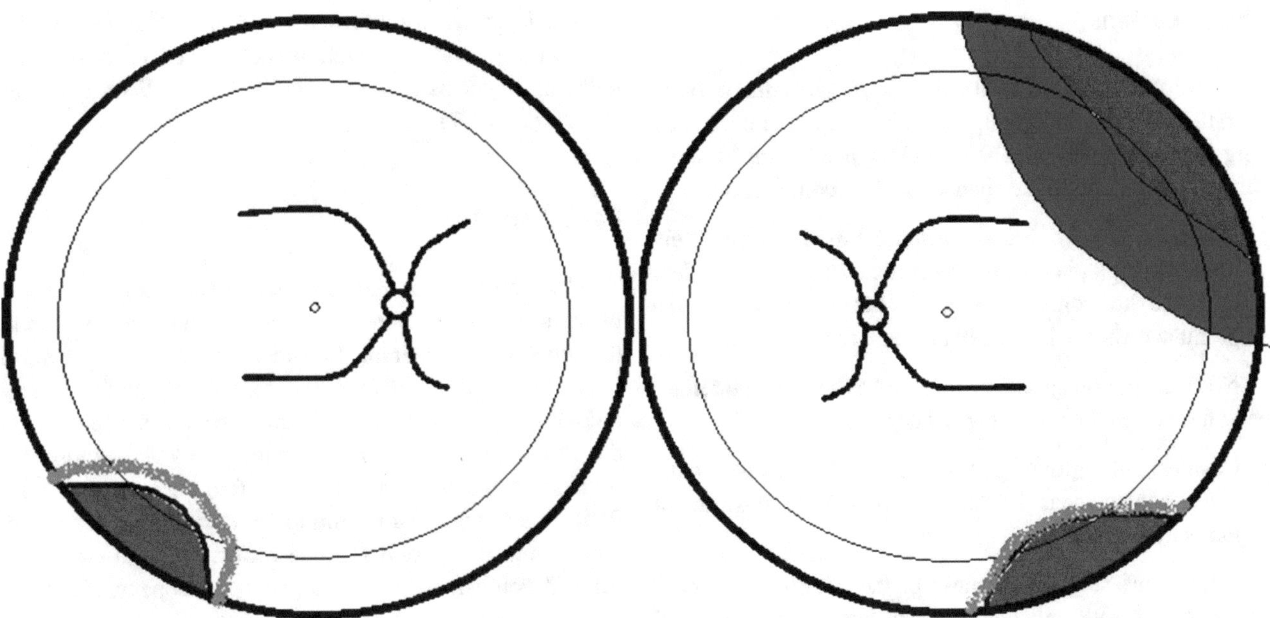

Fig. 9.5 A patient with multiple dialyses

Table 9.2 difficulty rating of surgery for retinal dialysis

Difficulty Rating	Moderate
Success rates	High
Complication rates	Low
When to use in training	Early

Cryotherapy

This requires confluence of the burns (see Plombage). Dialysis often extends from extraocular muscle insertion to extraocular muscle insertion (usually the inferior rectus to lateral rectus), therefore the retinopexy is over a large area. The dialysis, at its apex, often seems too far away from the indent internally to achieve a cryotherapy burn. However, it is usually possible to obtain all the burns required. Be particularly aware of which parts of the retina you have treated (avoid overlapping the burns too much), to limit the number of burns but still achieve confluence. It is important that the retina has been sealed along all the extent of the dialysis by the retinopexy because removal of the plombage postoperatively is sometimes required (to reverse complications from its anterior position, e.g. poor cosmesis or diplopia).

Marking the Break

For large dialysis, mark the ends of the break, or the position of any satellite dialysis, and the apex. The ends are usually at the muscle insertions, but it is important to know exactly where in case extension of the plombage under the muscle is required running the risk of postoperative diplopia (especially with the superior and inferior recti). The apex may extend further posteriorly than the ends of the dialysis requiring bowing of the plombage to ensure that the dialysis will fall onto the smallest plombage.

Plombage

Select a sponge that will cover the required area. A 3–4 mm sponge is preferred because it will be less prominent postoperatively than a 5 mm. However, the elevations of some dialyses are remarkably high and may require the latter. If the dialysis is small, two sutures will be sufficient, which with a 4 mm sponge is unlikely to compromise the optic nerve circulation (check it after suture tying in any case). Larger dialyses require three sutures, one at each end and one at the apex. Insert the sutures as usual placing the "marks" on the sclera centrally between the suture bites. Tie one of the sutures at one end of the plomb. Make sure you use a reef knot of some sort. Perform a paracentesis and remove approximately 0.15 mls of aqueous. This avoids occlusion of the optic nerve circulation. Tie the middle suture. The softer eye eases the production of a high indent at the apex. Finally, tie the last suture. Softening of the eye causes the plombage to produce an internal indent rather than being proud of the eye (resulting in poor cosmesis or disturbance the function of the extraocular muscles).

Checking the Indent

Check the optic nerve. View the indent, which should go past the ends of the dialysis slightly and judge that the dialysis will fall on to the apex of the indent or slightly onto the anterior border (remember parallax). Trim the ends of the indent and slope the ends 45° to help reduce the protrusion of the sponge at its ends. Check that Tenon's is not caught up in the sutures and sew up the conjunctiva.

Complications

The complications are as for non-drain procedures, however, the anterior placement of the plombage, the need for a long circumferential plombage, and the need to insert under vertical recti increase the chance of some complications.

- Diplopia. Surgery around the vertical recti is more likely to induce diplopia because the vertical fusion range is less than the horizontal. If diplopia occurs, removing the plombage early will usually alleviate the problem.

Note: the plombage can be removed as soon as the retinopexy has sealed the break, e.g. 10 days.

- Cosmesis, the plombage may be visible because of the anterior placement and the inferotemporal position of many dialyses.

Note: some surgeons because of the possibility of poor cosmesis use solid silicone explants but perform external drainage of SRF with its attendant risks.

- Trapped foveal SRF occurs because of the chronicity of the RRD.
- Failure of reattachment is rare if the indent is in the correct place, fish-mouthing (folding of the break on a circumferential indent) does not seem to happen. I have seen a dialysis held off the indent by two retinal cysts. The patient was re-operated with removal of the original indent and a radial plomb placed on the unattached area of the break between the two cysts.

Giant Retinal Dialysis

This is a rare presentation in which the dialysis is more than 90°. The presentation in my experience has occurred in patients with an odd traumatic history such as patients who may injure their own eyes, e.g. schizophrenia or patients who are under institutional care from neurological deficit (e.g. cerebral palsy). Non-drain surgery will not work in these and a PPV will be required. The PHM will need to be detached from the retina and the vitreous will removed over the break to gain access to the SRF through the dialysis. Take care when you have instruments at the site of the break because you are awfully close to the lens which can be damaged. Apply laser retinopexy and minimal cryotherapy, use a long-acting gas or silicone oil.

Dialysis and PVR

Subretinal bands are the commonest form of PVR in Dialysis. Mostly these will allow use of the non-drain procedure and settling of the RRD with minimal tenting of the retina. Occasionally more severe PVR is seen in grade C. This is exceedingly difficult to deal with and is usually seen with an odd presentation such as severe trauma and delay in diagnosis (e.g. in a child). Apply PVR techniques to treat (Chap. 7).

Par Ciliaris Tear

This is a rare form of dialysis in which the tear is in the pars plana. It occurs in severe blunt trauma and is usually seen in the superonasal quadrant. Consider the diagnosis in a child with a total shallow RRD of uncertain history (unfortunately a common presentation in children) which is of unknown duration. These breaks are difficult to see and diagnose and because of delay in presentation often accompanied with PVR. It is my only indication for an encircling explant, e.g. 360° 7 mm wide solid silicone explant with an encircling band. If you can see the break, apply retinopexy. If not use the explant on its own.

Surgical steps

- 360° conjunctival perimetry
- Sling all muscles.
- Search.
- Cryotherapy.
- Place four 5/0 polyester sutures spaced at 9 mm apart, one in each quadrant straddling the ora serrata.
- Insert the explant under the muscles and the sutures.
- Method 1.
  - Insert the 2 mm silicone band starting superotemporally and returning there.
  - Insert one end of the silicone band through a silicone sleeve, e.g. Watzke sleeve (place the sleeve on a curved artery clip and open the clip to expand the sleeve) then insert the other end of the band from the other direction. Close the forceps and slip off the sleeve.
  - Tighten the silicone band by pulling through about 1 cm.
- Method 2.
  - Suture the two ends of the solid silicone explant together (insert the needle and suture directly into the explant) with a nonabsorbable suture.
- Check you have a diffuse indent and the optic nerve is perfusing.
- Close.

Note: these retinas are difficult to fix a decision to perform PPV and oil must be taken very carefully. These eyes may have poor visual recovery, even if successful. They are cosmetically normal at presentation and relatively non-progressive because of shallow RRD and formed vitreous, therefore it may not be in your patient's best interests to pursue multiple operations with attendant cosmetic changes to the eye. Often these eyes are stable after surgery even with a persistent shallow total RRD and maintain some navigation vision. These young patients do not want the risk of an ugly phthisical eye from multiple operations.

Giant Retinal Tear

Clinical Features

(Fig. 9.6) A giant retinal tear (GRT) is defined as a tear of more than three clock hours of the retina (or 90°) with PVD with an incidence 0.091 per 100,000 in the UK [29], 1.5% of RRD [30]. The patients are often in the third to fifth decades of age, more often male and present early, frequently with the macula still on (55%) [29]. It is bilateral in 13%. The vitreous is detached from the posterior pole and is attached to the anterior portion of the retinal tear, thereby distinguishing a GRT from a dialysis. Because the posterior flap of the tear is not attached to the vitreous, this can fold over on itself onto the retina. In addition, there may be radial slits at either end of the tear extending posteriorly, which also aid the folding of the retina. There may be satellite U-shaped breaks elsewhere in the retina that should be searched for (Fig. 9.7).

Clinical features in GRT	
Sex	Females<males
Age	20–40 years
Refraction	Myopia
Bilaterality	13%
Onset	Fast
Vitreous	Detached
Retinal break type	More than 90 degrees
Retinal break size	Large
Retinal break position	Superior>inferior, temporal > nasal
Median number of breaks	1
Multiple breaks >1	15%
Fovea off	45%
Retinal degeneration	Lattice
PVR	Preretinal membranes
Surgery	Vitrectomy and long-acting gas or oil
Primary success rate	80–85%

A giant retinal tear may occur in isolation, usually in a myopic patient, but may also be present in hereditary vitreoretinal disorders such as Stickler's syndrome (14%) [31] or rarely in Marfan's syndrome [32]. In Sticker's syndrome, in particular, there is a risk of bilateral retinal tears up to 40%, and for this reason some surgeons advocate prophylactic 360° cryotherapy to the fellow eye [33]. A giant retinal tear can also occur as a result of trauma either penetrating or non-penetrating [34, 35]. It possible for the tear to appear during complicated anterior segment surgery when traction on the vitreous pulls on the vitreous base [36, 37]. A careless vitreoretinal surgeon may induce a GRT during insertion of instruments through the vitreous base at the pars plana.

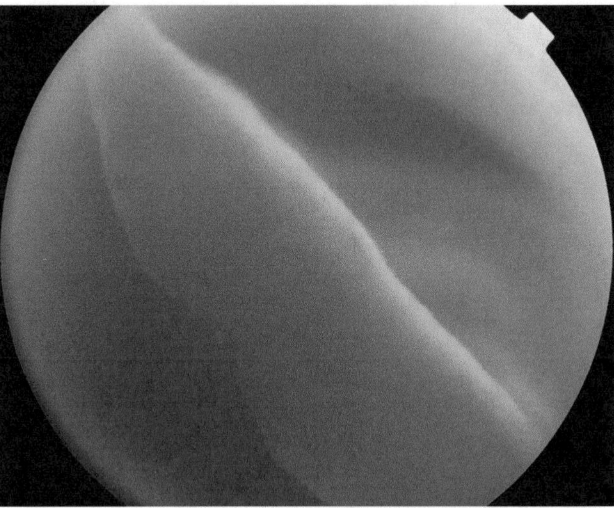

Fig. 9.6 Giant retinal tears can often fold over onto the posterior retina

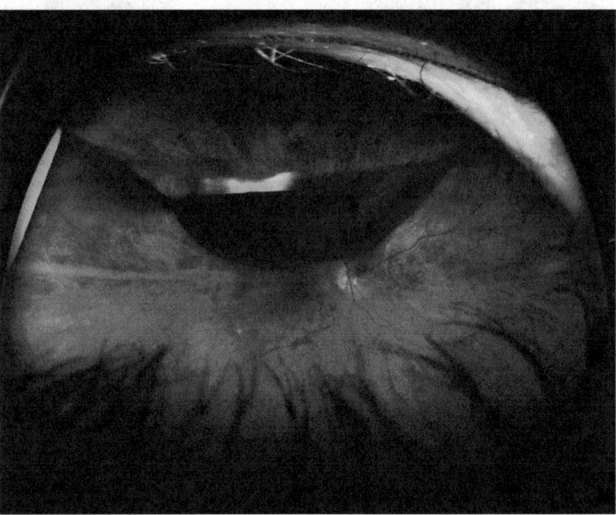

Fig. 9.7 A wide-angle view of a superior giant retinal tear

Stickler's Syndrome

(Figs. 9.8, 9.9, 9.10, 9.11, 9.12, 9.13, 9.14, 9.15, 9.16, and 9.17) This syndrome is characterised by myopia, paravascular pigmentary changes, dragging of the major vessels at the optic disc, "veils" or condensations of cortical vitreous around large lacunae or dehiscence's in the gel and multiple posterior vitreoretinal adhesions. Differentiation from the Wagner syndrome is dubious. Stickler's syndrome has an autosomal dominant inheritance and has highly variable penetrance. A possible genetic abnormality has been identified at COL2A1 [38–40]. Systemic associations are very variable and include high palate, characteristic facies with a flattened nasal bridge, short mandible and long philtre, and arthralgia [41]. Retinal detachments are related to posterior paravascu-

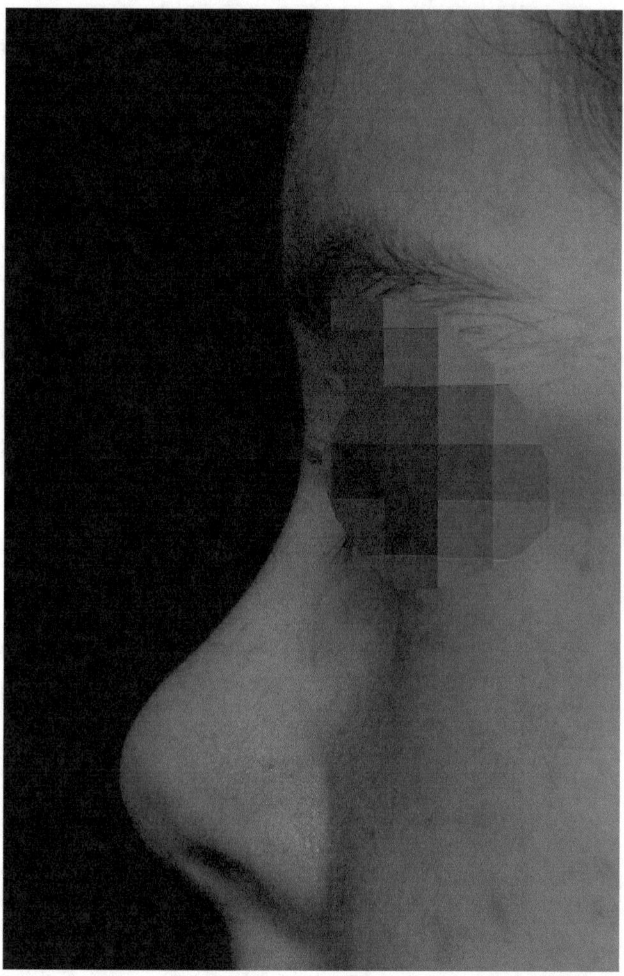

Fig. 9.8 The flattened nasal bridge typical of Stickler's syndrome

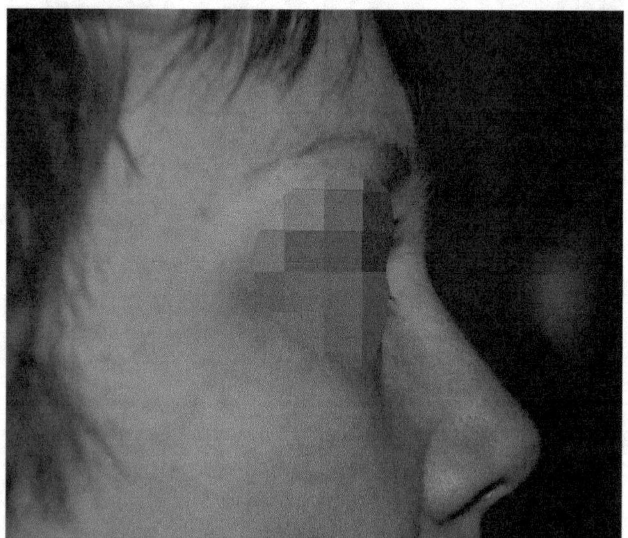

Fig. 9.9 The flattened nasal bridge in Stickler's syndrome

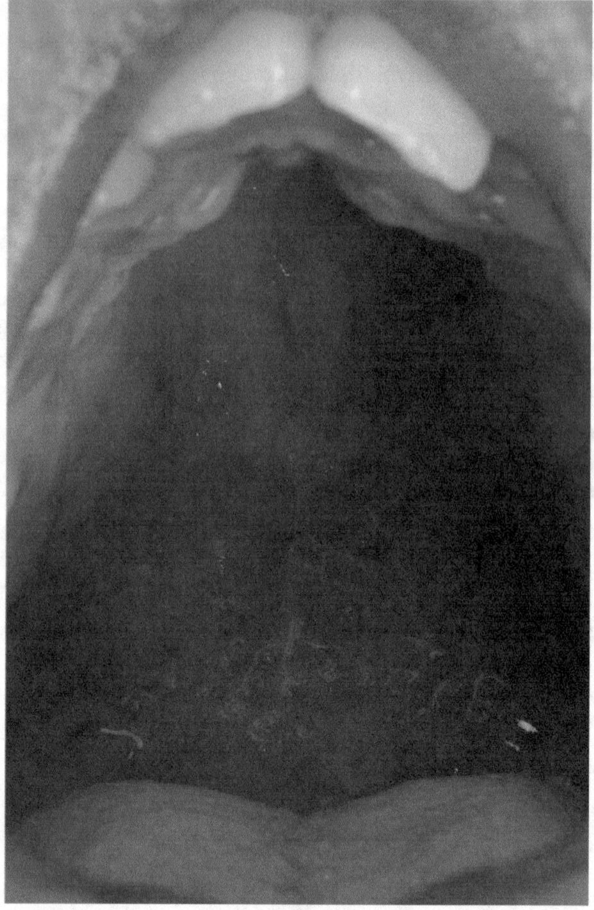

Fig. 9.10 A high arched palate in Stickler's syndrome

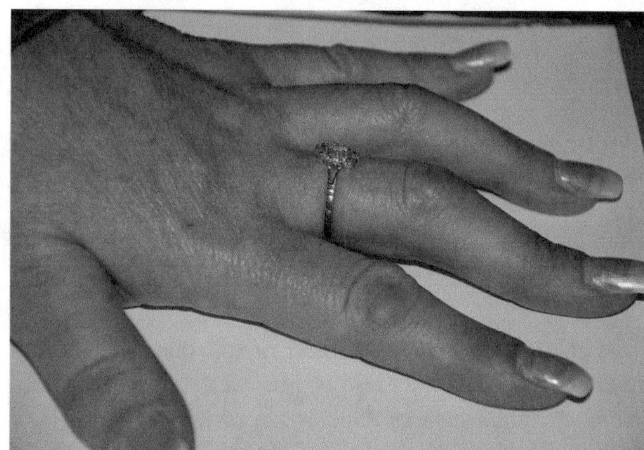

Fig. 9.11 Arthropathy in Stickler's syndrome

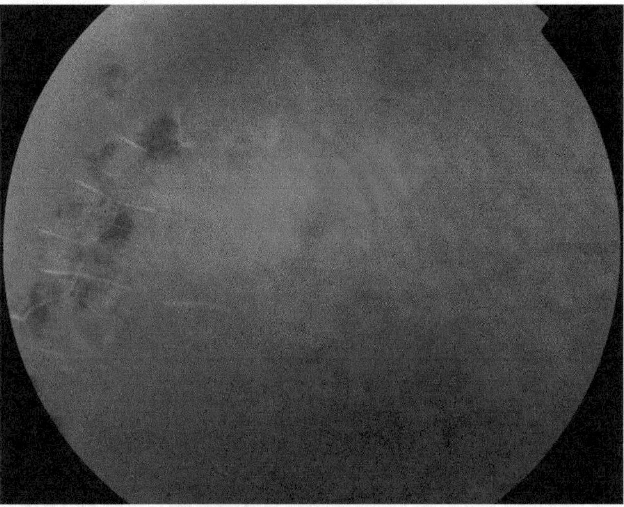

Fig. 9.12 Lattice degeneration in a patient with Stickler's syndrome/

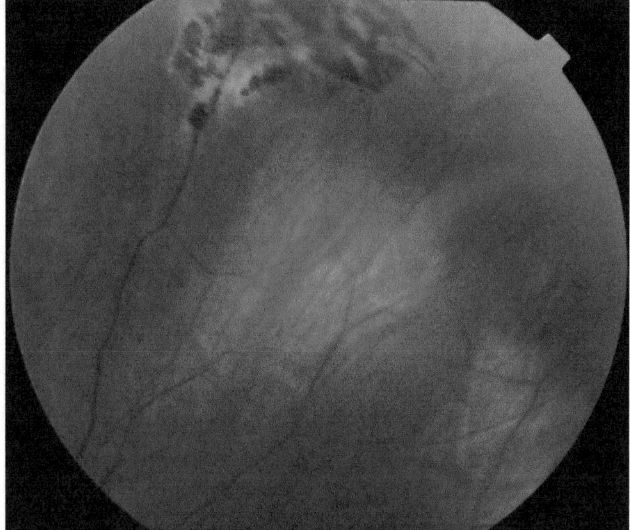

Fig. 9.13 Lattice is seen around a blood vessel typically in Stickler's syndrome

lar vitreoretinal adhesions or to radially orientated post-equatorial lattice degeneration. Bilateral giant retinal tears are common (Figs. 9.18 and 9.19).

Surgery for Giant Retinal Tear (Table 9.3)

Additional Surgical Steps.

1. Insert heavy liquids.
2. Apply laser retinopexy under heavy liquid tamponade.
3. Exchange silicone oil (air then gas if a small, 90-180°, superior GRT is present) for heavy liquid.
4. Apply further retinopexy as required.

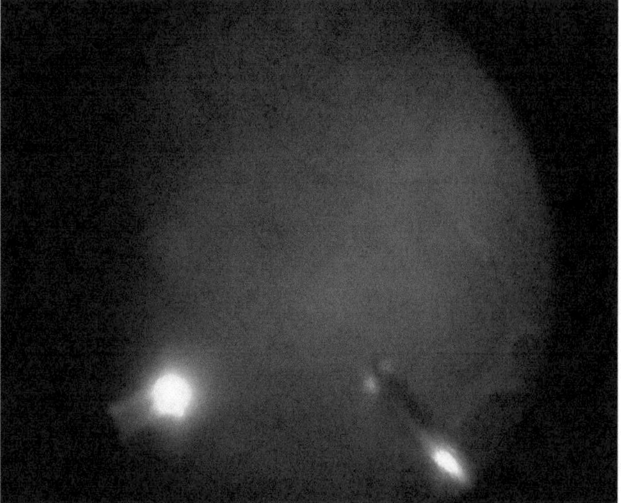

Fig. 9.14 The vitreous in Stickler's syndrome has veils of condensed vitreous within an otherwise optically empty vitreous cavity

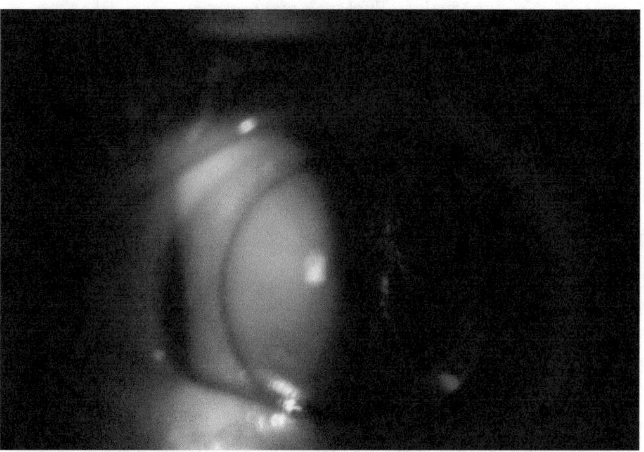

Fig. 9.15 Vitreous veils are seen in these images from a father and son with Stickler's syndrome

Vitrectomy has been used for many years for giant retinal tears [42–47] but recent innovations have considerably facilitated the manipulation of the retina.

Heavy Liquids

Insert heavy liquids (perfluorocarbon liquids) into the eye to unfold the flap of retina and to stabilise the retina [48–54]. Advance the heavy liquid up to the posterior edge of the tear: advancing over the tear risks allowing a droplet of heavy liquid to enter under the retina, however, if there is no traction on the edge of the tear this is unlikely. Use of heavy liquid minimises the risk of slippage of the retina (to 7% in one study [55]). Search 360° in case there are satellite U tears that need treatment as well. If the giant retinal tear is relatively posterior, you may be able to flatten the retina with the heavy

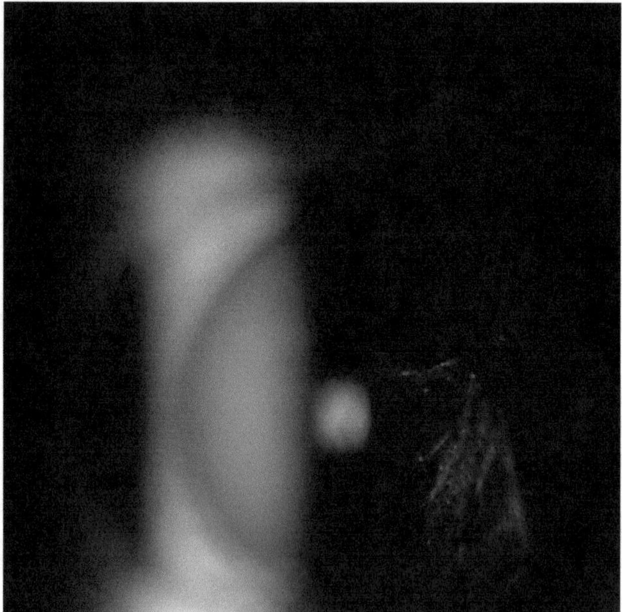

Fig. 9.16 Vitreous veils in Stickler's syndrome

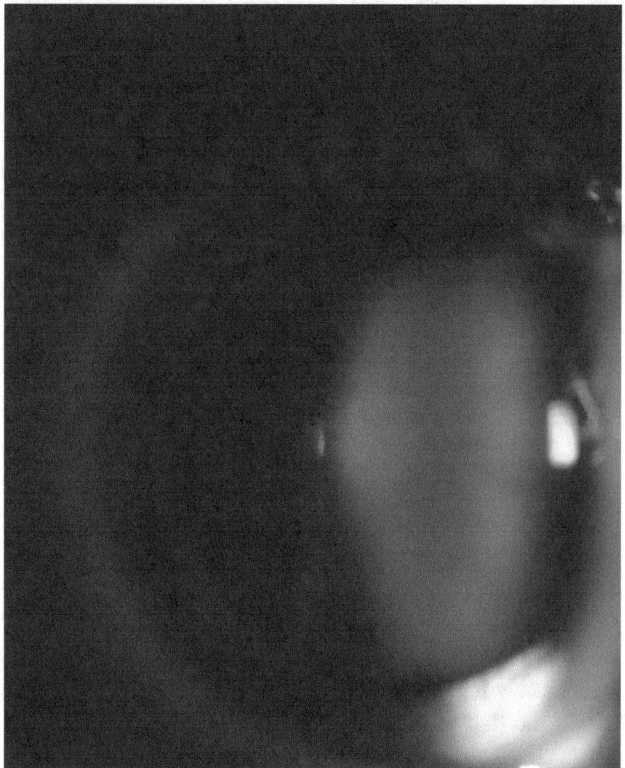

Fig. 9.17 Some vitreoretinal surgeons claim that there is a form of Stickler's syndrome which does not have optically clear vitreous but has a membrane in the anterior vitreous as in this image

liquids and apply laser therapy under heavy liquids. This will provide slightly improved optical properties over trying to do this under the silicone oil. However, occasionally the giant retinal tear is very anterior, and to fill the eye fully with heavy

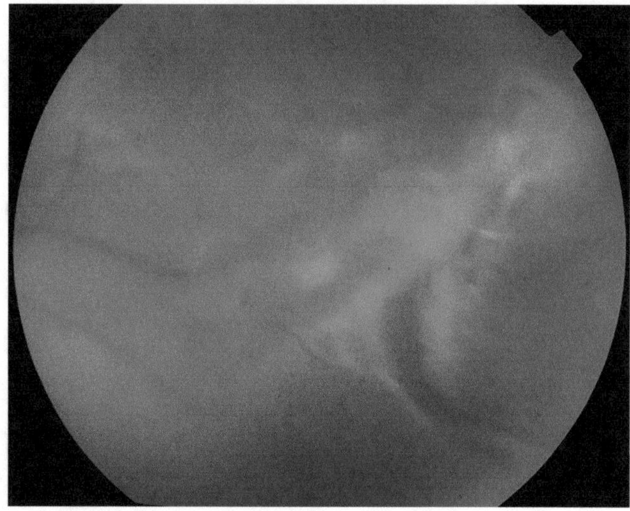

Fig. 9.18 A retinal tear near lattice in Stickler's syndrome

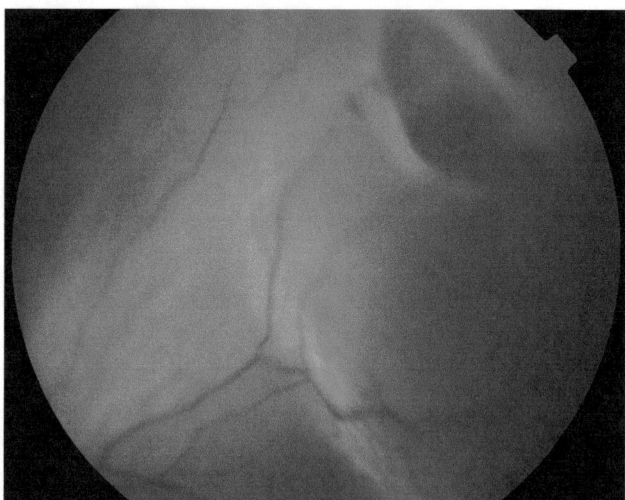

Fig. 9.19 A retinal tear in Stickler's syndrome

Table 9.3 difficulty rating of PPV for GRT

Difficulty Rating	Moderate
Success rates	High
Complication rates	Medium
When to use in training	Middle

liquids runs the risk of leaving bubbles of heavy liquid at the vitreous base. These will be seen by the patient postoperatively when lying supine (the bubbles sink onto the fovea) and may enter the anterior chamber and be droplets lying in the inferior angle (Figs. 9.20, 9.21, 9.22 and 9.23).

Retinopexy

Apply endolaser to the posterior edge of the giant retinal tear and around the ends, and anteriorly if the tear is posterior. If the tear is very anteriorly placed, apply laser to the edge,

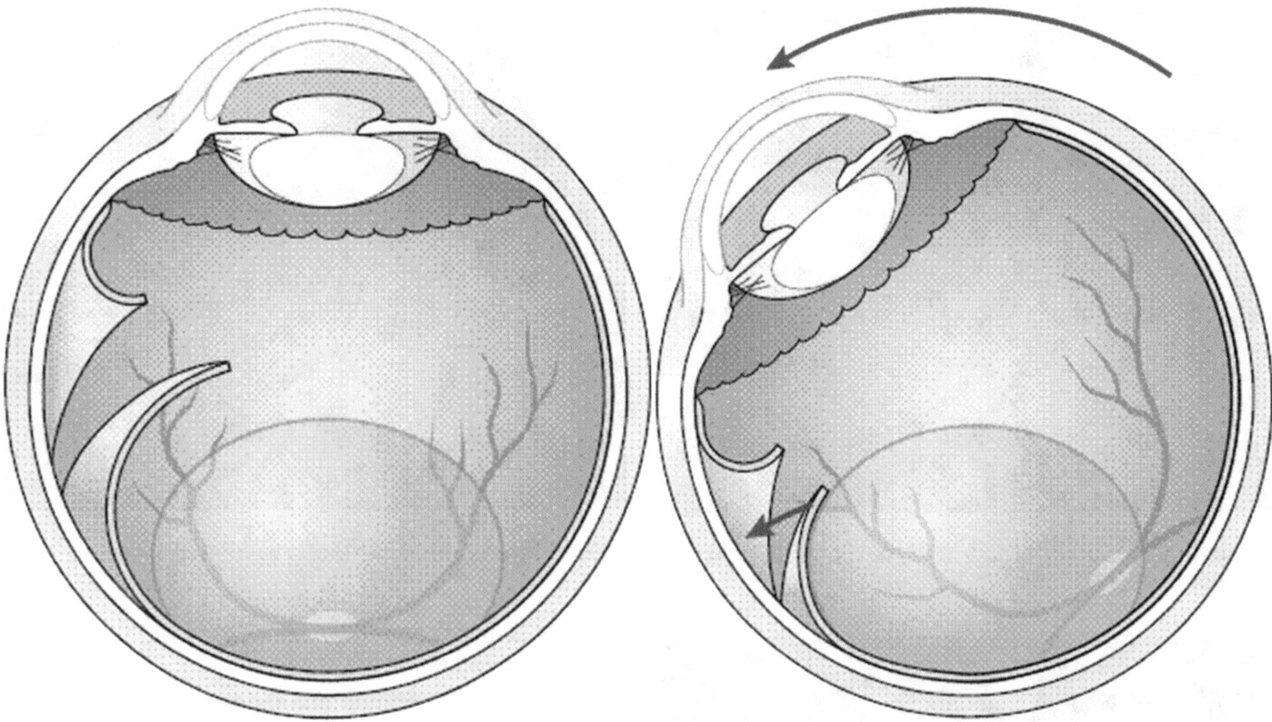

Fig. 9.20 Heavy liquids placed onto the retina can be rolled with the eye to unfold a GRT

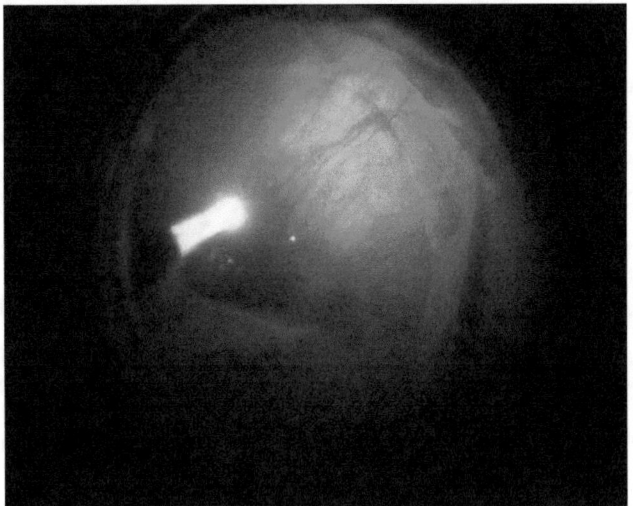

Fig. 9.21 The GRT can be flattened by the heavy liquid

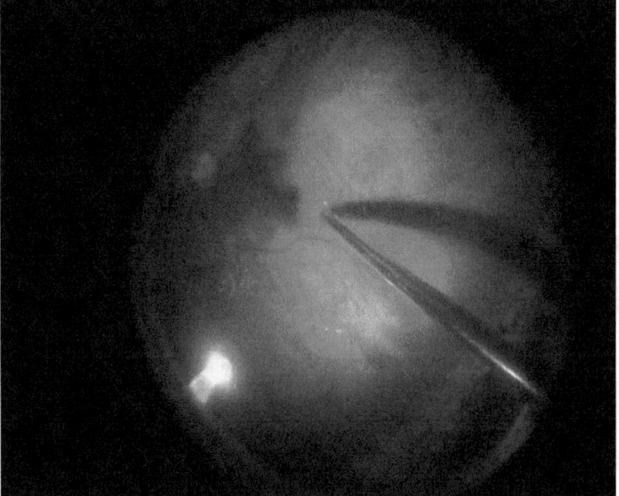

Fig. 9.22 Heavy liquid can be used to open the retina in GRT. Laser can be applied under the heavy liquid

around the ends, and up to the ora serrata, without applying laser to the anterior flap. Check that you have reached the ora serrata by indenting the retina after the laser.

The ends of the giant retinal tear and the anterior edge may be more difficult to treat because most of these patients are phakic.

There are three options that can be employed.

- One is to apply cryotherapy to the ends in the same manner as a retinectomy (one or two burns at each end should be enough). The cryotherapy probe has the advantage of allowing simultaneous indentation to push the peripheral retina into view. Its use as always should be kept to a minimum to avoid excessive dispersion of retinal pigment epithelial cells into the vitreous cavity thereby risking PVR [56].
- Use a curved laser probe and ask an assistant to indent the peripheral retina. This runs the risk of the assistant moving the indent during your retinopexy resulting in a retinal scrape.
- Alternatively perform trans-scleral illumination (Figs. 9.24 and 9.25).

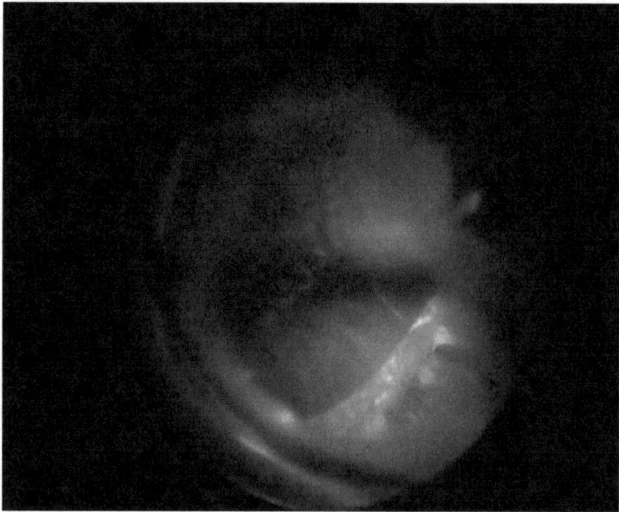

Fig. 9.23 Insert oil on top of the heavy liquid whilst draining residual SRF from the edge of the GRT

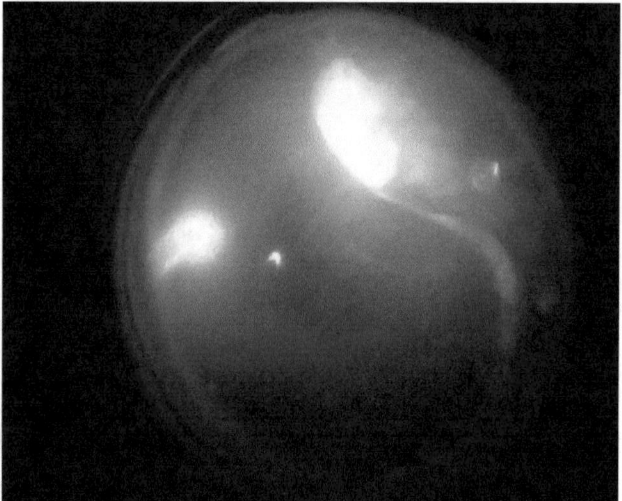

Fig. 9.24 In a phakic patient cryotherapy with indentation can be used to seal the ends of the tear

Trans-Scleral Illumination Technique

The surgeon performs indentation of the external sclera with the bullet fibre optic light, which will provide illumination of the retina through the sclera.

1. Before starting, identify with endo-illumination which retina has already lasered.
2. Establish the area which requires treatment.
3. Point the laser probe at the unlasered retina.
4. Remove the light pipe.
5. Press the light pipe onto the sclera to indent the appropriate retina.

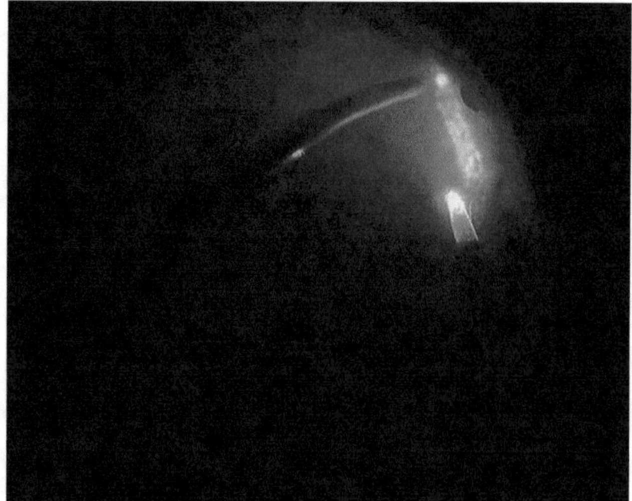

Fig. 9.25 Laser is applied to the posterior edge of the GRT

6. Laser around the anterior edge of the break.
7. Remove the laser probe.
8. With endo-illumination and indentation with a squint hook check that the retina has been treated correctly.

Note: using the bullet light pipe to indent prevents the problems of indentation using an assistant. However, the retinal laser burns are not well seen during this manoeuvre. The surgeon must remember where the treatment was placed by using retinal landmarks and subconscious awareness of the of the 3-dimensional structure of the eye.

Check the retina with endo-illumination, to make sure that the laser uptake has been adequate.

Silicone Oil or Long-Acting Gas Insertion

Perform an exchange of silicone oil for the heavy liquids, allowing the oil to enter the eye, whilst draining subretinal fluid and peripheral fluid from the giant retinal tear. The heavy liquids will contact the silicone oil, spreading a doughnut of subretinal fluid and vitreous cavity fluid to the periphery, which then can be drained at the edge of the giant retinal tear. Theoretically this manoeuvre is more effective with silicone oil / heavy liquid exchange than gas / heavy liquid exchange [57] therefore a direct oil / heavy exchange is recommended.

Eventually there is no subretinal fluid or vitreous cavity fluid to be drained, and the heavy liquids can be removed. Remember to remove the heavy liquid in one movement, thereby avoiding losing its location as the bubble of heavy liquid contracts. If a "stop and start" method is used, it is possible to lose sight of the heavy liquid especially as it gets smaller in size.

Surgical Pearl

How to Avoid and Tackle Slippage during Air/Perfluorocarbon Exchange in Giant Retinal Tear

In the case of Giant retinal tear, the first step of the surgery is to remove the vitreous and make the retina freely mobile. Moreover, the residual peripheral edge of the tear edge is also cut as far as possible to reduce the chances of PVR in the future. At this stage Perfluorocarbon liquid is injected and filled up to the brim to flatten the retina till beyond the edges of the tear. Once a good fill is achieved, a 360-degree laser barrage of 3 rows is carried out especially taking care that the edges of the tear are flat.

Now one could either do a direct PFCL-Silicon oil exchange or do a two-step exchange switching to air first and then silicon oil. I prefer the two-step approach. Whilst doing this exchange there is a chance that some fluid accumulates under the edges of the tear and leads to slippage and can create folds in the retina potentially leading to eventual failure of the surgery.

To avoid this slippage, one must carefully apply the following steps

1. When the air PFCL exchange starts one must use the cutter in aspiration mode just above the meniscus of PFCL and make sure that the space is totally devoid of fluid and is replaced with air.
2. Gradual aspiration of the PFCL should be done in the periphery near the edges of the giant tear as well as 360 degrees instead of going towards the disc as one would do for regular retinal detachments. Once again this should be done patiently, and 2–3 times circumvent the periphery with aspiration.
3. Once the PFCL meniscus reduces up to the edges of the tear, once again make sure that the edges are dry before aspirating the PFCL further.
4. Only when the edges are dry then the residual PFCL can be aspirated, finally going down till the last drop of PFCL is aspirated from the posterior pole.
5. Usually if one meticulously follows the above steps, the chances of slippage are almost nil. In case one does encounter a mild slippage at this stage, then the best way is to refill PFCL to iron out the fold and carefully retrace the above steps. (Another tip at this stage is that if the slippage starts, then one could stop aspirating further and inject silicon oil in the space above the PFCL and then in a graded way just do passive extrusion of the PFCL and then fill the rest of silicon oil. This graded step also irons out a mild slippage if it is starting to occur, however, this would not work if most of the PFCL is out and the slippage is significant. In that case of course you would need to refill PFCL as I mentioned earlier.)
6. After this, silicon oil is injected in the air-filled cavity.

Dr Manish Nagpal, Retina Foundation, Ahmedabad, India

Choice of Endotamponade

Many surgeons will use silicone oil as the preferred tamponade; however, if the GRT is less than 180° perfluorocarbon gas can be used [58, 59] especially if the GRT is superiorly located. Failure with gas can lead to a high risk of PVR whilst silicone oil can cause toxicity and other well-known complications. In studies no difference in outcomes has been seen between gas and oil and addition of scleral buckles does not add to success [30]. Attempts to use perfluorocarbon liquids for postoperative tamponade seem to be associated with reduced primary retinal reattachment rates of approximately 50% [60, 61]. Scleral buckling has also been used as an addition to PPV and intraocular tamponade but is usually not necessary in the primary procedure [62, 63].

Success Rates

These are high for reattachment of the retina at 87% primary and 95% secondary success [29, 30] although visual acuities are affected by epiretinal membrane and postoperative cataract.

Removal of the Silicone Oil

The silicone oil can be removed at two to four months after the surgery, at which point it is recommended to re-inspect the giant retinal tear internally and treat any portions of the tear which have retracted beyond the retinopexy or for which retinopexy has been inadequate.

The Other Eye

Some surgeons have advocated 360° laser retinopexy in the unaffected eye because of the risk of bilaterality of 13% overall and 40% in Sticklers syndrome [64, 65]. The evidence for treatment of the fellow eye is uncertain because of the structure of previous studies [66, 67]. Historically the reported bilateral rate of GRTs is high, especially in Stickler's syndrome (25-40%). Application of 360° cryotherapy has been reported to reduce this incidence to 6–10% in retrospective studies [33, 65]. If applied, the hope is that the cryotherapy will restrict movement of a giant retinal tear if it occurs anterior to the laser. However, the procedure does have some risks of its own, and therefore it is not universally recommended.

Retinal Detachment in High Myopes

See chapter **.

Retinoschisis Related Retinal Detachment

Clinical Features (Figs. 9.26, 9.27, 9.28, 9.29, 9.30, 9.31, 9.32, and 9.33)

The term retinoschisis refers to a process whereby fluid accumulates within the retinal neuroepithelium to form a large intraretinal cyst. The cyst cavity has an inner leaf and an outer leaf. Breaks may develop in one or both leaves. When fluid passes through an inner leaf break and then an outer leaf break, the outer layer detaches from the pigment epithelium and the schisis is said to have progressed to a retinal detachment. Occasionally the fluid in the schisis can enter the subretinal space through the outer leaf break (without an inner leaf break) and very slowly lift the retina giving a slow onset retinal detachment. This can on occasion be treated by laser to the outer leaf breaks causing slow resolution of the retinal detachment.

Retinoschises are classically divided into "infantile" and senile varieties.

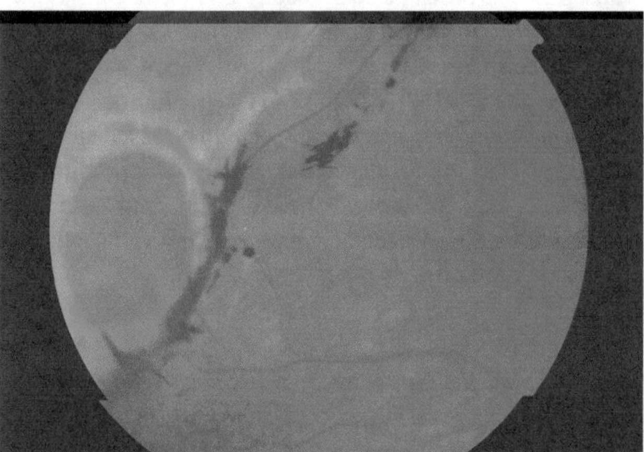

Fig. 9.26 Outer leaf breaks in retinoschisis can become pigmented

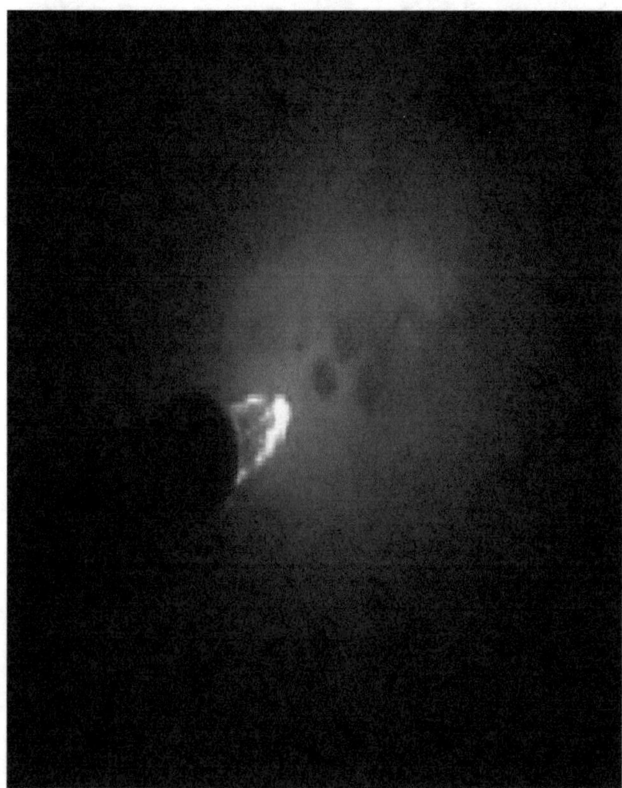

Fig. 9.27 Inner leaf breaks in a retinoschisis

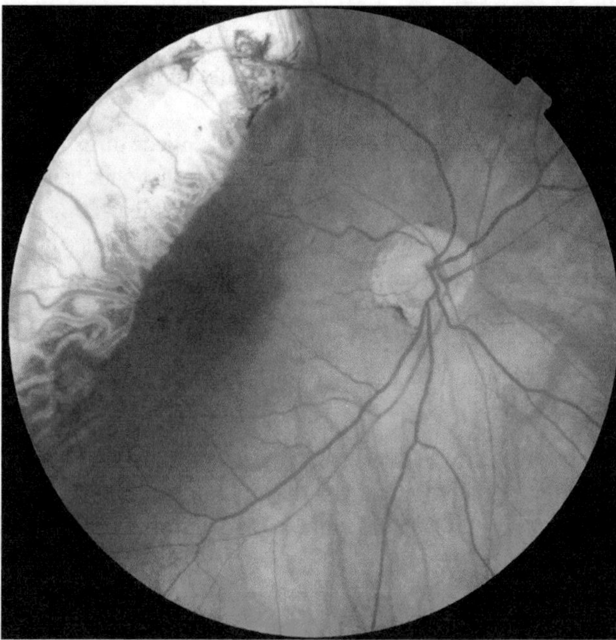

Fig. 9.28 The coloboma from deroofing of a retinoschisis RRD 10 years after the surgery

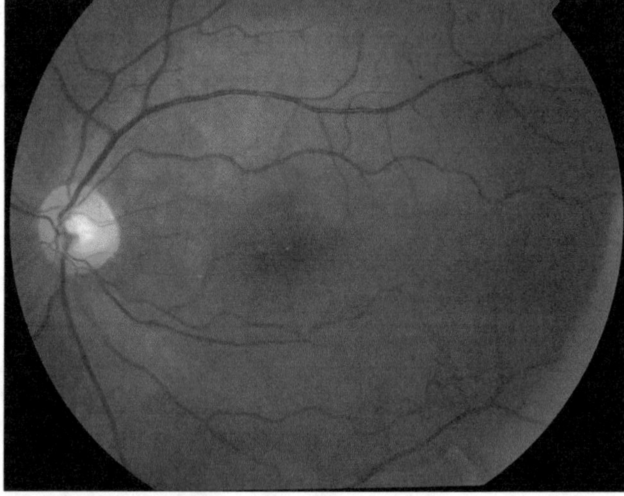

Fig. 9.29 The leading edge of a retinoschisis RD in which the SRF has come from the schisis cavity lifting the outer leaf breaks. There are no inner leaf breaks so that fluid accumulation is terribly slow

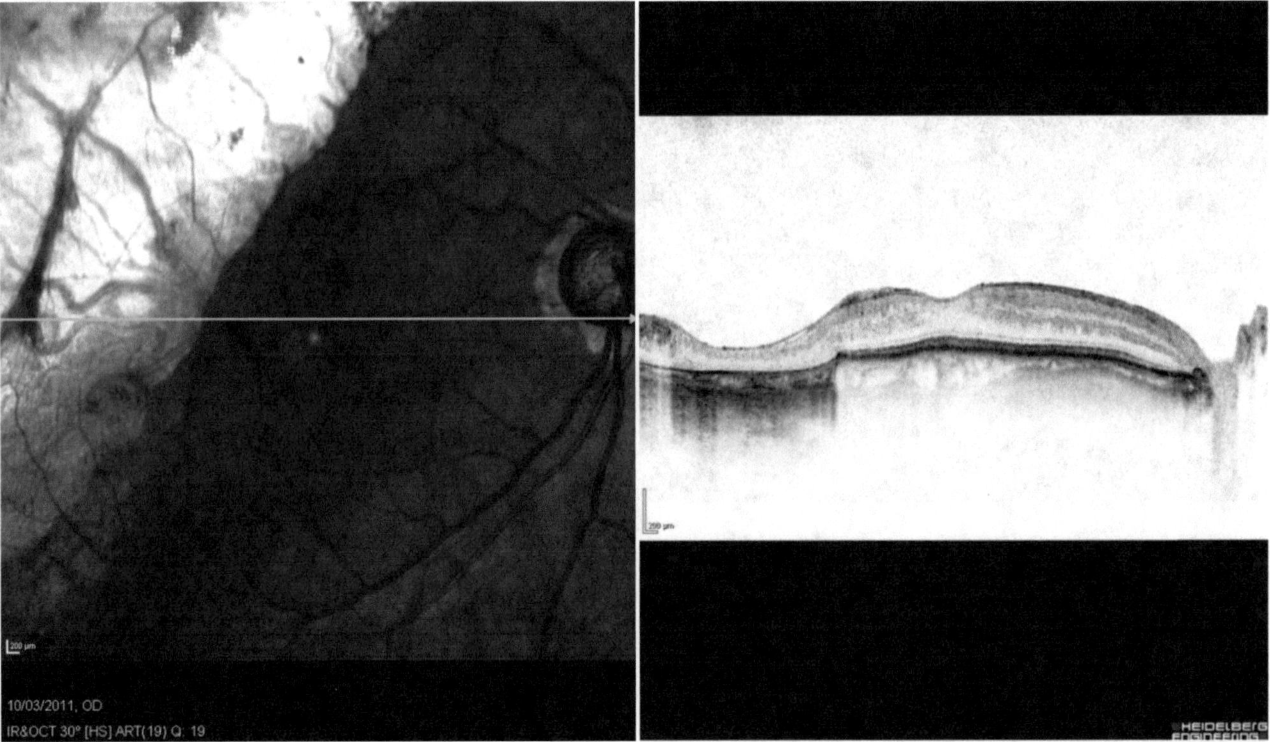

Fig. 9.30 A postoperative retinoschisis RRD in which the schisis was deroofed. The OCT of the fovea is seen ten years after surgery with 6/18 vision

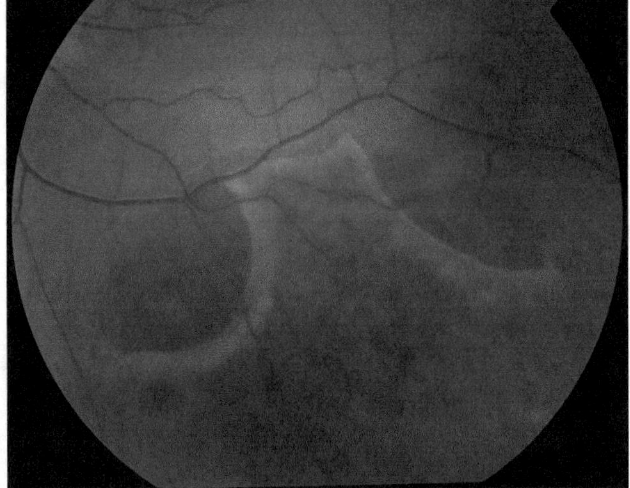

Fig. 9.31 Outer leaf breaks in retinoschisis

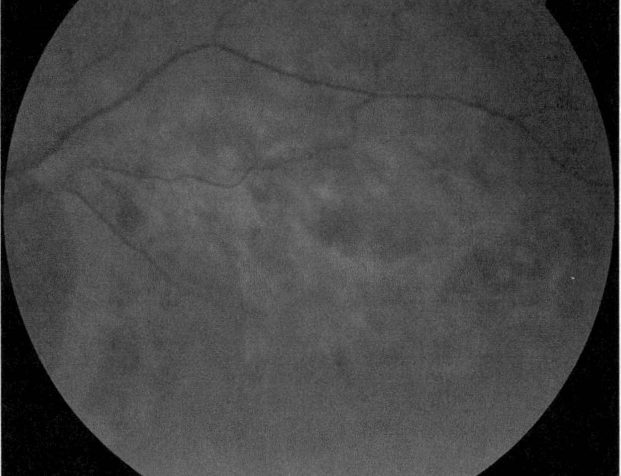

Fig. 9.32 Laser to the edge of the outer leaf breaks was enough to cause flattening of the retinal detachment over 18 months

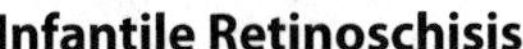

Infantile Retinoschisis

Infantile retinoschisis is a rare disorder with an "X-linked recessive" mode of inheritance, therefore affecting young males, and must be considered in the differential diagnosis when a young boy presents with retinal elevation. A common presentation is vitreous haemorrhage, whilst central vision may be impaired by associated foveal schisis. The inner leaf may be extremely thin because the split in the retina is at the level of the ganglion cells, with large breaks between the blood vessels. Progression to true rhegmatogenous retinal detachment is unusual. Resolution of the macular schisis with restoration of the foveal dip has been

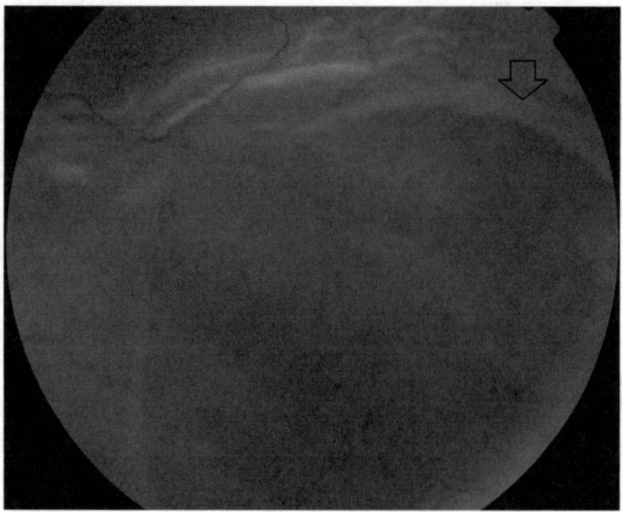

Fig. 9.33 A retinoschisis RRD showing the edge of an outer leaf break

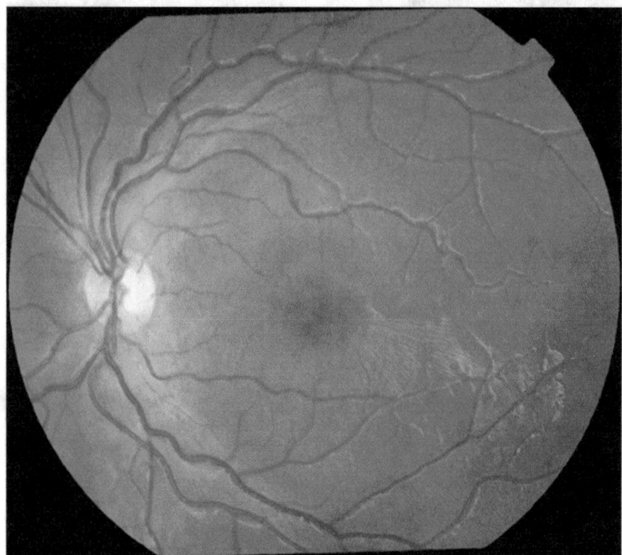

Fig. 9.34 Subtle cart-wheel maculopathy in XL schisis

described in a few patients after PPV [68] (Figs. 9.34, 9.35, and 9.36).

Senile Retinoschisis

Senile retinoschisis occurs after middle age, is usually bilateral, tends to be located inferotemporally and is frequently discovered during routine examination of the peripheral fundus or even during PPV for other pathologies (when the schisis can be ignored). It is probably commoner in hypermetropes. The split in the retina is in the outer plexiform layer and therefore the inner leaf is relatively thick. The outer leaf of the schisis often has a grey translucency with a mottled pattern. Outer leaf breaks tend to be large with rolled edges and may be pigmented, whilst inner leaf breaks are generally small and round. Most schisis will remain stable and no intervention is required unless RRD occurs [69–74].

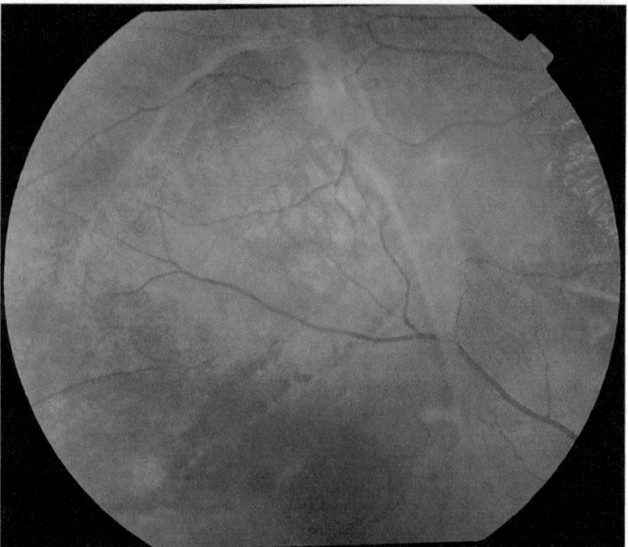

Fig. 9.35 XL retinoschisis has a very diaphanous inner layer. Occasionally these patients develop retinal detachment as shown here with OCT confirming SRF

Differentiation of Retinoschisis from Chronic Rhegmatogenous Retinal Detachment

Differentiation from chronic retinal detachment (usually atrophic round hole RRD) may be difficult and primarily relies on experience and the ability of the observer to differentiate detached retina from the thinner inner leaf. Other features help, however, see Table.

A demarcation line, often seen in chronic retinal detachment, may occasionally be seen in retinoschisis where haemorrhage into the cyst has occurred.

Laser photocoagulation applied to the outer wall of a retinoschisis produces a typical blanching retinal burn (in contrast, in a retinal detachment a poor reaction is seen because only retinal pigment epithelium is present on the outer wall) (Table 9.4).

Retinal Detachment in Retinoschisis

Occasionally a retinal detachment is seen advancing from the schisis, this advancing edge should consist of the full-thickness of the retina and not an increase in split retina, i.e. the schisis itself. The appearance of the retina should show a line where the thin inner leaf joins the thicker (and more opaque) full-thickness retina. OCT can be used to differentiate the schitic retina from the full-thickness elevated retina if the elevation is extending posteriorly.

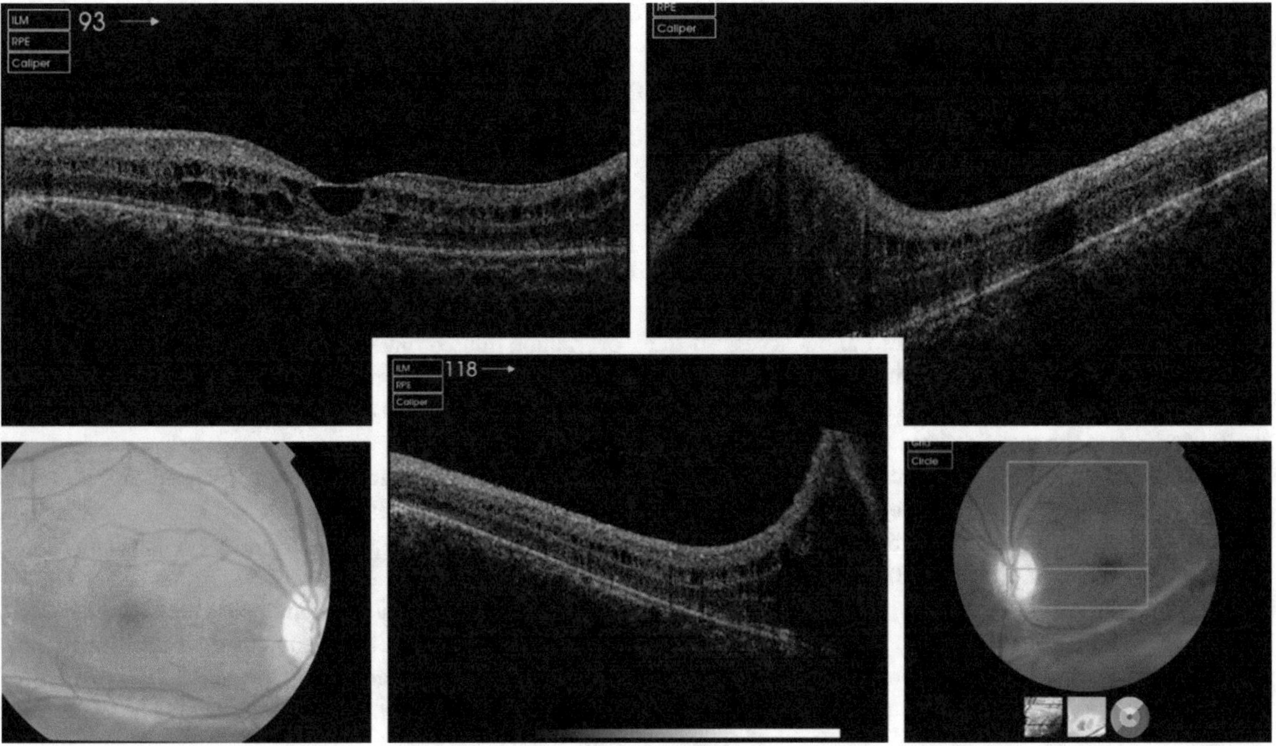

Fig. 9.36 XL retinoschisis with macular schisis and an encroaching peripheral schisis

Table 9.4 comparison between chronic RRD and retinoschisis

Retinoschisis	Chronic retinal detachment
Retina moves inward on indentation	Retina does not move inwards
Outer leaf breaks and retina on outer surface visible	Bare RPE on outer wall
Absolute visual field defect, patient cannot see indentor when placed in front of indirect ophthalmoscope illumination	Relative visual field defect, patient can see T bar of indentor
Patient unaware of visual field loss	Patient aware of area of field loss
Often hyperopic	Often myopic
No pigment in vitreous	Pigment in the vitreous
Usually no pigmented demarcation line (unless there has previously been a bleed into the cyst)	Demarcation line sometimes present
Typical laser burns can be produced in the outer wall (because of the presence of retina)	Laser burns cannot be produced

Two types are described:

- A slowly progressive elevation of the retina at the edge of the schisis thought to be from egress of the fluid in the cyst cavity through the outer leaf breaks and into the subretinal space. There is no communication from the vitreous cavity to the subretinal space because there are no inner leaf breaks. These can be observed. Lincoff in unpublished work has described resolution of these after 48 hrs of double eye padding reputably to reduce eye movements followed by laser to the outer breaks to prevent re-accumulation of fluid.
- More commonly there is a rapid onset RRD in a schisis which has inner and outer leaf breaks. Vitreous cavity fluid can enter the subretinal space producing a more rapid accumulation of SRF. These will require surgery.

Table 9.5 Difficulty rating of surgery for retinoschisis

Difficulty Rating	High
Success rates	Low
Complication rates	Medium
When to use in training	Late

Surgery (Table 9.5)

This is a surgical challenge. The principle of closure of retinal breaks either outer leaf or the inner leaf applies. The inner breaks are usually only a few and small. If the RRD is shallow and the inner holes can be closed onto a scleral indent, then a non-drain approach can be used.

Note: the holes must be flat on the indent (unlike RRD) for non-drain repair to work (as far as we know!).

These inner breaks do not respond to retinopexy and are reliant upon the effect of the indent alone.

More commonly the schisis is too elevated to buckle and a PPV is required [75–79]. The outer leaf breaks can then be flattened and treated with endolaser and internal tamponade. This often means extensive laser as the outer breaks are large and often their extent is not obvious.

Note: the retina of the outer leaf is fragile and liable to contract with heavy laser therefore apply carefully to avoid increasing the size of the outer breaks.

The inner retina is often slightly short but seems to settle if the outer leaf breaks are sealed. A deroofing method whereby the inner leaf is removed to allow access to the outer layer has been used but seems unnecessary. PVR if present results in a reduction in success rate. If the schisis itself extends into the macula visual recovery will not occur even with flattening of the retina because the nerve fibres in the retina have been severed. Juvenile XL retinoschisis rarely needs surgery but some have described surgical approaches [80–83] (Figs. 9.28, 9.29, 9.30, 9.31, 9.32, 9.37, 9.38 and 9.39).

Surgical Pearl

Check the Relatives' Retinas

In piecing the puzzle together, clinicians should always be cautious of avoiding bias even during examinations. In a difficult case it is easy to "imagine" signs to make the pieces fit. Always endeavour to look further. There are numerous hereditary conditions in which (sometimes), even a cursory examination of the relatives gives away the diagnosis. Conversely, anyone with an apparent hereditary condition should always receive genetic counselling and be alerted to inform the family members to have an eye examination.

A 2-year old boy was referred for not being able to focus on objects or ambulate independently. On examination anterior segments were normal with no RAPD, however, upon dilated fundoscopy it was immediately obvious that he had bilateral temporal giant retinal tears with a macula-involving RRD in the right eye and macula-sparing RD in the left.

Upon further questioning it was gleaned that he had 3 other brothers; an 8-year old who had had bilateral scleral buckles for RD 2 years prior and had cystic macular changes noted on prior OCT scans. The eldest brother had no significant history and a clinical examination was unremarkable. The youngest brother, age 6 months, had no known problems, however an examination revealed the presence of bilateral inferior retinoschises with no outer leaf breaks (Fig. 9.40).

This scenario illustrates the importance of taking a good family history, especially in children who may have atypical or late presentations thus making it difficult to discern subtle clinical signs. As in these cases, the findings in the siblings shed light on the primary aetiology in the index case thus

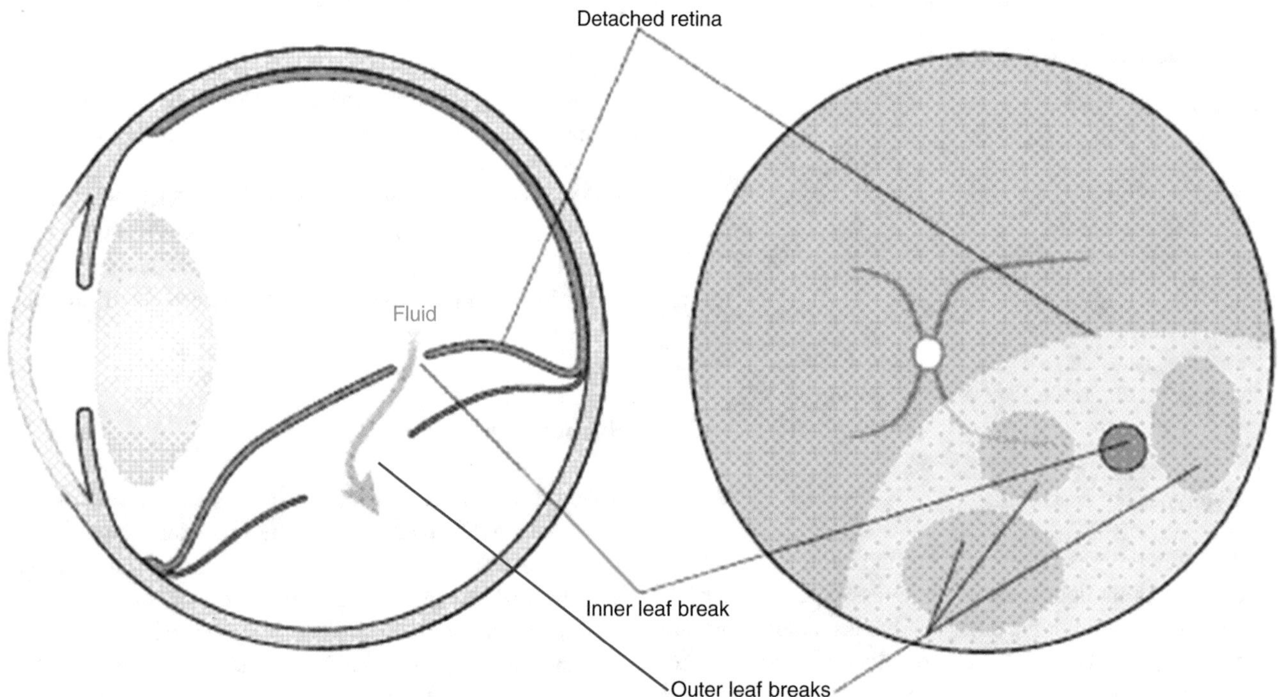

Fig. 9.37 Retinoschisis retinal detachments occur when a communication occurs between the vitreous cavity and the subretinal space. This happens when an inner leaf break is present in conjunction with outer leaf breaks, allowing fluid to pass from the vitreous cavity to the subretinal space

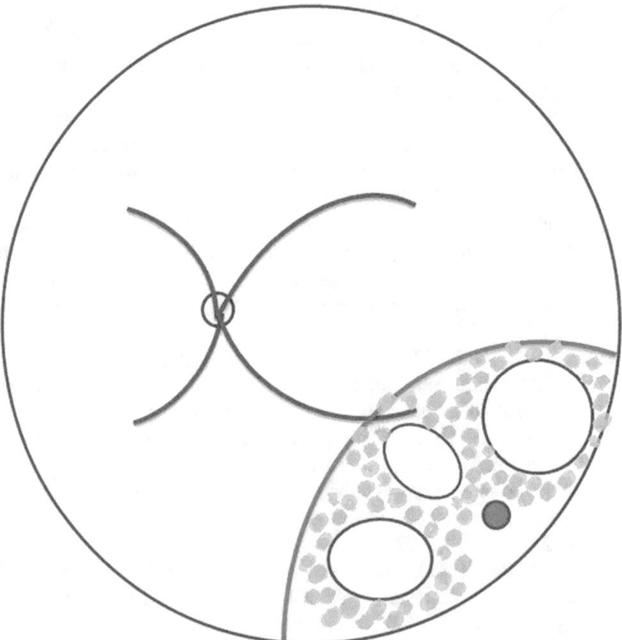

Fig. 9.38 Apply laser around the outer leaf holes in schisis RRD

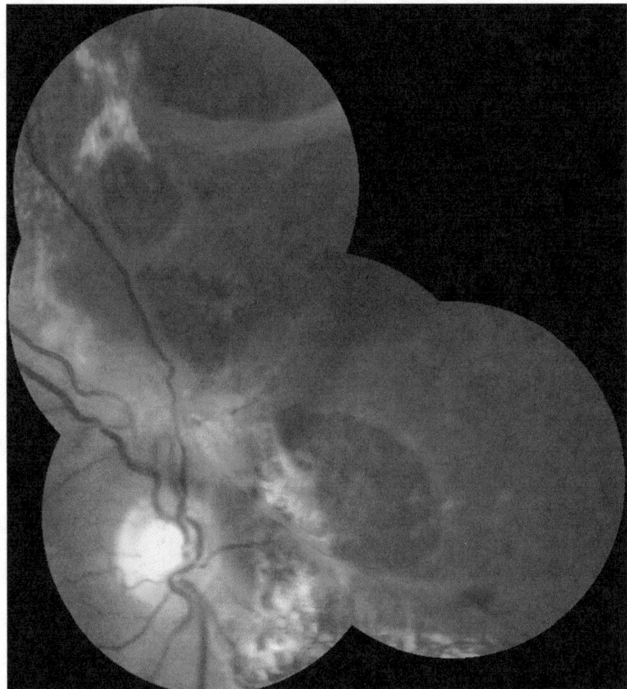

Fig. 9.39 This retinoschisis RRD has been reattached. There is extensive laser retinopexy to the outer leaf breaks

aiding in optimal management and providing the family with more precise and realistic prognostication. It is also imperative to ensure genetic counselling is undertaken to ensure other members of the family are screened and treated in a timely fashion.

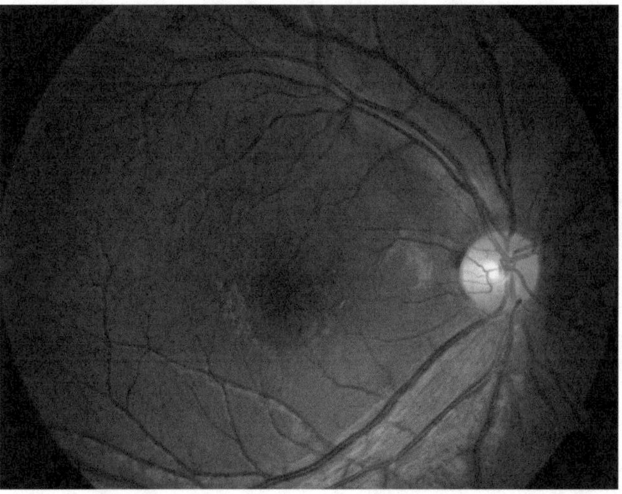

Fig. 9.40 A relative's macula shows signs of XLRS with spokes in the fovea

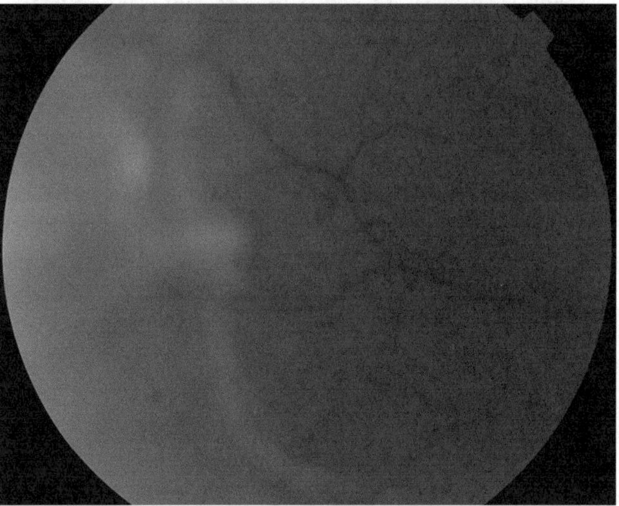

Fig. 9.41 A young chronic RRD treated with encirclage

Dr Manoharan Shunmugam, Pantai Hospital, Kuala Lumpur, Malaysia

Juvenile Retinal Detachment

Children occasionally present with RRD usually with a predisposing factor such as trauma, high myopia, Stickler's syndrome, previous intraocular surgery, familial exudative vitreoretinopathy, uveitis and previous retinopathy of prematurity [84, 85]. The frequency of bilateral vision threatening abnormalities in these patients is reportedly high at 89% [86]. PVR rates are also high (40%) because of slow presentation. Both final retinal reattachment rates and visual acuity outcomes are lower than for adult surgery.

Be aware that a pars ciliaris tear may be present in a shallow total RRD without a good history of trauma. (Fig. 9.41).

Atopic Dermatitis

This has been associated with RRD in 2.2% of patients in Japan [87] with a high incidence of cataract and PVR.

Refractive Surgery

Although RRD has been described associated with LASIK [88], the causal relationship remains uncertain with only 17 patients having RRD from 1 to 36 months after LASIK out of 31,739 patients treated in one study [89].

Congenital Cataract

Patients with prior surgery for congenital cataract may present with RRD. Employ the usual methods. PPV is often favoured because of the ability to deal with residual medial opacities.

Others

RRD can complicate many other conditions which are more fully described elsewhere in this text. Any condition which causes posterior vitreous detachment in the presence of vitreoretinal adhesions or which injures the retina by causing a full-thickness break can potentially cause RRD, such as:

- Uveitis.
- Trauma.
- Viral retinitis.
- Retinal vein occlusion.
- Von Hippel–Lindau disease.
- Sickle cell disease.
- Dropped nucleus.
- Needle stick injury.
- Vitreoretinal surgery.
- Retinopathy of prematurity.

Summary

Applying the principles of break closure, retinopexy and temporary support of the retina can be applied to a variety of rhegmatogenous retinal detachment presentations.

References

1. Gonzales CR, Gupta A, Schwartz SD, Kreiger AE. The fellow eye of patients with rhegmatogenous retinal detachment. Ophthalmology. 2004;111(3):518–21.
2. Ung T, Comer MB, Ang AJ, Sheard R, Lee C, Poulson AV, et al. Clinical features and surgical management of retinal detachment secondary to round retinal holes. Eye (Lond). 2005;19(6):665–9. https://doi.org/10.1038/sj.eye.6701618.
3. Williams KM, Dogramaci M, Williamson TH. Retrospective study of rhegmatogenous retinal detachments secondary to round retinal holes. Eur J Ophthalmol. 2012;22(4):635–40. https://doi.org/10.5301/ejo.5000080.
4. Gonzales CR, Gupta A, Schwartz SD, Kreiger AE. The fellow eye of patients with phakic rhegmatogenous retinal detachment from atrophic holes of lattice degeneration without posterior vitreous detachment. Br J Ophthalmol. 2004;88(11):1400–2. https://doi.org/10.1136/bjo.2004.043240.
5. Javitt JC, Vitale S, Canner JK, Krakauer H, McBean AM, Sommer A. National outcomes of cataract extraction. I. Retinal detachment after inpatient surgery. Ophthalmology. 1991;98(6):895–902.
6. Javitt JC, Tielsch JM, Canner JK, Kolb MM, Sommer A, Steinberg EP. National outcomes of cataract extraction. Increased risk of retinal complications associated with Nd:YAG laser capsulotomy. The cataract patient outcomes research team. Ophthalmology. 1992;99(10):1487–97.
7. Sheu SJ, Ger LP, Ho WL. Late increased risk of retinal detachment after cataract extraction. Am J Ophthalmol. 2010;149(1):113–9. https://doi.org/10.1016/j.ajo.2009.08.006.
8. Boberg-Ans G, Villumsen J, Henning V. Retinal detachment after phacoemulsification cataract extraction. J Cataract Refract Surg. 2003;29(7):1333–8.
9. Boberg-Ans G, Henning V, Villumsen J, la Cour M. Longterm incidence of rhegmatogenous retinal detachment and survival in a defined population undergoing standardized phacoemulsification surgery. Acta Ophthalmol Scand. 2006;84(5):613–8. https://doi.org/10.1111/j.1600-0420.2006.00719.x.
10. Erie JC, Raecker ME, Baratz KH, Schleck CD, Robertson DM. Risk of retinal detachment after cataract extraction, 1980-2004: a population-based study. Trans Am Ophthalmol Soc. 2006;104:167–75.
11. Lois N, Wong D. Pseudophakic retinal detachment. Surv Ophthalmol. 2003;48(5):467–87.
12. Bradford JD, Wilkinson CP, Fransen SR. Pseudophakic retinal detachments. The relationships between retinal tears and the time following cataract surgery at which they occur. Retina. 1989;9(3):181–6.
13. Mahroo OA, Dybowski R, Wong R, Williamson TH. Characteristics of rhegmatogenous retinal detachment in pseudophakic and phakic eyes. Eye (Lond). 2012;26(8):1114–21. https://doi.org/10.1038/eye.2012.112.
14. Menezo JL, Frances J, Reynolds RS. Number and shape of tears in aphakic retinal detachment: its relationship with different surgical techniques of cataract extraction. Mod Probl Ophthalmol. 1977;18:457–63.
15. Snyder WB, Bernstein I, Fuller D, Hutton WL, Vaiser A. Retinal detachment and pseudophakia. Ophthalmology. 1979;86(2):229–41.
16. Ramos M, Kruger EF, Lashkari K. Biostatistical analysis of pseudophakic and aphakic retinal detachments. Semin Ophthalmol. 2002;17(3-4):206–13.
17. McDonnell PJ, Patel A, Green WR. Comparison of intracapsular and extracapsular cataract surgery. Histopathologic study of eyes obtained postmortem. Ophthalmology. 1985;92(9):1208–25.
18. Tuft SJ, Minassian D, Sullivan P. Risk factors for retinal detachment after cataract surgery: a case-control study. Ophthalmology. 2006;113(4):650–6. https://doi.org/10.1016/j.ophtha.2006.01.001.
19. Yoshida A, Ogasawara H, Jalkh AE, Sanders RJ, McMeel JW, Schepens CL. Retinal detachment after cataract surgery. Surgical results. Ophthalmology. 1992;99(3):460–5.
20. Phillips CI. Distribution of breaks in Aphakic and "senile" eyes with retinal detachments. Br J Ophthalmol. 1963;47:744–52.

21. Kennedy CJ, Parker CE, McAllister IL. Retinal detachment caused by retinal dialysis. Aust NZJ Ophthalmol. 1997;25(1):25–30.
22. Qiang Kwong T, Shunmugam M, Williamson TH. Characteristics of rhegmatogenous retinal detachments secondary to retinal dialyses. Can J Ophthalmol. 2014;49(2):196–9. https://doi.org/10.1016/j.jcjo.2013.12.013.
23. Kinyoun JL, Knobloch WH. Idiopathic retinal dialysis. Retina. 1984;4(1):9–14.
24. Verdaguer TJ, Rojas B, Lechuga M. Genetical studies in nontraumatic retinal dialysis. Mod Probl Ophthalmol. 1975;15:34–9.
25. Ross WH. Retinal dialysis: lack of evidence for a genetic cause. Can J Ophthalmol. 1991;26(6):309–12.
26. Zion VM, Burton TC. Retinal dialysis. Arch Ophthalmol. 1980;98(11):1971–4.
27. Katsura H, Hida T. Atopic dermatitis. Retinal detachment associated with atopic dermatitis. Retina. 1984;4(3):148–51.
28. Ahmad A, Pruett RC. The fundus in mongolism. Arch Ophthalmol. 1976;94(5):772–6.
29. Ang GS, Townend J, Lois N. Epidemiology of giant retinal tears in the United Kingdom: the British Giant retinal tear epidemiology eye study (BGEES). Invest Ophthalmol Vis Sci. 2010;51(9):4781–7. https://doi.org/10.1167/iovs.09-5036.
30. Shunmugam M, Ang GS, Lois N. Giant retinal tears. Surv Ophthalmol. 2014;59(2):192–216. https://doi.org/10.1016/j.survophthal.2013.03.006.
31. Billington BM, Leaver PK, McLeod D. Management of retinal detachment in the Wagner-stickler syndrome. Trans Ophthalmol Soc UK. 1985;104(Pt 8):875–9.
32. Sharma T, Gopal L, Shanmugam MP, Bhende PS, Agrawal R, Shetty NS, et al. Retinal detachment in Marfan syndrome: clinical characteristics and surgical outcome. Retina. 2002;22(4):423–8.
33. Wolfensberger TJ, Aylward GW, Leaver PK. Prophylactic 360 degrees cryotherapy in fellow eyes of patients with spontaneous giant retinal tears. Ophthalmology. 2003;110(6):1175–7.
34. Duguid IG, Leaver PK. Giant retinal tears resulting from eye gouging in rugby football. Br J Sports Med. 2000;34(1):65–6.
35. Aylward GW, Cooling RJ, Leaver PK. Trauma-induced retinal detachment associated with giant retinal tears. Retina. 1993;13(2):136–41.
36. McLeod D. Giant retinal tears after central vitrectomy. Br J Ophthalmol. 1985;69(2):96–8.
37. Aaberg TM Jr, Rubsamen PE, Flynn HW Jr, Chang S, Mieler WF, Smiddy WE. Giant retinal tear as a complication of attempted removal of intravitreal lens fragments during cataract surgery. Am J Ophthalmol. 1997;124(2):222–6.
38. Richards AJ, Meredith S, Poulson A, Bearcroft P, Crossland G, Baguley DM, et al. A novel mutation of COL2A1 resulting in dominantly inherited Rhegmatogenous retinal detachment. Invest Ophthalmol Vis Sci. 2005;46(2):663–8.
39. Richards AJ, Martin S, Yates JR, Scott JD, Baguley DM, Pope FM, et al. COL2A1 exon 2 mutations: relevance to the stickler and Wagner syndromes. Br J Ophthalmol. 2000;84(4):364–71.
40. Snead MP, Yates JR. Clinical and molecular genetics of stickler syndrome. J Med Genet. 1999;36(5):353–9.
41. Spallone A. Stickler's syndrome: a study of 12 families. Br J Ophthalmol. 1987;71(7):504–9.
42. Vidaurri-Leal J. de BS, Michels RG. Surgical treatment of giant retinal tears with inverted posterior retinal flaps. Am J Ophthalmol. 1984;98(4):463–6.
43. Leaver PK, Cooling RJ, Feretis EB, Lean JS, McLeod D. Vitrectomy and fluid/silicone-oil exchange for giant retinal tears: results at six months. Br J Ophthalmol. 1984;68(6):432–8.
44. Peyman GA, Rednam KR, Seetner AA. Retinal microincarceration with penetrating diathermy in the management of giant retinal tears. Arch Ophthalmol. 1984;102(4):562–5.
45. Michels RG, Rice TA, Blankenship G. Surgical techniques for selected giant retinal tears. Retina. 1983;3(3):139–53.
46. Federman JL, Shakin JL, Lanning RC. The microsurgical management of giant retinal tears with trans-scleral retinal sutures. Ophthalmology. 1982;89(7):832–9.
47. Scott JD. Giant retinal tears. Mod Probl Ophthalmol. 1979;20:275–8.
48. Kreiger AE, Lewis H. Management of giant retinal tears without scleral buckling. Use of radical dissection of the vitreous base and perfluoro-octane and intraocular tamponade. Ophthalmology. 1992;99(4):491–7.
49. Glaser BM, Carter JB, Kuppermann BD, Michels RG. Perfluoro-octane in the treatment of giant retinal tears with proliferative vitreoretinopathy. Ophthalmology. 1991;98(11):1613–21.
50. Chang S, Lincoff H, Zimmerman NJ, Fuchs W. Giant retinal tears. Surgical techniques and results using perfluorocarbon liquids. Arch Ophthalmol. 1989;107(5):761–6.
51. Millsap CM, Peyman GA, Mehta NJ, Greve MD, Lee KJ, Ma PE, et al. Perfluoroperhydrophenanthrene (Vitreon) in the management of giant retinal tears: results of a collaborative study. Ophthalmic Surg. 1993;24(11):759–63.
52. Mathis A, Pagot V, Gazagne C, Malecaze F. Giant retinal tears. Surgical techniques and results using perfluorodecalin and silicone oil tamponade. Retina. 1992;12(3 Suppl):S7–10.
53. Scott IU, Murray TG, Flynn HW Jr, Feuer WJ, Schiffman JC. Outcomes and complications associated with giant retinal tear management using perfluoro-n-octane. Ophthalmology. 2002;109(10):1828–33.
54. Chang S. Low viscosity liquid fluorochemicals in vitreous surgery. Am J Ophthalmol. 1987;103(1):38–43.
55. Meffert S, Peyman GA. Intraoperative complications of perfluoroperhydrophenanthrene: subretinal perfluorocarbon, retinal slippage and residual perfluorocarbon. Vitreon Study Group Can J Ophthalmol. 1999;34(5):272–80.
56. Glaser BM, Vidaurri-Leal J, Michels RG, Campochiaro PA. Cryotherapy during surgery for giant retinal tears and intravitreal dispersion of viable retinal pigment epithelial cells. Ophthalmology. 1993;100(4):466–70.
57. Wong D, Williams RL, German MJ. Exchange of perfluorodecalin for gas or oil: a model for avoiding slippage. Graefes Arch Clin Exp Ophthalmol. 1998;236(3):234–7.
58. Batman C, Cekic O. Vitrectomy with silicone oil or long-acting gas in eyes with giant retinal tears: long-term follow-up of a randomized clinical trial. Retina. 1999;19(3):188–92.
59. Verstraeten T, Williams GA, Chang S, Cox MS Jr, Trese MT, Moussa M, et al. Lens-sparing vitrectomy with perfluorocarbon liquid for the primary treatment of giant retinal tears. Ophthalmology. 1995;102(1):17–20.
60. Kertes PJ, Wafapoor H, Peyman GA, Calixto N Jr, Thompson H. The management of giant retinal tears using perfluoroperhydrophenanthrene. A multicenter case series. Vitreon collaborative study group. Ophthalmology. 1997;104(7):1159–65.
61. Banker AS, Freeman WR, Vander JF, Flores-Aguilar M, Munguia D. Use of perflubron as a new temporary vitreous substitute and manipulation agent for vitreoretinal surgery. Wills eye hospital Perflubron study group. Retina. 1996;16(4):285–91.
62. Ie D, Glaser BM, Sjaarda RN, Thompson JT, Steinberg LE, Gordon LW. The use of perfluoro-octane in the management of giant retinal tears without proliferative vitreoretinopathy. Retina. 1994;14(4):323–8.
63. Hoffman ME, Sorr EM. Management of giant retinal tears without scleral buckling. Retina. 1986;6(4):197–204.
64. Ambresin A, Wolfensberger TJ, Bovey EH. Management of giant retinal tears with vitrectomy, internal tamponade, and peripheral 360 degrees retinal photocoagulation. Retina. 2003;23(5):622–8.
65. Ang A, Poulson AV, Goodburn SF, Richards AJ, Scott JD, Snead MP. Retinal detachment and prophylaxis in type 1 stickler syndrome. Ophthalmology. 2008;115(1):164–8. https://doi.org/10.1016/j.ophtha.2007.03.059.

66. Ang GS, Townend J, Lois N. Interventions for prevention of giant retinal tear in the fellow eye. Cochrane Database Syst Rev. 2009;2:CD006909. https://doi.org/10.1002/14651858.CD006909.pub2.
67. Fincham GS, Pasea L, Carroll C, McNinch AM, Poulson AV, Richards AJ, et al. Prevention of retinal detachment in stickler syndrome: the Cambridge prophylactic cryotherapy protocol. Ophthalmology. 2014;121(8):1588–97. https://doi.org/10.1016/j.ophtha.2014.02.022.
68. Ikeda F, Iida T, Kishi S. Resolution of retinoschisis after vitreous surgery in X-linked retinoschisis. Ophthalmology. 2008;115(4):718–22 e1. https://doi.org/10.1016/j.ophtha.2007.05.047.
69. Byer NE. Clinical study of senile retinoschisis. Arch Ophthalmol. 1968;79(1):36–44.
70. Byer NE. Long-term natural history study of senile retinoschisis with implications for management. Ophthalmology. 1986;93(9):1127–37.
71. Byer NE. The natural history of senile retinoschisis. Trans Am Acad Ophthalmol Otolaryngol. 1976;81(3 Pt 1):458–71.
72. Byer NE. The natural history of senile retinoschisis. Mod Probl Ophthalmol. 1977;18:304–11.
73. Byer NE. Perspectives on the management of the complications of senile retinoschisis. Eye. 2002;16(4):359–64.
74. Byer NE. Spontaneous regression of senile retinoschisis. Arch Ophthalmol. 1972;88(2):207–9.
75. Hoerauf H, Joachimmeyer E, Laqua H. Senile schisis detachment with posterior outer layer breaks. Retina. 2001;21(6):602–12.
76. Aslan O, Batman C, Cekic O, Ozalp S. The use of perfluorodecalin in retinal detachments with retinoschisis. Ophthalmic Surg Lasers. 1998;29(10):818–21.
77. Ambler JS, Gass JD, Gutman FA. Symptomatic retinoschisis-detachment involving the macula. Am J Ophthalmol. 1991;112(1):8–14.
78. Ambler JS, Gutman FA. Retinal detachment and retinoschisis. Ophthalmology. 1991;98(1):1.
79. Sneed SR, Blodi CF, Folk JC, Weingeist TA, Pulido JS. Pars plana vitrectomy in the management of retinal detachments associated with degenerative retinoschisis. Ophthalmology. 1990;97(4):470–4.
80. Rosenfeld PJ, Flynn HW Jr, McDonald HR, Rubsamen PE, Smiddy WE, Sipperley JO, et al. Outcomes of vitreoretinal surgery in patients with X-linked retinoschisis. Ophthalmic Surg Lasers. 1998;29(3):190–7.
81. Ferrone PJ, Trese MT, Lewis H. Vitreoretinal surgery for complications of congenital retinoschisis. Am J Ophthalmol. 1997;123(6):742–7.
82. Trese MT, Ferrone PJ. The role of inner wall retinectomy in the management of juvenile retinoschisis. Graefes Arch Clin Exp Ophthalmol. 1995;233(11):706–8.
83. Regillo CD, Tasman WS, Brown GC. Surgical management of complications associated with X-linked retinoschisis. Arch Ophthalmol. 1993;111(8):1080–6.
84. Weinberg DV, Lyon AT, Greenwald MJ, Mets MB. Rhegmatogenous retinal detachments in children: risk factors and surgical outcomes. Ophthalmology. 2003;110(9):1708–13.
85. Akabane N, Yamamoto S, Tsukahara I, Ishida M, Mitamura Y, Yamamoto T, et al. Surgical outcomes in juvenile retinal detachment. Jpn J Ophthalmol. 2001;45(4):409–11.
86. Fivgas GD, Capone A Jr. Pediatric rhegmatogenous retinal detachment. Retina. 2001;21(2):101–6.
87. Hida T, Tano Y, Okinami S, Ogino N, Inoue M. Multicenter retrospective study of retinal detachment associated with atopic dermatitis. Jpn J Ophthalmol. 2000;44(4):407–18.
88. Farah ME, Hofling-Lima AL, Nascimento E. Early rhegmatogenous retinal detachment following laser in situ keratomileusis for high myopia. J Refract Surg. 2000;16(6):739–43.
89. Arevalo JF, Ramirez E, Suarez E, Cortez R, Antzoulatos G, Morales-Stopello J, et al. Rhegmatogenous retinal detachment in myopic eyes after laser in situ keratomileusis. Frequency, characteristics, and mechanism. J Cataract Refract Surg. 2001;27(5):674–80.

10 Proliferative Vitreoretinopathy

Contents

Introduction

Proliferative vitreoretinopathy (PVR) is a cellular proliferation producing "epiretinal membranes" in rhegmatogenous retinal detachment. Primary RRDs which have been present for weeks or months are likely to develop PVR. At presentation the rate of PVR in all patients with RRD varies depending on the ease of access to health care, where prompt surgery is available PVR rates of 5% are expected; however, where there is delay in receiving surgery PVR rates are much higher, e.g. 53% in South America [1] and 17.5% in East Africa [2]. Failed surgery increases the risk of postoperative PVR which has been reported in 5% of RRDs with U tears, 18% with paravascular tears, and 25% of giant retinal tears [3].

The onset of the proliferative response is variable with some eyes producing a response after short duration and others with chronic detachment remaining free from proliferation. Other conditions with retinal detachment are also at high risk of PVR such as severe ocular trauma and some inflammatory conditions, e.g. acute retinal necrosis (ARN). Eyes with vascular conditions von Hippel–Lindau, vasculi-

T. H. Williamson, *Vitreoretinal Surgery*, https://doi.org/10.1007/978-3-030-68769-4_10

tis, or ARN with leaking blood vessels are very vulnerable to PVR probably because growth factors are high in the eye to stimulate migration, differentiation, and multiplication of RPE cells.

Pathogenesis

(Fig. 10.1) The retinal pigment epithelial cell appears to be the main source of the proliferation [4] although Muller cells and inflammatory cells are also implicated [5, 6]. These cells are dispersed into the vitreous cavity through a retinal break. They change into myofibroblasts by the action of growth hormones and cytokines released because of the breakdown of the blood retinal barrier from ischaemia. The ischaemia is induced by the separation of the retina from the choroidal blood supply. Types 1 and 3 collagens are laid down and the cells contract in a similar fashion to a normal wound healing response.

To stimulate PVR there needs to be

- Retinal break to allow access of the RPE to the vitreous cavity.
- Breakdown of the blood retinal barrier which results secondarily from.
  - The presence of the retinal detachment.
  - Surgical interventions like cryopexy and laserpexy.
  - Vascular abnormalities.

Note: Contraction of a wound on a planar surface usefully closes the wound by drawing the wound edges together.

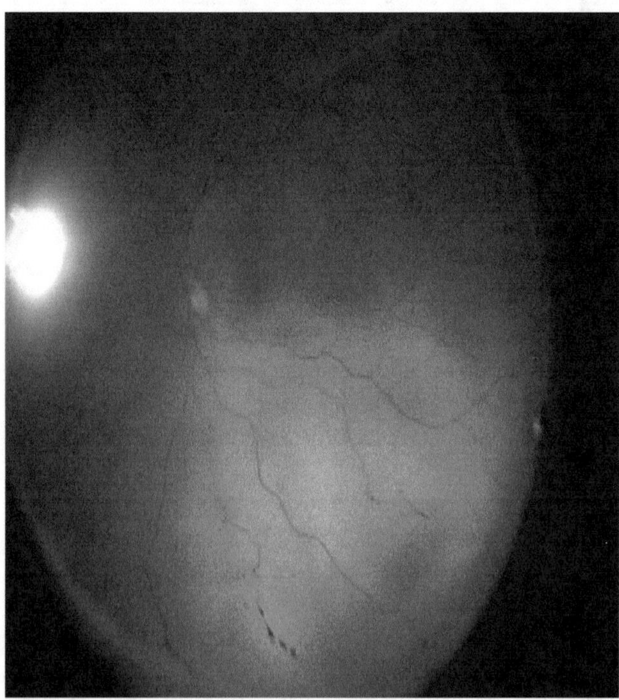

Fig. 10.1 Activation of RPE cells can be seen by clumping of the cells on retinal blood vessels

However, the same process is detrimental on the inside surface of a sphere such as the eye where the contraction tends to drag tissue (in this case the neurosensory retina) into the centre of the sphere, exacerbating the retinal detachment process.

In addition, the retina becomes shortened and stiffened (between its anchor points the optic disc and the ora serrata) by the PVR process. The surface area of retina is not large enough to allow it to reattach to the inner surface of the posterior segment of the eye.

Clinical Features

Introduction

PVR is characterised by shortening, stiffening, and folding of the retina progressing to a funnel retinal detachment which is immobile. Fibrosis can be seen on the inner and outer surfaces of the retina. PVR has the effect of reopening existing tears, creating new tears especially at the site of previous retinopexy but will also induce RD in eyes in which no open tears are found [7]. Patients who have preoperative PVR are at risk of developing more severe postoperative PVR [8].

Grading (Figs. 10.2, 10.3, 10.4, and 10.5)

The response can be usefully graded [9].

A. Clumping of retinal pigment epithelial cells and stiffening of the vitreous.
B. Partial thickness folding of the inner retina.
C. Full-thickness fixed folding of the retina, commencing as localised star folds, and progressing to an open funnel formation and then a closed funnel in the final stages. C proliferative vitreoretinopathy is quantified by locating the area of folding either anterior (A) or posterior (P) to the equator and by indicating the number of clock hours of retina involved (1–12) (Figs. 10.6, 10.7, 10.8, 10.9, 10.10, 10.11, 10.12, 10.13, 10.14, 10.15, and 10.16).

Occasionally the proliferation is predominantly subretinal [10] producing fibrous strands which elevate the retina like the guy ropes of a tent or even "purse string" the retina around the optic disc (Table 10.1) (Fig. 10.17).

Risk of PVR (Figs. 10.18, 10.19, and 10.20)

PVR is particularly likely to occur if the patient has any of the following.

- RRD for a prolonged period [1].
- choroidal detachment [11],

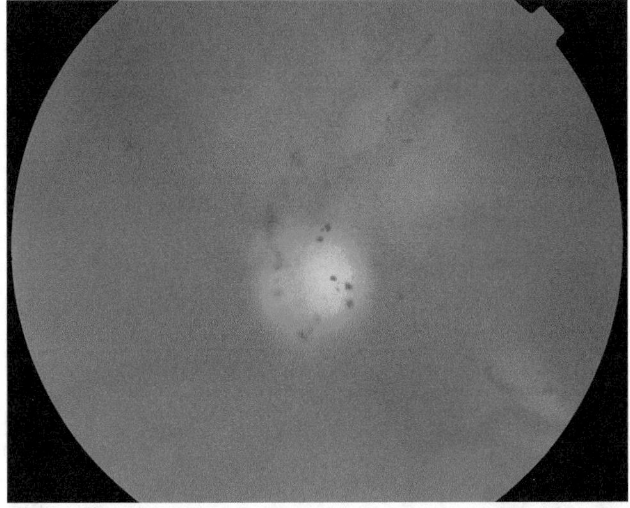

Fig. 10.2 Clusters of RPE cells can be seen in the vitreous of this patient with RRD indicating Grade A PVR

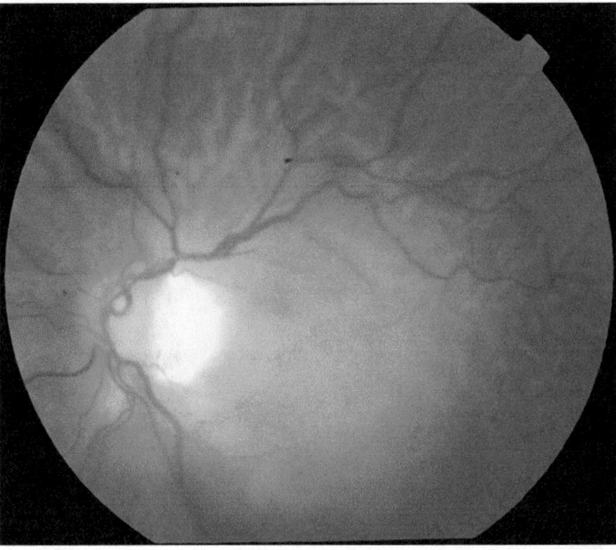

Fig. 10.4 B PVR, diffuse partial thickness wrinkling is shown on the retina indicating Grade B PVR in this patient

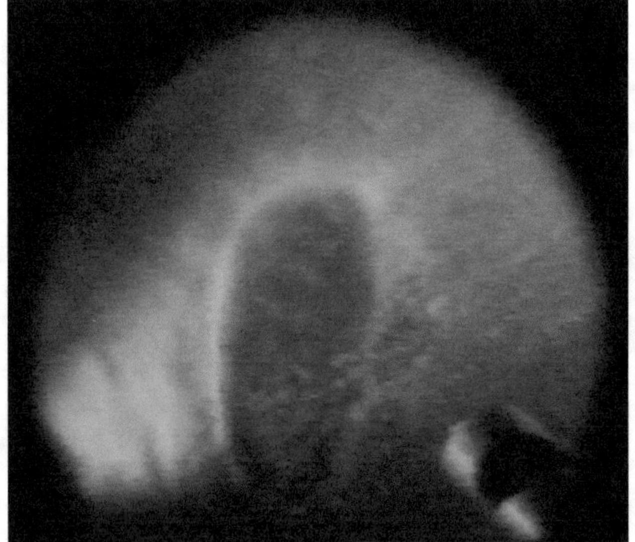

Fig. 10.3 Grade A PVR is diagnosed by stiffening of the vitreous clumps of pigmentation in the gel

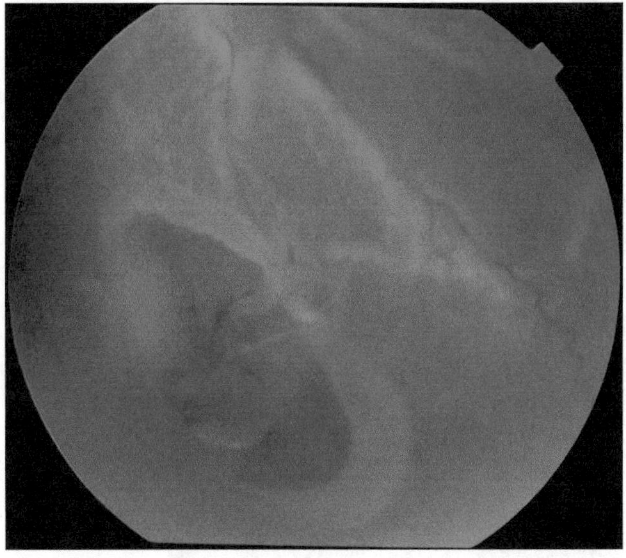

Fig. 10.5 A rolled edge to a retinal tear is an early sign of PVR

- previous surgery or cryotherapy which may aid the dispersion of the RPE cells [12] and their stimulation by growth hormones. A difference in risk between cryotherapy and laser has been hard to determine [13] though most surgeons regard cryotherapy as more inflammatory and therefore more likely to stimulate PVR.
- pre-existing PVR,
- aphakia [14],
- vitreous haemorrhage, the effect on PVR formation is uncertain but there is an belief that this may increase the risk of PVR [15].
- vascular abnormalities such as retina telangiectasia or angiomas,
- uveitis,
- trauma (Figs. 10.21, 10.22, and 10.23).

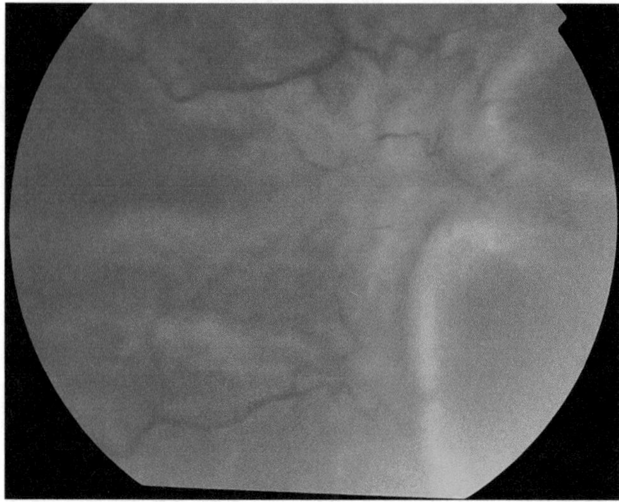

Fig. 10.6 This patient has CP2 PVR, but the membranes are very poorly formed and may be difficult to remove with forceps. The membranes can be stretched by insertion of heavy liquid to relieve the tension on the retina

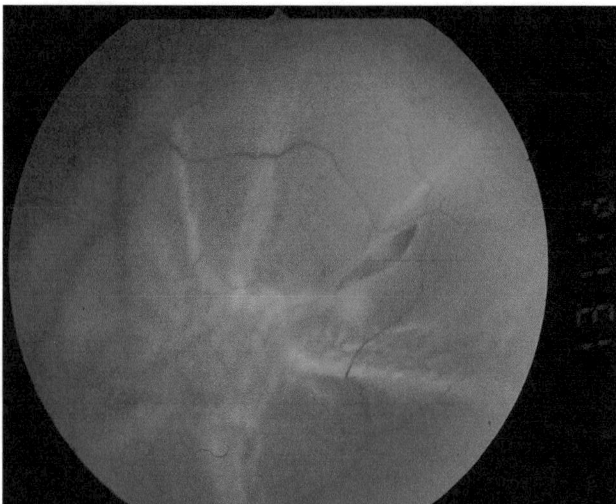

Fig. 10.7 CP2: In this patient, a small focus of PVR is present over a previously failed non-drain retinal detachment repair

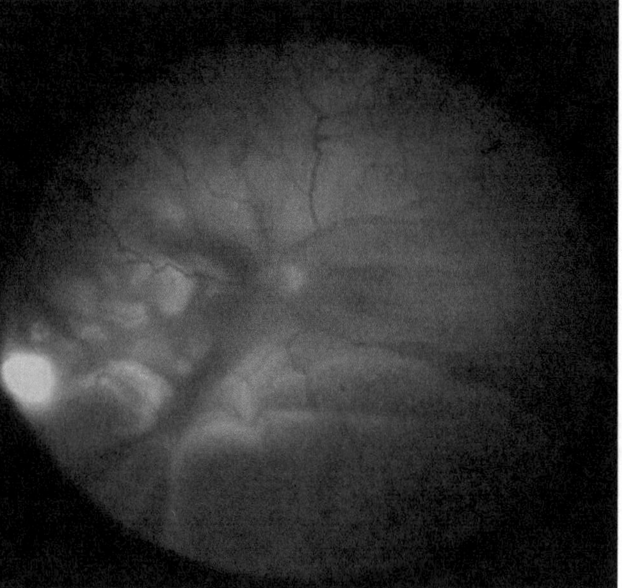

Fig. 10.8 This patient has PVR grade CP4 mostly on the nasal side which is early in its evolution and can present immature membranes which are friable difficult to remove. Stretching out the retina with heavy liquids helps open out the retina

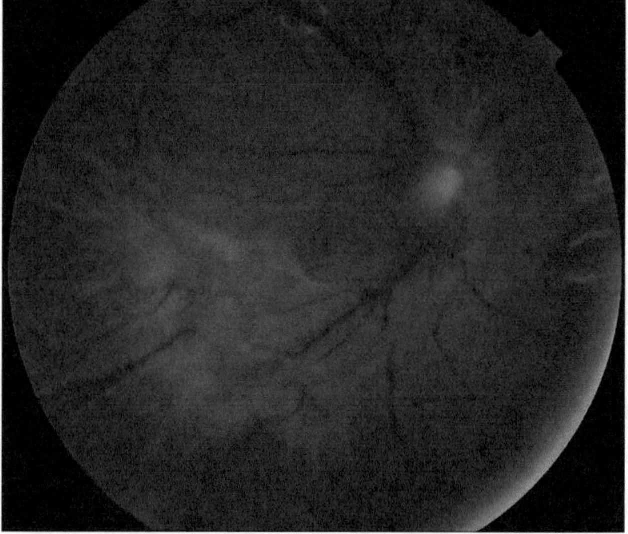

Fig. 10.9 CP4: In this patient there is a focal PVR

Surgery

Surgery for PVR varies from performing conventional operations to retinectomy of the inferior retina.

Mild PVR

(approximately C1–2) (Table 10.2)

Perform a Non-Drain Procedure.

Or

PPV with additional surgical steps.

- Stain with Trypan blue.
- Insert heavy liquids.
- Peel PVR membranes.
- Use long-acting tamponade.

When dealing with PVR from C1 to C2, if the retinal breaks are far away from the PVR, for example, you have a

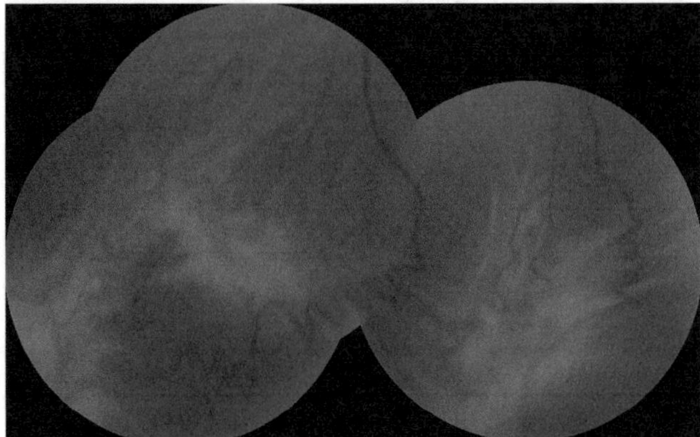

Fig. 10.10 CP6: This patient shows full-thickness retinal folds over an extent of the retina of approximately 6 o'clock hours

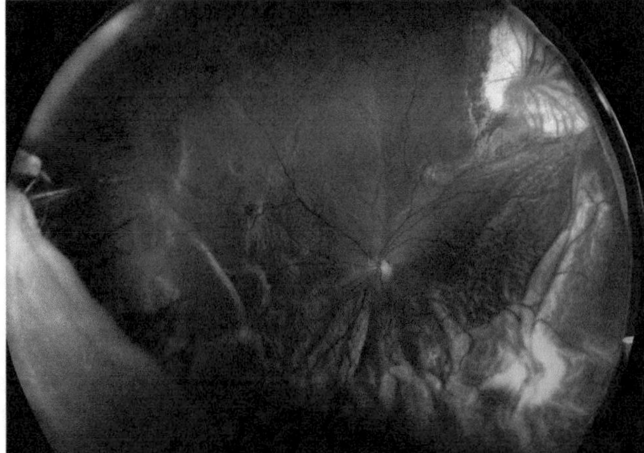

Fig. 10.11 A postoperative RRD with CP6 PVR requires urgent surgery to restrict the PVR process

superior horseshoe break with inferior CP2 PVR, often all that is required is to close the break, e.g. a plombage can be placed on the tear. The normal physiological mechanisms will overcome the shortening to the retina from the PVR.

If the PVR is any more than this, however, you will have to perform a vitrectomy, and attempt to peel any retinal membrane from the surface of the retina to allow the retina to open up and reattach itself to the back of the eye.

Use trypan blue dye to visualise the membranes and grasp with serrated forceps. Note: Insert heavy liquids onto the posterior retina to stabilise the retina and act as counter traction as you pull on the membranes.

Unfortunately, early membranes are often friable and difficult to remove. In this case stretch and open out the contraction from the membranes using heavy liquid. The eye is primed to produce scar tissue and the surgical intervention may induce further PVR formation, therefore C2F6 gas or even silicone oil may be required.

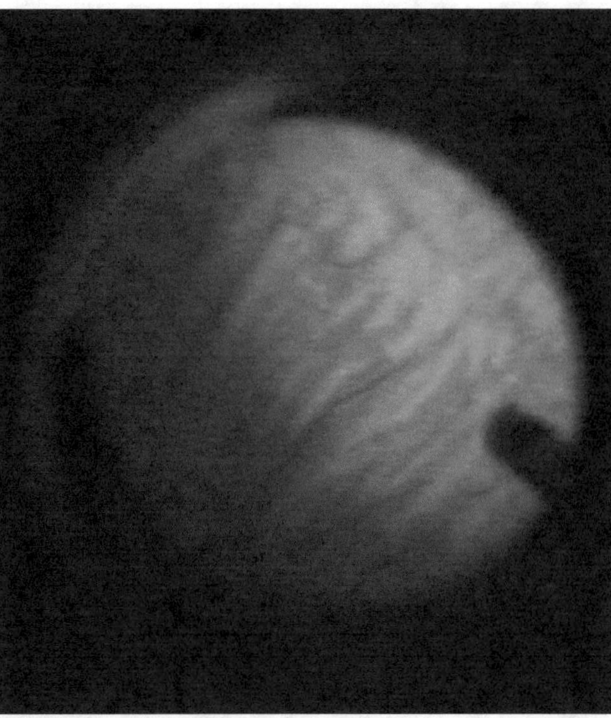

Fig. 10.12 CA8: Anterior PVR is shown by shortening of the anterior retina with full-thickness retina folds

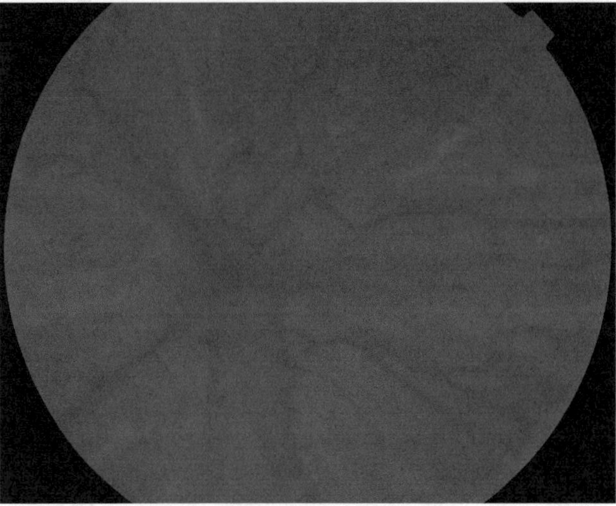

Fig. 10.13 CP 12 PVR or a closed posterior funnel is present on this patient with RRD

Moderate PVR

(diffuse grade B, C3–5) (Table 10.3)

PPV with additional surgical steps.

Stain with Trypan blue.

Insert heavy liquids.

Peel PVR membranes.

Use silicone oil or long-acting gas (Fig. 10.24).

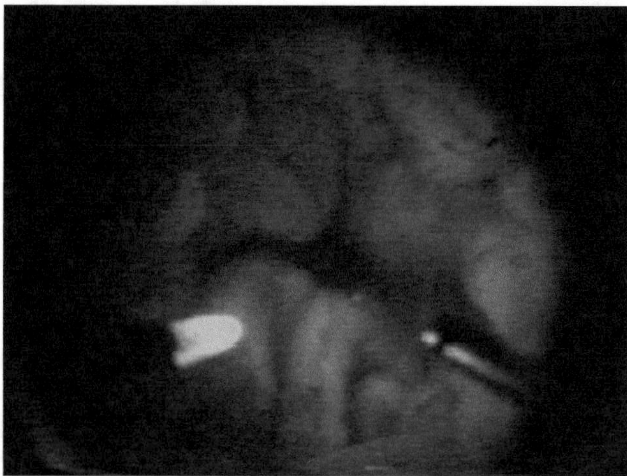

Fig. 10.14 CP12: In this patient with severe PVR, the PVR is almost complete with a funnel retinal detachment

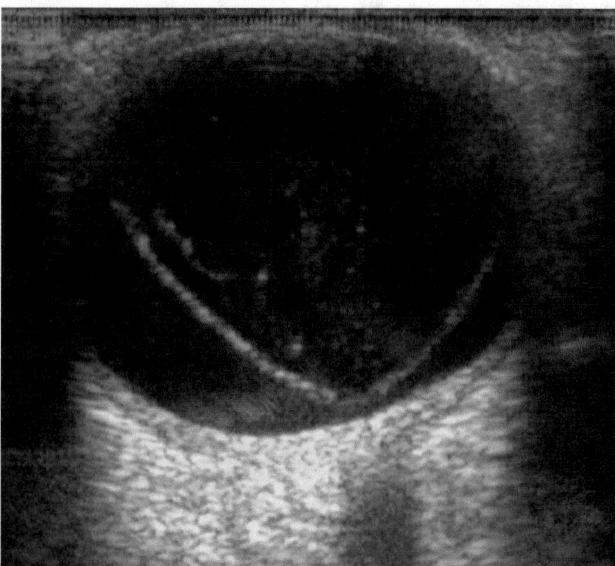

Fig. 10.15 An open funnel RRD from PVR on ultrasound, CP12

With levels of PVR C3–5 peeling the membrane may be enough. Stabilise the retina with a heavy liquid, e.g. perfluoro-n-octane [16]. This acts as a counterweight when pulling on the membranes otherwise the retina will be pulled with the membrane and there is a risk of tearing. Use Trypan blue stain to see the membrane more easily, and use either serrated forceps, or forceps with a sharp tip, to elevate the membrane. It is often easiest to engage the membrane in the centre of a star fold. Thereafter deal with any breaks and fill the eye with silicone oil to allow reattachment of the retina. Leave the oil in until the proliferative process has had a chance to stop, usually requiring a few months. Superior

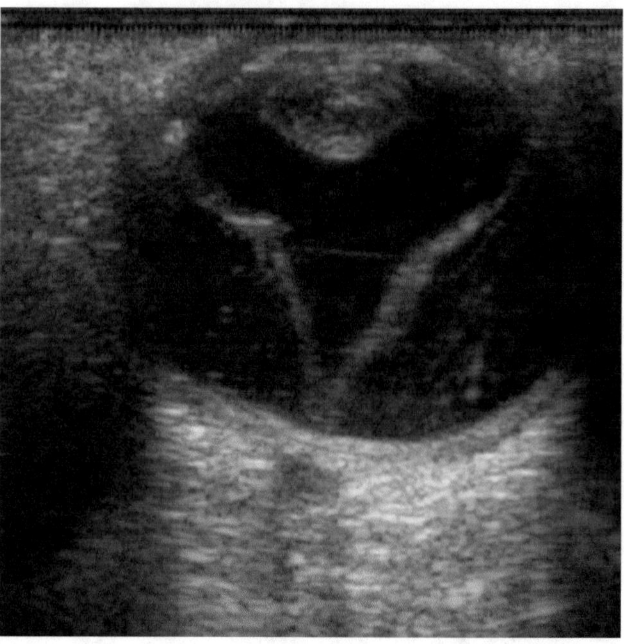

Fig. 10.16 A closed "funnel" RRD from PVR on ultrasound, CP12 and CA12

Table 10.1 Grading PVR

Proliferative Vitreoretinopathy		
Grading		
A	Vitreous haze, pigment clumps, pigment clusters on inferior retina	
B	Inner retinal wrinkling, retinal stiffness, rolled break edges, vitreous stiffness	
CP 1–12	Full-thickness retinal folds or subretinal strands posterior to the equator (described as 1–12 clock hours of involvement)	
CA 1–12	Full thickness retinal folds or subretinal strands anterior to the equator (described as 1–12 clock hours of involvement), anterior displacement, condensed vitreous strands	
Descriptive terms		
Type	Usual location	Features
Focal	Posterior	Star folds in the retina
Diffuse	Posterior	Confluent retinal folding
Subretinal	Posterior	Fibrous strands, linear and purse string around the optic disc Fibrous sheets
Circumferential	Anterior	Contraction of the retina inwards at the posterior edge of the vitreous base
Anterior displacement	Anterior	Anterior traction on the retina at the vitreous base. Ciliary body detachment and epiciliary membrane. Iris retraction.

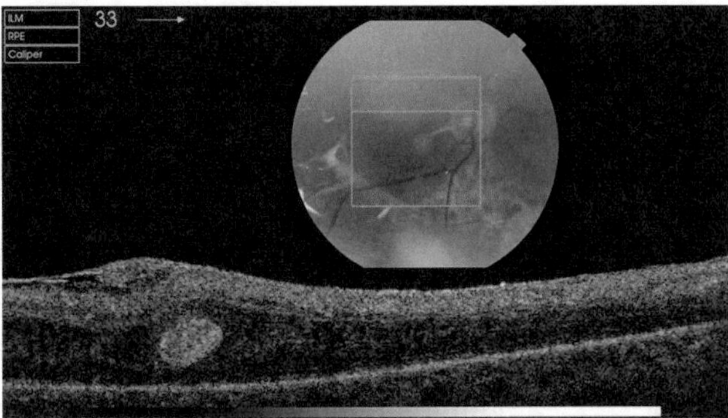

Fig. 10.17 Intraretinal PVR membrane

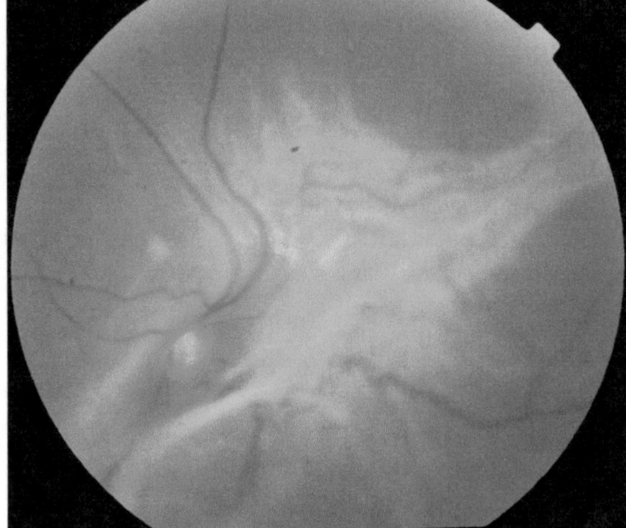

Fig. 10.18 A subretinal band of fibrosis can "purse string" the retina around the optic disc

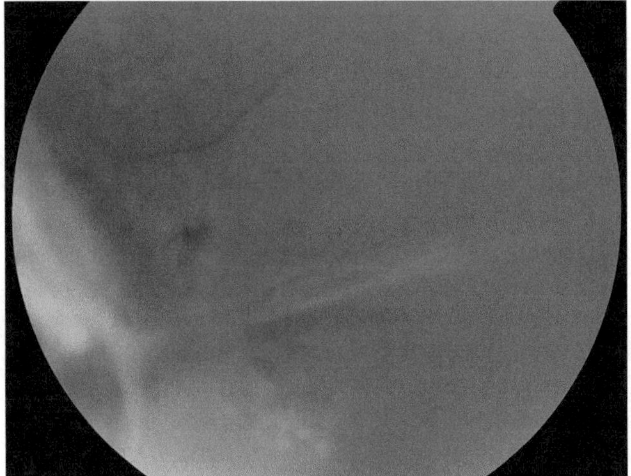

Fig. 10.19 PVR in the periphery is causing a fold in the retina in the macula

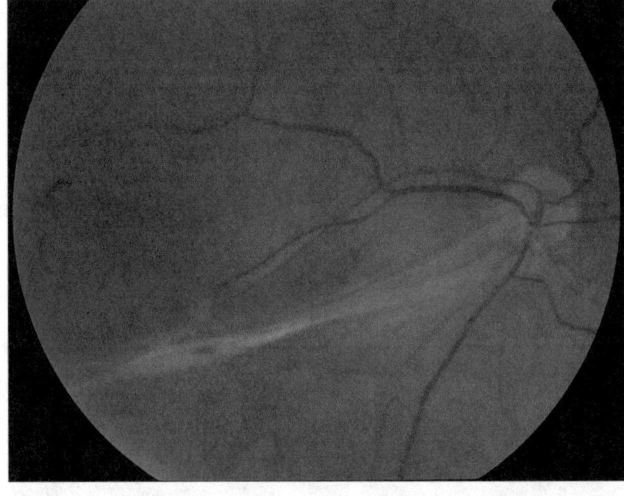

Fig. 10.20 CA PVR is causing the fold posteriorly

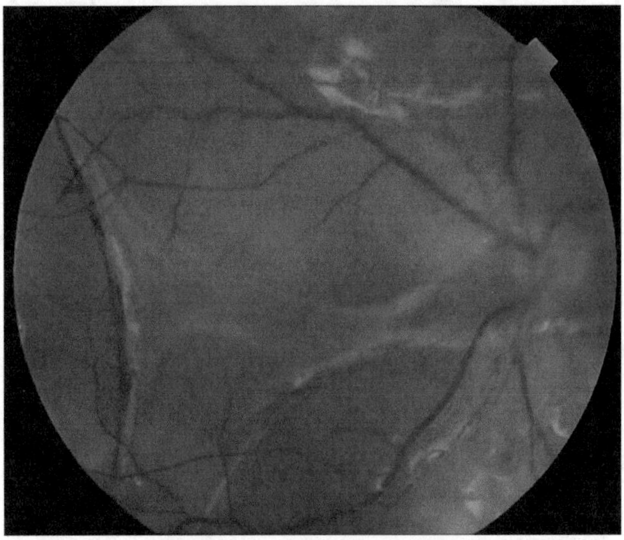

Fig. 10.21 Severe subretinal fibrosis postoperatively

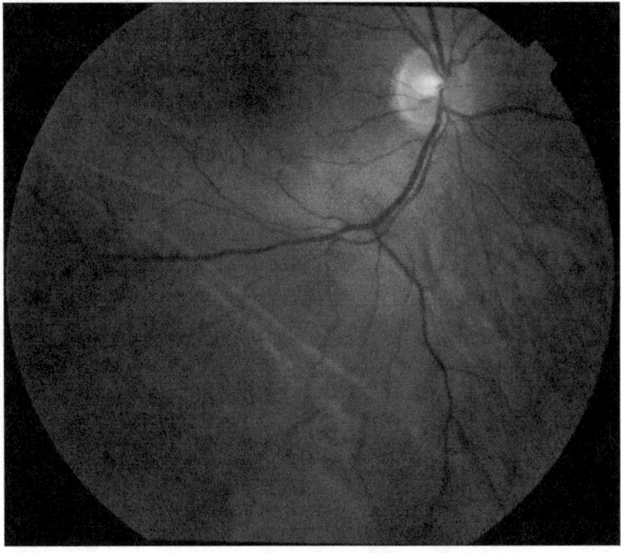

Fig. 10.22 Subretinal fibrosis in a chronic retinal detachment

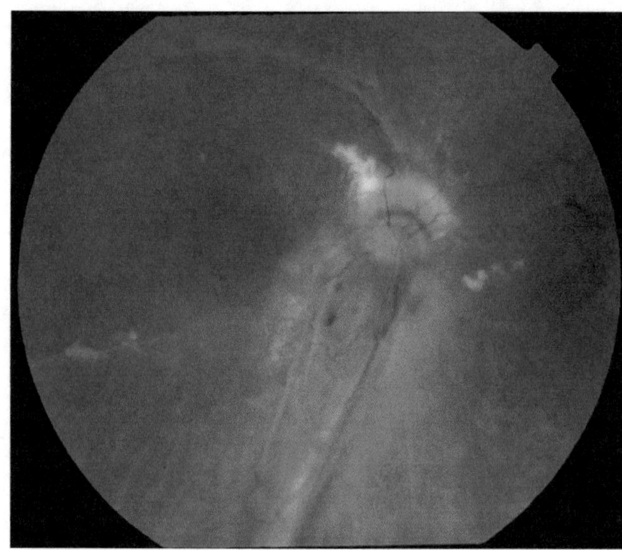

Fig. 10.23 This patient has a purse string subretinal band which is anchored in the periphery and is dragging retina downwards over the surface of the disc. Another instance of retina pulled over the disc surface is in "dragged disc", e.g. retinopathy of prematurity. The surgeon must be aware that retina overlies the disc and care must be taken when draining residual vitreous cavity fluid off the optic nerve head during PPV in these patients because the retina can be aspirated into the flute needle tip

Table 10.2 Difficulty rating for surgery for mild PVR

Difficulty Rating	Low
Success rates	Moderate
Complication rates	Low
When to use in training	Middle

Table 10.3 Difficulty rating for surgery for moderate PVR

Difficulty Rating	Moderate
Success rates	Moderate
Complication rates	Medium
When to use in training	Late

holes can be treated with silicone oil. The management of inferior breaks is controversial. The placement of an inferior indentation in a silicone eye may prevent adequate inferior silicone oil fill and may create a space behind the indent where shortening of the retina can easily form. I now do not use inferior buckles with moderate PVR and rely on the silicone oil fill on its own. Surprisingly, the inferior holes can flatten in this situation allowing silicone oil removal. This is despite the lack of inferior tamponade on the breaks from the oil (see sphere within a sphere in Appendix). If the inferior retina does not flatten, proceed to retinectomy [17, 18] (Figs. 10.25 and 10.26).

Remove the silicone oil at 3 to 4 months, to avoid long-term oil induced complications (Figs. 10.27 and 10.28).

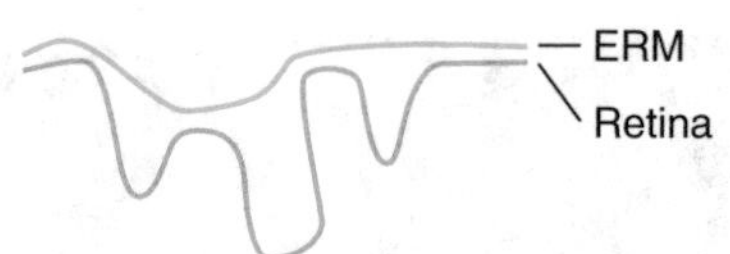

Fig. 10.24 Membrane (green) on the retina (orange) causes full-thickness folds, by removing the membrane, the retina can be unfolded and therefore its length increased again, improving the chances of re-attaching it to the curve to the eye

Severe PVR

(C6–8) (Table 10.4)

Additional surgical steps.

Operation 1

- Stain with Trypan blue.
- Insert heavy liquids.
- Peel PVR membranes.
- Flatten the macula.
- Close breaks if possible, with tamponade superiorly and indentation inferiorly and apply retinopexy.
- Insert silicone oil.

Operation 2.

- Peel PVR membranes.
- Diathermy blood vessels.
- Incise along retinectomy.
- Remove the redundant anterior retina.
- Check for folds and perform radial cuts in the retina if required.
- Top up the silicone oil.
- Apply laser retinopexy (with cryopexy to the apices if required).

Operation 3

- Remove the silicone oil.

In more severe PVR, and depending on the location of retinal breaks, and in grade B PVR where there is a diffuse shortening of the retina without the ability to remove surface membrane, a three-stage approach is recommended. At the first operation, perform a vitrectomy and peel as much membrane as possible. Heavy liquid will allow opening of the retina peroperatively [19]. However, shortening of the retina itself is likely to prevent the retina from re-settling on the back of the eye fully. Heavy liquid will "flatter" the appearance of reattachment of the retina because of its high density and may cause an underestimation of the degree of residual traction. Do not be tempted to perform a retinectomy at this stage, as in the early stages of the PVR process, when cyto-

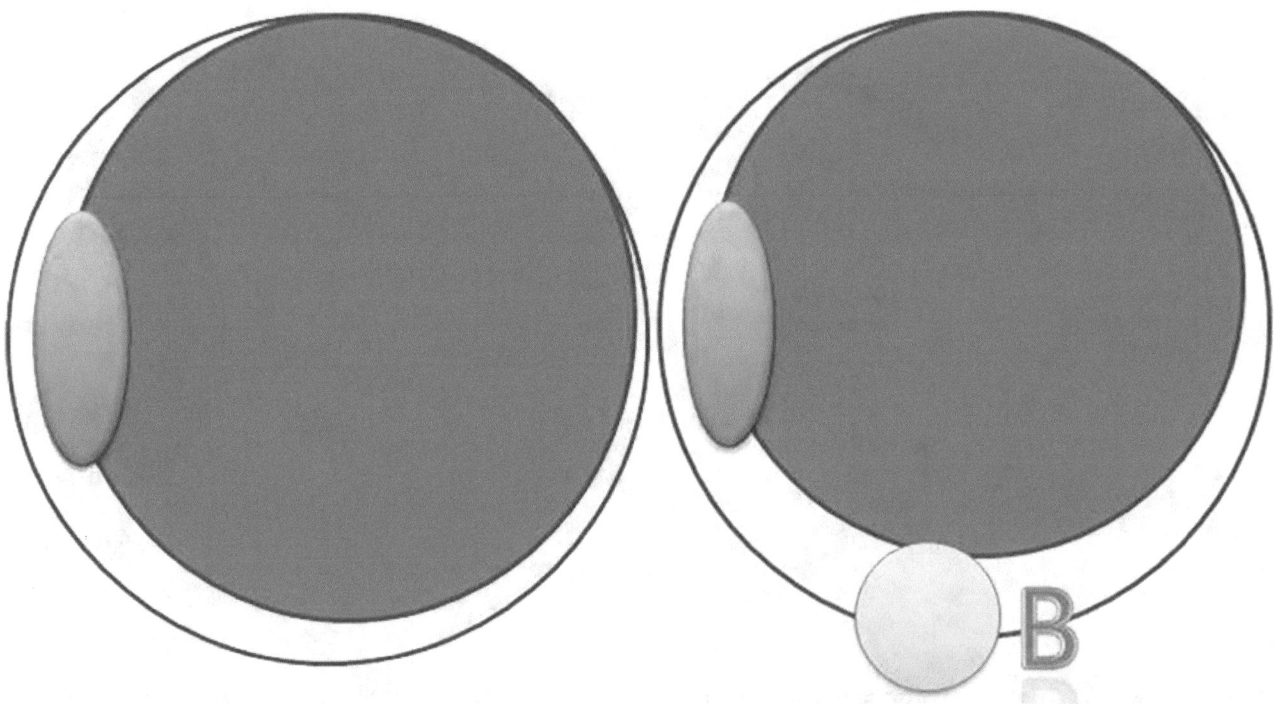

Fig. 10.25 Adding an inferior indent to try to close inferior breaks in a patient with moderate PVR often results in more shortened retina, elevated inferior breaks probably because the oil bubble cannot fill the inferior vitreous cavity at B. It is better to allow the oil to fill the eye after stretching or removing the PVR. Surprisingly, the breaks often close, most likely from reduced fluid currents inferiorly

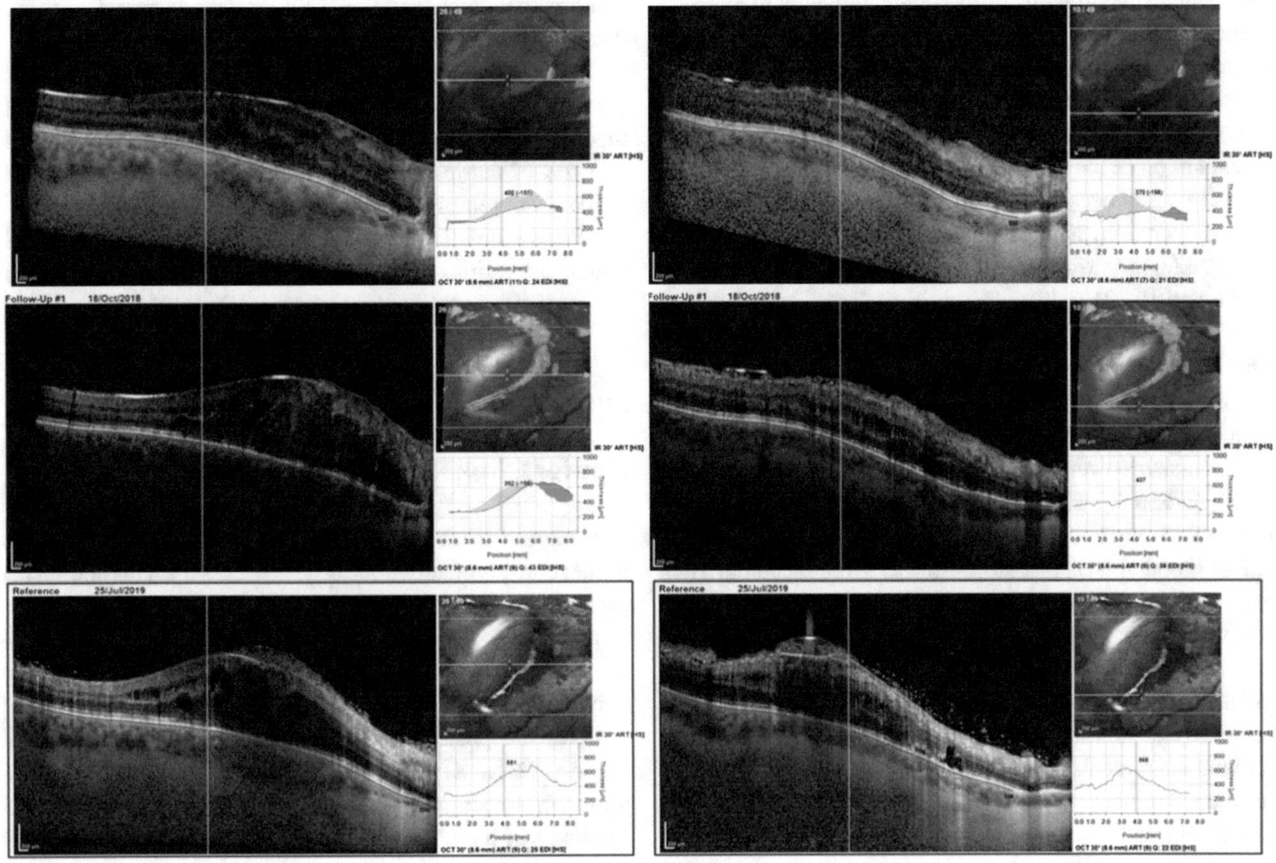

Fig. 10.26 Progression of macular changes in PVR despite a flat retina

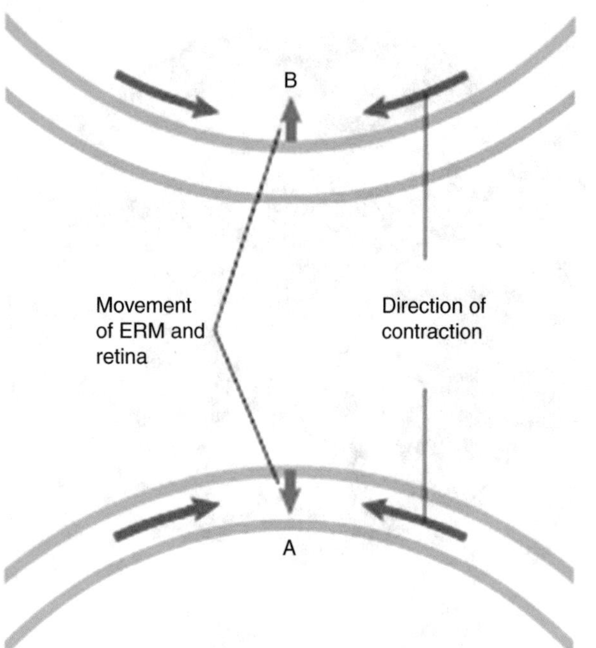

Fig. 10.27 Indentation under an area of contraction from PVR membrane (shown in green) here can be used to aid attachment of the retina at that site. However, the system only works if the PVR is on the apex of the indent Point A. If the PVR is also present at Point B, the indent will cause lifting of the retina

kines and growth factors are still present, and cells are still activated, there is a risk that the retinectomy will end up as a "roller-blind" contraction of the retina, in which the inferior retina rolls up through the macula. This is irredeemable. Therefore, fill the eye up with oil, which, in most circumstances, will flatten two thirds of the retina, leaving the inferior retina detached because of its shortening. With the macula in place the retina can be left for three to six months for the PVR process to become quiescent. Then perform a second operation, cut the inferior retina as far peripherally as is possible to perform a retinectomy (Figs. 10.29, 10.30, 10.31, and 10.32).

The Relieving Retinectomy

The edges of the retinectomy should at least reach the 8 and 4 o'clock meridians and will have to go at least one clock hour into non-scarred retina on each upper aspect. (Figs. 10.33, 10.34, and 10.35) Therefore, it is common to have a retinectomy which is 150° to 180°. First, diathermy the peripheral retinal blood vessels that are visible to avoid bleeding. Then use a vertical cutting scissor to fashion the retinectomy, cutting through the diathermy points. At this stage, the infusion can be attached to balanced salt solution to keep the eye inflated. Any oil that leaks from the eye will be replaced by balanced salt solution, and this will help provide some space for your instruments. If the eye is full of oil, there is less space for the instruments to cut the retina which makes the operation technically more demanding. Use the vitreous cutter to remove the anterior retina. Try and remove the entire anterior retina, as any remnants will cause retinal neovascularisation and iris neovascularisation [20] or may contract causing detachment of the ciliary body and hypotony.

Note it may be useful to use a chandelier light pipe so that the peripheral retina can be removed with the cutter whilst indenting the eye with a squint hook in the other hand. There is a risk of cutting the choroid and causing bleeding if the retina is not removed under direct observation.

Once completed, insert oil through the infusion line, and flatten the retina. A method where the laser application is delayed till post-surgery has been described [21] (Fig. 10.36).

Surgical Pearl

Tips for Large Retinectomies

In advanced PVR with circumferential contraction, a large retinectomy, typically inferiorly, is necessary. This should be performed after removal of as much preretinal proliferation as possible posterior to the vitreous base. Extended dissection within the vitreous base is rarely effective in relieving circumferential traction.

Once the posterior retina is mobilised, perfluorocarbon liquid (PFCL) is used to stabilise and protect the macula prior to retinectomy. This allows the surgeon to assess the adequacy of the posterior dissection and to identify areas of

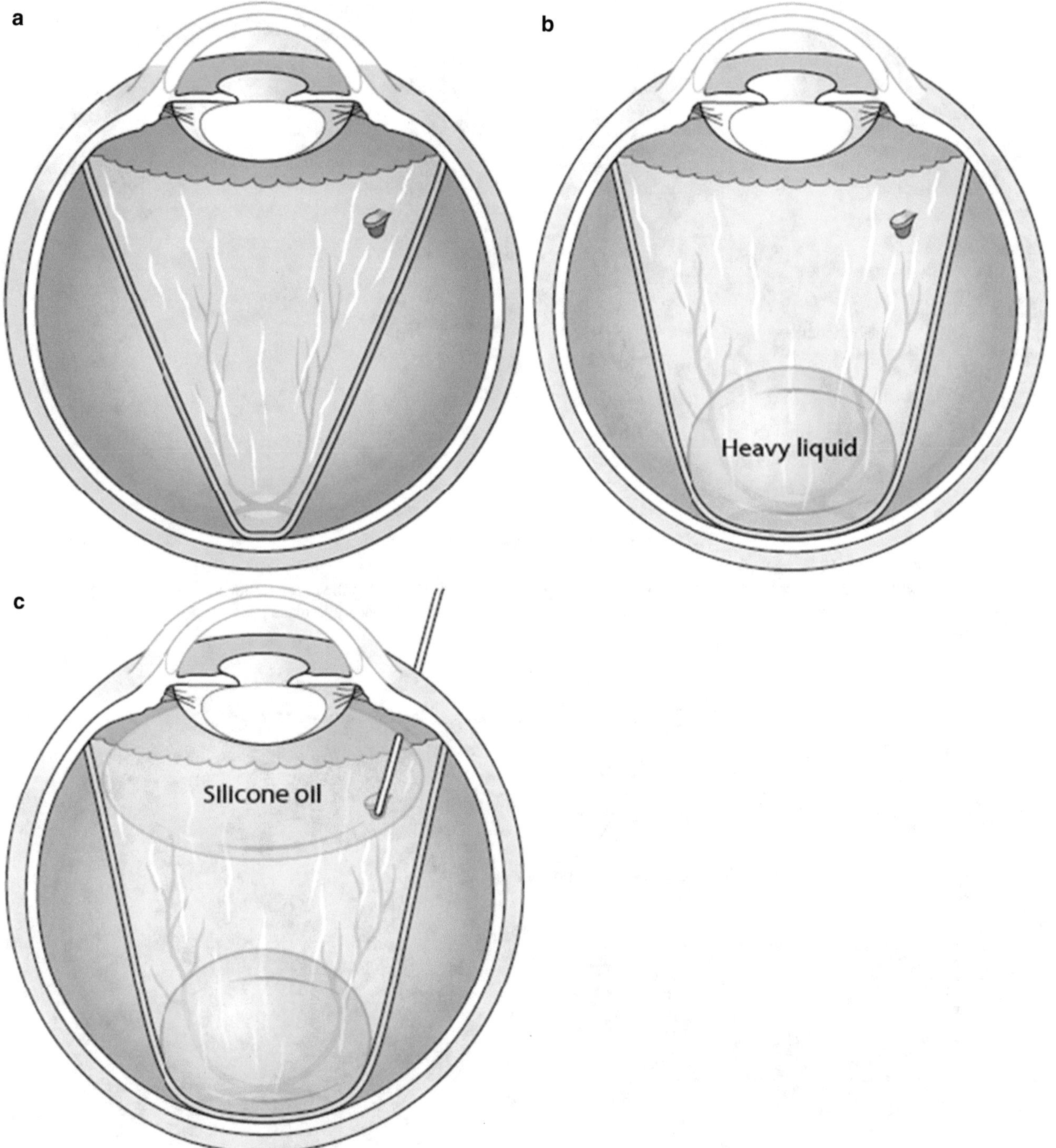

Fig. 10.28 Heavies are useful in patients with PVR to stabilise the posterior retina. Oil can be inserted on top of the heavies whilst draining through the retinal break. As the oil bubble increases, the heavy liquid is compressed by the oil which pushes the peripheral retina flat. The SRF can be drained from the meniscus between the oil and heavy liquids

Table 10.4 Difficulty rating for surgery for severe PVR

Difficulty Rating	High
Success rates	Low
Complication rates	High
When to use in training	Late

residual traction requiring further dissection. It also minimises the risk of retinal rotation with large retinectomies. Additional PFCL is injected until the retina does not further reattach.

At this point, the retinectomy is initiated just posterior to the vitreous base and extended circumferentially whilst

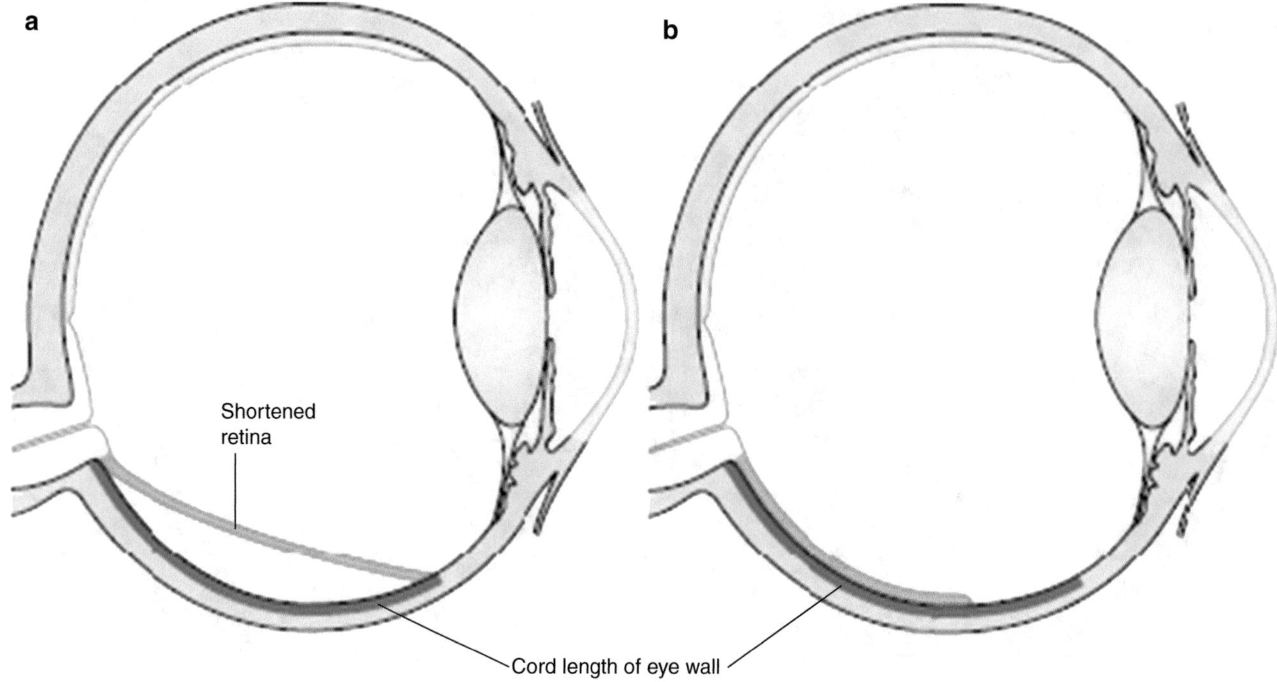

Fig. 10.29 PVR will shorten the cord length of the retina. The orange line, indicating the retina, cannot return to the circumference of the posterior pole (the blue line), if it is anchored at both points anteriorly and posteriorly. By cutting the retina (relieving retinectomy), the retina can be allowed to slip back into place

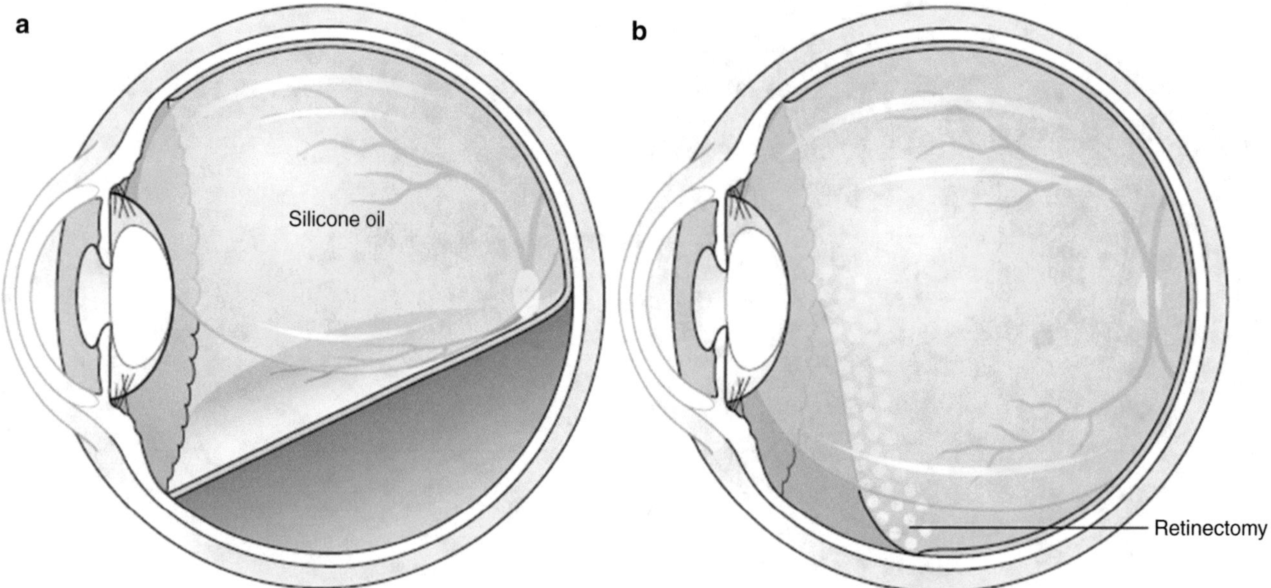

Fig. 10.30 Silicone oil insertion can be used in conjunction with inferior retinectomies. It is probable that the oil does not tamponade the whole extent of the retinectomy. However, the oil allows satisfactory adhesion of the retinectomy scar, probably because a thin layer of fluid is present between the oil and the retinectomy, which prevents subretinal fluid accumulation

observing the effect of the PFCL. Typically, the retinectomy is performed under high infusion pressure of 60 mmHg without any diathermy and extended above the midline temporally and nasally. If the posterior flap of the retinectomy is still curled, further resection with radial incision every 2 to 3 clock hours is performed. Once adequate relaxation is obtained, further PFCL is added beyond the retinectomy edge. If the retina is now flat, one row of continuous laser is applied to the edge of the retinectomy and extended circumferentially and superiorly beyond the extent of the retinec-

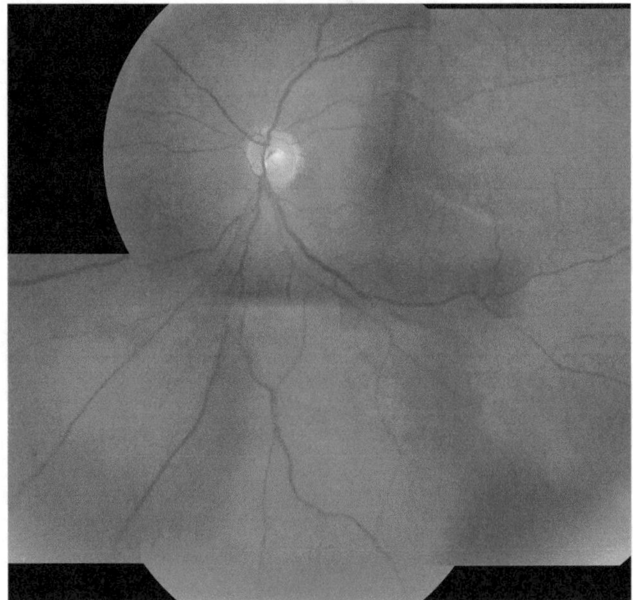

Fig. 10.31 After the first operation for reattachment of most of the retina in moderate PVR there will be persistent inferior SRF, but the macula should be flat

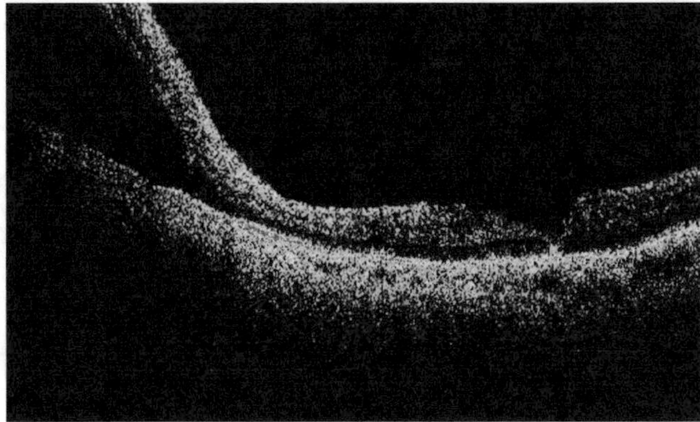

Fig. 10.32 This OCT shows a flat macula under oil with inferior RRD

tomy. Any bleeding from the retinectomy edge is cauterised with confluent laser.

An air fluid exchange is then performed first removing the residual infusion fluid before removing the PFCL and completely drying the edge of the retinectomy. The radial relaxations facilitate the drying. Silicone oil is then injected beginning posteriorly over the nerve then extending anteriorly over the retinectomy until an adequate fill is obtained.

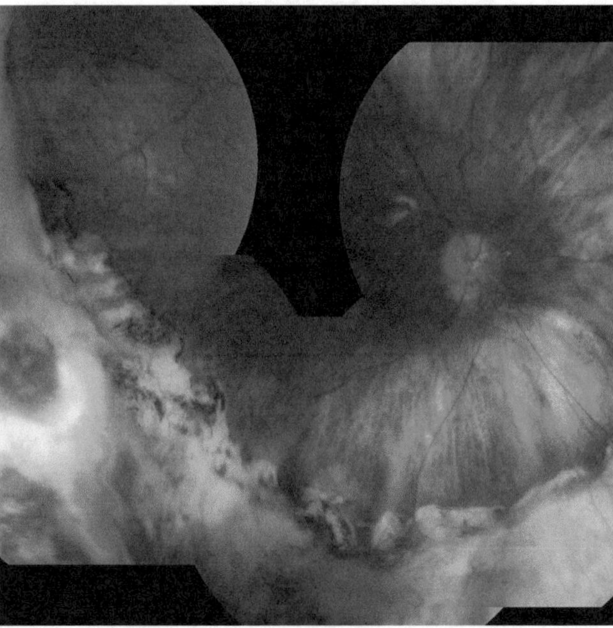

Fig. 10.33 Retinectomies performed early can produce extensive scarring because the PVR process is still active

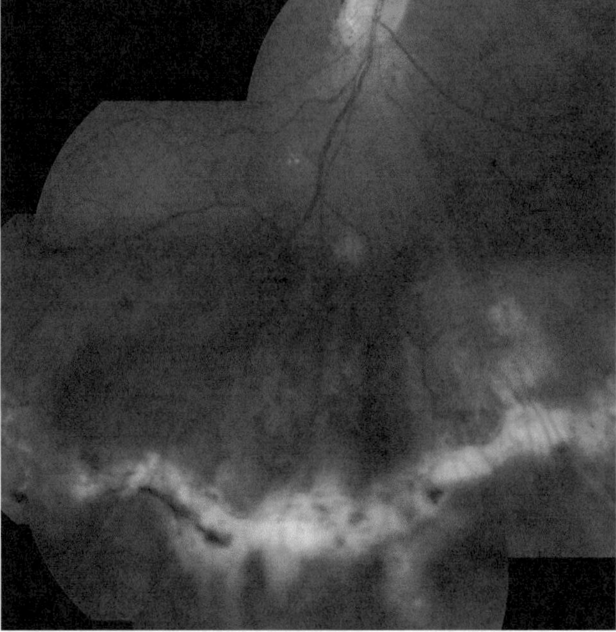

Fig. 10.34 Using a sequence of surgeries with delay before the retinectomy may produce a cleaner retinectomy edge which is less likely to fail

George A Williams, Neuroscience Center Building, Royal Oak, Michigan, USA

Radial Retinotomy

Sometimes there will be circumferential shortening of the retina, seen as folding of the retina inferior to the disc, perhaps passing through the macula horizontally. You will now need to perform a radial retinotomy. This is best performed between the inferotemporal arcade and the inferonasal arcade (this avoids the major retinal blood vessels and avoids cutting across too many retinal nerve fibres) passing up towards the disc and may even reach almost as far as the disc, depending on the shortening that is present. This allows the

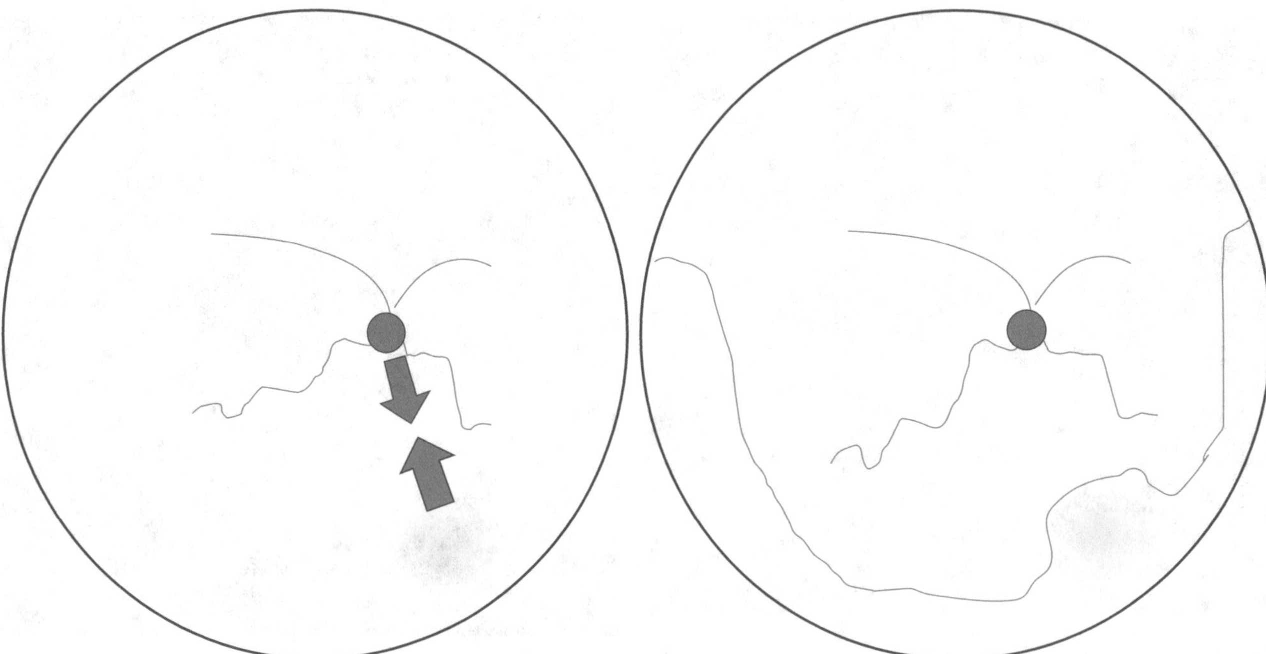

Fig. 10.35 If there is a point of adhesion inferiorly, e.g. an old retinopexy scar, the retinectomy should be taken posterior to the scar to relieve the shortened retina as indicated by the arrows. Failure to do so causes persistent elevation of the retina between the scar and the optic disc postoperatively

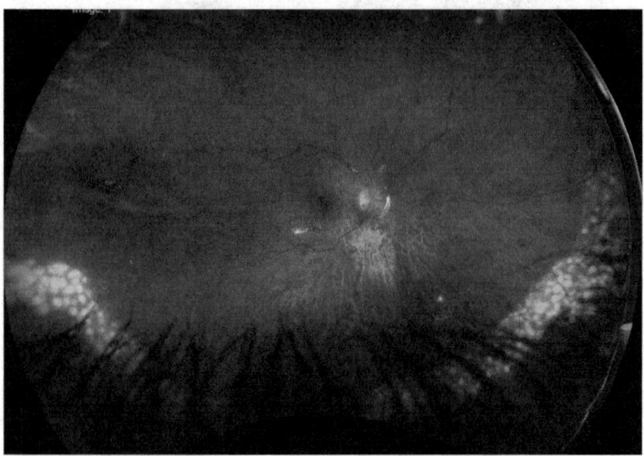

Fig. 10.36 A recent inferior 180-degree retinectomy

retina to open out like the petal of a flower and reduces the chances of any folds. Sometimes a small radial retinotomy will be needed at the temporal upper end of the retinectomy (Figs. 10.37, 10.38, 10.39, and 10.40).

Silicone Oil Injection

Now continue to flatten the retina, whilst injecting oil, and aspirating aqueous fluid from the inferior margin of the retinectomy. Take care not to engage the retinectomy in the fluid needle by increasing the pressure only slightly in the eye, and then aspirating. Do not inflate the silicone continuously, as there is a lag time for the silicone to enter the eye (because of its viscosity) which may not be anticipated during aspiration of the fluid, thereby risking incarceration of the retina into the flute needle end. If this eventuality occurs, remove your light pipe so that some oil comes out through the sclerotomy and this will usually be enough to release the pressure; by pressing the bulb of a finger into the flute needle, or using a back-flush flute, the retina will extrude. If in a severe case, this is not possible, disconnect the flute needle from the shaft, and attach a syringe to the end of the fluid needle to eject the retina.

Surgical Pearl

Avoiding Retinal Slippage during Vitrectomy Surgery for Retinal Detachment

Retinal slippage occurs when aqueous is displaced posteriorly under the retina in the context of vitreous surgery. The displaced aqueous can cause retinal folds and even displacement of the fovea. Retinal slippage typically occurs during an incoming bubble of endotamponade (such as air or silicone oil) and is more common in cases of retinal detachment with large breaks, giant retinal tears, and any surgeries involving large retinotomies/retinectomies. Despite advances in vitreous surgery, avoidance of retinal slippage remains a challenge.

It has been reported that slippage is less common when direct exchange of perfluorocarbon liquid (PFCL) for sili-

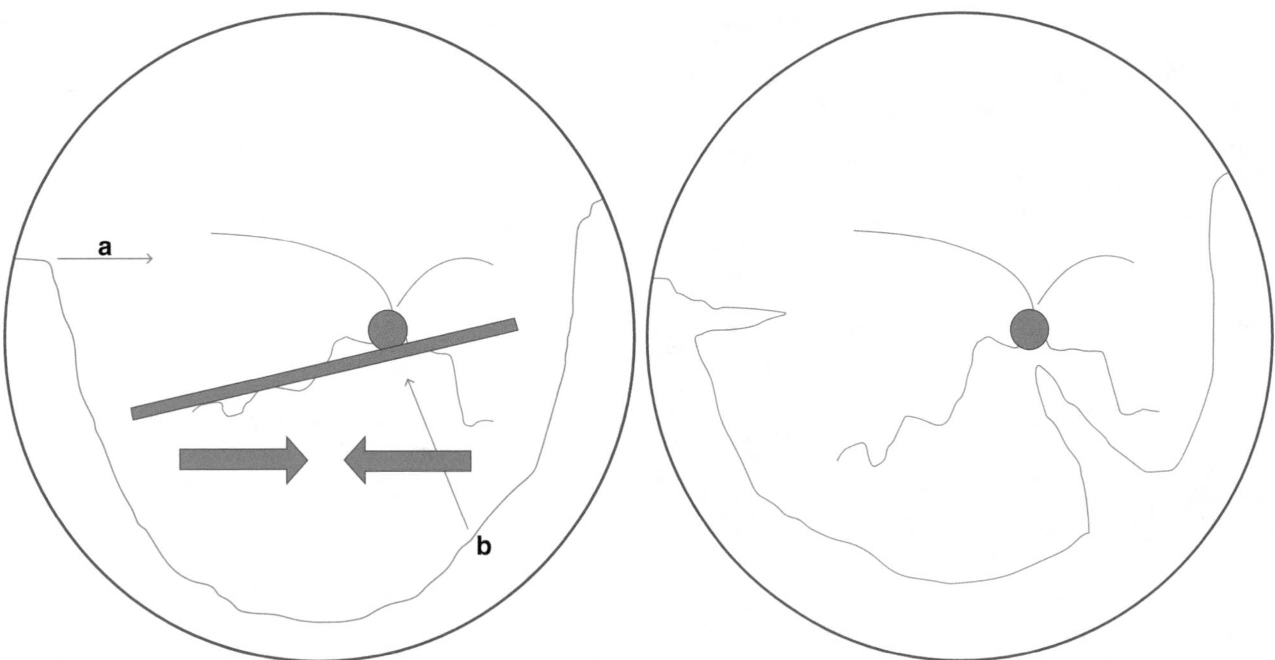

Fig. 10.37 After the circumferential retinotomy a fold of retina under the optic nerve head indicates circumferential shortening of the retina, thick arrows. This can be relieved by a small radial retinotomy temporally (**a**) and a longer retinotomy inferonasally (**b**) to create a petaloid shape to the inferior retina

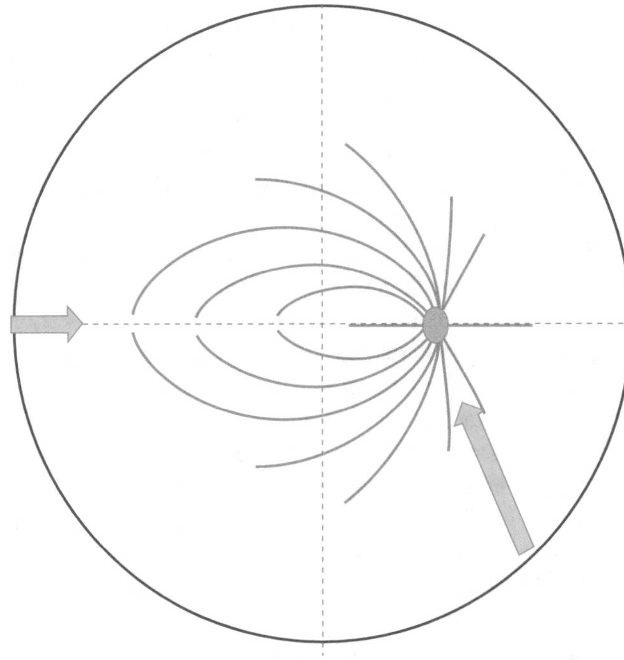

Fig. 10.38 When incising for a radial retinotomy use the direction of the arrows to minimise the number of nerve fibres cut during the retinotomy thereby reducing visual field loss

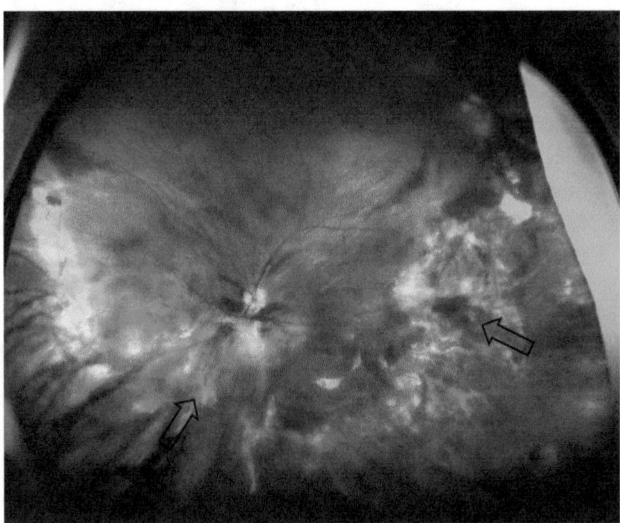

Fig. 10.39 This patient presented with CA12 CP12 PVR and has had a large retinectomy with two radial cuts (arrows) to open out the retina as seen in this early postoperative image

cone oil is performed [22]. This is also supported by observation made using a model eye chamber that showed the aqueous phase was excluded from the interface in order for the silicone oil to achieve lower surface energies [23].

We have previously described an enhanced technique of direct perfluorocarbon exchange for silicone oil to prevent retinal slippage by elimination of all aqueous from the vitreous cavity [24]. Here are the surgical tips:

1. After completion of vitreous shaving and removal of all epiretinal and subretinal membranes, PFCL is injected into the vitreous cavity.
2. After the retina is flattened by PFCL, chorioretinal adhesion is created by either laser or/and cryotherapy.

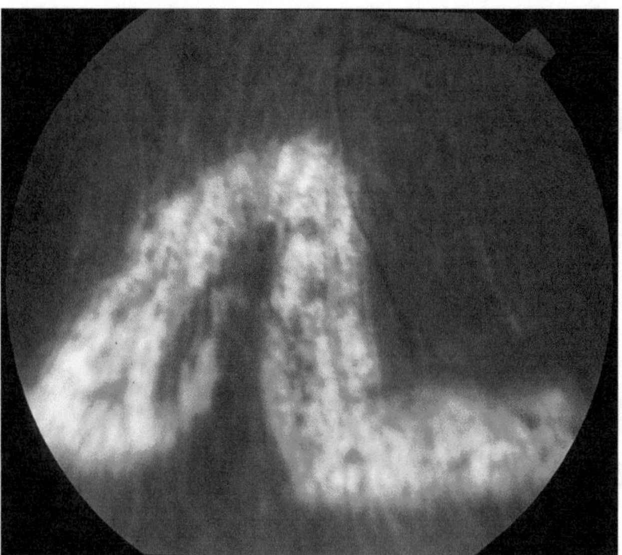

Fig. 10.40 A retinectomy edge is shown. A radial cut has been made because of circumferential shortening of the retina to allow reattachment of the retina without folding through the macula

3. To "overfill" the entire vitreous cavity, more PFCL is injected.
4. However, there is always some BSS in the infusion tubing (up to 0.2 ml) that will be pushed into the vitreous cavity during the start of direct PFCL/silicone oil exchange. Any amount of BSS if displaced posteriorly can cause slippage.
5. To ensure no aqueous in the system, the infusion cannula was disconnected temporarily whilst continuing PFCL injection. This allows PFCL to fill up the entire tubing and displace all aqueous in the tubing. "Overfilling" is thus achieved.
6. Infusion cannula was then connected directly to the silicone oil driving syringe in the viscous fluid injection system.
7. Direct exchange of PFCL and silicone oil was performed as normal.

Kenneth K.W. Li, United Christian Hospital, Kowloon, Hong Kong, China

Applying laser

Having flattened the retina; apply three rows of laser to the posterior edge of the retinectomy, and around any radial retinectomy. In an aphakic or pseudophakic eyes it should be possible to laser close to the ora serrata at the upper ends of the retinectomy. Sometimes there is a need to indent the ends of the retinectomy from the outside through the sclera with the light pipe (see Chapter 6). This will transilluminate the retina and allows visualisation of the edge of the retinectomy and where the ora serrata is to apply laser. The laser burns are not seen whilst being applied, and the surgeon must keep a mental note of which part of the retina has already been treated.

In a phakic eye, however, this may not be possible without touching the back of the lens and damaging the lens, and therefore it is recommended that two or three cryotherapy burns are applied to the top edge of the retinectomy, thereby sealing the top edge. Cryotherapy allows indentation whilst visualising from the inside and applying only a few burns minimises any re-activation of the PVR process.

Note: At the end of the silicone oil insertion, on closing the eye, keep the eye relatively soft, 10 mmHg.

A hard eye indicates an overfill causing raised intraocular pressure postoperatively. Remove some silicone oil in the immediate 1–2-week postoperative period.

Now that the retinectomy has been created, leave the eye for another 3 to 6 months, to allow the retinectomy to seal, and to allow any re-activation of the PVR to cease.

ROSO Plus

Then return to the eye to perform a silicone oil removal. It is recommended to re-inspect the retinectomy at this stage, by using a vitrectomy approach at the same operation (removal of oil and vitrectomy procedure, ROSO plus). Once the oil has been removed inspect the retina to look for any return of retinal detachment. Occasionally, if there is a problem at the edge of the retinectomy, a shallow retinal detachment will appear which must then be dealt with by further surgery, usually involving gas tamponade if the SRF is superior. If there is SRF inferiorly, there is a 6 times higher chance of recurrent retinal detachment and it is recommended to reinsert silicone oil. The inferior retinal detachment can be dealt with by further retinectomy.

Problem areas in the retinectomy include the upper ends where, if the retinectomy was not performed high enough, there may be shortening of the retina in an antero-posterior tangent, and elevation of the ends of the retinectomy. You will need to cut the retinectomy further superiorly to overcome the shortening, and to get into healthy elastic retina, and then retinopexy the edge of the new cut. Occasionally a small one- or two-millimetre edge of the retinectomy is elevated allowing fluid to enter the subretinal space; this will be a thicker area of the retinectomy edge, often being pulled posteriorly through the retinopexy scar. These can easily be dealt with by applying further retinopexy posterior to the extension of this part of the retinectomy.

Very Severe PVR

(C9–12) (Table 10.5)

Additional surgical steps.

- Insert heavy liquids.
- Stain with Trypan blue.

Table 10.5 Difficulty rating for surgery for very severe PVR

Difficulty Rating	Very High
Success rates	Low
Complication rates	High
When to use in training	Late

- Peel PVR membranes.
- Diathermy blood vessels.
- Incise along retinectomy for 350° initially.
- Remove the redundant anterior retina.
- Check for folds and perform radial cuts in the retina if required.
- Insert silicone oil and cut remaining 10°.
- Apply laser retinopexy (Figs. 10.41 and 10.42).

Finally, occasionally very severe PVR may be encountered, where there is a closed funnel anteriorly/posteriorly, such as CA12/CP12. There is no option in these eyes but to perform a large retinectomy. Perform a vitrectomy, open out the funnel as far as possible with the heavy liquids placed over the disc, remove any PVR membrane as before. Perform a retinectomy, usually 360°, and often one or two radial retinotomy cuts to allow the retina to open. Thereafter insert oil on top of the heavy liquids; remove the aqueous layer first, allowing the oil to contact the heavy liquid, which will further open out the retina. Make sure all the aqueous is removed before removing the heavy liquid, so that the heavy liquid can be pushed posteriorly, allowing subretinal fluid to be pushed laterally, and aspirated. Once the retina has opened out, apply three rows of laser to the posterior edge of the retinectomy. There is a risk, of course, in this scenario, that the PVR process will overcome the tamponading effect of the silicone oil, and that the retina rolls up. The patient should know that the prognosis for this eye is poor, and that the surgery is only to preserve some vision of a low grade.

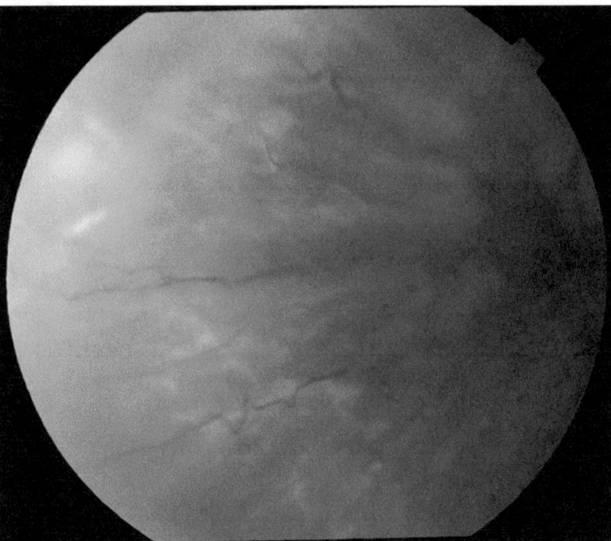

Fig. 10.41 This patient had CP12 and CA12 PVR after only 2 months of RRD with an open funnel configuration. The eye required a PPV with membrane peel and 270-degree retinectomy with silicone oil insertion

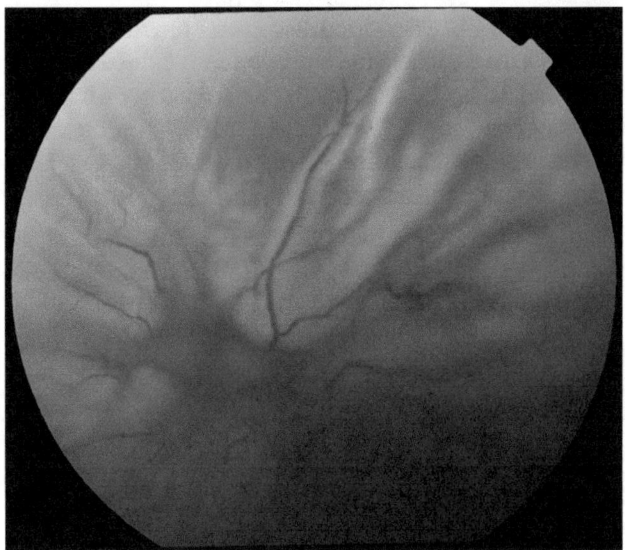

Fig. 10.42 Posterior PVR in this patient

Choice of Endotamponade

Silicone Oil or Perfluoro Propane Gas

Both long-acting tamponade agents have been used in PVR [25, 26]. The silicone oil study suggested that success rates of 61–73% can be achieved with either agent. Although for patients without previous surgery gas was slightly better at achieving surgical attachment there was also a higher chance of hypotony, 31% versus 18% [27]. In most circumstances opt for silicone oil insertion to avoid a catastrophic postoperative retinal detachment with severe PVR leading to hypotony and phthisis.

Heavy Oils

These may be used to treat inferior retinectomy or inferior retinal breaks. The oils currently available are not very dense and so their effect on inferior PVR is poor. In addition, PVR occurs in the superior retina in the postoperative period often exacerbating the problem. Extraction of the oil is more difficult than routine silicone oil because the heavy oil:

- may separate into its components,
- tends to stick to the retina.

The oil does not float; therefore, it cannot be removed passively and must be actively aspirated by an 18-gauge cannula. A metal cannula is recommended because plastic or silicone causes the oil to stick to the tip of the cannula.

It may be better to use conventional oil the properties of which are well established and the results predictable. Heavy oil has not shown better results than routine oil [26]. Some have tried temporary heavy liquids for inferior PVR. These liquids are pro-inflammatory however [28].

Removal of Subretinal Bands

In severe PVR subretinal bands may prevent reattachment of the retina. The bands are usually attached to the choroid in the periphery and may have subretinal attachments along their course. These attachments will usually break when the band is pulled (Figs. 10.43 and 10.44).

To remove make a retinotomy adjacent to the band to allow you to grasp the band with forceps. There are two methods:

Unimanual—it is not safe to pull the band towards the sclerotomies because the band will put pressure on the rim of the sclerotomy and cause it to enlarge. In addition, these bands can be long, and you will run out of space in the eye to pull it. Instead roll the forceps in your fingers as if rolling spaghetti on a fork to gradually roll up the band without any displacement of the position of the forceps tips.

Bimanual—Insert a chandelier system to provide illumination. Make a retinotomy. Use two pairs of forceps one in each hand. Grasp the membrane at the retinotomy with a pair of forceps and pull a short distance then regrasp the membrane at the retinotomy site with the other forceps and pull a short distance. Repeat the "hand over hand" approach until the adhesions break and the band has been removed.

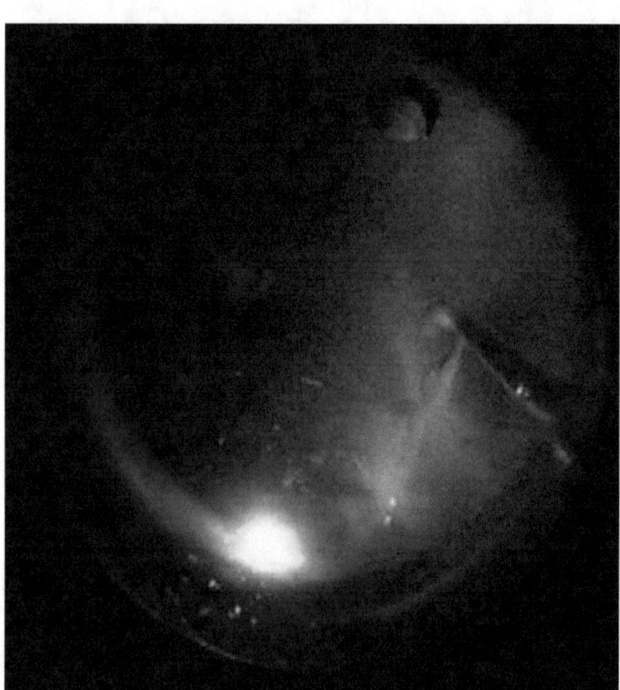

Fig. 10.43 A subretinal band is removed through a retinotomy, by rolling the fibrosis onto the instrument (like spaghetti on to a fork) the band is removed without traction on the retinotomy and without movement of the instrument spatially within the eye

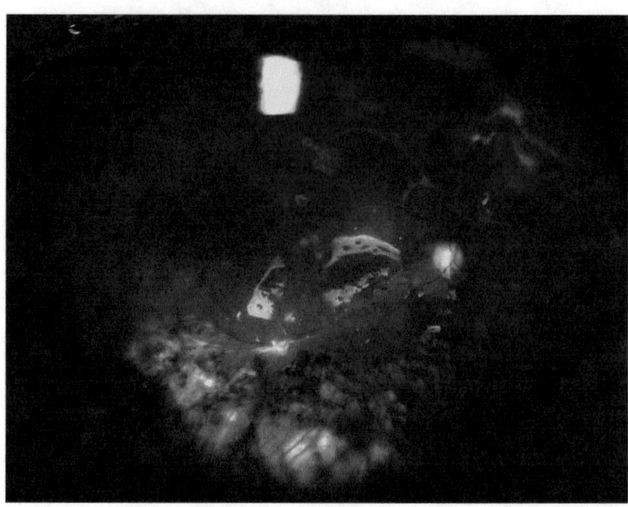

Fig. 10.44 A persistent RRD under oil with shallow SRF and subretinal bands, this will be difficult to fix because the extensive inferior laser will force a very posterior retinectomy. In addition, the subretinal fibrosis will not be easy to remove from under the retina

Note: Always keep retinotomies as superiorly placed in the eye as possible to allow tamponade postoperatively.

Adjunctive Therapies

Adjunctive therapies such as Daunomycin, dexamethasone, and a combination of Heparin and 5 Fluorouracil have been investigated to try to reduce redetachment rates but without success in patients with established PVR [29–33]. The latter was found to be effective in reducing the risk of developing PVR in patients with retinal detachment with a high risk of PVR but reoperation rates were unaffected [34]. Others have suggested washing out any RPE cells in the vitreous cavity after retinopexy to try to reduce the postoperative risk of PVR [35].

Success Rates

The aim for these cases is to achieve reattached retina with silicone oil removed. Success rates are usually stubbornly low in patients with PVR with single operations approximately 62–65% [16, 36–38] or multiple operations 68%–84% [16, 39] despite a variety of methods used [40] and even poorer if silicone oil removal is a requirement of success, e.g. 51%–81% [30, 41]. Patients who achieve a reattached retina with the one operation have significantly better visual outcomes [42] but this is often not achievable. The visual outcome is only a 24–45% chance of 20/200 vision or better [25, 39]. Patients with anterior PVR have poorer outcomes than those with posterior PVR [43]. There is a risk of sight threatening complications in the other eye of these patients (50%) which helps justify the surgery in the eye despite poor success rates [44].

Quiram et al. 2007 have reported a high success rate of 93% reattached retina with primary retinotomy with a mean of 1.8 operations prior to retinotomy. However, 42% of the patients in their study did not achieve silicone oil removal despite a mean follow up of 25 months which was reflected in frequent postoperative silicone oil induced complications. It is best to remove the oil because of the attendant complications of glaucoma, band keratopathy, and central visual loss.

The cause of failure of surgery is usually further PVR formation [45] with reoperations required at 2 months. Using a three-operation approach (planned delayed relieving retinotomy, PDRR) may increase success rates for retinal reattachment without permanent silicone oil insertion in the patients to 89% and contribute to a high success rate for PVR in general with 85% reattached retina without silicone oil tamponade for all cases of PVR.

A possible disadvantage of the PDRR method is the delay in attaching some of the retina thereby delaying the recovery of the neuroretina. If the macula is off after stage one, proceed to stage two early, e.g. two months. Luckily, the inferior retina lost during retinectomy serves superior visual field which is less used than the inferior visual field (Figs. 10.45 and 10.46).

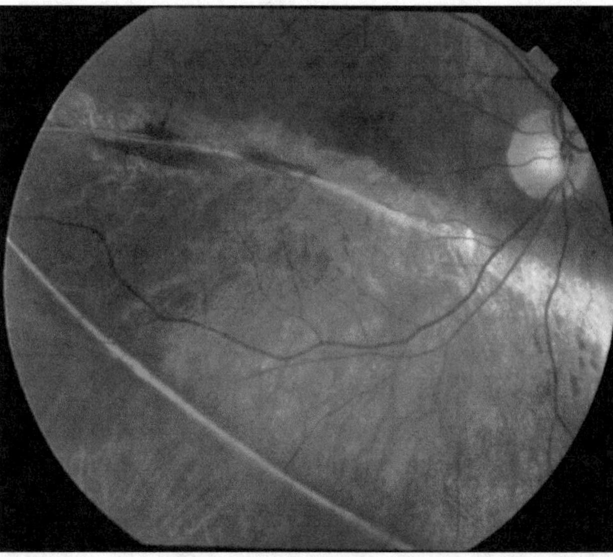

Fig. 10.45 A subretinal band is seen in this patient tenting up the retina with a concave configuration. No action is required

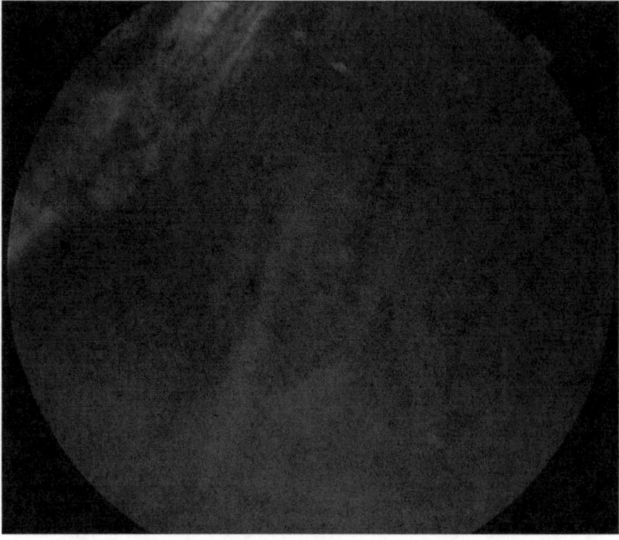

Fig. 10.46 This patient has not had any specific action taken for inferior PVR, approximately CA2; because no retinal break is present the normal physiological processes are able to maintain a flat retina. Observation of this retina postoperatively showed that the retinal detachment did not recur, and the patient avoided further surgery

Postoperative Complications

- Cataract.
  - There is at least a 92% chance of cataract formation.
- Hypotony.
  - Is associated with the presence of anterior PVR. It is claimed excision of the anterior PVR can help restore the IOP [46, 47].
- Macular Pucker.
  - Occurs in 15% of eyes with PVR postoperatively [48], can be removed at the time of silicone oil removal.
- Cystoid macular oedema.
  - This is common in patients with poor visual recovery after PVR surgery but a flat retina. It tends to be refractory to treatment. It is not clear if this is from the effects of retinectomy or the proliferative process [49].
- Retinal distortion and displacement (Figs. 10.47 and 10.48).

The retina after retinectomy is tangentially shorter causing more retinal receptors per area and therefore micropsia. In addition, the retina may not be evenly spread and therefore distortion created. On occasion the patient who attains better visual acuity for the two previous reasons may not like the disruption of vision in the operated eye and its effect of disruption in the other eye.

Complications of Silicone Oil Use (see Chap. 2) (Fig. 10.49).

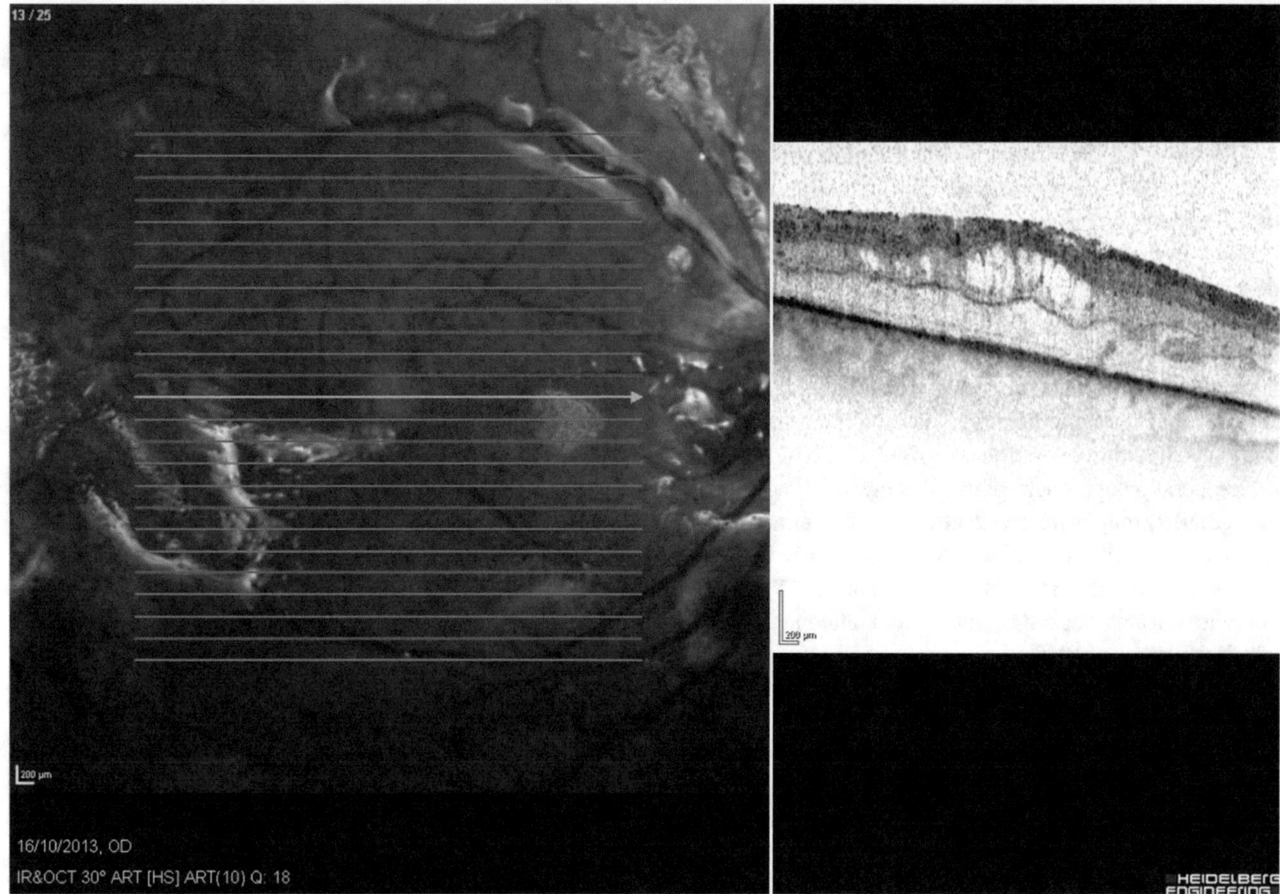

Fig. 10.47 CMO in a patient with retinectomy is unfortunately common

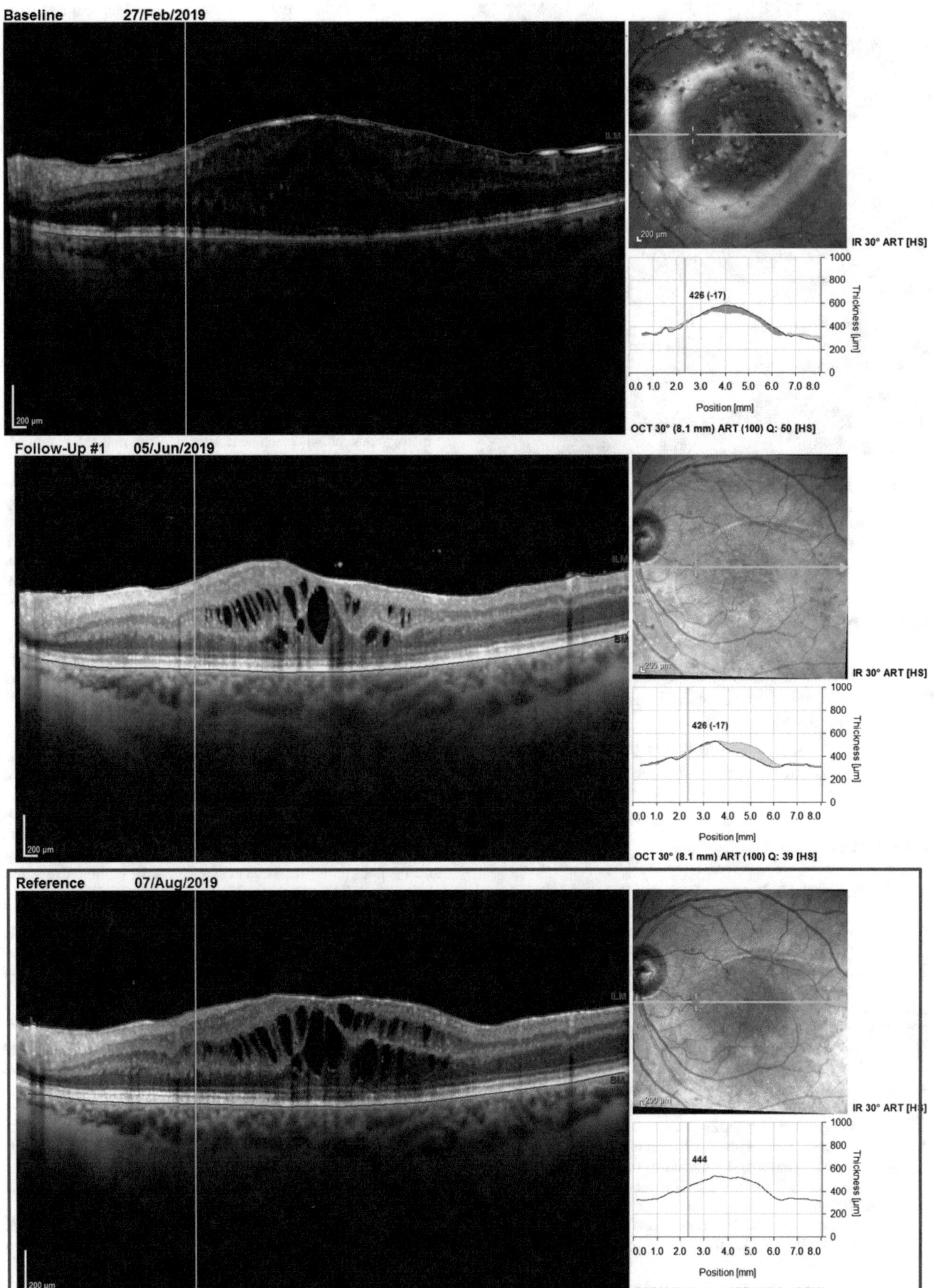

Fig. 10.48 CMO in a patient with retinectomy and PVR. It is not clear whether it is the retinectomy or the PVR which stimulates the CMO. It does not seem to be responsive to topical medication

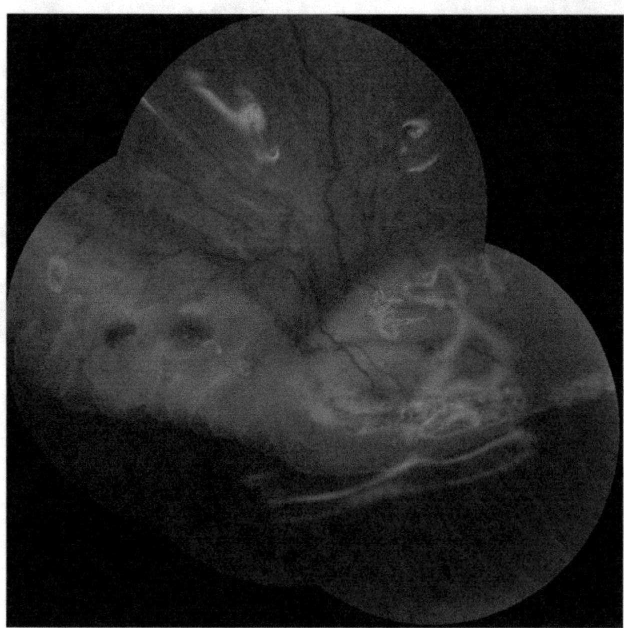

Fig. 10.49 Just under 2% of retinectomies may produce a catastrophic folding of the inferior retina from activation of the PVR process in the postoperative period (approximately 2–4 months) which leads to HM or perception of light vision

Summary

A variety of surgical methods are applied to the treatment of PVR. In the more severe cases it is useful to prepare the patient for the likelihood of three operations, one to flatten most of the retina, a second to flatten the remaining retina, and a final procedure to remove silicone oil.

References

1. Tseng W, Cortez RT, Ramirez G, Stinnett S, Jaffe GJ. Prevalence and risk factors for proliferative vitreoretinopathy in eyes with rhegmatogenous retinal detachment but no previous vitreoretinal surgery. Am J Ophthalmol. 2004;137(6):1105–15.
2. Yorston DB, Wood ML, Gilbert C. Retinal detachment in East Africa. Ophthalmology. 2002;109(12):2279–83.
3. Bonnet M, Fleury J, Guenoun S, Yaniali A, Dumas C, Hajjar C. Cryopexy in primary rhegmatogenous retinal detachment: a risk factor for postoperative proliferative vitreoretinopathy? Graefes Arch Clin Exp Ophthalmol. 1996;234(12):739–43.
4. Glaser BM, Cardin A, Biscoe B. Proliferative vitreoretinopathy. The mechanism of development of vitreoretinal traction. Ophthalmology. 1987;94(4):327–32.
5. Charteris DG. Proliferative vitreoretinopathy: revised concepts of pathogenesis and adjunctive treatment. Eye (Lond). 2020;34(2):241–5. https://doi.org/10.1038/s41433-019-0699-1.
6. Mudhar HS. A brief review of the histopathology of proliferative vitreoretinopathy (PVR). Eye (Lond). 2020;34(2):246–50. https://doi.org/10.1038/s41433-019-0724-4.
7. Moisseiev J, Glaser BM. New and previously unidentified retinal breaks in eyes with recurrent retinal detachment with proliferative vitreoretinopathy. Arch Ophthalmol. 1989;107(8):1152–4.
8. Kon CH, Asaria RH, Occleston NL, Khaw PT, Aylward GW. Risk factors for proliferative vitreoretinopathy after primary vitrectomy: a prospective study. Br J Ophthalmol. 2000;84(5):506–11.
9. Machemer R, Aaberg TM, Freeman HM, Irvine AR, Lean JS, Michels RM. An updated classification of retinal detachment with proliferative vitreoretinopathy. Am J Ophthalmol. 1991;112(2):159–65.
10. Lewis H, Aaberg TM, Abrams GW, McDonald HR, Williams GA, Mieler WF. Subretinal membranes in proliferative vitreoretinopathy. Ophthalmology. 1989;96(9):1403–14.
11. Cowley M, Conway BP, Campochiaro PA, Kaiser D, Gaskin H. Clinical risk factors for proliferative vitreoretinopathy. Arch Ophthalmol. 1989;107(8):1147–51.
12. Glaser BM, Vidaurri-Leal J, Michels RG, Campochiaro PA. Cryotherapy during surgery for giant retinal tears and intravitreal dispersion of viable retinal pigment epithelial cells. Ophthalmology. 1993;100(4):466–70.
13. Bentivoglio M, Valmaggia C, Scholl HPN, Guber J. Comparative study of endolaser versus cryocoagulation in vitrectomy for rhegmatogenous retinal detachment. BMC Ophthalmol. 2019;19(1):96. https://doi.org/10.1186/s12886-019-1099-9.
14. Bhardwaj G, Walker RJE, Ezra E, Mirza Z, Muqit MMK. A 21-year study of vitreoretinal surgery for Aphakic retinal detachment: long-term surgical outcomes and complications. Ophthalmol Retina. 2019;3(9):784–90. https://doi.org/10.1016/j.oret.2019.04.002.
15. Duquesne N, Bonnet M, Adeleine P. Preoperative vitreous hemorrhage associated with rhegmatogenous retinal detachment: a risk factor for postoperative proliferative vitreoretinopathy? Graefes Arch Clin Exp Ophthalmol. 1996;234(11):677–82.
16. Han DP, Rychwalski PJ, Mieler WF, Abrams GW. Management of complex retinal detachment with combined relaxing retinotomy and intravitreal perfluoro-n-octane injection. Am J Ophthalmol. 1994;118(1):24–32.
17. Deaner JD, Aderman CM, Bonafede L, Regillo CD. PPV, Retinectomy, and silicone oil without scleral buckle for recurrent RRD from proliferative vitreoretinopathy. Ophthalmic Surg Lasers Imaging Retina. 2019;50(11):e278–e87. https://doi.org/10.3928/23258160-20191031-15.
18. Storey P, Alshareef R, Khuthaila M, London N, Leiby B, DeCroos C, et al. Pars plana vitrectomy and scleral buckle versus pars plana vitrectomy alone for patients with rhegmatogenous retinal detachment at high risk for proliferative vitreoretinopathy. Retina. 2014;34(10):1945–51. https://doi.org/10.1097/IAE.0000000000000216.
19. Coll GE, Chang S, Sun J, Wieland MR, Berrocal MH. Perfluorocarbon liquid in the management of retinal detachment with proliferative vitreoretinopathy. Ophthalmology. 1995;102(4):630–8.
20. Bourke RD, Cooling RJ. Vascular consequences of retinectomy. Arch Ophthalmol. 1996;114(2):155–60.
21. Veckeneer M, Maaijwee K, Charteris DG, van Meurs JC. Deferred laser photocoagulation of relaxing retinotomies under silicone oil tamponade to reduce recurrent macular detachment in severe proliferative vitreoretinopathy. Graefes Arch Clin Exp Ophthalmol. 2014;252(10):1539–44. https://doi.org/10.1007/s00417-014-2605-7.
22. Mathis A, Pagot V, Gazagne C, Malecaze F. Giant retinal tears. Surgical techniques and results using perfluorodecalin and silicone oil tamponade. Retina. 1992;12(3 Suppl):S7–10.
23. Wong D, Williams RL, German MJ. Exchange of perfluorodecalin for gas or oil: a model for avoiding slippage. Graefes Arch Clin Exp Ophthalmol. 1998;236(3):234–7.

24. Li KK, Wong D. Avoiding retinal slippage during macular translocation surgery with 360 retinotomy. Graefes Arch Clin Exp Ophthalmol. 2008;246(5):649–51. https://doi.org/10.1007/s00417-007-0677-3.
25. Vitrectomy with silicone oil or perfluoropropane gas in eyes with severe proliferative vitreoretinopathy: results of a randomized clinical trial. Silicone study report 2. Arch Ophthalmol. 1992;110(6):780–92.
26. Schwartz SG, Flynn HW Jr, Lee WH, Wang X. Tamponade in surgery for retinal detachment associated with proliferative vitreoretinopathy. Cochrane Database Syst Rev. 2014;2:Cd006126. https://doi.org/10.1002/14651858.CD006126.pub3.
27. Barr CC, Lai MY, Lean JS, Linton KL, Trese M, Abrams G, et al. Postoperative intraocular pressure abnormalities in the silicone study. Silicone study report 4. Ophthalmology. 1993;100(11): 1629–35.
28. Sigler EJ, Randolph JC, Calzada JI, Charles S. Pars plana vitrectomy with medium-term postoperative perfluoro-N-octane for recurrent inferior retinal detachment complicated by advanced proliferative vitreoretinopathy. Retina. 2013;33(4):791–7. https://doi.org/10.1097/IAE.0b013e31826a6978.
29. Wiedemann P, Hilgers RD, Bauer P, Heimann K. Adjunctive daunorubicin in the treatment of proliferative vitreoretinopathy: results of a multicenter clinical trial. Daunomycin Study Group Am J Ophthalmol. 1998;126(4):550–9.
30. Charteris DG, Aylward GW, Wong D, Groenewald C, Asaria RH, Bunce C. A randomized controlled trial of combined 5-fluorouracil and low-molecular-weight heparin in management of established proliferative vitreoretinopathy. Ophthalmology. 2004;111(12):2240–5.
31. Stern WH, Lewis GP, Erickson PA, Guerin CJ, Anderson DH, Fisher SK, et al. Fluorouracil therapy for proliferative vitreoretinopathy after vitrectomy. Am J Ophthalmol. 1983;96(1):33–42.
32. Blumenkranz M, Hernandez E, Ophir A, Norton EW. 5-fluorouracil: new applications in complicated retinal detachment for an established antimetabolite. Ophthalmology. 1984;91(2):122–30.
33. Banerjee PJ, Quartilho A, Bunce C, Xing W, Zvobgo TM, Harris N, et al. Slow-release dexamethasone in proliferative vitreoretinopathy: a prospective, randomized controlled clinical trial. Ophthalmology. 2017;124(6):757–67. https://doi.org/10.1016/j.ophtha.2017.01.021.
34. Asaria RH, Kon CH, Bunce C, Charteris DG, Wong D, Khaw PT, et al. Adjuvant 5-fluorouracil and heparin prevents proliferative vitreoretinopathy: results from a randomized, double-blind, controlled clinical trial. Ophthalmology. 2001;108(7):1179–83.
35. Vidaurri-Leal J, de BS, Michels RG. Surgical treatment of giant retinal tears with inverted posterior retinal flaps. Am J Ophthalmol. 1984;98(4):463–6.
36. Stolba U, Binder S, Velikay M, Datlinger P, Wedrich A. Use of perfluorocarbon liquids in proliferative vitreoretinopathy: results and complications. Br J Ophthalmol. 1995;79(12):1106–10.
37. Fisher YL, Shakin JL, Slakter JS, Sorenson JA, Shafer DM. Perfluoropropane gas, modified panretinal photocoagulation, and vitrectomy in the management of severe proliferative vitreoretinopathy. Arch Ophthalmol. 1988;106(9):1255–60.
38. Cox MS, Trese MT, Murphy PL. Silicone oil for advanced proliferative vitreoretinopathy. Ophthalmology. 1986;93(5):646–50.
39. Scott IU, Flynn HW Jr, Murray TG, Feuer WJ. Outcomes of surgery for retinal detachment associated with proliferative vitreoretinopathy using perfluoro-n-octane: a multicenter study. Am J Ophthalmol. 2003;136(3):454–63.
40. Iverson DA, Ward TG, Blumenkranz MS. Indications and results of relaxing retinotomy. Ophthalmology. 1990;97(10):1298–304.
41. Lam RF, Cheung BT, Yuen CY, Wong D, Lam DS, Lai WW. Retinal redetachment after silicone oil removal in proliferative vitreoretinopathy: a prognostic factor analysis. Am J Ophthalmol. 2008;145(3):527–33. https://doi.org/10.1016/j.ajo.2007.10.015.
42. Scott IU, Flynn HW, Lai M, Chang S, Azen SP. First operation anatomic success and other predictors of postoperative vision after complex retinal detachment repair with vitrectomy and silicone oil tamponade. Am J Ophthalmol. 2000;130(6):745–50.
43. Diddie KR, Azen SP, Freeman HM, Boone DC, Aaberg TM, Lewis H, et al. Anterior proliferative vitreoretinopathy in the silicone study. Silicone study report number 10. Ophthalmology. 1996;103(7):1092–9.
44. Schwartz SD, Kreiger AE. Proliferative vitreoretinopathy: a natural history of the fellow eye. Ophthalmology. 1998;105(5):785–8.
45. Lewis H, Aaberg TM. Causes of failure after repeat vitreoretinal surgery for recurrent proliferative vitreoretinopathy. Am J Ophthalmol. 1991;111(1):15–9.
46. Lewis H, Verdaguer JI. Surgical treatment for chronic hypotony and anterior proliferative vitreoretinopathy. Am J Ophthalmol. 1996;122(2):228–35.
47. O'Connell SR, Majji AB, Humayun MS, De Juan E. The surgical management of hypotony. Ophthalmology. 2000;107(2):318–23.
48. Cox MS, Azen SP, Barr CC, Linton KL, Diddie KR, Lai MY, et al. Macular pucker after successful surgery for proliferative vitreoretinopathy. Silicone study report 8. Ophthalmology. 1995;102(12):1884–91.
49. Benson SE, Schlottmann PG, Bunce C, Xing W, Charteris DG. Optical coherence tomography analysis of the macula after vitrectomy surgery for retinal detachment. Ophthalmology. 2006;113(7):1179–83. https://doi.org/10.1016/j.ophtha.2006.01.039.

Macular Hole

11

Contents

T. H. Williamson, *Vitreoretinal Surgery*, https://doi.org/10.1007/978-3-030-68769-4_11

Introduction

The macula is a common site of symptomatic retinal pathology requiring vitreoretinal intervention. Posterior vitreous detachment is implicated in the production of most common macular disorders (Figs. 11.1 and 11.2).

Idiopathic Macular Hole

Clinical Features

Introduction

Age-related macular hole is a dehiscence of the neuroretina at the fovea, which occurs in middle-aged or elderly patients, and more often in females (3.321 females:1 male, with 7.8/100000 population) [1]. They are bilateral in 12–13% in 2 years after presentation in one eye [2]. The risk of surgery to the fellow eye is 7.5% in 10 years [3]. Patients present with blurred vision or distortion. In the early stages (grade 1) the patient notices a small central grey patch without distortion of the image. Distortion becomes a feature as the fovea dehisces and the photoreceptors are moved outwards onto the rim of the hole (grades 2 and 3). Typically, the features at the centre of an image (e.g. the nose and mouth of a face) are smaller, giving the appearance that the centre of someone's face is "scrunched up". The receptors are on the perimeter of the hole and spread out by the dehiscence. The brain, therefore, receives fewer signals than it should in the centre of the macula and interprets this as a falsely small image centrally. Eventually the receptors at the edge of the hole will stop functioning (grades 3 and 4) and the patient will only perceive a central scotoma (Figs. 11.3, 11.4, and 11.5).

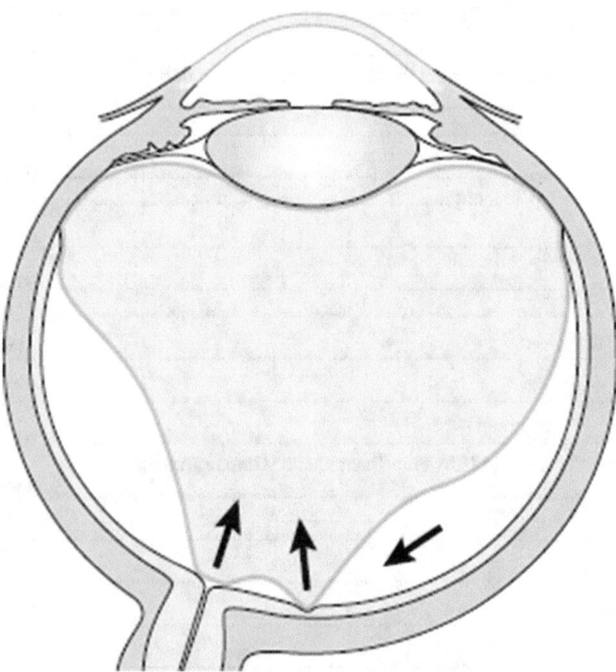

Fig. 11.1 The vitreous has attachments at the vitreous base and weaker attachments at the disc and fovea. These are vulnerable to damage during PVD

Watzke Allen Test

The phenomena of distortion and loss of vision are exploited in the Watzke Allen test [4]. This involves shining a thin line of light (usually vertically) via the slit lamp biomicroscope over the macular hole, whilst asking the patient to describe whether the line of light is straight or has a narrowing (waist) or gap (break) centrally [4]. A straight line indicates an intact fovea, whilst a narrowing or a gap is seen in macular holes [5]. A narrowing indicates separated but functioning foveal receptors and a break loss of function of those receptors. If you place the beam on the edge of the hole, a kink is perceived with the apex pointing towards the hole.

Vitreous detachment stimulates the dehiscence of the fovea. Indeed, a subclinical separation of the vitreous is visible on optical coherence tomography (OCT) of the macula and can sometimes be seen clinically, evidenced by the presence of a prefoveal operculum in the early stages. The operculum does not consist of full-thickness retina but is made up of glial tissue and a few neural tissue remnants or receptors [6, 7] (Figs. 11.6, 11.7, 11.8, 11.9, 11.10, 11.11, 11.12, and 11.13).

Grading

It is useful to use the grading system devised by Gass to describe macular holes because these have been shown to relate to surgical success rates and visual outcome.

Grade 1	The hole commences as a foveal intraretinal cyst [8] (1A) or ring of cysts (1B), seen as a central yellow spot or ring of spots [9–11] at which point the patient may be asymptomatic or have mild blur or distortion.
Grade 2	A small crescentic or round hole less than 400 μm.
Grade 3	A large round hole of more than 400 μm diameter
Grade 4	A hole with an associated posterior vitreous detachment.

Note: The grading system Gass devised relates to ophthalmoscopy and not to OCT findings, therefore a micro separation of the vitreous, with or without an operculum, in an eye with a full-thickness break would be graded as 3 not a grade 4.

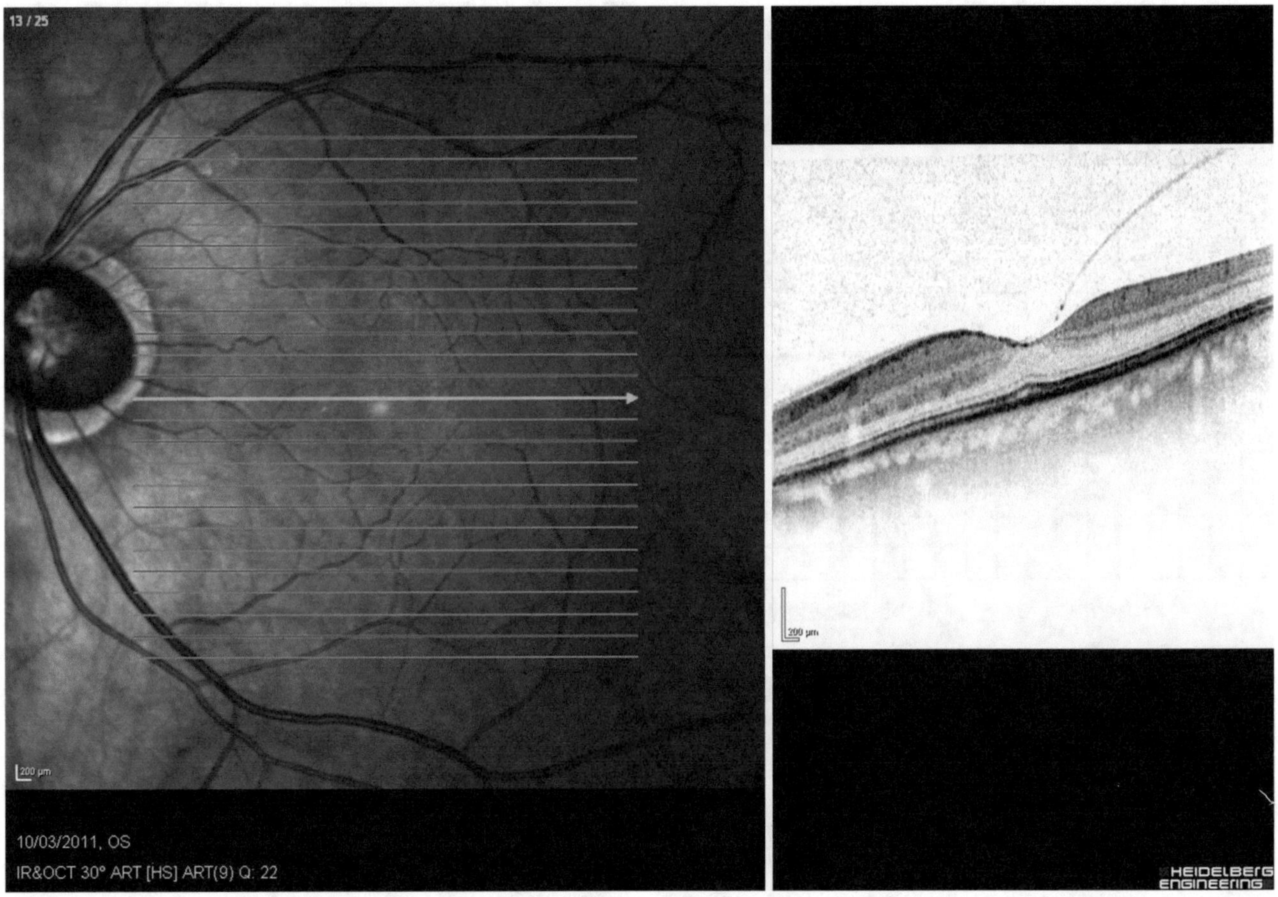

Fig. 11.2 Vitreous separation may start temporally but attachments at the fovea are stronger commencing the process of macular hole formation

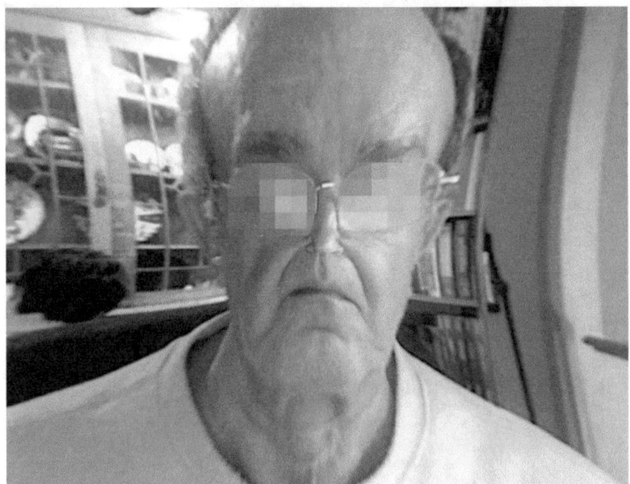

Fig. 11.3 A patient's representation of the distortion of their face created by their own macular hole because the central receptors are spread around the edge of the hole the central image is minified

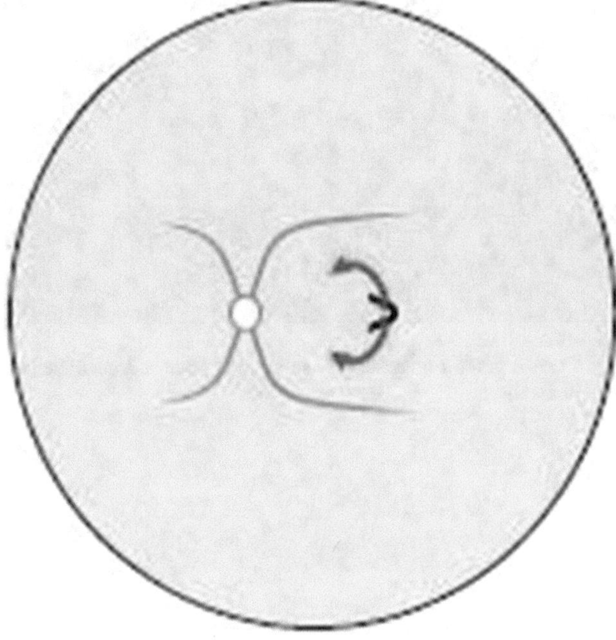

Fig. 11.4 An early macular hole may show traction on OCT indicating tearing towards the disc

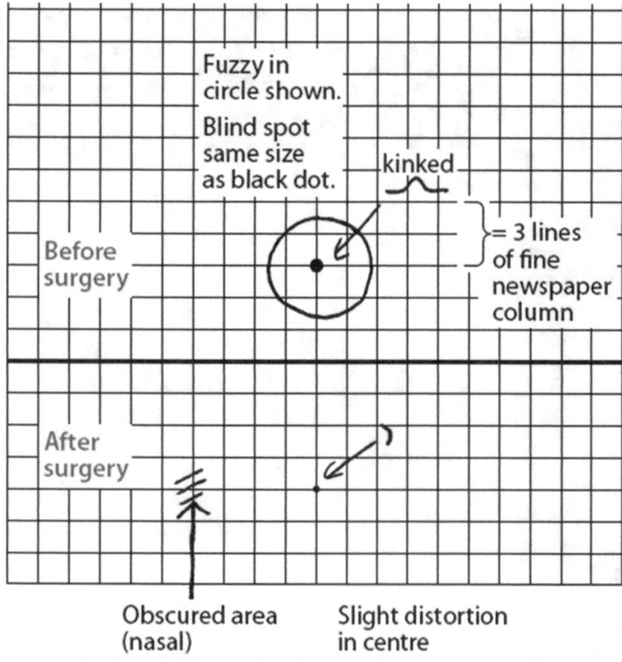

Fig. 11.5 A patient's description of their symptoms before and after macular hole surgery

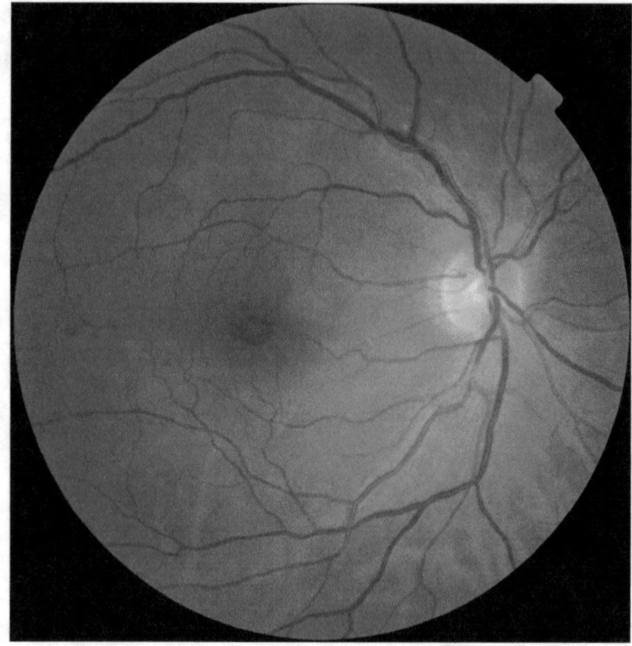

Fig. 11.7 A grade 1a macular hole

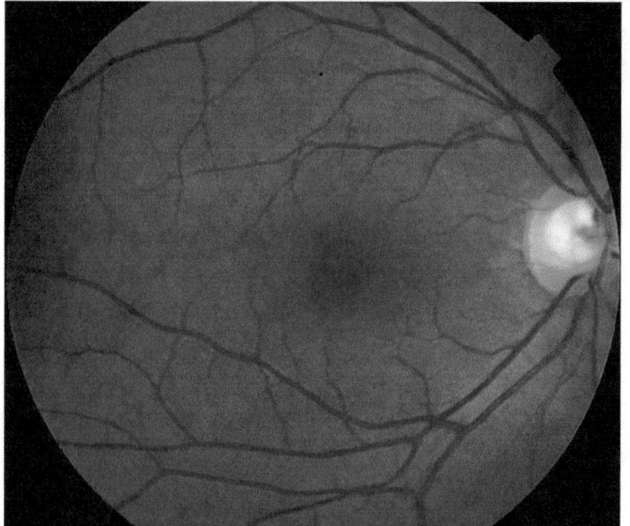

Fig. 11.6 A grade 1 hole is a very subtle sign often as a small yellow spot in the fovea

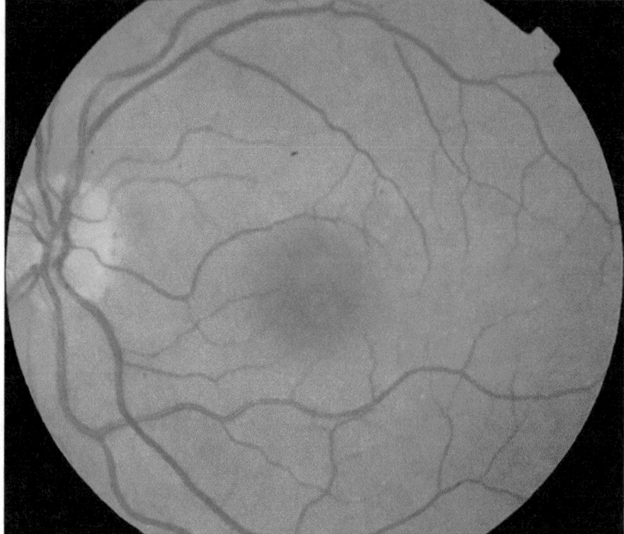

Fig. 11.8 Grade 1b, a ring of yellow spots

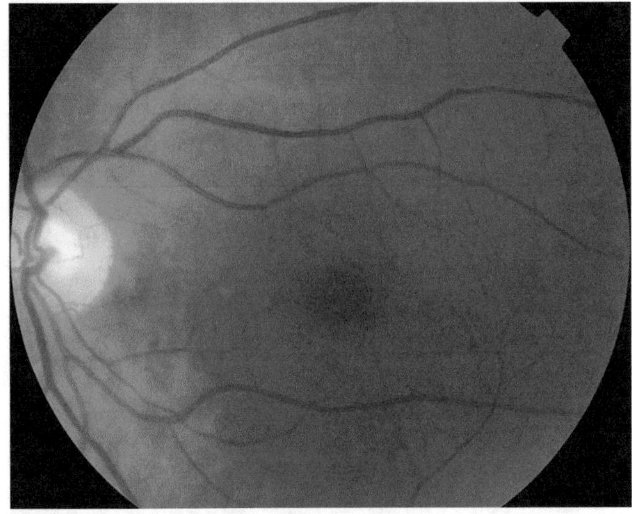

Fig. 11.9 A grade 1b hole with an incomplete ring of spots

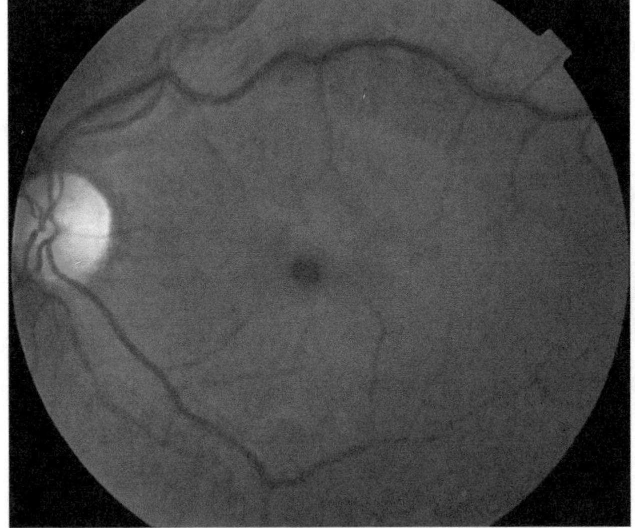

Fig. 11.10 A grade 2, vitreous attached and hole diameter less than 400 μm

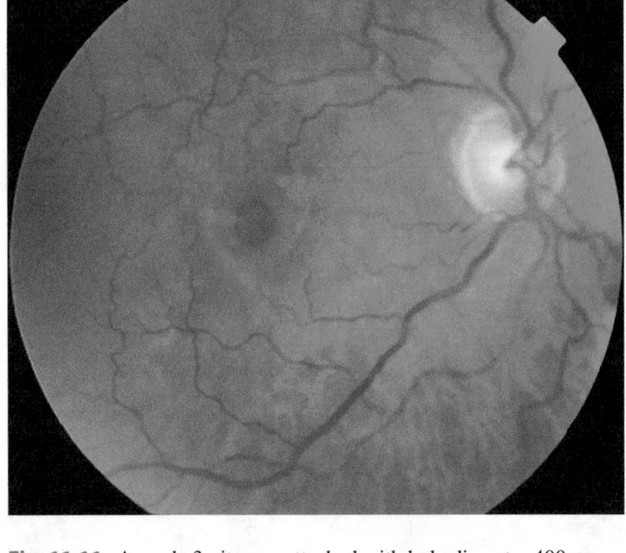

Fig. 11.11 A grade 3 vitreous attached with hole diameter 400 μm or more. This hole has some surrounding retinal thickening and subretinal fluid

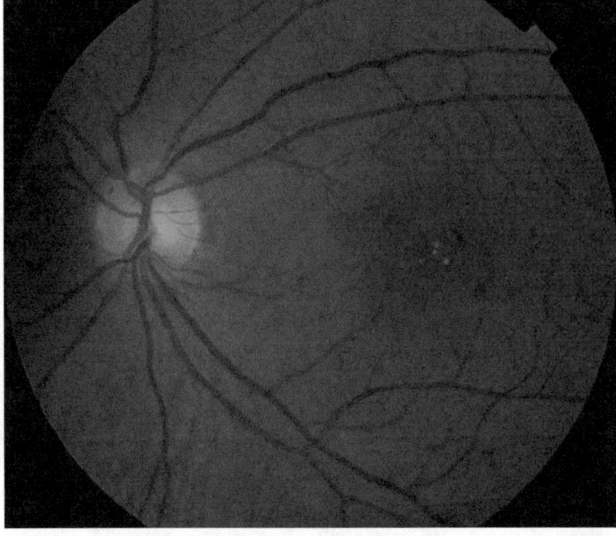

Fig. 11.12 A longstanding macular hole with yellow flecks in its base

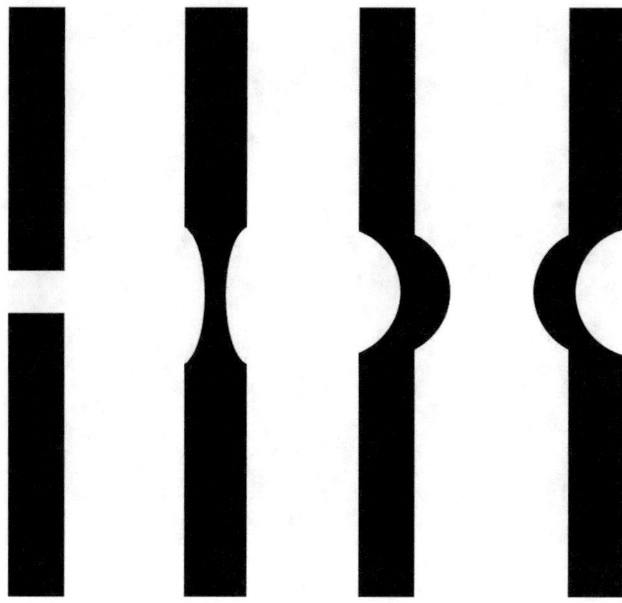

Fig. 11.13 Different patterns of abnormality are seen in Watzke Allen test including a break, central narrowing and bowing of this slit lamp beam. The first two are associated with macular hole. The second two are associated with epiretinal membrane, but this abnormality can also be demonstrated on the edge of macular holes

OCT can be used to measure the width of the hole at its narrowest separation to discriminate grades 2 and 3. More recently surgeons are relying on the size of the hole to determine outcome. The minimal inner diameter of the hole is a particularly good indicator of surgical closure rate. Up to 500 microns hole closure rates can be over 95%. After this size closure rates fall drastically unless other adjuncts are added to surgery such as ILM flap methods. The basal diameter (where the receptors meet the RPE) is a good indicator of visual outcome with large gaps of 1000 microns doing less well for visual recovery.

Natural History (Figs. 11.14, 11.15, 11.16, and 11.17) (Figs. 11.18 and 11.19) Grade 1 holes progress to full-thickness holes in approximately 40% of cases [12].

Grade 1 holes with poorer vision have a higher chance of progressing [13].

Grade 2 holes have 74% chance of proceeding to stage 3 or 4 in 6 to 12 months [14] (Figs. 11.20, 11.21, 11.22, 11.23, 11.24, 11.25, 11.26, 11.27, and 11.28).

(Figs. 11.29 and 11.30) At five years without treatment there is a 75% chance of 20/200 vision or worse [2, 15].

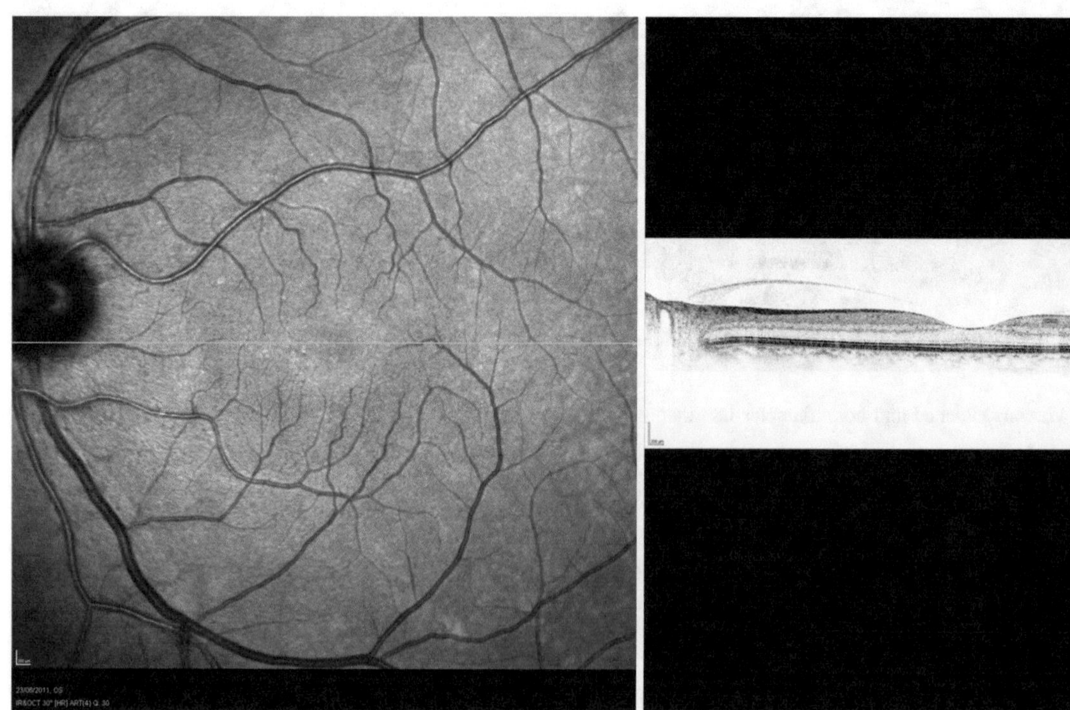

Fig. 11.14 When examining the risk to the fellow eye of a patient with macular hole any sign of traction from the posterior hyaloid on the fovea as in this patient (which has been named as grade 0 macular hole) increases the risk of progression to full-thickness macular hole to 40%. In absence of this sign risk of progression is low

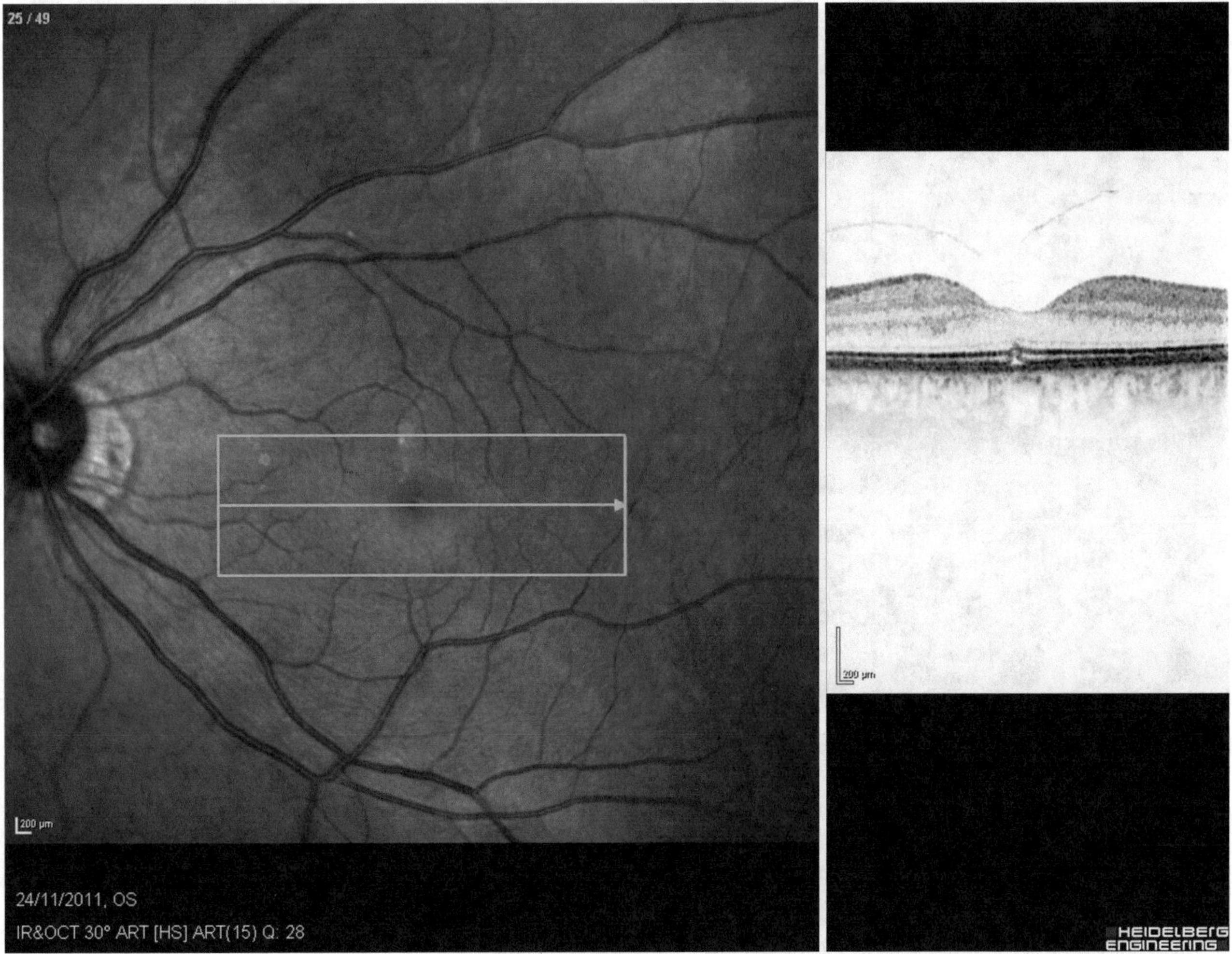

Fig. 11.15 Mild foveal disruption is present from vitreo-foveal traction. The vitreous separated without progression to macular hole

Spontaneous closure can occur especially with grade 2 holes, 11.5%; [16] reducing in grades 3 and 4 holes to 4% [17].

Optical Coherence Tomography

OCT is essential for confirming the diagnosis and to help determine the risk to the other eye [18, 19]. Optical coherence tomography (OCT) images also aid the discrimination of partial thickness and pseudoholes (from epiretinal membrane) from full-thickness macular holes.

In the grade 1 hole the posterior hyaloid pulls on the fovea causing an intraretinal cyst.

In the grade 2 hole the retina ruptures producing a small full-thickness hole often with the vitreous still attached to one edge which causes an eccentric opening of the roof of the hole by traction from the posterior hyaloid [20].

In a grade 3 hole the vitreous is often separated (but too close to the retina to see biomicroscopically) whilst the hole has enlarged.

The occult separation of the vitreous detectable on OCT is seen in 74% of grades 2 and 3 holes and is attached to the disc margin in 33% [20, 21]. The visible membrane on the posterior hyaloid probably consists of vitreous cortex with fragments of ILM [22]. The fellow eye shows separation of the vitreous on OCT in 31%.

Grade 0 macular holes have been described as a vitreous separation on OCT but with persistent attachment to the fovea. Grade 0 is present in 29% of the contralateral eyes of patients with macular holes. 46% of eyes with Grade 0 progress to macular hole at 2 years compared with 6% in those with no vitreous attachments [23].

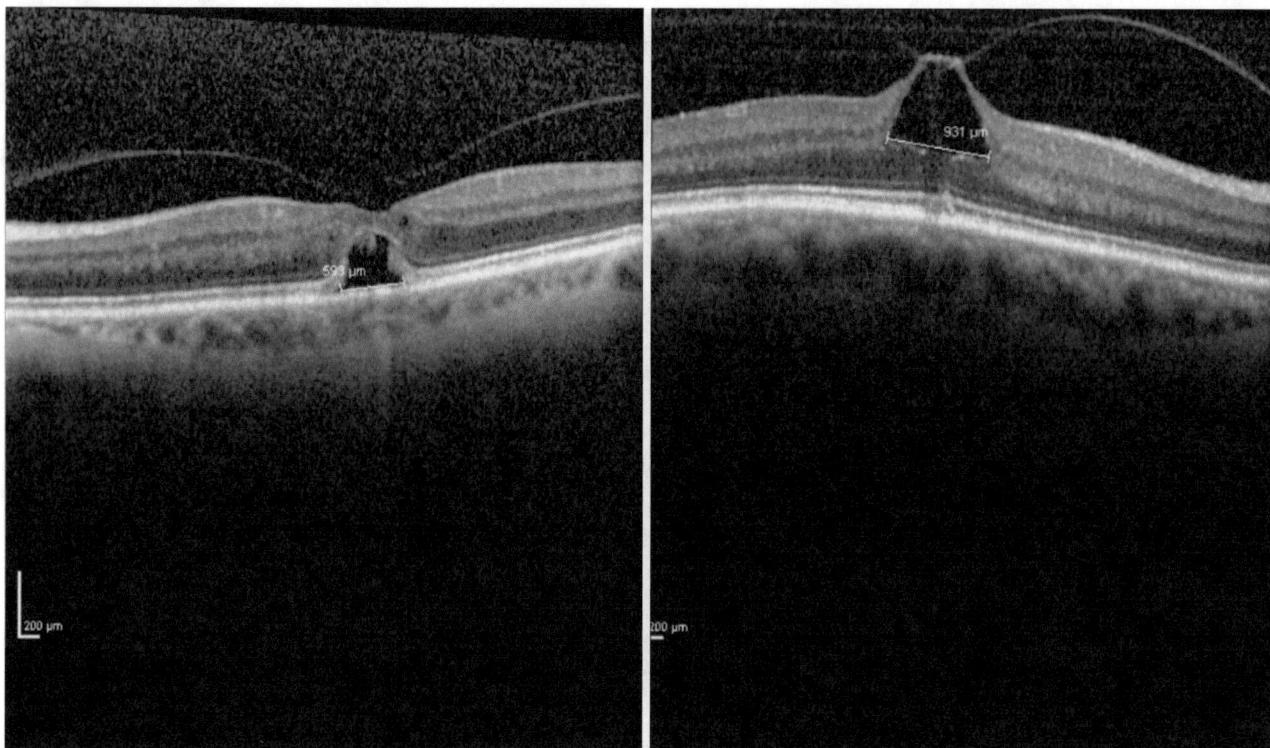

Fig. 11.16 Two types of grade 1 macular hole

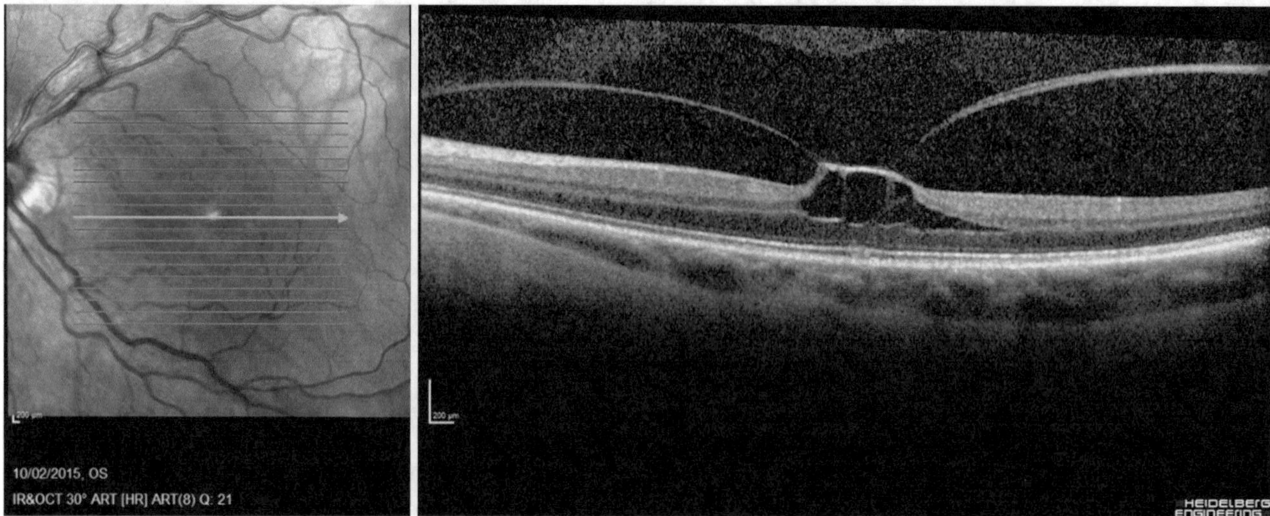

Fig. 11.17 Grade 1 hole in the fellow eye of a patient with MH

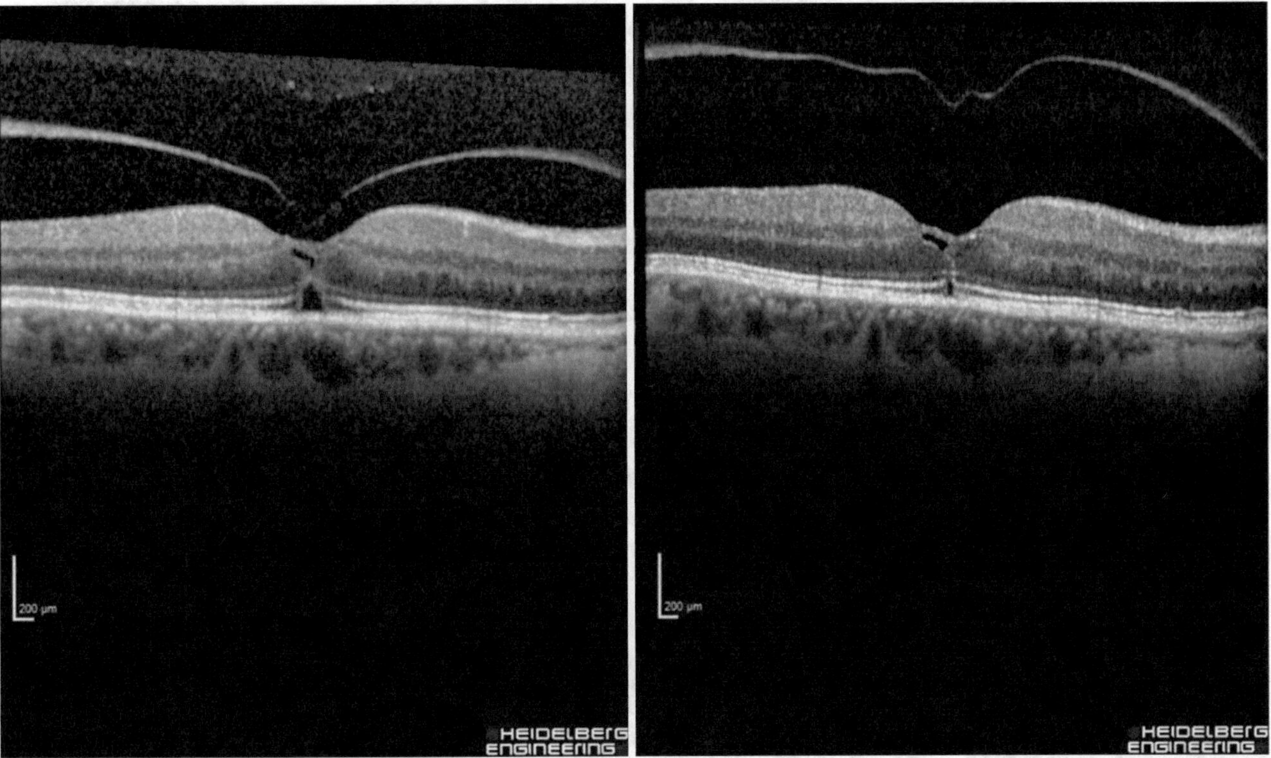

Fig. 11.18 Spontaneous resolution of a grade 1 MH

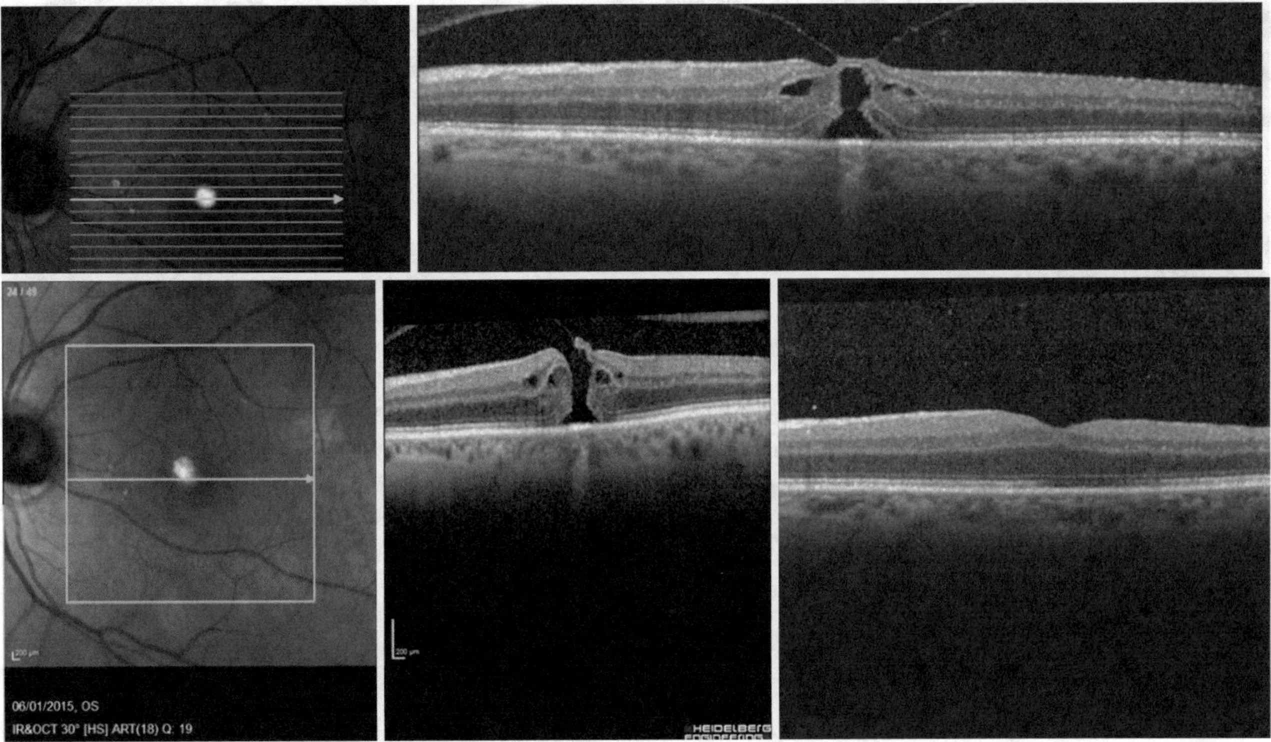

Fig. 11.19 Progression of MH 1 to 2 and postoperative closure

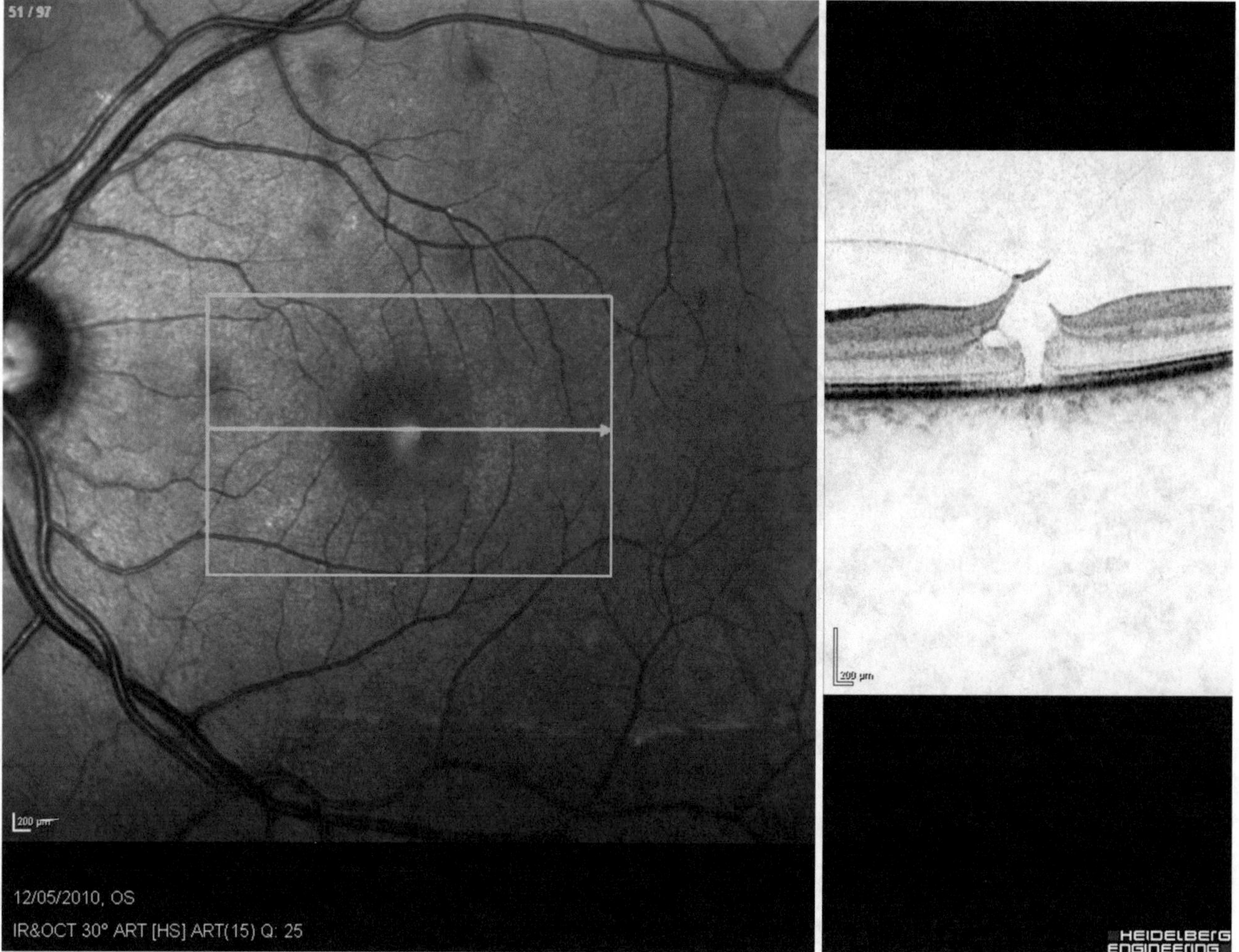

Fig. 11.20 A grade 2 hole with traction of vitreous and its closure after PPV and gas

FEA Mathematical Modelling of Full-Thickness Macular Hole

Mahmut Dogramaci

For the purposes of mathematical modelling of full-thickness macular holes, the process of macular hole formation could be divided in to two steps. The first step involves vitreomacular traction and the second step involves peripheral retraction of internal limiting membrane.

Step 1: Vitreomacular traction.

Vitreomacular tractions pull the internal limiting membrane that overlies the fovea in a direction perpendicular to the retina. Finite element analysis of the fovea under such circumstances reveals the following details (Fig. 11.31).

1. Enhanced stress levels at the internal limiting membrane result in a tear and subsequent operculum formation over the fovea. This process leads to loss of support provided by internal limiting membrane, which has an important impact on neuroretinal strength at the centre of the fovea. Neuroretinal structures are primarily laid in either vertical or horizontal directions. Vertically aligned structures, namely photoreceptors and bipolar cells, provide resistance against vertical loads, whilst horizontal aligned structures, namely nerve fibre layer, internal limiting membrane, horizontal cells, and bipolar cells, provide resistance against horizontal loads. Out of all the horizontal structures, internal limiting membrane is the only layer that bridges over centre of fovea, therefore a rip in the internal limiting membrane at these areas results in total loss of resistance to horizontal loads [24].
2. Persistent vertical strain leads to plastic deformation and intraretinal fluid accumulation in perifoveal neuroretinal layers with a subsequent weakening in resistance against horizontal loads.

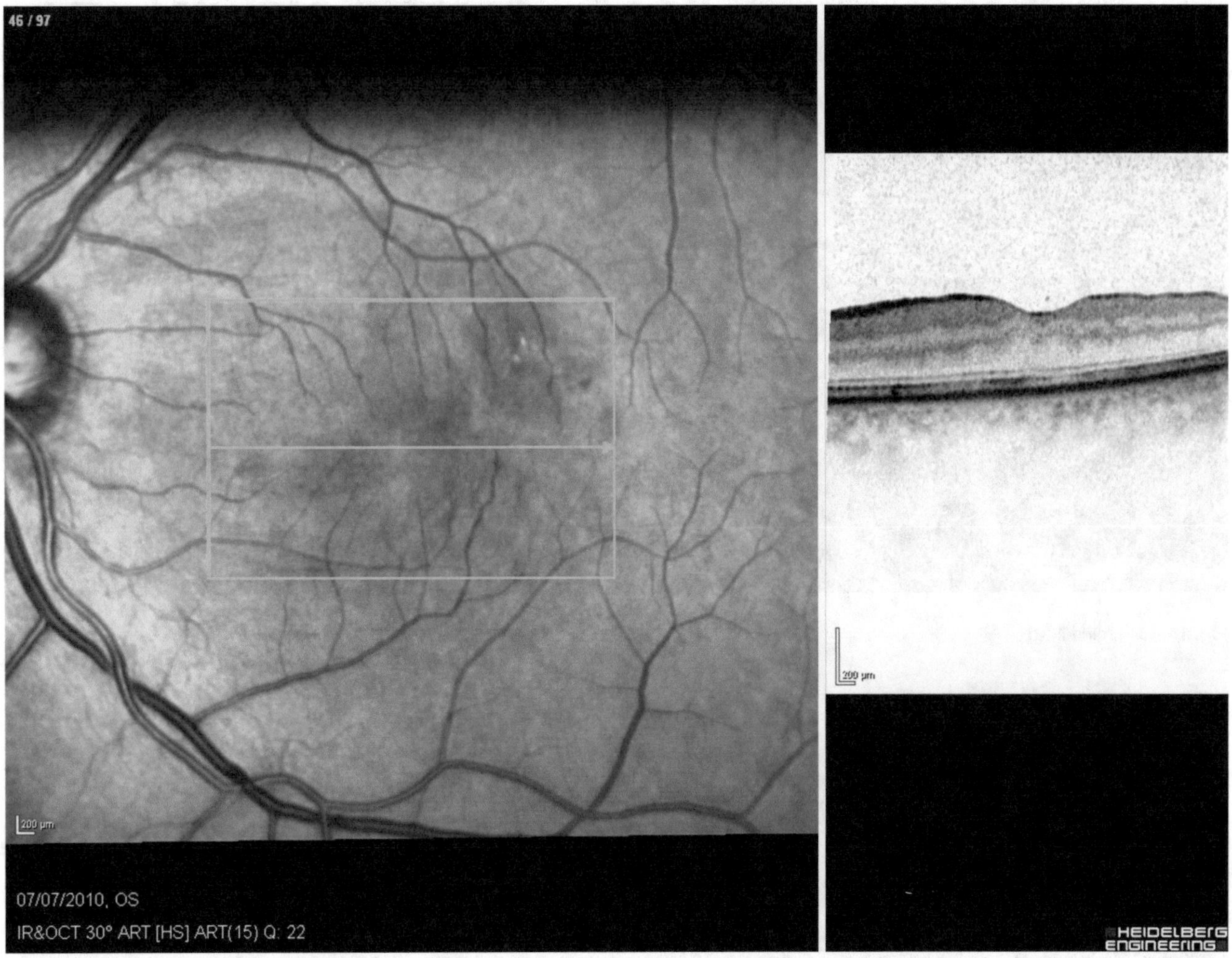

46 / 97
200 µm
07/07/2010, OS
IR&OCT 30° ART [HS] ART(15) Q: 22
200 µm
HEIDELBERG ENGINEERING

Fig. 11.21 The hole has closed. The shadow from the gas can be seen at the top of the scan

200 µm
HEIDELBERG ENGINEERING
200 µm

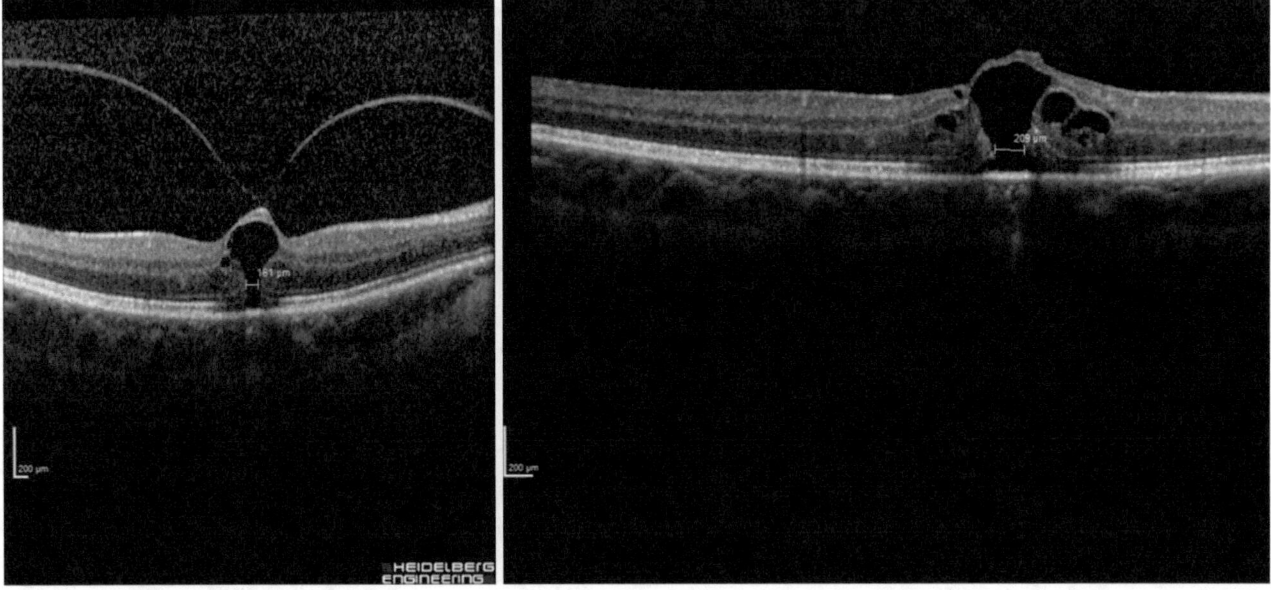

Fig. 11.22 Although the MH has an inner surface the fovea is opened. These should be operated upon

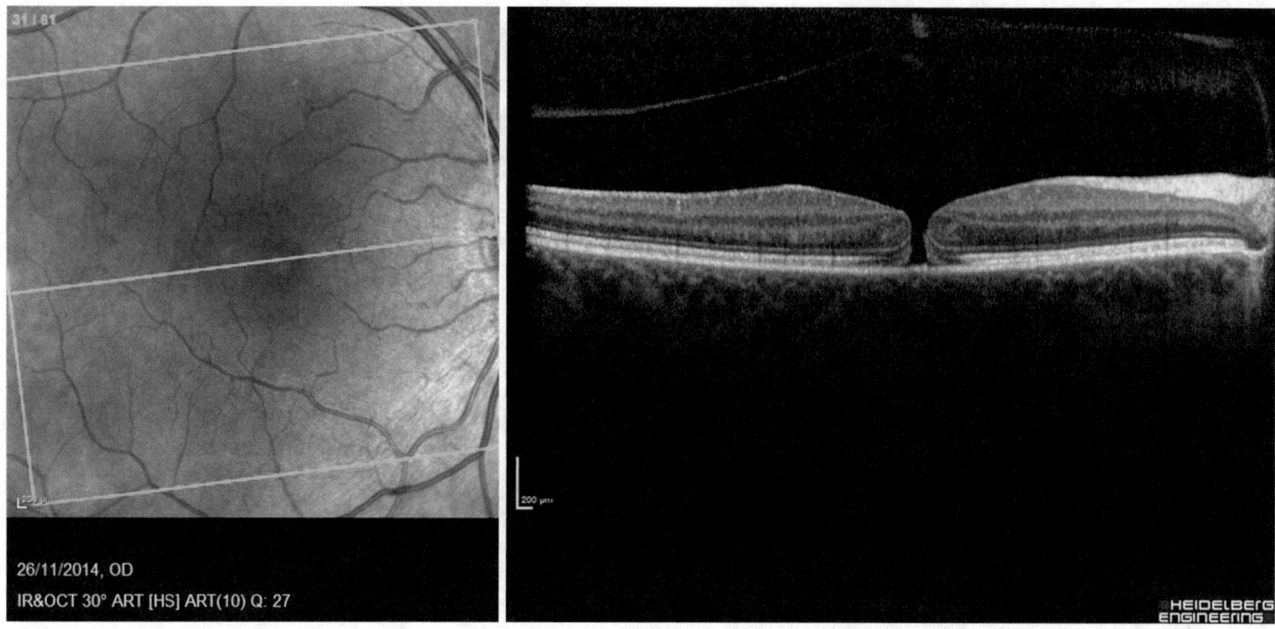

Fig. 11.23 Grade 2 MH

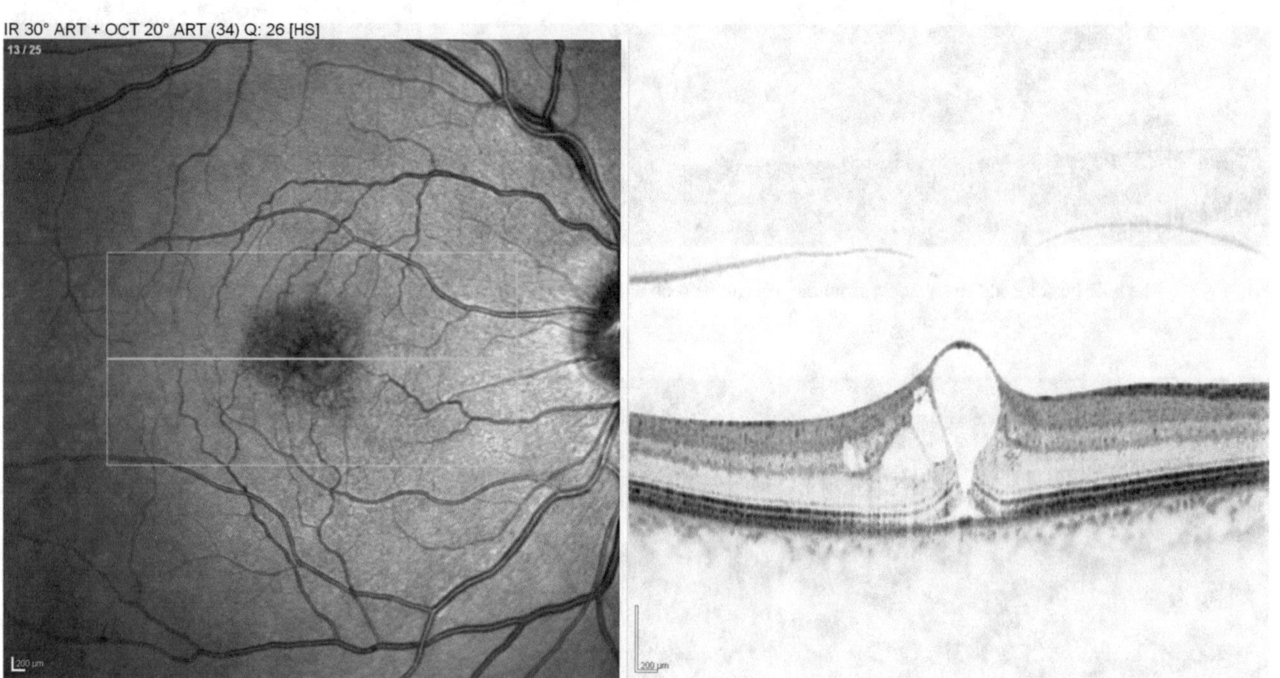

Fig. 11.24 An exceedingly early grade 2 macular hole seen on HD OCT.

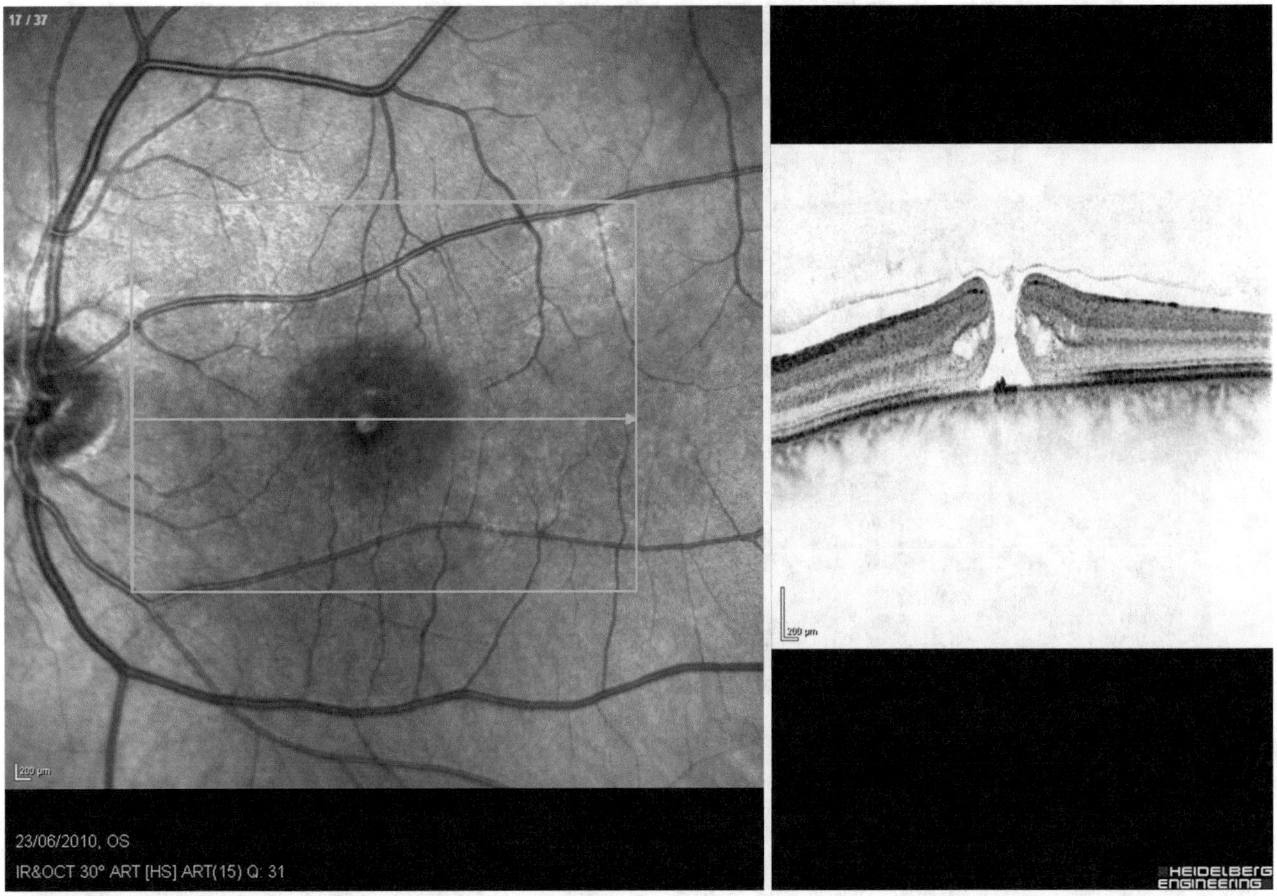

Fig. 11.25 A grade 2 macular hole on HD OCT showing cystoid spaces beginning to appear at the edge of the hole

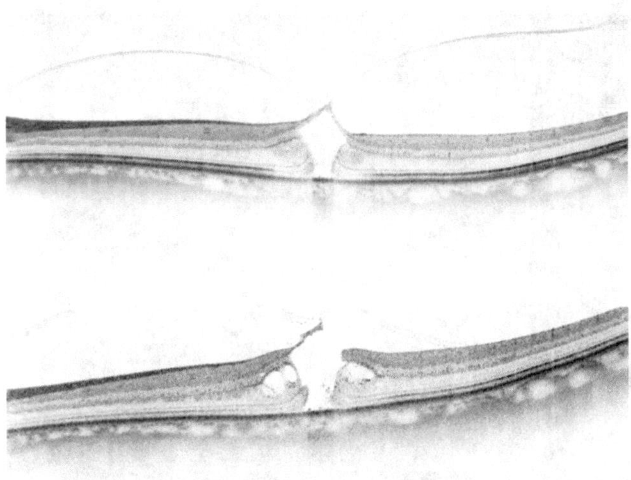

Fig. 11.26 A grade 2 hole progresses from outer retina dehiscence to full-thickness hole

3. Separation of photoreceptors from the pigment epithelium layer. This separation further weakens the resistance of the parafoveal neuroretinal rim against horizontal loads.

Step 2: Internal limiting membrane retraction.

Careful observations during internal limiting membrane peel procedures suggest that internal limiting membrane retracts when freed from its adhesions to underlying tissues. When the fovea is exposed to vitreomacular traction and lost both its resistance to horizontal loads and its adherence to underlying pigment epithelium, the perifoveal internal limiting membrane can retract pulling the foveal edges both sideways and upward (Fig. 11.32).

Finite element analysis showed that the size and the height of the macular hole are dependent on the size of the gap in the internal limiting membrane, elasticity of perifoveal neu-

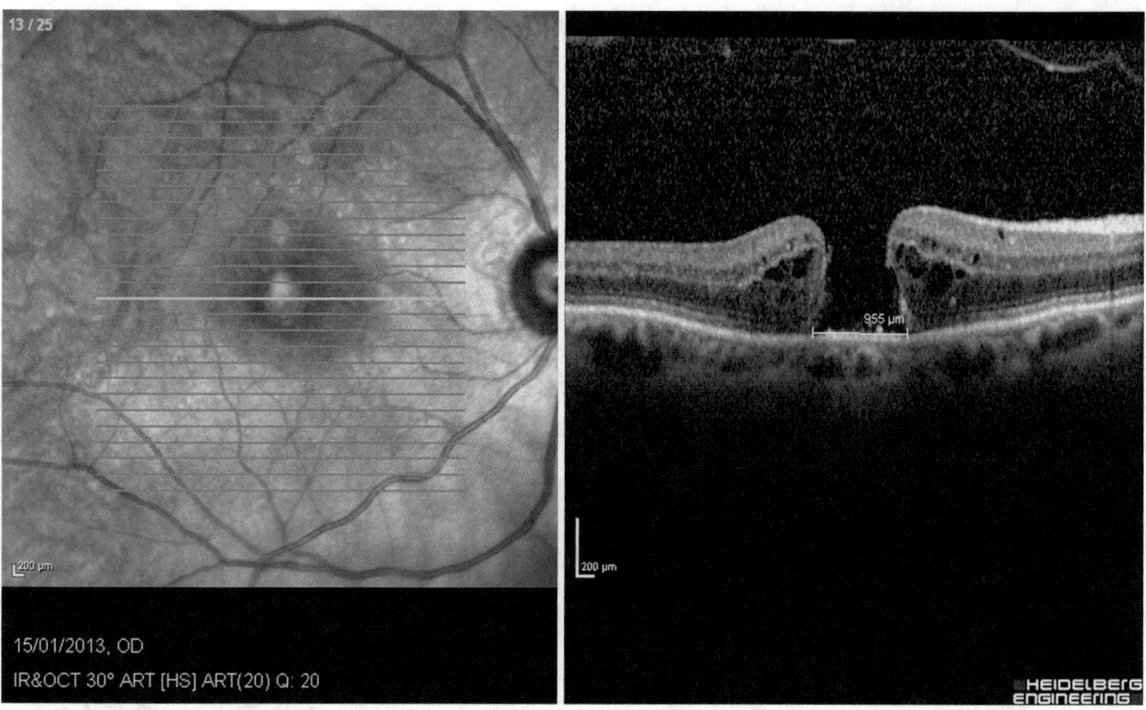

Fig. 11.27 Large MH grade 3. Grading the hole helps predict outcome but size also matters with large holes closing less often (above 500 microns minimum internal diameter) with less visual recovery

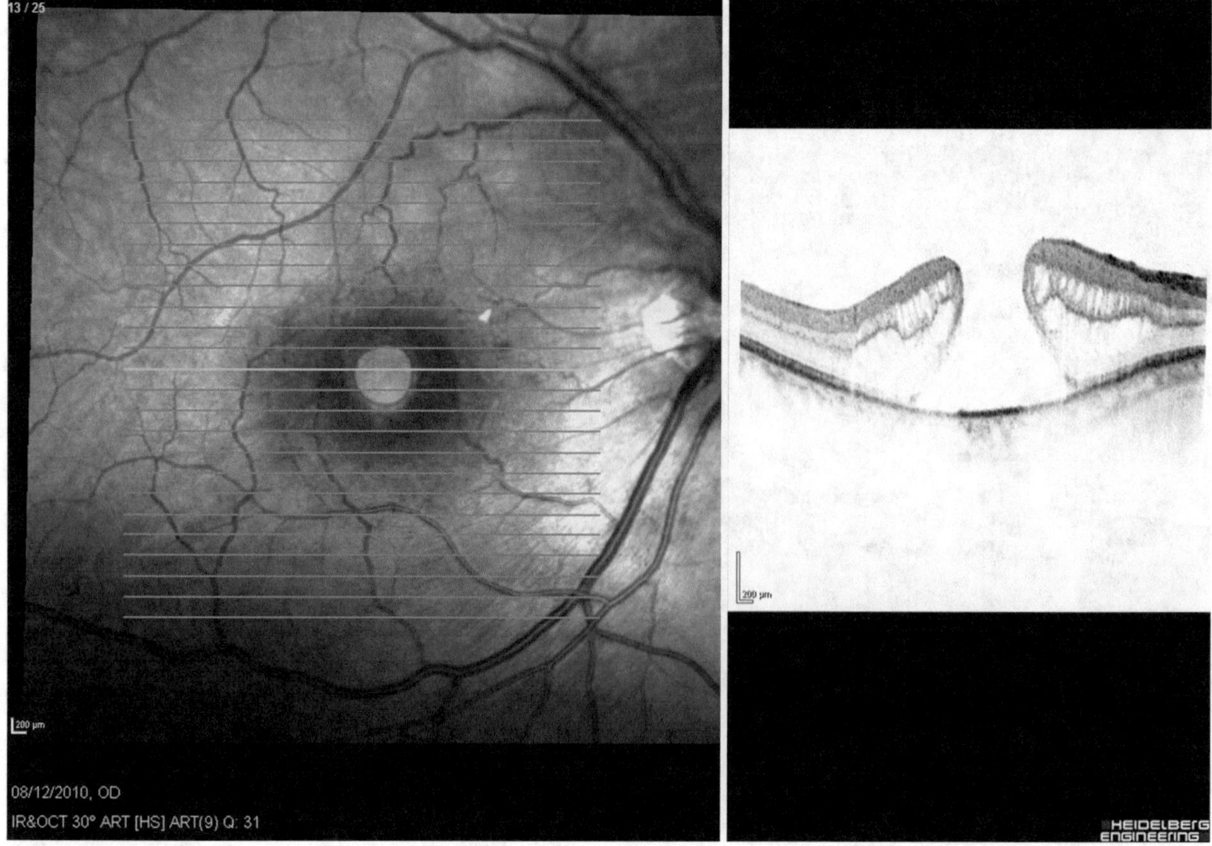

Fig. 11.28 A large grade 4 macular hole

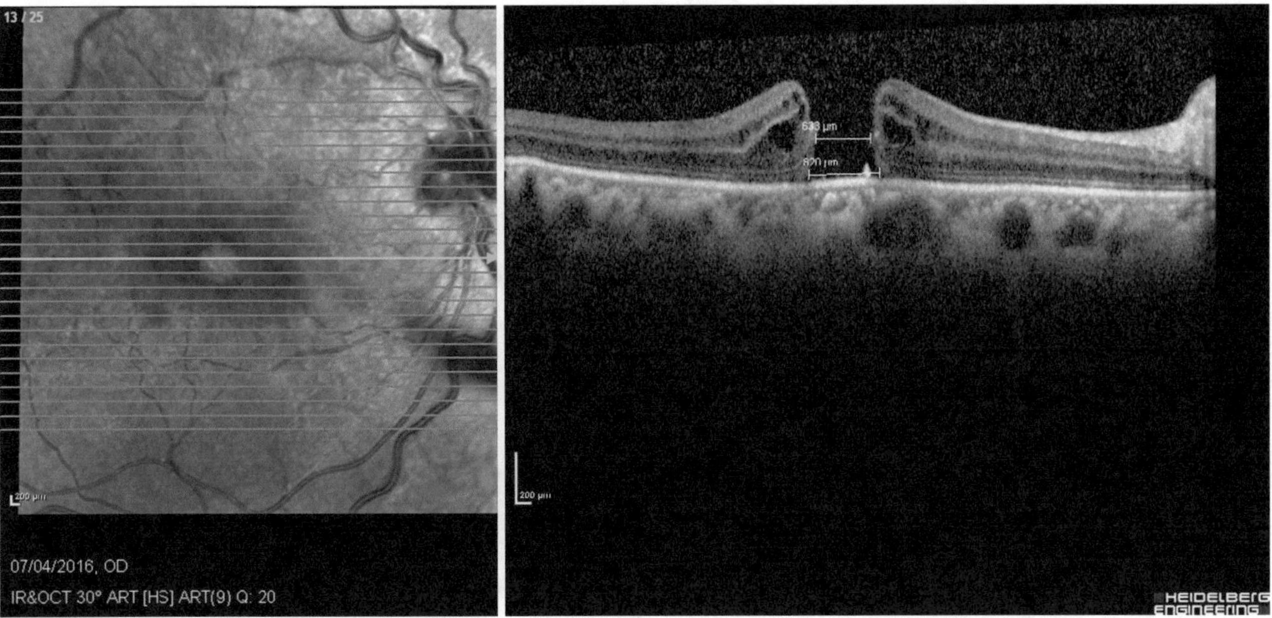

Fig. 11.29 A large grade 4 macular hole

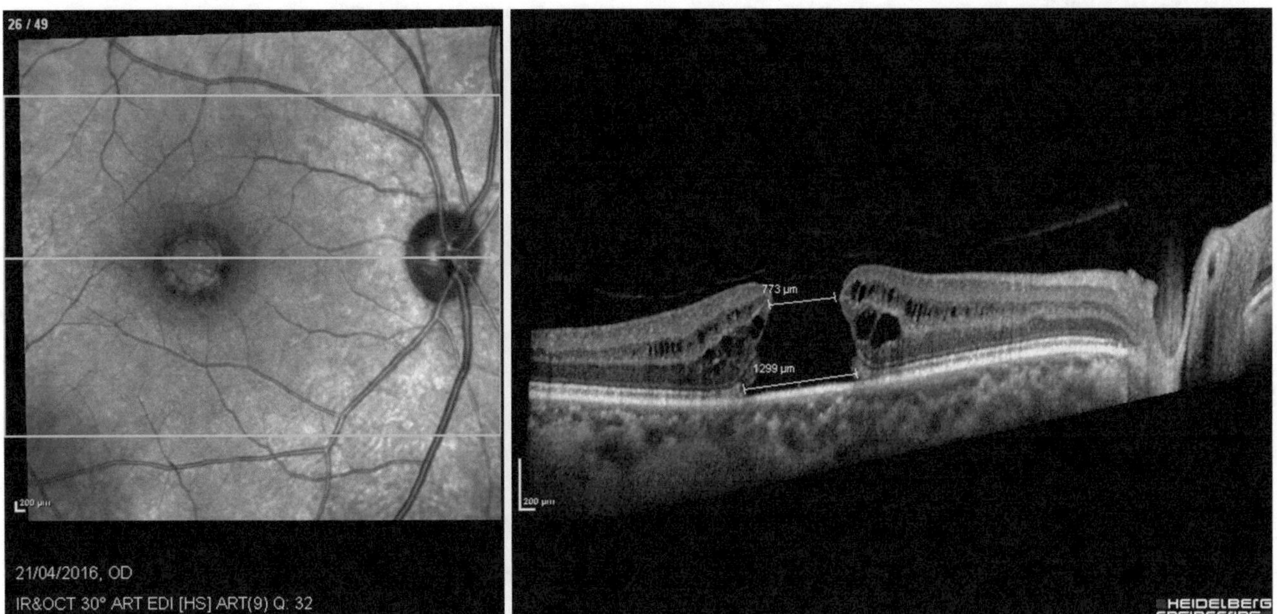

Fig. 11.30 A large hole. The wide separation at the base will indicate poor visual recovery

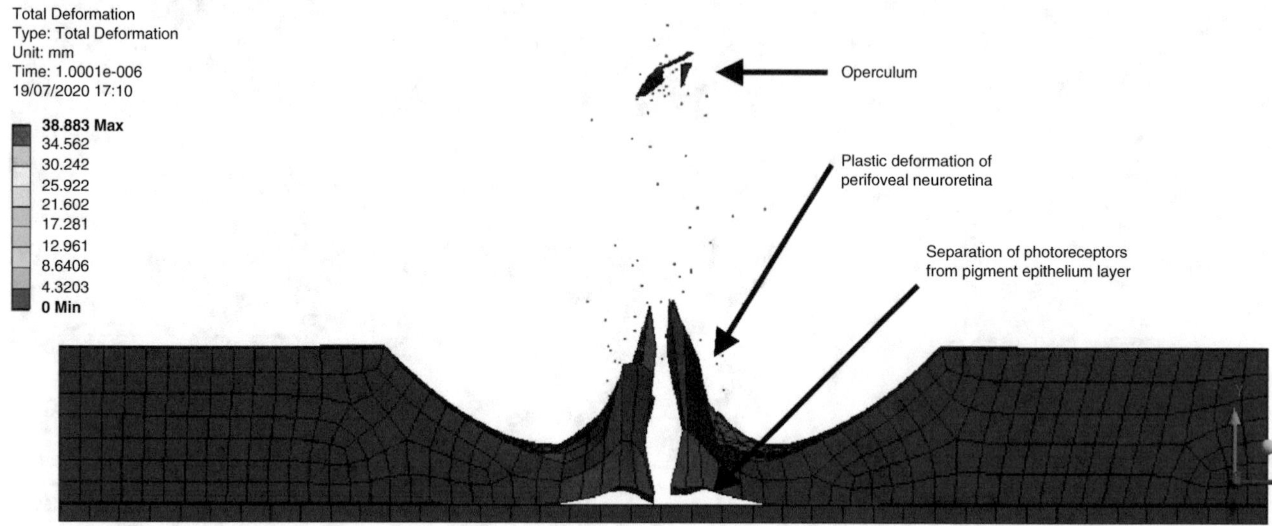

Fig. 11.31 FEA of macular hole traction

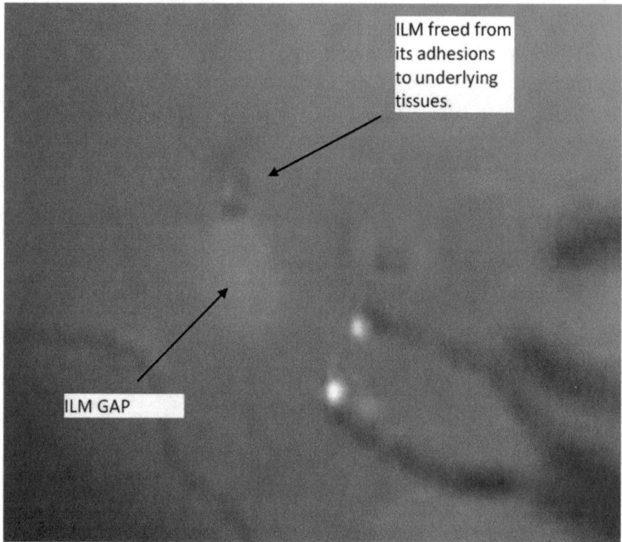

Fig. 11.32 ILM peeling during surgery

roretina, and force of retraction. With smaller gaps in internal limiting membrane, more elastic retina and higher retraction force being associated with larger and more elevated holes (Fig. 11.33).

Perifoveal retraction of internal limiting membrane also explains the role of internal limiting membrane peel procedure in closing macular holes. Removing the perifoveal internal limiting membrane is likely to alleviate the influence of retraction imposed over the loosely attached retina. If enough retinal elasticity is maintained in the perifoveal neuroretina and the effect of internal limiting membrane retraction is eliminated, the macular hole can close. However, if perifoveal neuroretina showed plastic deformation and little elastic strength, or if the hole is too large, then internal limiting membrane peel procedure will fail to close the hole. Perifoveal internal limiting membrane retraction also explains, why opercula observed in OCT images of stage 2 macular holes are often shorter than the gap created by their removal.

Surgery (Table 11.1)

Additional surgical steps.

- Peel posterior hyaloid membrane off retina (in grades 2 and 3 holes).
- Stain the internal limiting membrane (ILM) with brilliant blue.
- Remove ILM.
- Insert air.
- Insert long-acting gas.

In macular hole surgery vitrectomy is performed [25]. A gas bubble is inserted to tamponade the hole. During the first week the patient may have the inconvenience of positioning their face towards the ground, allowing the bubble to float against the hole. Many other manoeuvres have been added to this procedure to try to maximise the chances of hole closure, such as dissection of the internal limiting membrane from the retina or application of autologous platelets to the hole

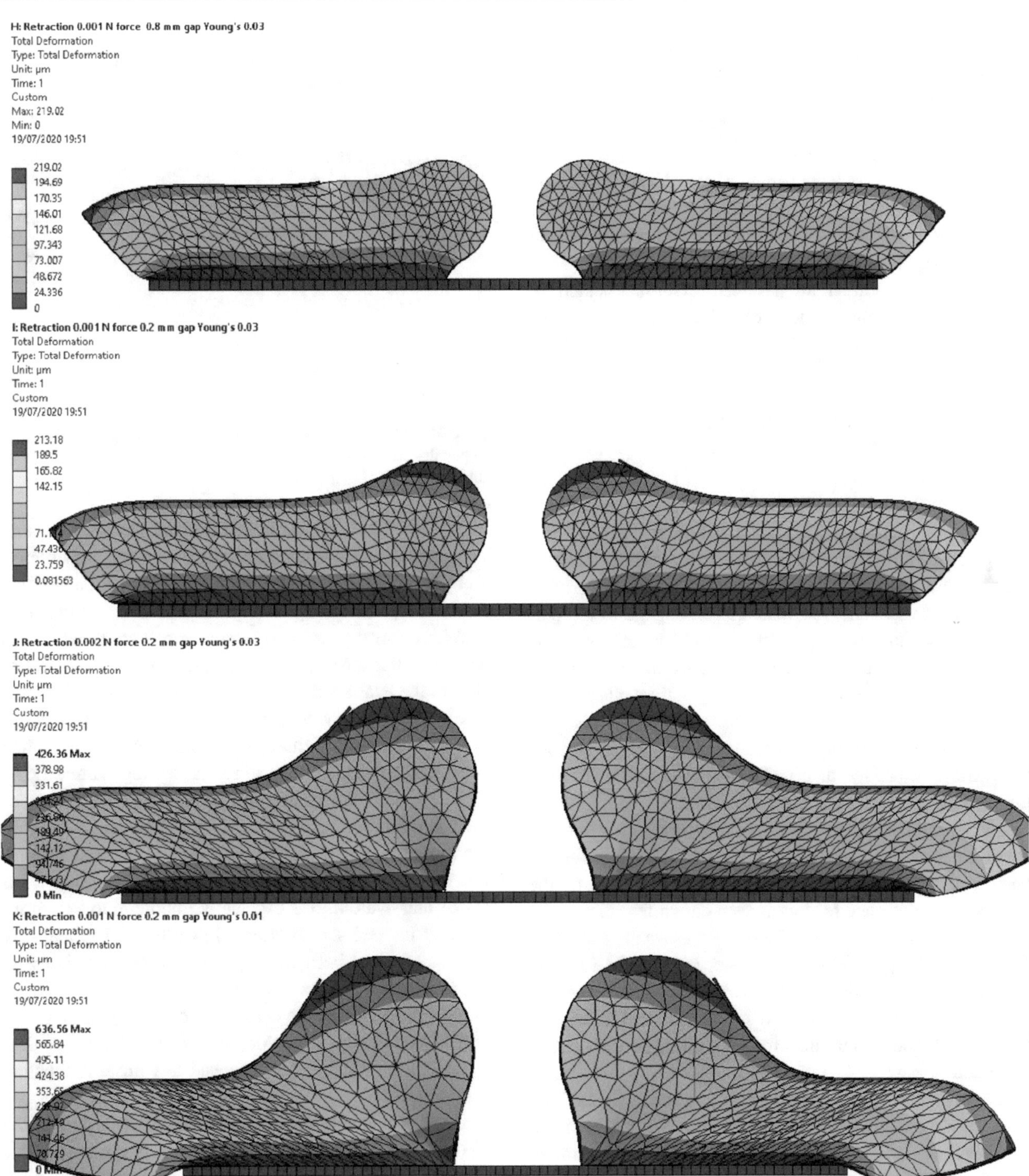

Fig. 11.33 The stress applied to the tissue is illustrated by increased red and shows the effects of ILM gap and force of the retraction on the anatomy of the hole

Table 11.1 Difficulty rating of PPV for macular hole

Difficulty Rating	Moderate
Success rates	High
Complication rates	Low
When to use in training	Middle

(platelets obtained from the patient's blood by spinning, separation, and aliquoting). Successful closure of the hole arrests progression to a stage 4 hole and frequently reduces the distorting effects of the hole and improves vision.

Once the core vitrectomy has been performed detach the posterior hyaloid from the retina in all macular holes except grade 4.

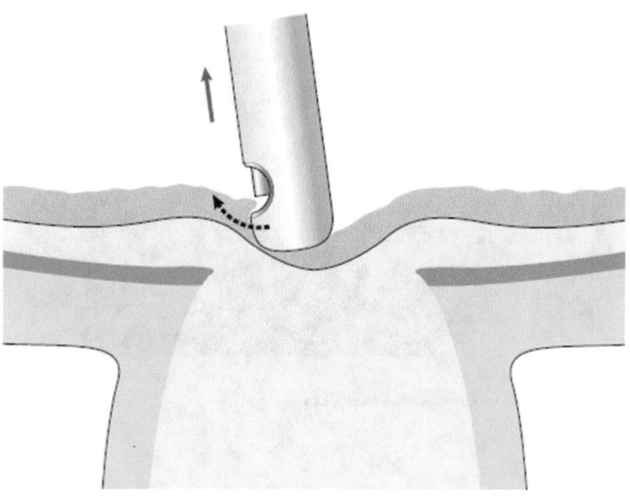

Fig. 11.34 When starting the posterior hyaloid peel, go to the edge of the optic disc, try to engage the posterior hyaloid and then elevate away from the disc

Peeling the Posterior Hyaloid Membrane (Figs. 11.34, 11.35, 11.36, and 11.37)

(Fig. 11.38) Detect preoperatively whether the posterior hyaloid has detached or not. This will save time and anxiety during the operation. Remove as much vitreous as possible over the optic disc. If there is too much cortical vitreous overlying the hyaloid membrane, the vitreous will engage in the port and shred without pulling up the hyaloid membrane. The membrane needs to be engaged to start the detachment process. Use the vitrectomy cutter on aspiration, place the tip near the optic disc so that it is almost touching the disc and aspirate on 300–600 mmHg vacuum. Allow a moment for the hyaloid to engage then move the cutter one millimetre tangentially over the optic nerve rim taking care not to touch the nerve or retina. Then move the cutter tip towards the centre of the eye. Keep trying different parts of the optic nerve head until suddenly a ring indicating the juncture of the attached and detached hyaloid is seen circumferential to the disc margin. OCT shows that the hyaloid is usually separated from the underlying retina. It is easier to raise the PHM in macular hole than other conditions which do not have this micro separation. The PHM will still be attached to the surface of the blood vessels; therefore, it is easier to lift between the blood vessels.

Observe the ring of vitreous separation and again aspirate over the nerve, this time pull further into the centre of the eye, see the ring increases in size as the vitreous detachment spreads to the equator of the globe. Early in this process create a hole in the elevated posterior hyaloid membrane to allow vitreous cavity fluid to enter between the PHM and the retinal surface. This breaks the "vacuum" between the PHM and the retina and aids elevation of the rest of the PHM to the periphery.

Note: Make a hole in the centre of the posterior hyaloid to allow fluid to enter between the PHM and the retina (Fig. 11.39).

It should now be possible to see the posterior hyaloid floating in the vitreous cavity. Continue the detachment process by aspirating the hyaloid into the four quadrants of the eye. If this is not working or the instruments are getting close to the lens, use the cutter to remove the central membrane, place the cutter through the hole, and aspirate the posterior aspect of the hyaloid in each quadrant and lift the membrane towards the periphery. Stop before the insertion of the vitreous base because the vitreous will not detach any further, forcing it anteriorly will cause retinal tearing. Similarly, do not pull through abnormal vitreoretinal attachments such as lattice degeneration because traction on these will cause retinal tears. Instead trim the vitreous around these adhesions. Once the posterior hyaloid has been detached remove the vitreous and hyaloid. It is especially important to search for breaks by internal search after surgical PVD. The tears are often easy to find because they are of moderate size with often a ragged appearance and may bleed.

In stage 4 holes the posterior hyaloid will present a distinct peripheral edge, if you do not detect such an edge then the hyaloid is probably not detached and posterior suction should be tried.

Note: Occasionally the PHM is difficult to elevate off the disc (usually in conditions other than macular hole). In this case stain the vitreous with membrane blue to help its visualisation, trim it down so that there is minimal cortical gel. Repeat the aspiration with the cutter, increase the vacuum to 300 or 500 mmHg. Rarely you may need to grasp the vitreous with forceps; however, it is possible to damage the retina by touching it with the instrument or by pressure from the instrument tip transmitted to the retina through the residual cortical gel. It is however not acceptable to leave the PHM on the retina as later separation will occur with the risk of retinal

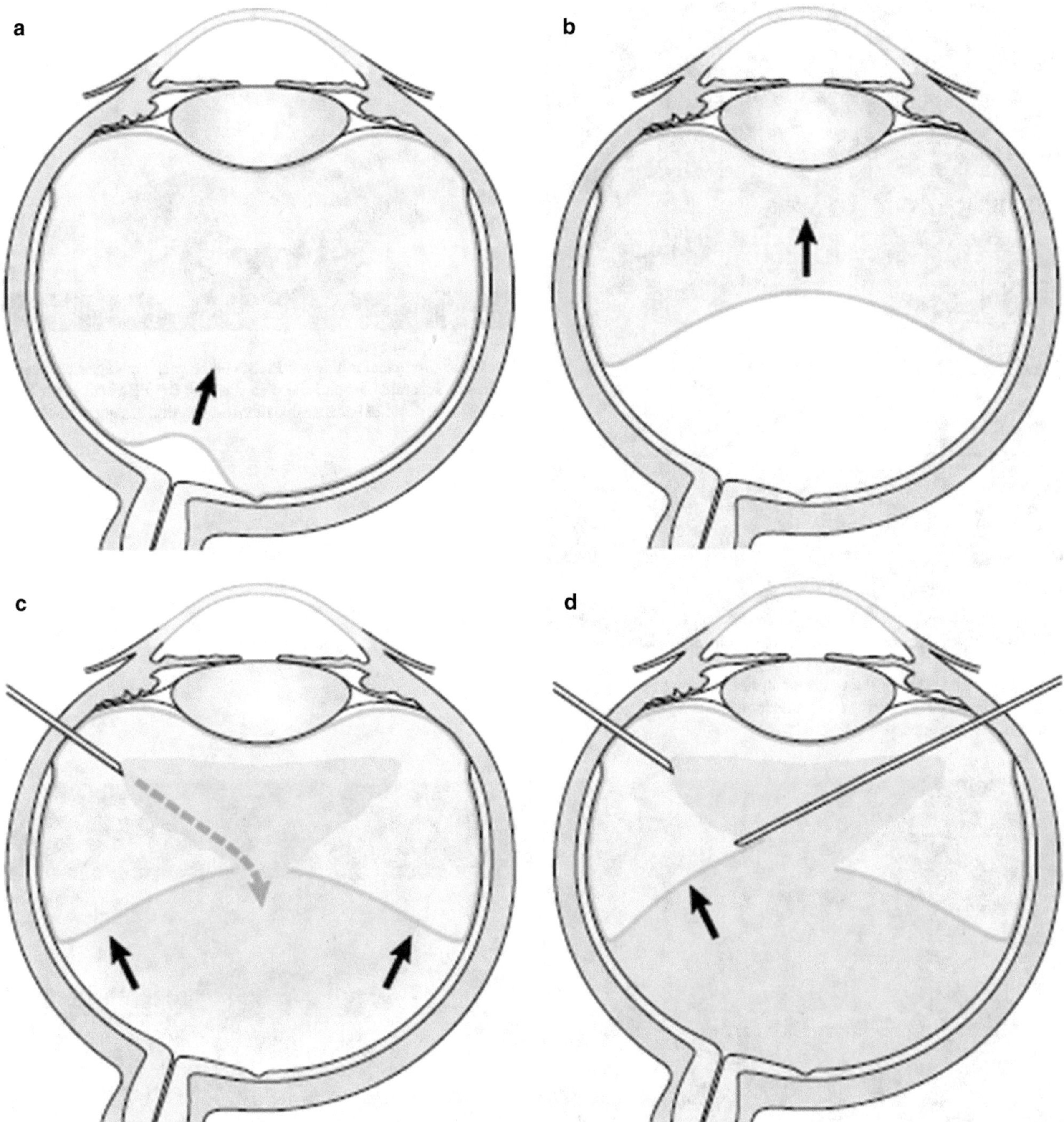

Fig. 11.35 Peel a posterior vitreous detachment in the centre of the eye going towards the back of the lens (**a**) then (**b**). Once the core of the vitreous has been removed the infusion fluid has access to behind the posterior hyaloid membrane. By making a hole in the posterior hyaloid membrane the fluid can pass through (**c**). This will aid dissection of the posterior hyaloid membrane by the infusion fluid. Once the PVD is more established an instrument such as a cutter can be inserted through the hole and the membrane elevated along an axis tangentially to the retina, in each quadrant (**d**). Commencing the PVD peel is safe. Commencing the posterior vitreous hyaloid is performed at the optic disc. Pull perpendicularly away from the disc to commence the peel. A ring of attachment is seen around the disc. This will expand as the hyaloid detaches and this should be watched more to confirm elevation of the membrane

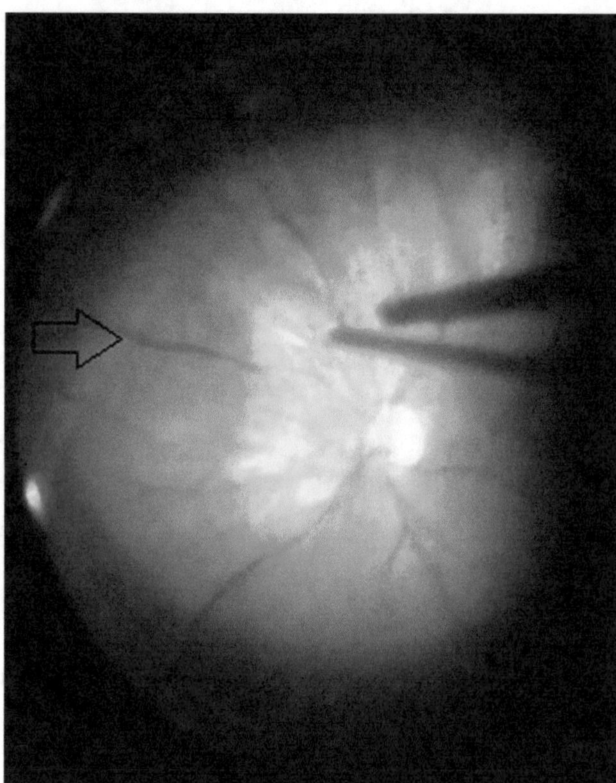

Fig. 11.36 The edge of the posterior hyaloid (arrow) peeling off the retina can be observed during PVD induction and is a good guide to the extent of PVD produced

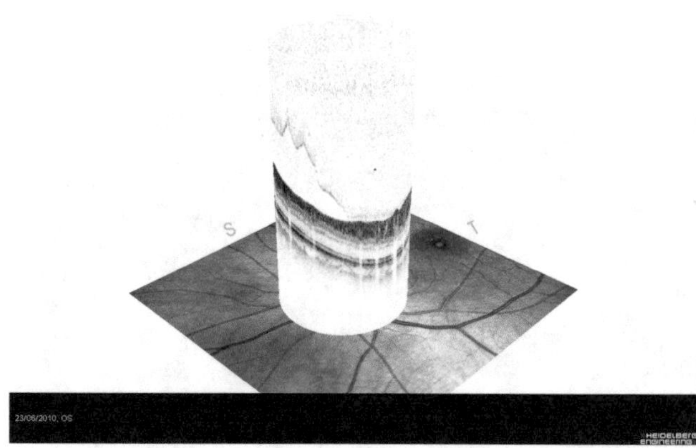

Fig. 11.37 In macular hole the PHM can be easily engaged because it is already separated around the disc. Peeling the PHM off other eyes may be more difficult because this micro separation has not yet occurred

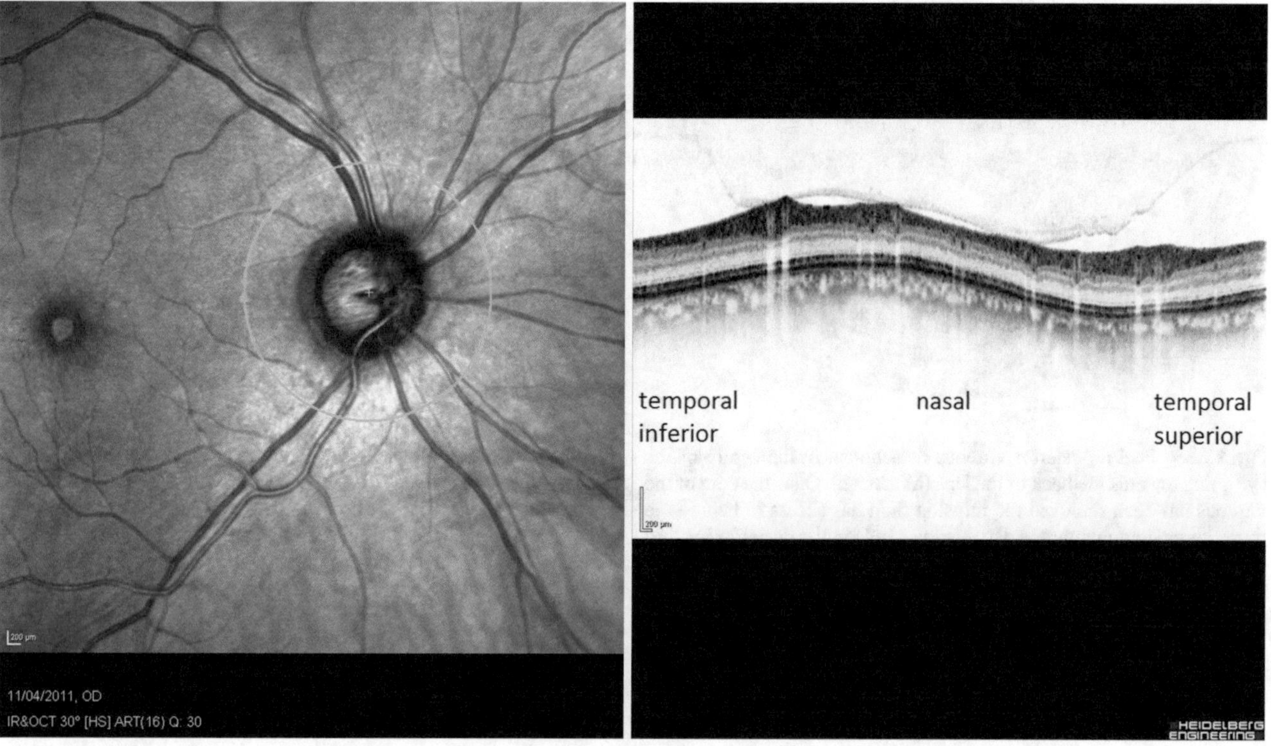

Fig. 11.38 The vitreous remains attached on the blood vessels and is separated less from the retina on the nasal side

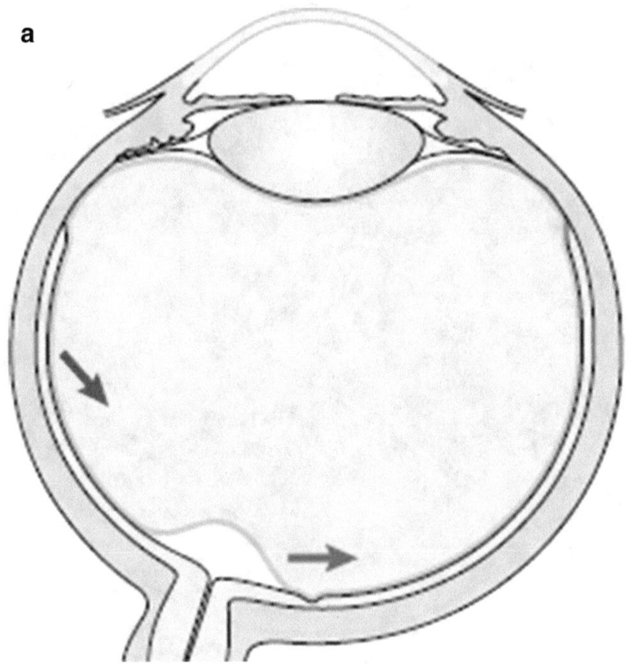

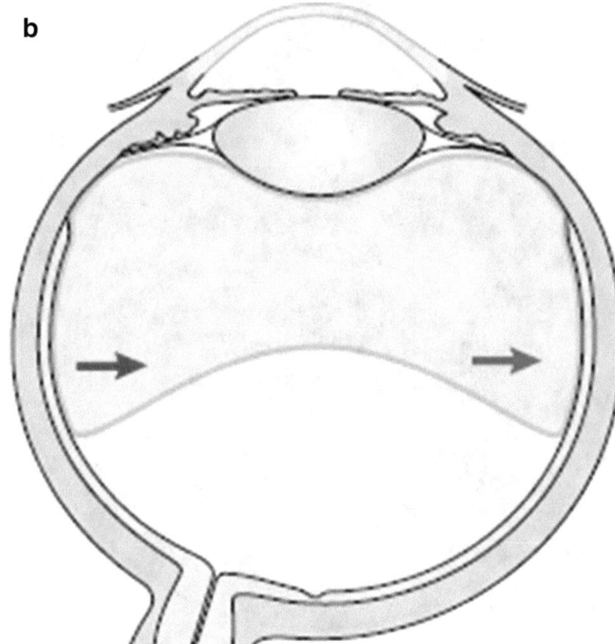

Fig. 11.39 Do not pull the membrane as shown by the blue arrows as this will cause traction on the opposite retina, red arrows, and if there are any retinal adhesions may increase the chance of retinal tear formation (**a**). Similarly, when the PVD peel is just started, do not pull tangentially across the retina as this runs the risk of producing forces at the vitreous base which could tear (**b**)

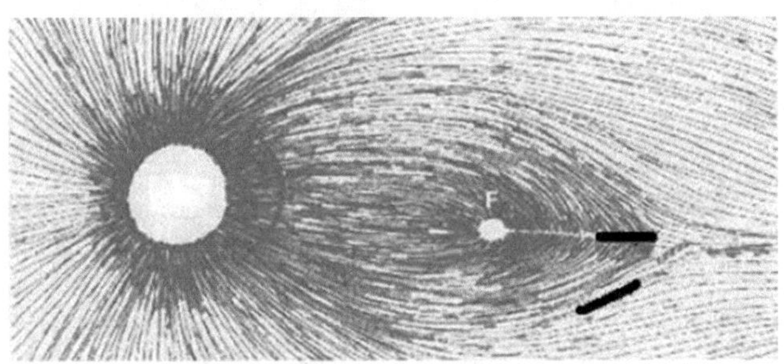

Fig. 11.40 When commencing the ILM peel, incise as shown in order to minimise damage to the nerve fibres in the nerve fibre layer

tear formation and RRD, therefore every effort must be made to achieve vitreous separation (Figs. 11.40, 11.41, 11.42, 11.43, and 11.44).

ILM Peel

Many methods have been described to facilitate macular hole closure. The method favoured here is internal limiting membrane (ILM) peel which can improve success rates from 89% to 94% [26–28]. Insert Brilliant Blue onto the macula to allow staining of the ILM. Leave on the retina for 30 seconds and remove with a flute. Aim the injection onto the retina just temporal to the macular hole allowing the dye to flow back over the hole. Do not aim at the hole as the dye can enter the subretinal space with potential toxicity to the RPE. You can aim the dye at the tip of the light pipe to break up the flow of the dye, thereby avoiding a jet of dye hitting the retina. Dye at velocity can penetrate the retina and go into the subretinal space.

The dye provides a blue stain to the ILM allowing removal. Brilliant Blue appears to be less toxic than Indocyanine Green and is now recommended. During the peel Brilliant Blue can be re-injected to help see the edge of the ILM, again inject over undisturbed retina and allow the dye to flow over the macula. The dye can particularly penetrate damaged retina entering the subretinal space if injected with force. Any cut ILM edge will stain more intensely facilitating detection of the ILM.

Note: A previous technique prior to the availability of Brilliant Blue was to insert indocyanine green dye, 0.5 mg/ml, onto the macula and allow to stain the ILM [27] briefly (enough time to change the instruments to the aspirating flute needle). Diluting the ICG in 5% Dextrose allows a denser mixture than in BSS, therefore the dye sits on the macula without dispersing into the vitreous cavity. Removal with a flute is then rapid and easy. ICG provides a superior stain of the ILM but is less favoured because of toxicity. ICG has been implicated in retinal pigment epithelial toxicity [29–31] resulting in less visual improvement despite improved hole closure [32, 33]. The agent has been shown to persist in the eye up to 8 months after insertion [34, 35]. Some have suggested that ICG induces a different cleavage plane for ILM dissection [36] which may cause damage to retinal ganglion

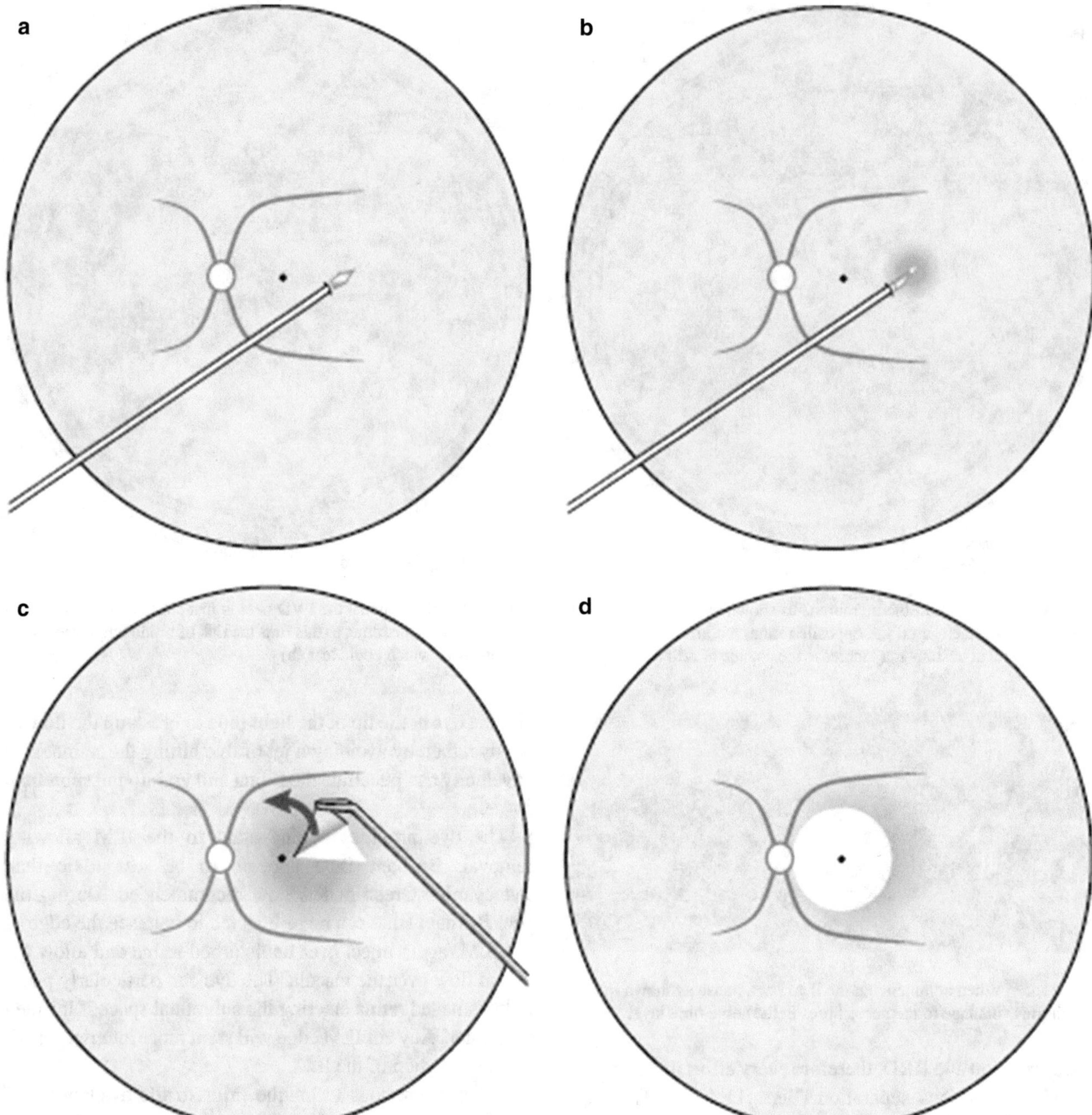

Fig. 11.41 To start the ILM peel, perform a slight incision of the ILM temporal to the fovea with a blade or the tip of the forceps by piching the ILM. In this area you are less likely to slice nerve fibres and cause small paracentral scotoma (**a** and **b**). Alternatively, use a diamond dusted brush to start the ILM peel. Once the ILM is lifted, remove it further in the fashion of the capsulorhexis going around the fovea in a circular fashion (**c** and **d**). To maintain an intact ILM during peeling firstly pull perpendicularly to the edge of attachment of the ILM to the retina and secondly readjust the forceps every so often so that you are grasping the membrane close to the edge of attachment. Angled forceps allow you to see the point at which to grasp the ILM. Be careful that you intermittently check the position of the heel of the forceps to avoid damaging retina with this whilst you are distracted by the ILM peel

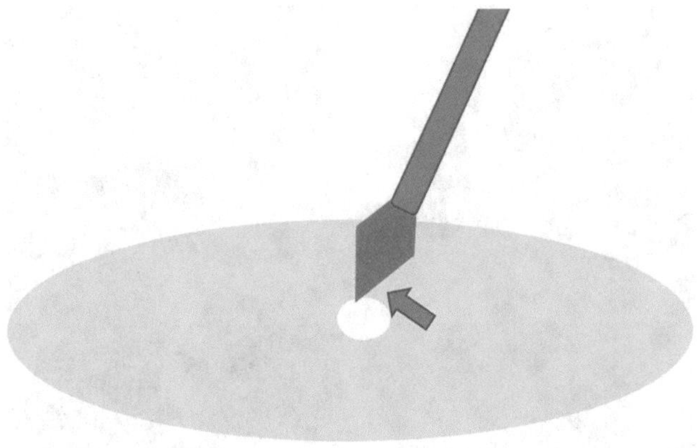

Fig. 11.42 When starting an ILM peel you can use the flat edge of the MVR blade to scrape the surface, because the ILM is relatively stiff this will induce a small hole to appear providing an edge to allowing forceps to grasp the ILM. The ILM is so close to the underlying nerve fibres that trying to insert a blade under the ILM to start lifting is exceedingly difficult and should be avoided

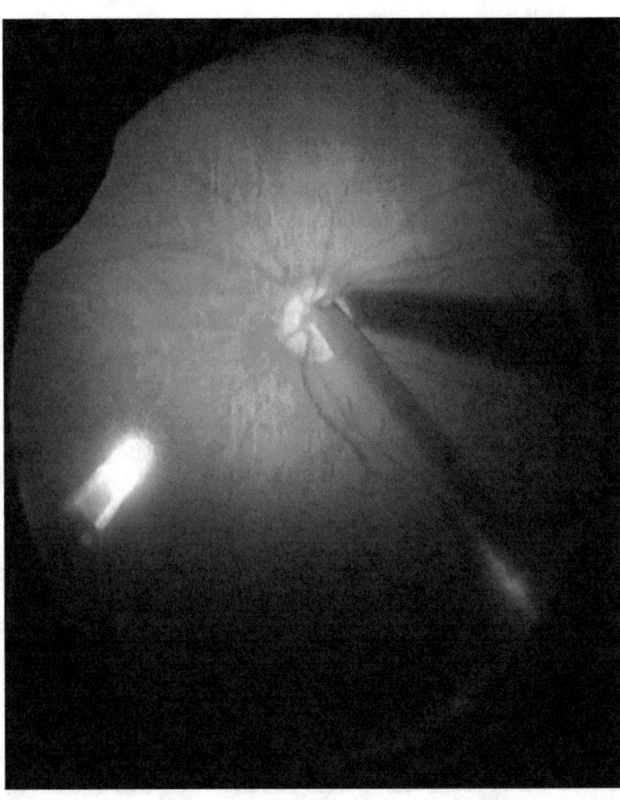

Fig. 11.44 Aspirate on the disc to engage the PHM. Watch the PHM peel from the retina. When applying any dyes to the macula, apply the dye away from the fovea in the first instance to avoid damage to the retinal pigment epithelium and to avoid insertion of the dye underneath the retina. Using a contact lens provides high magnification and enhanced depth perception to incise the ILM. Peel the ILM, search the peripheral retina, and fill with gas

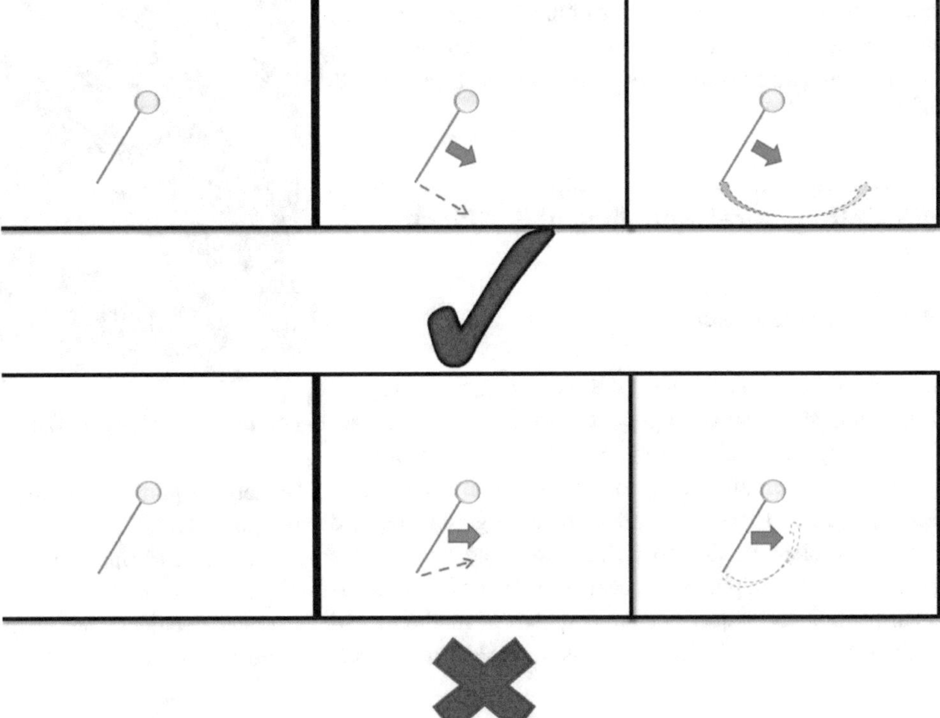

Fig. 11.43 When peeling the ILM pull in a perpendicular motion to the edge of the torn ILM this encourages the ILM to tear around the hole in a circumferential way as the top graphic shows. Do not pull the edge over the hole or the ILM will tear towards the hole as shown in the bottom graphic reducing the quantity of ILM that you will remove and requiring a regrip of the ILM at another site

cells [37]. If used the concentration and duration of application of the dye should be kept to a minimum [38].

The aim is to make a small slit in the ILM temporal and radial to the fovea with the MVR blade.

- Pinch technique: Use the end gripping forceps to "pinch" the surface of the retina. A small amount of pressure is required to engage the ILM. Pull up s short distance to rip the ILM, disengage in case you have some inner retina in the forceps to avoid ripping the more elastic retina (stiff ILM will rip first). Hopefully, you now have an edge of ILM to regrasp.
- Needle method: It is easier to see the end of your needle than the posterior edge of forceps. Stroke the needle tip across the ILM till a rip is created.
- Diamond duster: The diamond duster grabs the surface of the retina like sandpaper on wet tissue paper and induces a tear in the ILM.

The slit should be visible now as an orange colour between the two edges of a blue ILM. Using fine end gripping forceps to grasp an edge of the ILM and detach the ILM in a circular fashion (like performing a capsulorhexis in cataract surgery) around the fovea. Clear at least one to two-disc diameters of ILM from around the fovea. These manoeuvres can be performed using the IVS; however, if you are having trouble place a disposable contact lens onto the cornea (the stereo inverter is disengaged). The contact lens reduced the field of view considerably but provides better stereopsis. The commencement of the ILM peel is easier because the ILM can be grasped without injury to the underlying nerve fibre layer. Digital 3D systems such as the Ngenuity allow enhanced stereopsis through artificial widening of the displacement of the two images. They are useful particularly in macular surgery for discriminating layers (Figs. 11.45, 11.46, 11.47, 11.48, 11.49, and 11.50).

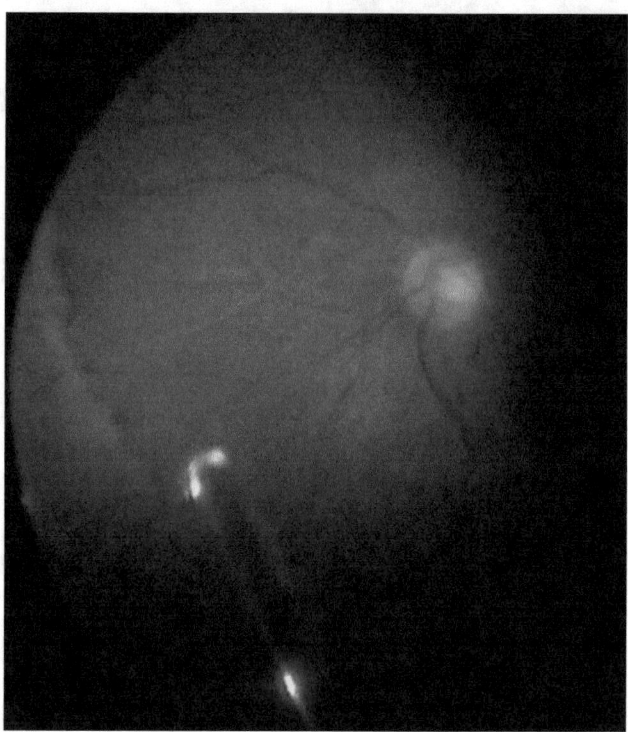

Fig. 11.45 The juncture of the attached and detached posterior hyaloid membrane can be seen

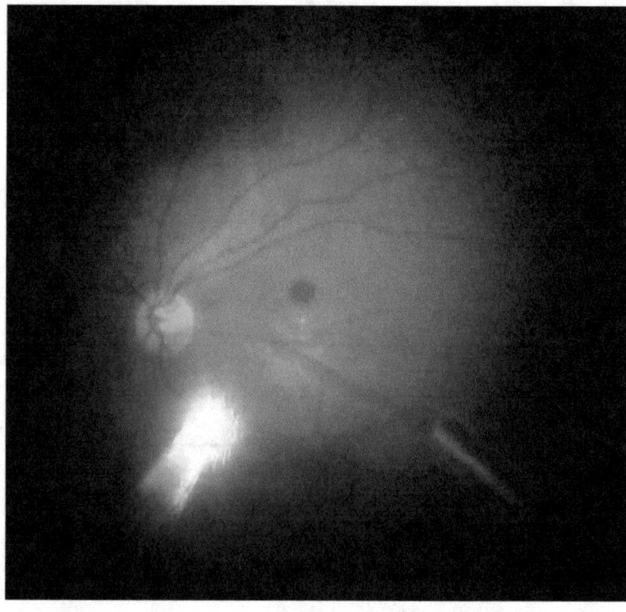

Fig. 11.46 ICG is a good stain but is associated with retinal toxicity

FEA Mathematical Modelling of ILM Pinch Peeling

Mahmut Dogramaci

Internal limiting membrane peel is a common surgical approach in vitreoretinal surgery, it is primarily used in macular hole repair, but also has been tried in other vitreoretinal pathologies. Internal limiting membrane has a smooth surface, therefore, to peel the membrane surgeons need to induce sufficient friction to be able to grasp and lift the membrane. One approach to achieve sufficient friction is pinch peeling technique. For the purposes of mathematical modelling pinch peeling technique is divided in to 3 steps, namely ripple creation, ripple elevation, and tear propagation.

Step 1: ILM ripple creation.

This step entails pressing forceps blades against the ILM to create two dents, one against each blade. Denting the ILM increases friction between the ILM and forceps blades by

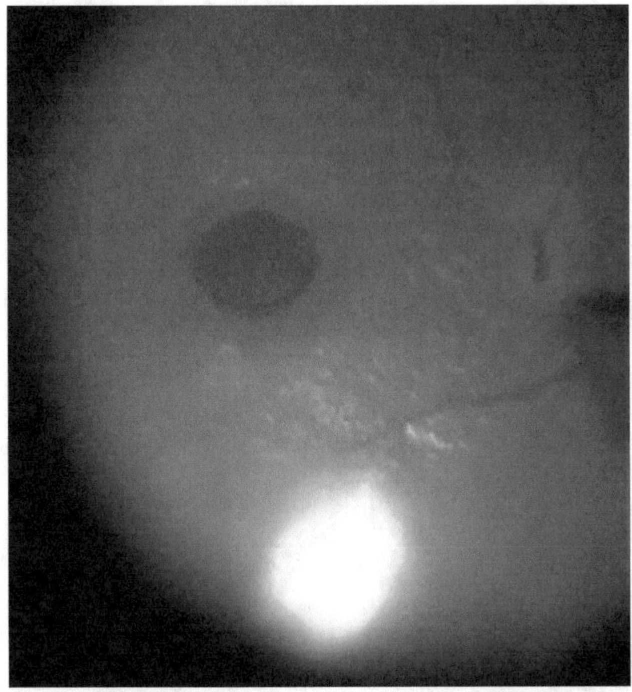

Fig. 11.47 Start the peel temporally

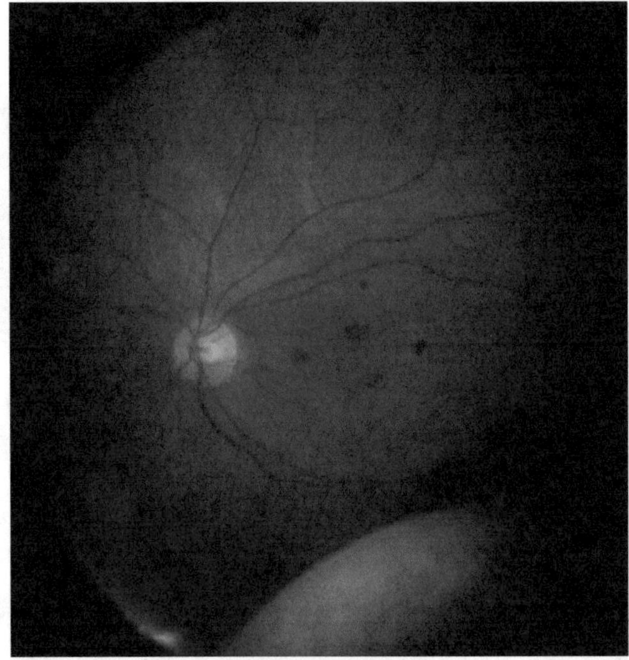

Fig. 11.49 Search for peripheral retinal breaks

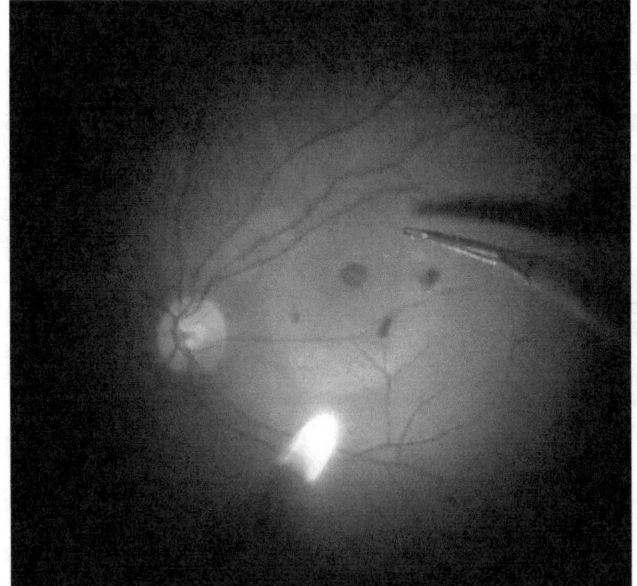

Fig. 11.48 Peel circumferentially around the fovea

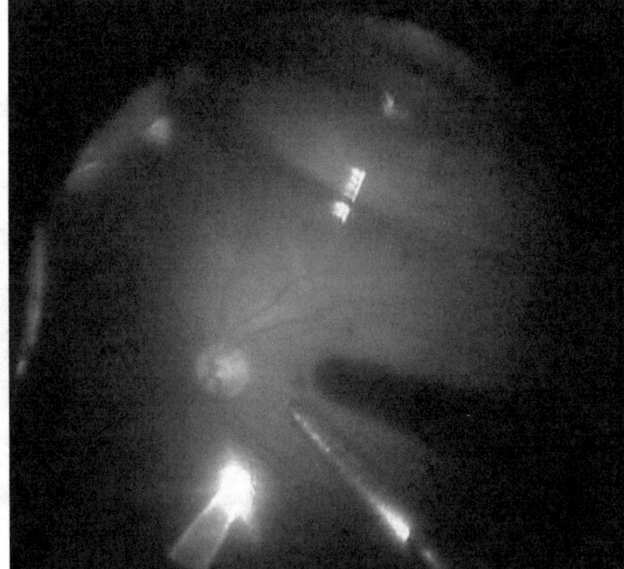

Fig. 11.50 Perform a fluid / air exchange

increasing contact pressure and contact surface area. Once the denting creates enough friction between the blades and the ILM, the surgeon starts to move the blades towards each other by closing the forceps. If enough friction exists to resist slippage of the blades over the ILM, an ILM ripple will be generated. Finite element analysis shows that deep denting generates more friction but equally results in higher stress values in the ILM. High stress in the ILM from excessive denting would lead to premature penetration of the ILM with possible neuroretinal tissue damage (Fig. 11.51).

Furthermore, ILM ripples are not always of good quality, finite element analysis reveals 4 possible configurations of ripples depending on the bite size, sharpness, and alignment of the blades. The ripples are described as single ripple configuration, if only one ripple is generated, or multiple ripple configuration, if multiple ripples of equal heights are generated. A herniated ripple is a multiple ripple configuration, but

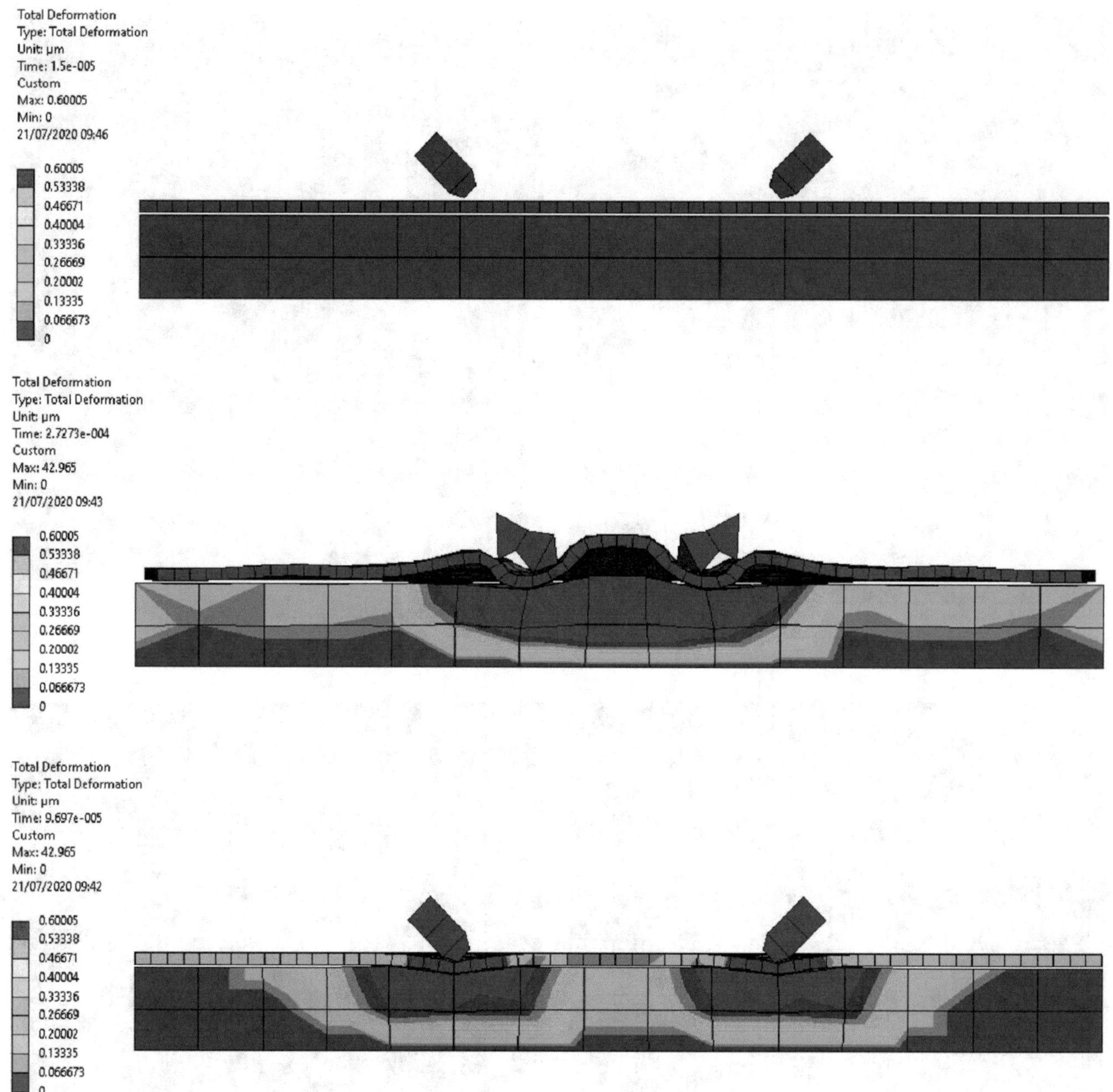

Fig. 11.51 Finite element analysis of sub-steps of ripple creation. Top: Cross-section of forceps blades, ILM, and neuroretina. Middle: pressing forceps blades against the ILM to create two dents, one against each blade. Bottom: moving the blades towards each other by closing the forceps leading to ripple formation

the ripples are of different heights. Finally, inverted ripple configuration term is used when a groove, instead of a ripple, is formed between the two blades. According to finite element analysis results, single ripple configuration of a maximum height is the most efficient configuration that facilitates successful ripple compression and elevation (Fig. 11.52).

Step 2: Ripple compression and elevation.

Once a good quality ripple is generated, the surgeon compresses the ripple between the two blades of the forceps. Unlike denting, compression induces friction that resists ILM slippage when the forceps are pulled up. Finite element analysis shows that high compression forces generate more friction but equally results in higher stress values in the ILM. Excessive stress in the ILM would lead to premature

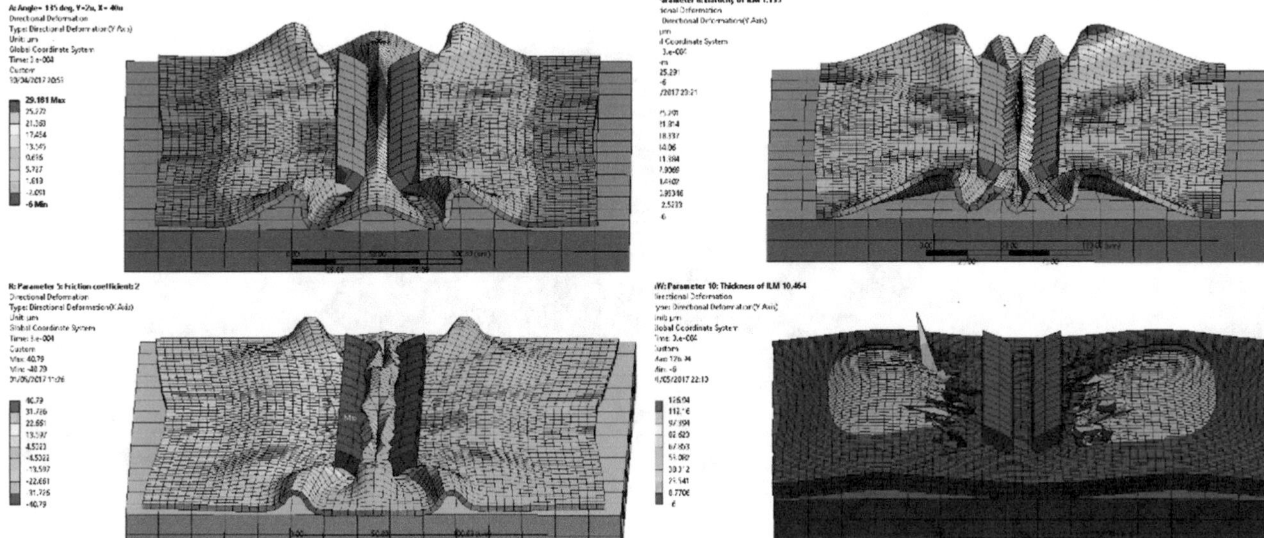

Fig. 11.52 Finite element analysis reveals 4 possible configurations of ripples depending on the bite size, sharpness, and alignment of the blades. Top left: a single ripple configuration showing only one ripple. Top right: A multiple ripple configuration showing multiple ripples of equal heights. Bottom left: A herniated ripple configuration showing multiple ripples of different heights. Bottom right: an inverted ripple configuration showing a groove, instead of a ripple, between the two blades of the forceps

tear and eventual slippage of the ILM during ripple elevation (Fig. 11.53).

Step 3: Tear induction and propagation.

Ripple compression and elevation generates stress in the ILM, and when the threshold is crossed, high stress levels result in a linear tear formation, that is perpendicular to the direction of the load. Such tears originate at maximum stress points, which are usually at the point of contact between the sharpest part of forceps blade and the ILM, leading to an immediate drop of stress values at these points (Fig. 11.54). If the elevation of compressed ripple continues, the linear tear will propagate in a direction that is perpendicular to the load applied and curves towards the closest free edge [39]. A surgeon can only control the direction of tear by carefully constructing the initial tear plane and by controlling the angle at which he pulls the membrane and also generate a large flap by adjusting the direction of the load to reduce the turning of the tear edge (Fig. 11.55).

Surgical Pearl

A Little PFCL Bubble Injection to Protect RPE and Prevent the Dye under the Retina during Macular Hole Surgery: The Roll over Technique

Whilst a surgeon is going to operate upon full-thickness macular hole, a useful surgical trick is the injection of a small bubble of perfluorocarbon liquid (PFCL) to protect the RPE from the dye. The bubble must be small so that after dye injection all the macula area is stained. To increase the staining effect (with both instruments, optic fibre and vitrectome in the vitreous chamber), gently rotate the eyeball in one direction (clockwise or counter clockwise) so that the PFCL bubble can massage the dye onto the retinal surface obtaining a strong stain of epiretinal membranes and/or ILM but always protecting the RPE from the dye.

Then using the vitrectome (cutter off) or a Charles cannula, the dye can be carefully removed. At this point the surgeon chooses to continue PFCL injection into the eye and perform ILM peeling under PFCL control or removes it completely performing a standard ILM peeling under BSS.

Stanislao Rizzo, Alfonso Savastano, Policlinico Gemelli, Rome, Italy

Insert air and exchange with 20% C_2F_6. Silicone oil has been used where gas is undesirable, e.g. when air travel is necessary [40]. This is not recommended routinely because of the need for a second operation for oil removal and the risks of oil induced complications (Fig. 11.56). SF_6 has been used for shorter duration of gas but often with more intense posturing (Figs. 11.56, 11.57, 11.58, 11.59, and 11.60).

Trypan blue also stains the ILM (and also epiretinal membranes) but less well [41]. Other agents such as autologous serum [16, 42], autologous platelets [43], and transforming growth factor-beta 2 [44, 45] have been tried without proven success over ILM peel (Figs. 11.61 and 11.62).

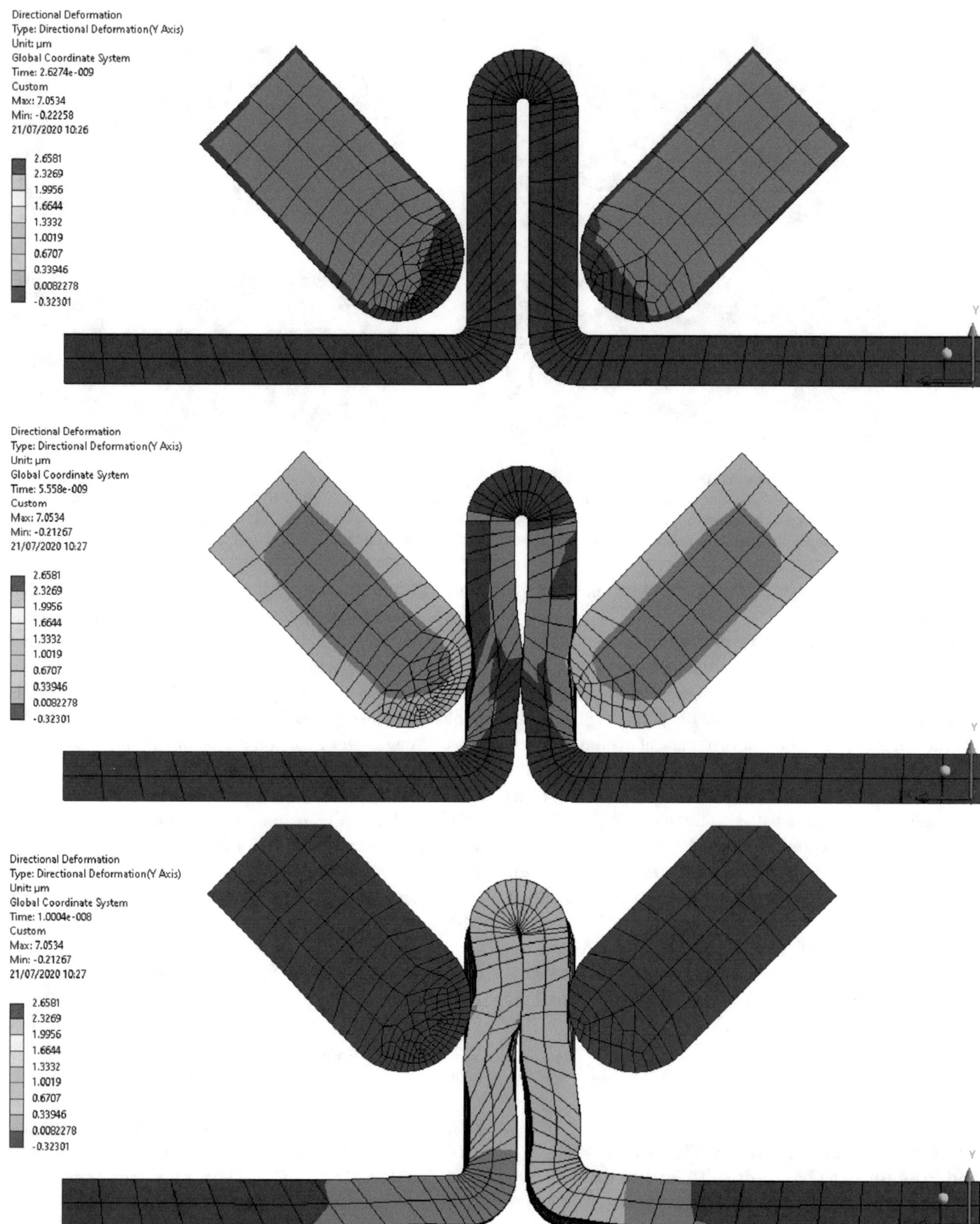

Fig. 11.53 Finite element analysis of ripple compression and elevation. Top: a well-formed ripple, Middle: compression application, bottom: ripple elevation

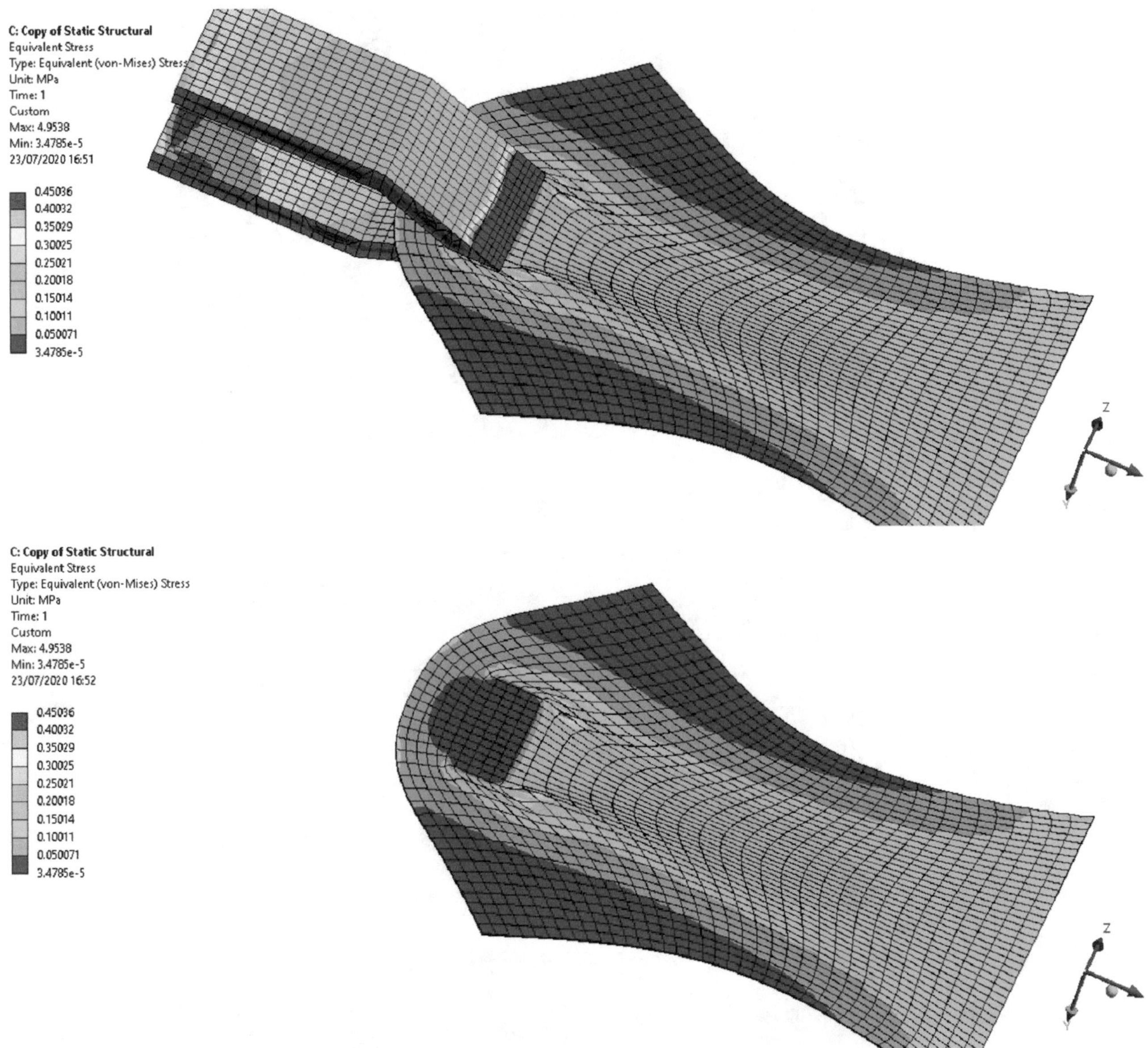

Fig. 11.54 High stress areas are located at points of contact between the sharpest part of forceps blade and the internal limiting membrane, tears usually originate at these points. Top: finite element analysis of a forceps grasping an internal limiting membrane. Bottom: Stress distribution in the internal limiting membrane that is pulled by forceps blades

ILM Flap

Large macular holes and redo holes can be encouraged close more often by adding a membrane to overly or fill the hole. The most popular system is to use the ILM as a flap overlying the macular hole at the end of the peel. The easiest way to do this is to peel the ILM around the hole but leave an area of persistent attachment to the edge of the hole, usually on the temporal side, creating a tongue of ILM which can be folded over the hole. This is held there by the gas bubble. Occasionally the hole is so big that you may wish to insert the ILM into the hole [46]. It can be tucked into the hole. Do this with care as the RPE is delicate and must not be compressed [47, 48].

The ILM flap appears to increase closure rates of large macular holes. Restoration of the foveal architecture is rare but by reducing cystoid spaces and causing some contraction of the edges of the hole the vision is improved to moderate levels, some use ILM flaps routinely but this is unnecessary and leads to a less tidy inner surface of the retina. In redo operations the ILM is usually already removed and a free flap is required. This can be taken from outside the area of the previous peel or from the arcades. Keeping the flap in place is more difficult as there is no attachment and you may

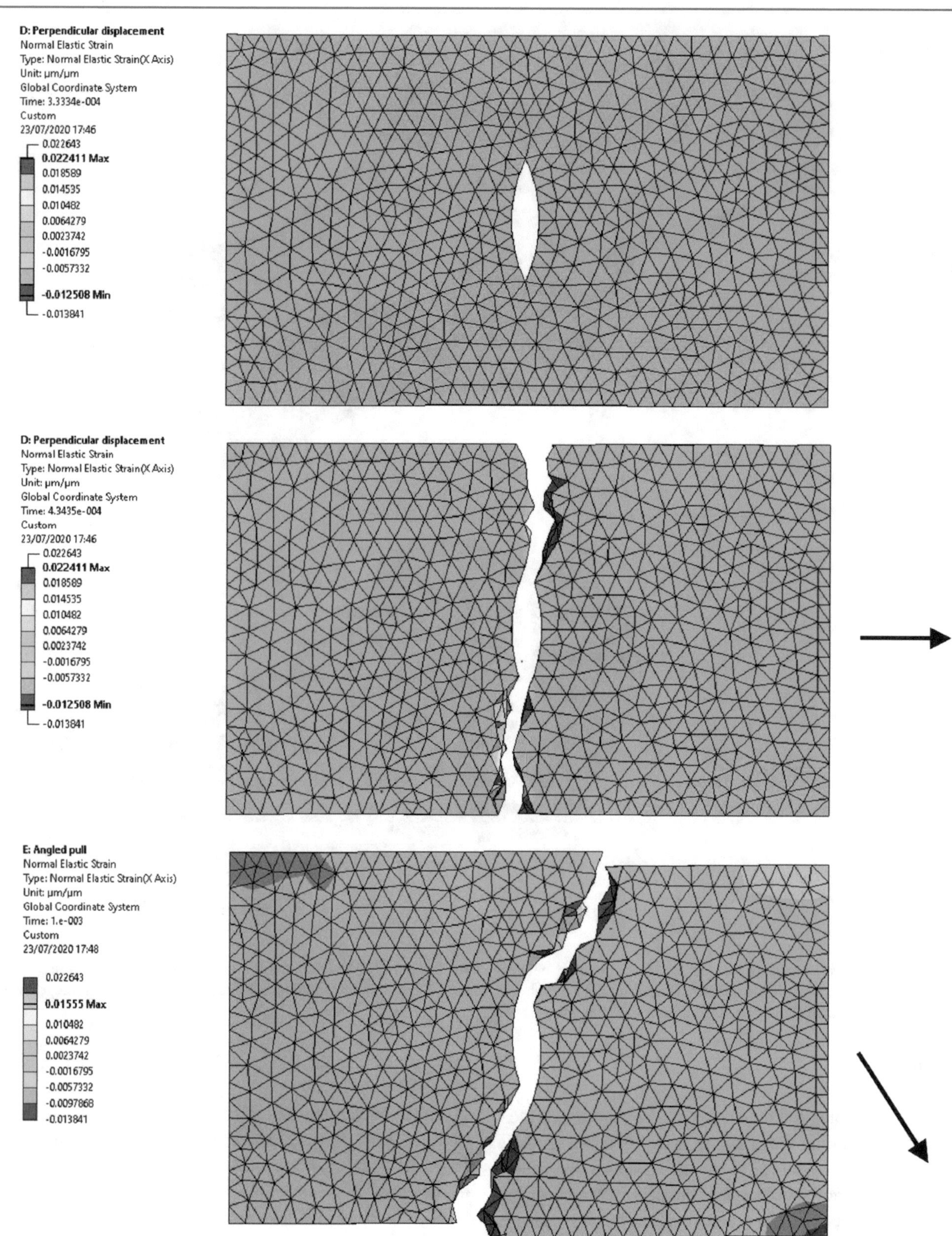

Fig. 11.55 A linear tear will propagate perpendicular to the direction of the load applied and curves towards the closest free edges. Top: Finite element analysis of a linear tear in the middle of a membrane. The left edge of the membrane is fixed, and the right edge is pulled towards the right. Middle: Right edge of the membrane is pulled towards the right in a direction perpendicular to the plane of the initial tear, as a response the tear has extended towards the upper and lower free edges of the membrane. Bottom: Right edge of the membrane is pulled right and downward in an angled direction in relation to the plane of the initial tear, as a response the tear has extended towards the upper and lower free edges of the membrane but this time in an angled direction making the extension almost perpendicular to the direction of the pull applied on the right edge of the membrane

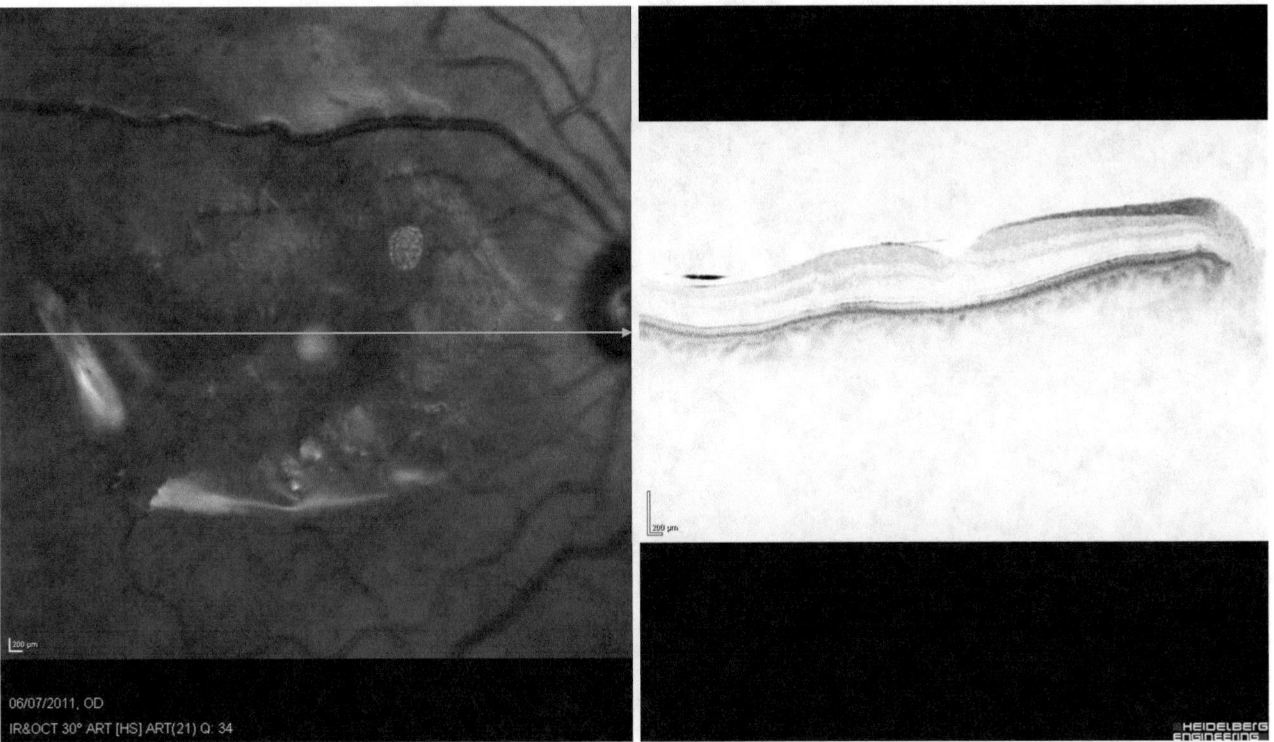

Fig. 11.56 A postoperative OCT of a macular hole with oil tamponade showing closure of the hole and contact of the oil on the foveal margin

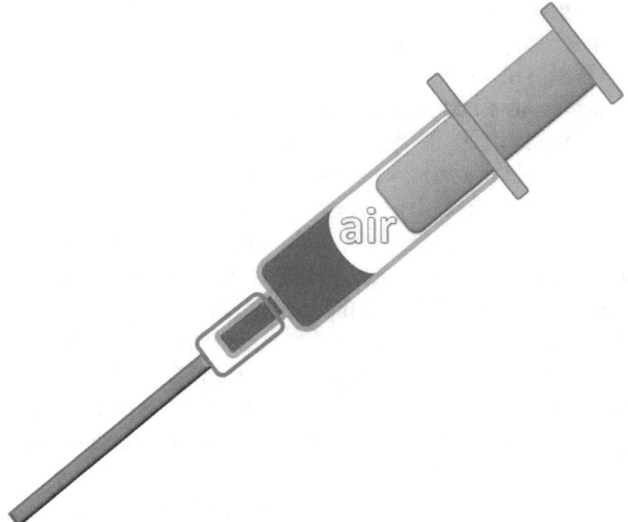

Fig. 11.57 Occasionally the plungers of syringes will stick to the sides of the syringe. The surgeon increases the force on the plunger to make it move and there is a sudden release of the plunger and rapid injection of fluid, e.g. dye. This risks a jet of dye hitting the retina and entering the subretinal space. To overcome this draw a small amount of air into the syringe, the compressible air cushions the effect of sudden force on the plunger (in effect acting as a damper) preventing a sudden injection of the fluid

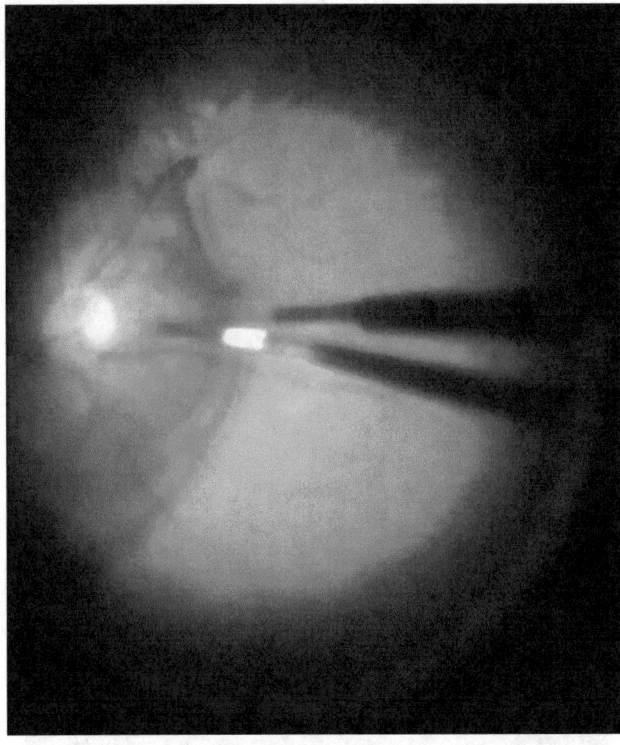

Fig. 11.58 Inject brilliant blue dye away from the fovea and allow to fall back over the fovea. Injecting directly over the fovea risks insertion of subretinal dye which is potentially toxic

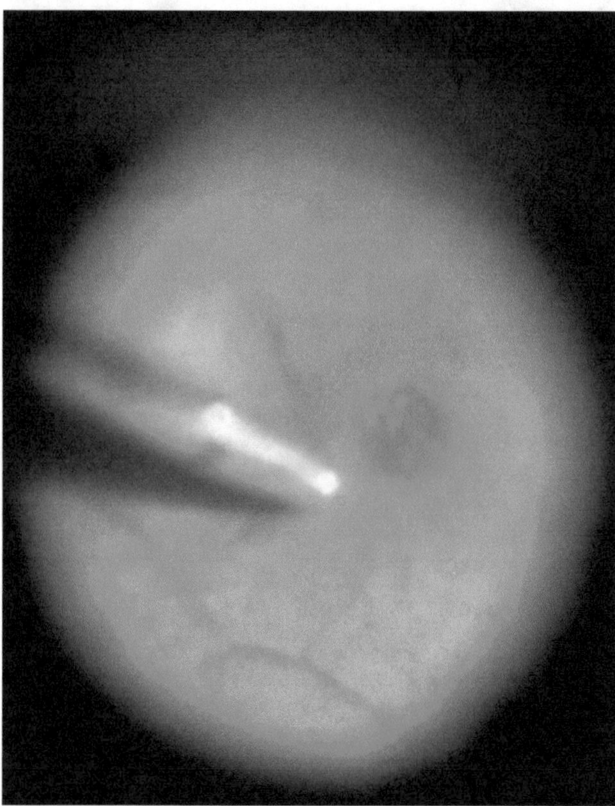

Fig. 11.59 Peeling the ILM with brilliant blue stain

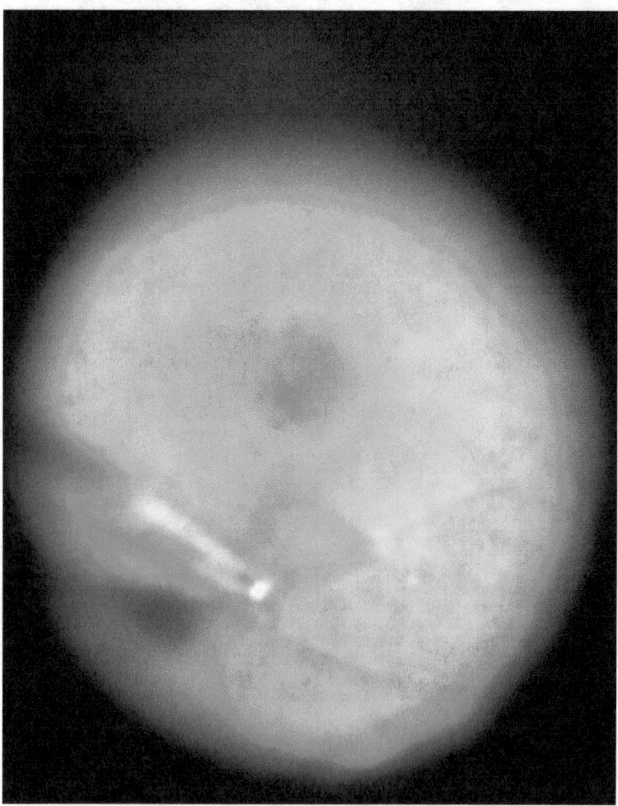

Fig. 11.60 Peeling the membrane

need to use some HPMC to allow it to stick whilst you insert the air to splint the flap. Intraoperative OCT is useful for monitoring the flap [49] (Figs. 11.63, 11.64, 11.65, 11.66, 11.67, 11.68, and 11.69).

Surgical Pearl

The Inverted Internal Limiting Membrane Flap Technique

As the inverted ILM flap technique has become more popular globally, its indications have grown from its initial role to treat large macular holes to now being successfully used to treat all macular holes regardless of size, origin, or associated maculopathies. Furthermore, stuffing an optic disc pit with ILM results in good anatomical and functional results when treating optic disc pit associated maculopathy. It has also spawned various new techniques such as autologous ILM flap transplants and amniotic membrane transplants.

Perhaps one of the most interesting aspects of the inverted ILM flap technique is that it never prohibits the surgeon from trying it and later electing to use the classical approach of complete ILM peeling if the surgeon feels that this would be the more appropriate treatment in a specific case or recurrence.

My surgical pearls for operating with the inverted ILM flap technique would include the following:

Peel with care. You must peel up to the margins of the macular hole and take care to ensure that the flap remains attached to the underlying macular tissue at the point where it is folded backwards over the macular hole.

Peel one or two flaps. Personally, I always now create two flaps. First, in one smooth, slow movement I peel an ILM flap a little bit wider than the size of the macular hole from the upper temporal side of the macular hole, keep hold if it so that it remains flat and does not curl, and invert it to cover the macular hole. I create a second flap from the temporal side and fold this back over the first one so that the hole is completely covered and the ILM flaps are flat against the retina. I never introduce the ILM flap into the hole in primary surgery. I then place a very tiny amount of viscoelastic material on top of the flaps to anchor them in place. Use as little viscoelastic as possible—it is only an adjuvant to help prevent the flap from reapproximating!

Use a flute needle for fluid/air exchange. Place the tip of the flute at the lower boundary of the optic nerve. In this way, the fluid will flow towards the needle across the flap (hinged on the temporal side) and help to keep the flaps in the correct position. When fluid/air exchange is finished, repeat it. And then do it again! Several times, until the retina is completely dry—it is particularly important to ensure that fluid/air exchange is as thorough and complete as possible!

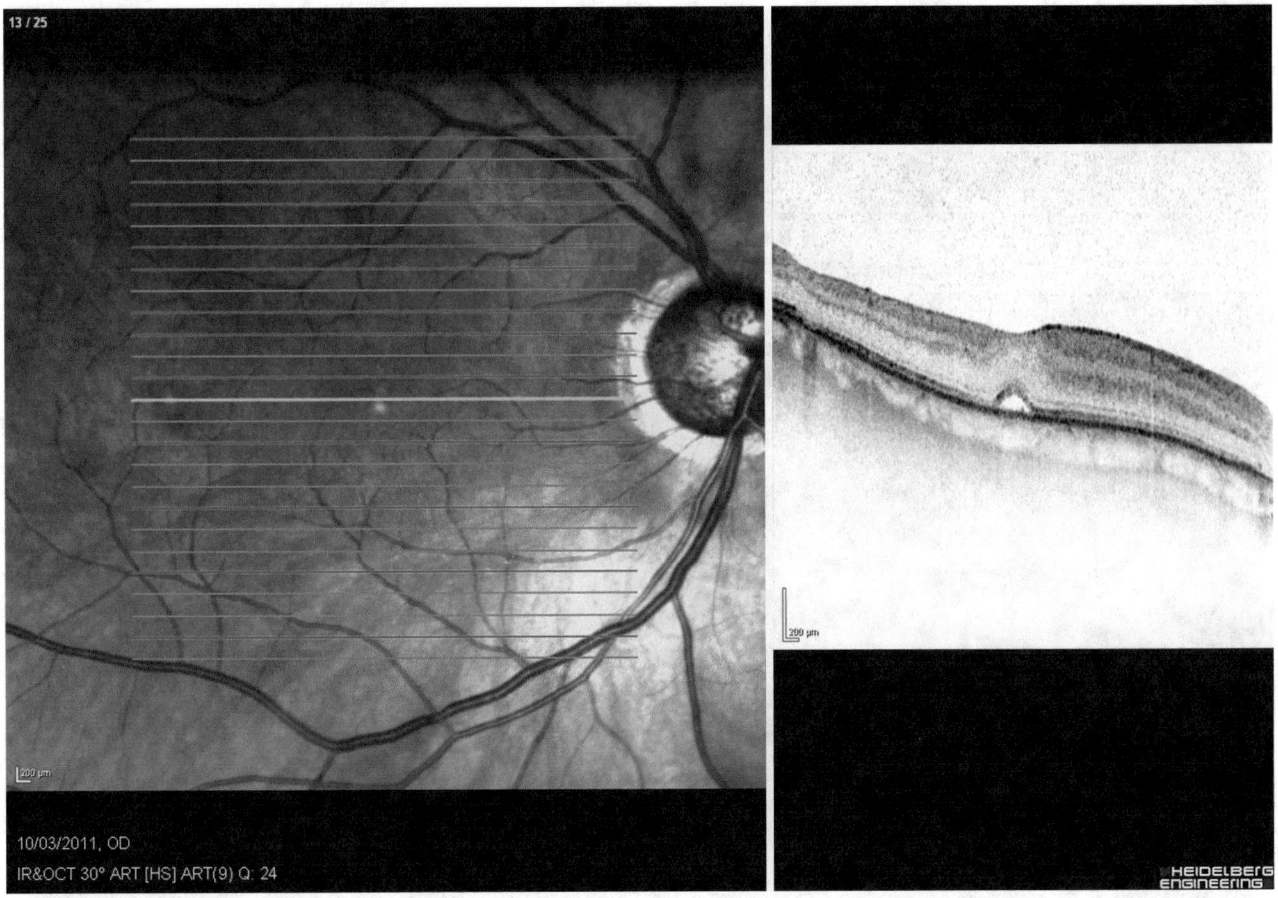

Fig. 11.61 Early hole closure often shows an outer retinal cyst which disappears in a few weeks

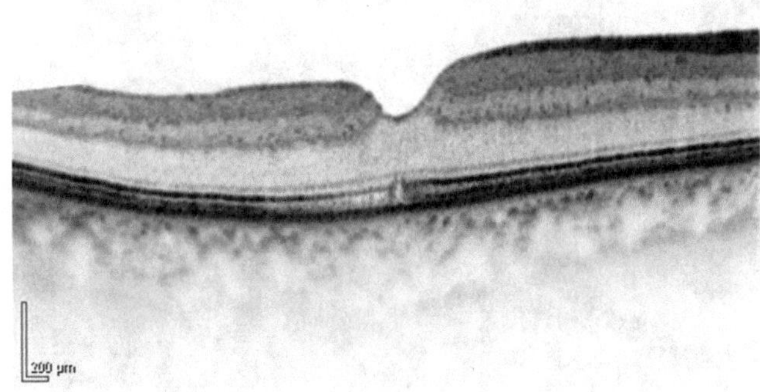

Fig. 11.62 A postoperative HD OCT of a grade 2 macular hole with 20/300 vision

Professor Jerzy Nawrocki, Professor Zofia Michalewska, Ophthalmic Clinic "Jasne Blonia", Lodz, Poland

Other Adjunctive Methods

The macular hole contains a thick viscous fluid which can be aspirated from the hole. As you do this you may see the edges of the hole loosen and contract. Some have used this as a method to contract the hole and increase closure rates [50]. I often aspirate the contents of a hole which look a stiff.

Amniotic membrane introduced through a sclerotomy has been used as a flap instead of ILM. Autologous platelets (spun from a blood sample taken at the time of surgery) were one of the original ways used to create a membrane on the hole [51]. Detaching the retina at the macula allows the retina to loosen and encourages closure of large holes [52]. The retina is detached using a 40-gauge needle to raise a bleb of SRF. The SRF is forced into the macula by inserting air into the eye. An autologous retinal transplant taken from peripheral retina has been used to plug large macular holes with claimed improvement in vision [53].

Choice of Tamponade

Usually a long-acting gas bubble is used such as C3F8 or C2F6 (I prefer C2F6 which will last 5 weeks but the macula can be seen at 3 weeks), shorter duration gas such as SF6 may also be used but may need more rigorous posturing postoperatively. Silicone oil has been inserted [40] and heavy oil with face up posture tried with successful closure [54]. Oil use requires further surgery by ROSO which can be avoided by gas insertion. Injection of an expansile gas bubble (0.5 ml of 100% SF6) can induce a PVD in 95% with a

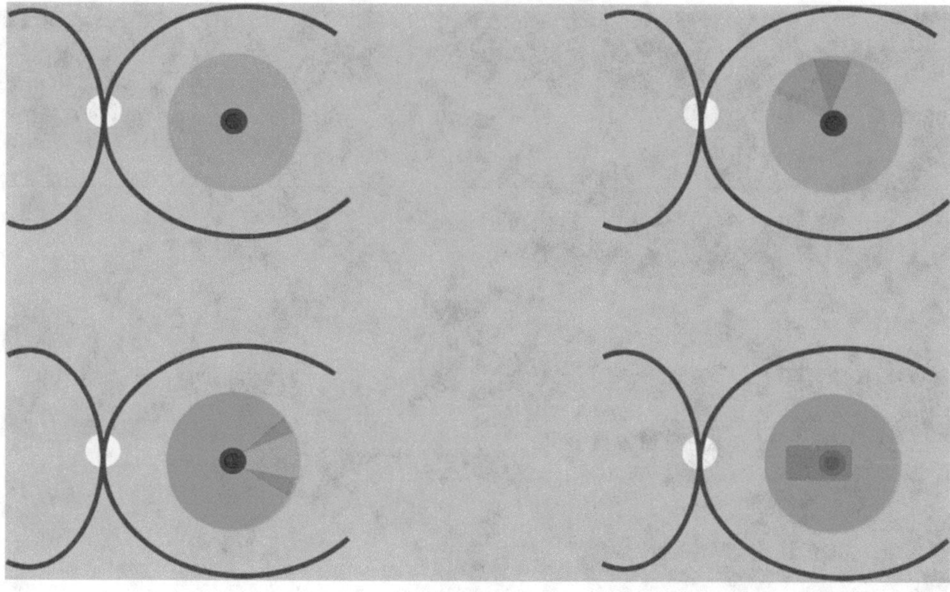

Fig. 11.63 Stain the ILM with brilliant blue. Peel around the macular hole but leave tongue of ILM attached to the edge of the hole. Then fold the flap created over the hole

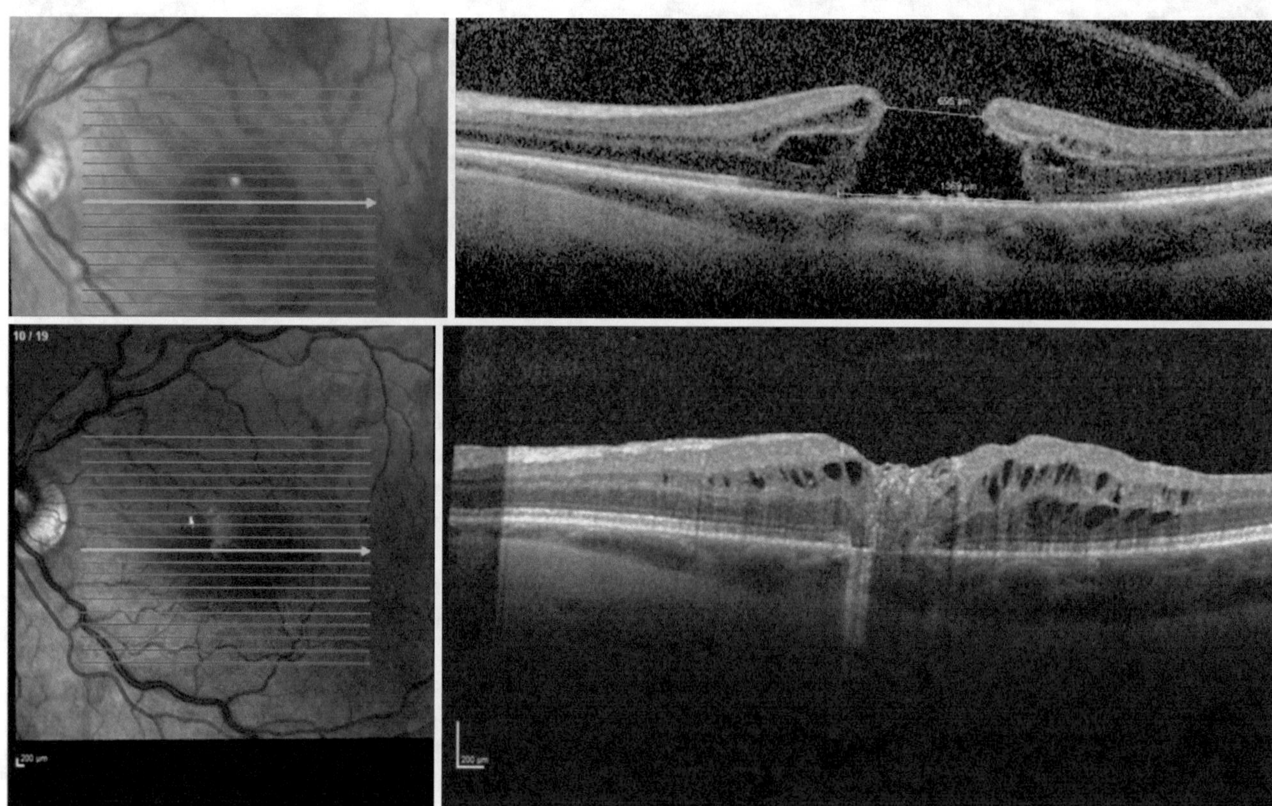

Fig. 11.64 The minimal internal diameter is related to the ability to close the hole and the basal diameter (next to the RPE) is related to visual outcome. This exceptionally large hole was closed by ILM flap

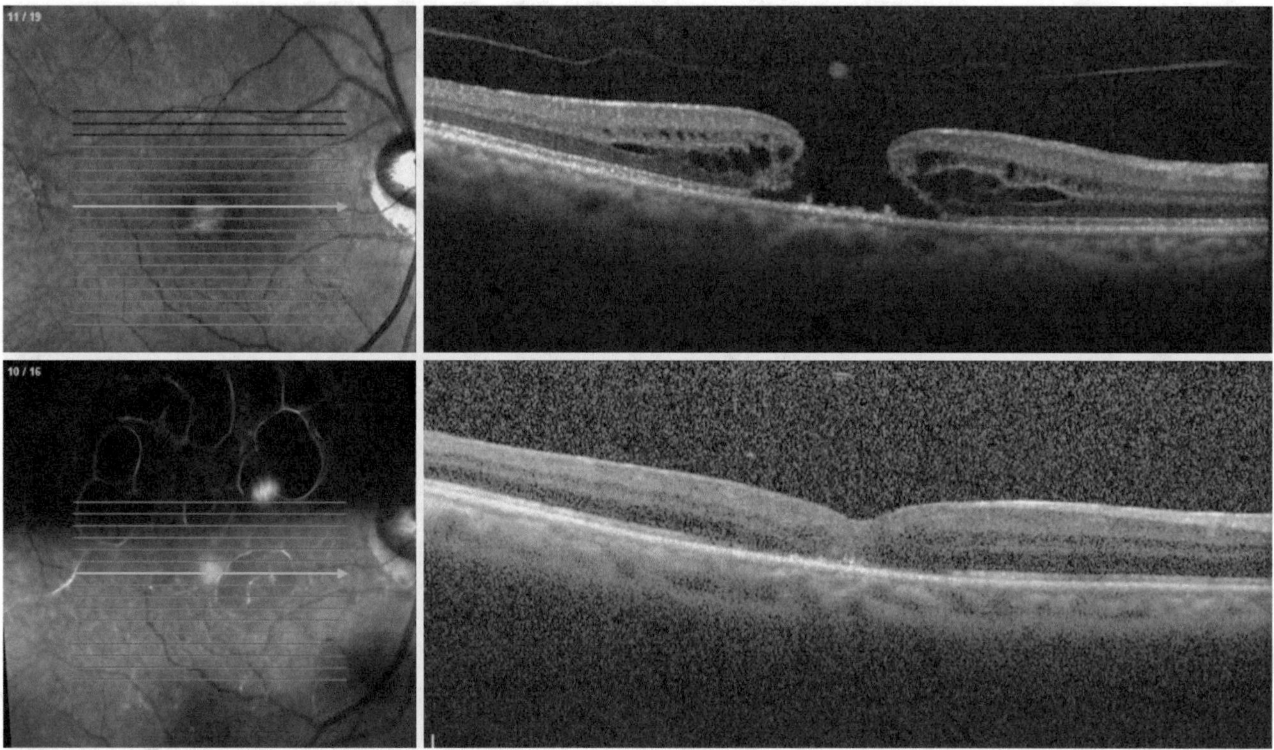

Fig. 11.65 Early closure of a large hole using an ILM flap

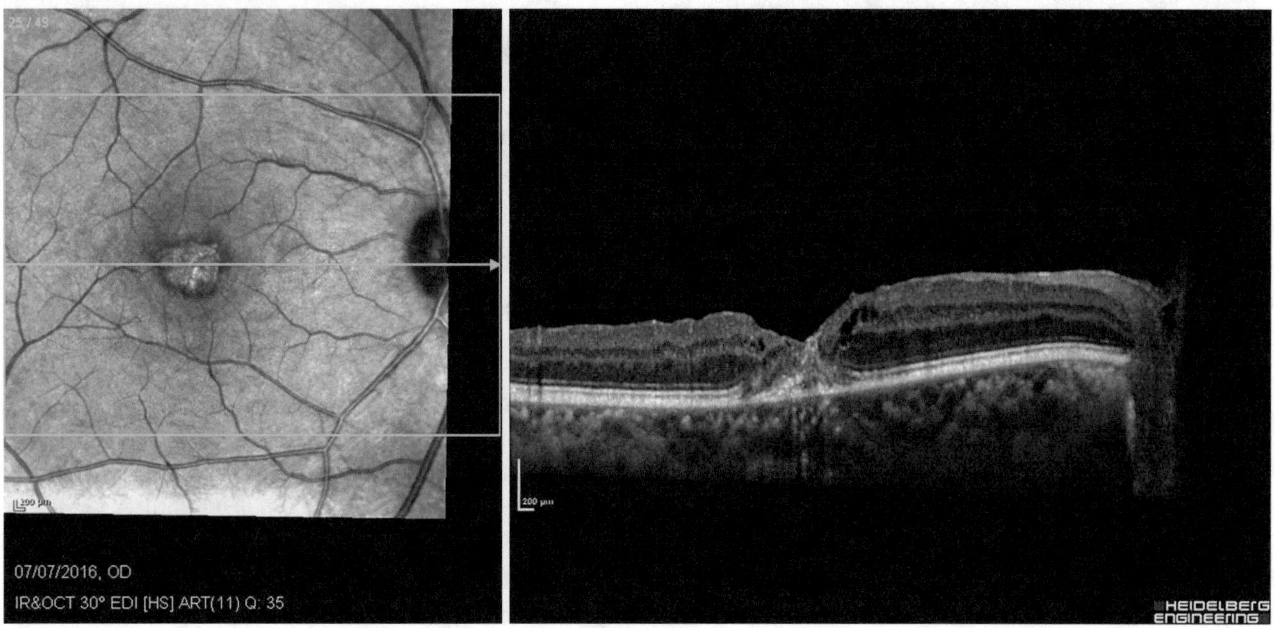

Fig. 11.66 A MH treated by ILM flap

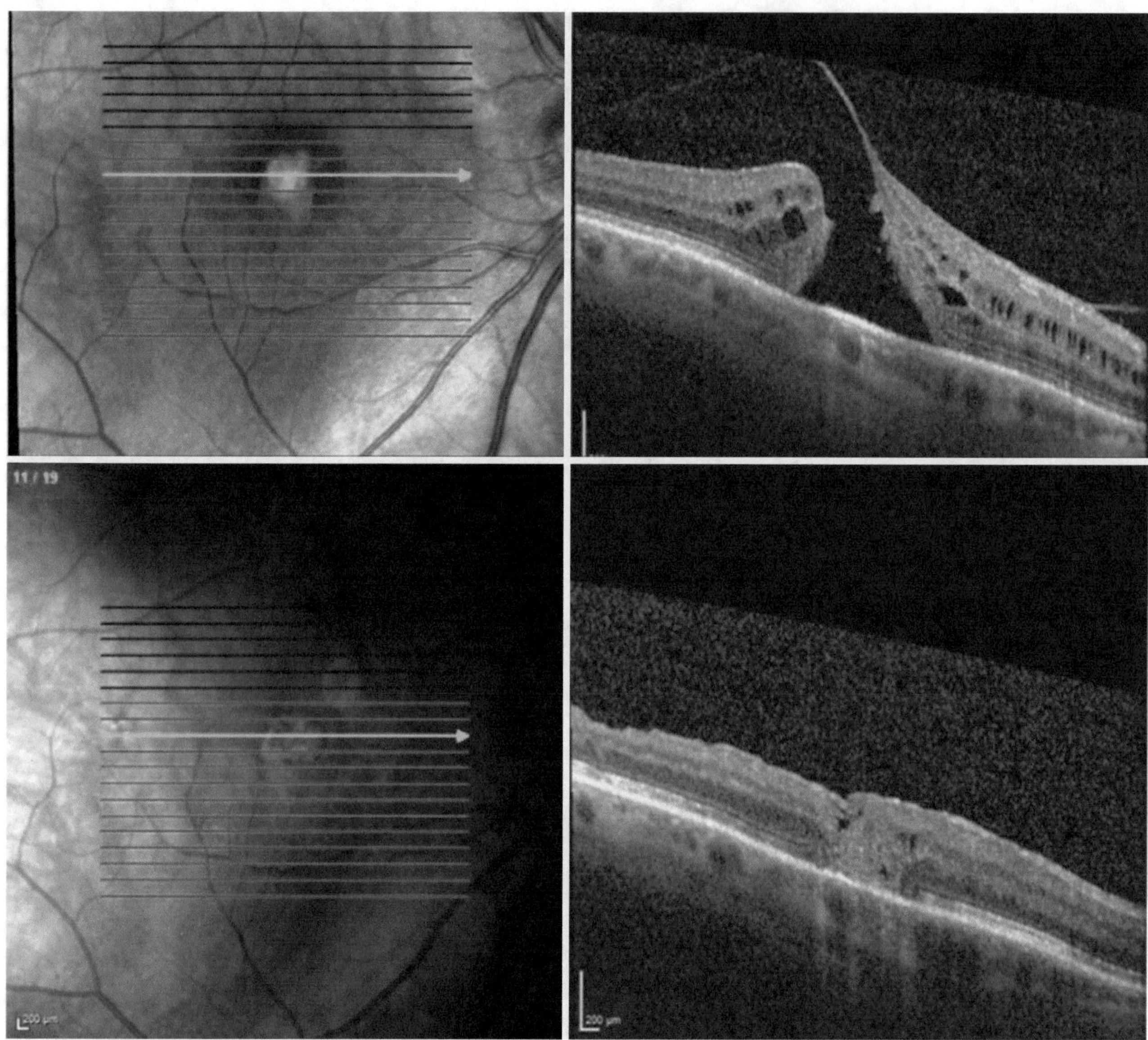

Fig. 11.67 Closure of a large hole by ILM inserted into the hole. There is improved vision from loss of the cystoid space, flattening of the rim, and partial contraction of the hole

grade 2 hole closure rate of 50% in a non-vitrectomised eye [55]. PPV and air and OCT of a face down patient (face down to allow OCT scan without reflections) has revealed that 54.5% of holes are closed in 24 hrs and 75.6% closed at 40 hrs postoperatively [56]. In this study the inner retina closed first followed by the outer retina (Figs. 11.70, 11.71, and 11.72).

PostOperative Posturing of the Patient

It is uncertain whether posturing is necessary to increase the hole closure rate after surgery but very short-term tamponade agents such as air appear to have reduced success rates of 53% [57] suggesting that tamponade is important. A randomised controlled study from France has shown that there is a significant increase in success rates for larger holes (grade 3) if a reduced regime of posturing is employed, 8 hours a day for 5 days, with overall success rates of 97.5% if posturing is used and 87.5% if it is not [58]. A regime of daytime posturing 50 minutes in the hour for 3 hours in the morning and 3 hours in the afternoon for seven days is often used if posturing is required. Posturing face down is easiest with the use of a specially fabricated frame. Most patients find the posturing particularly bothersome at night and this can be abandoned. Posturing compensates for the effects of any operative error in the gas mix which might reduce the bubble size or duration. For this reason, I ask the patient to look at the level of the skirting board for 7 days. They are encouraged to put the television on the floor, to read on their

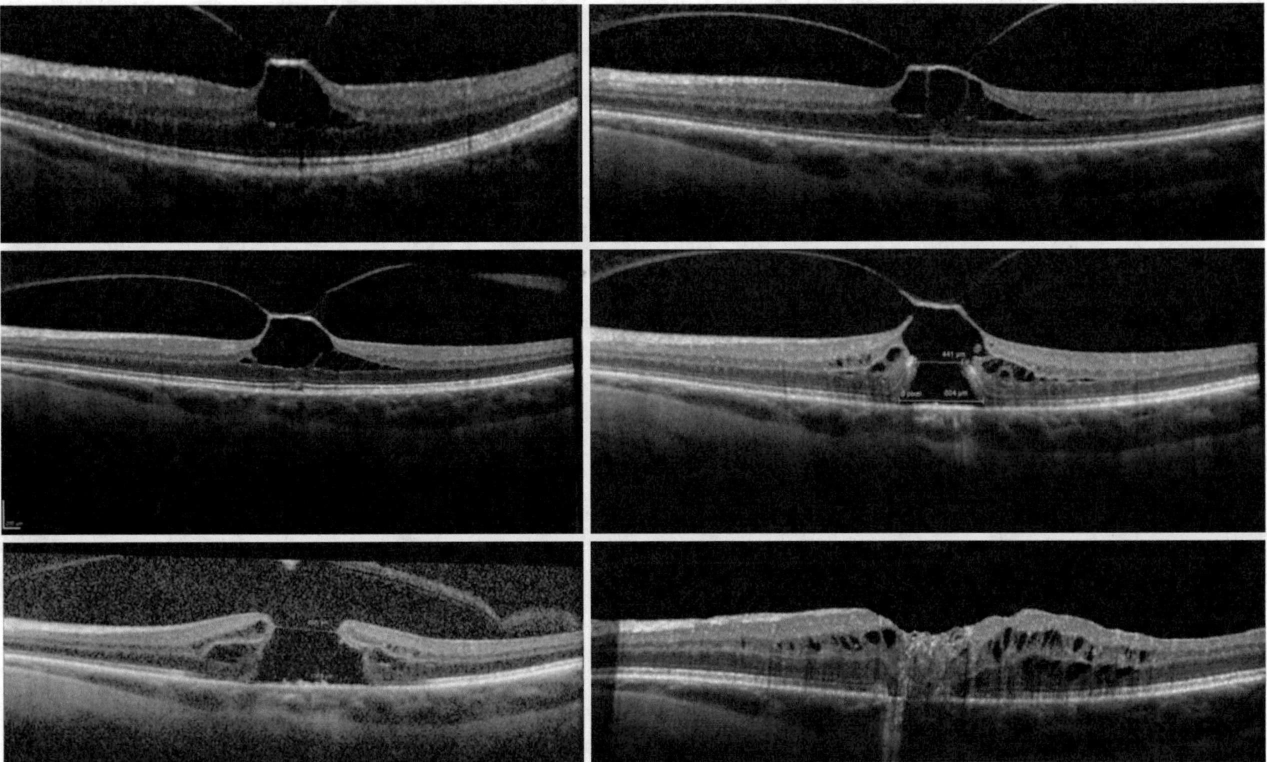

Fig. 11.68 Progression of a large MH preoperatively treated with ILM flap, note the plug of ILM in the hole

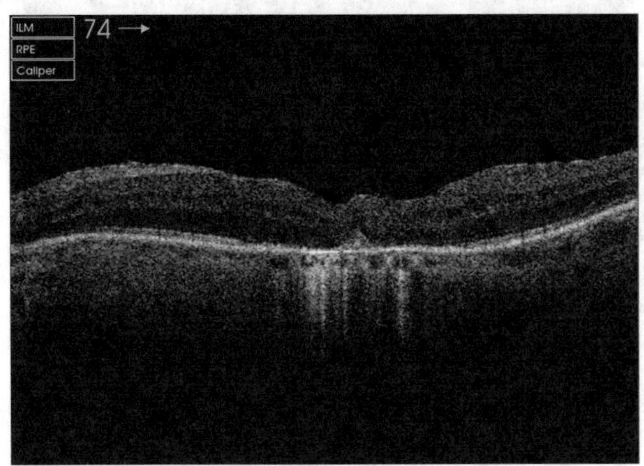

Fig. 11.69 MH closure after reverse ILM flap

laps and not to sleep face up. This has helped when on a couple of occasions, I have had a poor gas bubble size. Most holes close in the first few days. I do not posture after 7 days.

Combined PhacoEmulsification and IOL

Cataract is common after PPV and gas for macular hole. For this reason, cataract surgery is often combined with PPV. Not all vitrectomy surgeons perform phacoemulsification; therefore, four protocols have been performed.

- Separate planned operations:
  - Cataract extraction then PPV.
  - PPV then cataract extraction.
- Combined operation of simultaneous cataract extraction and PPV.
- PPV then cataract extraction when symptomatic.

Simultaneous cataract extraction and PPV is favoured here because of the rapid visual rehabilitation of the patient and the need for only one surgical episode. Surgery in this way produces increased flare (and increased risk of posterior synaechiae) and some risk of iris capture because the gas bubble may tilt the newly implanted IOL. Delaying the cataract surgery seems to run an increased risk of CMO formation, presumably from easier access of prostaglandins to the macula in an empty vitreous cavity. Also be aware that the thickening of the retina at the edge of the hole can result in a falsely short axial length with some biometry systems creating a myopic error after IOL implantation (Fig. 11.73).

Posturing

The conventional process was to ask the patient to posture postoperatively for 2 weeks. Most have abandoned this with apparently insignificant effects on outcome especially for

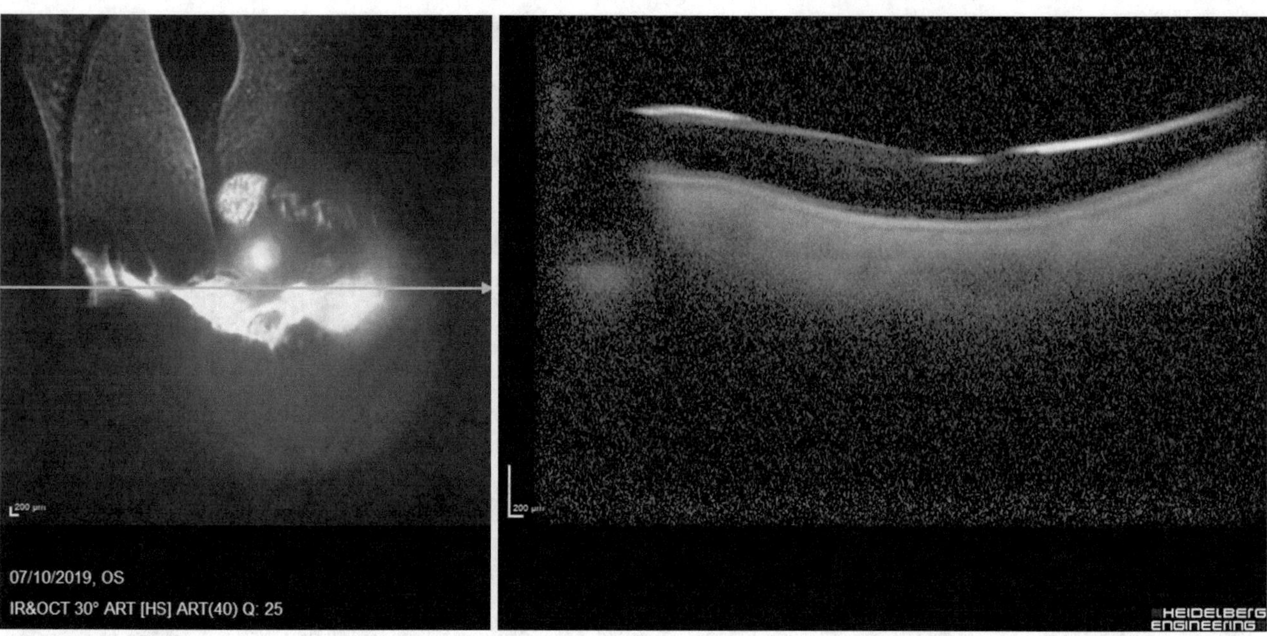

Fig. 11.70 Gas up against an early closure of a macular hole

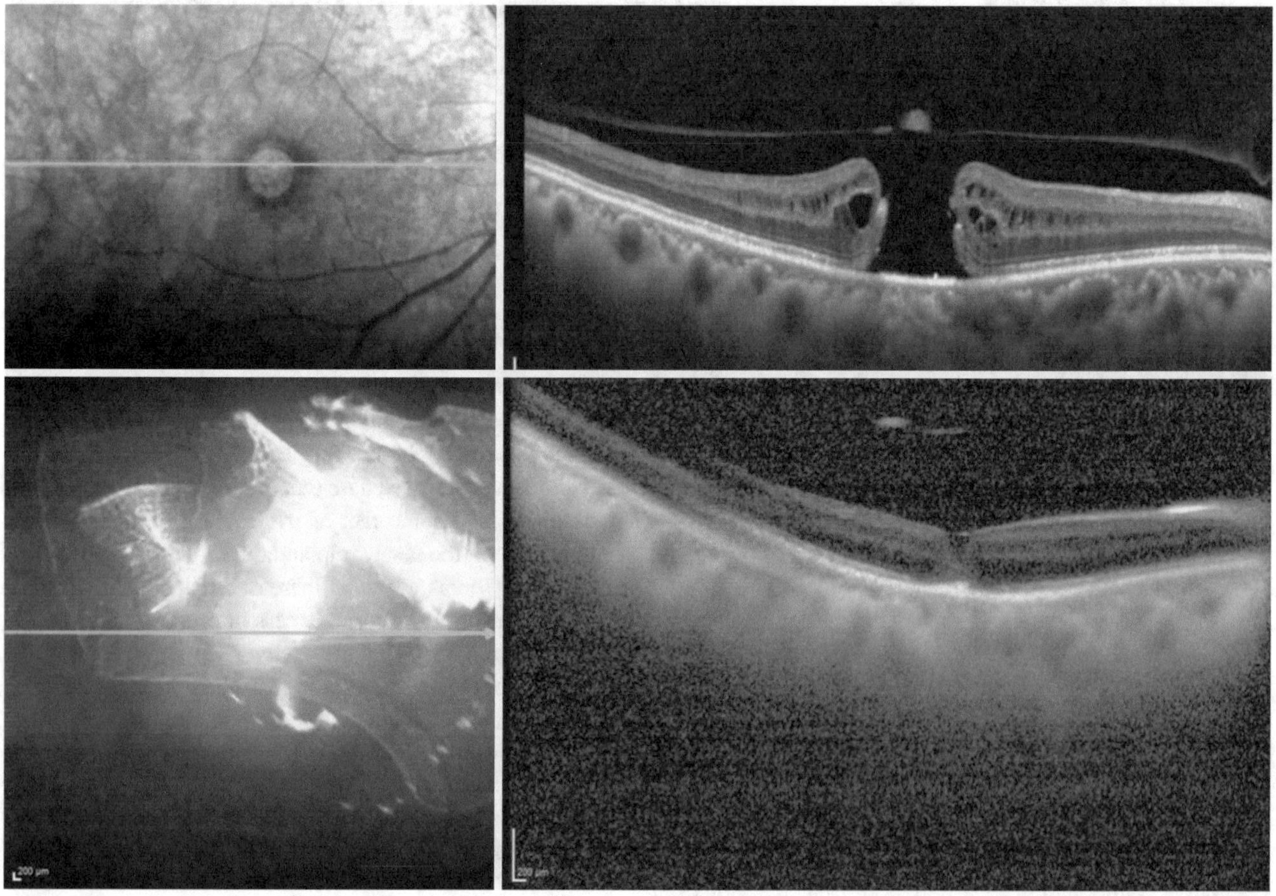

Fig. 11.71 MHs close early in the first few days and this can be detected on occasion by OCT through the gas bubble

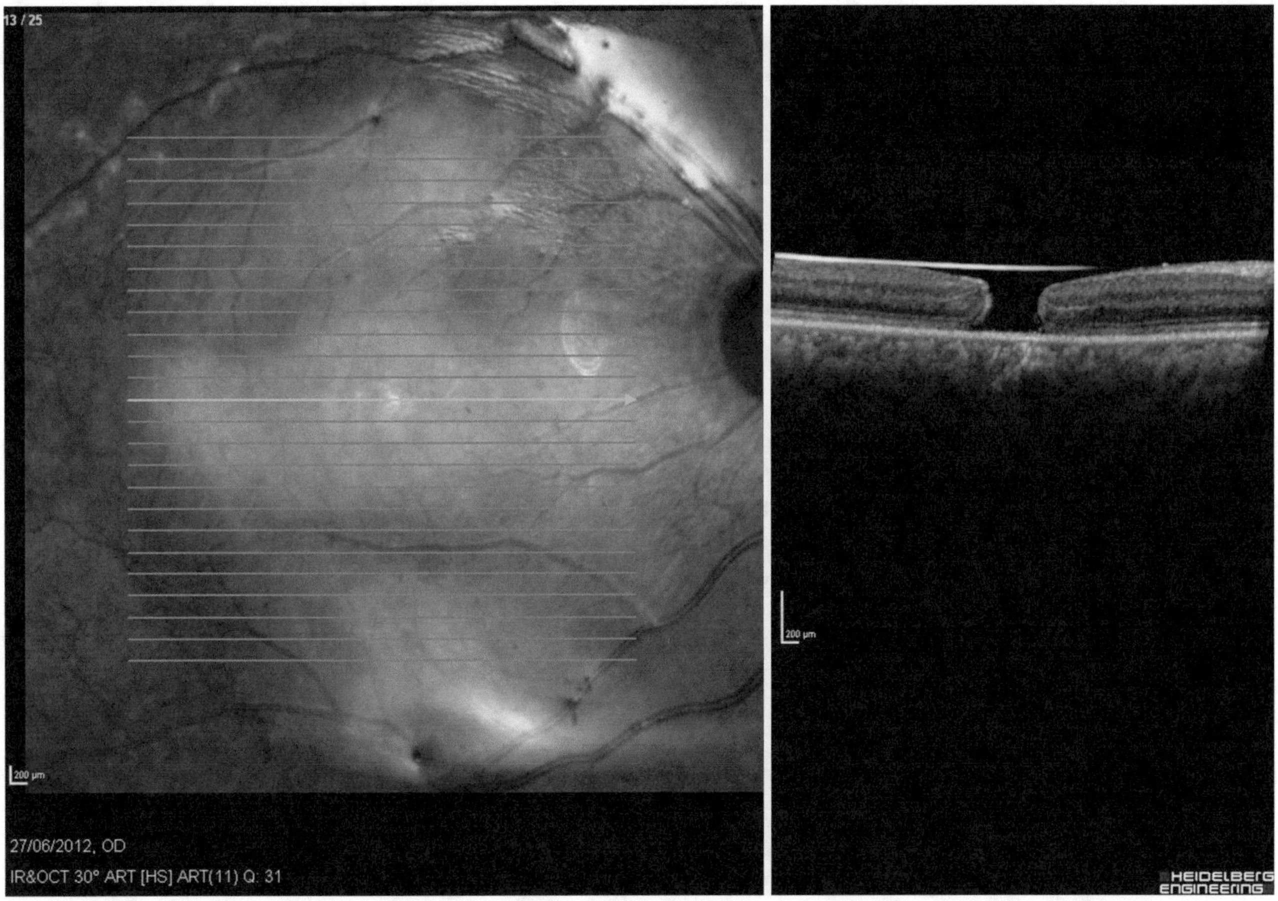

Fig. 11.72 Contact of an oil bubble with a MH

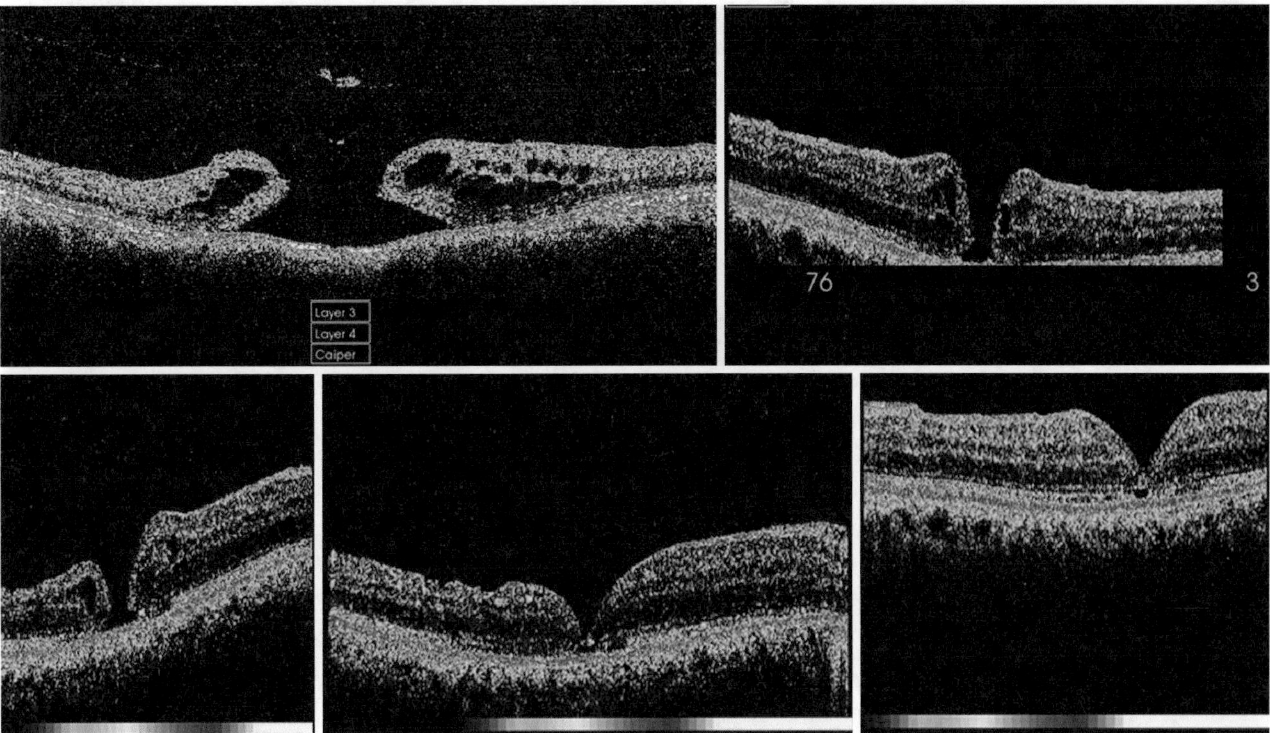

Fig. 11.73 A large macular hole initially reduced in size after PPV and gas but took 1 year to finally close after the surgery with recovery of 20/60 vision

small holes [59]. I ask the patient to look at the level of the skirting board, put their television on the floor or read a book on their lap. This keeps the eye at 45 degrees. This is enough to make sure that the hole remains in contact with the gas bubble even if for some reason there is an under fill of gas postoperatively. The patient should be asked to avoid sleeping on their back at night. This is only required for 7 days because most holes have already closed in the first week.

Specific Complications

These are varied [60–63].

Cataract nuclear sclerosis progression is almost 100% with a 76% chance of requiring cataract surgery [64]. The high rate of cataract postoperatively has led some surgeons to perform the cataract extraction at the time of vitrectomy surgery [65]. Indeed, this is my preferred practice (see Chap. 2).

Retinal pigment epithelial changes 33%.

Retinal breaks during surgery 12.7% with PVD induction and 3.1% without PVD induction [66].

RRD up to 6.6–14% [67] and is higher when the posterior hyaloid is peeled in stages 2 and 3 holes than in stage 4 (PVD already present) but is 2% in more recent analysis [68].

Macular hole reopening has been described in 11% [69] especially in those who have postoperative cataract extraction, but this is now rare with ILM peeling routinely.

Choroidal neovascularisation rarely.

Iatrogenic eccentric full-thickness macular holes have been associated with ILM peel and require no treatment [70].

Visual field loss (Figs. 11.74, 11.75, 11.76, 11.77, and 11.78).

Visual Field Loss

Visual field loss [71] has been described with arcuate or paracentral scotomata or peripheral loss in as many as 23% of patients [72] and attributed to loss of nerve fibres at the time of posterior hyaloid peel [71, 73] or dehydration of the

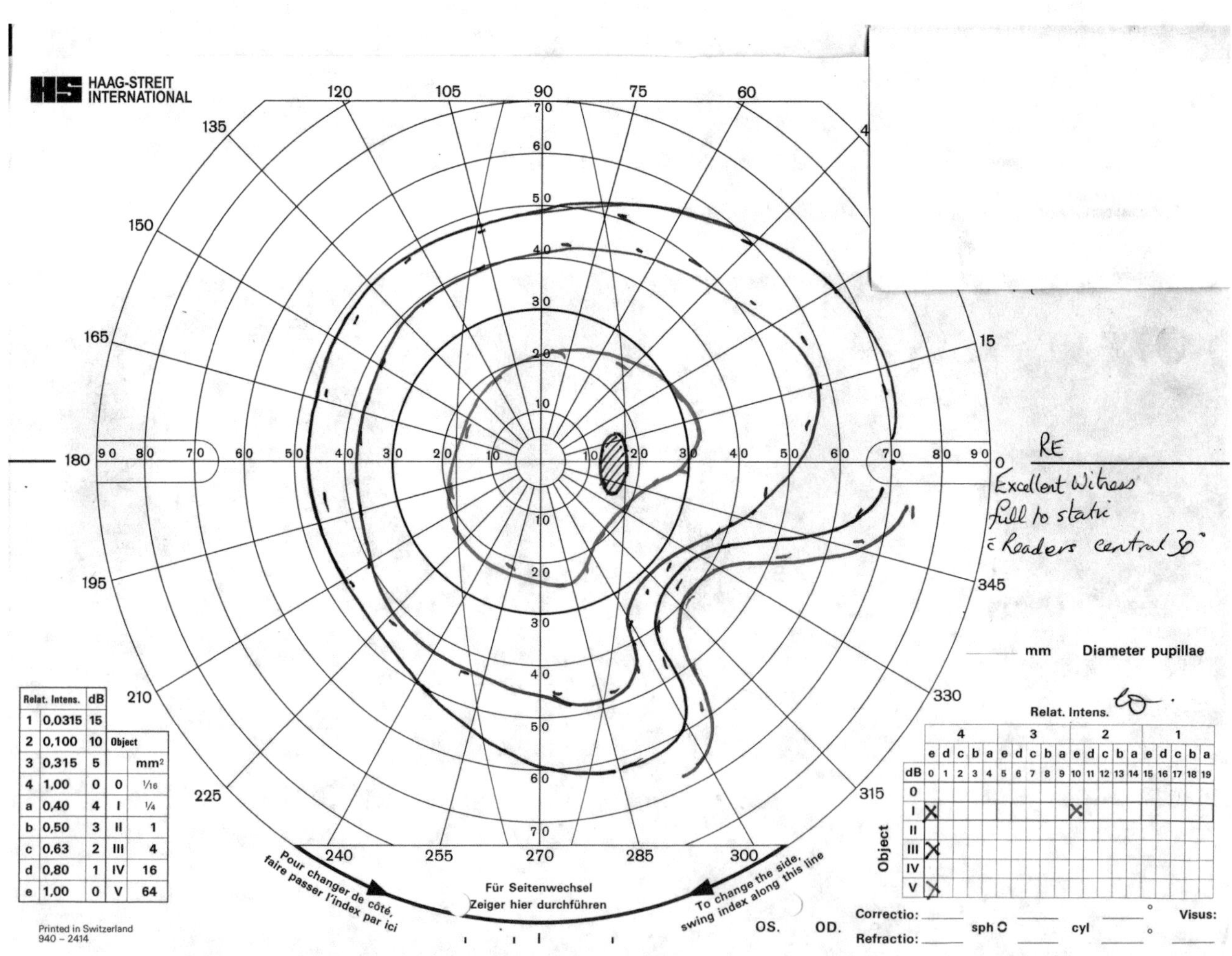

Fig. 11.74 An example of visual field loss after macular hole surgery. Visual field loss has been described after macular hole surgery often in an arcuate or segmental pattern

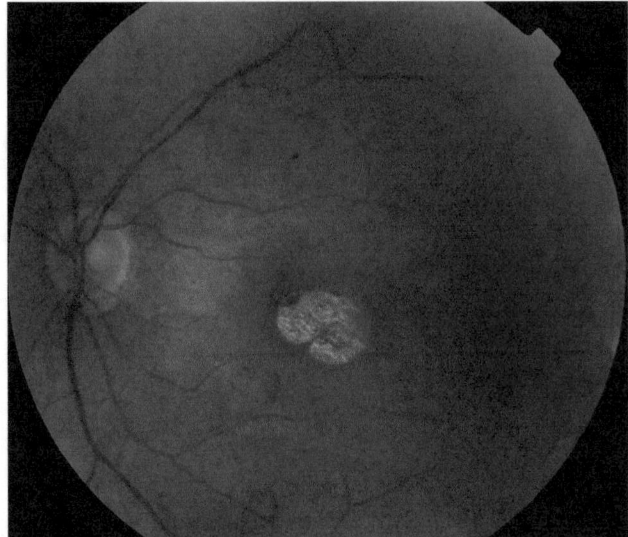

Fig. 11.75 This patient, unfortunately, had subretinal ICG during ICG injection. This has resulted in an area of retinal pigment epithelial damage, thankfully away from the fovea which retains 20/30 vision

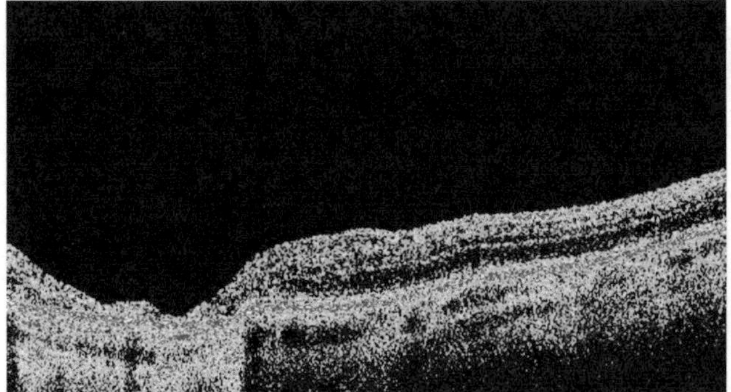

Fig. 11.76 Atrophy is seen on OCT

nerve fibre layer of the retina during air fluid exchange [74] or to a variety of changes such as RPE degeneration, choroidal filling delay, or epiretinal membrane [75]. Nasal visual field loss has been attributed to ICG usage [76] (Figs. 11.64, 11.79, 11.80, and 11.81).

Success Rates

These depend on the mix of grades of macular hole and the duration of the symptoms and vary from 80 to 100% for hole closure [16, 27, 77, 78]. The macular retina moves inward after closure of the hole [79].

- Treatment of grade 1 holes to try to help prevent progression has shown no benefit [12, 80].
- In groups with stage 2, success is 88% [81] hole closure with 60% achieving 20/50 or better.
- With stages 3 and 4, the success rate is less at 69% [17] hole closure and 60% with 20/80 or better.

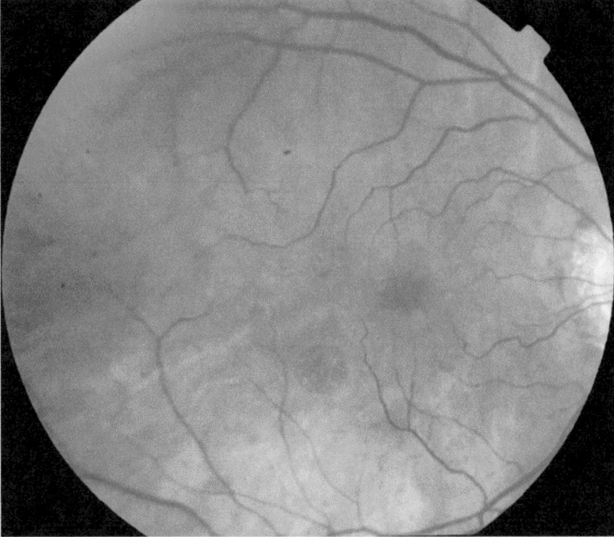

Fig. 11.77 On occasion, in the postoperative period, paracentral holes are seen in the retina because of macular hole surgery. The origin of these holes is uncertain but may be related to ILM peeling. The foveal architecture has been restored after this macular hole surgery, but a full-thickness paracentral hole is demonstrated

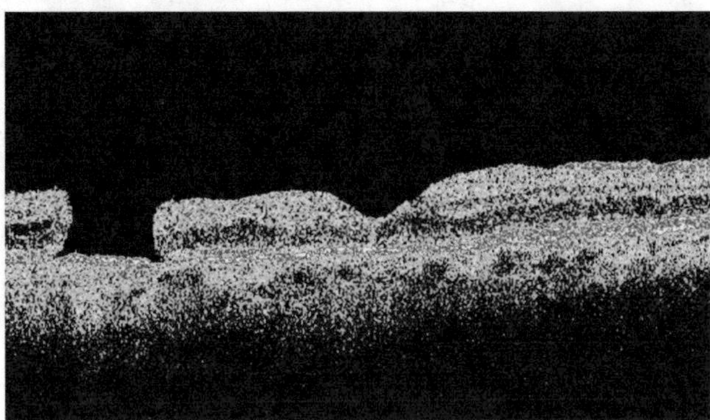

Fig. 11.78 OCT shows a full thickness retinal defect

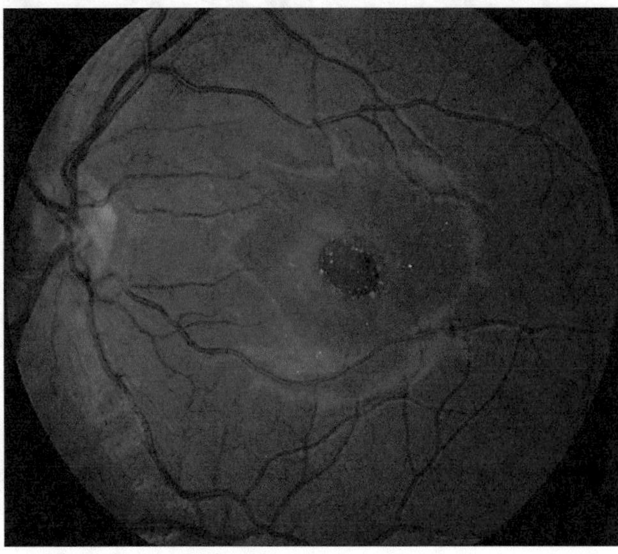

Fig. 11.79 A traumatic macular hole

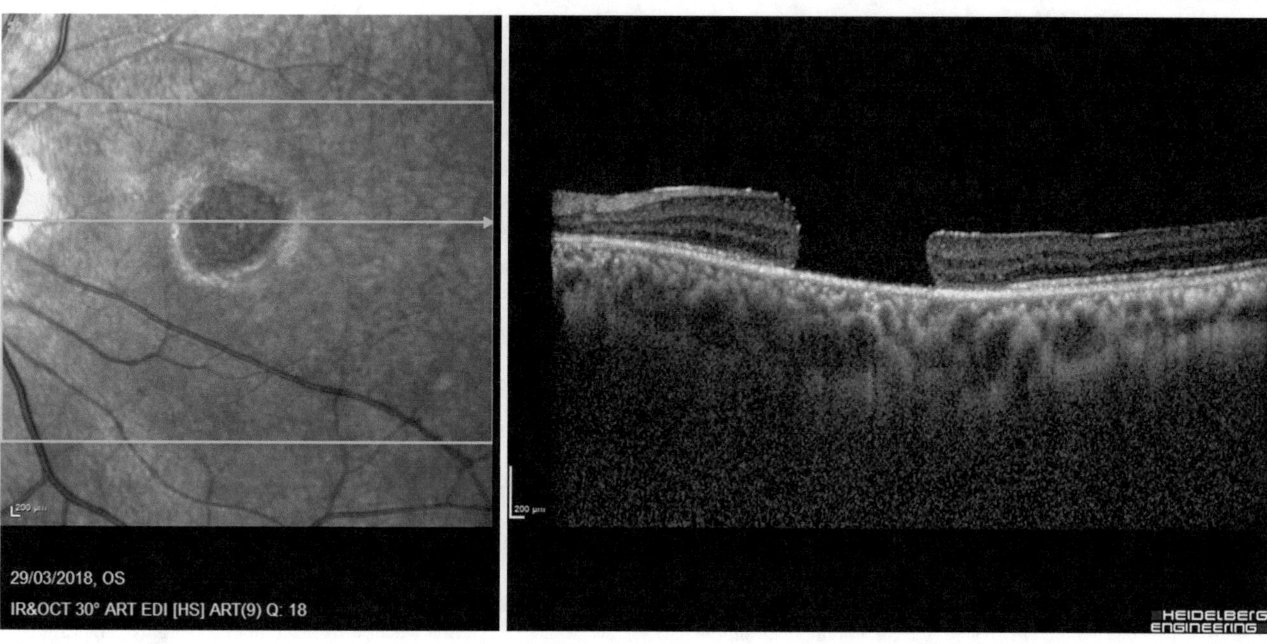

Fig. 11.80 A traumatic MH

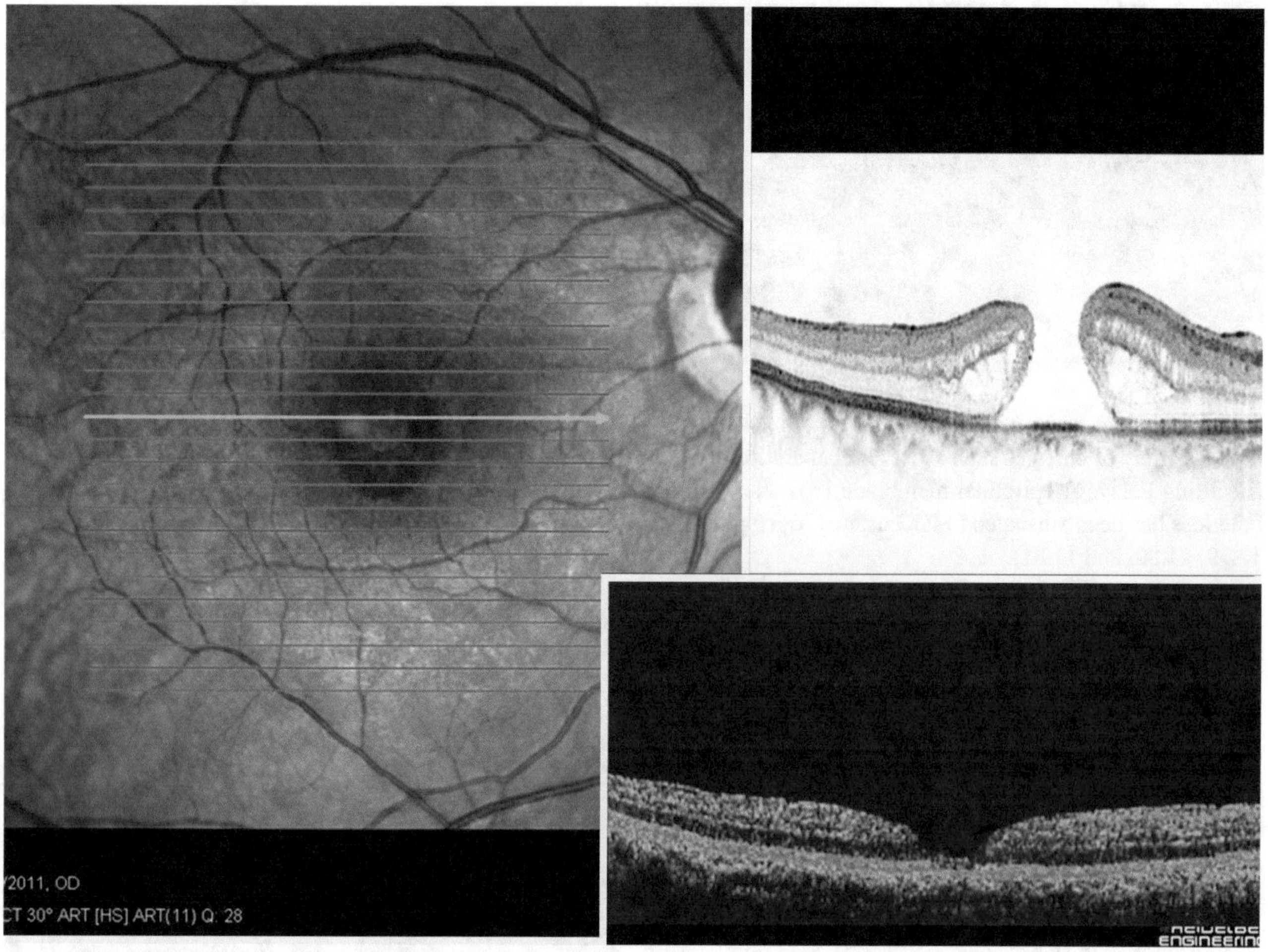

Fig. 11.81 A macular hole which was closed by surgery but reopened years later

- Smaller holes under 400 μm (measured on OCT) have an increased chance of closure 94% compared with 56% for those 400 μm or larger [82].
- Partly the hole may be closed by a glial cell plug thought to come from the Muller cells [45].
- In patients with macular holes of more than one year's duration the use of ILM peel has been associated with success rates of 81% [83] but success rates can be much lower at 47% [84].
- Those patients with better postoperative vision have thicker fovea's on OCT [85].
- Larger initial holes are more prone to late reopening.
- Traumatic macular holes can be closed after operation in 96% [86].
- Visual outcome is improved by reduced age, increased preoperative visual acuity, and reduced hole size [87].
- Visual acuity improves over years from surgery [88].
- Afro-Caribbean race is associated with larger hole at presentation and poorer outcome [89] (Figs. 11.64, 11.82, 11.83, 11.84, 11.85, 11.86, 11.87, 11.88, 11.89, 11.90, 11.91, and 11.92).

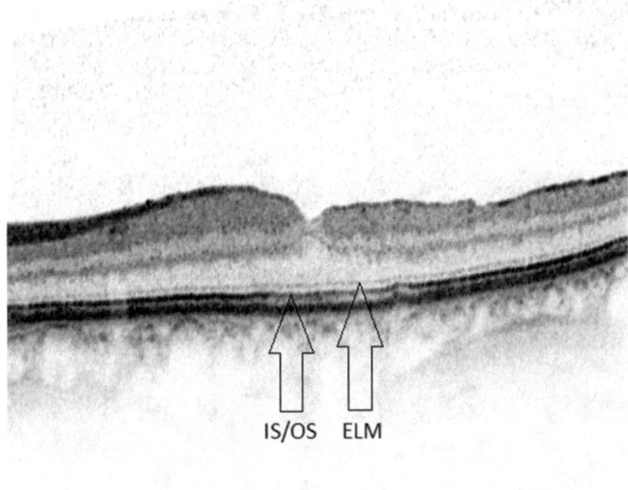

Fig. 11.82 The recovery of the lines indicating the external limiting membrane (ELM) and the inner segment/outer segment juncture (IS/OS) are good prognostic factors for improved visual recovery after macular hole repair, as in this eye postoperatively

Reoperation

Reoperation for failed surgery occurs in 4% [68] has a success rate for closure of 74% if performed within 2 months of the initial surgery [90, 91]. Patients in whom the hole was closed and then reopened postoperatively are more likely to achieve closure of the hole with reoperation than those in whom the hole has never closed [91]. ILM does not appear to regenerate [92] and should therefore be absent in the peeled area on reoperation. Patients with a cuff of fluid visible on OCT are more likely to close after reoperation than those with a flat rim around the macular hole [93]. Patients achieve better vision with reoperation [94] (Fig. 11.93).

Surgical Pearl

Repeat Surgery for Macular Hole Using the Inverted ILM Flap Technique or Human Amniotic Membrane

I treat all macular hole cases with the temporal inverted ILM flap technique regardless of their origin, size, or associated maculopathy. This means every case is dealt with according to its unique needs and I believe the functional and anatomical results are better. However, there are rare occasions where the macular hole fails to close after initial surgery. The majority of these are caused by the flap reapproximating during fluid/air exchange or after surgery has ended. They can almost always be corrected by repositioning the flap over the macular hole during a second intervention.

Even rarer are the cases where the flap is lost and cannot be recovered during second surgery. What options do we then have? If the first surgical approach had been made using the temporal ILM flap technique, enough ILM still remains next to the macular hole (attached up to the hole margins) for the surgeon to create a new flap from the nasal side. This would be the ideal solution.

Perhaps we are dealing with a case initially operated elsewhere and the previous surgeon had performed classical ILM peeling and careful staining reveals that there is no viable ILM next to the macular hole from which we can create an attached inverted flap. What then? We might find that there is some remaining ILM further away from the macular hole that is of sufficient size to cover the hole. We can peel as large a piece as possible and form an autologous “free flap”.

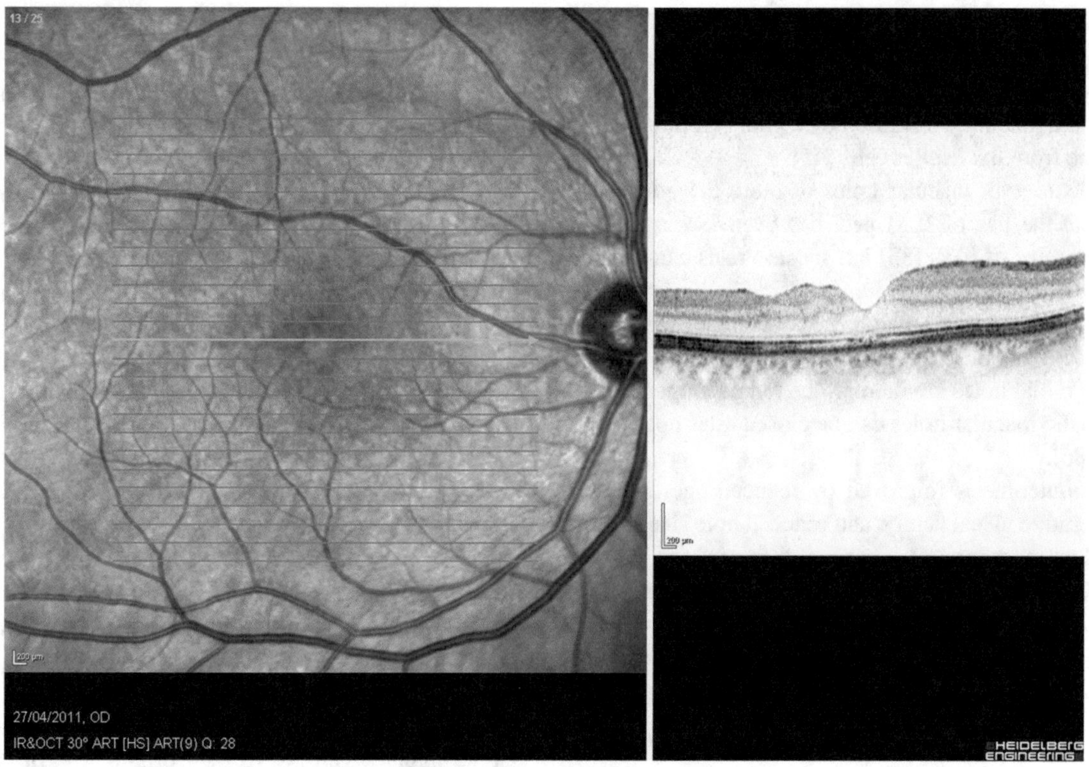

Fig. 11.83 In this postoperative macular hole at 5 weeks the IS/OS junction (ellipsoid) is still disrupted, and vision is 20/70, time is required for the retina to remodel and for the vision to improve over 6 to 12 months. Notice the corrugation on the macula temporal to the fovea, a common feature after macular hole surgery and associated with poorer nasal paracentral vision in these eyes (this is more problematic in the left eye where the nasal paracentral visual field is used when reading words)

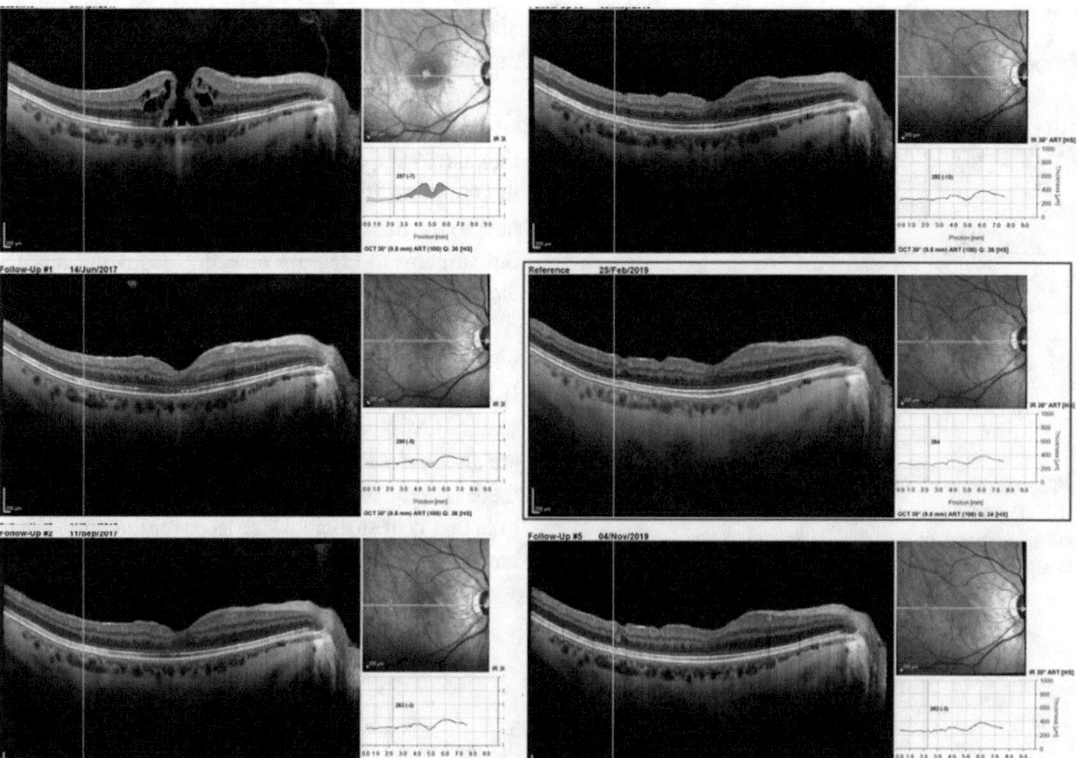

Fig. 11.84 MH surgery and postoperative recovery

HEIDELBERG ENGINEERING

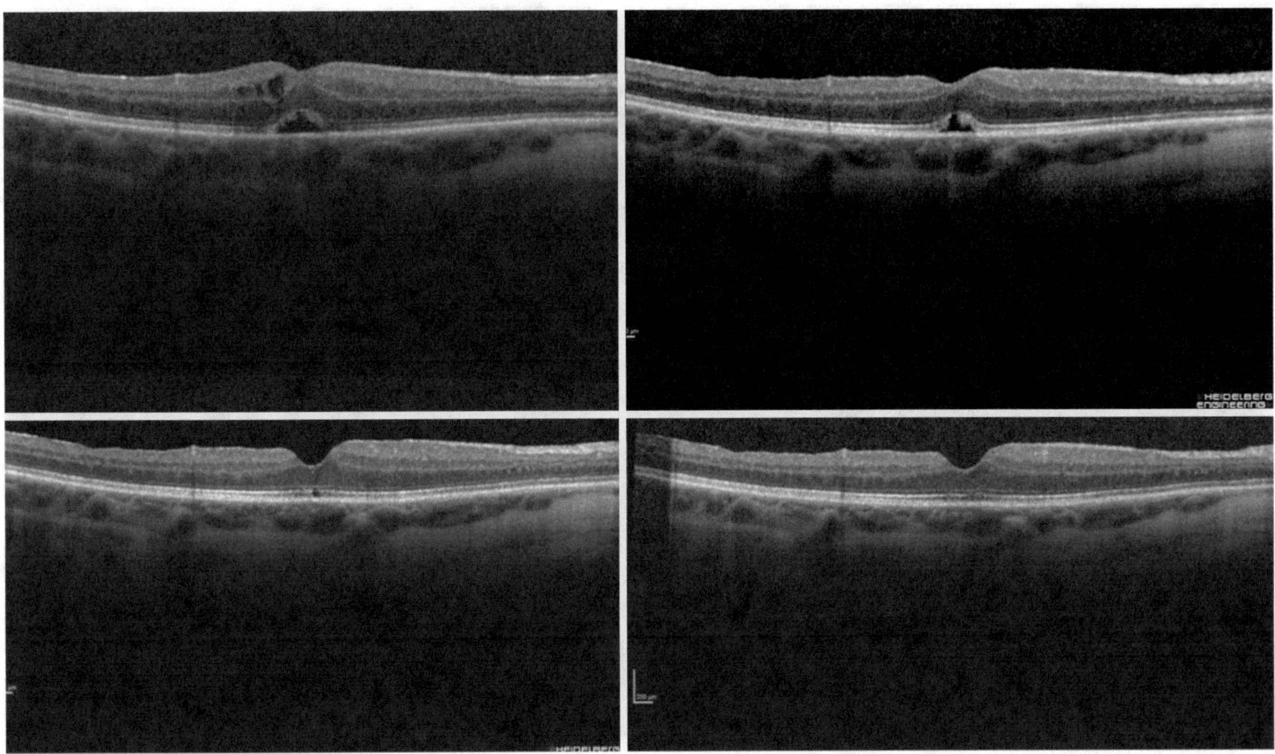

Fig. 11.85 In the postoperative period it is common to have a delayed closure of the outer retina over a few months

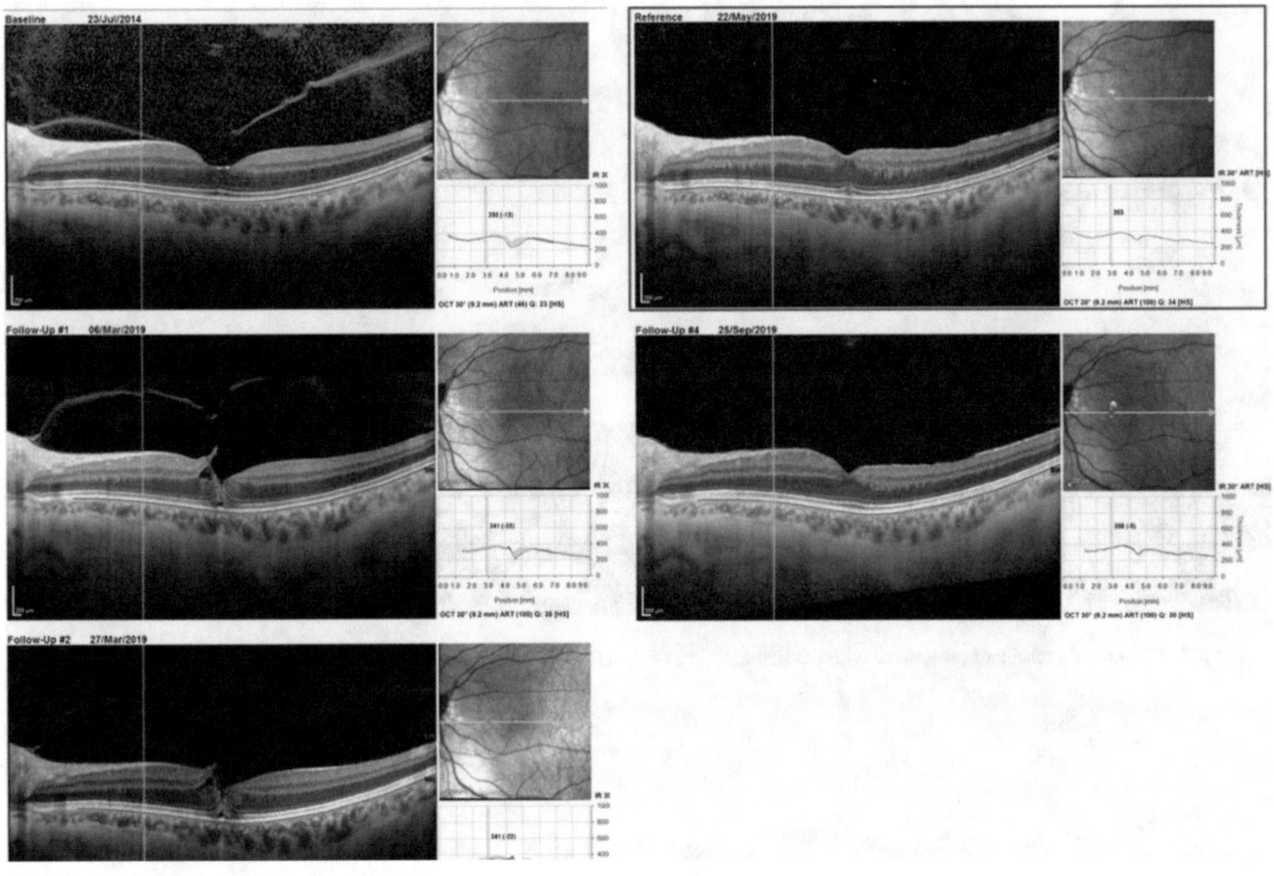

Baseline 23/Jul/2014
Reference 22/May/2019
Follow-Up #1 06/Mar/2019
Follow-Up #4 25/Sep/2019
Follow-Up #2 27/Mar/2019

Fig. 11.86 Small MH progression and closure

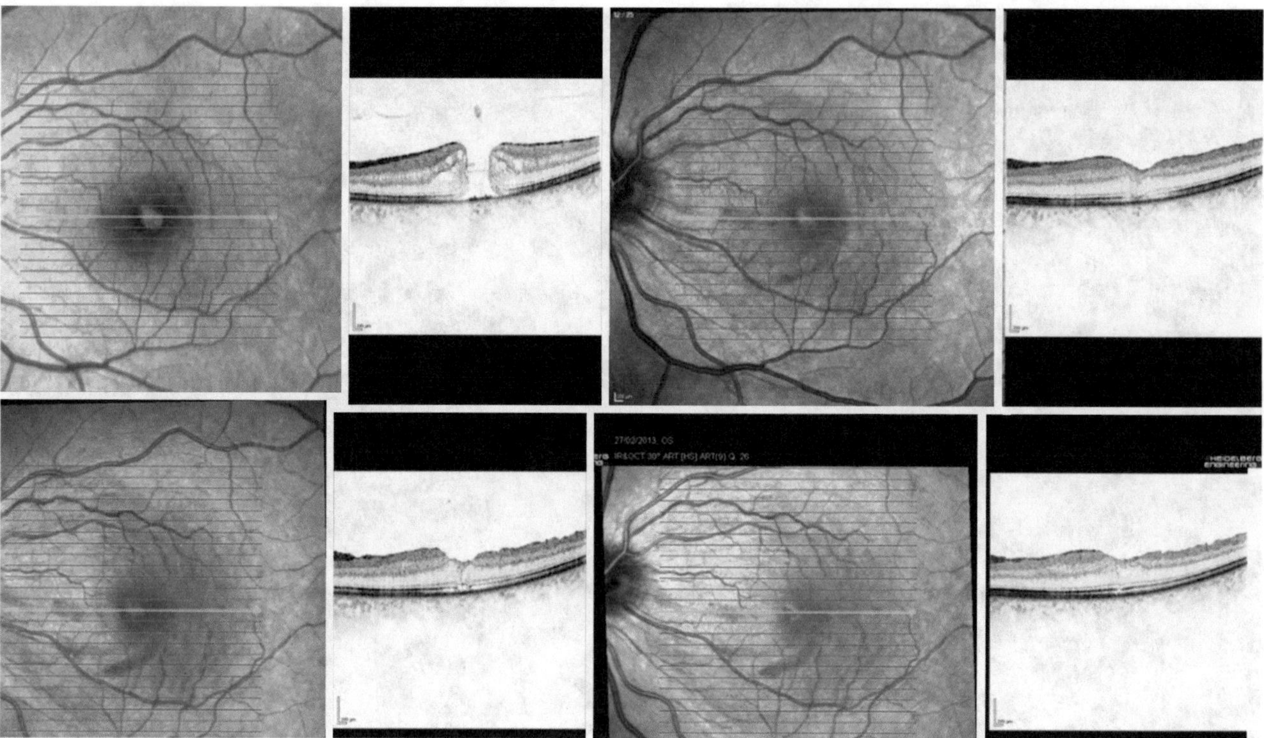

Fig. 11.87 Closure of a macular hole postoperatively

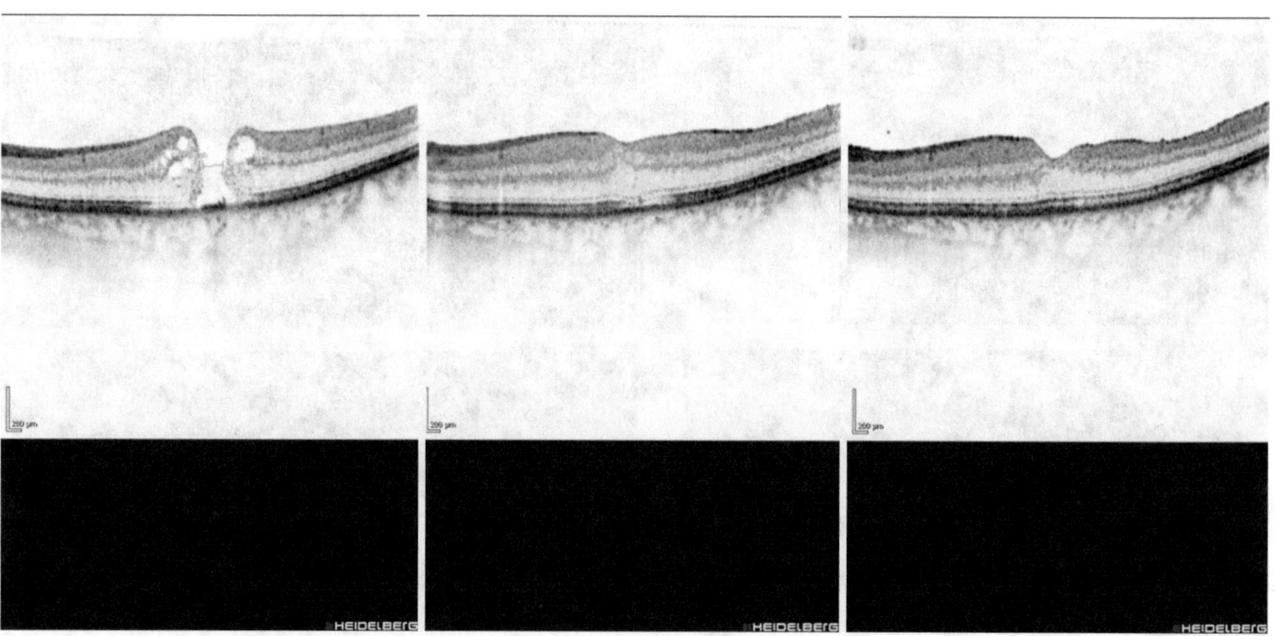

Fig. 11.88 Closure of a macular hole grade 2 with gradual recovery of the ellipsoid layer

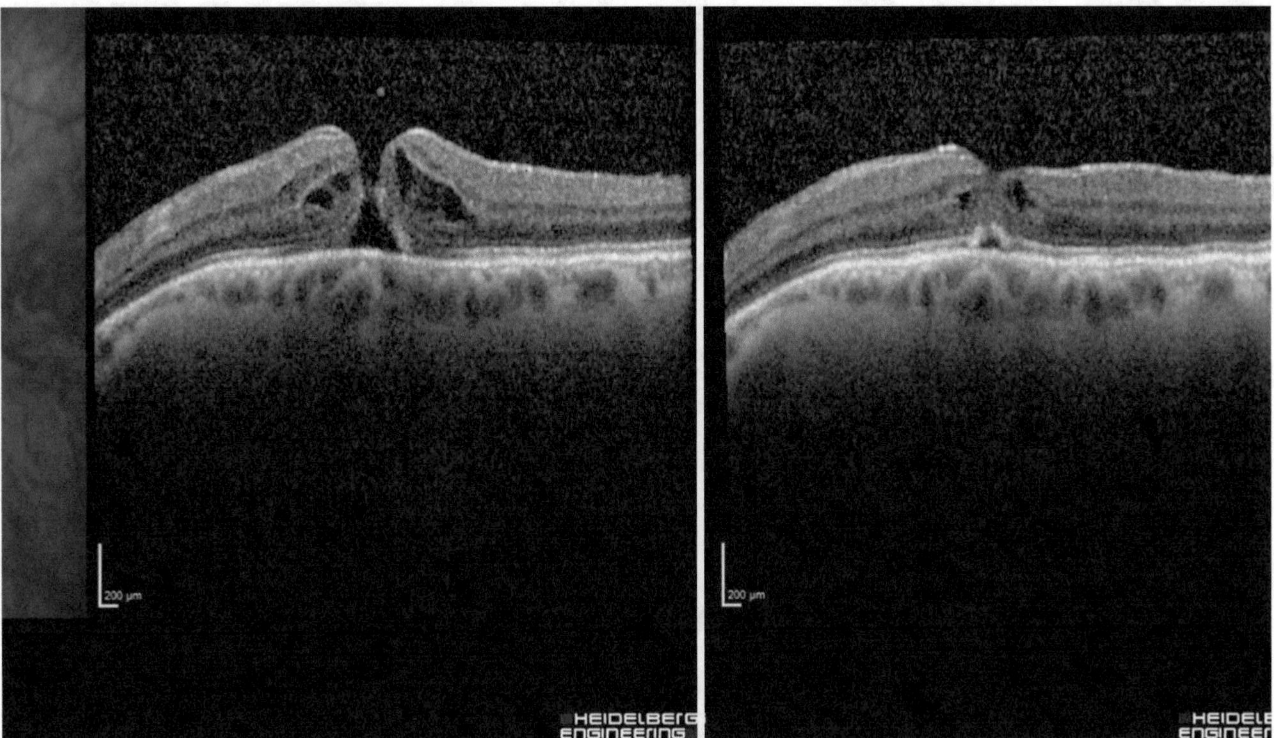

Fig. 11.89 A closed grade 2 macular hole after surgery

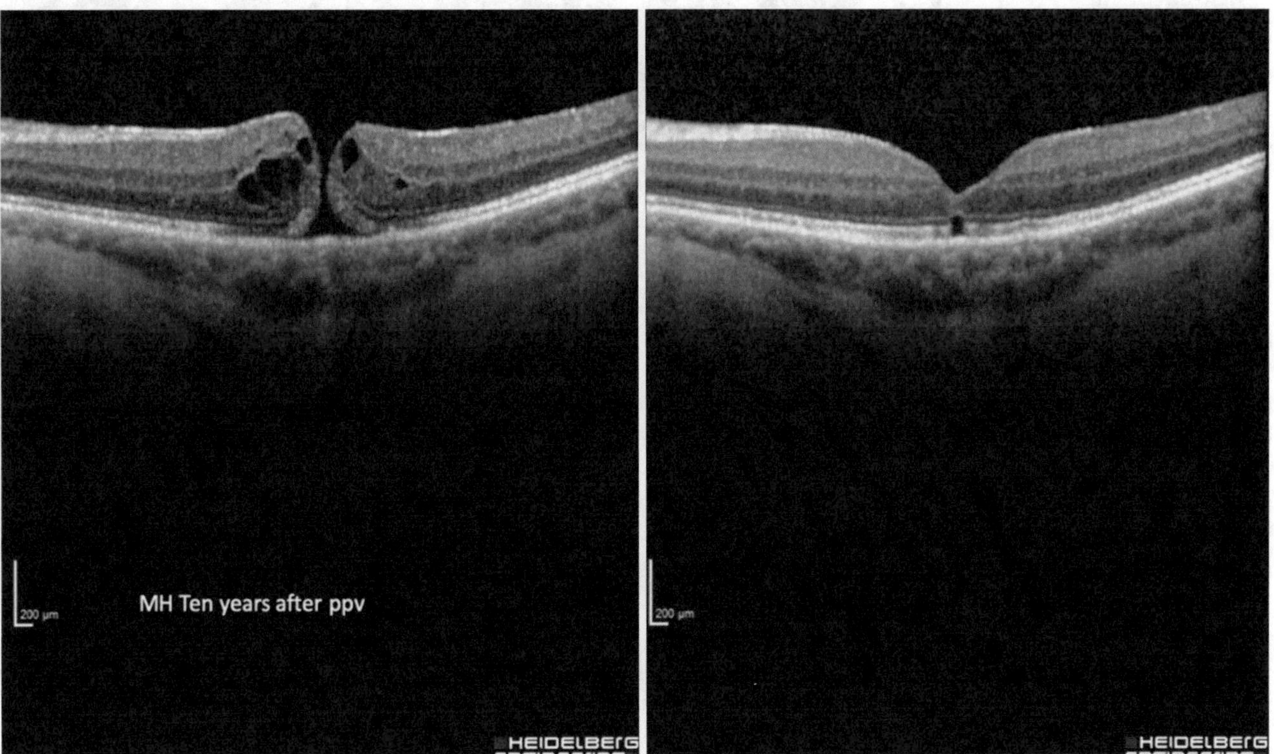

Fig. 11.90 MH closure with an early small defect that usually resolves

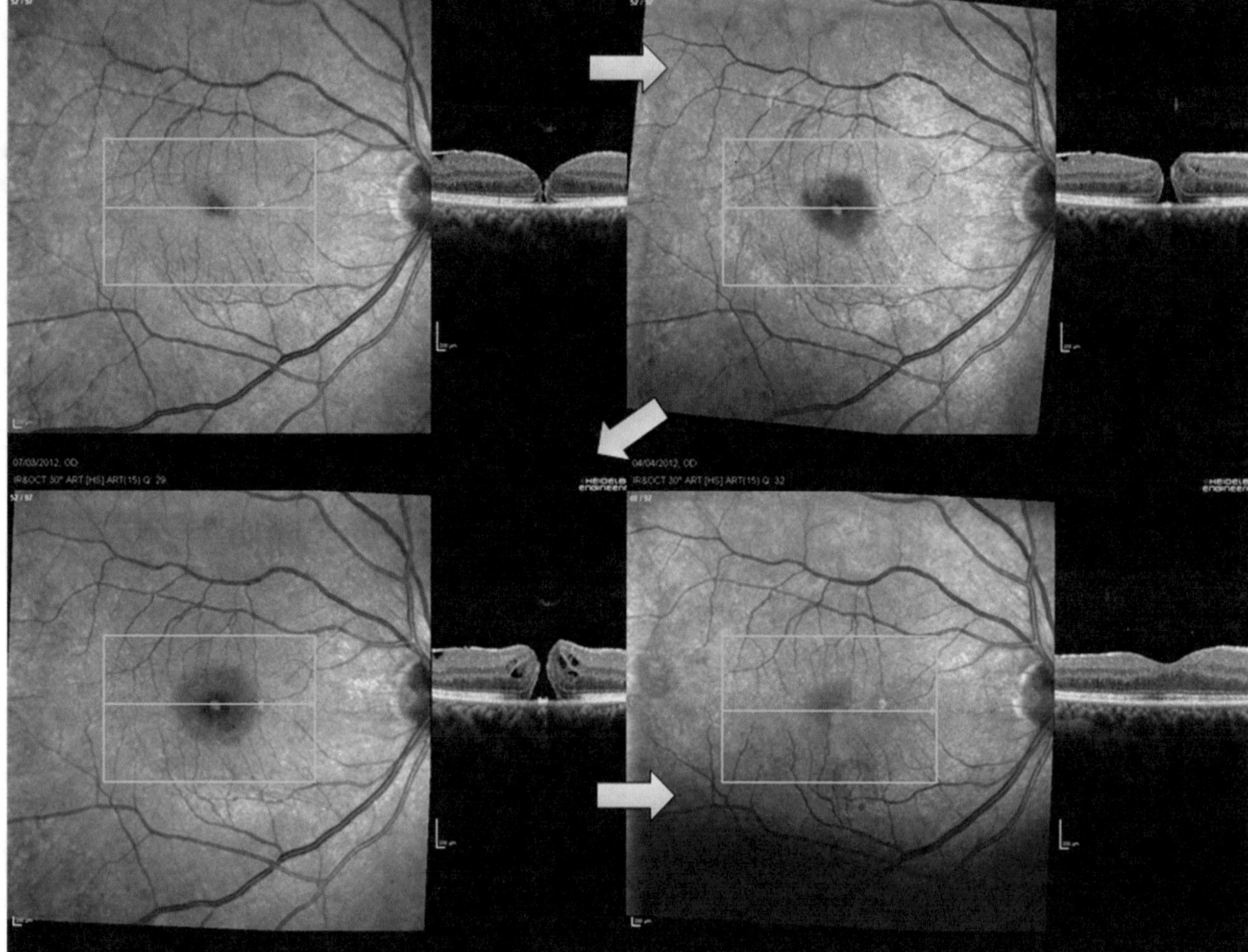

Fig. 11.91 MH evolution and after vitrectomy

We transplant this and lay it over the hole on top of the retina. Viscoelastic material is particularly useful in keeping the flap in position during the very complete and thorough fluid/air exchange that completes the surgery.

Remember, the aim of the inverted ILM flap technique is to allow gliosis to occur underneath the flap as this will enable retinal tissue to fill the hole and the photoreceptors are in contact with the retinal epithelium so all of the layers repair. Although we believe that trying to introduce the flap into the macular hole may cause additional trauma there are occasions when only a small amount of ILM can be harvested for an autologous free flap. In this case, or perhaps also if it proves extremely difficult to keep the flap in place over the macular hole, the ILM flap may be inserted into the macular hole.

What should we do when there is no viable ILM and we cannot create an autologous flap? Human amniotic membrane can be used to close the macular hole. The aim is just the same as when creating an ILM flap, we want to cover the macular hole with a suitably sized flap. Amniotic membrane is, however, thicker, and more rigid than ILM and tends to adhere to surgical instruments (whereas ILM tends to "stick" to the retinal pigment epithelium). Thus, manoeuvring the amniotic membrane flap in place on top of the hole and making it stay there can be quite difficult. One solution is to perform the flap manoeuvres after first performing complete fluid/air exchange. Having made sure that no fluid remains it is relatively easy to introduce the amniotic membrane and place it over the macular hole on the surface of the retina as our manoeuvres will not cause any currents, which can disturb the flap in an eye with fluid. The eye can remain filled with gas, or silicone oil can be used as an adjuvant to keep the flap in place if the surgeon is concerned about it possibly moving.

Professor Jerzy Nawrocki, Professor Zofia Michalewska, Ophthalmic Clinic "Jasne Blonia", Lodz, Poland

Secondary Macular Holes

Contusion injury to the eye can result in secondary macular holes [95] which have a high spontaneous closure rate (50%)

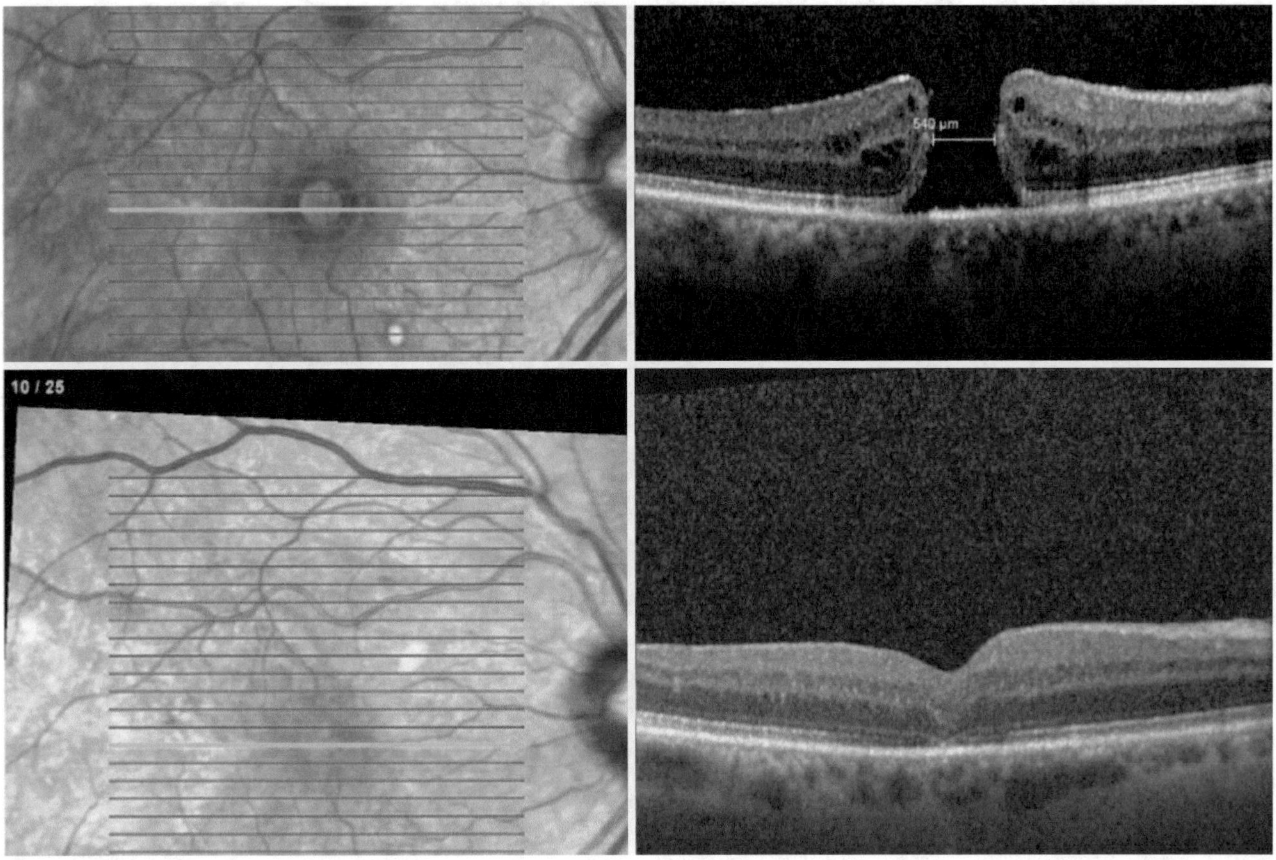

Fig. 11.92 Postoperative closure of a grade 4 hole by PPV and ILM peel alone

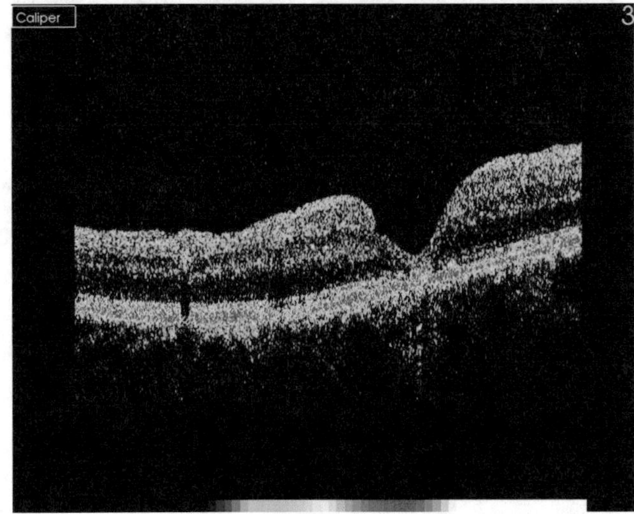

Fig. 11.93 Although the hole is closed in this patient the fovea is very thin and is related to poor visual recover of 20/200

in the first few months, therefore it is recommended to wait 4 months from the trauma before surgical intervention [96]. Traumatic macular holes can be associated with the production of retinal detachment [97].

Rhegmatogenous retinal detachment may produce a secondary macular hole and Yag laser injury has been associated with hole formation [98]. Holes may appear in other retinal pathologies such as sickle cell retinopathy and Von Hippel–Lindau disease.

Lamellar and Partial Thickness Holes

On some occasions macular holes will not penetrate through the whole retina, producing a partial thickness hole with mild reduction of vision. Some are seen in the fellow eyes of macular hole patients. They are often associated with ERM discovered on OCT or found if surgery is performed. The ERM looks different on OCT often with a thicker less dense cross-section. During surgery the ERM feels different and has the consistency more of inner retina than typical ERM [99]. This can be disconcerting to the surgeon performing the operation (Figs. 11.94, 11.95, 11.96, 11.97, and 11.98).

Lamellar holes should be discriminated from pseudoholes which are holes in an ERM over the fovea with underlying intact retina [100–106]. Surgical intervention will improve the anatomical appearance of the hole but as yet good data on

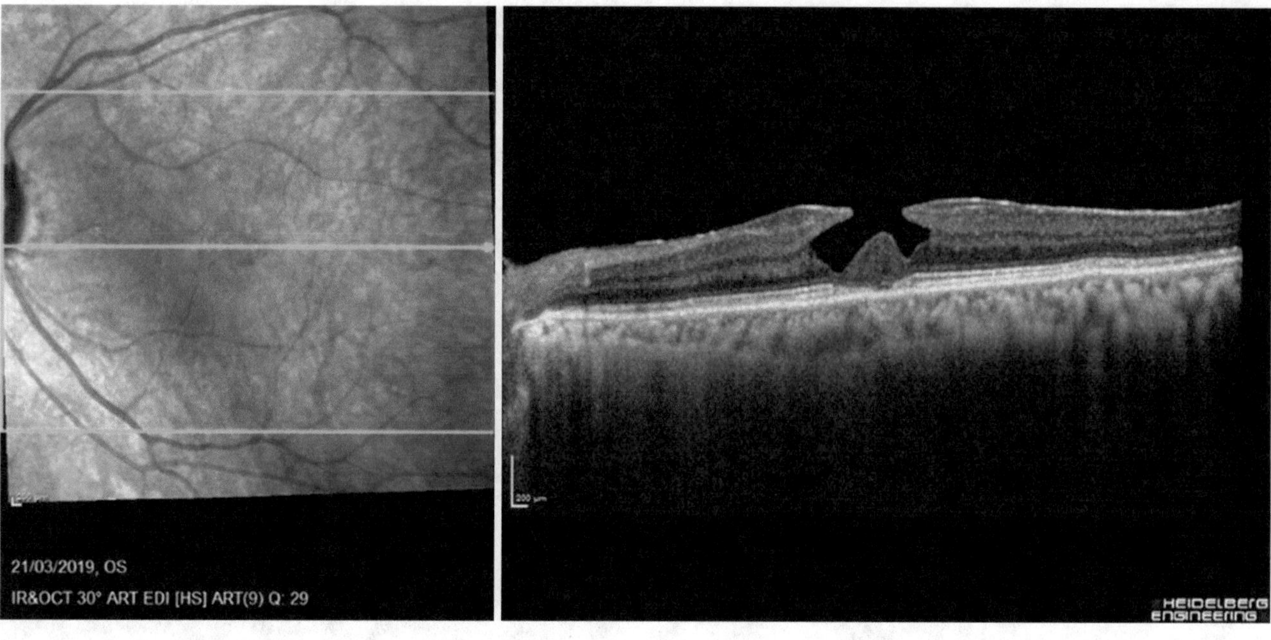

Fig. 11.94 An omega shaped MH with gelatinous ERM

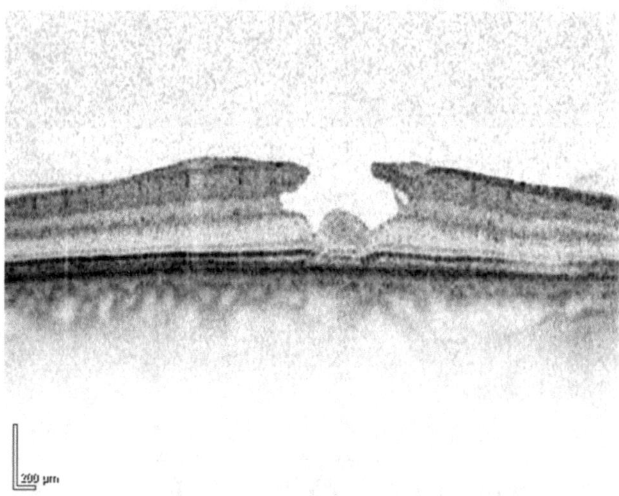

Fig. 11.95 Lamellar macular holes can be associated with ERM

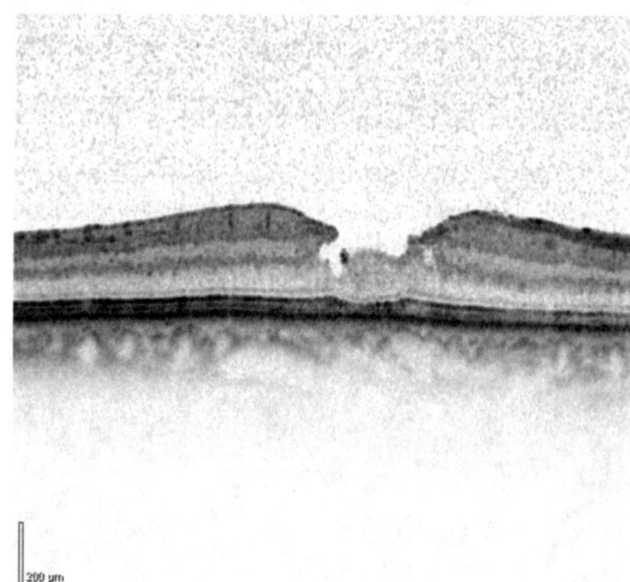

Fig. 11.96 Removal of the ERM causes resolution of the hole (5 days post op in this case)

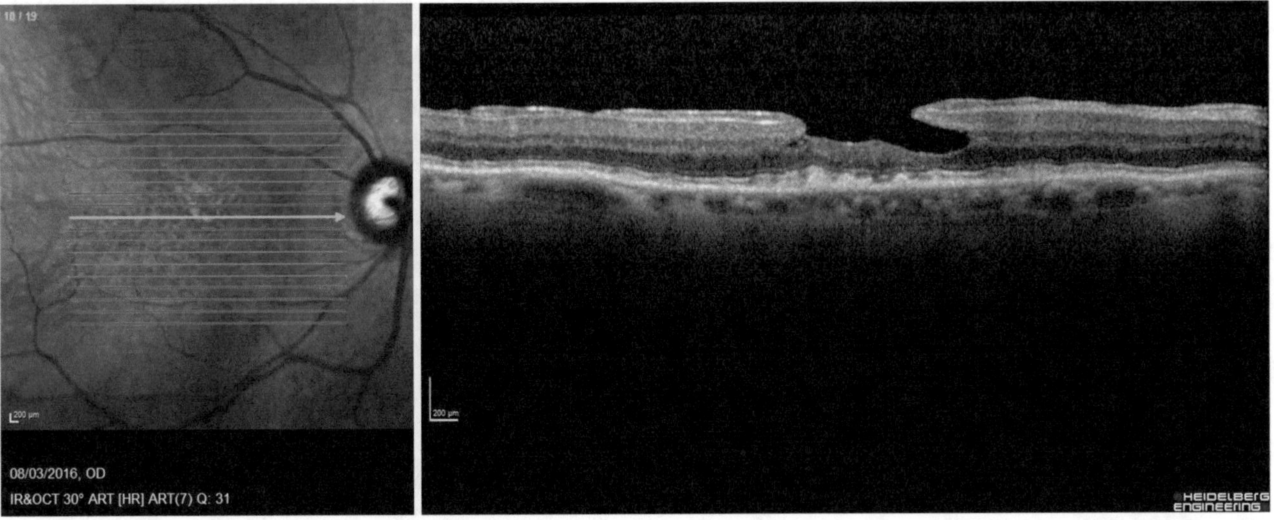

Fig. 11.97 A lamellar hole with a typical accompanying gelatinous ERM

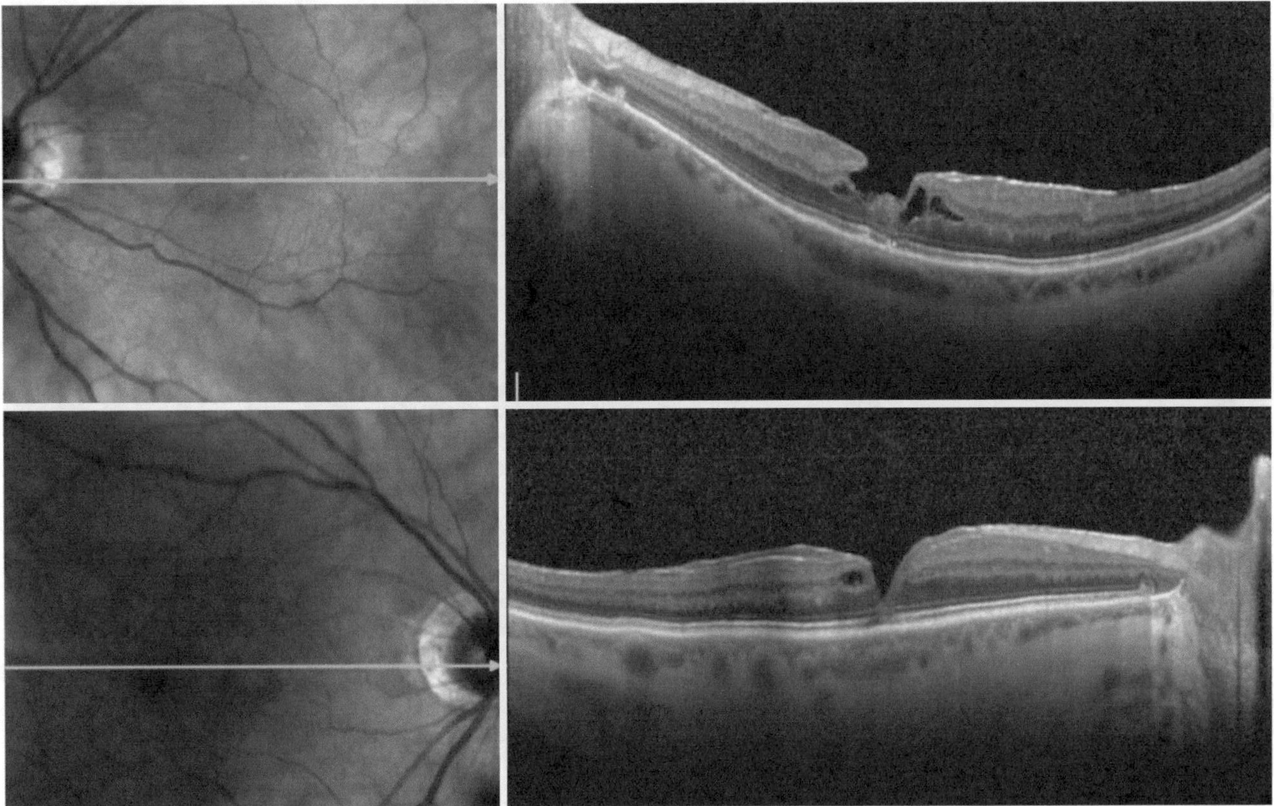

Fig. 11.98 A low density epiretinal membrane showing a double layer is associated with lamellar holes. During surgery these can be removed but the consistency is different to routine ERM. Often it feels as if you are removing tissue with similar characteristics to retina itself

surgical outcomes is not available although visual improvement has been shown the influence of removal of the ERM on visual recovery needs to be determined [106]. PPV has been combined with ERM peel and ILM peel in these eyes. Left alone the patient often experiences further slow deterioration of vision over years to the 20/120. Lamellar holes have also been described after chronic cystoid macular oedema in diabetes or after cataract surgery and associated with idiopathic retinal telangiectasia [2, 102–104].

Micro Plasmin

Enzymatic vitreolysis showed promise as a method of inducing vitreal separation in the MIVI trials with a role for treating grade 0, grade 1, and grade 2 macular holes. 125 microg micro plasmin can be injected intravitreally to induce separation in up to 44% of patients with vitreomacular adhesion [107]. Real life use of the agent has not borne out the early optimism with increased side effects such as retinal detachment, severe visual loss (usually temporary), and ERG changes.

Summary

PPV is established as the treatment of macular hole. Variations in technique exist relating to intraocular dyes, duration of gas tamponade, and use of posturing, but success rates are high if the operation is performed early in the disease process.

References

1. McCannel CA, Ensminger JL, Diehl NN, Hodge DN. Population-based incidence of macular holes. Ophthalmology. 2009;116(7):1366–9. https://doi.org/10.1016/j.ophtha.2009.01.052.
2. Lewis ML, Cohen SM, Smiddy WE, Gass JD. Bilaterality of idiopathic macular holes. Graefes Arch Clin Exp Ophthalmol. 1996;234(4):241–5.
3. Fajgenbaum MAP, Wong RS, Laidlaw DAH, Williamson TH. Vitreoretinal surgery on the fellow eye: a retrospective analysis of 18 years of surgical data from a tertiary center in England. Indian J Ophthalmol. 2018;66(5):681–6. https://doi.org/10.4103/ijo.IJO_1176_17.
4. Watzke RC, Allen L. Subjective slitbeam sign for macular disease. Am J Ophthalmol. 1969;68(3):449–53.
5. Tanner V, Williamson TH. Watzke-Allen slit beam test in macular holes confirmed by optical coherence tomography. Arch Ophthalmol. 2000;118(8):1059–63.
6. Ezra E, Fåriss RN, Possin DE, Aylward WG, Gregor ZJ, Luthert PJ, et al. Immunocytochemical characterization of macular hole opercula. Arch Ophthalmol. 2001;119(2):223–31.
7. Ezra E, Munro PM, Charteris DG, Aylward WG, Luthert PJ, Gregor ZJ. Macular hole opercula. Ultrastructural features and clinicopathological correlation. Arch Ophthalmol. 1997;115(11):1381–7.
8. Haouchine B, Massin P, Gaudric A. Foveal pseudocyst as the first step in macular hole formation: a prospective study by optical coherence tomography. Ophthalmology. 2001;108(1):15–22.
9. Gass JD. Idiopathic senile macular hole. Its early stages and pathogenesis. Arch Ophthalmol. 1988;106(5):629–39.
10. Gass JD. Reappraisal of biomicroscopic classification of stages of development of a macular hole. Am J Ophthalmol. 1995;119(6):752–9.
11. Johnson RN, Gass JD. Idiopathic macular holes. Observations, stages of formation, and implications for surgical intervention. Ophthalmology. 1988;95(7):917–24.
12. de BS. Vitrectomy for prevention of macular holes. Results of a randomized multicenter clinical trial. Vitrectomy for prevention of macular hole study group. Ophthalmology. 1994;101(6):1055–1059.
13. Kokame GT. de BS. Visual acuity as a prognostic indicator in stage I macular holes. The vitrectomy for prevention of macular hole study group. Am J Ophthalmol. 1995;120(1):112–4.
14. Kim JW, Freeman WR, El-Haig W, Maguire AM, Arevalo JF, Azen SP. Baseline characteristics, natural history, and risk factors to progression in eyes with stage 2 macular holes. Results from a prospective randomized clinical trial. Vitrectomy for macular hole study group. Ophthalmology. 1995;102(12):1818–28.
15. Casuso LA, Scott IU, Flynn HW Jr, Gass JD, Smiddy WE, Lewis ML, et al. Long-term follow-up of unoperated macular holes. Ophthalmology. 2001;108(6):1150–5.
16. Ezra E, Gregor ZJ. Surgery for idiopathic full-thickness macular hole: two-year results of a randomized clinical trial comparing natural history, vitrectomy, and vitrectomy plus autologous serum: Morfields macular hole study group RAeport no. 1. Arch Ophthalmol. 2004;122(2):224–36.
17. Freeman WR, Azen SP, Kim JW, El-Haig W, Mishell DR, Bailey I. Vitrectomy for the treatment of full-thickness stage 3 or 4 macular holes. Results of a multicentered randomized clinical trial. The vitrectomy for treatment of macular hole study group. Arch Ophthalmol. 1997;115(1):11–21.
18. Hee MR, Izatt JA, Swanson EA, Huang D, Schuman JS, Lin CP, et al. Optical coherence tomography of the human retina. Arch Ophthalmol. 1995;113(3):325–32.
19. Tanner V, Chauhan DS, Jackson TL, Williamson TH. Optical coherence tomography of the vitreoretinal interface in macular hole formation. Br J Ophthalmol. 2001;85(9):1092–7.
20. Chauhan DS, Antcliff RJ, Rai PA, Williamson TH, Marshall J. Papillofoveal traction in macular hole formation: the role of optical coherence tomography. Arch Ophthalmol. 2000;118(1):32–8.
21. Ito Y, Terasaki H, Suzuki T, Kojima T, Mori M, Ishikawa K, et al. Mapping posterior vitreous detachment by optical coherence tomography in eyes with idiopathic macular hole. Am J Ophthalmol. 2003;135(3):351–5.
22. Smiddy WE, Michels RG, de BS, de la CZ, Green WR. Histopathology of tissue removed during vitrectomy for impending idiopathic macular holes. Am J Ophthalmol. 1989;108(4):360–4.
23. Chan A, Duker JS, Schuman JS, Fujimoto JG. Stage 0 macular holes: observations by optical coherence tomography. Ophthalmology. 2004;111(11):2027–32.
24. Kolb H, Nelson RF, Ahnelt PK, Ortuño-Lizarán I, Cuenca N. The Architecture of the Human Fovea. Webvision: The Organization of the Retina and Visual System [Internet]. University of Utah Health Sciences Center; 2020.
25. Kelly NE, Wendel RT. Vitreous surgery for idiopathic macular holes. Results of a pilot study. Arch Ophthalmol. 1991;109(5):654–9.
26. Tognetto D, Grandin R, Sanguinetti G, Minutola D, Di Nicola M, Di Mascio R, et al. Internal limiting membrane removal during macular hole surgery: results of a multicenter retrospective study.

Ophthalmology. 2006;113(8):1401–10. https://doi.org/10.1016/j.ophtha.2006.02.061.

27. Da Mata AP, Burk SE, Riemann CD, Rosa RH Jr, Snyder ME, Petersen MR, et al. Indocyanine green-assisted peeling of the retinal internal limiting membrane during vitrectomy surgery for macular hole repair. Ophthalmology. 2001;108(7):1187–92.
28. Sheidow TG, Blinder KJ, Holekamp N, Joseph D, Shah G, Grand MG, et al. Outcome results in macular hole surgery: an evaluation of internal limiting membrane peeling with and without indocyanine green. Ophthalmology. 2003;110(9):1697–701.
29. Engelbrecht NE, Freeman J, Sternberg P Jr, Aaberg TM Sr, Aaberg TM Jr, Martin DF, et al. Retinal pigment epithelial changes after macular hole surgery with indocyanine green-assisted internal limiting membrane peeling. Am J Ophthalmol. 2002;133(1):89–94.
30. Ho JD, Tsai RJ, Chen SN, Chen HC. Cytotoxicity of indocyanine green on retinal pigment epithelium: implications for macular hole surgery. Arch Ophthalmol. 2003;121(10):1423–9.
31. Ho JD, Tsai RJ, Chen SN, Chen HC. Removal of sodium from the solvent reduces retinal pigment epithelium toxicity caused by indocyanine green: implications for macular hole surgery. Br J Ophthalmol. 2004;88(4):556–9.
32. Ando F, Sasano K, Ohba N, Hirose H, Yasui O. Anatomic and visual outcomes after indocyanine green-assisted peeling of the retinal internal limiting membrane in idiopathic macular hole surgery. Am J Ophthalmol. 2004;137(4):609–14.
33. Gass CA, Haritoglou C, Schaumberger M, Kampik A. Functional outcome of macular hole surgery with and without indocyanine green-assisted peeling of the internal limiting membrane. Graefes Arch Clin Exp Ophthalmol. 2003;241(9):716–20.
34. Weinberger AW, Kirchhof B, Mazinani BE, Schrage NF. Persistent indocyanine green (ICG) fluorescence 6 weeks after intraocular ICG administration for macular hole surgery. Graefes Arch Clin Exp Ophthalmol. 2001;239(5):388–90.
35. Ciardella AP, Schiff W, Barile G, Vidne O, Sparrow J, Langton K, et al. Persistent indocyanine green fluorescence after vitrectomy for macular hole. Am J Ophthalmol. 2003;136(1):174–7.
36. Haritoglou C, Gandorfer A, Gass CA, Schaumberger M, Ulbig MW, Kampik A. Indocyanine green-assisted peeling of the internal limiting membrane in macular hole surgery affects visual outcome: a clinicopathologic correlation. Am J Ophthalmol. 2002;134(6):836–41.
37. Horio N, Horiguchi M. Effect on visual outcome after macular hole surgery when staining the internal limiting membrane with indocyanine green dye. Arch Ophthalmol. 2004;122(7):992–6.
38. Sippy BD, Engelbrecht NE, Hubbard GB, Moriarty SE, Jiang S, Aaberg TM Jr, et al. Indocyanine green effect on cultured human retinal pigment epithelial cells: implication for macular hole surgery. Am J Ophthalmol. 2001;132(3):433–5.
39. Hosoi A, Arao Y, Kawada H. Transverse crack growth behavior considering free-edge effect in quasi-isotropic CFRP laminates under high-cycle fatigue loading. Compos Sci Technol. 2009;69(9):1388–93.
40. Goldbaum MH, McCuen BW, Hanneken AM, Burgess SK, Chen HH. Silicone oil tamponade to seal macular holes without position restrictions. Ophthalmology. 1998;105(11):2140–7.
41. Lee KL, Dean S, Guest S. A comparison of outcomes after indocyanine green and trypan blue assisted internal limiting membrane peeling during macular hole surgery. Br J Ophthalmol. 2005;89(4):420–4.
42. Banker AS, Freeman WR, Azen SP, Lai MY. A multicentered clinical study of serum as adjuvant therapy for surgical treatment of macular holes. Vitrectomy for macular hole study group. Arch Ophthalmol. 1999;117(11):1499–502.
43. Wachtlin J, Jandeck C, Potthofer S, Kellner U, Foerster MH. Long-term results following pars plana vitrectomy with platelet concentrate in pediatric patients with traumatic macular hole. Am J Ophthalmol. 2003;136(1):197–9.
44. Lansing MB, Glaser BM, Liss H, Hanham A, Thompson JT, Sjaarda RN, et al. The effect of pars plana vitrectomy and transforming growth factor-beta 2 without epiretinal membrane peeling on full-thickness macular holes. Ophthalmology. 1993;100(6):868–71.
45. Rosa RH Jr, Glaser BM, de la CZ, Green WR. Clinicopathologic correlation of an untreated macular hole and a macular hole treated by vitrectomy, transforming growth factor-beta 2, and gas tamponade. Am J Ophthalmol. 1996;122(6):853–63.
46. Rossi T, Gelso A, Costagliola C, Trillo C, Costa A, Gesualdo C, et al. Macular hole closure patterns associated with different internal limiting membrane flap techniques. Graefes Arch Clin Exp Ophthalmol. 2017;255(6):1073–8. https://doi.org/10.1007/s00417-017-3598-9.
47. Michalewska Z, Michalewski J, Adelman RA, Nawrocki J. Inverted internal limiting membrane flap technique for large macular holes. Ophthalmology. 2010;117(10):2018–25. https://doi.org/10.1016/j.ophtha.2010.02.011.
48. Rizzo S, Tartaro R, Barca F, Caporossi T, Bacherini D, Giansanti F. Internal limiting membrane peeling versus inverted flap technique for treatment of full-thickness macular holes: a comparative study in a large series of patients. Retina. 2018;38(Suppl 1):S73–s8. https://doi.org/10.1097/iae.0000000000001985.
49. Inoue M, Itoh Y, Koto T, Kurimori HY, Hirakata A. Intraoperative OCT findings may predict postoperative visual outcome in eyes with idiopathic macular hole. Ophthalmol Retina. 2019;3(11):962–70. https://doi.org/10.1016/j.oret.2019.05.022.
50. Iovino C, Caminiti G, Miccoli M, Nasini F, Casini G, Peiretti E. Comparison of inverted flap and subretinal aspiration technique in full-thickness macular hole surgery: a randomized controlled study. Eur J Ophthalmol. 2018;28(3):324–8. https://doi.org/10.5301/ejo.5001040.
51. Gaudric A, Massin P, Paques M, Santiago PY, Guez JE, Le Gargasson JF, et al. Autologous platelet concentrate for the treatment of full-thickness macular holes. Graefes Arch Clin Exp Ophthalmol. 1995;233(9):549–54.
52. Wong R, Howard C, Orobona GD. Retina expansion technique for macular hole apposition report 2: efficacy, closure rate, and risks of a macular detachment technique to close large full-thickness macular holes. Retina. 2018;38(4):660–3. https://doi.org/10.1097/IAE.0000000000001705.
53. Grewal DS, Charles S, Parolini B, Kadonosono K, Mahmoud TH. Autologous retinal transplant for refractory macular holes: multicenter international collaborative study group. Ophthalmology. 2019;126(10):1399–408. https://doi.org/10.1016/j.ophtha.2019.01.027.
54. Schurmans A, Van Calster J, Stalmans P. Macular hole surgery with inner limiting membrane peeling, Endodrainage, and heavy silicone oil tamponade. Am J Ophthalmol. 2008; https://doi.org/10.1016/j.ajo.2008.09.003.
55. Mori K, Saito S, Gehlbach PL, Yoneya S. Treatment of stage 2 macular hole by intravitreous injection of expansile gas and induction of posterior vitreous detachment. Ophthalmology. 2007;114(1):127–33. https://doi.org/10.1016/j.ophtha.2006.07.001.
56. Eckardt C, Eckert T, Eckardt U, Porkert U, Gesser C. Macular hole surgery with air tamponade and optical coherence tomography-based duration of face-down positioning. Retina. 2008;28(8):1087–96. https://doi.org/10.1097/IAE.0b013e318185fb5f.
57. Thompson JT, Glaser BM, Sjaarda RN, Murphy RP, Hanham A. Effects of intraocular bubble duration in the treatment of macular holes by vitrectomy and transforming growth factor-beta 2. Ophthalmology. 1994;101(7):1195–200.
58. Guillaubey A, Malvitte L, Lafontaine PO, Jay N, Hubert I, Bron A, et al. Comparison of face-down and seated position after idio-

pathic macular hole surgery: a randomized clinical trial. Am J Ophthalmol. 2008;146(1):128–34. https://doi.org/10.1016/j.ajo.2008.02.029.

59. Xia S, Zhao XY, Wang EQ, Chen YX. Comparison of face-down posturing with nonsupine posturing after macular hole surgery: a meta-analysis. BMC Ophthalmol. 2019;19(1):34. https://doi.org/10.1186/s12886-019-1047-8.
60. Banker AS, Freeman WR, Kim JW, Munguia D, Azen SP. Vision-threatening complications of surgery for full-thickness macular holes. Vitrectomy for macular hole study group. Ophthalmology. 1997;104(9):1442–52.
61. Chang TS, McGill E, Hay DA, Ross WH, Maberley AL, Sibley LM, et al. Prophylactic scleral buckle for prevention of retinal detachment following vitrectomy for macular hole. Br J Ophthalmol. 1999;83(8):944–8.
62. Cheng L, Azen SP, El-Bradey MH, Scholz BM, Chaidhawangul S, Toyoguchi M, et al. Duration of vitrectomy and postoperative cataract in the vitrectomy for macular hole study. Am J Ophthalmol. 2001;132(6):881–7.
63. Park SS, Marcus DM, Duker JS, Pesavento RD, Topping TM, Frederick AR Jr, et al. Posterior segment complications after vitrectomy for macular hole. Ophthalmology. 1995;102(5):775–81.
64. Thompson JT, Glaser BM, Sjaarda RN, Murphy RP. Progression of nuclear sclerosis and long-term visual results of vitrectomy with transforming growth factor beta-2 for macular holes. Am J Ophthalmol. 1995;119(1):48–54.
65. Lahey JM, Francis RR, Fong DS, Kearney JJ, Tanaka S. Combining phacoemulsification with vitrectomy for treatment of macular holes. Br J Ophthalmol. 2002;86(8):876–8.
66. Chung SE, Kim KH, Kang SW. Retinal breaks associated with the induction of posterior vitreous detachment. Am J Ophthalmol. 2009;147(6):1012–6. https://doi.org/10.1016/j.ajo.2009.01.013.
67. Guillaubey A, Malvitte L, Lafontaine PO, Hubert I, Bron A, Berrod JP, et al. Incidence of retinal detachment after macular surgery: a retrospective study of 634 cases. Br J Ophthalmol. 2007;91(10):1327–30. https://doi.org/10.1136/bjo.2007.115162.
68. Vaziri K, Schwartz SG, Kishor KS, Fortun JA, Moshfeghi AA, Smiddy WE, et al. Rates of reoperation and retinal detachment after macular hole surgery. Ophthalmology. 2016;123(1):26–31. https://doi.org/10.1016/j.ophtha.2015.09.015.
69. Bhatnagar P, Kaiser PK, Smith SD, Meisler DM, Lewis H, Sears JE. Reopening of previously closed macular holes after cataract extraction. Am J Ophthalmol. 2007;144(2):252–9. https://doi.org/10.1016/j.ajo.2007.04.041.
70. Rubinstein A, Bates R, Benjamin L, Shaikh A. Iatrogenic eccentric full thickness macular holes following vitrectomy with ILM peeling for idiopathic macular holes. Eye. 2004.
71. Ezra E, Arden GB, Riordan-Eva P, Aylward GW, Gregor ZJ. Visual field loss following vitrectomy for stage 2 and 3 macular holes. Br J Ophthalmol. 1996;80(6):519–25.
72. Paques M, Massin P, Santiago PY, Spielmann AC, Gaudric A. Visual field loss after vitrectomy for full-thickness macular holes. Am J Ophthalmol. 1997;124(1):88–94.
73. Haritoglou C, Ehrt O, Gass CA, Kristin N, Kampik A. Paracentral scotomata: a new finding after vitrectomy for idiopathic macular hole. Br J Ophthalmol. 2001;85(2):231–3.
74. Welch JC. Dehydration injury as a possible cause of visual field defect after pars plana vitrectomy for macular hole. Am J Ophthalmol. 1997;124(5):698–9.
75. Yonemura N, Hirata A, Hasumura T, Negi A. Fundus changes corresponding to visual field defects after vitrectomy for macular hole. Ophthalmology. 2001;108(9):1638–43.
76. Kanda S, Uemura A, Yamashita T, Kita H, Yamakiri K, Sakamoto T. Visual field defects after intravitreous administration of indocyanine green in macular hole surgery. Arch Ophthalmol. 2004;122(10):1447–51.
77. Da Mata AP, Burk SE, Foster RE, Riemann CD, Petersen MR, Nehemy MB, et al. Long-term follow-up of indocyanine green-assisted peeling of the retinal internal limiting membrane during vitrectomy surgery for idiopathic macular hole repair. Ophthalmology. 2004;111(12):2246–53.
78. Dori D, Thoelen AM, Akalp F, Bernasconi PP, Messmer EP. Anatomic and functional results of vitrectomy and long-term intraocular tamponade for stage 2 macular holes. Retina. 2003;23(1):57–63.
79. Rodrigues IA, Lee EJ, Williamson TH. Measurement of retinal displacement and Metamorphopsia after Epiretinal membrane or macular hole surgery. Retina. 2016;36(4):695–702. https://doi.org/10.1097/IAE.0000000000000768.
80. Smiddy WE, Michels RG, Glaser BM, de BS. Vitrectomy for impending idiopathic macular holes. Am J Ophthalmol. 1988;105(4):371–6.
81. Ruby AJ, Williams DF, Grand MG, Thomas MA, Meredith TA, Boniuk I, et al. Pars plana vitrectomy for treatment of stage 2 macular holes. Arch Ophthalmol. 1994;112(3):359–64.
82. Ip MS, Baker BJ, Duker JS, Reichel E, Baumal CR, Gangnon R, et al. Anatomical outcomes of surgery for idiopathic macular hole as determined by optical coherence tomography. Arch Ophthalmol. 2002;120(1):29–35.
83. Stec LA, Ross RD, Williams GA, Trese MT, Margherio RR, Cox MS Jr. Vitrectomy for chronic macular holes. Retina. 2004;24(3):341–7.
84. Jaycock PD, Bunce C, Xing W, Thomas D, Poon W, Gazzard G, et al. Outcomes of macular hole surgery: implications for surgical management and clinical governance. Eye. 2004;
85. Villate N, Lee JE, Venkatraman A, Smiddy WE. Photoreceptor layer features in eyes with closed macular holes: optical coherence tomography findings and correlation with visual outcomes. Am J Ophthalmol. 2005;139(2):280–9.
86. Johnson RN, McDonald HR, Lewis H, Grand MG, Murray TG, Mieler WF, et al. Traumatic macular hole: observations, pathogenesis, and results of vitrectomy surgery. Ophthalmology. 2001;108(5):853–7.
87. Gupta B, Laidlaw DA, Williamson TH, Shah SP, Wong R, Wren S. Predicting visual success in macular hole surgery. Br J Ophthalmol. 2009;93(11):1488–91. https://doi.org/10.1136/bjo.2008.153189.
88. Elhusseiny AM, Schwartz SG, Flynn HW Jr, Smiddy WE. Long-term outcomes after macular hole surgery. Ophthalmol Retina. 2019; https://doi.org/10.1016/j.oret.2019.09.015.
89. Chandra A, Lai M, Mitry D, Banerjee PJ, Flayeh H, Negretti G, et al. Ethnic variation in primary idiopathic macular hole surgery. Eye (Lond). 2017;31(5):708–12. https://doi.org/10.1038/eye.2016.296.
90. Johnson RN, McDonald HR, Schatz H, Ai E. Outpatient postoperative fluid-gas exchange after early failed vitrectomy surgery for macular hole. Ophthalmology. 1997;104(12):2009–13.
91. Valldeperas X, Wong D. Is it worth reoperating on macular holes? Ophthalmology. 2008;115(1):158–63. https://doi.org/10.1016/j.ophtha.2007.01.039.
92. Mittleman D, Green WR, Michels RG, de la CZ. Clinicopathologic correlation of an eye after surgical removal of an epiretinal membrane. Retina. 1989;9(2):143–7.
93. Hillenkamp J, Kraus J, Framme C, Jackson TL, Roider J, Gabel VP, et al. Retreatment of full-thickness macular hole: predictive value of optical coherence tomography. Br J Ophthalmol. 2007;91(11):1445–9. https://doi.org/10.1136/bjo.2007.115642.
94. Yek JTO, Hunyor AP, Campbell WG, McAllister IL, Essex RW. Australian, et al. outcomes of eyes with failed primary surgery for idiopathic macular hole. Ophthalmol Retina. 2018;2(8):757–64. https://doi.org/10.1016/j.oret.2017.10.012.
95. Ismail R, Tanner V, Williamson TH. Optical coherence tomography imaging of severe commotio retinae and associated macular hole. Br J Ophthalmol. 2002;86(4):473–4.

96. Yamashita T, Uemara A, Uchino E, Doi N, Ohba N. Spontaneous closure of traumatic macular hole. Am J Ophthalmol. 2002;133(2):230–5.
97. Chen YP, Chen TL, Chao AN, Wu WC, Lai CC. Surgical management of traumatic macular hole-related retinal detachment. Am J Ophthalmol. 2005;140(2):331–3.
98. Sakaguchi H, Ohji M, Kubota A, Otori Y, Hayashi A, Kusaka S, et al. Amsler grid examination and optical coherence tomography of a macular hole caused by accidental Nd:YAG laser injury. Am J Ophthalmol. 2000;130(3):355–6.
99. Dell'omo R, Virgili G, Rizzo S, De Turris S, Coclite G, Giorgio D, et al. Role of lamellar hole-associated Epiretinal proliferation in lamellar macular holes. Am J Ophthalmol. 2017;175:16–29. https://doi.org/10.1016/j.ajo.2016.11.007.
100. Spaide RF. Closure of an outer lamellar macular hole by vitrectomy: hypothesis for one mechanism of macular hole formation. Retina. 2000;20(6):587–90.
101. Haouchine B, Massin P, Tadayoni R, Erginay A, Gaudric A. Diagnosis of macular pseudoholes and lamellar macular holes by optical coherence tomography. Am J Ophthalmol. 2004;138(5):732–9. https://doi.org/10.1016/j.ajo.2004.06.088.
102. Patel B, Duvall J, Tullo AB. Lamellar macular hole associated with idiopathic juxtafoveolar telangiectasia. Br J Ophthalmol. 1988;72(7):550–1.
103. Unoki N, Nishijima K, Kita M, Oh H, Sakamoto A, Kameda T, et al. Lamellar macular hole formation in patients with diabetic cystoid macular edema. Retina. 2009; https://doi.org/10.1097/IAE.0b013e3181a4d2d9.
104. Gass JD. Lamellar macular hole: a complication of cystoid macular edema after cataract extraction. Arch Ophthalmol. 1976;94(5):793–800.
105. Hirakawa M, Uemura A, Nakano T, Sakamoto T. Pars plana vitrectomy with gas tamponade for lamellar macular holes. Am J Ophthalmol. 2005;140(6):1154–5. https://doi.org/10.1016/j.ajo.2005.07.022.
106. Garretson BR, Pollack JS, Ruby AJ, Drenser KA, Williams GA, Sarrafizadeh R. Vitrectomy for a symptomatic lamellar macular hole. Ophthalmology. 2008;115(5):884–6 e1. https://doi.org/10.1016/j.ophtha.2007.06.029.
107. de Smet MD, Gandorfer A, Stalmans P, Veckeneer M, Feron E, Pakola S, et al. Microplasmin intravitreal administration in patients with vitreomacular traction scheduled for vitrectomy: the MIVI I trial. Ophthalmology. 2009;116(7):1349–55 e1-2. https://doi.org/10.1016/j.ophtha.2009.03.051.

Macular Pucker and Vitreomacular Traction

12

Contents

Clinical Features (Figs. 12.1 and 12.2)

(Fig. 12.3) Idiopathic epiretinal membrane formation in the macula is also stimulated by posterior vitreous detachment giving the clinical entities of macular pucker or cellophane maculopathy. It is postulated that the PVD damages the internal limiting membrane stimulating microglial cells proliferation and fibrosis [1, 2]. Some ERMs have the vitreous attached, however. Myofibroblastic activity may be present [3] and may be commoner in younger patients [4]. The incidence of ERMs of any sort in the macula is described as 29% over the age of 45 years and increased in the Chinese population [5, 6]. ERM can appear in proliferative vitreoretinopathy from RRD in which case the cell of origin is likely to be the RPE cell.

(Figs. 12.4, 12.5, 12.6, and 12.7) The patient notices a reduction of vision accompanied by distortion of images and macropsia (increased image size) as the membrane pulls the retina centrally. The membrane can be a reflective sheet (cellophane) or as a thick opaque membrane which is drawing the retinal arcades together. A pseudohole in the central membrane can sometimes be detected and distinguished from a hole in the retina (macular hole) by a negative Watzke Allen test [7, 8] and by OCT. Vitreomacular traction is present when the vitreous separation is incomplete and an area of attachment of the epiretinal membrane to the posterior hyaloid membrane remains. The membrane is associated with the presence of mild CMO on FFA in the early stages progressing to severe retinal thickening and large cystoid spaces.

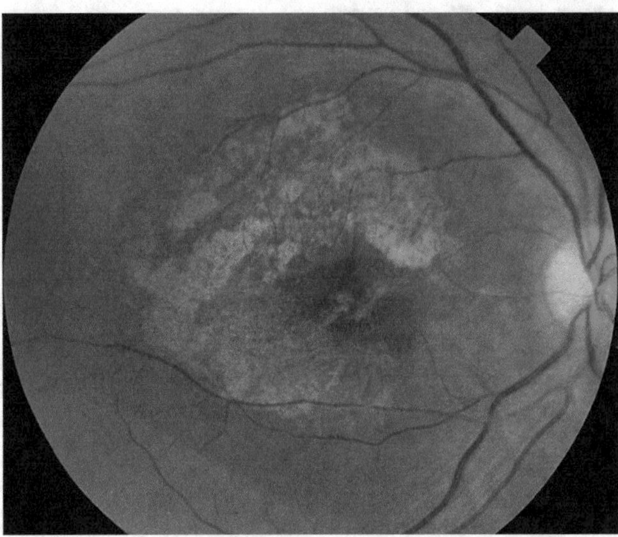

Fig. 12.1 A diffuse membrane can be described as cellophane maculopathy. This is part of the spectrum of epiretinal membrane formation from posterior vitreous detachment in middle-aged and elderly individuals

T. H. Williamson, *Vitreoretinal Surgery*, https://doi.org/10.1007/978-3-030-68769-4_12

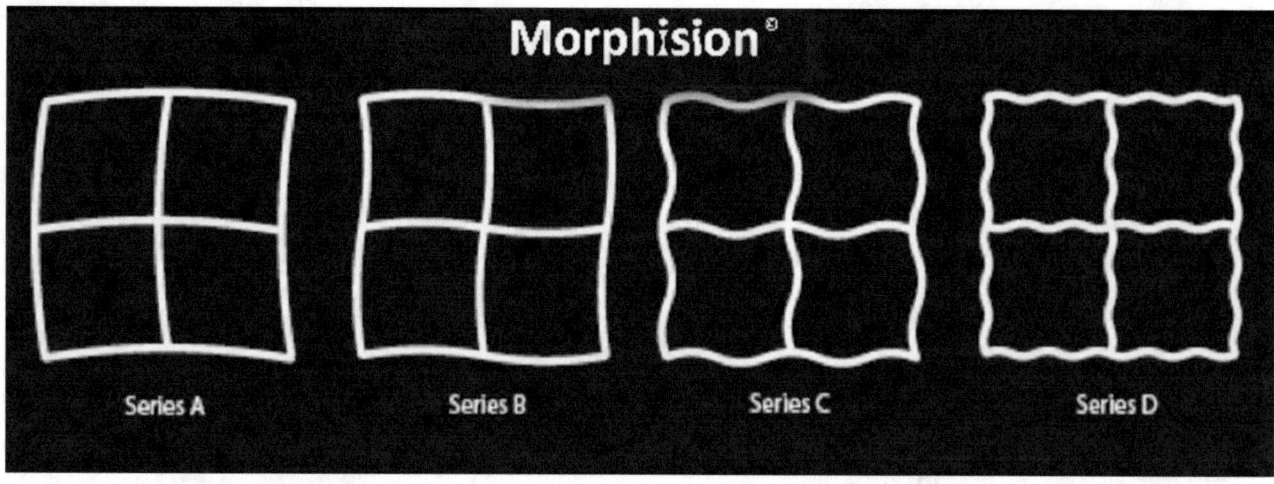

Fig. 12.2 Use Morphision which uses sinusoidal patterns to measure and monitor distortion in these patients

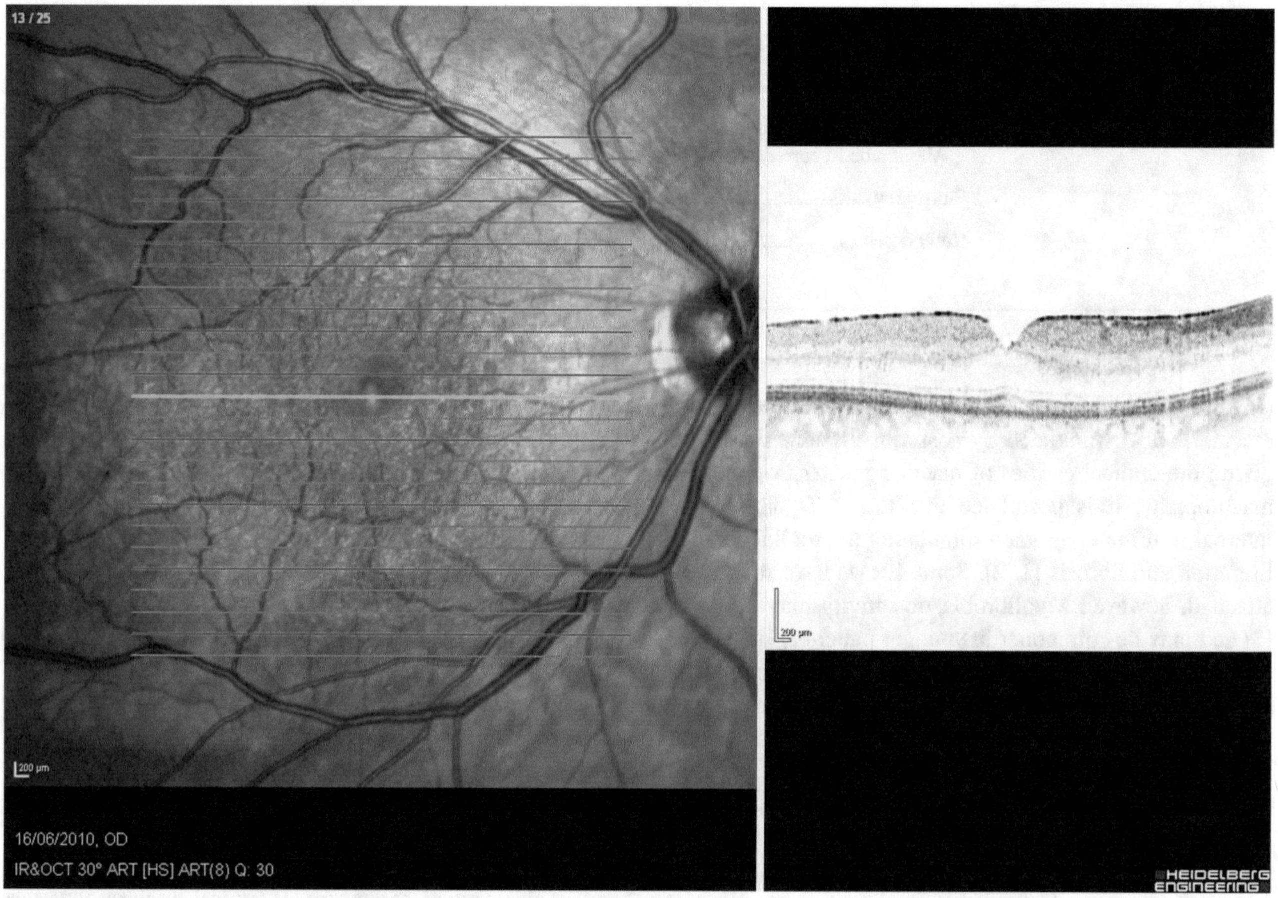

Fig. 12.3 Cellophane maculopathy can be seen coincidentally in many patients without symptoms

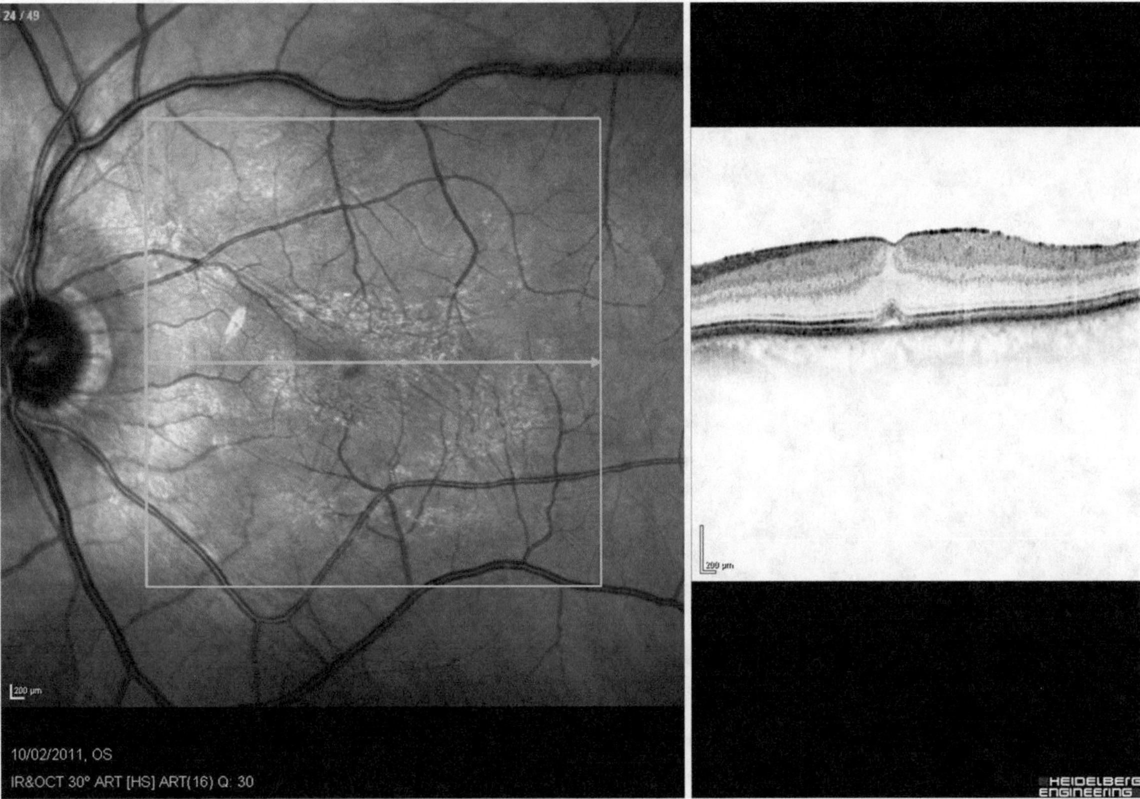

Fig. 12.4 Cellophane starts to distort the fovea and flatten the foveal dip

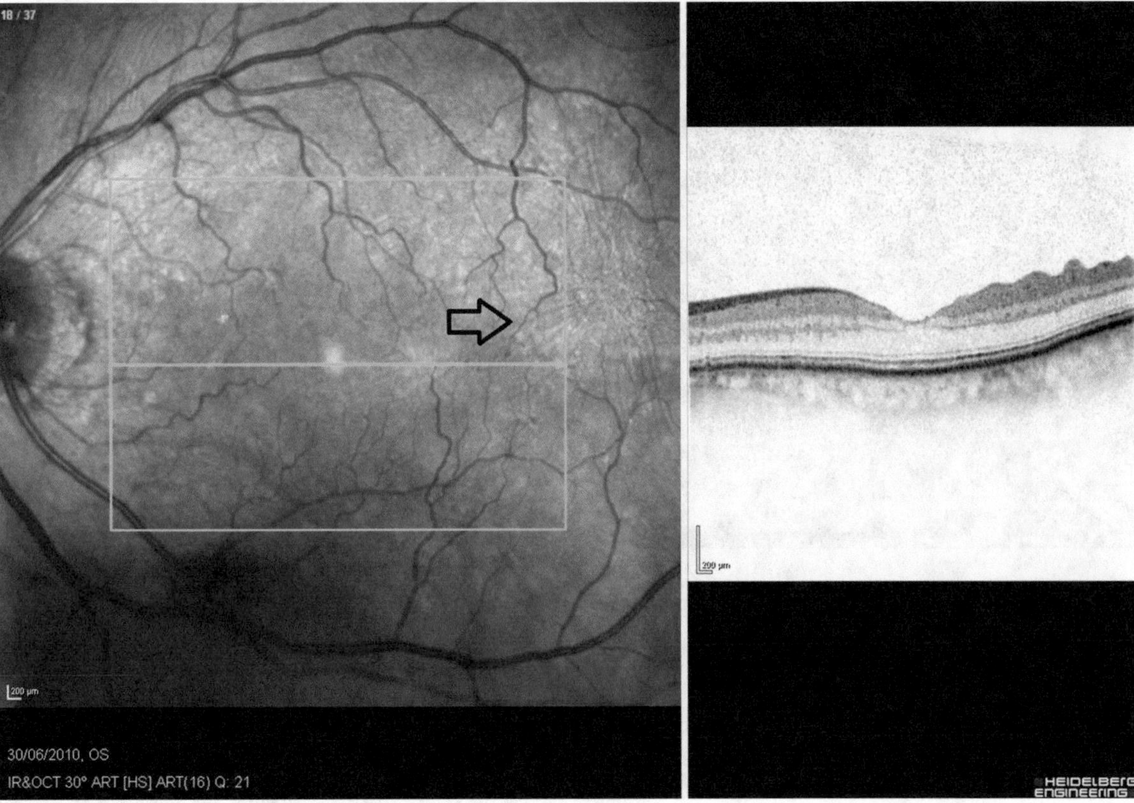

Fig. 12.5 Although most ERM are stable after presentation some can progress with reduction in vision. This ERM has gradually grown across the macula over 1 year

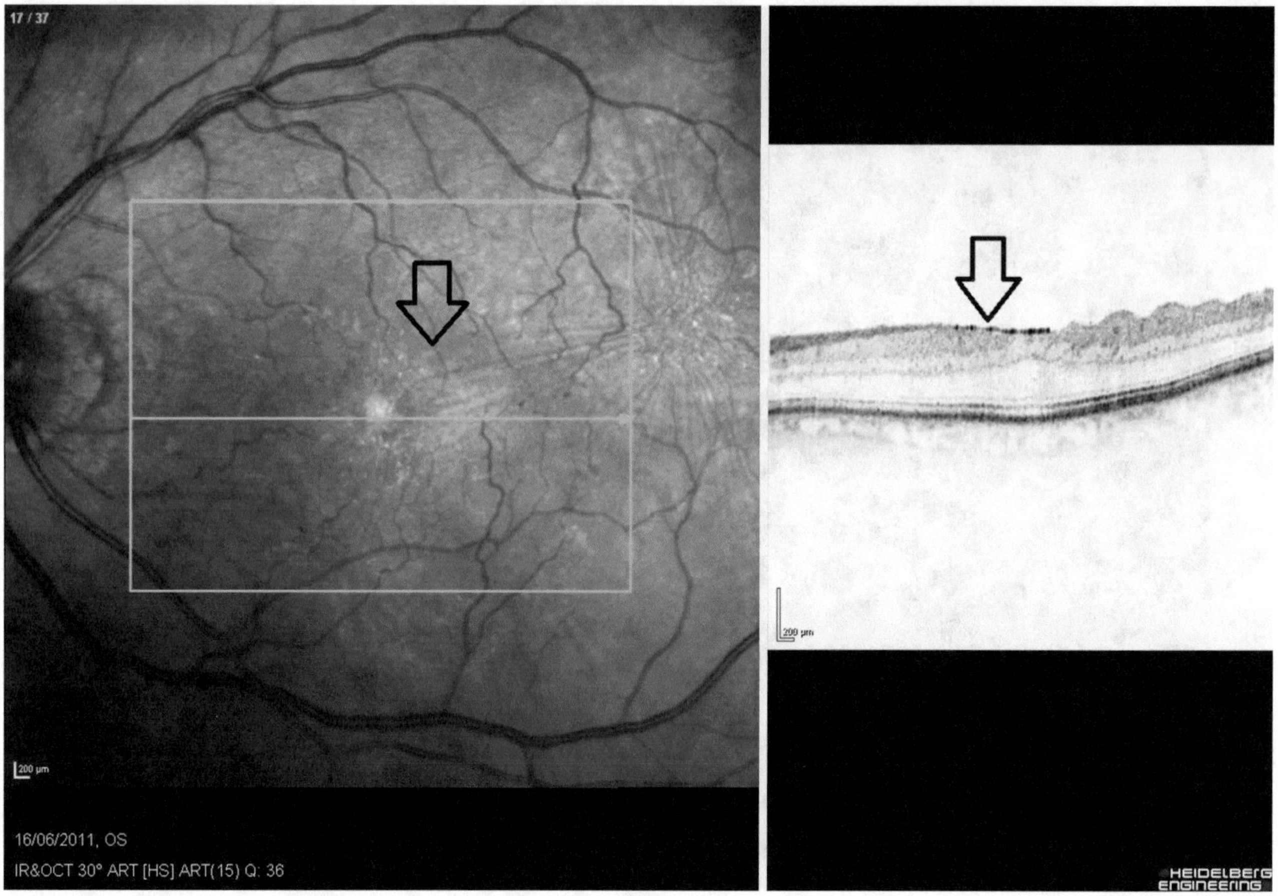

Fig. 12.6 The ERM has grown over the fovea

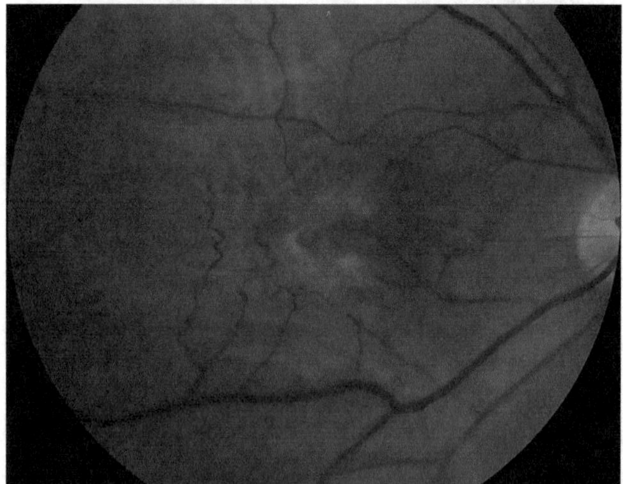

Fig. 12.7 A severe ERM causing pucker of the macula

The risk of surgery in 10 years to the other eye is 9% [9] (Figs. 12.8, 12.9, 12.10, 12.11, and 12.12).

Young patients often have an attached PHM and more often show spontaneous separation of the ERM because the vitreous separates taking the ERM with it [10]. A PVD is not always seen [11] (Figs. 12.13, 12.14, 12.15, 12.16, 12.17, 12.18 and 12.19).

Other Conditions

Mild vitreous shrinkage with a taught posterior hyaloid membrane that is still attached to the retina may be partly responsible for cystoid macular oedema in diabetic maculopathy or uveitis (Figs. 12.20, 12.21, 12.22, and 12.23).

Secondary Macular ERM

Macular pucker can occur after retinal tear or retinal detachment [12] seen in approximately 7–10% [13, 14] and is more commonly seen in PVR. A six month prevalence of 15% has been described after surgery for PVR by vitrectomy and gas or silicone oil [15]. Post-mortem studies suggest much higher prevalence most of which must be subclinical [16]. The ERM in RRD can occur relatively rapidly with symptoms deteriorating over weeks [17]. In RRD the ERM is

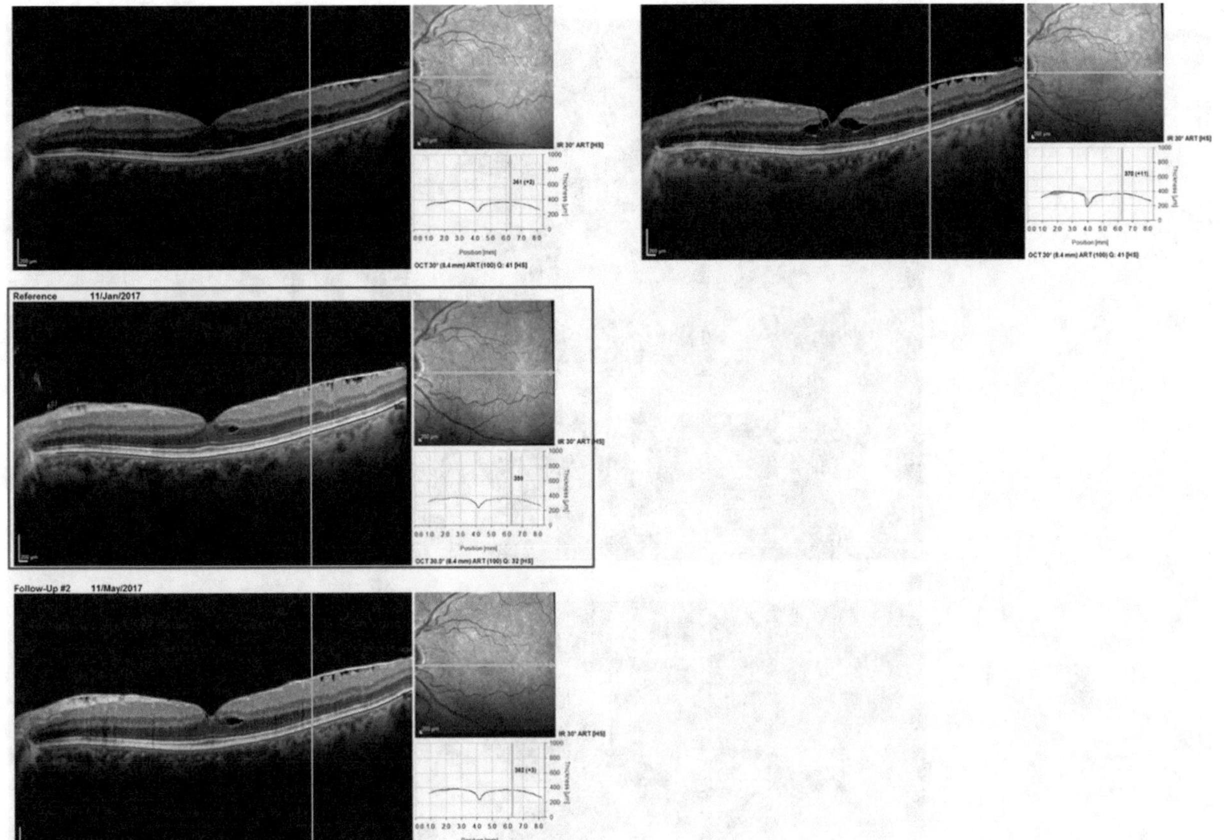

Fig. 12.8 Progressive growth of an ERM causing foveal disruption

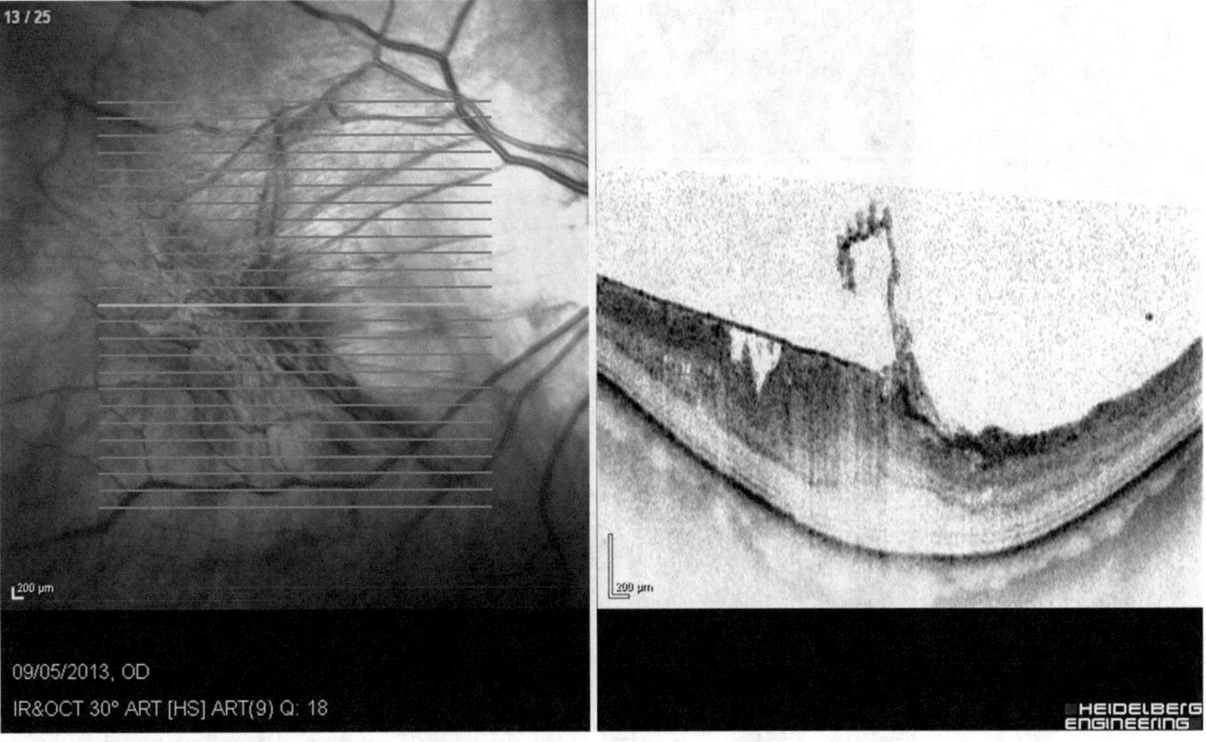

Fig. 12.9 ERM with a rolled edge

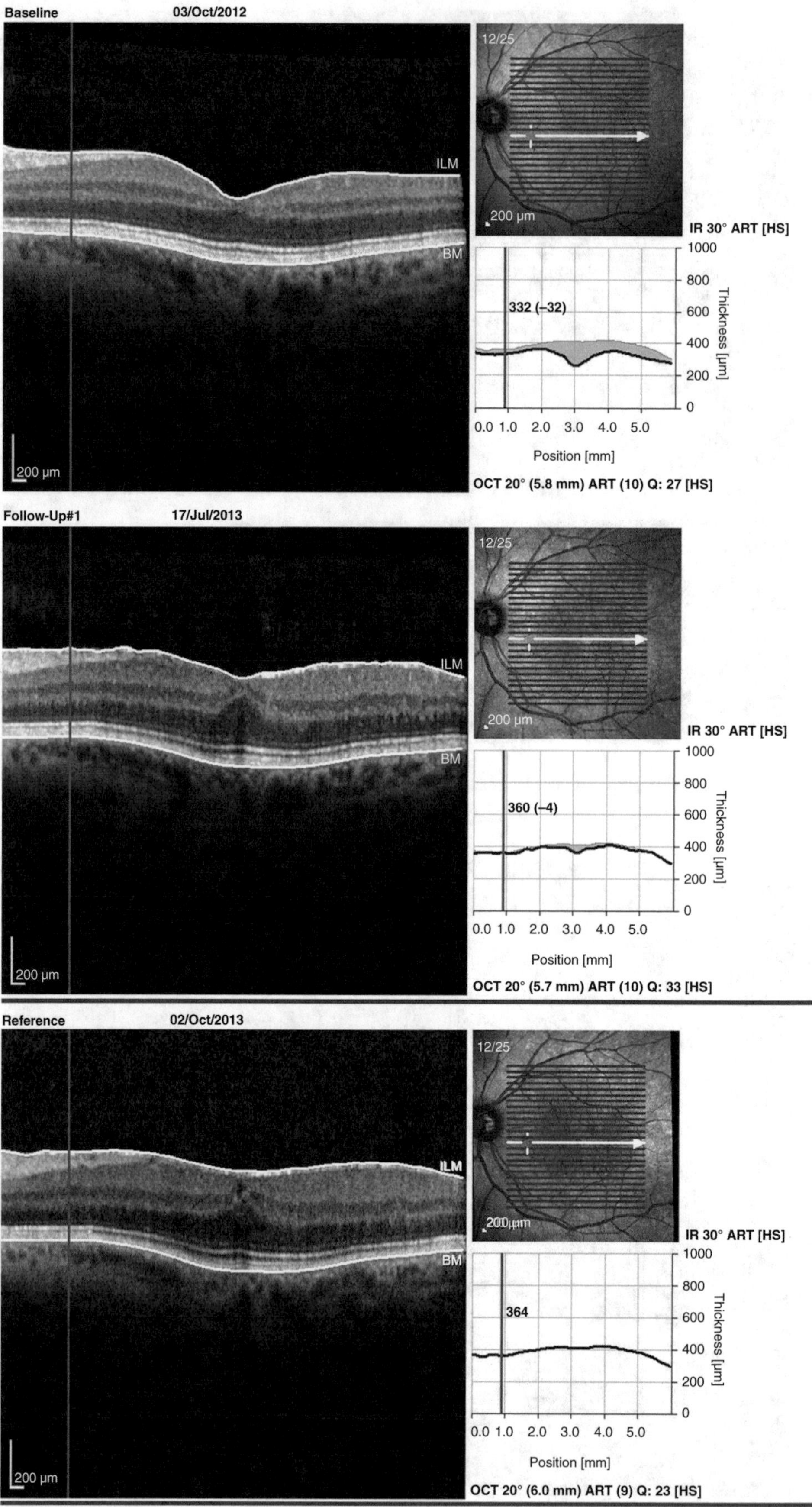

Fig. 12.10 Gradual development of an ERM

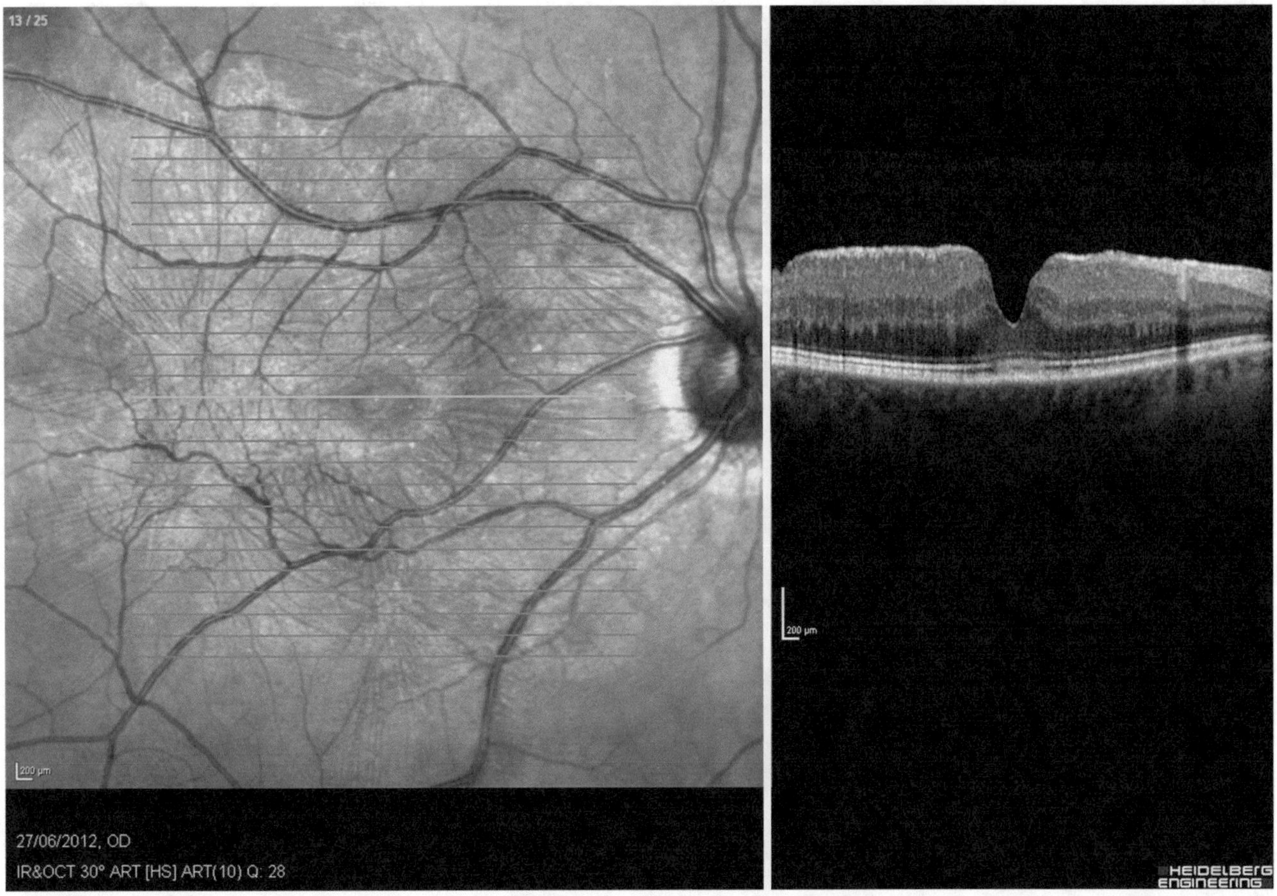

Fig. 12.11 ERM with a pseudohole

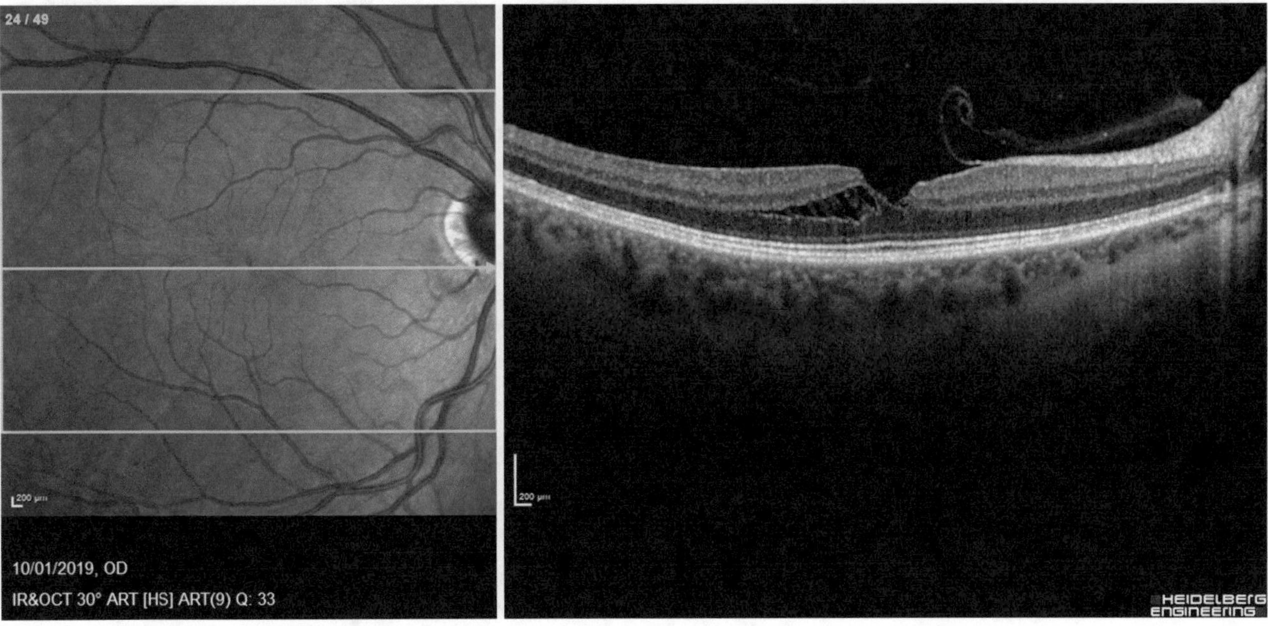

Fig. 12.12 Some of the ILM has spontaneously peeled and rolled in this eye

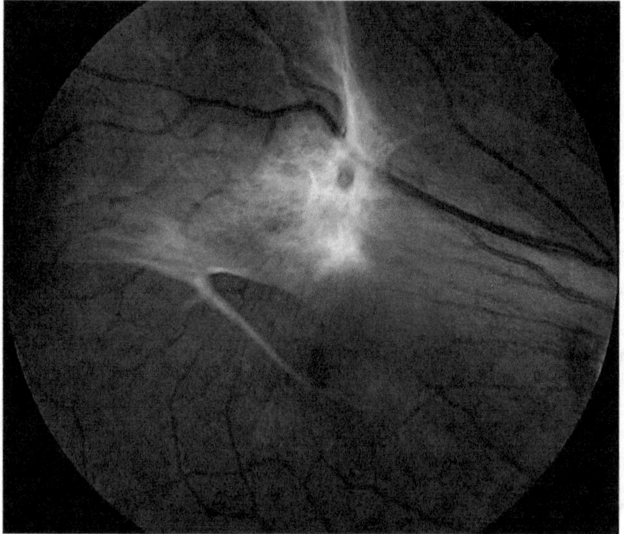

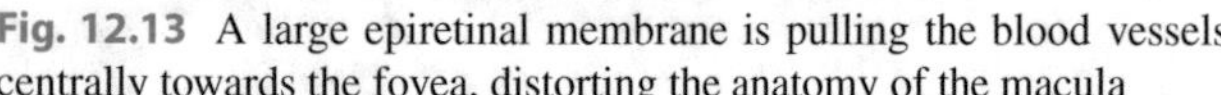

Fig. 12.13 A large epiretinal membrane is pulling the blood vessels centrally towards the fovea, distorting the anatomy of the macula

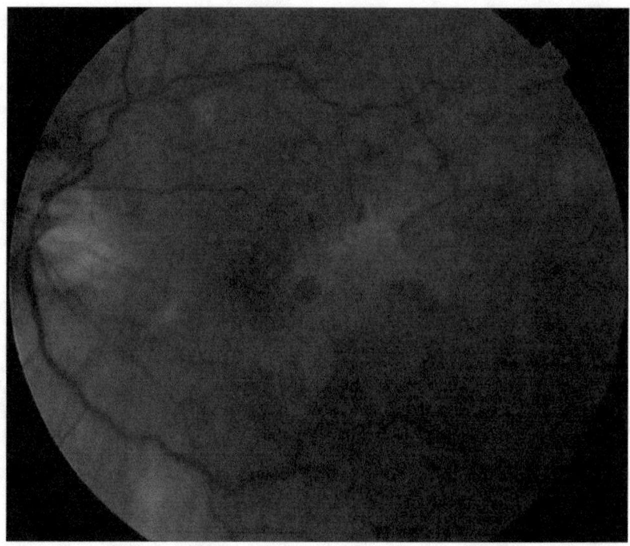

Fig. 12.15 An epiretinal membrane is shown with a pseudohole over the fovea

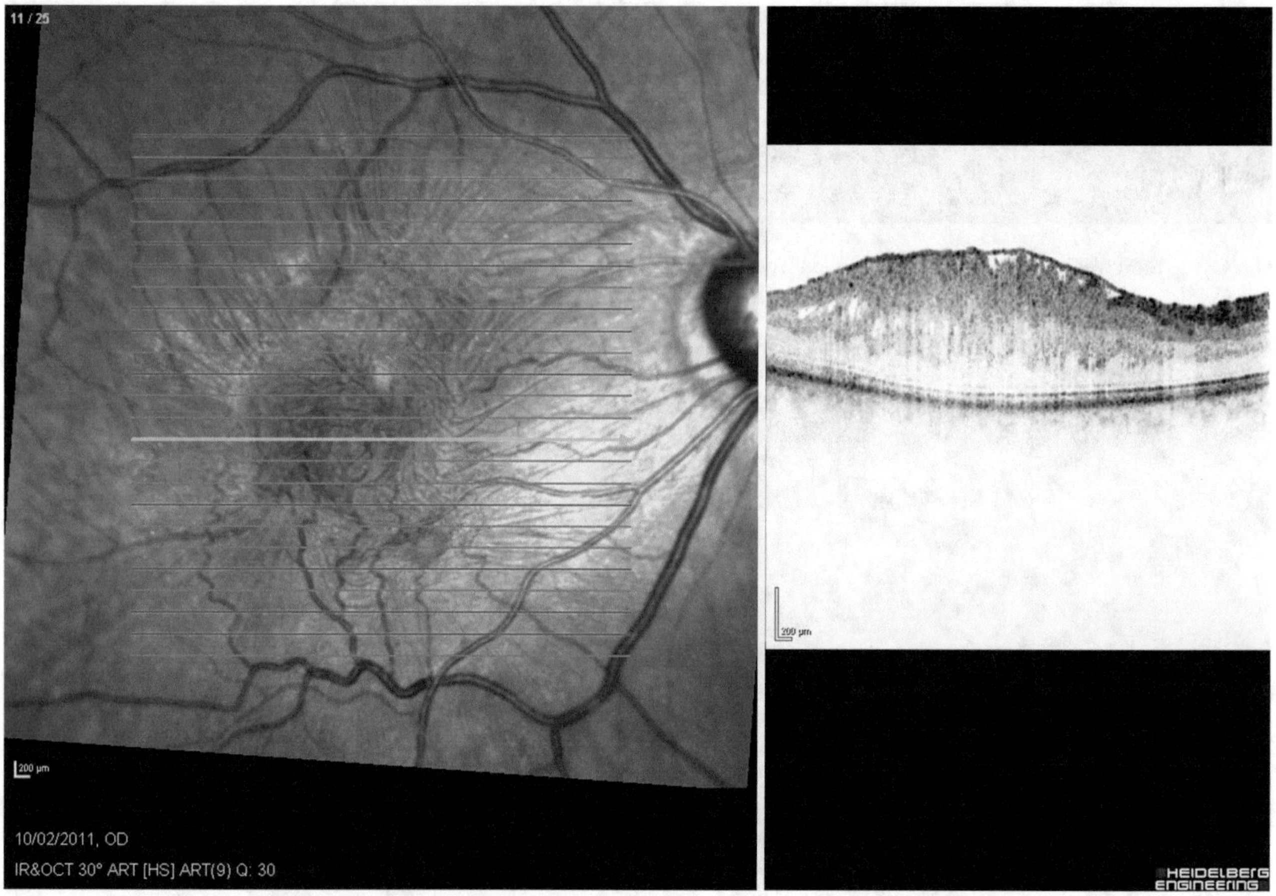

Fig. 12.14 The OCT shows thickening and wrinkling of the retina from an ERM. Pegs of attachment of the ERM to the retinal can be seen

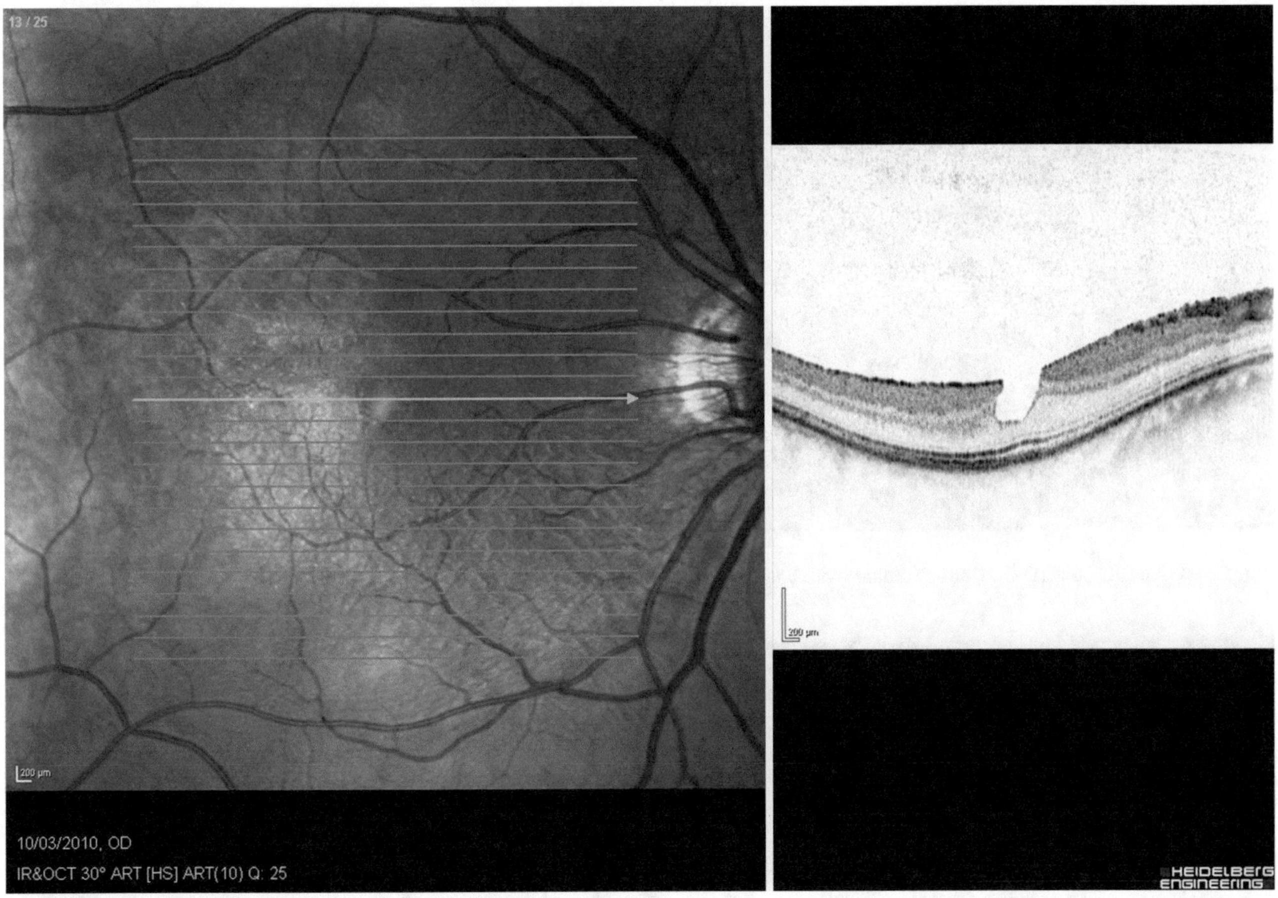

Fig. 12.16 A mild cellophane ERM with pseudohole, vision was 20/20

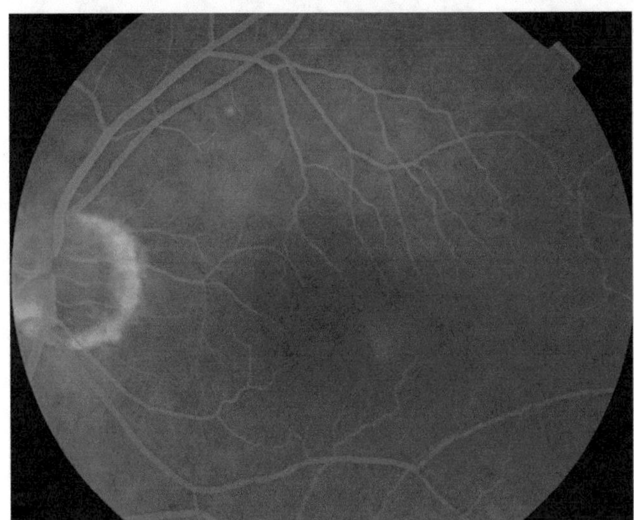

Fig. 12.17 ERM on the macula will produce mild CMO in some cases, seen on FFA

more often associated with pigmented cells, histologically of RPE origin [18].

In some cases, the ERM is secondary to branch retinal vein occlusion (BRVO) in which case it is worth checking an FFA to assess the perifoveal arcade. If this is not complete, this may indicate a poorer prognosis for vision postoperatively.

ERM can appear secondary to uveitis.

If the hyaloid is incompletely removed at vitrectomy in patients with vitreoschisis such as in surgery for diabetic retinopathy, ERM may occur.

ERM can occur in patients with peripheral retinal angiomata, e.g. Von Hippel–Lindau disease or idiopathic acquired angiomata [19, 20] (Figs. 12.24, 12.25, 12.26, 12.27, 12.28, 12.29, 12.30, 12.31, 12.32, and 12.33).

In sickle cell disease ERM is seen in 4% [21].

Candida endophthalmitis also stimulates ERM in some patients [22].

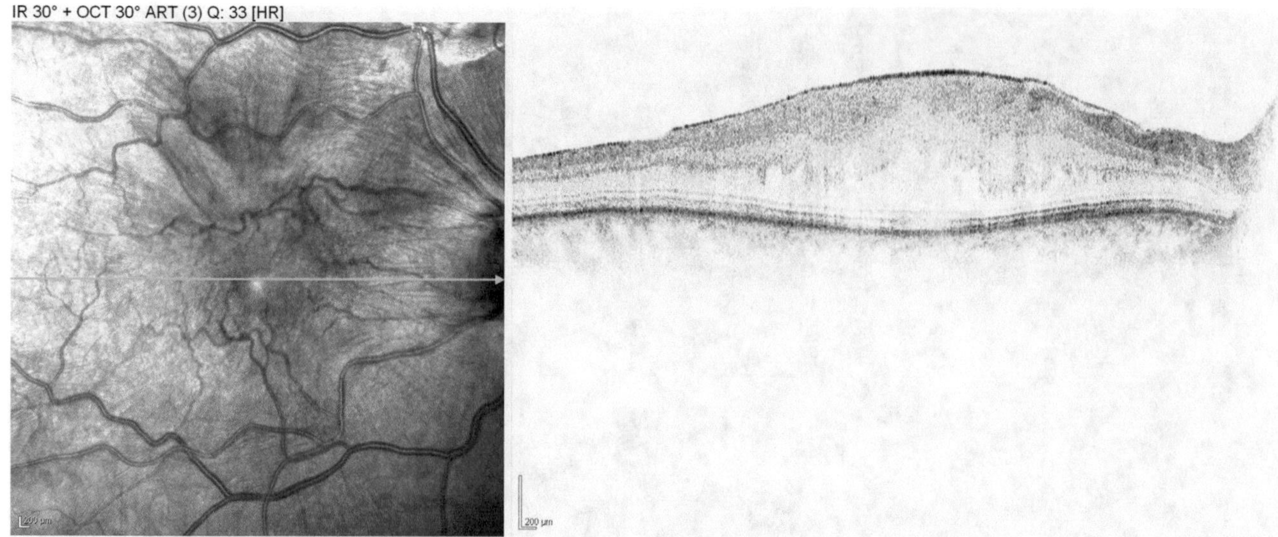

Fig. 12.18 An ERM on HD OCT notice retinal wrinkling on the SLO scan and thickening of the retina on OCT.

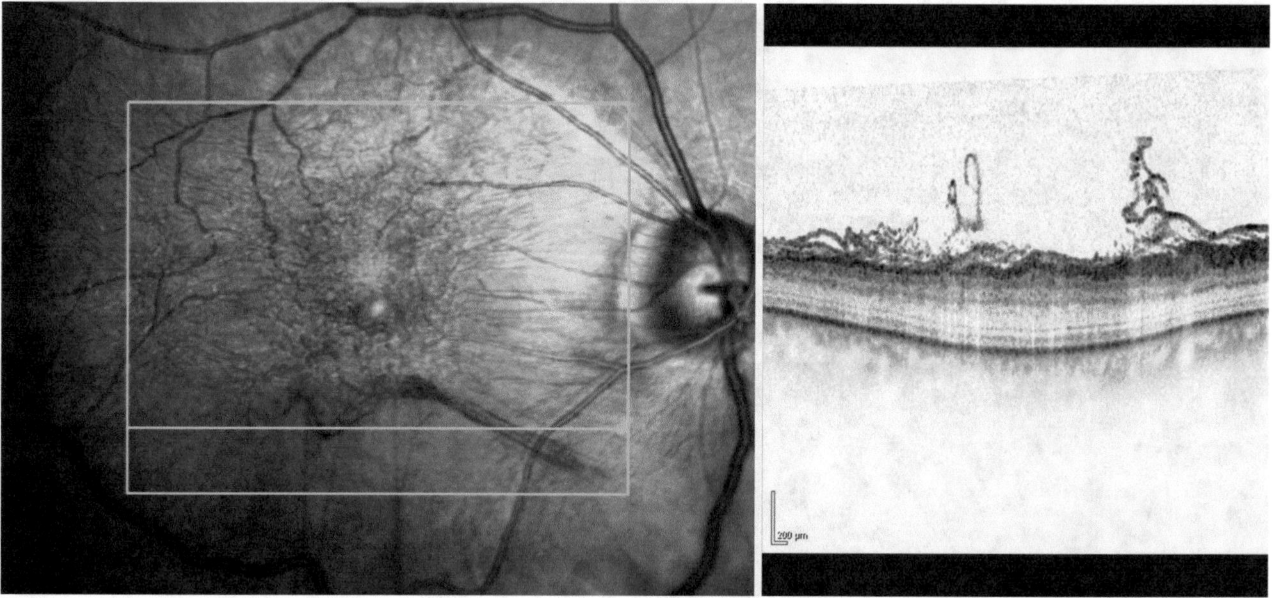

Fig. 12.19 This ERM has a rolled edge which will be easily grasped during surgery. Notice the elastic membrane has rolled at its lifted edge

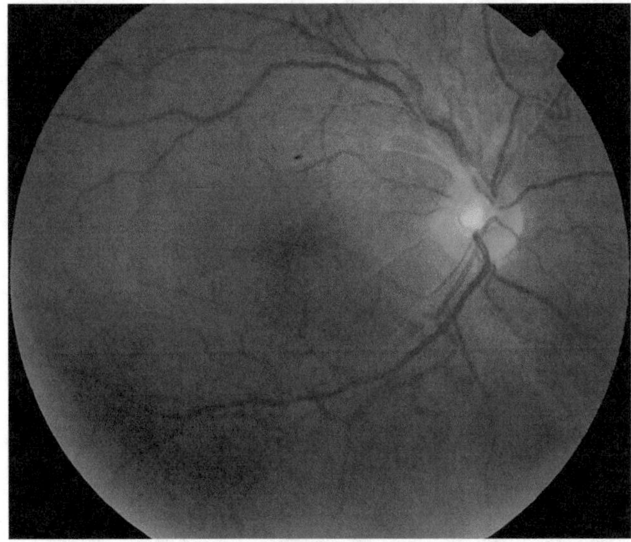

Fig. 12.20 In young patients, spontaneous separation of the ERM is common. With the ERM visible on the PHM of the PVD

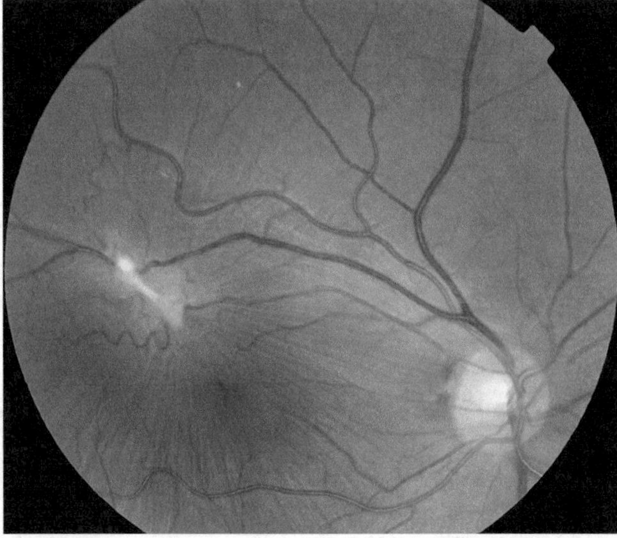

Fig. 12.22 This macular lesion was seen coincidentally with macular striae in a patient of 13 years of age

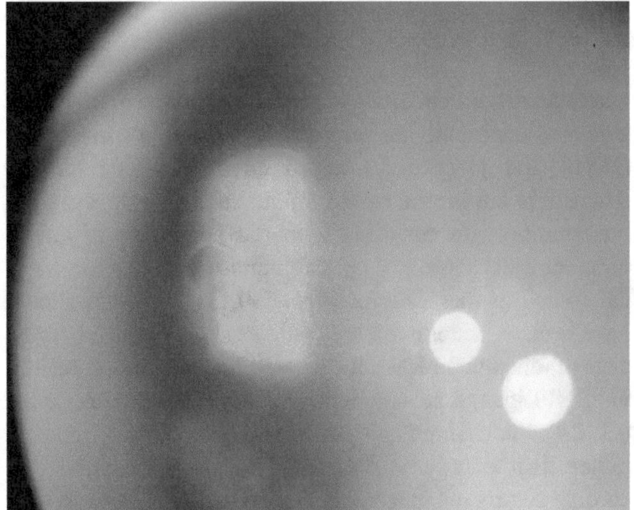

Fig. 12.21 Later the ERM separates with the formation of PVD

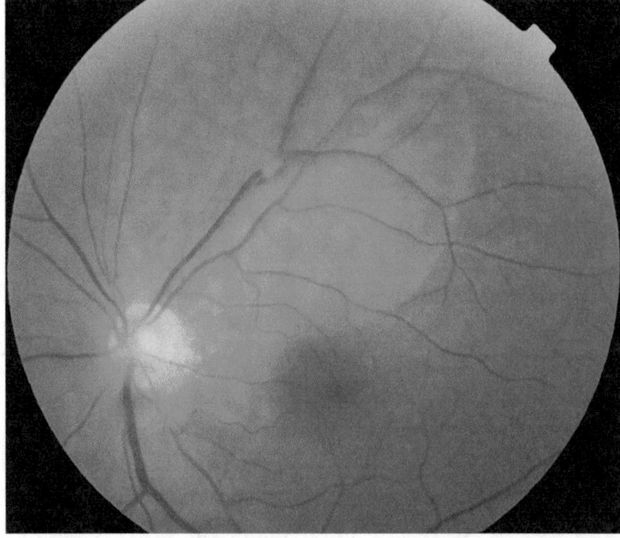

Fig. 12.23 This eye was observed with an area of chronic shallow elevation of the retina from vitreomacular traction without progression. Usually VM traction is associated with ERM of the macula but no ERM had developed in this eye

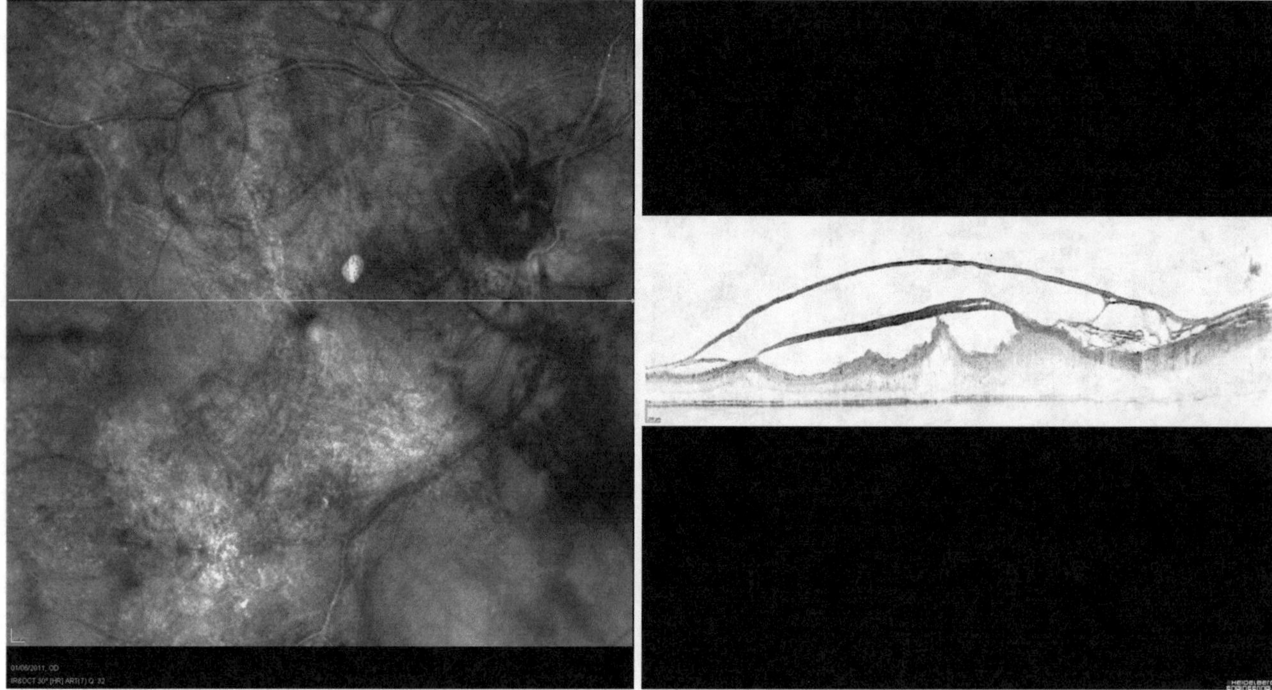

Fig. 12.24 Extensive ERM and traction in an eye which has received plaque radiotherapy for peripheral angiomata

Combined hamartoma and FEVR may be associated with ERM in young patients [23] (Figs. 12.34 and 12.35).

Surgical Pearl

Intraretinal Changes

Epiretinal membranes (ERM) consist of non-vascularized fibrocellular tissue, formed by cellular metaplasia and proliferation at the vitreoretinal interface, found with a prevalence varied from 1.02% to 26.1% [24–26]. The ERM is clinically classified as idiopathic, if no secondary causes are identified [27]. We will describe the intraretinal changes in presence of epiretinal traction in idiopathic and diabetic ERM.

In idiopathic ERM, it is hypothesised that microscopic breaks of internal limiting membrane (ILM) following an anomalous posterior vitreous detachment (PVD) allow the migration of glial cells on the retinal surface and their subsequent proliferation with the interposition of the remnants of native vitreous between the ILM and the epiretinal tissue [28]. Histopathologic analysis has shown that myofibroblasts are the main cellular component of ERM [29]. The ILM is formed by the footplates and the basal membrane of the Müller cells, with consequent close correlation between epiretinal and intraretinal modifications. Müller cells are glial cells that regulate retinal homeostasis and support structurally the foveola thanks to their binding of the photoreceptors. Müller cells in the parafoveal region show a "z-shaped" anatomical configuration and their horizontal part of the z-shaped contribute anatomically to the Henle's fibre layer (HNL) and physical to a protective "damping effect"; whereas in the central foveal Müller cells display a straight configuration, the central bouquet (CB), resulting in a more efficient transmission of optical impulse, but also mechanical forces to the photoreceptors [30, 31]. Recently, there have been a greater number of studies showing that, in presence of idiopathic ERMs, the inner retinal alterations, mainly in RNFL-ganglion cell–inner plexiform layer complex (GCCx), thickening is responsible for functional symptoms rather than outer retinal damage to photoreceptors. The chronic centripetal tangential traction and/or anteroposterior traction may induce an activation of Müller cells and astrocyte with reactive gliosis, characterised by hypertrophy, proliferation, and upregulation of glial fibrillary acidic protein (GFAP) [32–35]Recently, it has also been proved, by analysing the differences in the vitreous cytokine profiles in ERM eyes with and without ectopic inner foveal layers (EIFL), that the eyes with EIFL had increased vitreous levels of macrophage markers, supporting the hypothesis that the activation of glial cell proliferation contributes to EIFL formation [36]. The hypertrophy of the macroglia (Müller cells and astrocyte) aims to protect the neuronal cells from the damage induced by the traction. Such intraretinal gliosis, described as EIFL, extends from the INL and IPL across the central fovea [32]. (Fig. 12.36).

The chronic tractional stress exerted by ERM mechanically displaces the inner retinal layers centripetally and the

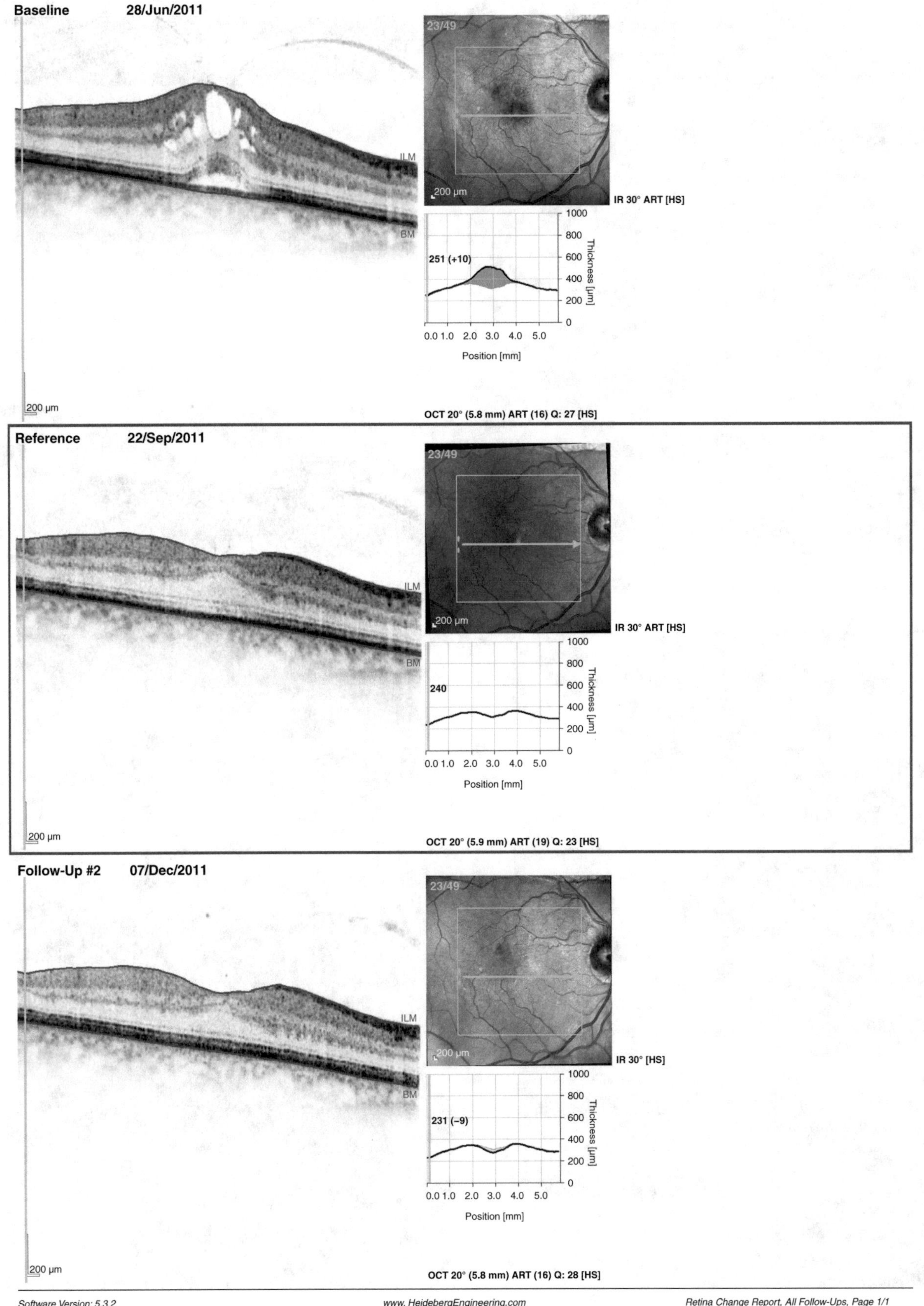

Fig. 12.25 Vitreomacular traction after phaco cataract surgery can spontaneously resolve after separation of the vitreous therefore it is worth waiting two months to see if this will occur before operating

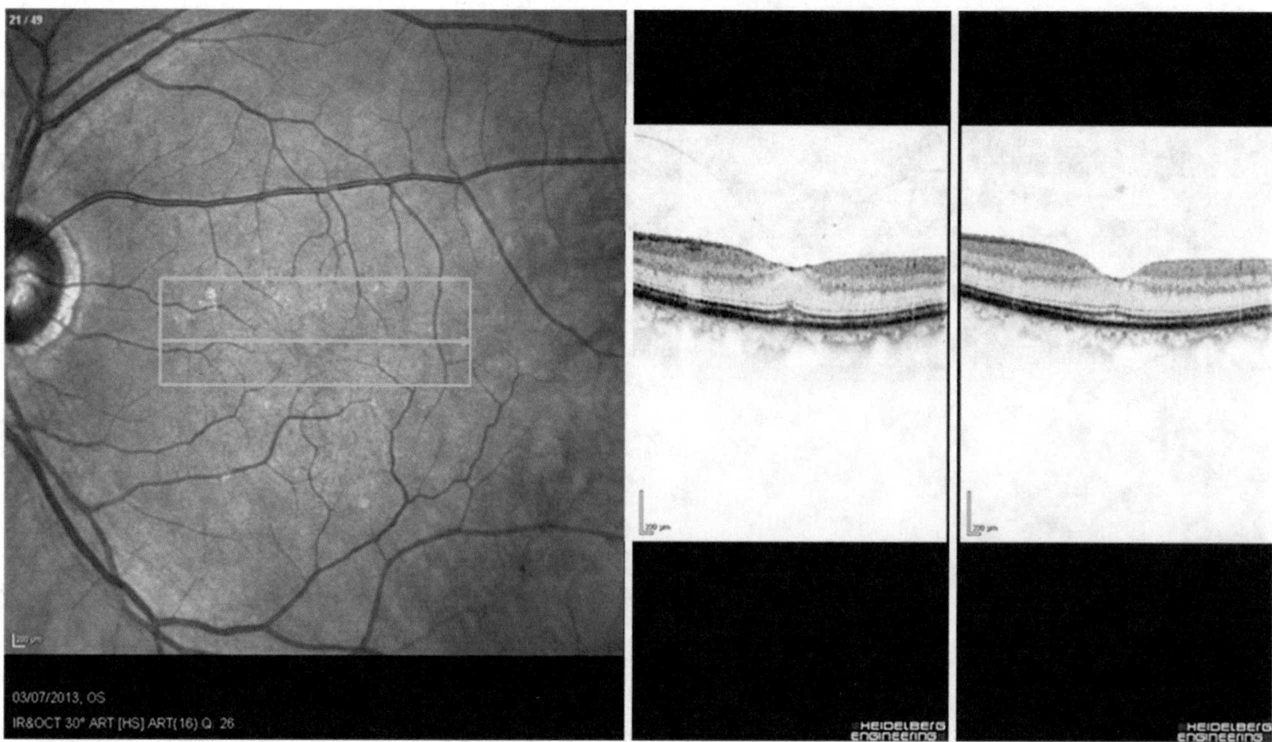

Fig. 12.26 VMA spontaneous resolution

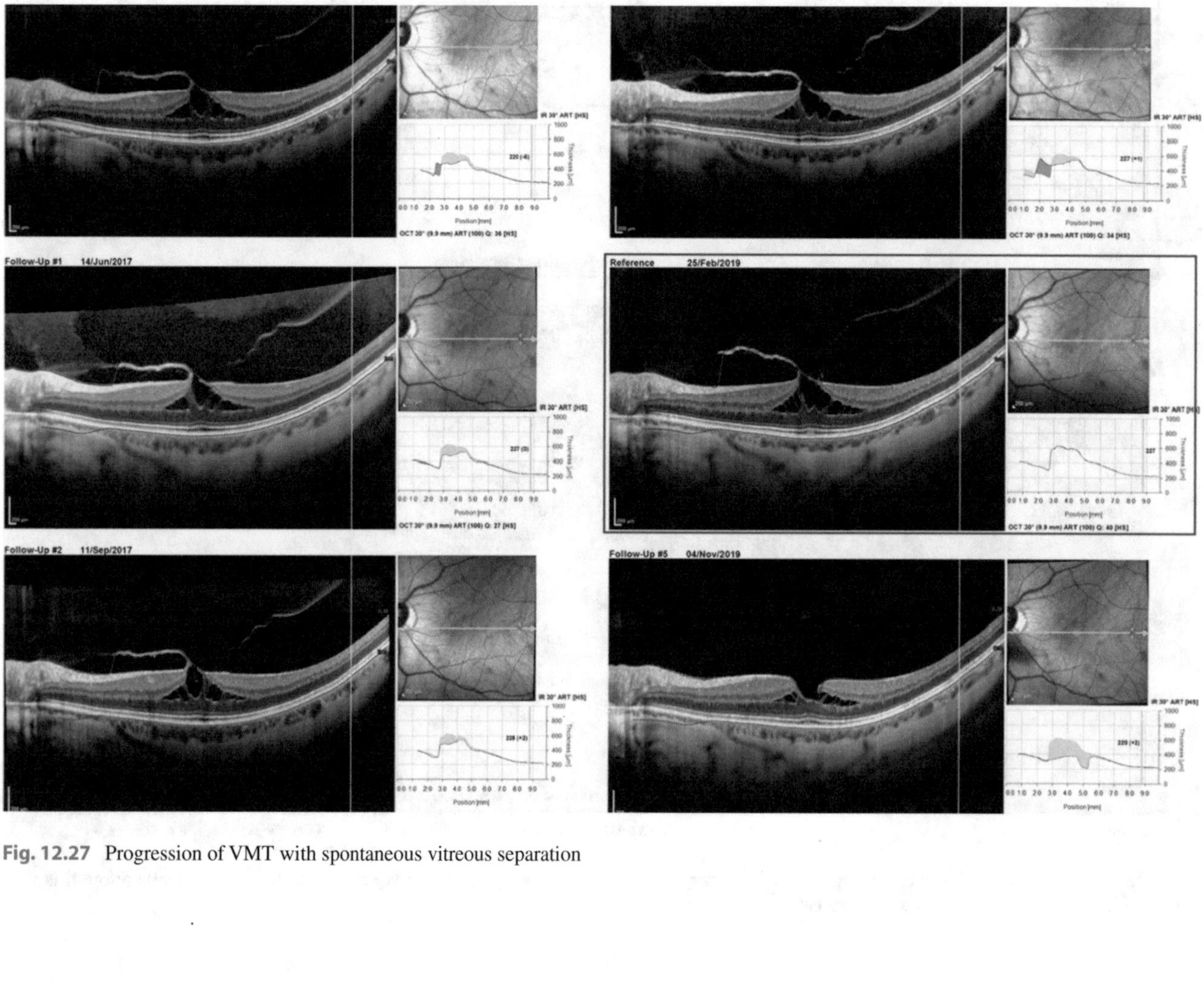

Fig. 12.27 Progression of VMT with spontaneous vitreous separation

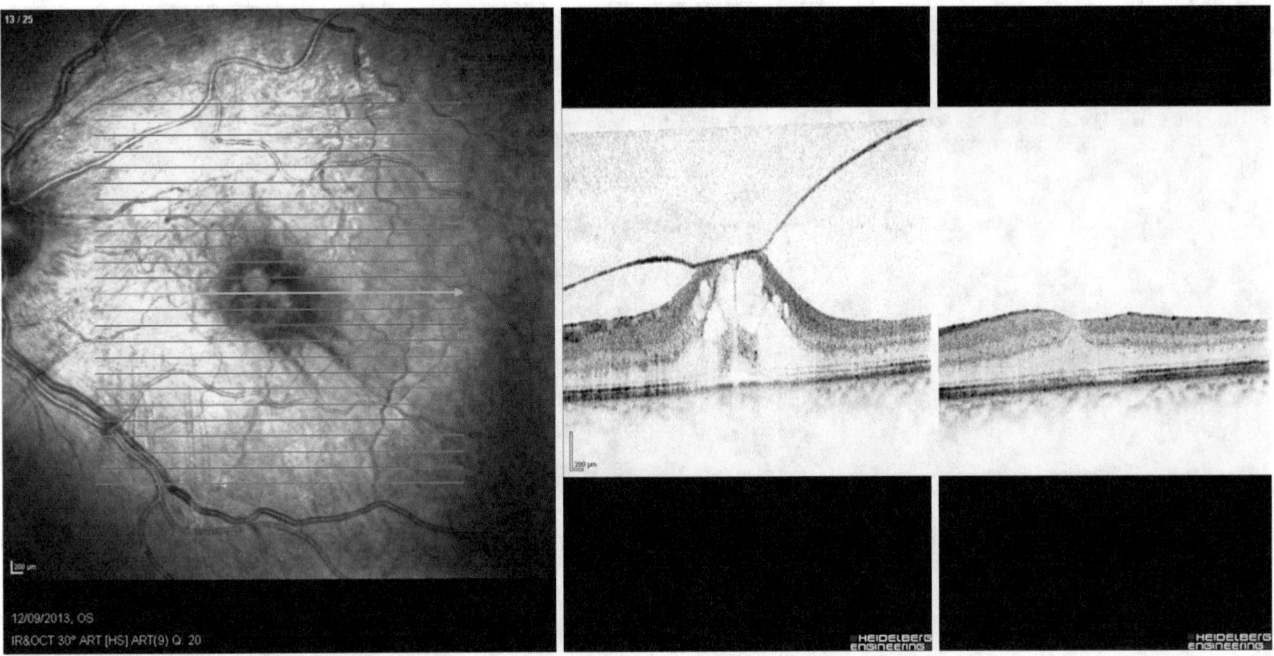

Fig. 12.28 VMT before and after surgery

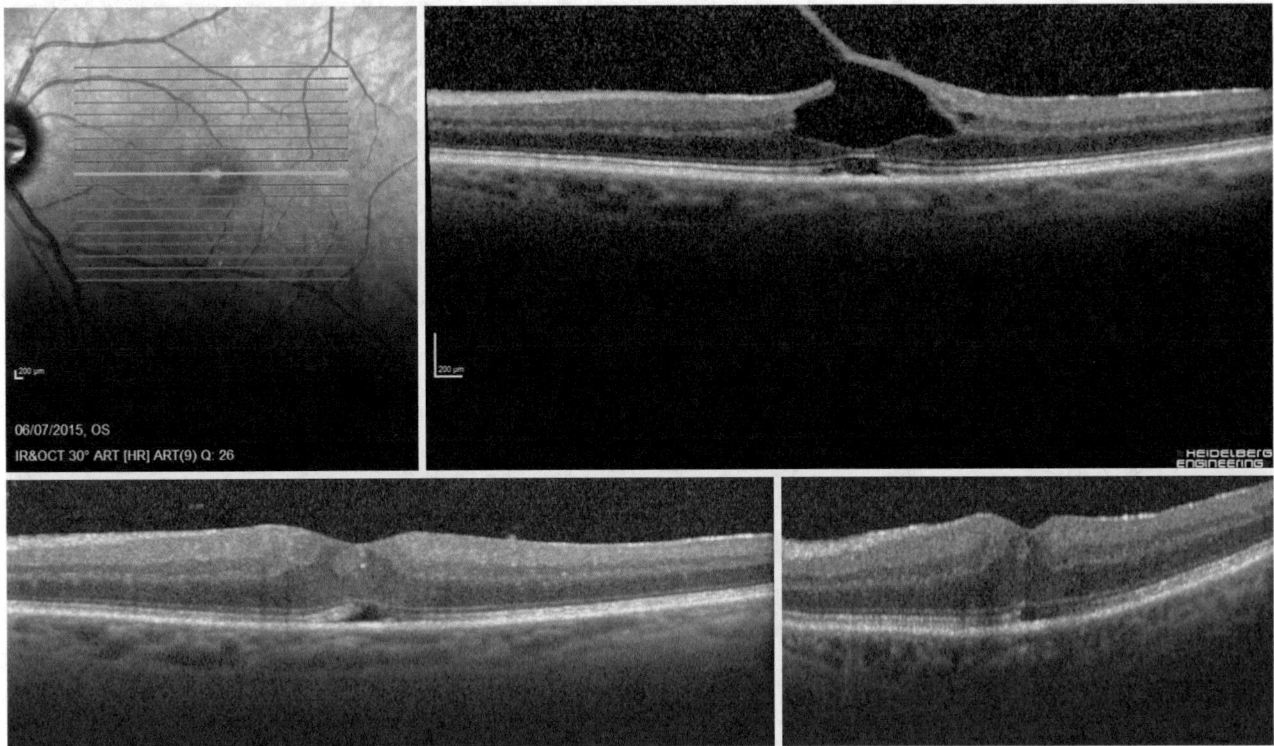

Fig. 12.29 VMT before and after surgery

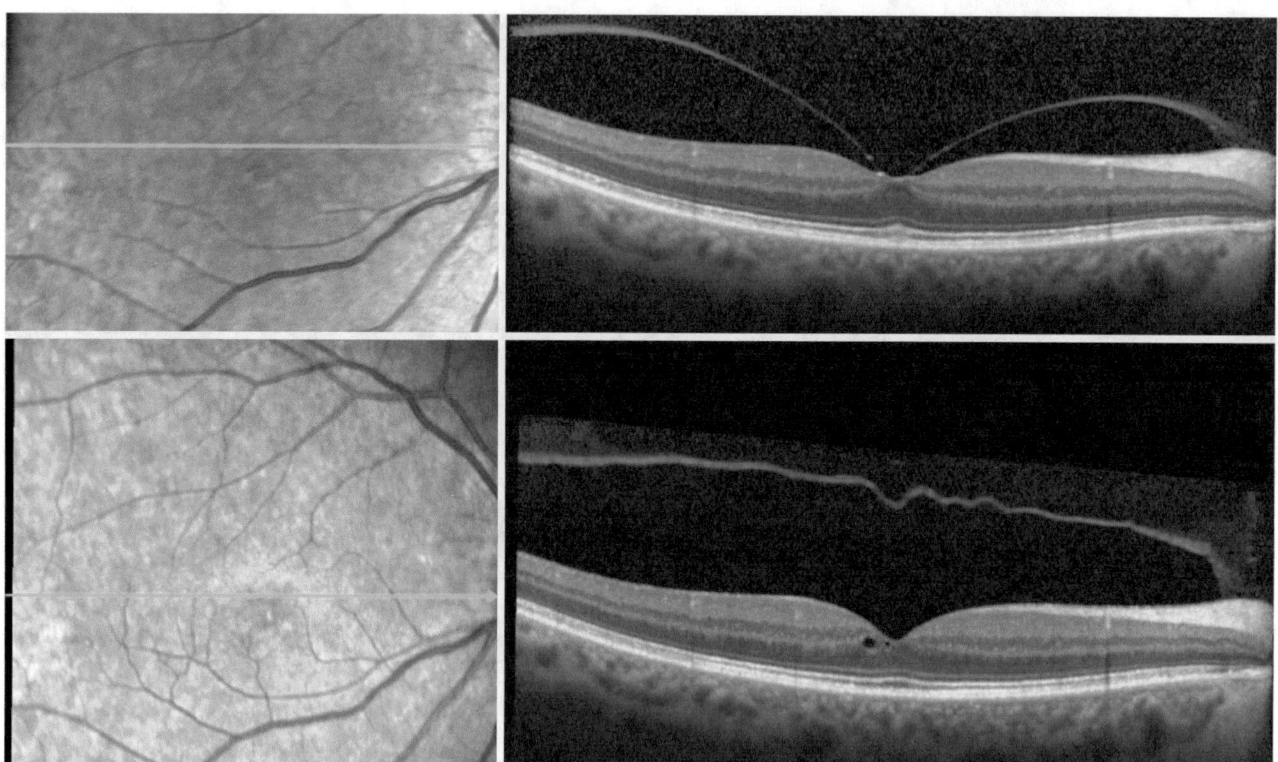

Fig. 12.30 VMT separation spontaneously

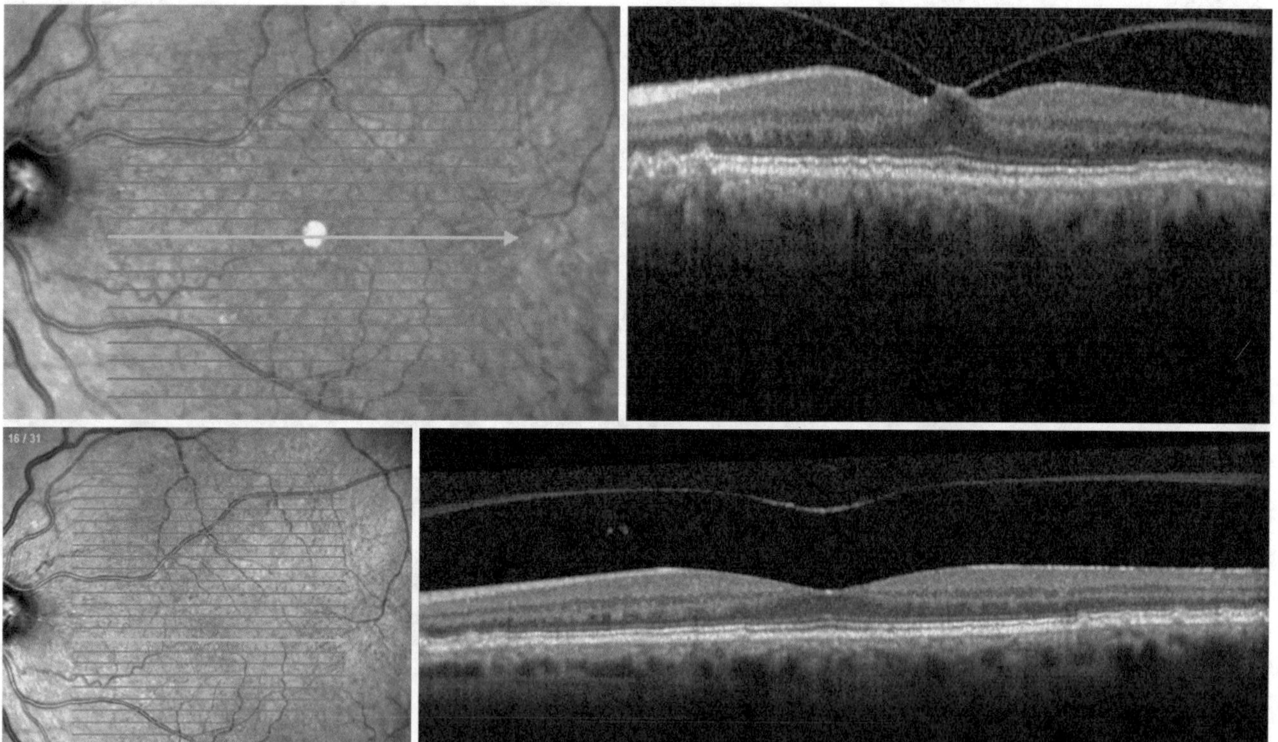

Fig. 12.31 Spontaneous separation of VMT

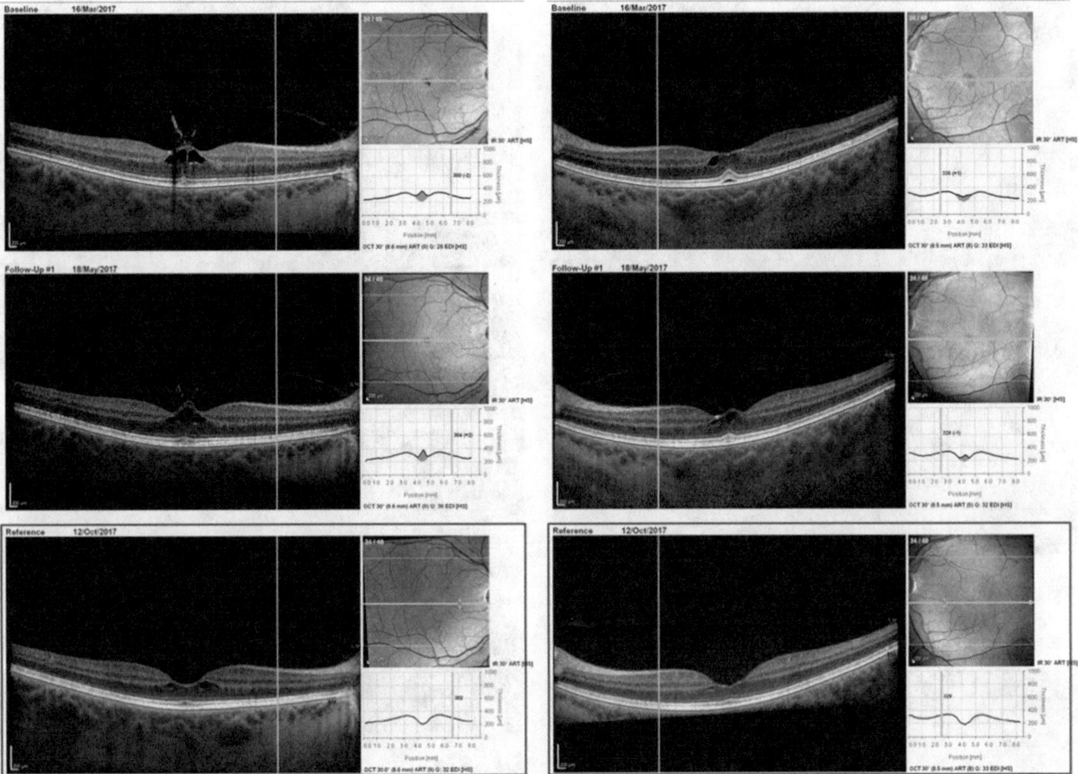

Fig. 12.32 Bilateral spontaneous resolution of VMT

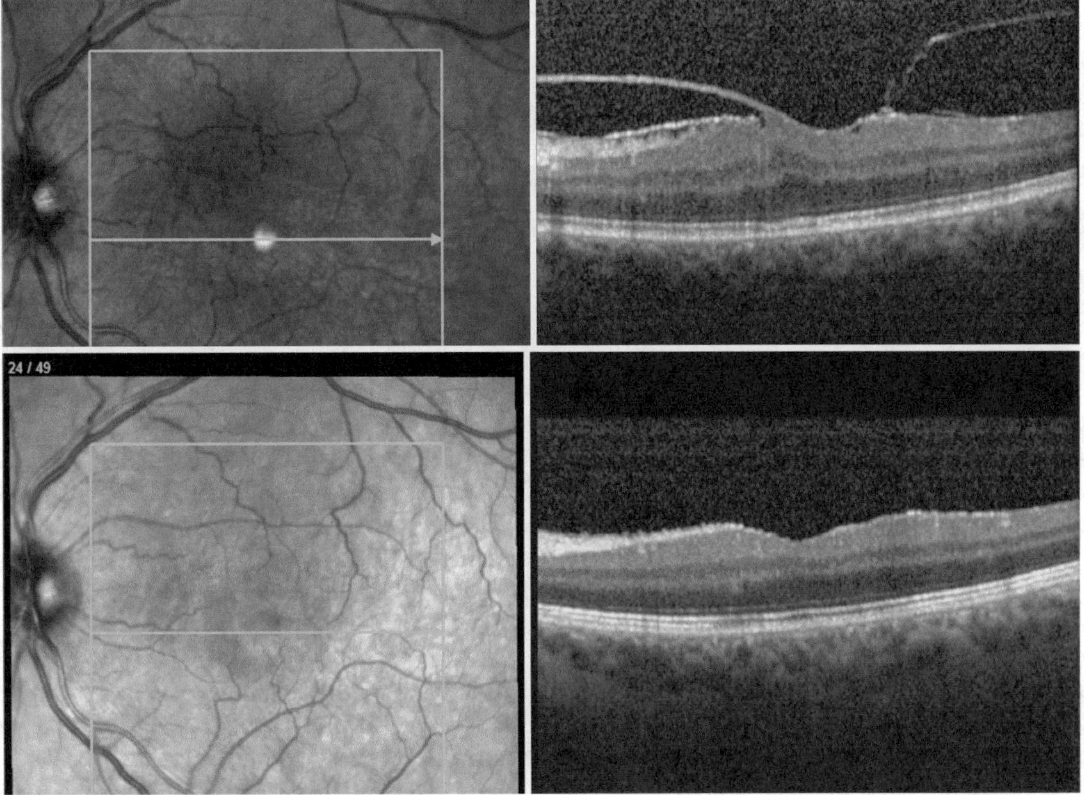

Fig. 12.33 VMT and ERM before and after surgery

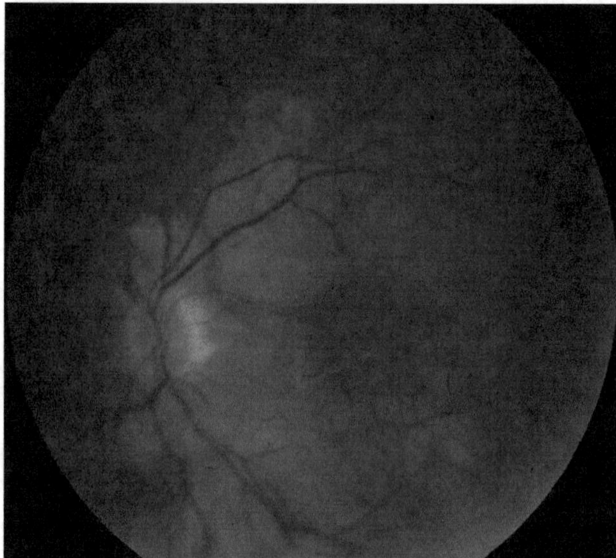

Fig. 12.34 The membrane has been removed from this macula

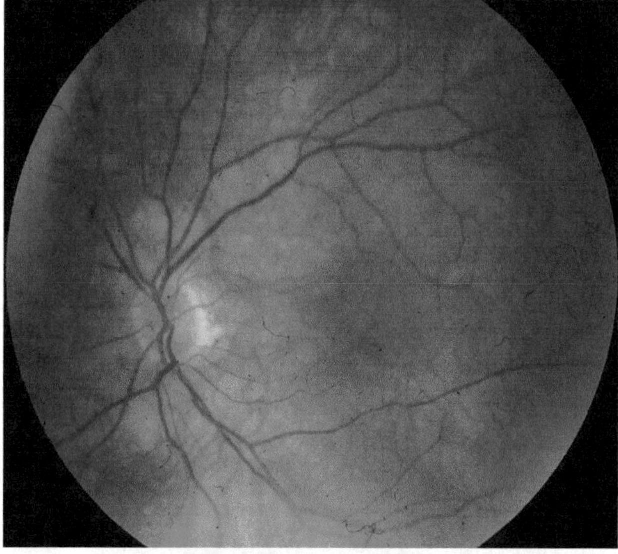

Fig. 12.35 The macula postoperatively

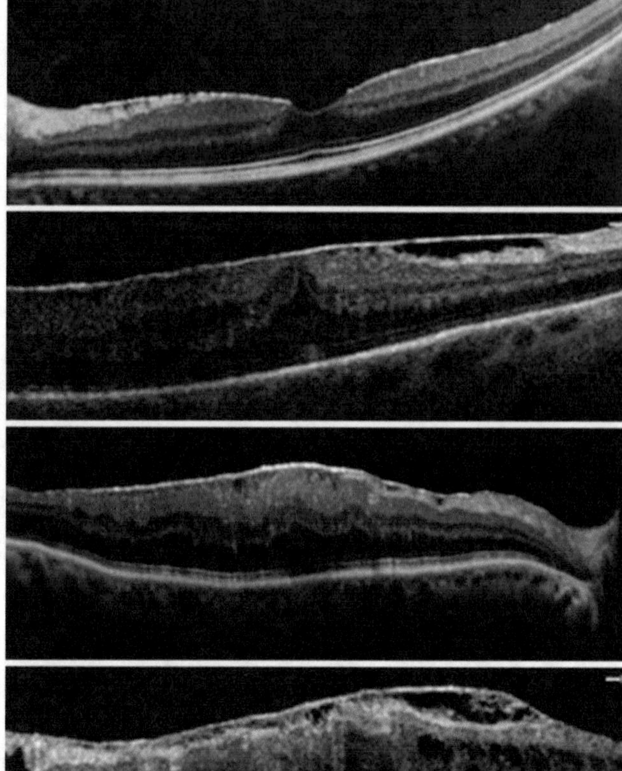

Fig. 12.36 Classification of epiretinal traction based on intraretinal changes. (**a**) Stage 1: wrinkling of retinal surface, presence of foveal pit, well-defined intraretinal layer. (**b**) Stage 2: ERM, absence of foveal pit, enlargement of outer nuclear layer. (**c**) Stage 3: ERM, absence of foveal pit, presence of inner ectopic foveal layer with intraretinal gliosis. (**d**) Stage 4: ERM, absence of foveal pit, presence of wider inner ectopic foveal layer with intraretinal gliosis / fibrosis

superficial and deep vascular plexus. A classification of ERM based on intraretinal changes has been recently proposed by Govetto et al. [32]. This intermediate filament strengthens the Müller cells-ILM bond, acting as a bridge, due to its interaction with cytoskeleton, surface receptors, and the proteins of extracellular matrix. Regarding the symptoms, metamorphopsia is mainly associated with INL thickness, and the reduction in BCVA is significantly associated with the presence of EIFL [37]. The negative correlation between EIFL thickness and BCVA suggests that the EIFL acts as a physical barrier, between the afferent light and photoreceptors, reducing the light that runs on the Müller, which has also a fibre optic function. The extent of this optical obstruction increases with increasing EIFL thickness. It has also been hypothesised that if the epiretinal traction is incident mainly on the CB, the chronic forces can induce different changes as the cotton ball sign, foveolar detachment and acquired vitelliform lesion, subsequent stages of CB abnormalities. The presence of the EIFL may be protective against CB abnormalities. The foveal straight Müller cells may play an integral role in the transmission of mechanical forces to the central foveal cones leading to a spectrum of CB abnormalities. (Fig. 12.37) The presence of EIFL may be protective against the development of tractional CB abnormalities [38].

On the other side, in diabetic epiretinal membrane, intraretinal cysts were significantly more common intraretinal findings than EILF. In diabetic retinopathy there are an inner neuroretinal degeneration due to micro-vasculopathy and a high glucose (HG)-induced mitochondrial dysfunction that promote the apoptosis of Müller cells, compromising their

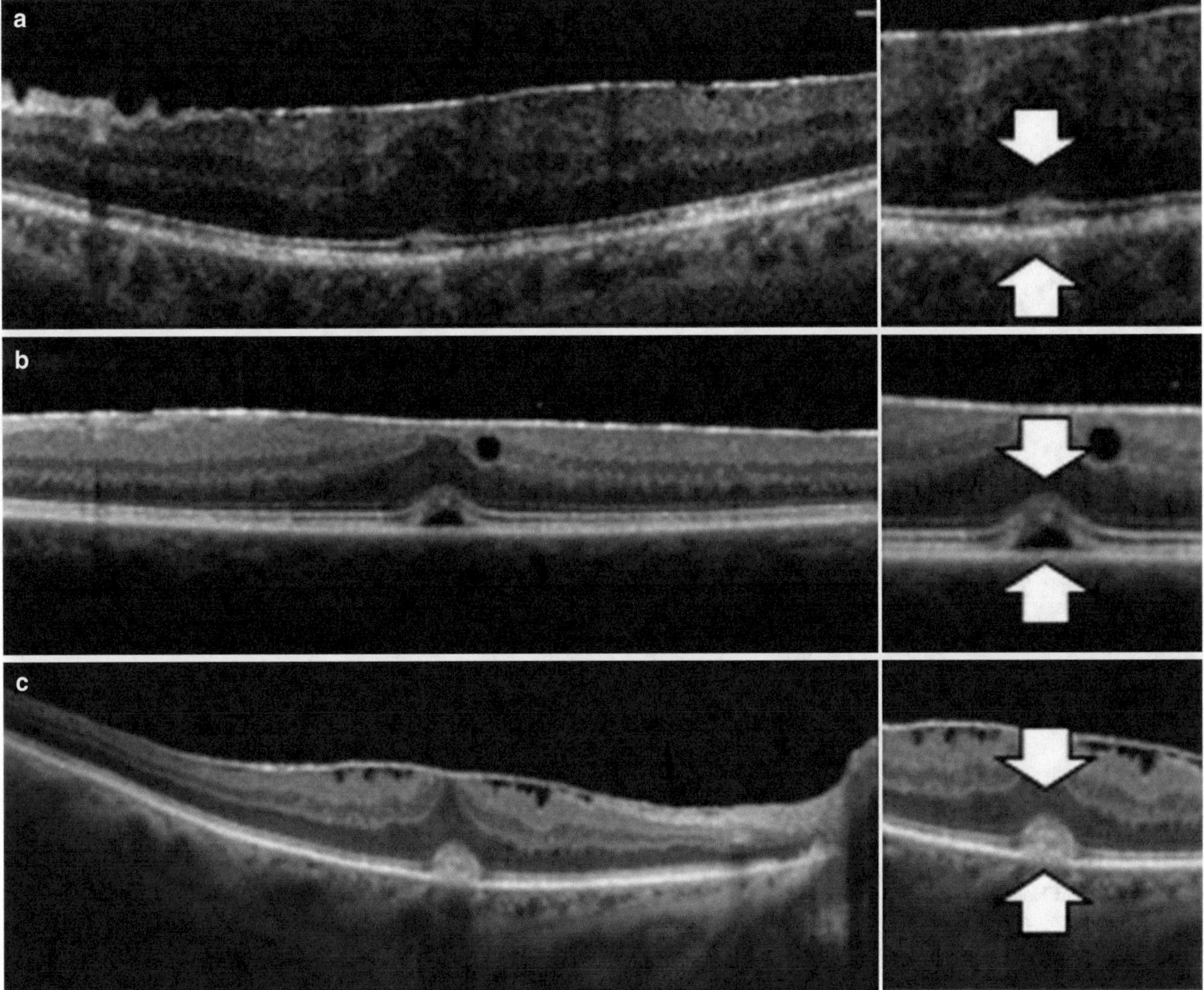

Fig. 12.37 Cotton ball (CB) sign. (**a**) Stage 2 ERM associated with small CB between the external limiting membrane (ELM) and ellipsoid zone (EZ). (**b**) Stage 2 ERM associated with thicker CB. ELM and EZ are still preserved and associated with subretinal fluid under the interdigitation zone. (**c**) Stage 2 ERM associated with acquired vitelliform lesion between the EZ and retinal pigment epithelium. The ELM is preserved, whereas the EZ appears disrupted

protective role towards neurons. Since the Müller cells play an important role in the maintenance of the inner blood retinal barrier (BRB) and in retinal VEGF production, this can contribute to increased vascular permeability. It has been hypnotised that in diabetic EMRs the injury and loss of Müller cells may result, under traction, in less reactive intraretinal gliosis with consequent absence of EIFL. This results in a greater percentage of intraretinal cysts, with postoperative enlargement of deep capillary free zone network. All the above-mentioned conditions in diabetic retinopathy may make macula and perifoveal capillary plexus more sensitive to the mechanical damage of Müller cells induced by ILM peeling. The consequent deep capillary ischemia and macular non-perfusion contribute to disrupt the outer retina [39, 40].

Finally, we would like to draw attention to the differences on OCT structural cross-section and enface scans in tractional and exudative diabetic maculopathy [20].

In tractional disorders, mechanical forces physically separate and displace mainly the horizontal part of Müller cells processes at the level of HNL. Therefore, the interstitial fluid flows freely within such anatomical "spaces" showing as schisis on OCT, maintained by and independent from Starling's equation. We can describe, in cross-section OCT scans, hyperreflective columnar elements corresponding to "verticalized" HNL.

The enface OCT scans morphology shows radially oriented Müller cell processes extending from the foveal centre (Fig. 12.38) as "spoke wheel" [20].

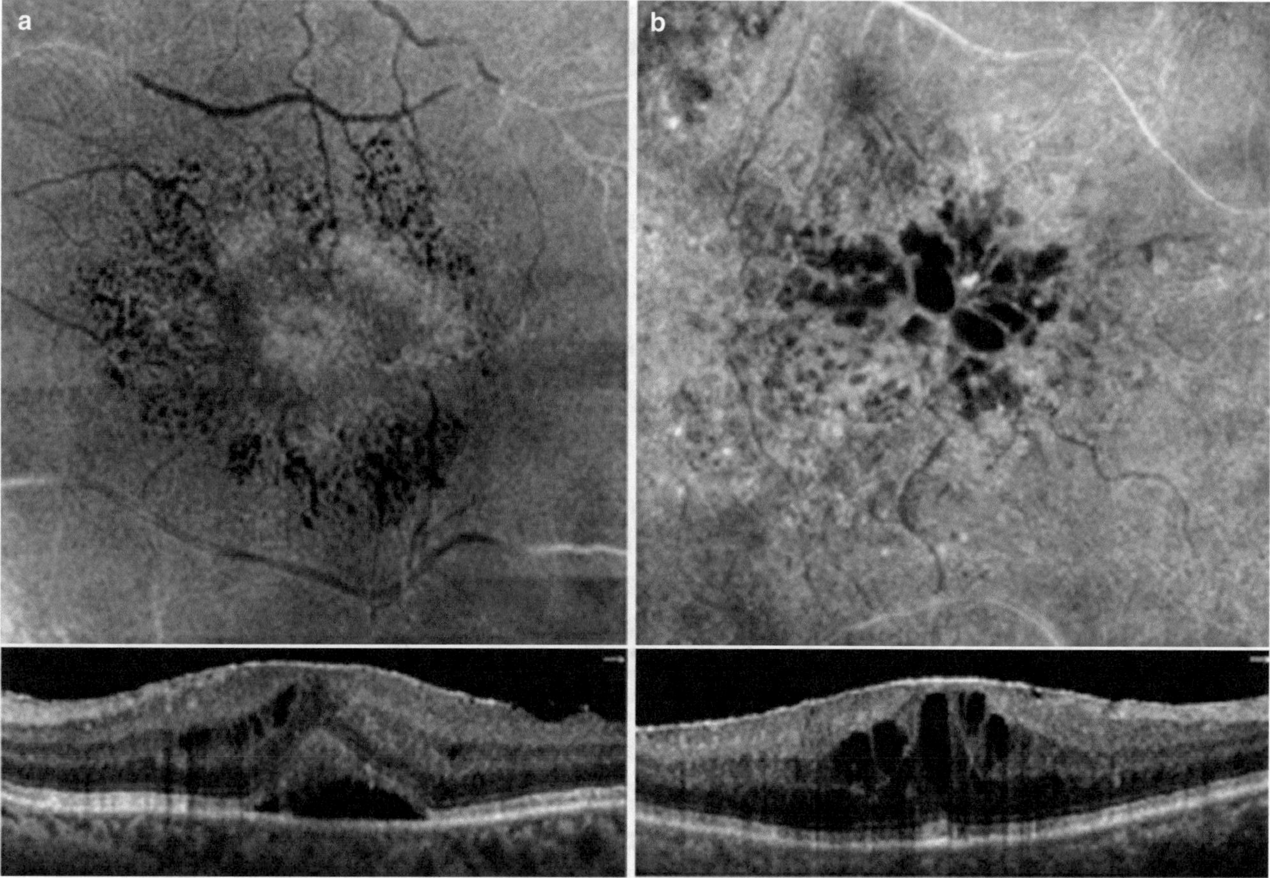

Fig. 12.38 Enface OCT segmentation including in the inner nuclear, outer nuclear and Henle's fibre layers. In presence of prevalent tractional disorders, the enface OCT scans morphology shows radially oriented Müller cell processes extending from the foveal centre as "spoke wheel" (**a**); whereas in case of prevalent exudative disorders, it shows cystoid spaces with characteristic petaloid pattern due to the structural damage of Müller cells and to the increase of capillary permeability (**b**)

In exudative disorders, we describe cross-section OCT scans hypo-reflective cystoid spaces in both the INL and HFL. The enface OCT scans morphology shows cystoid spaces with characteristic petaloid pattern due to the structural damage of Müller cells and to the increase of capillary permeability (i.e. Starling's law) and deep retinal capillary plexus involvement [20]. (Fig.12.38b) This analysis has significant implications in the daily clinical practice, as the management of tractional and exudative intraretinal cystoid spaces may require different therapeutic strategies.

Mario R Romano, Department of Biomedical Sciences, Humanitas University, Rozzano, Milano, Italy

Surgery (Table 12.1)

Additional surgical steps.

Stain the ERM with trypan and brilliant blue combined.
Peel off the ERM.
Re-stain the to detect residual ERM and the ILM.
Peel the ILM (Figs. 12.39 and 12.40).

Table 12.1 Difficulty rating for PPV for macular pucker

Difficulty Rating	Easy
Success rates	Moderate
Complication rates	Low
When to use in training	Early

In cellophane maculopathy, vitreomacular traction or macular pucker, pars plana vitrectomy is employed to access epiretinal membranes, allowing their surgical dissection and removal. This is often effective in reducing distortion and improving vision and is one of the easier procedures in vitreoretinal surgery [41].

Perform the usual vitrectomy, if the hyaloid is not detached peel it off watching to see if the ERM comes with it. Apply combined trypan and brilliant blue dyes. Leave for 30 seconds on the retina (enough time to switch over to the contact lens). Always loosen the syringe plunger by injecting a drop or two of dye outside of the eye. When commencing the injection of dye, point the dye needle tip at the light pipe so that if there is a sudden ingress of dye it is blocked by the

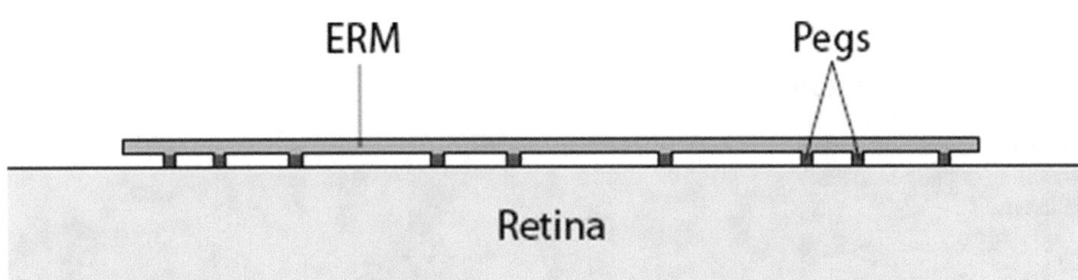

Fig. 12.39 ERMs have pegs of attachment to the retina

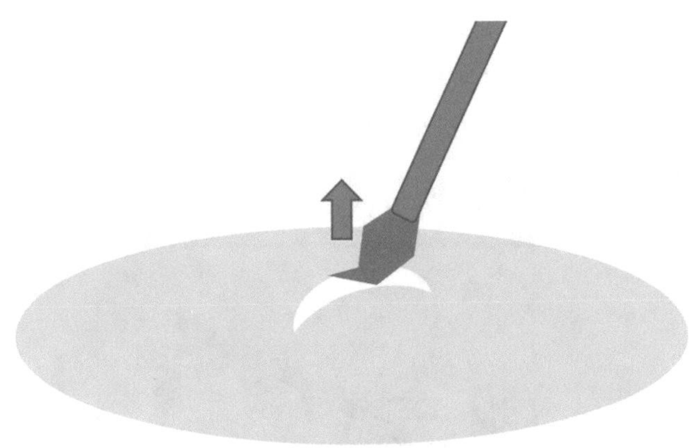

Fig. 12.40 Use a bent MVR blade to lift the ERM to provide an edge. Scraping the ERM as per ILM peel does not create a hole or edge in the ERM because the ERM is elastic and will stretch with the movement of the blade, however there is usually a virtual space between the ERM and the underlying ILM which can allow passage of a blade to commence lifting

light pipe and does not penetrate into the retina with a risk of going subretinally.

Note: Subretinal dye may be toxic. Thankfully, the blue dyes seem to be quite safe but indocyanine green is very toxic to the RPE and will lead to vision loss.

Use a contact lens to increase the magnification and depth perception but be aware of the reduction in visual field. The last makes it difficult to find the light pipe and forceps. Great care must be taken moving those inside the eye when visualising with a contact lens.

In small gauge surgery, use the forceps to grasp the ERM (You can use a bent needle to start the lift if necessary) in this circumstance it helps to grasp an edge if available to get started. Pull the membrane off the retina, trying not to tear the membrane, whilst observing the retina to avoid damage from the traction. Usually by adjusting the angle of the traction the membrane can be removed as one sheet. If there is a particularly strong attachment to the retina do not pull away from the site of attachment instead pull the membrane from around the attachment 360° and then over the top of it. The membrane is often much more extensive than expected sometimes spreading beyond the arcades. If a patch of ILM stains (i.e. it is not covered by the ERM), this is often a good place to start the peel. Pinch the ILM with the forceps as for a macular hole (see later chapter) and then peel into the area of ERM.

Re-stain the macula with the dye. Removal of the ILM helps to ensure removal of all the ERM which can on occasion be multi-layered. In addition, ILM removal reduces the chance of recurrence of the ERM postoperatively. It does not seem to influence vision.

Vitreomacular traction is a variant of epiretinal membrane and can be dealt with in a similar fashion.

The main aim is to relieve traction on the fovea. Do not leave membrane near to the fovea, i.e. clear at least 2-disc diameters around the fovea. You may however safely leave membrane from the arcades outward.

Occasionally a PVD is not present and must be induced. Sometimes the ERM will come with the vitreous but always check the retina with stain as there may still be ERM on the retina (Figs. 12.41, 12.42, 12.43 and 12.44).

Trypan blue stains ERM well and ILM poorly [42–46]. Indocyanine green has been used as an adjunct but has been associated with poorer visual acuity results and is best avoided [47]. As I usually remove the ILM routinely using a combination dye of brilliant blue and Trypan blue is useful.

Pucker can be removed at the time of silicone oil removal in cases of PVR often an ERM is more adherent to the retina in this pathology than in idiopathic ERM [48] (Figs. 12.45, 12.46, 12.47, and 12.48).

Success Rates

Vision can be improved in 80-86% [47, 49] and to 20/60 or better in 75%. Those with shorter duration, better presenting vision, thinner membranes and no retinal elevation, less disruption of the ellipsoid layer and thicker ganglion cell inner plexiform layer do better [50, 51]. Even if vision does not improve quality of life, scores are improved after surgery by reduction of distortion [52]. In general, patients can expect a 2 line improvement from where they start, therefore, to get better vision you need to start with better vision, however this needs balanced with the risks of surgery [53, 54]. The macula remodels after surgery by spreading out from the fovea [55]. (Figs. 12.49 and 12.50).

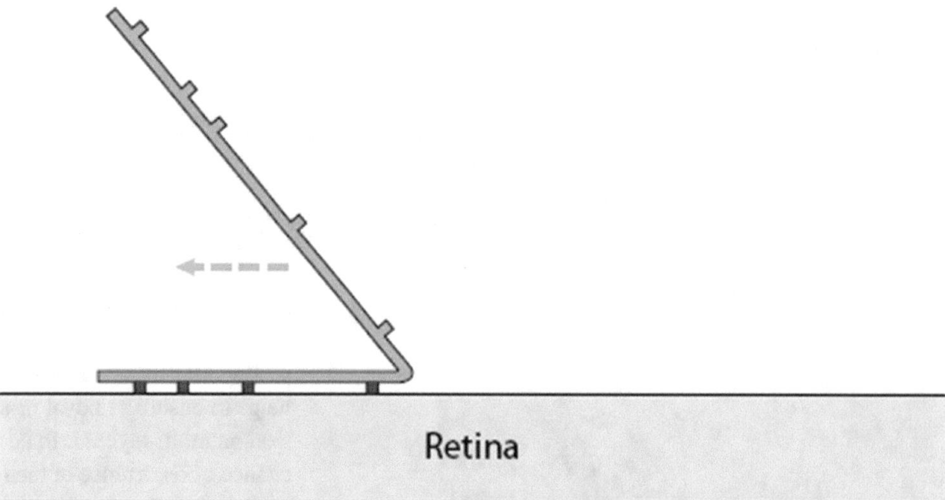

Fig. 12.41 By peeling the membrane back upon itself, most of the force is applied to the small pegs of attachment of the membrane, rather than providing traction onto the retina itself

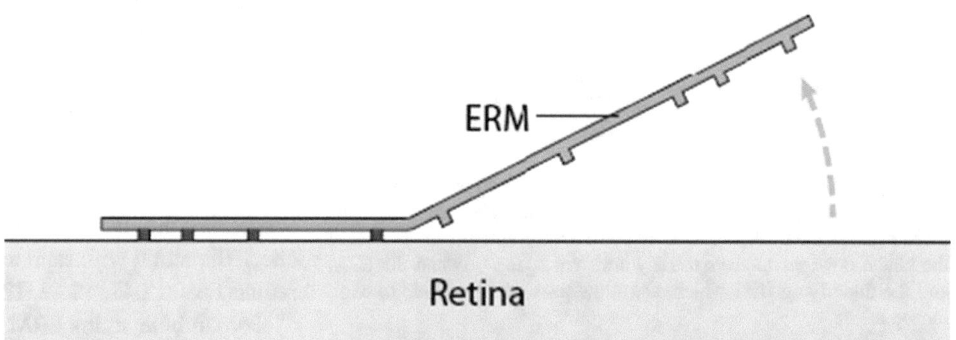

Fig. 12.42 By peeling the membrane upwards there is a force applied to the edge of the retina, which should be avoided

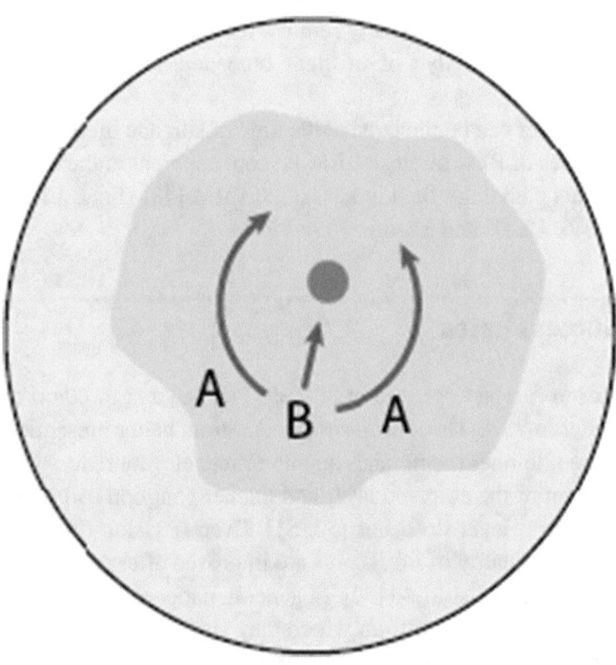

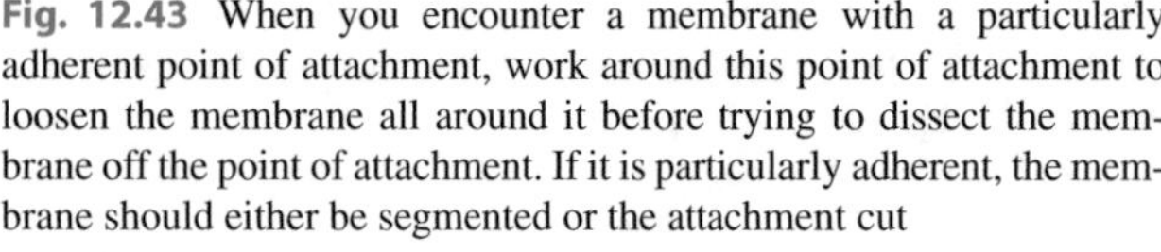

Fig. 12.43 When you encounter a membrane with a particularly adherent point of attachment, work around this point of attachment to loosen the membrane all around it before trying to dissect the membrane off the point of attachment. If it is particularly adherent, the membrane should either be segmented or the attachment cut

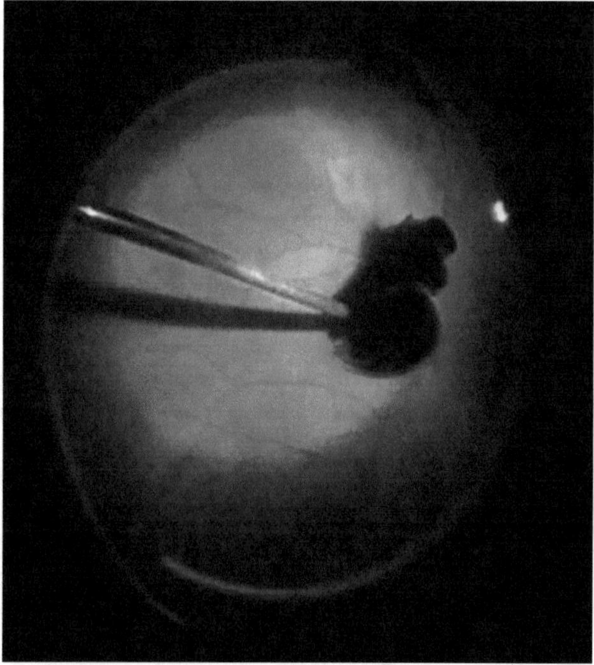

Fig. 12.44 Trypan blue can be used to stain the ERM or as a weak stain of the ILM. Aim the dye away from the macula and allow the dye to fall back onto the macula. This avoids the risk of injection of dye under the retina if there is a sudden burst of dye during the commencement of the injection

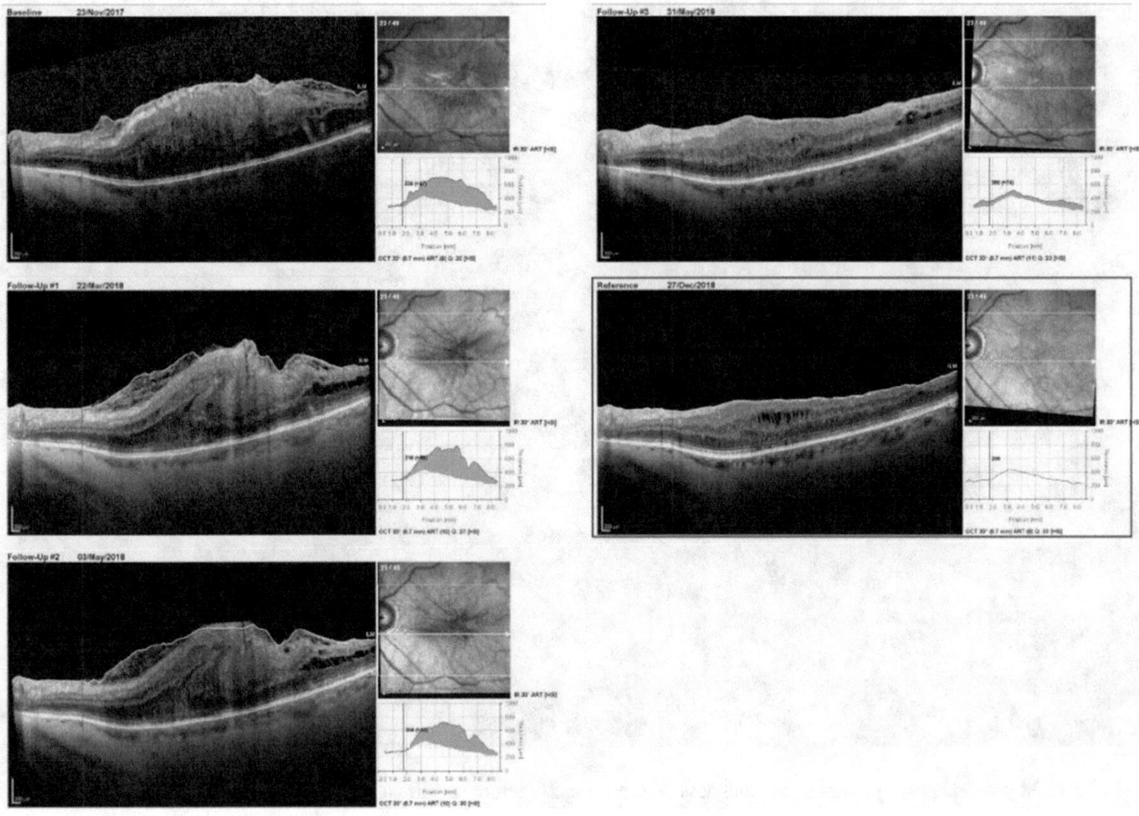

Fig. 12.45 ERM progression preoperatively on the left column and postoperatively on the right column

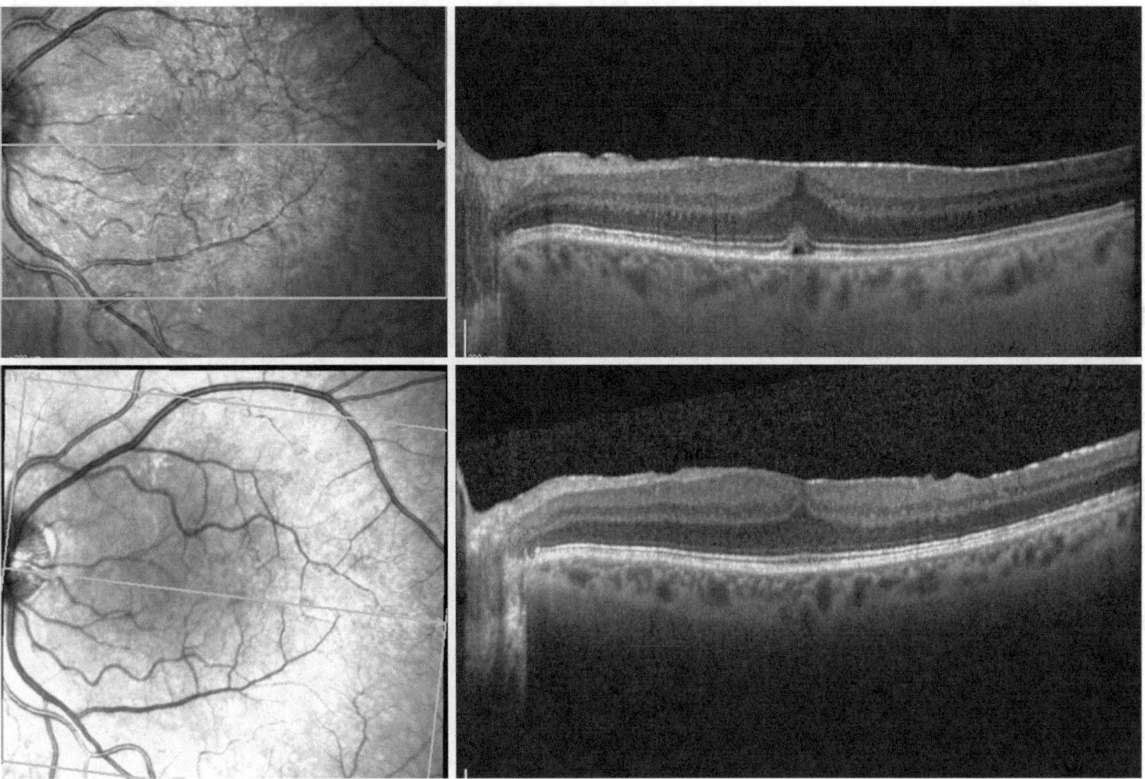

Fig. 12.46 An ERM peel pre- and postoperatively with good visual recovery

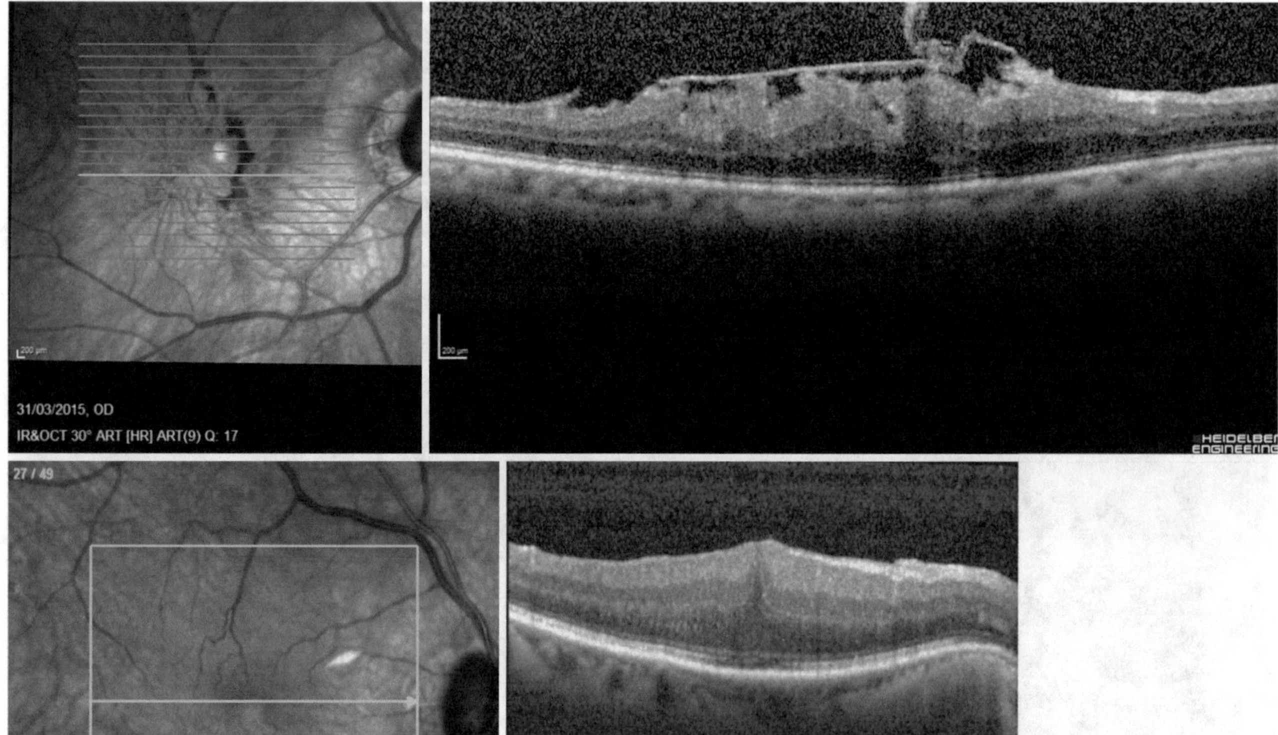

Fig. 12.47 An ERM pre- and post-op. The retinal thickness does not usually return to normal

Specific Complications

- Cataract appears in 47–80% [56, 57] for this reason many surgeons will combine PPV with phacoemulsification cataract surgery rather than wait for the cataract to develop. This approach is recommended.
- Damage to the internal limiting membrane and nerve fibre layer may result [58, 59]. Therefore, it is prudent to remove the ILM as well during surgery.
- Persistent cystoid macular oedema often unresponsive to IVTA or topical nonsteroidal anti-inflammatories.
- Myopic postoperative refraction may occur because the elevation of the retina in the macula by an ERM may lead to a short axial length during biometry and the use of an overly powerful IOL. See the example of measurements from a patient who developed an ERM and who had prior biometry measurements. The result of ERM on biometry is unpredictable. It is therefore difficult to introduce a correction factor. The patient should be warned about the variation. Leaving the cataract operation to after the vitrectomy does not seem to help [60] (Figs. 12.51 and 12.52).

	Before ERM	After ERM development
Axial length (mm)	23.93	23.27
Keratometry (D)	42.27	42.27
IOL suggested power (D)	21.0	23.0
Predicted refraction (D)	0	−0.06
Refraction (D) at time of biometry	0	+0.25

- Retinal tear and retinal detachment [61] may occur in 2.5% although this is less commonly reported than for macular hole in which the posterior hyaloid membrane must be detached [62]. If PVD is induced, retinal tears have been described in 32.1% compared to 2.1% in those without induction of PVD [63]. Often old retinal tears are found at the time of surgery. These have occurred at the time of posterior vitreous detachment commonly more than a year before presentation. They can be treated with retinopexy and air inserted (they may be safe without tamponade, but inserting air has minimal impact on the rate of visual recovery) (Figs. 12.53, 12.54, 12.55 and 12.56).

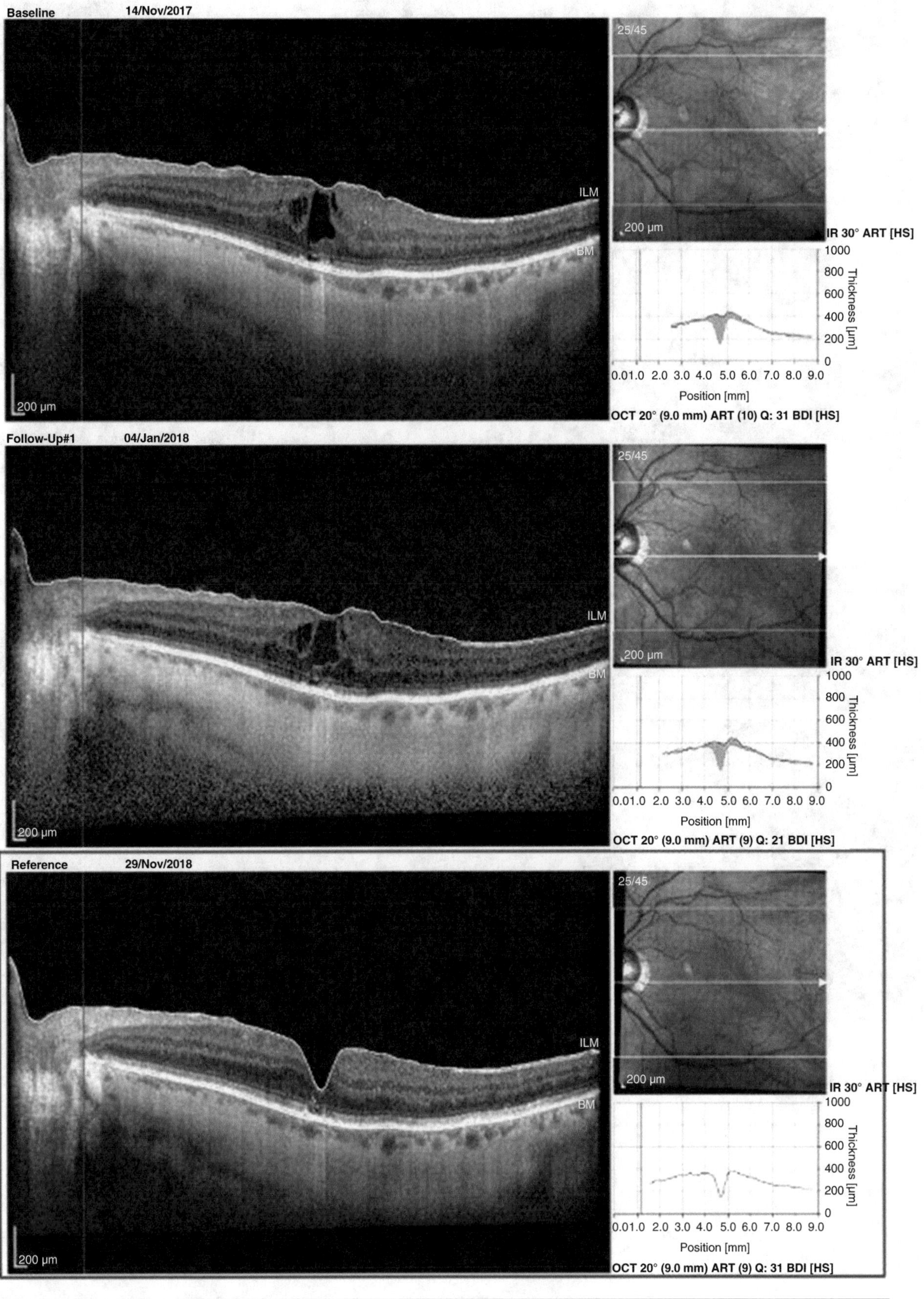

Fig. 12.48 Spontaneous resolution or ERM occurs in approximately 3% of cases

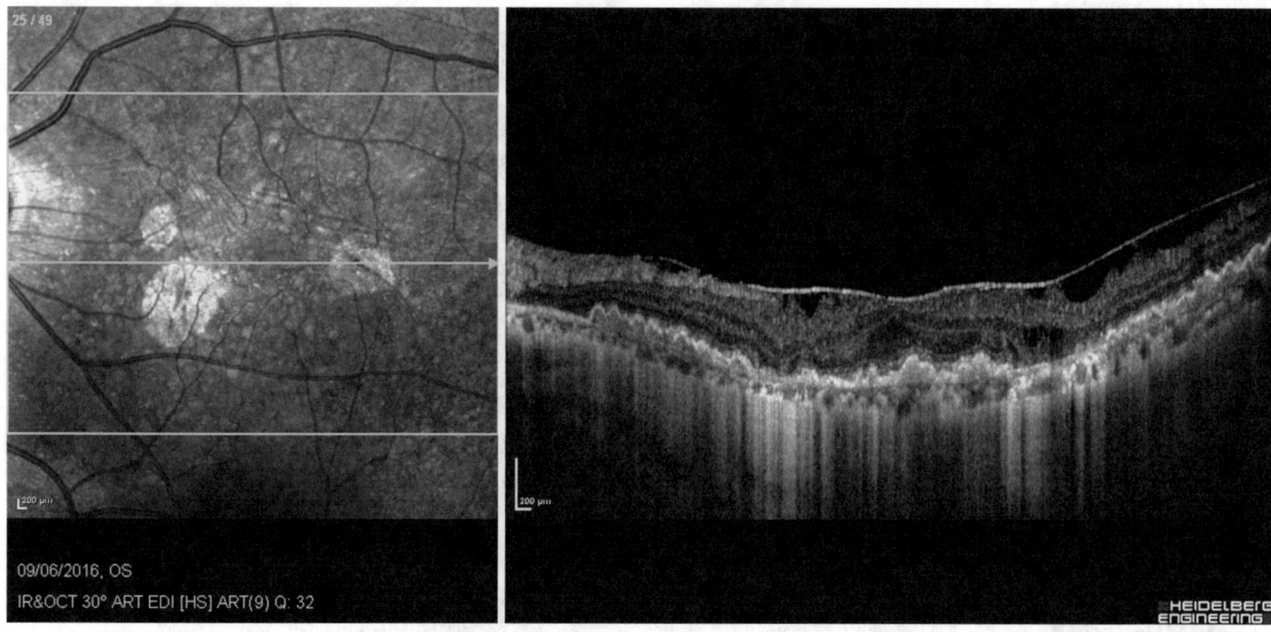

Fig. 12.49 Surgery on ERM with underlying age macular degeneration has lower success rates for improving vision

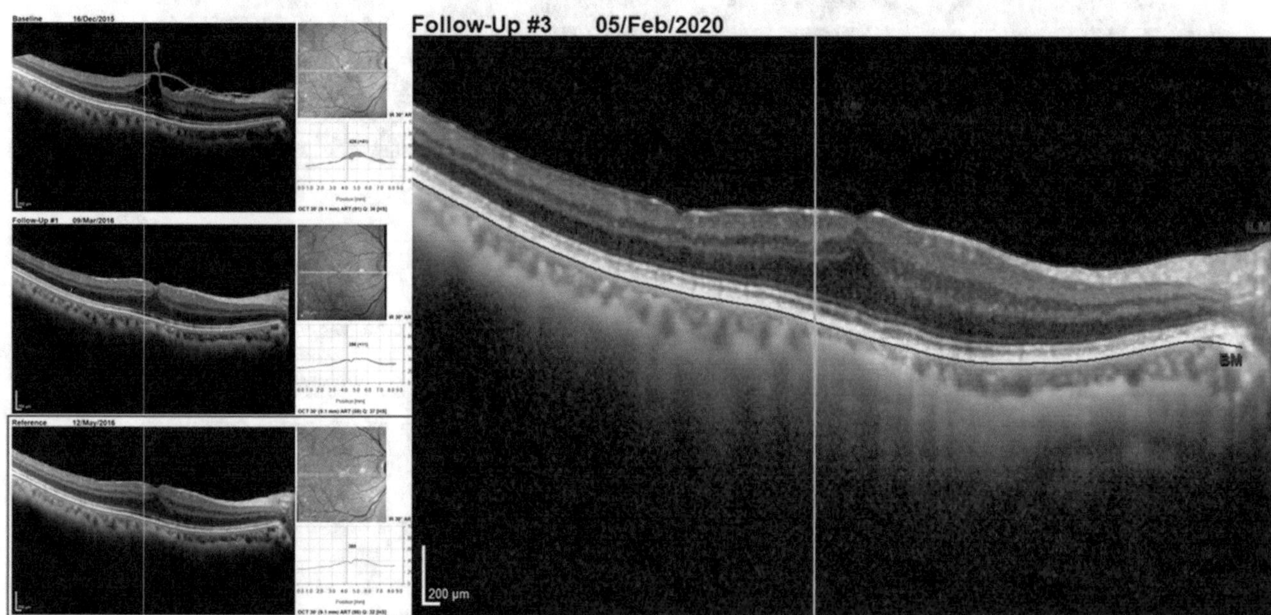

Fig. 12.50 The retina heals very slowly. In this patient there is improvement in the ellipsoid layer over 3 years after ERM surgery with accompanying increase in visual acuity

Membrane Recurrence

This has been shown to occur in 4–20% of cases [64–66] but will respond to repeated surgery. Removal of the ILM has been reported to reduce recurrence [66] and is now my routine practice. After surgery recurrence appears to be more common in secondary ERM, e.g. in patients with retinal angiomata (30%) [67] and in uveitis [68]. A small group of ERMs, 3%, may spontaneously disappear over time. ERM are usually stable one year after their occurrence however an occasional ERM can change and progress (Figs. 12.57, 12.58, and 12.59).

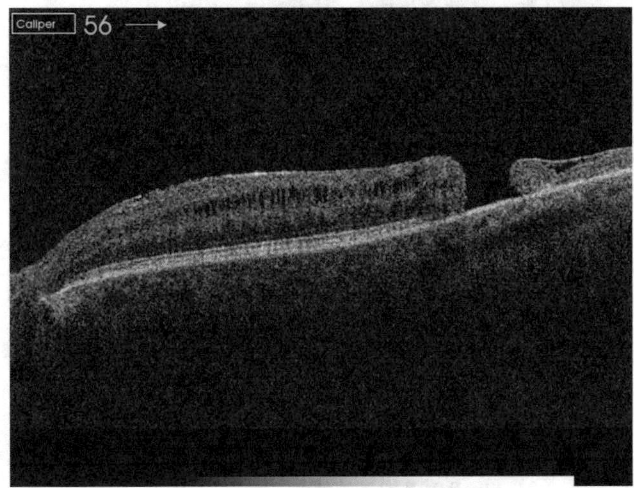

Fig. 12.51 A paracentral macular hole after peel surgery. This can be left alone and does not detach

Summary

Epiretinal membranes are usually easily removed however surprises can occur. Visual results can also be unpredictable with distortion improving more often that visual acuity. Operating with good vision achieves better outcomes but the unpredictability of surgery can lead to an occasional bed outcome.

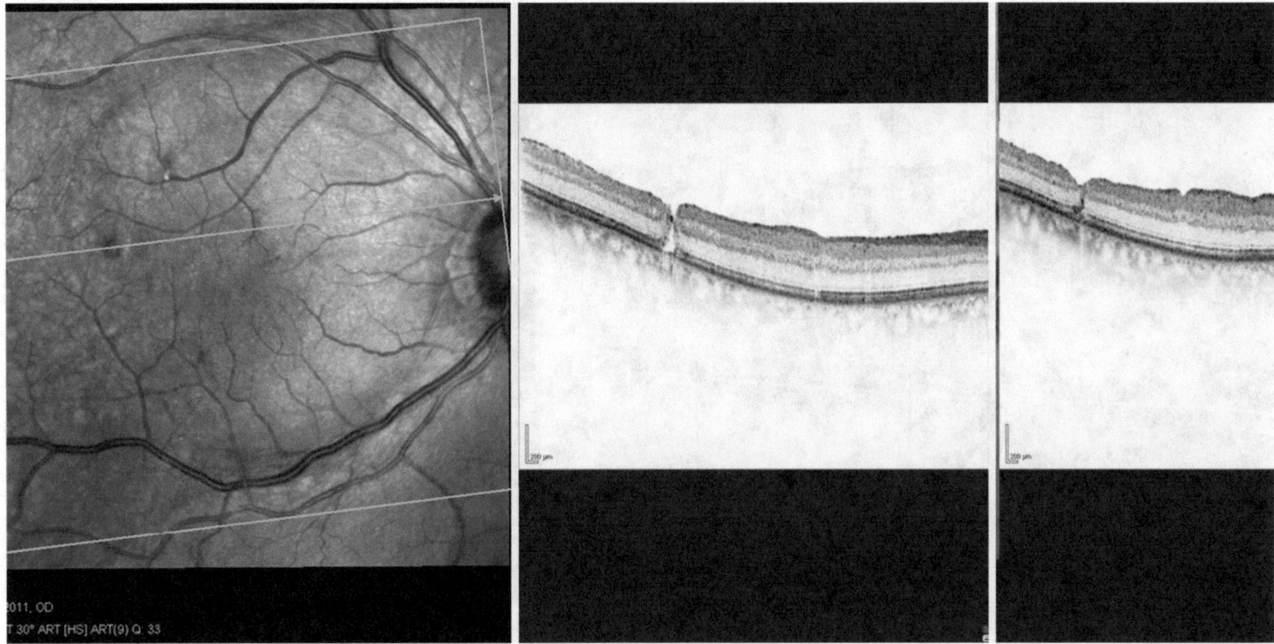

Fig. 12.52 An eccentric hole in the macula after ERM peel which eventually closed spontaneously

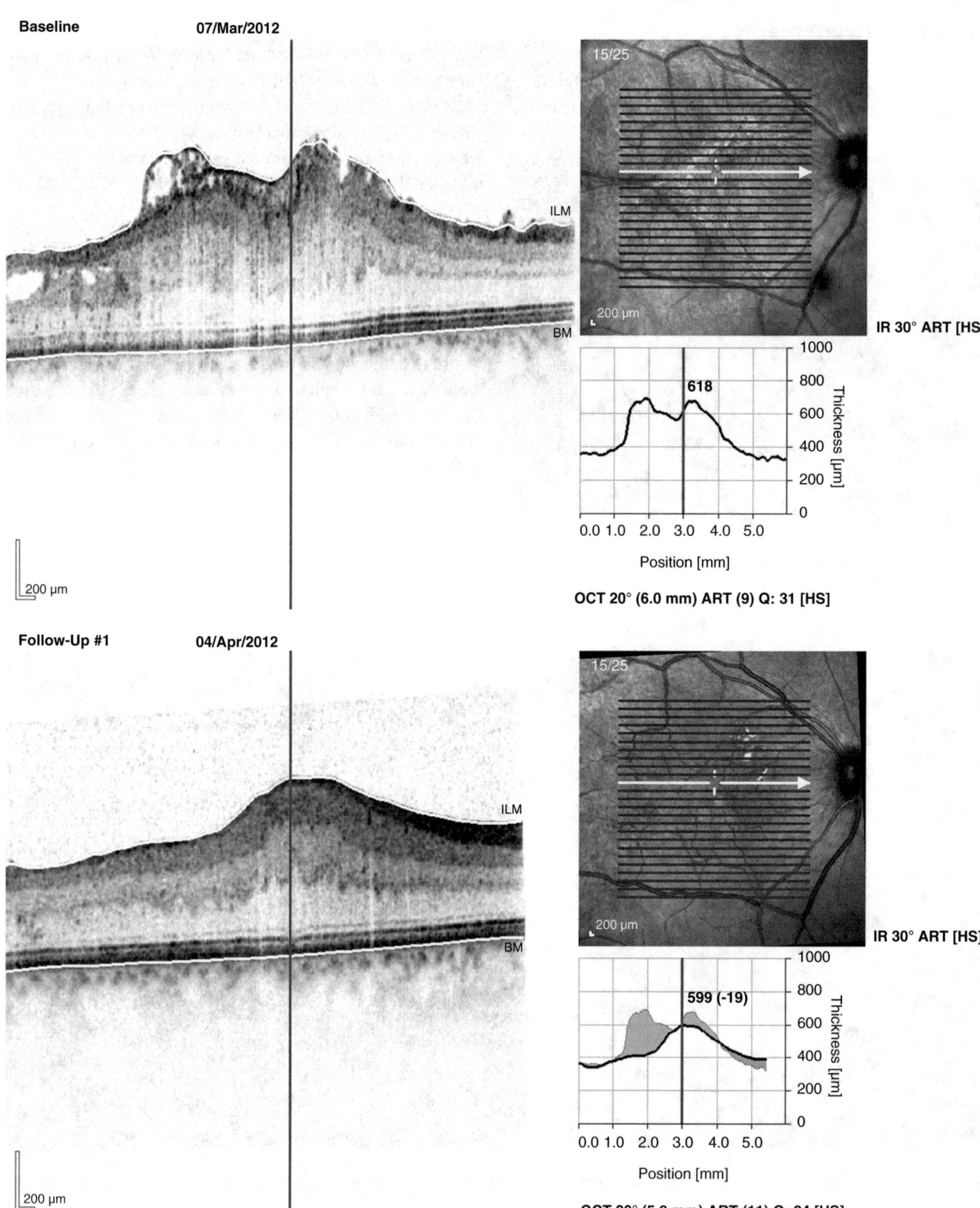

Fig. 12.53 ERM before and after surgery

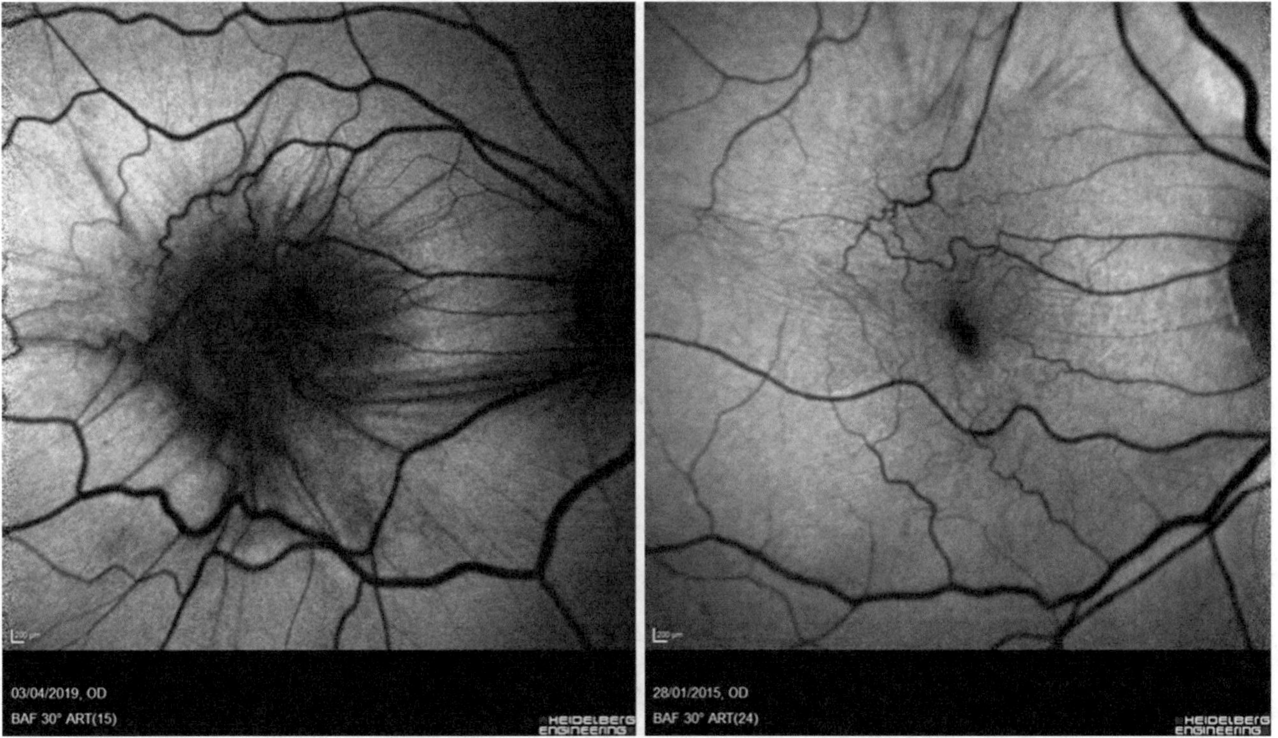

Fig. 12.54 Distortion before and after surgery for ERM

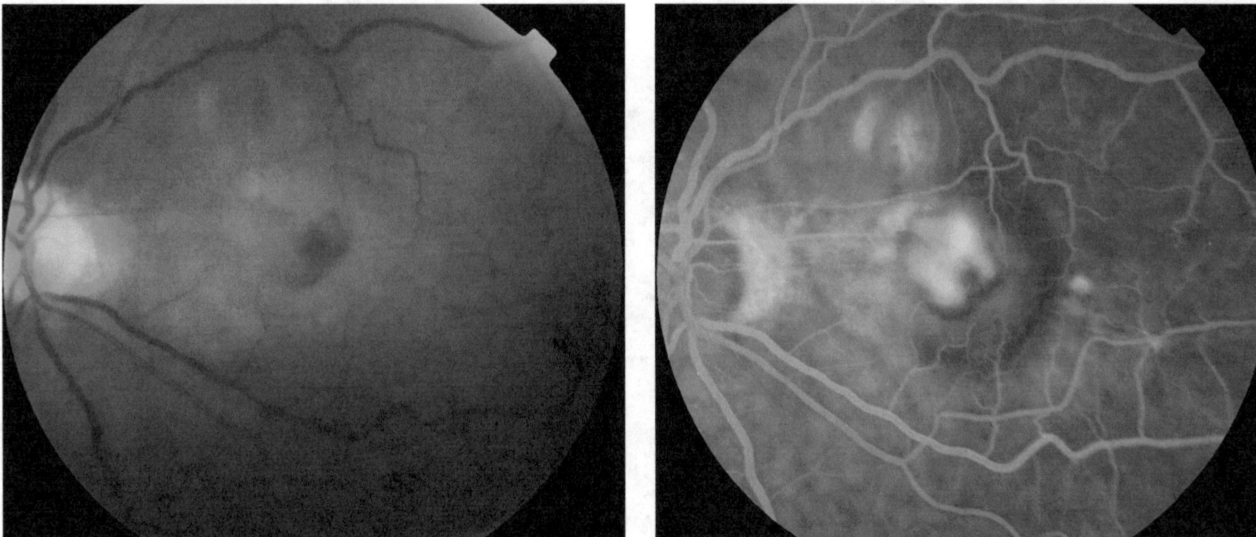

Fig. 12.55 Damage to the macula after removal of ERM has caused a secondary CNV to form

Fig. 12.56 FFA of the CNV

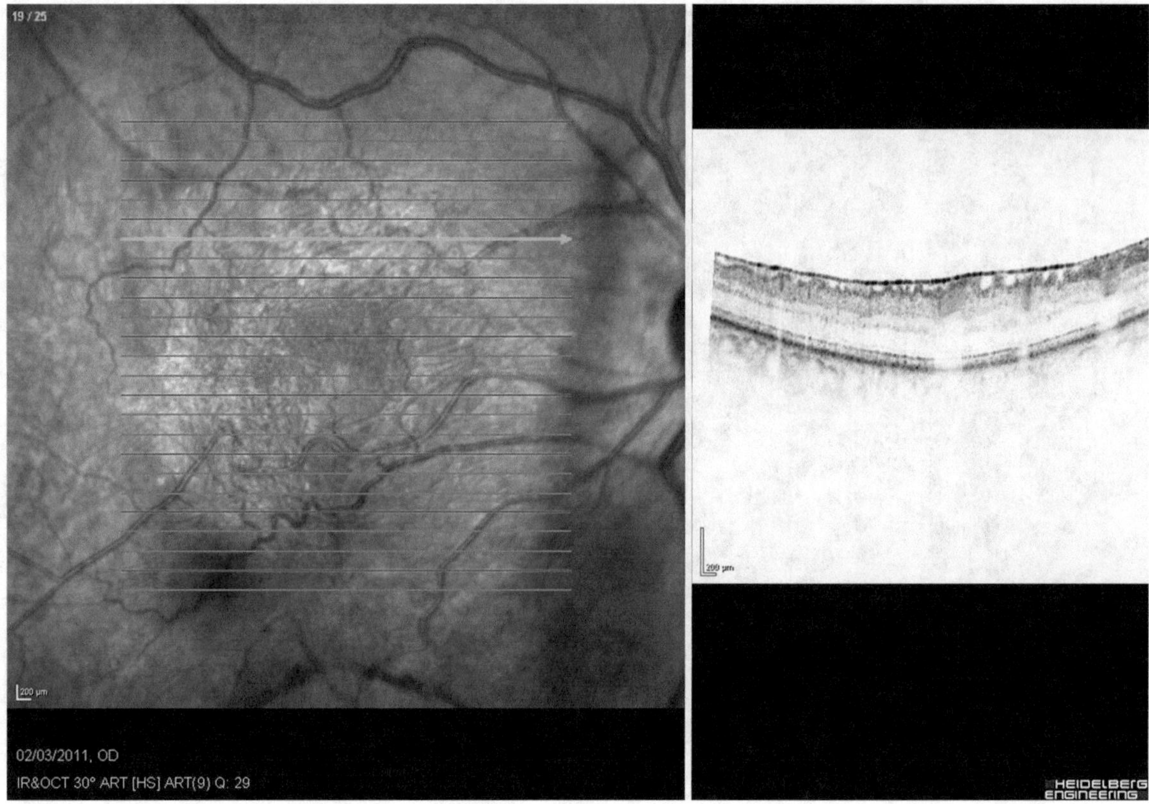

Fig. 12.57 ERM can recur after surgery, removing the ILM may reduce recurrence

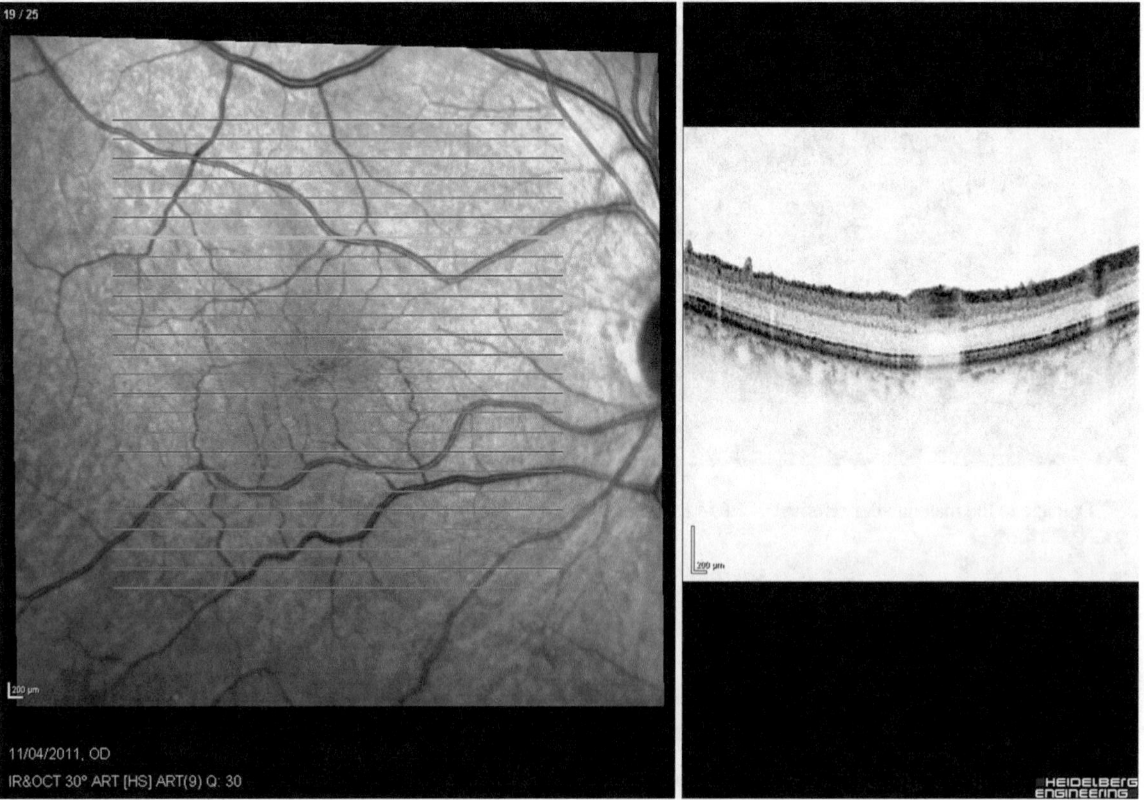

Fig. 12.58 The macula without ERM postoperatively

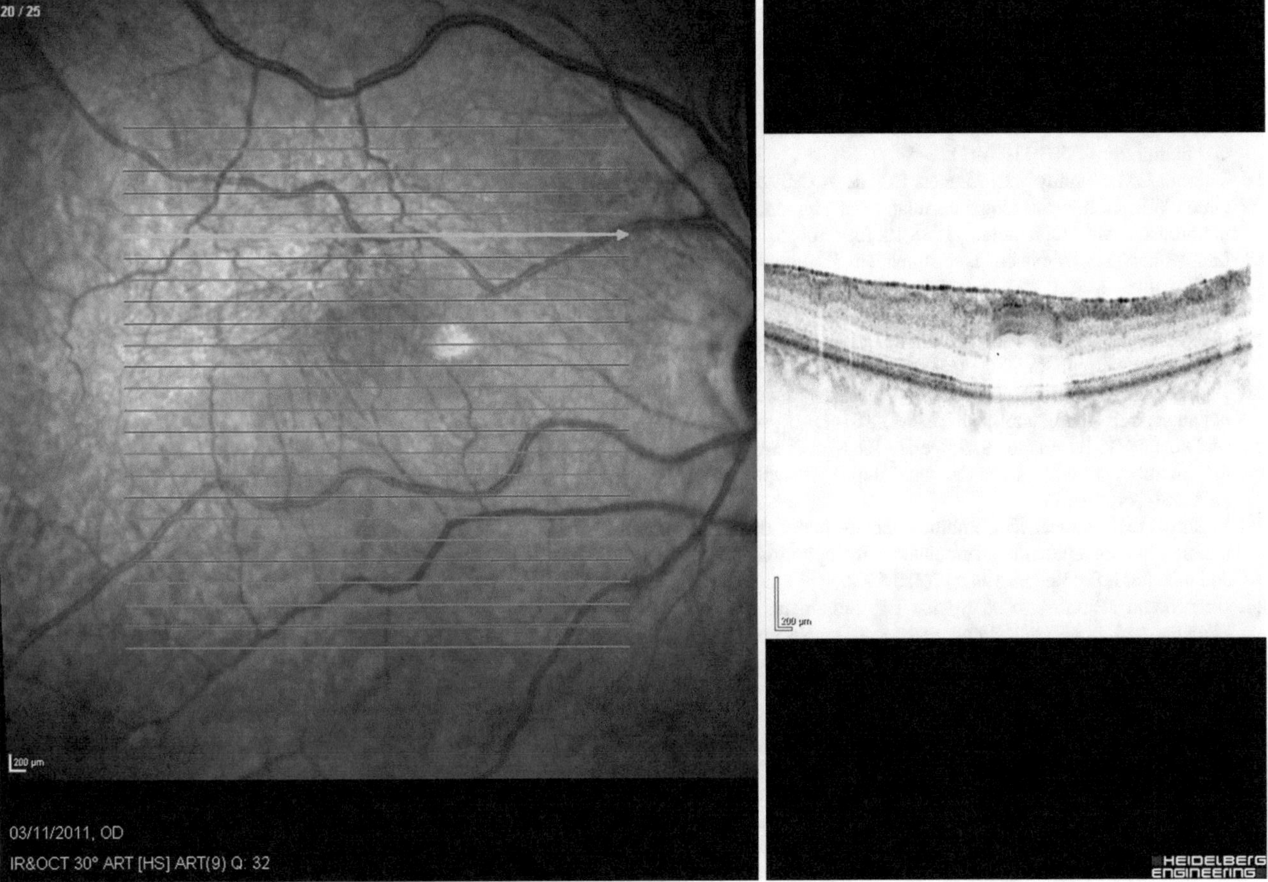

Fig. 12.59 The ERM returns over time

References

1. Messmer EM, Heidenkummer HP, Kampik A. Ultrastructure of epiretinal membranes associated with macular holes. Graefes Arch Clin Exp Ophthalmol. 1998;236(4):248–54.
2. Snead DR, Cullen N, James S, Poulson AV, Morris AH, Lukaris A, et al. Hyperconvolution of the inner limiting membrane in vitreomaculopathies. Graefes Arch Clin Exp Ophthalmol. 2004;242(10):853–62.
3. De Juan E, Jr., Lambert HM, Machemer R. Recurrent proliferations in macular pucker, diabetic retinopathy, and retrolental fibroplasialike disease after vitrectomy. Graefes Arch Clin Exp Ophthalmol. 1985;223(4):174–83.
4. Smiddy WE, Michels RG, Gilbert HD, Green WR. Clinicopathologic study of idiopathic macular pucker in children and young adults. Retina. 1992;12(3):232–6.
5. Ng CH, Cheung N, Wang JJ, Islam AF, Kawasaki R, Meuer SM, et al. Prevalence and risk factors for epiretinal membranes in a multi-ethnic United States population. Ophthalmology. 2011;118(4):694–9. https://doi.org/10.1016/j.ophtha.2010.08.009.
6. Klein R, Klein BE, Wang Q, Moss SE. The epidemiology of epiretinal membranes. Trans Am Ophthalmol Soc. 1994;92:403–25. discussion 25–30
7. Allen AW Jr, Gass JD. Contraction of a perifoveal epiretinal membrane simulating a macular hole. Am J Ophthalmol. 1976;82(5):684–91.
8. Martinez J, Smiddy WE, Kim J, Gass JD. Differentiating macular holes from macular pseudoholes. Am J Ophthalmol. 1994;117(6):762–7.
9. Fajgenbaum MAP, Wong RS, Laidlaw DAH, Williamson TH. Vitreoretinal surgery on the fellow eye: a retrospective analysis of 18 years of surgical data from a tertiary center in England. Indian J Ophthalmol. 2018;66(5):681–6. https://doi.org/10.4103/ijo.IJO_1176_17.
10. Desatnik H, Treister G, Moisseiev J. Spontaneous separation of an idiopathic macular pucker in a young girl. Am J Ophthalmol. 1999;127(6):729–31.
11. Meyer CH, Rodrigues EB, Mennel S, Schmidt JC, Kroll P. Spontaneous separation of epiretinal membrane in young subjects: personal observations and review of the literature. Graefes Arch Clin Exp Ophthalmol. 2004;242(12):977–85. https://doi.org/10.1007/s00417-004-0934-7.
12. de Bustros S, Rice TA, Michels RG, Thompson JT, Marcus S, Glaser BM. Vitrectomy for macular pucker. Use after treatment of retinal tears or retinal detachment. Arch Ophthalmol. 1988;106(6):758–60.
13. Lobes LA Jr, Burton TC. The incidence of macular pucker after retinal detachment surgery. Am J Ophthalmol. 1978;85(1):72–7.
14. Ishida Y, Iwama Y, Nakashima H, Ikeda T, Emi K. Risk factors, onset, and progression of Epiretinal membrane after 25-gauge pars Plana vitrectomy for Rhegmatogenous retinal detachment. Ophthalmol Retina. 2019; https://doi.org/10.1016/j.oret.2019.10.004.
15. Cox MS, Azen SP, Barr CC, Linton KL, Diddie KR, Lai MY, et al. Macular pucker after successful surgery for prolifera-

tive vitreoretinopathy. Silicone study report 8. Ophthalmology. 1995;102(12):1884–91.

16. Wilson DJ, Green WR. Histopathologic study of the effect of retinal detachment surgery on 49 eyes obtained post mortem. Am J Ophthalmol. 1987;103(2):167–79.
17. Sheard RM, Sethi C, Gregor Z. Acute macular pucker. Ophthalmology. 2003;110(6):1178–84.
18. Cherfan GM, Smiddy WE, Michels RG, de la CZ, Wilkinson CP, Green WR. Clinicopathologic correlation of pigmented epiretinal membranes. Am J Ophthalmol. 1988;106(5):536–45.
19. Laatikainen L, Immonen I, Summanen P. Peripheral retinal angiomalike lesion and macular pucker. Am J Ophthalmol. 1989;108(5):563–6.
20. Machemer R. Peripheral retinal angiomalike lesion and macular pucker. Am J Ophthalmol. 1990;109(2):244.
21. Carney MD, Jampol LM. Epiretinal membranes in sickle cell retinopathy. Arch Ophthalmol. 1987;105(2):214–7.
22. McDonald HR, de Bustros S, Sipperley JO. Vitrectomy for epiretinal membrane with Candida chorioretinitis. Ophthalmology. 1990;97(4):466–9.
23. Mason JO III, Kleiner R. Combined hamartoma of the retina and retinal pigment epithelium associated with epiretinal membrane and macular hole. Retina. 1997;17(2):160–2.
24. Hubschman JP, Govetto A, Spaide RF, Schumann R, Steel D, Figueroa MS, et al. Optical coherence tomography-based consensus definition for lamellar macular hole. Br J Ophthalmol. 2020; https://doi.org/10.1136/bjophthalmol-2019-315432.
25. Bu SC, Kuijer R, Li XR, Hooymans JM, Los LI. Idiopathic epiretinal membrane. Retina. 2014;34(12):2317–35. https://doi.org/10.1097/IAE.0000000000000349.
26. Cheung N, Tan SP, Lee SY, Cheung GCM, Tan G, Kumar N, et al. Prevalence and risk factors for epiretinal membrane: the Singapore epidemiology of eye disease study. Br J Ophthalmol. 2017;101(3):371–6. https://doi.org/10.1136/bjophthalmol-2016-308563.
27. Romano MR, Comune C, Ferrara M, Cennamo G, De Cilla S, Toto L, et al. Retinal changes induced by Epiretinal tangential forces. J Ophthalmol. 2015;2015:372564. https://doi.org/10.1155/2015/372564.
28. Kritzenberger M, Junglas B, Framme C, Helbig H, Gabel VP, Fuchshofer R, et al. Different collagen types define two types of idiopathic epiretinal membranes. Histopathology. 2011;58(6):953–65. https://doi.org/10.1111/j.1365-2559.2011.03820.x.
29. Compera D, Entchev E, Haritoglou C, Scheler R, Mayer WJ, Wolf A, et al. Lamellar hole-associated Epiretinal proliferation in comparison to Epiretinal membranes of macular Pseudoholes. Am J Ophthalmol. 2015;160(2):373–84. e1. https://doi.org/10.1016/j.ajo.2015.05.010.
30. Govetto A, Hubschman JP, Sarraf D, Figueroa MS, Bottoni F, dell'omo R, et al. The role of Muller cells in tractional macular disorders: an optical coherence tomography study and physical model of mechanical force transmission. Br J Ophthalmol. 2020;104(4):466–72. https://doi.org/10.1136/bjophthalmol-2019-314245.
31. Lu YB, Iandiev I, Hollborn M, Korber N, Ulbricht E, Hirrlinger PG, et al. Reactive glial cells: increased stiffness correlates with increased intermediate filament expression. FASEB J. 2011;25(2):624–31. https://doi.org/10.1096/fj.10-163790.
32. Govetto A, Lalane RA 3rd, Sarraf D, Figueroa MS, Hubschman JP. Insights into Epiretinal membranes: presence of ectopic inner foveal layers and a new optical coherence tomography staging scheme. Am J Ophthalmol. 2017;175:99–113. https://doi.org/10.1016/j.ajo.2016.12.006.
33. Romano MR, Cennamo G, Amoroso F, Montorio D, Castellani C, Reibaldi M, et al. Intraretinal changes in the presence of epiretinal traction. Graefes Arch Clin Exp Ophthalmol. 2017;255(1):31–8. https://doi.org/10.1007/s00417-016-3413-z.
34. Romano MR, Ilardi G, Ferrara M, Cennamo G, Allegrini D, Pafundi PC, et al. Intraretinal changes in idiopathic versus diabetic epiretinal membranes after macular peeling. PLoS One. 2018;13(5):e0197065. https://doi.org/10.1371/journal.pone.0197065.
35. Bringmann A, Pannicke T, Grosche J, Francke M, Wiedemann P, Skatchkov SN, et al. Muller cells in the healthy and diseased retina. Prog Retin Eye Res. 2006;25(4):397–424. https://doi.org/10.1016/j.preteyeres.2006.05.003.
36. Baek J, Park HY, Lee JH, Choi M, Lee JH, Ha M, et al. Elevated M2 macrophage markers in Epiretinal membranes with ectopic inner foveal layers. Invest Ophthalmol Vis Sci. 2020;61(2):19. https://doi.org/10.1167/iovs.61.2.19.
37. Govetto A, Virgili G, Rodriguez FJ, Figueroa MS, Sarraf D, Hubschman JP. Functional and anatomical significance of the ectopic inner foveal layers in eyes with idiopathic epiretinal membranes: surgical results at 12 months. Retina. 2019;39(2):347–57. https://doi.org/10.1097/IAE.0000000000001940.
38. Govetto A, Bhavsar KV, Virgili G, Gerber MJ, Freund KB, Curcio CA, et al. Tractional abnormalities of the central foveal bouquet in Epiretinal membranes: clinical Spectrum and pathophysiological perspectives. Am J Ophthalmol. 2017;184:167–80. https://doi.org/10.1016/j.ajo.2017.10.011.
39. Tien T, Zhang J, Muto T, Kim D, Sarthy VP, Roy S. High glucose induces mitochondrial dysfunction in retinal Muller cells: implications for diabetic retinopathy. Invest Ophthalmol Vis Sci. 2017;58(7):2915–21. https://doi.org/10.1167/iovs.16-21355.
40. Reichenbach A, Bringmann A. New functions of Muller cells. Glia. 2013;61(5):651–78. https://doi.org/10.1002/glia.22477.
41. Michels RG. Vitreous surgery for macular pucker. Am J Ophthalmol. 1981;92(5):628–39.
42. Haritoglou C, Gandorfer A, Schaumberger M, Priglinger SG, Mueller AJ, Gass CA, et al. Trypan blue in macular pucker surgery: an evaluation of histology and functional outcome. Retina. 2004;24(4):582–90.
43. Haritoglou C, Eibl K, Schaumberger M, Mueller AJ, Priglinger S, Alge C, et al. Functional outcome after trypan blue-assisted vitrectomy for macular pucker: a prospective, randomized, comparative trial. Am J Ophthalmol. 2004;138(1):1–5.
44. Li K, Wong D, Hiscott P, Stanga P, Groenewald C, McGalliard J. Trypan blue staining of internal limiting membrane and epiretinal membrane during vitrectomy: visual results and histopathological findings. Br J Ophthalmol. 2003;87(2):216–9.
45. Stalmans P, Feron EJ, Parys-Van GR, Van LA, Melles GR, Veckeneer M. Double vital staining using trypan blue and infracyanine green in macular pucker surgery. Br J Ophthalmol. 2003;87(6):713–6.
46. Teba FA, Mohr A, Eckardt C, Wong D, Kusaka S, Joondeph BC, et al. Trypan blue staining in vitreoretinal surgery. Ophthalmology. 2003;110(12):2409–12.
47. Haritoglou C, Gandorfer A, Gass CA, Schaumberger M, Ulbig MW, Kampik A. The effect of indocyanine-green on functional outcome of macular pucker surgery. Am J Ophthalmol. 2003;135(3):328–37.
48. Korobelnik JF, Hannouche D, D'Hermies F, Egot S, Frau E, Chauvaud D, et al. Silicone oil removal combined with macular pucker dissection: a retrospective review of 14 cases. Retina. 1998;18(3):228–32.
49. Trese MT, Chandler DB, Machemer R. Macular pucker. I. Prognostic criteria. Graefes Arch Clin Exp Ophthalmol. 1983;221(1):12–5.
50. de Bustros S, Thompson JT, Michels RG, Rice TA, Glaser BM. Vitrectomy for idiopathic epiretinal membranes causing macular pucker. Br J Ophthalmol. 1988;72(9):692–5.
51. Lee EK, Yu HG. Ganglion cell-inner plexiform layer thickness after epiretinal membrane surgery: a spectral-domain optical coherence tomography study. Ophthalmology. 2014;121(8):1579–87. https://doi.org/10.1016/j.ophtha.2014.02.010.
52. Ghazi-Nouri SM, Tranos PG, Rubin GS, Adams ZC, Charteris DG. Visual function and quality of life following vitrec-

tomy and epiretinal membrane peel surgery. Br J Ophthalmol. 2006;90(5):559–62.

53. Dawson SR, Shunmugam M, Williamson TH. Visual acuity outcomes following surgery for idiopathic epiretinal membrane: an analysis of data from 2001 to 2011. Eye (Lond). 2014;28(2):219–24. https://doi.org/10.1038/eye.2013.253.
54. Jackson TL, Donachie PH, Williamson TH, Sparrow JM, Johnston RL. The royal college of ophthalmologists' national ophthalmology database study of vitreoretinal surgery: report 4. Epiretinal Membrane Retina. 2015;35(8):1615–21. https://doi.org/10.1097/IAE.0000000000000523.
55. Rodrigues IA, Lee EJ, Williamson TH. Measurement of retinal displacement and Metamorphopsia after Epiretinal membrane or macular hole surgery. Retina. 2016;36(4):695–702. https://doi.org/10.1097/IAE.0000000000000768.
56. Cherfan GM, Michels RG, de BS, Enger C, Glaser BM. Nuclear sclerotic cataract after vitrectomy for idiopathic epiretinal membranes causing macular pucker. Am J Ophthalmol. 1991;111(4):434–8.
57. De BS, Thompson JT, Michels RG, Enger C, Rice TA, Glaser BM. Nuclear sclerosis after vitrectomy for idiopathic epiretinal membranes. Am J Ophthalmol. 1988;105(2):160–4.
58. Maguire AM, Smiddy WE, Nanda SK, Michels RG, de la CZ, Green WR. Clinicopathologic correlation of recurrent epiretinal membranes after previous surgical removal. Retina. 1990;10(3):213–22.
59. Trese M, Chandler DB, Machemer R. Macular pucker. II. Ultrastructure. Graefes Arch Clin Exp Ophthalmol. 1983;221(1):16–26.
60. Manvikar SR, Allen D, Steel DH. Optical biometry in combined phacovitrectomy. J Cataract Refract Surg. 2009;35(1):64–9. https://doi.org/10.1016/j.jcrs.2008.09.020.
61. Michels RG, Gilbert HD. Surgical management of macular pucker after retinal reattachment surgery. Am J Ophthalmol. 1979;88(5):925–9.
62. Guillaubey A, Malvitte L, Lafontaine PO, Hubert I, Bron A, Berrod JP, et al. Incidence of retinal detachment after macular surgery: a retrospective study of 634 cases. Br J Ophthalmol. 2007;91(10):1327–30. https://doi.org/10.1136/bjo.2007.115162.
63. Chung SE, Kim KH, Kang SW. Retinal breaks associated with the induction of posterior vitreous detachment. Am J Ophthalmol. 2009;147(6):1012–6. https://doi.org/10.1016/j.ajo.2009.01.013.
64. Michels RG. Vitrectomy for macular pucker. Ophthalmology. 1984;91(11):1384–8.
65. Grewing R, Mester U. Results of surgery for epiretinal membranes and their recurrences. Br J Ophthalmol. 1996;80(4):323–6.
66. Park DW, Dugel PU, Garda J, Sipperley JO, Thach A, Sneed SR, et al. Macular pucker removal with and without internal limiting membrane peeling: pilot study. Ophthalmology. 2003;110(1):62–4.
67. McDonald HR, Schatz H, Johnson RN, Abrams GW, Brown GC, Brucker AJ, et al. Vitrectomy in eyes with peripheral retinal angioma associated with traction macular detachment. Ophthalmology. 1996;103(2):329–35.
68. Verbraeken H. Therapeutic pars plana vitrectomy for chronic uveitis: a retrospective study of the long-term results. Graefes Arch Clin Exp Ophthalmol. 1996;234(5):288–93.

Choroidal Neovascular Membrane

13

Contents

Age-Related Macular Degeneration

Clinical Features (Figs. 13.1, 13.2, and 13.3)

Choroidal neovascular membranes (CNVs) most commonly occur with age-related macular degeneration (ARMD). Features of "dry" AMD include hard drusen, soft drusen, retinal pigment epithelial disruption and geographic atrophy.

- Patients with extensive small drusen, non-extensive intermediate size drusen, or pigment abnormalities have only a 1.3% 5-year probability of progression to advanced AMD according to the AREDs study [1].
- Those with extensive intermediate size drusen, at least 1 large druse, non-central geographic atrophy in 1 or both eyes, or advanced AMD or vision loss due to AMD in 1 eye, are at a risk of vision loss from advanced AMD in up to 50% (large drusen with pigmentary changes) after 5 years [2].

Simplified AREDs scoring system

- 1 or more large drusen (> or = 125 microns, width of a large vein at disc margin) in an eye = 1 risk factor
- Any pigment abnormality in an eye = 1 risk factor.
- Risk factors summed across both eyes.
- The 5-year risk of developing advanced AMD in at least one eye.
  - 0 factor 0.5%
  - 1 factor 3%
  - 2 factors 12%
  - 3 factors 25%
  - 4 factors 50%.
- If no large drusen but intermediate drusen present in both eyes = 1 risk factor.

This risk can be reduced by taking a cocktail of high dose vitamins (commercially available in combination preparations) such as 500 mg vitamin C, 400 IU vitamin E, and

T. H. Williamson, *Vitreoretinal Surgery*, https://doi.org/10.1007/978-3-030-68769-4_13

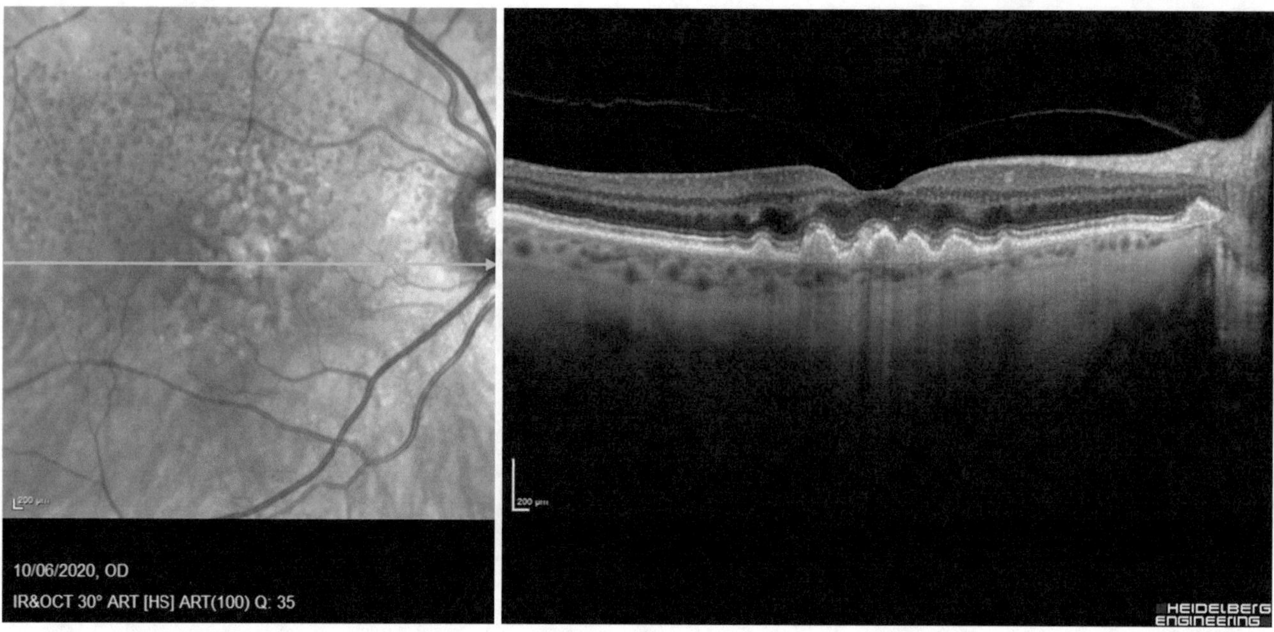

Fig. 13.1 High risk drusen for conversion to CNV

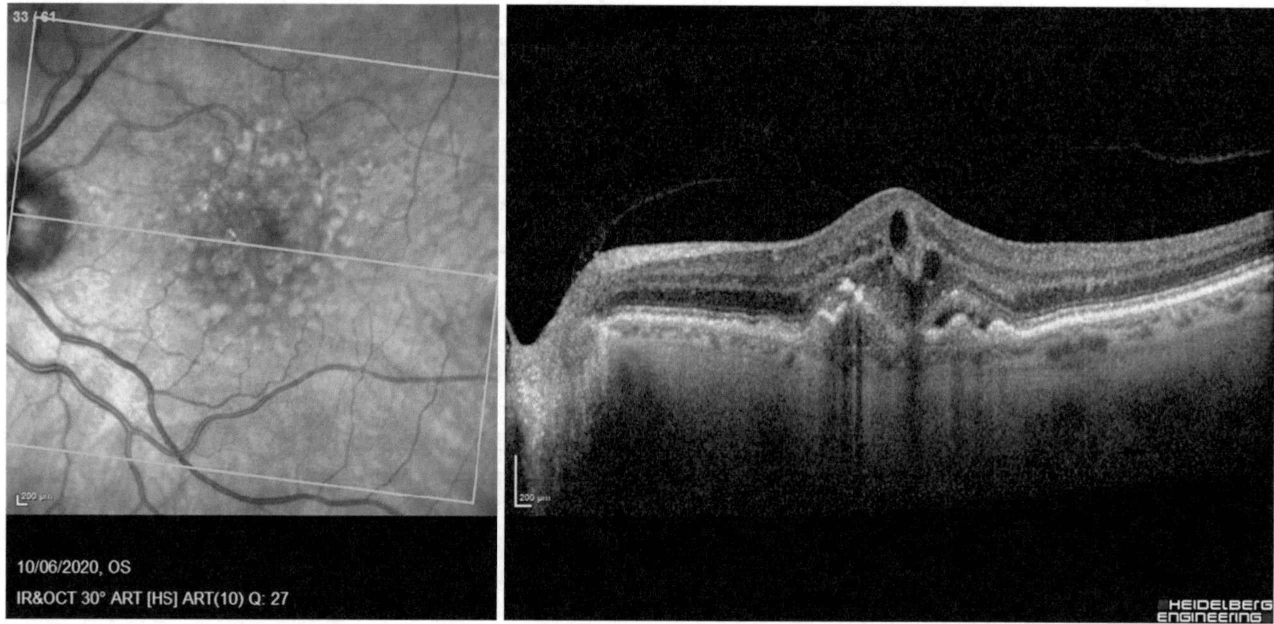

Fig. 13.2 An early CNV in AMD. There is subretinal and intraretinal fluid. Vitreomacular adhesion (VMA) is often seen in AMD, its significance is uncertain

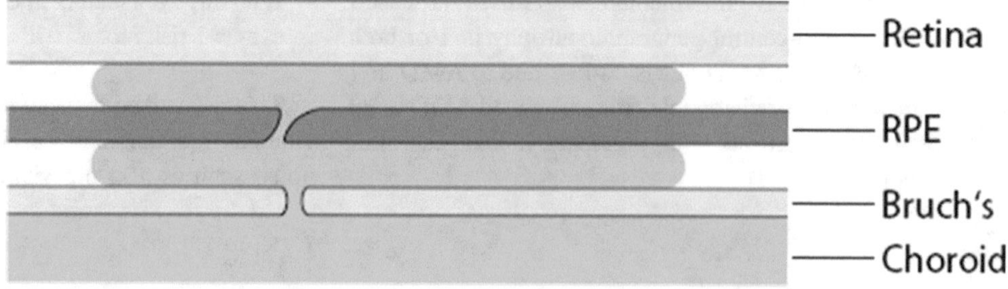

Fig. 13.3 Type 1 CNV is associated with age-related macular degeneration, presenting in all layers of the retina: sub-RPE in occult membrane, subneuroretina in classic membrane and possibly in the retina in retinal angiomatous proliferation (RAP)

15 mg beta carotene (to be avoided in smokers or ex-smokers of less than 10 years because of an increased risk of lung carcinoma) and zinc, 80 mg, as zinc oxide and copper, 2 mg, as cupric oxide [1]. This cocktail has been shown to reduce the chance of advancement in patients with high risk characteristics by approximately 30%.

Patients with CNV already in one eye are at particular risk of progressing to "wet" ARMD with CNV production. The CNV cause distortion and loss of vision with serous elevation of the retina, subretinal haemorrhage and finally disciform scar formation.

The CNV are usually classified on fluorescein angiography into:

- Classic, fluorescein appears early and the CNV is thought to be beneath the neuroretina.
- Non-classic, fluorescein is indistinct and slower in appearance, CNV thought to be under the RPE.
- Mixed can be either predominantly classic or non-classic.

The frequent bilaterality of the condition results in a high proportion of patients who are technically blind, with severe loss of central vision. For this reason, surgical approaches have been tried. However, these are much less commonly used since the effectivity of anti-VEGF treatments bevacizumab [3], pegaptanib [4], ranibizumab [5–7], and aflibercept has been proven. The last two are now established as the therapies of choice for CNV from AMD.

Vitreomacular traction is more common in eyes with exudative AMD (38%) compared with nonexudative AMD (10%) and PVD is less common (21% and 68%, respectively) suggesting to some investigators a role for the vitreous in exudative AMD [8] (Fig. 13.4) (Table 13.1).

There may be situations where the surgery can be of use

- Vitreous haemorrhage from CNV with associated subretinal haemorrhage.
- Pneumatic displacement of submacular haemorrhage.
- Failure of anti-VEGF regimes (Fig. 13.5).

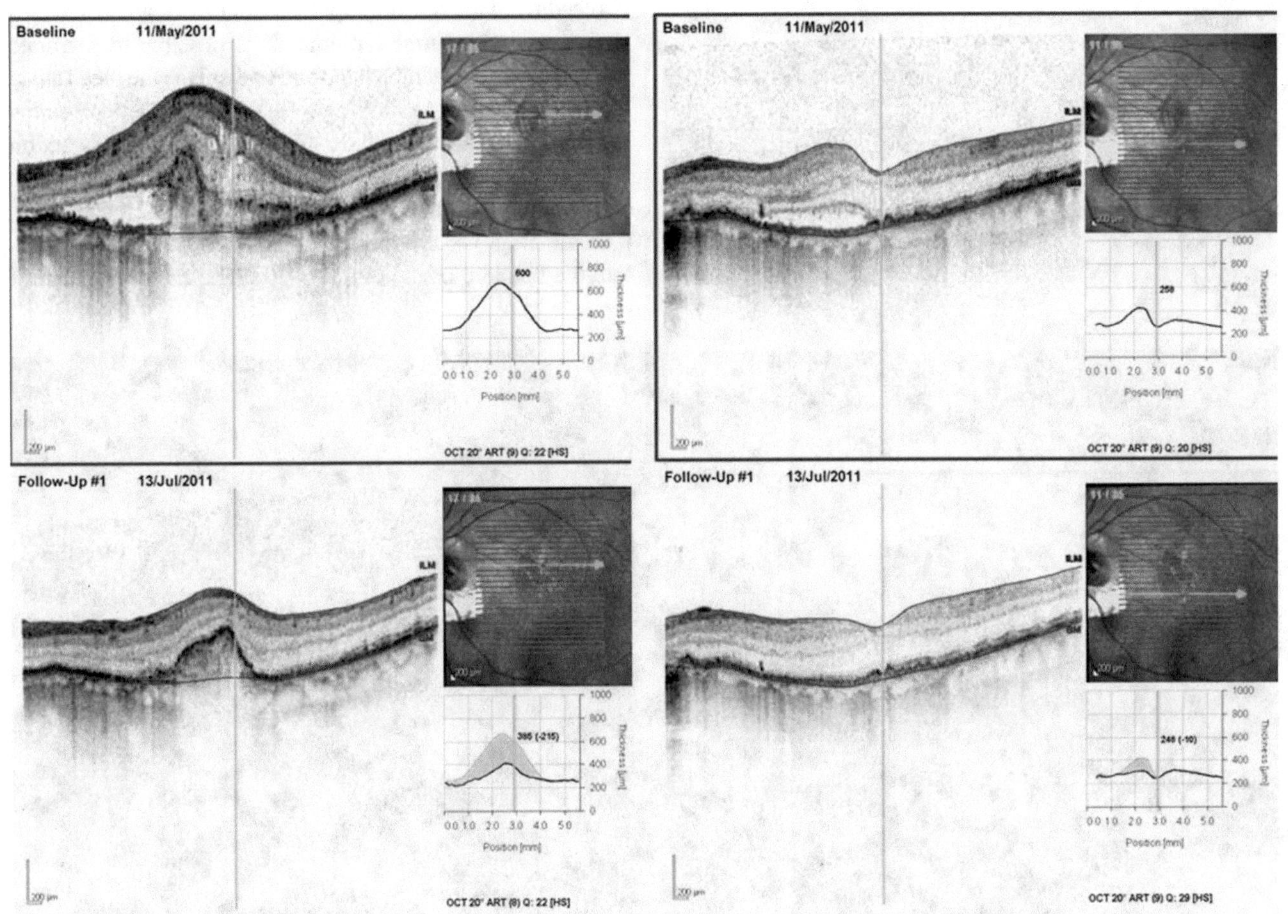

Fig. 13.4 A CNV shrunken with resolution of fluid leakage after Ranibizumab injection, resulting in 20/20 vision

Vitreous Haemorrhage and CNV

A patient with sudden onset vitreous haemorrhage with evidence of a large subretinal craggy mass on ultrasound is very likely to have suffered a subretinal bleed from a CNV from AMD [13]. The subretinal haemorrhage is usually in the macular area but occasionally is due to a peripheral CNV and the macula is clear of blood. Removing the vitreous haemorrhage is useful to restore peripheral vision. The haemorrhage is often very thick and may be altered to an ochre colour as seen in severe bleeds. The vitreous may or may not be detached. If attached, separate it from the retina as in macular hole surgery. If there are large bullae of subretinal haemorrhage, there is a temptation to remove some of the subretinal blood via retinectomy, however, this is often not very effective in removing the blood as fibrinous mass has a "cottage cheese" consistency and cannot be washed out. The retinectomies may allow fluid blood to egress in the postoperative period causing severe hyphaema and the potential for raised IOP and corneal staining. A larger 180° retinectomy will allow access to the blood for removal but runs the risk of postoperative PVR and visual recovery is unlikely to be much improved after prolonged surgery. If the subretinal blood is localised leave it in situ, in most circumstances it will not spread allowing the patient to achieve vision from unaffected parts of the retina. Subretinal rTPA and pneumatic displacement can be attempted, see below (Figs. 13.6, 13.7, and 13.8).

Often these patients are on antiplatelet or anticoagulation therapy which increases the chance of a large bleed [14]. Examine the other eye for evidence of AMD.

Preoperative injection of intravitreal tissue plasminogen activator can be used to try to liquefy the clot [15] (Figs. 13.9 and 13.10).

Table 13.1 Intravitreal injections

Drug	Structure	Dosage	Route of Administration
Ranibizumab (Lucentis) [5–7]	Antibody fragment binds to VEGF A	0.5 mg/0.05 ml	Intravitreal
Aflibercept (Eylea) [9–12]	Decoy receptor for VEGF (A and B) and anti-placental growth factor (PGF)	2.0 mg/0.05 ml	Intravitreal
Bevacizumab (Avastin)	Complete immunoglobulin binds to VEGF A	1.25 mg/0.05 ml	Intravitreal

Pneumatic Displacement of Subretinal Haemorrhage

A bleed from a CNV may spread under the macula giving a rise to a large central scotoma. It is possible to facilitate resorption of the haemorrhage and to displace the bleed away from the fovea by performing a PPV and gas. The patient is required to posture upright to allow the gas bubble to act on the haemorrhage displacing it inferiorly. There is a debate whether either intravitreal tissue plasminogen activator (tPA, 0.05 ml, 50 µg) or subretinal tPA should be injected to facilitate the breakup of the clot [16–20]. The molecular size of

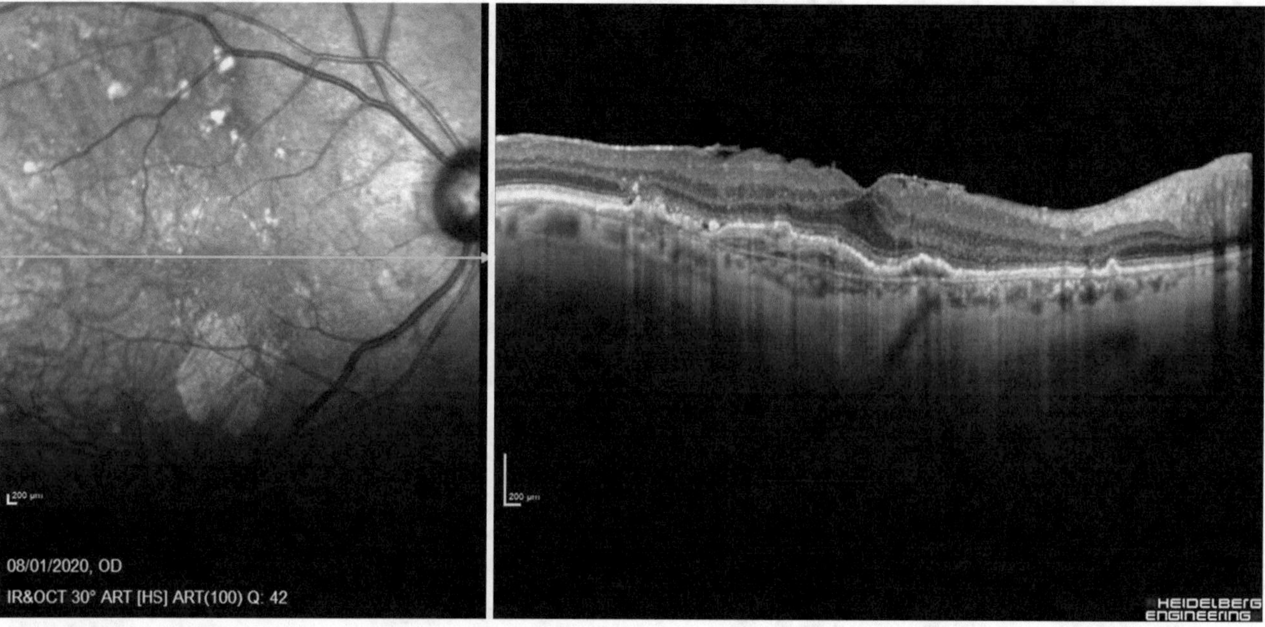

Fig. 13.5 A CNV treated with Anti-VEGF with no current fluid leakage

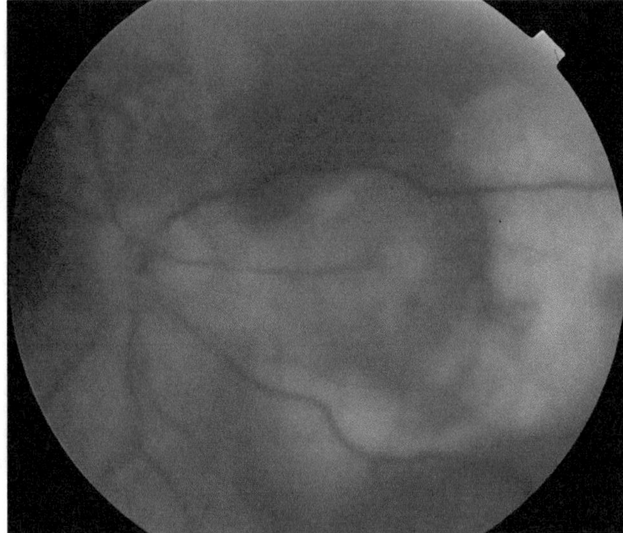

Fig. 13.6 Very large subretinal bleeds from CNV can cause severe vitreous haemorrhage. These are usually obvious on ultrasound as a crenated posterior mass

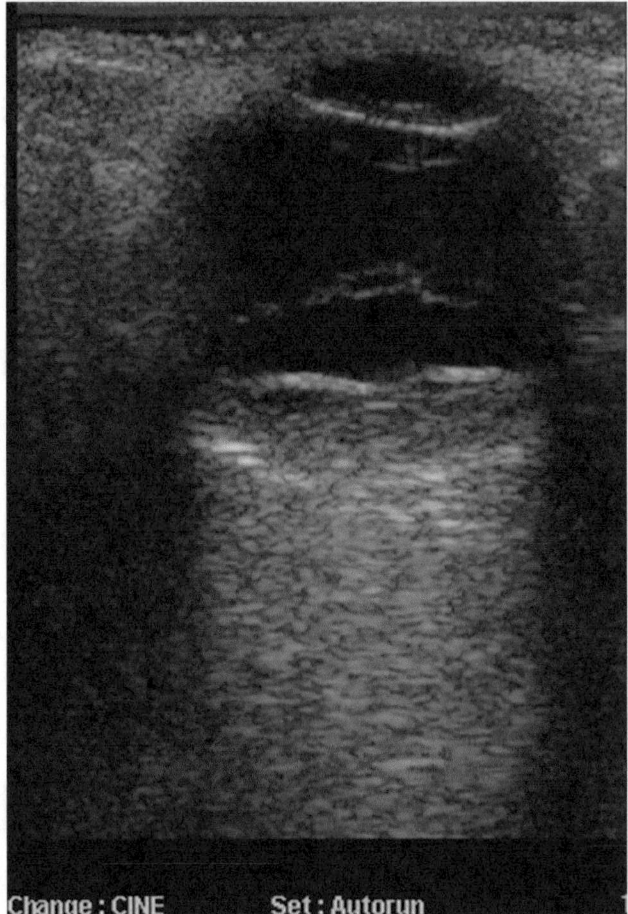

Fig. 13.7 An ultrasound of a patient with vitreous haemorrhage from subretinal bleed and age-related CNV, note the PVD and large craggy mass at the posterior pole

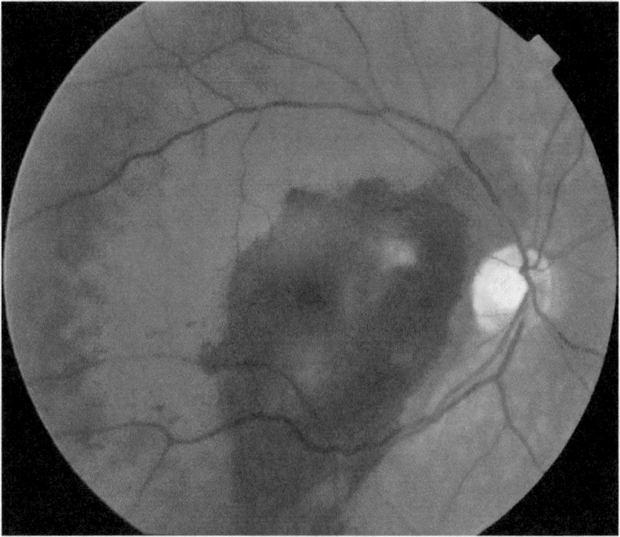

Fig. 13.8 Subretinal blood can occur from a number of reasons including Type I choroidal neovascular membranes and macular aneurysms. Often the blood will break through the retina, as seen in this case, into the posterior vitreous gel

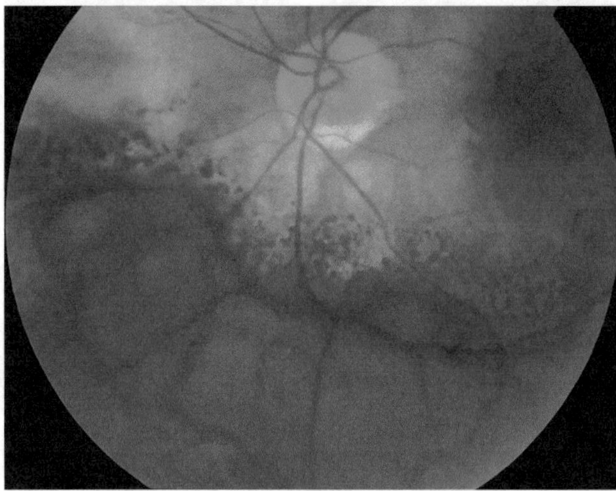

Fig. 13.9 An eccentric CNV caused a vitreous haemorrhage after a subretinal haemorrhage which did not affect the macula

tPA is like bevacizumab which can cross the retina in AMD. Any agent injected into the vitreous cavity in a vitrectomised eye, however, tends to have a shorter half-life because of more rapid clearance of the drug in the fluid filled vitreous cavity in comparison to the gel filled cavity. If injecting tPA into the subretinal space, the drug can be inserted using a 40-gauge needle to raise a bleb of fluid under the retina. This is my preferred option at a dose of 50microgram in 0.1 ml. As with any injection under the macula, take care that the pressure rise in the subretinal space does not "blow" a hole in the fovea, the weakest point in the macula. Usually there is a site of slight serous elevation on

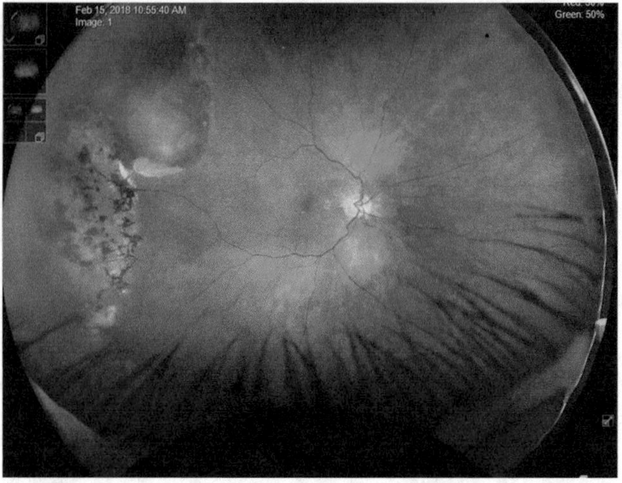

Fig. 13.10 A peripheral CNV caused a vitreous haemorrhage treated by vitrectomy

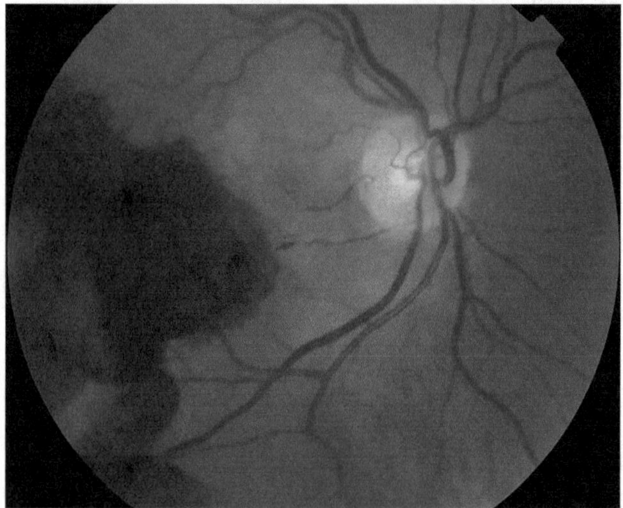

Fig. 13.11 Some CNV in ARMD will bleed into the subretinal space, a PPV and gas insertion (with or without subretinal tissue plasminogen activator, TPa) can displace the blood away from the fovea thereby increasing vision despite a persistent CNV. This sequence of images shows the preoperative status and sequential improvement in the retinal appearance over months

the edge of the haemorrhagic mass into which the drug can be inserted with ease. Raise a bleb of injected drug under the retina (Figs. 13.11, 13.12, 13.13, 13.14, and 13.15).

Surgery for Failed Anti-VEGF Therapy

Introduction (Fig. 13.16)

Surgical approaches have been applied to subfoveal CNV. The most established strategy has been 360° macular translocation [21–23]. Success rates are reportedly 33% improvement in vision but the usual benefit is for reading

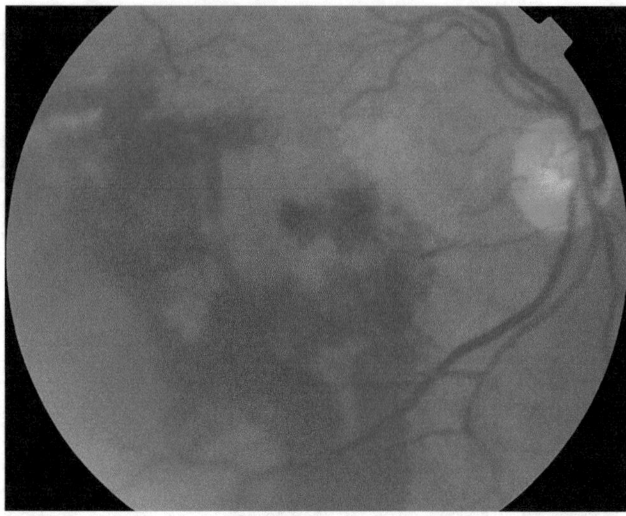

Fig. 13.12 Early postoperative view with displacement of the blood

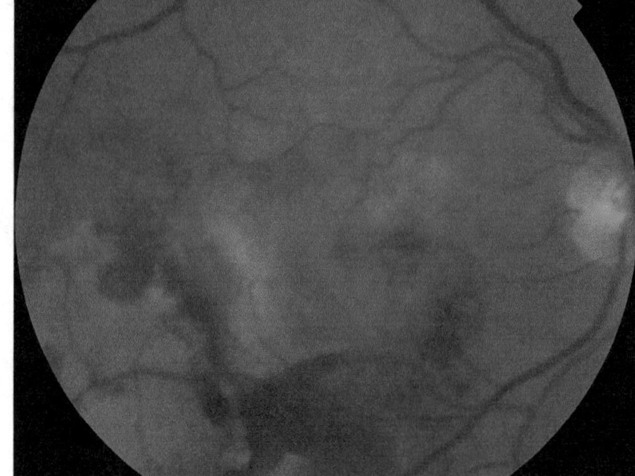

Fig. 13.13 The blood disperses

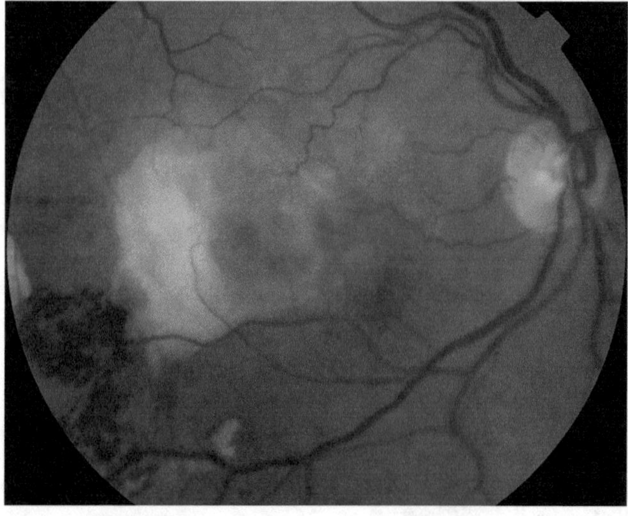

Fig. 13.14 Finally the CNV fibroses

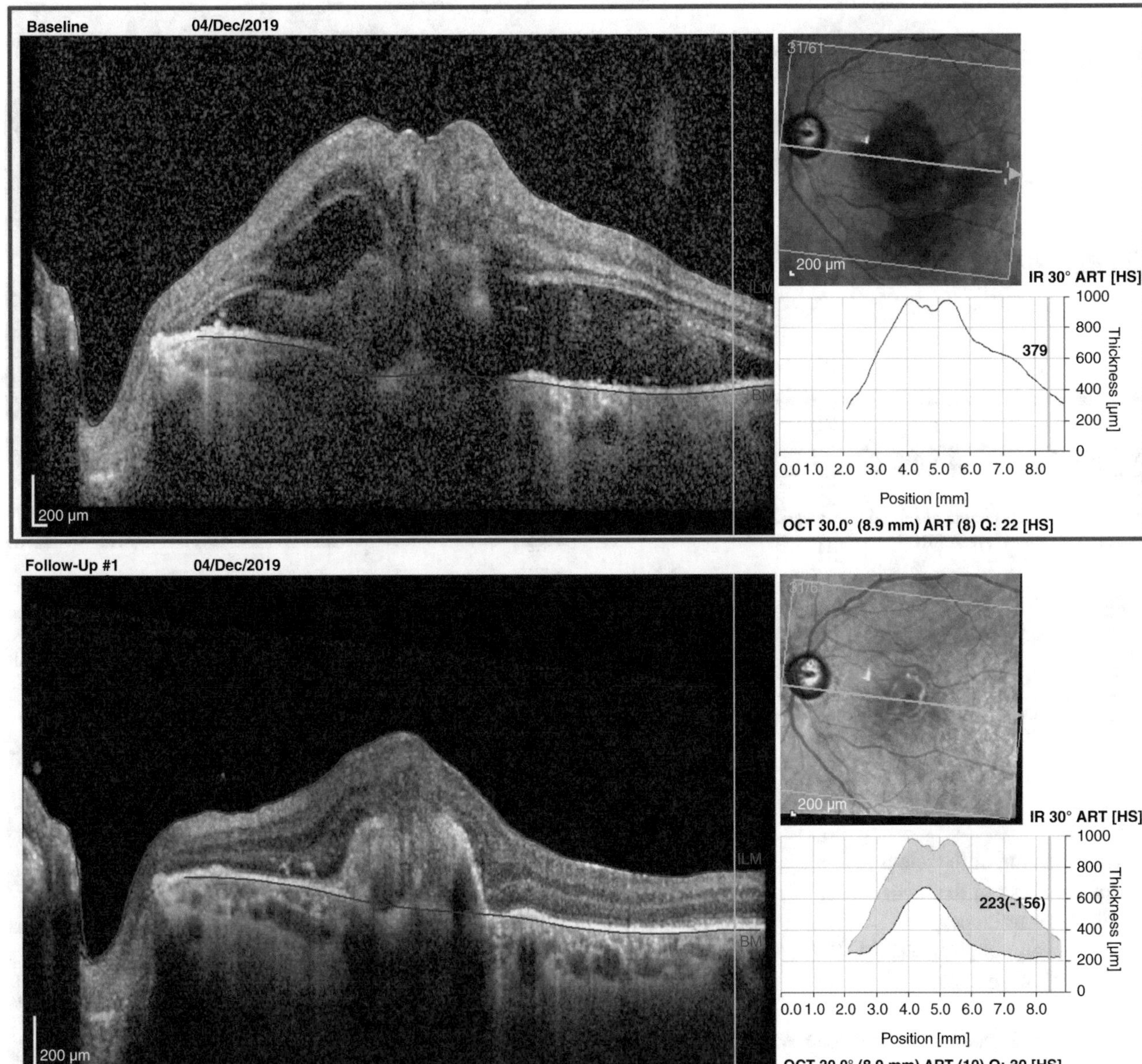

Fig. 13.15 Pneumatic displacement has moved blood from the macula in this patient with a subfoveal CNV

speed [24, 25] with 10% recurrence. Translocation for geographic atrophy has been complicated by the rapid return of the atrophy in the translocated macula [26].

Various other methods such as limited macular translocation and transplant of an RPE and choroidal patch are of unproven benefit [27–35]. Removal of peripapillary CNV on its own is of doubtful benefit [36]. Clinicopathological studies of eyes with surgically removed CNV reveal breaks in Bruch's membrane and persistent sub-RPE CNV [37].

In most circumstances the monthly injection of ranibizumab is the current treatment of choice for CNV from AMD. However, the long-term dosage regimes for these agents are not well understood and combination therapy with intravitreal steroid and PDT are being investigated to try to reduce the need for years of repeated injections. In those patients with loss of vision in their second affected eye who are not responsive to these agents there may still be a role for 360° macular translocation surgery.

360° Macular Translocation (Table 13.2)

Additional surgical steps.

- Phacoemulsification of the lens with IOL.
- Artificial inducement of retinal detachment via infusion of fluid through a retinotomy.
- Removal of the CNV.

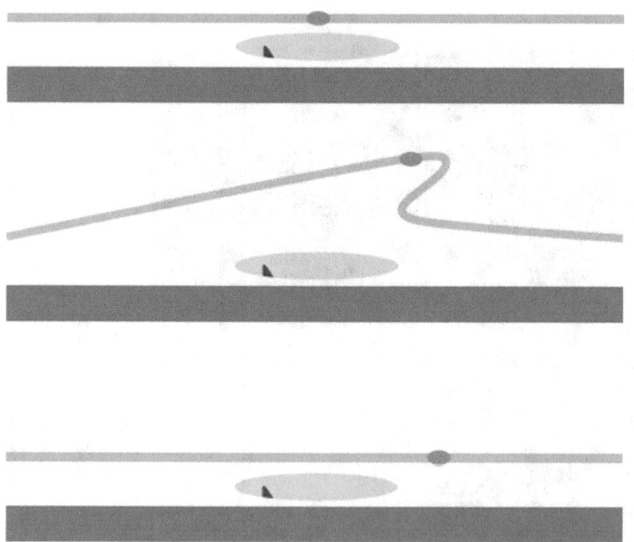

Fig. 13.16 The principle of retinal translocation is to move the fovea onto an undamaged area of RPE

Table 13.2 difficulty rating for 360° macular translocation

Difficulty Rating	Very Difficult
Success rates	Low
Complication rates	High
When to use in training	Late

- Drainage of subretinal fluid and insertion of heavy liquids.
- Translocation of the retina.
- Reattachment of the retina.
- 360° laser retinopexy
- Silicone oil tamponade (Figs. 13.17, 13.18, 13.19, 13.20, 13.21, 13.22, and 13.23).

Perform a phacoemulsification cataract extraction. Set up the PPV using a shortened infusion cannula preferably. Perform the PPV with close removal of the peripheral gel at the vitreous base with indentation if required.

Note: It is especially important not to create an iatrogenic break as this will create difficulty during the induction of the retinal detachment by the loss of infusion fluid through the break.

Insert a high gauge (40G) cannula through the retina at the equator. Inject fluid gradually increasing the pressure until retinal bullae are formed. Use air injection to spread the SRF to attached retina and then replace with fluid. Repeat until the entire retina is detached. Perform a 360° retinectomy as anteriorly as possible. Remove the CNV. Use a small bubble of "light heavy" liquids to open out the retina again.

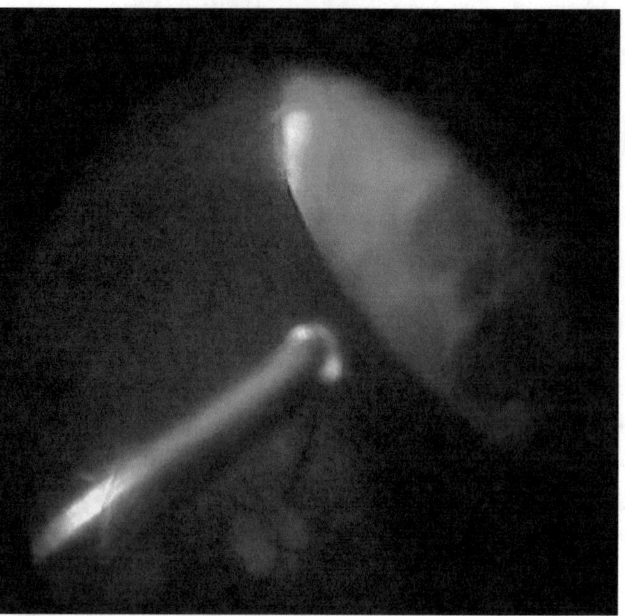

Fig. 13.17 For 360° macular translocation after cataract extraction and lens implantation trim the vitreous base with a high speed cutter. With a 40 gauge cannula create a retinal detachment and then spread the SRF with fluid air exchange. Create the 360° retinectomy, dissect off the CNV, rotate the retina, laser the retinectomy, and insert silicone oil

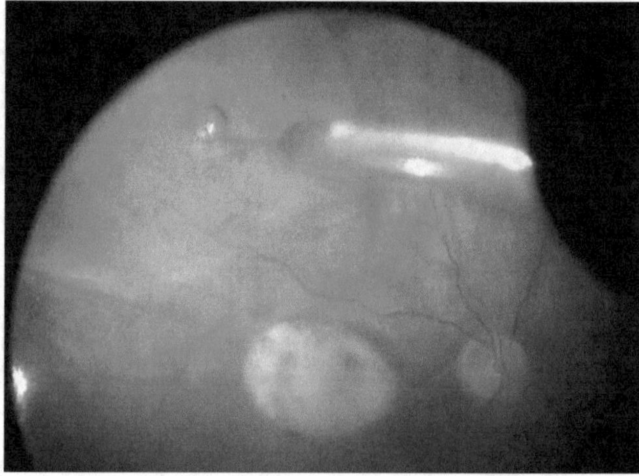

Fig. 13.18 Subretinal injection of fluid via 40 guage needle

Rotate the retina by gentle traction with a diamond dusted silicone tipped manipulator so that the fovea reaches healthy RPE. Use additional "light heavy" liquids to reattach the retina completely. Apply laser retinopexy to the 360° retinectomy. Exchange the liquid for the silicone oil and close.

At a second operation (3-6 months) the silicone oil is removed, and the extraocular muscles moved to compensate for torsional displacement of the image.

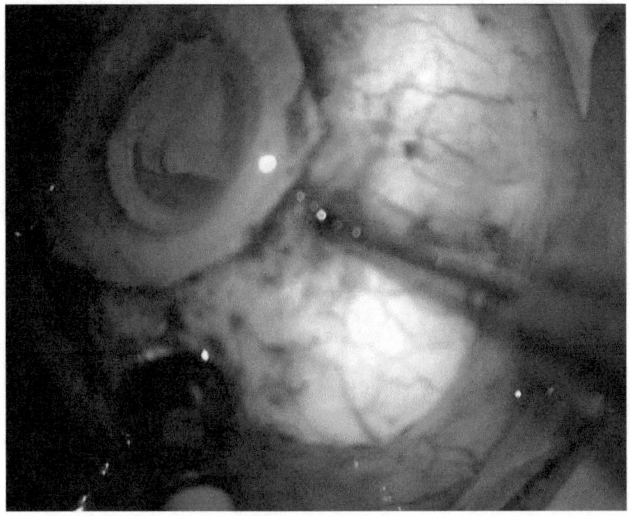

Fig. 13.19 Cutting the peripheral retina

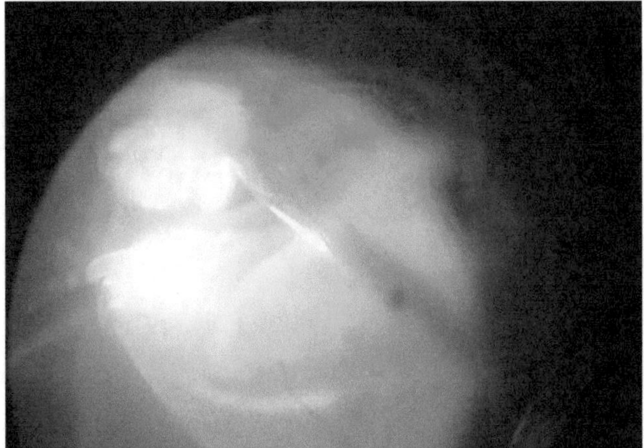

Fig. 13.20 Folding the retina over and removing the CNV

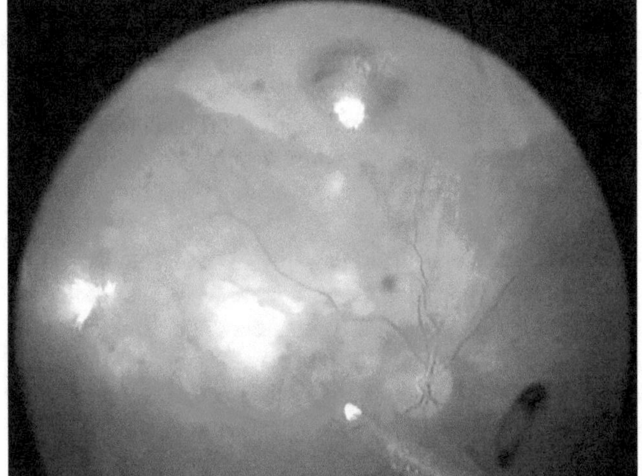

Fig. 13.21 Insertion of heavy liquid and rotation of the retina

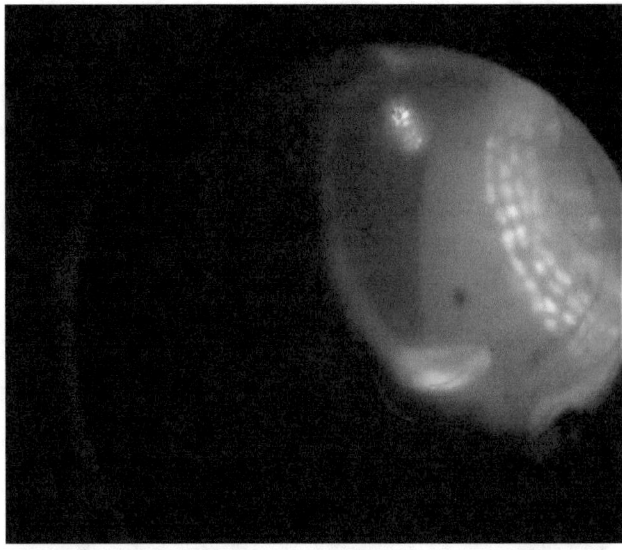

Fig. 13.22 Laser application to the retinectomy

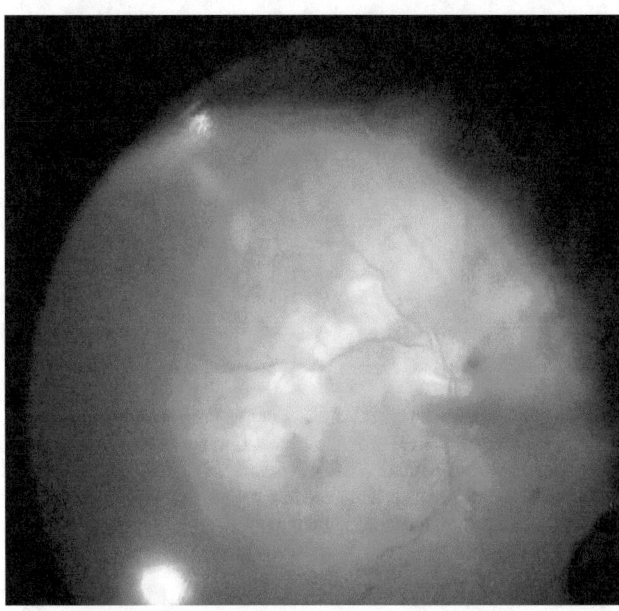

Fig. 13.23 Insertion of silicone oil with the fovea rotated off the area of RPE damage from the CNV

Specific Complications

- Retinal detachment associated with proliferative vitreoretinopathy in approximately 10%–20% [38, 39].
- Diplopia 6%.
- Recurrent CNV 10%.
- Choroidal haemorrhage.
- Macular hole and pucker.
- Severe hypotony has also been described [40].

Success Rates (Figs. 13.24, 13.25, 13.26, and 13.27)

The surgery does not significantly improve vision from preoperatively but does improve reading speed and quality of life scores [41–44].

Choroidal Neovascular Membrane Not from ARMD

Introduction

These occur in a variety of conditions and most often have a more benign clinical course. The CNV are often smaller and self-limiting. Surgical removal is possible with immediate restoration of vision or reduction in distortion but with a high chance of recurrence of approximately 30%. Intravitreal injections are effective in these conditions and therefore surgical cases are now rare.

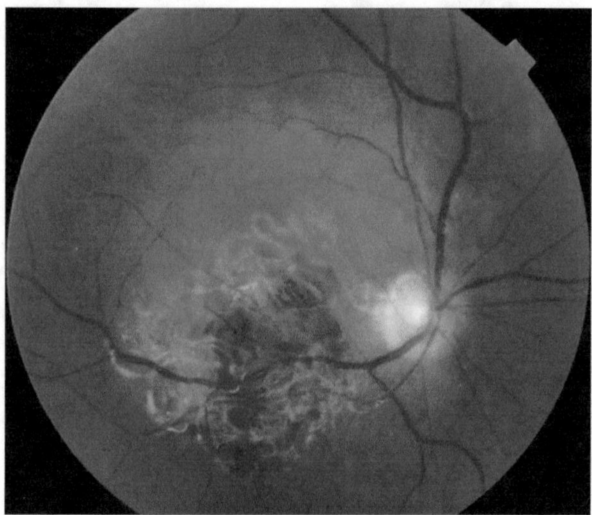

Fig. 13.24 The retina has been moved in this patient, the fovea is now situated over healthy RPE providing 20/120, picture one. Retinal pigment epithelial transplantation techniques are being investigated but are still experimental and not established as a means of improving vision in age-related macular degeneration picture 2

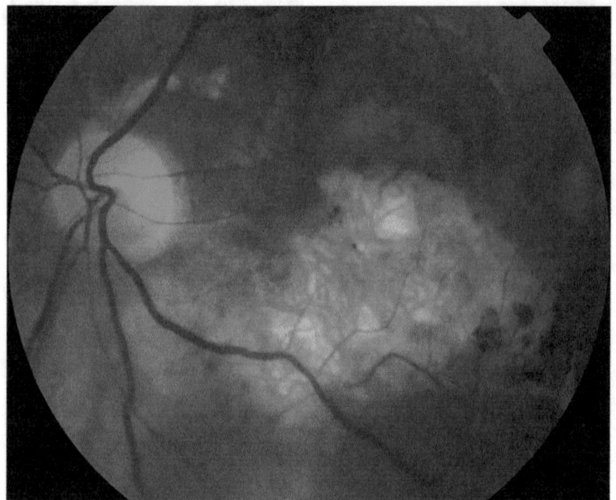

Fig. 13.25 Recurrences after 360 MT are common and usually occur on the foveal side of the scar, a colour, and FFA image are shown

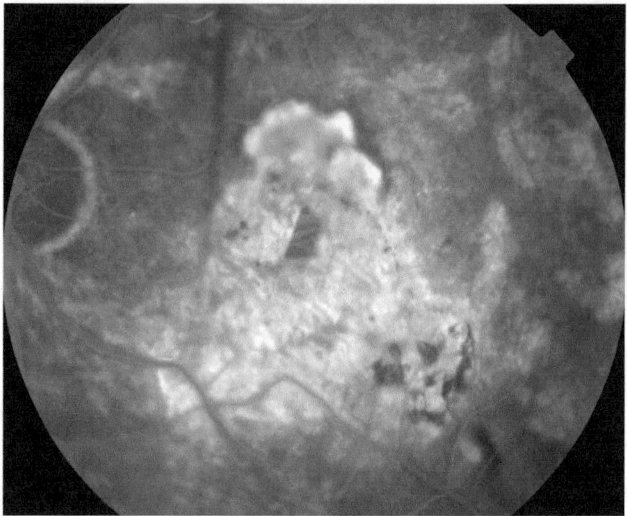

Fig. 13.26 FFA of the recurrent CNV

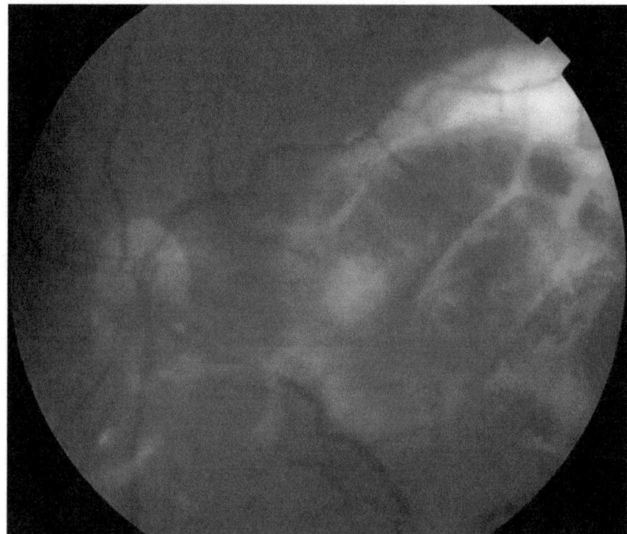

Fig. 13.27 The RPE has been cut and moved into the area of defect left by removal of a CNV

Presumed ocular histoplasmosis [45–47] (also called punctate inner choroidopathy or multifocal inner choroidopathy in some countries), uveitis, choroidal rupture [48], juxtafoveolar telangiectasia [49], central serous chorioretinopathy [50] or macular surgery [51] can all be associated with CNV which will respond to surgical removal. However, a randomised trial has shown no benefit of surgery over observation [52]. Angioid streaks and myopia [53–55] may produce CNV but surgical removal is less successful (Figs. 13.28, 13.29, 13.30, 13.31, 13.32, 13.33, 13.34, 13.35 and 13.36).

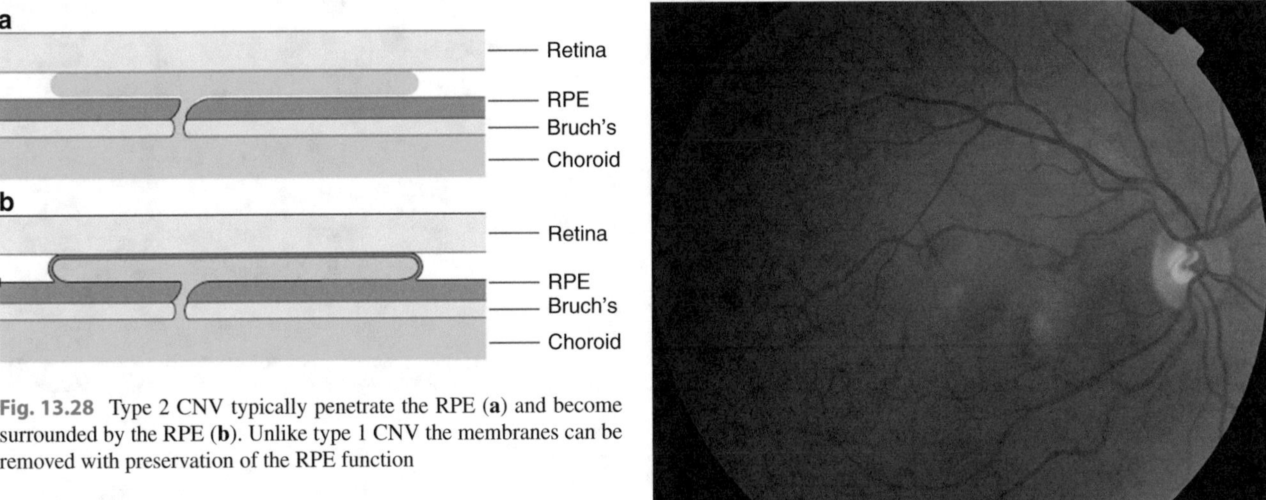

Fig. 13.28 Type 2 CNV typically penetrate the RPE (**a**) and become surrounded by the RPE (**b**). Unlike type 1 CNV the membranes can be removed with preservation of the RPE function

Fig. 13.29 Spontaneous idiopathic type 2 CNV can occur and can be treated with intravitreal anti-VEGF therapy although spontaneous resolution occurs in 50%

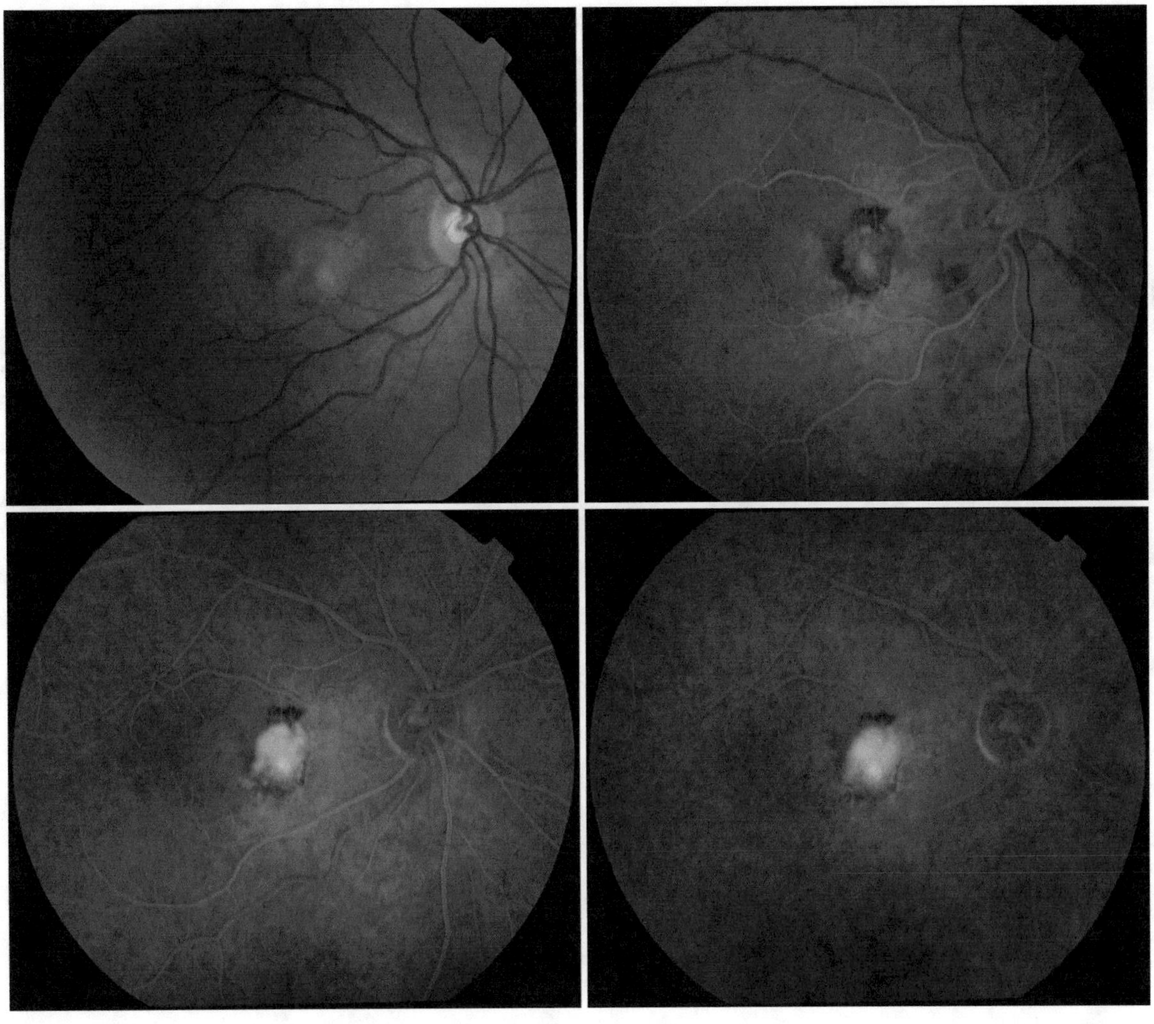

Fig. 13.30 FFA of the type 2 CNV

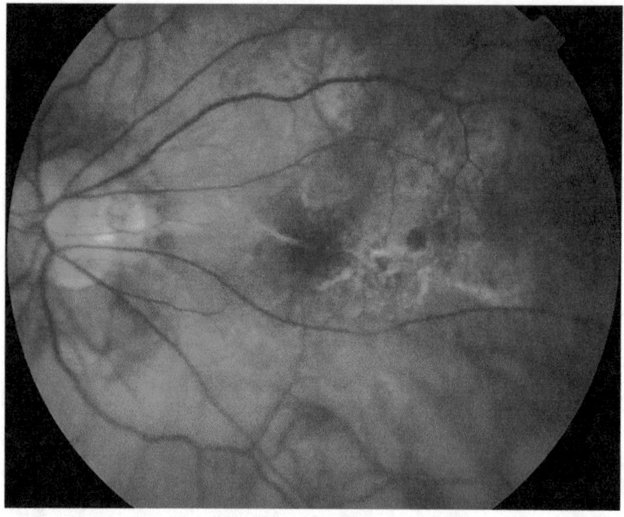

Fig. 13.31 There is a Foster Fuch's spot temporal to the fovea in this high myope signifying a subretinal bleed from a small type 2 CNV. Most of these resolve with maintenance of stable vision. Note the lacquer cracks (splits in Descemet's membrane) a risk factor for CNV

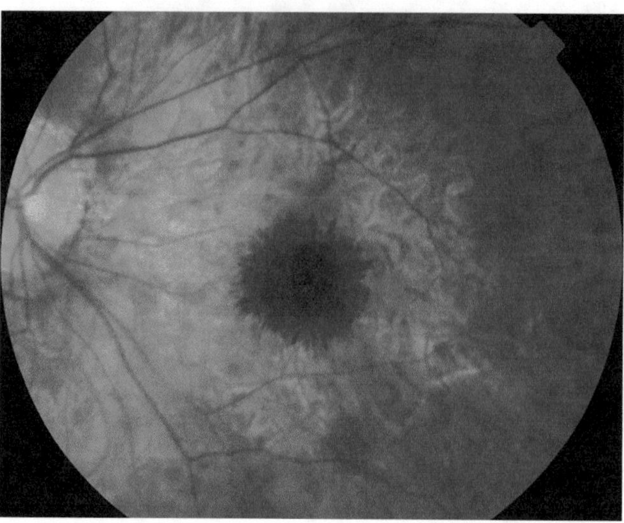

Fig. 13.32 Myopic CNV are often mixed type 1 and 2 and can produce subfoveal haemorrhage. Anti-VEGF therapy can be tried but visual loss may persist

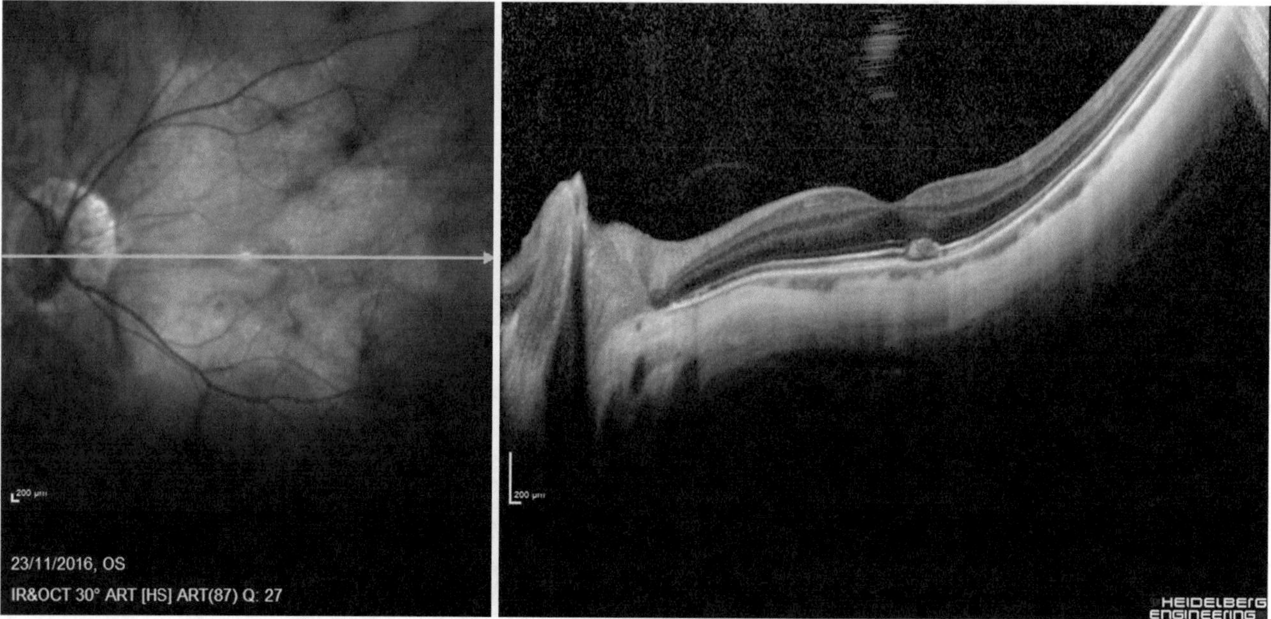

Fig. 13.33 A small CNV near the fovea in a high myope, which is inactive and shrinking

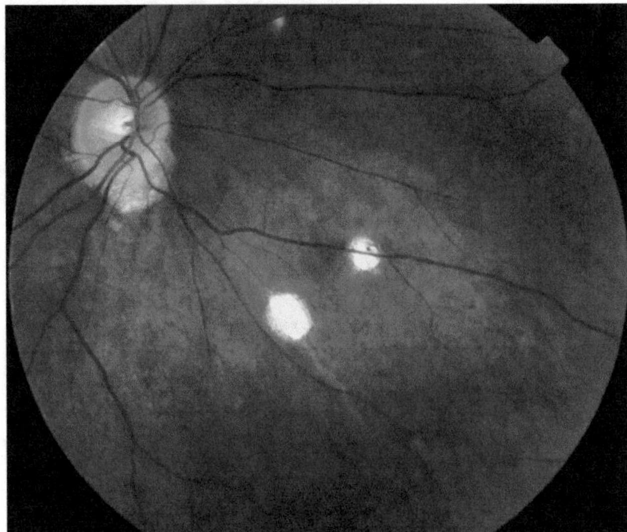

Fig. 13.34 PIC is often associated with neovascular membrane formation of Type II. These can respond to surgery by removal but recurrence is unfortunately common. Membranes vary in size, but the best for removal are small, well circumscribed, pigmented lesions as opposed to more diffuse web shaped lesions

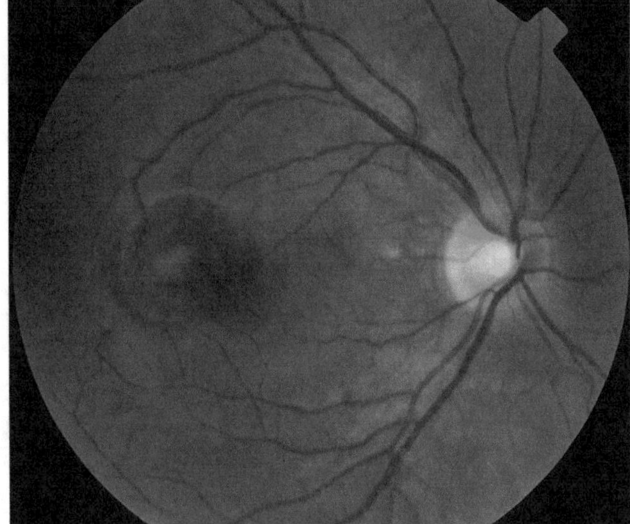

Fig. 13.35 Serous elevation around this small neovascular membrane distorts the fovea and reduces vision. Removal of the membrane will cause resolution of the serous elevation and improvement in the visual acuity

Surgery (Table 13.3)

Additional surgical steps

- Create a retinotomy in the macula, temporal to the fovea.
- Insert subretinal forceps.
- Loosen and grasp the CNV.
- Extract the CNV through the retinotomy.

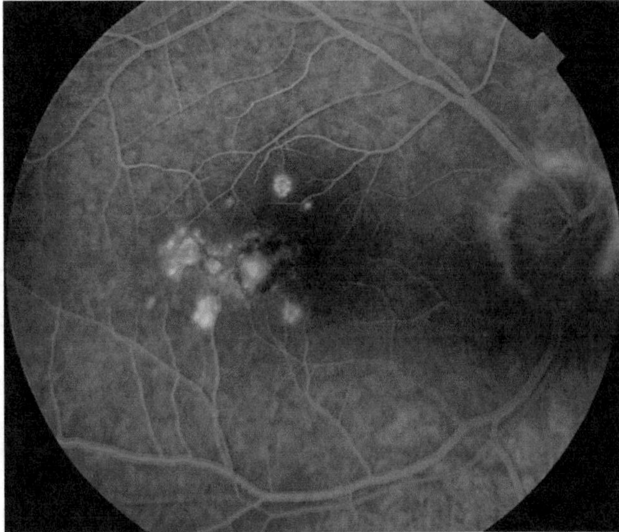

Fig. 13.36 A fluorescein angiogram of PIC

Table 13.3 difficulty rating for PPV for type 2 CNV

Difficulty Rating	Moderate
Success rates	Low
Complication rates	Low
When to use in training	Late

Access the retina via a PPV. Usually the posterior hyaloid membrane requires detachment because these patients are young. With a bent MVR blade incise the retina in the macula just temporal to the CNV to access the subneuroretinal space. Insert subretinal forceps (angled with delicate long prongs). With the forceps closed sweep under and over the CNV to loosen attachments. With slightly open forceps press down on the anterior surface of the CNV (this avoids grasping the retina whilst inserting the CNV tissue) and close the forceps. Extract the CNV through the retinotomy. Even quite large CNV will pass through the retinotomy, which has some inherent elasticity. The membranes can have retinal attachments. Care must be exercised during removal that the retina does not tear. Bleeding is usually slight because there is low blood flow in the CNV. Tamponade and laser retinopexy are not required and the PPV can be closed.

Surgical Pearl

Nano Subretinal Gateway Device for Subretinal Delivery without Vitrectomy

With the advent of gene therapy and expected future expansion of precise drug, gene, and possible stem cell delivery to the subretinal space, the Nano Subretinal Gateway Device (NSGD) was developed to deliver medicine to the subretinal space without pars plana vitrectomy (PPV). The objective would be to reduce any complications related to PPV and detaching the hyaloid, preserving the vitreous, and achieving the goal of delivering the medicine to the target location.

Vitreoretinal surgeons are trained to use subretinal cannulas to displace subretinal haemorrhage. Controlling eye movement with good visualisation of the macular area can easily be achieved since the instruments and light pipe are introduced through scleral cannulas. This may not be as easy with the NSGD, which has a very thin needle-like tip, introduced through pars plana but with no scleral cannulas.

Here are some tricks to help better visualisation of the macular area to achieve safer delivery to target site:

1. A chandelier is needed in those cases for visualisation. The chandelier should be positioned at the opposite quadrant to where the NSGD will be introduced; for example, if the surgeon is right-handed, the device is introduced supero-temporally in the right eye, and the chandelier should be inferonasal. This allows symmetry of instruments being introduced to try and keep the eye in primary position for a better view of the posterior pole.
2. Controlling the patient's eye movement through the chandelier also helps keeping the eye steady with a good focus on the macula. This can be through a utility forceps or similar instruments to hold the cannula of the chandelier in place or even by holding the chandelier with the left hand for a better control.
3. Automated infusion through the machine with a foot pedal control can also prevent any fine movement of the surgeon's hand to keep the NSGD in perfect location for precise steady delivery. A pressure of 8-10 PSI is ideal for subretinal delivery and should be checked by the surgeon before automated infusion [56].

Tamer H. Mahmoud, Beaumont Neuroscience Center Building, Royal Oak, Michigan, USA

Summary

Vitrectomy surgery has uses in specific situations in AMD, but anti-VEGF therapy is the mainstay of therapy.

References

1. A randomized, placebo-controlled, clinical trial of high-dose supplementation with vitamins C and E, beta carotene, and zinc for age-related macular degeneration and vision loss: AREDS report no. 8. Arch Ophthalmol. 2001;119(10):1417-36.
2. Ferris FL, Davis MD, Clemons TE, Lee LY, Chew EY, Lindblad AS, et al. A simplified severity scale for age-related macular degeneration: AREDS report no. 18. Arch Ophthalmol. 2005;123(11):1570–4. https://doi.org/10.1001/archopht.123.11.1570.
3. Avery RL, Pieramici DJ, Rabena MD, Castellarin AA, Nasir MA, Giust MJ. Intravitreal bevacizumab (Avastin) for neovascular age-related macular degeneration. Ophthalmology. 2006;113(3):363–72.
4. Chakravarthy U, Adamis AP, Cunningham ET Jr, Goldbaum M, Guyer DR, Katz B, et al. Year 2 efficacy results of 2 randomized controlled clinical trials of pegaptanib for neovascular age-related macular degeneration. Ophthalmology. 2006;113(9):1508–25.
5. Rosenfeld PJ, Rich RM, Lalwani GA. Ranibizumab: Phase III clinical trial results. Ophthalmol Clin N Am. 2006;19(3):361–72.
6. Rosenfeld PJ, Brown DM, Heier JS, Boyer DS, Kaiser PK, Chung CY, et al. Ranibizumab for neovascular age-related macular degeneration. N Engl J Med. 2006;355(14):1419–31. https://doi.org/10.1056/NEJMoa054481.
7. Brown DM, Kaiser PK, Michels M, Soubrane G, Heier JS, Kim RY, et al. Ranibizumab versus verteporfin for neovascular age-related macular degeneration. N Engl J Med. 2006;355(14):1432–44. https://doi.org/10.1056/NEJMoa062655.
8. Robison CD, Krebs I, Binder S, Barbazetto IA, Kotsolis AI, Yannuzzi LA, et al. Vitreomacular adhesion in active and end-stage age-related macular degeneration. Am J Ophthalmol. 2009;148(1):79–82. e2. https://doi.org/10.1016/j.ajo.2009.01.014.
9. Kaiser PK, Singer M, Tolentino M, Vitti R, Erickson K, Saroj N, et al. Long-term safety and visual outcome of intravitreal Aflibercept in Neovascular age-related macular degeneration: VIEW 1 extension study. Ophthalmol Retina. 2017;1(4):304–13. https://doi.org/10.1016/j.oret.2017.01.004.
10. Waldstein SM, Simader C, Staurenghi G, Chong NV, Mitchell P, Jaffe GJ, et al. Morphology and visual acuity in Aflibercept and Ranibizumab therapy for Neovascular age-related macular degeneration in the VIEW trials. Ophthalmology. 2016;123(7):1521–9. https://doi.org/10.1016/j.ophtha.2016.03.037.
11. Talks JS, Lotery AJ, Ghanchi F, Sivaprasad S, Johnston RL, Patel N, et al. First-year visual acuity outcomes of providing Aflibercept according to the VIEW study protocol for age-related macular degeneration. Ophthalmology. 2016;123(2):337–43. https://doi.org/10.1016/j.ophtha.2015.09.039.
12. Schmidt-Erfurth U, Kaiser PK, Korobelnik JF, Brown DM, Chong V, Nguyen QD, et al. Intravitreal aflibercept injection for neovascular age-related macular degeneration: ninety-six-week results of the VIEW studies. Ophthalmology. 2014;121(1):193–201. https://doi.org/10.1016/j.ophtha.2013.08.011.
13. Orth DH, Flood TP. Management of breakthrough vitreous hemorrhage from presumed extramacular subretinal neovascularization. Retina. 1982;2(2):89–93.
14. Kuhli-Hattenbach C, Fischer IB, Schalnus R, Hattenbach LO. Subretinal hemorrhages associated with age-related macular degeneration in patients receiving anticoagulation or antiplatelet therapy. Am J Ophthalmol. 2010;149(2):316–21 e1. https://doi.org/10.1016/j.ajo.2009.08.033.
15. Oshima Y, Ohji M, Tano Y. Pars plana vitrectomy with peripheral retinotomy after injection of preoperative intravitreal tissue plasminogen activator: a modified procedure to drain massive subretinal haemorrhage. Br J Ophthalmol. 2007;91(2):193–8. https://doi.org/10.1136/bjo.2006.101444.
16. Gopalakrishan M, Giridhar A, Bhat S, Saikumar SJ, Elias A. N S. pneumatic displacement of submacular hemorrhage: safety, efficacy, and patient selection. Retina. 2007;27(3):329–34. https://doi.org/10.1097/01.iae.0000231544.43093.40.
17. Ohji M, Saito Y, Hayashi A, Lewis JM, Tano Y. Pneumatic displacement of subretinal hemorrhage without tissue plasminogen activator. Arch Ophthalmol. 1998;116(10):1326–32.
18. Hesse L, Meitinger D, Schmidt J. Little effect of tissue plasminogen activator in subretinal surgery for acute hemorrhage in age-related macular degeneration. Ger J Ophthalmol. 1996;5(6):479–83.

19. Singh RP, Patel C, Sears JE. Management of subretinal macular haemorrhage by direct administration of tissue plasminogen activator. Br J Ophthalmol. 2006;90(4):429–31. https://doi.org/10.1136/bjo.2005.085001.
20. Stanescu-Segall D, Balta F, Jackson TL. Submacular hemorrhage in neovascular age-related macular degeneration: a synthesis of the literature. Surv Ophthalmol. 2016;61(1):18–32. https://doi.org/10.1016/j.survophthal.2015.04.004.
21. Machemer R, Steinhorst UH. Retinal separation, retinotomy, and macular relocation: II. A surgical approach for age-related macular degeneration? Graefes Arch Clin Exp Ophthalmol. 1993;231(11):635–41.
22. Machemer R, Steinhorst UH. Retinal separation, retinotomy, and macular relocation: I. experimental studies in the rabbit eye. Graefes Arch Clin Exp Ophthalmol. 1993;231(11):629–34.
23. Eckardt C, Eckardt U, Conrad HG. Macular rotation with and without counter-rotation of the globe in patients with age-related macular degeneration. Graefes Arch Clin Exp Ophthalmol. 1999;237(4):313–25.
24. Bdel-Meguid A, Lappas A, Hartmann K, Auer F, Schrage N, Thumann G, et al. One year follow up of macular translocation with 360 degree retinotomy in patients with age related macular degeneration. Br J Ophthalmol. 2003;87(5):615–21.
25. Wong D, Stanga P, Briggs M, Lenfestey P, Lancaster E, Li KK, et al. Case selection in macular relocation surgery for age related macular degeneration. Br J Ophthalmol. 2004;88(2):186–90.
26. Khurana RN, Fujii GY, Walsh AC, Humayun MS, De Juan E, Jr., Sadda SR. Rapid recurrence of geographic atrophy after full macular translocation for nonexudative age-related macular degeneration. Ophthalmology. 2005;112(9):1586–91.
27. van Meurs JC, Hofland LJ, van Hagen PM, Mooy CM, Baarsma GS, et al. Autologous peripheral retinal pigment epithelium translocation in patients with subfoveal neovascular membranes. Br J Ophthalmol. 2004;88(1):110–3.
28. Stanga PE, Kychenthal A, Fitzke FW, Halfyard AS, Chan R, Bird AC, et al. Retinal pigment epithelium translocation after choroidal neovascular membrane removal in age-related macular degeneration. Ophthalmology. 2002;109(8):1492–8.
29. Lappas A, Foerster AM, Weinberger AW, Coburger S, Schrage NF, Kirchhof B. Translocation of iris pigment epithelium in patients with exudative age-related macular degeneration: long-term results. Graefes Arch Clin Exp Ophthalmol. 2004;242(8):638–47.
30. Angunawela RI, Williamson TH, Khan MA, Chong V. Choroidal translocation with a pedicle following excision of a type 1 choroidal neovascular membrane. Br J Ophthalmol. 2005;89(3):386.
31. Thomas MA, Grand MG, Williams DF, Lee CM, Pesin SR, Lowe MA. Surgical management of subfoveal choroidal neovascularization. Ophthalmology. 1992;99(6):952–68.
32. Phillips SJ, Sadda SR, Tso MO, Humayan MS, De Juan E, Binder S. Autologous transplantation of retinal pigment epithelium after mechanical debridement of Bruch's membrane. Curr Eye Res. 2003;26(2):81–8.
33. Fujii GY, De Juan E, Humayun MS, Chang TS. Limited macular translocation for the management of subfoveal choroidal neovascularization after photodynamic therapy. Am J Ophthalmol. 2003;135(1):109–12.
34. Pieramici DJ, De Juan E, Fujii GY, Reynolds SM, Melia M, Humayun MS, et al. Limited inferior macular translocation for the treatment of subfoveal choroidal neovascularization secondary to age-related macular degeneration. Am J Ophthalmol. 2000;130(4):419–28.
35. Joussen AM, Heussen FM, Joeres S, Llacer H, Prinz B, Rohrschneider K, et al. Autologous translocation of the choroid and retinal pigment epithelium in age-related macular degeneration. Am J Ophthalmol. 2006;142(1):17–30.
36. Bains HS, Patel MR, Singh H, Marcus DM. Surgical treatment of extensive peripapillary choroidal neovascularization in elderly patients. Retina. 2003;23(4):469–74.
37. Grossniklaus HE, Wilson DJ, Bressler SB, Bressler NM, Toth CA, Green WR, et al. Clinicopathologic studies of eyes that were obtained postmortem from four patients who were enrolled in the submacular surgery trials: SST report no. 16. Am J Ophthalmol. 2006;141(1):93–104. https://doi.org/10.1016/j.ajo.2005.07.076.
38. Aisenbrey S, Lafaut BA, Szurman P, Grisanti S, Luke C, Krott R, et al. Macular translocation with 360 degrees retinotomy for exudative age-related macular degeneration. Arch Ophthalmol. 2002;120(4):451–9.
39. Pertile G, Claes C. Macular translocation with 360 degree retinotomy for management of age-related macular degeneration with subfoveal choroidal neovascularization. Am J Ophthalmol. 2002;134(4):560–5.
40. Ichibe M, Yoshizawa T, Funaki S, Funaki H, Ozawa Y, Tanaka Y, et al. Severe hypotony after macular translocation surgery with 360-degree retinotomy. Am J Ophthalmol. 2002;134(1):139–41.
41. Fujikado T, Asonuma S, Ohji M, Kusaka S, Hayashi A, Ikuno Y, et al. Reading ability after macular translocation surgery with 360-degree retinotomy. Am J Ophthalmol. 2002;134(6):849–56.
42. Cahill MT, Stinnett SS, Banks AD, Freedman SF, Toth CA. Quality of life after macular translocation with 360 degrees peripheral retinectomy for age-related macular degeneration. Ophthalmology. 2005;112(1):144–51.
43. Lai JC, Lapolice DJ, Stinnett SS, Meyer CH, Arieu LM, Keller MA, et al. Visual outcomes following macular translocation with 360-degree peripheral retinectomy. Arch Ophthalmol. 2002;120(10):1317–24.
44. Mruthyunjaya P, Stinnett SS, Toth CA. Change in visual function after macular translocation with 360 degrees retinectomy for neovascular age-related macular degeneration. Ophthalmology. 2004;111(9):1715–24.
45. Atebara NH, Thomas MA, Holekamp NM, Mandell BA, Del Priore LV. Surgical removal of extensive peripapillary choroidal neovascularization associated with presumed ocular histoplasmosis syndrome. Ophthalmology. 1998;105(9):1598–605.
46. Melberg NS, Thomas MA, Dickinson JD, Valluri S. Managing recurrent neovascularization after subfoveal surgery in presumed ocular histoplasmosis syndrome. Ophthalmology. 1996;103(7):1064–7.
47. Lit ES, Kim RY, Damico DJ. Surgical removal of subfoveal choroidal neovascularization without removal of posterior hyaloid: a consecutive series in younger patients. Retina. 2001;21(4):317–23.
48. Gross JG, King LP, De Juan E, Jr., Powers T. Subfoveal neovascular membrane removal in patients with traumatic choroidal rupture. Ophthalmology. 1996;103(4):579–85.
49. Berger AS, McCuen BW, Brown GC, Brownlow RL Jr. Surgical removal of subfoveal neovascularization in idiopathic juxtafoveolar retinal telangiectasis. Retina. 1997;17(2):94–8.
50. Cooper BA, Thomas MA. Submacular surgery to remove choroidal neovascularization associated with central serous chorioretinopathy. Am J Ophthalmol. 2000;130(2):187–91.
51. Ng EW, Bressler NM, Boyer DS, De Juan E. Iatrogenic choroidal neovascularization occurring in patients undergoing macular surgery. Retina. 2002;22(6):711–8.
52. Hawkins BS, Miskala PH, Bass EB, Bressler NM, Childs AL, Mangione CM, et al. Surgical removal vs observation for subfoveal choroidal neovascularization, either associated with the ocular histoplasmosis syndrome or idiopathic: II. Quality-of-life findings from a randomized clinical trial: SST group H trial: SST report no. 10. Arch Ophthalmol. 2004;122(11):1616–28.
53. Ruiz-Moreno JM. de lV. Surgical removal of subfoveal choroidal neovascularisation in highly myopic patients. Br J Ophthalmol. 2001;85(9):1041–3.

54. Uemura A, Thomas MA. Subretinal surgery for choroidal neovascularization in patients with high myopia. Arch Ophthalmol. 2000;118(3):344–50.
55. Uemura A, Thomas MA. Visual outcome after surgical removal of choroidal neovascularization in pediatric patients. Arch Ophthalmol. 2000;118(10):1373–8.
56. Wood EH, Rao P, Mahmoud TH. Nanovitreoretinal subretinal gateway device to displace submacular hemorrhage: access to the subretinal space without vitrectomy. Retina. 2019; https://doi.org/10.1097/IAE.0000000000002669.

Diabetic Retinopathy 1

14

Contents

Introduction

There are several conditions which stimulate neovascularisation of the retina with subsequent complications such as vitreous haemorrhage and tractional retinal detachment from pathological separation of the vitreous. The most common is severe diabetic retinopathy but also retinal vein occlusion, sickle cell retinopathy, and retinal vasculitis.

Diabetic Retinopathy

Introduction

The complications of diabetic retinopathy remain despite major advances in screening of the population and clinical management of patients. Retinal laser photocoagulation is the mainstay of therapy [1–3] and reduces the chance of sight loss by 50%. Even so, the vitreoretinal surgeon is likely to have to treat many patients with diabetic vitreous haemorrhage or tractional retinal detachment with a reported 5% vitrectomy rate in diabetic retinopathy over 5 years [4]. Furthermore, the incidence of diabetes is increasing relentlessly negating the effects of improved diabetic control or prompt laser therapy. The increase in the use of PPV for the complications of diabetes is supported by the increased recording of the use of PPV with endolaser photocoagulation by 86% in Medicare fee data from the USA from 1997 to 2007 [5]. The risk of bilateral surgery in patients with VH or TRD in DMR is 30% [6].

Diabetic Retinopathy Grading (Table 14.1, Figs. 14.1 and 14.2)

Ischemic diabetic retinopathy characteristically affects the mid-peripheral retina outside the major temporal vascular arcades and nasal to the optic disc. Neovascularisation generally develops near the posterior limit of the ischemia, i.e. at the optic disc and along the major vascular arcades. Vascular tissue, arising from intraretinal venules, grows out through the inner limiting membrane and proliferates within the most cortical part of the vitreous gel as a vascularised epiretinal membrane (flat new vessels). The vessels do not grow into the central gel except occasionally within Cloquet's canal. The membranes incarcerate the gel on which they are proliferating, resulting in vitreoretinal adhesion. The vitreous may stiffen and shrink secondarily to the retinopathy increasing traction on blood vessels and membranes or the vitreous may detach rupturing blood vessels (Figs. 14.3, 14.4, 14.5, 14.6, and 14.7).

T. H. Williamson, *Vitreoretinal Surgery*, https://doi.org/10.1007/978-3-030-68769-4_14

Table 14.1 Diabetic retinopathy grading

Grade	Retinal features
No diabetic retinopathy	Nil
Mild non-proliferative retinopathy (NPDR)	Microaneurysms only
Moderate NPDR	More than "microaneurysms only" and less than severe NPDR
Severe NPDR	Any of the following: More than 20 microaneurysms in each quadrant Venous beading in more than 2 quadrants Intraretinal microvascular abnormalities in more than 1 quadrant No proliferation
Proliferative	Low risk, flat new vessels elsewhere High risk, raised new vessels elsewhere or disc new vessels

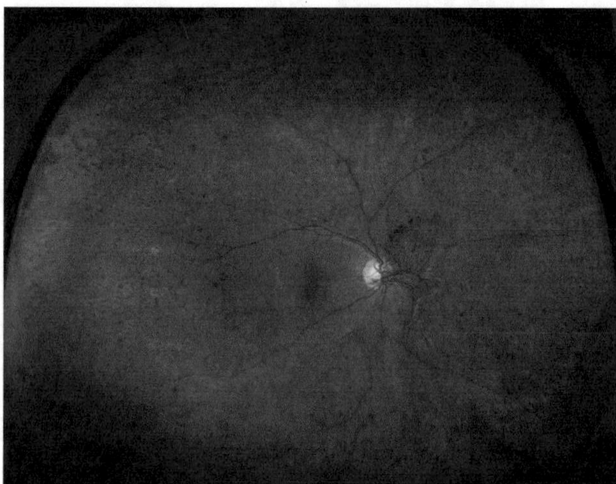

Fig. 14.1 NVD are present on this disc despite PRP

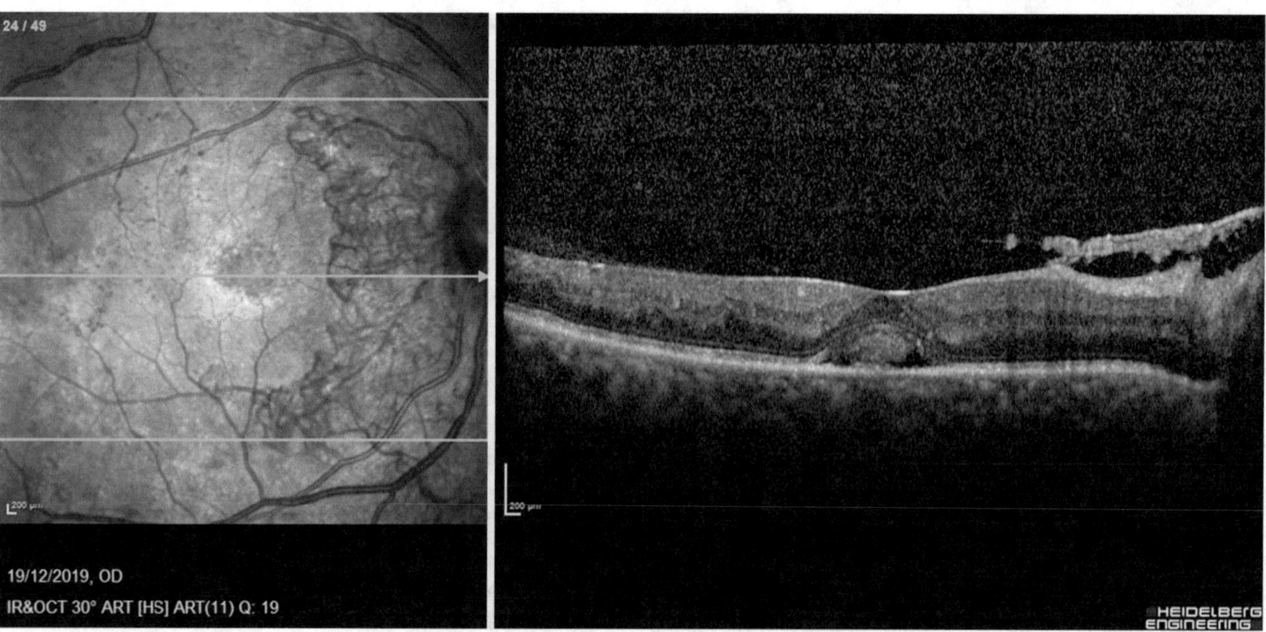

Fig. 14.2 Disc neovascularisation in DMR, notice the pegs of attachment

Diabetic Vitreous Haemorrhage (Figs. 14.8, 14.9, 14.10, 14.11, and 14.12)

Progression to Vitreous Haemorrhage and Tractional Retinal Detachment

(Fig. 14.13) In general progression to vitreous haemorrhage or retinal detachment can be seen as a sign of failure in the systems of screening to detect diabetic retinopathy early, monitoring and treatment of the retinopathy but also in the care of the patients diabetes, blood pressure, and other factors such as serum lipids by the diabetic physician and the patient themselves. The DRS and EDTRS demonstrated reduction in sight loss by 50–70% but not elimination of sight loss [1–3] because these patients develop maculopathy (the commonest cause of reduction in central vision), vitreous haemorrhage, and tractional retinal detachment. Rates of progression to vitrectomy are reduced by good control of blood sugar, hypertension, and lipids, timely and early PRP which reduce risk of PPV from 4% to 2.3% in the EDTRS [3]. Neovascularisation needs scaffold to grow on; therefore, PVD is protective. Most of these patients are too young to have spontaneous PVD and have had laser therapy which may reduce the chance of PVD due to vitreoretinal adhesion at laser scars. Progression to PPV has been calculated at 5% over 5 years [3]. The prevalence of PPV in the diabetic population in South London has been estimated as 5 per thousand diabetic patients (Figs. 14.14 and 14.15).

Demographics	
Male	54.1%
Type 1	36.8%
Type 2	63.2%
Insulin requiring	71.4%
Ethnicity	
Afro-Caribbean	31.4%
Caucasian	53.5%
Southeast Asian	11.4%

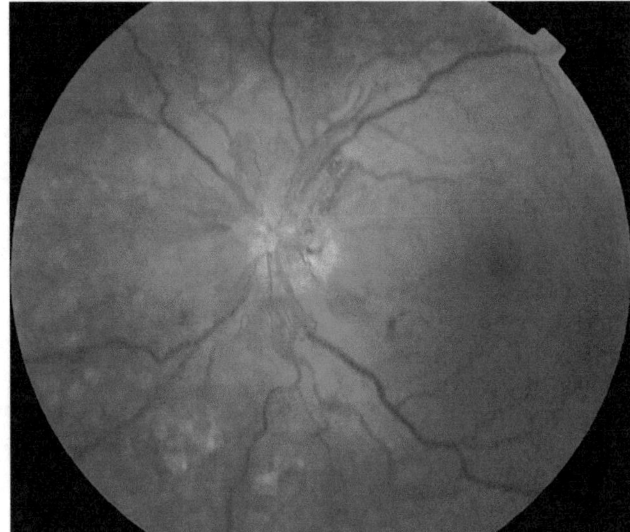

Fig. 14.3 Retinal neovascularisation requires a scaffold upon which to grow, i.e. the vitreous. In the left eye in which the vitreous is present extensive NVD are seen whilst in the right eye which has had PPV there is no structure (vitreous) upon which the vessels can grow

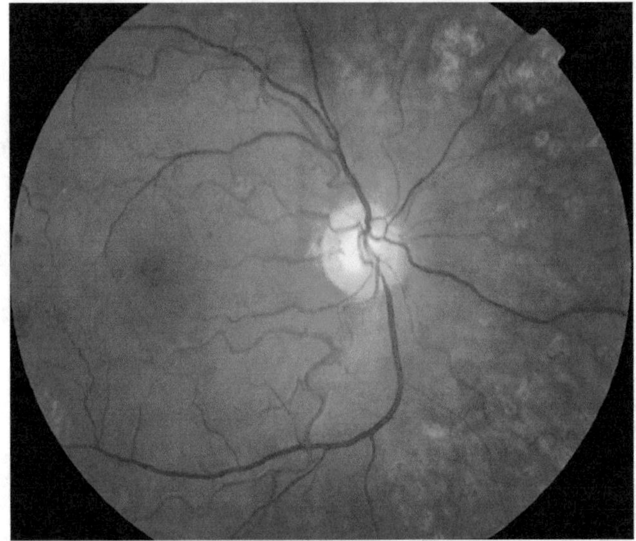

Fig. 14.4 Right eye with no vitreous does not have DNV

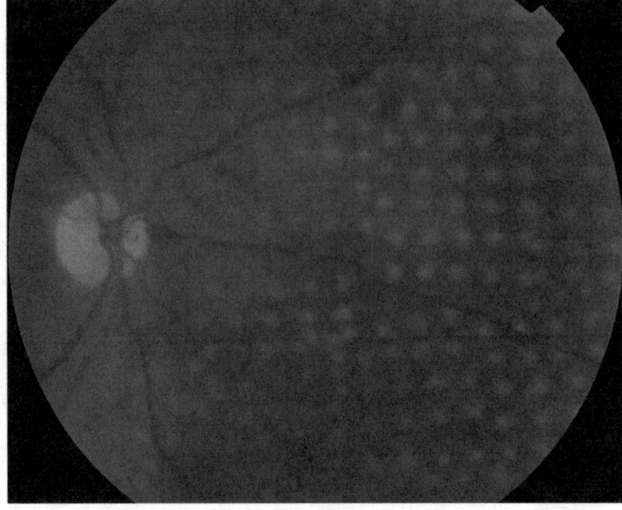

Fig. 14.5 Panretinal photocoagulation by pattern scan laser application

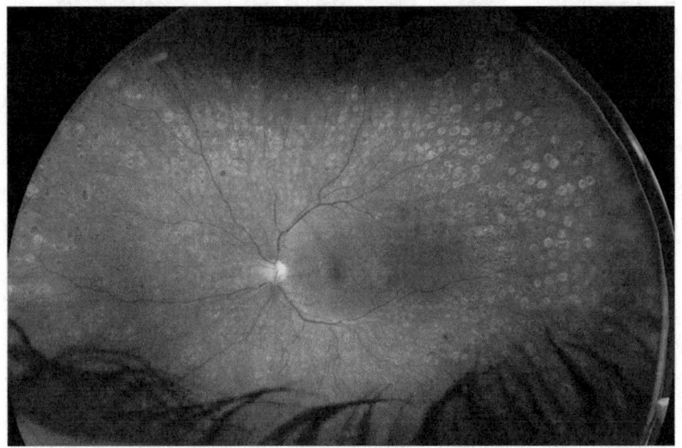

Fig. 14.6 Panretinal photocoagulation

Baseline Demographic Information in South London, UK.

Clinical Features

This is by far the commonest cause of haemorrhage into the vitreous cavity. The haemorrhage can occur into the gel or retrohyaloid space or rarely subretinal space (the last usually in association with tractional retinal detachment). Subretinal haemorrhage is associated with a poor visual outcome [7]. Severe retrohyaloid haemorrhage may cause the posterior vitreous face to bulge forward in bullae. Often diabetic haemorrhaging occurs spontaneously, i.e. from action of the vitreous on the new blood vessels, but occasionally haemor-

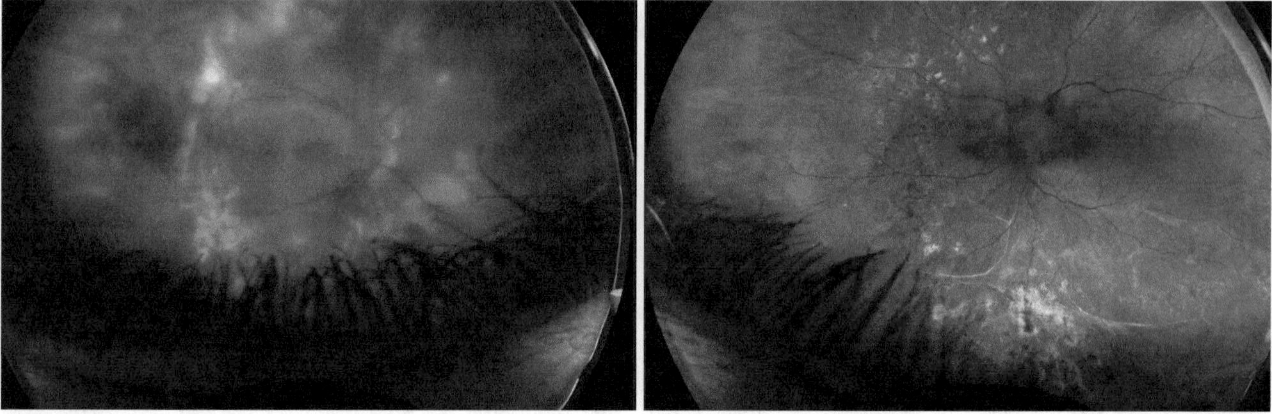

Fig. 14.7 A diabetic patient with vitreous haemorrhage in the right eye and subretinal bands in the left eye

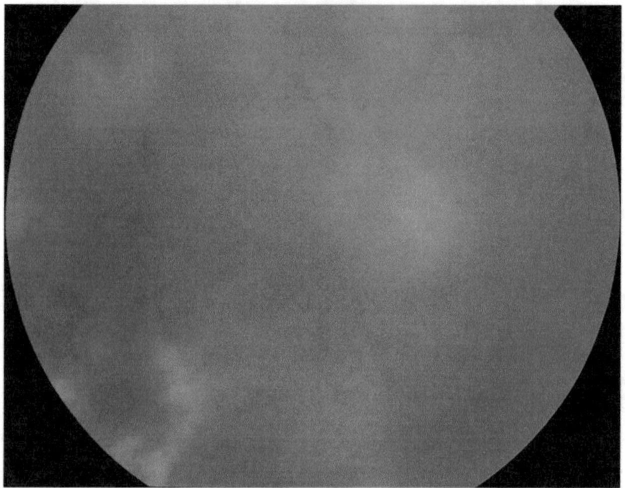

Fig. 14.8 Diffuse vitreous haemorrhage in diabetic retinopathy, visualisation with the indirect will reveal more detail in the retina than a 90D lens and the slit lamp

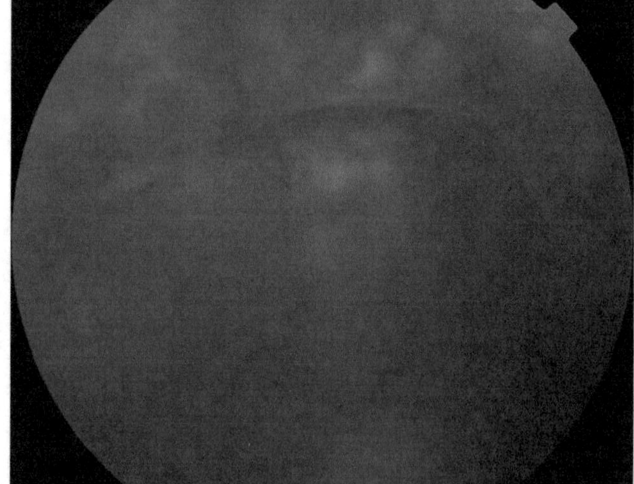

Fig. 14.10 A mature blood vessel is under traction by the vitreous causing it to haemorrhage. Laser will not regress this blood vessel and only removal of the vitreous will prevent recurrent bleeds

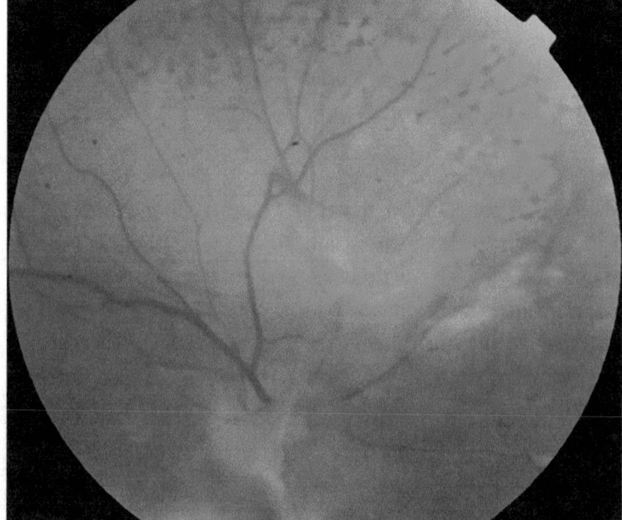

Fig. 14.9 Vitreous haemorrhage can be caused by neovascularisation or by avulsed blood vessels as in this patient

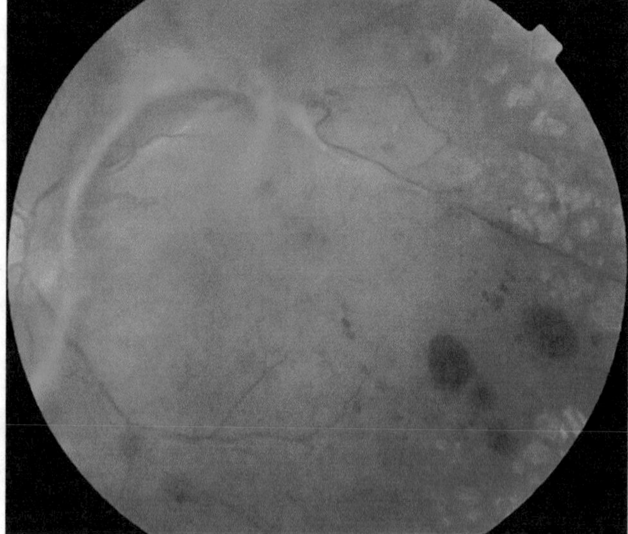

Fig. 14.11 The vitreous is applying traction to this blood vessel which may be a cause of recurrent haemorrhaging. Occasionally the blood vessel may be pulled out of the surface of the retina

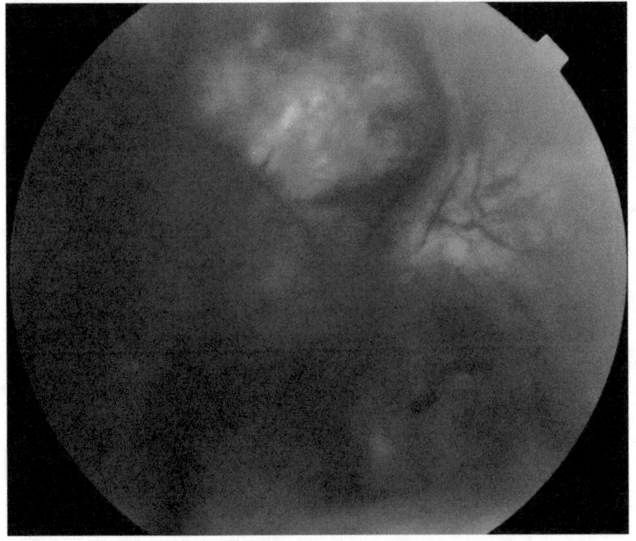

Fig. 14.12 Vitreous haemorrhage from neovascularisation of the optic disc

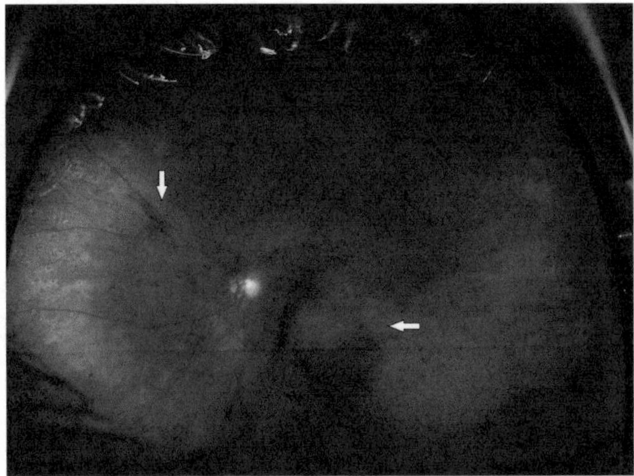

Fig. 14.13 A diabetic eye with NVE (vertical arrow) and central vitreous haemorrhage (horizontal arrow)

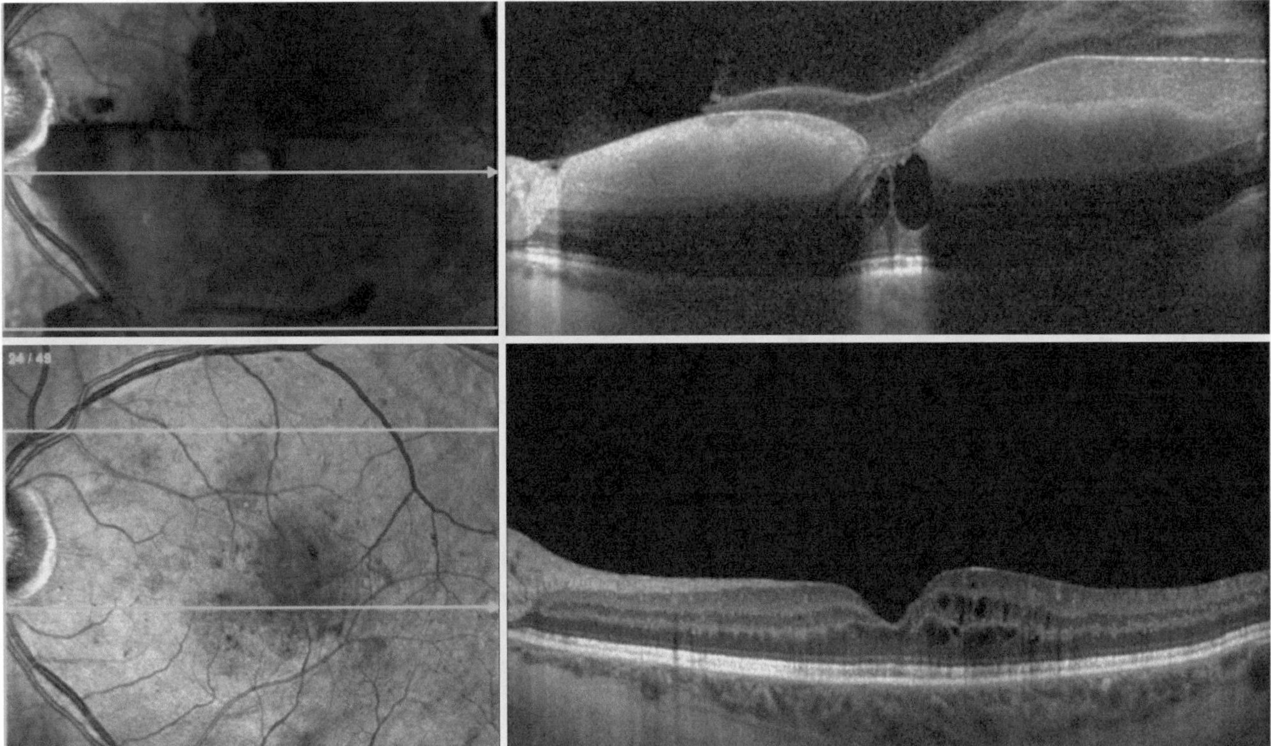

Fig. 14.14 A subhyaloid haemorrhage in DMR. Notice how it has put the fovea under traction. This is relieved after surgery

rhage happens during vigorous isometric exertion. Approximately 50% of the haemorrhages will clear spontaneously over three months. Untreated neovascularisation may progress over this time risking further haemorrhage, TRD, or neovascular glaucoma. Type one diabetics are particularly at risk of further complications if left too long before surgery [8, 9] and early intervention is recommended. If waiting for clearance, it is important to monitor the intraocular pressure for erythroclastic glaucoma and to perform repeated ultrasound examinations for retinal detachment (Fig. 14.16).

Note. If you cannot see the retina because of medial opacities, it is a good practice to always perform ultrasound. It is extremely useful to have an ultrasound in the outpatients' area and to be able to perform your own ultrasounds.

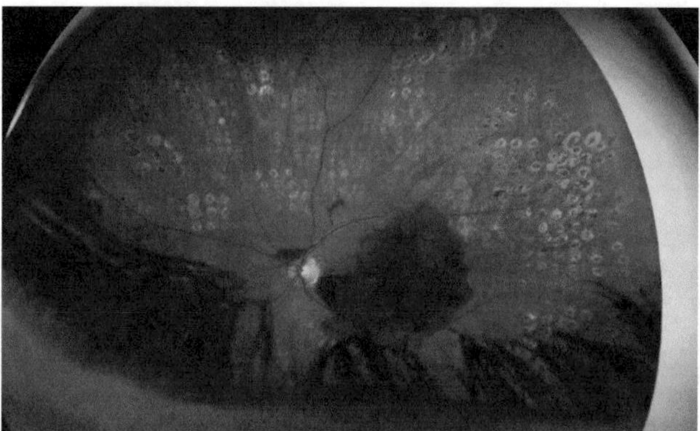

Fig. 14.15 Subhyaloid haemorrhage over the macula in DMR

Causes of vitreous haemorrhage.

- Active NV
- Inactive NV
- Vessel avulsion
- Traction from vitreous
- Pathological shrinkage of the vitreous
- Mobility of the vitreous
- PVD
- Acutely raised BP

PRP	PPV
Active NV and view rapidly clearing	Non-clearing VH
	Inadequate or no PRP
	INV
	For visual rehabilitation
	Associated TRD
	Recurrent VH

When to do more PRP and when to perform PPV in patients with vitreous haemorrhage (Fig. 14.17).

Indicators for Early Surgical Intervention

Iris neovascularisation	Urgent
No previous PRP	Urgent
Erythroclastic glaucoma	Soon
Type 1 diabetes	Soon

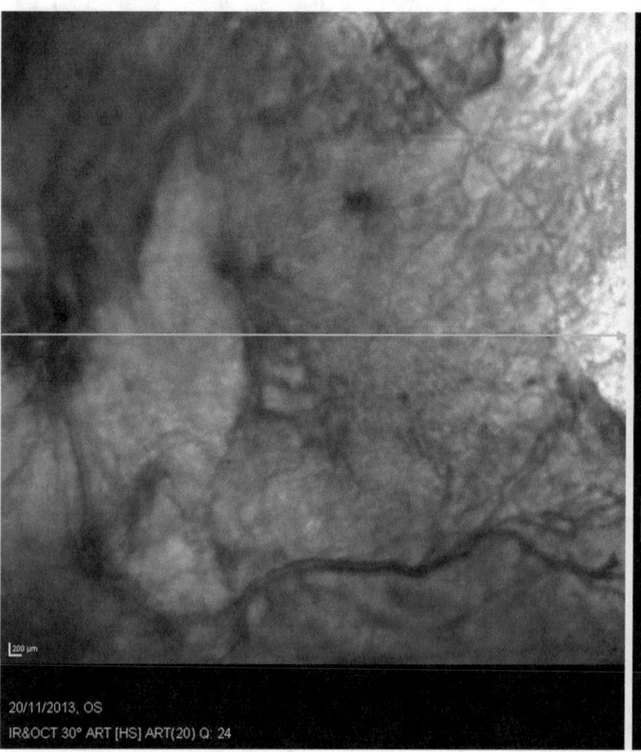

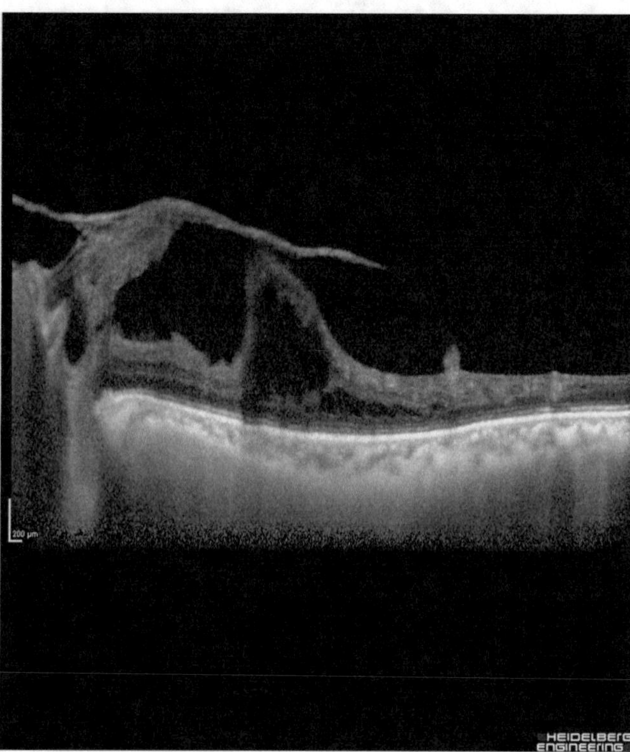

Fig. 14.16 Tractional elevation of the retina. Note the pegs of attachment

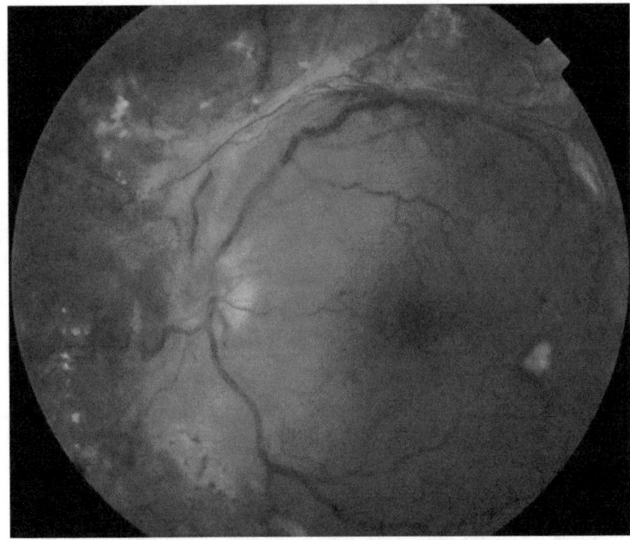

Fig. 14.17 Tractional membranes often follow the vascular arcades

B scan ultrasound examination is important to determine where the blood is situated, whether there is tractional retinal detachment, rhegmatogenous retinal detachment, or posterior vitreous detachment and is accurate in 90% of cases [10]. Adhesion of the vitreous to the retina can be seen at the sites of neovascularisation often on the vascular arcades or at the optic disc. The extent of the vitreoretinal adhesion should be assessed to guide the surgeon on the complexity of the surgery. The role of vitrectomy in the management of the complications of diabetic retinopathy has been established for many years [11–13]. The success rates of PPV are now high enough to offer surgery early in the clinical course of the haemorrhage without waiting for spontaneous clearance of the bleed.

In some circumstances if the vitreous haemorrhage is mild further laser can be applied to try to regress the neovascularisation without PPV. Some patients will bleed despite extensive PRP because of the presence of established neovascularisation which although gliosed has the capacity to bleed because of movement of attached gel or because the patient has an avulsed retinal blood vessel. These patients will not respond to further laser and will require PPV. The role of anti-VEGF injections in the treatment of vitreous haemorrhage has yet to be clarified although claims of more rapid regression of haemorrhage with injection alone have been made [14].

Surgery (Table 14.2)

Additional Surgical Steps.

- Remove the core vitreous and make a perforation in the posterior hyaloid.
- Remove any retrohyaloid haemorrhage through the perforation.

Table 14.2 Difficulty rating for PPV for diabetic vitreous haemorrhage

Difficulty Rating	Low
Success rates	High
Complication rates	Low
When to use in training	Early

- Remove the remaining vitreous.
- Apply panretinal photocoagulation.

Although vitreous haemorrhage from DMR may clear spontaneously after some months, pars plana vitrectomy is frequently required to rehabilitate the patient and can be associated with better visual prognosis [15]. The operation is more urgent in young diabetics to prevent irreversible loss of vision [8]. Preoperatively it is useful to determine with ultrasound whether the vitreous is fully detached or partially adherent to the retina, or whether there is TRD or neovascularisation. A fully detached vitreous promises an operation, which should be quick to perform with a good prognosis for visual recovery, whereas extensive TRD indicates a longer operation with a poorer prognosis.

If the media are clear subhyaloid blood can sometimes be treated with Yag laser [16, 17] without the need for vitrectomy. More often vitrectomy is required. During surgery, remove the central gel and then make a hole in the posterior hyaloid membrane. Remove the subhyaloid blood by placing a flute tip or the cutter on aspiration in the hole. This allows rapid removal of the subhyaloid blood without allowing it to enter the anterior vitreous cavity to spoil your view. Once the subhyaloid blood is removed the retina can be identified and the remaining gel removed with the reassurance that the retina is not detached and at risk of injury from cutter. Peripheral gel should be removed as much as possible as blood will leach out peroperatively and postoperatively causing vitreous cavity haemorrhage and occasionally erythroclastic glaucoma (raised IOP from clogging of the trabecular meshwork with macrophages laden with red blood cell break down products).

Note: When removing blood from the vitreous base, usually, a very thin layer of clear gel at the vitreous base is encountered before hitting the retina. This can be used as a guide to how close to the retina you are cutting. In very severe haemorrhages this clear zone may be absent.

Pan retinal photocoagulation is applied to prevent iris neovascularisation (INV) because the removal of the gel allows easy access of the neovascular factors to the anterior segment, especially in aphakic eyes, increasing the risk of INV [18, 19].

When using a blunt instrument near the retina, e.g. removing preretinal blood, apply the instrument close to the retina in an antero-posterior fashion in a "daub" like movement. Come away from the retina before moving to a new location.

The reason for doing this is that it is difficult to cause an injury to the retina with a blunt instrument if it is moved directly onto the retina without moving laterally. If it is moved laterally whilst touching the retina, resulting in a "scrape", there is a high chance of causing a tear.

The spherical shape of the eye means that an anterior movement of the instrument tip must accompany any lateral movement of an instrument to avoid striking the retina. Be aware of these principles when:

- Removing blood from the surface of the retina with a flute needle.
- Applying endolaser panretinal photocoagulation.
- Peeling epiretinal membranes.

Detaching the Posterior Hyaloid Membrane

Isolate and trim or dissect off any neovascularisation. Try not to leave any significant amount of tissue on the disc or elsewhere because these sites become small foci of contraction which may wrinkle the retina and fovea. Endodiathermy is usually unnecessary as the neovascularisation is of small calibre and low flow allowing rapid plugging with clot.

Preoperative Anti-VEGF

Intravitreal Bevacizumab can be inserted into the 3–7 days prior to surgery. This is not routinely necessary unless you anticipate the need to dissect active neovascularisation, in which case the blood vessels can be shrunk prior to surgery. I tend to use anti-VEGF only for patients with extensive neovascularisation or with TRD and active neovascularisation. Reduced rates of postoperative bleeding have been claimed with the use of anti-VEGF [20].

Surgical Pearl

When to Operate in Diabetic Vitreous Haemorrhage?

The Diabetic Retinopathy Vitrectomy Study demonstrated only modest improvements in visual outcomes from early vitrectomy in patients with proliferative diabetic retinopathy and vitreous haemorrhage.

Current conventional management of a patient with vitreous haemorrhage secondary to PDR, with no macular involving TRD, has been to start PRP immediately where possible or in cases where there is no fundus view, to wait until the vitreous haemorrhage clears such that scatter retinal laser photocoagulation can be applied. Vitrectomy in these patients has often been deferred until PRP has been completed in the outpatient setting, or once it is deemed that no further PRP can be applied or if the haemorrhage has failed to clear sufficiently to allow any PRP. In practical terms however, completion of laser PRP in patients with vitreous haemorrhage is often delayed and can take as long as six months whilst waiting for the blood to clear. Multiple sessions of PRP, often performed in small sectors at a time due to constraints imposed by a poor view of the retina from residual vitreous haemorrhage, necessitate frequent visits to the clinic and are inconvenient and costly to patients, accompanying carers, and the health service. This time also represents a significant delay in the visual rehabilitation of the patient during which loss of employment and income may ensue.

The rationale for early vitrectomy in cases of severe PDR and vitreous haemorrhage is that it removes the scaffold on which the fibrovascular proliferation grows, thus reducing the incidence of recurrent vitreous haemorrhage and future tractional retinal detachments. With improvements in vitreoretinal surgical techniques, in particular the introduction of the endolaser which allows the completion of a full laser PRP at the time of surgery, the outcomes of diabetic vitrectomy have improved significantly compared to 20 years ago when the first randomised controlled trial was done to evaluate its efficacy. For many vitreoretinal surgeons, the reduced risk profile of vitrectomy has lowered the threshold for surgical intervention in clinical practice. Increasingly VR surgeons are deviating from the conventional indications for vitrectomy and intervening within weeks of patients presenting with vitreous haemorrhage on a background of active PDR. By doing so, surgery is often technically less difficult and reduces the risk of surgical complications compared to deferring surgery which may result in progression of diabetic retinopathy because of inadequate laser treatment.

Ms Louisa Wickham, Moorfields Eye Hospital, London, UK

Specific Complications

Immediate vitreous haemorrhage after vitrectomy is common at about 30% of cases [21]. Some patients (10%) will have persistent haemorrhage and will need a vitrectomy to washout the vitreous cavity haemorrhage. This is a quick and safe operation. You can top up the laser at the same time. Be careful of erythroclastic glaucoma if you are observing the eye for spontaneous clearance. If you can see a blurred image of the optic disc or blood vessels through the haemorrhage, it is highly likely that the eye will clear within 2-3 weeks without surgery. Late vitreous cavity haemorrhage can occur and there has been much debate on the likely cause. The haemorrhage in a fluid filled eye clears more rapidly than in a vitreous filled eye (Figs. 14.18, 14.19, 14.20, 14.21, 14.22, 14.23, and 14.24).

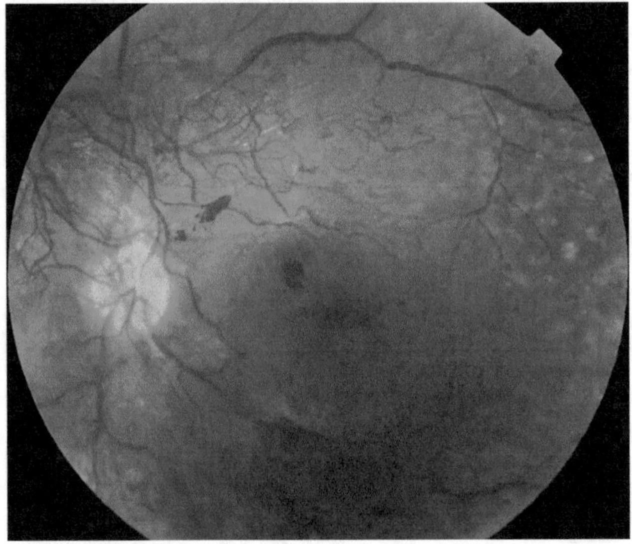

Fig. 14.18 In this patient, excessive neovascularisation is seen superior to the disc in the left eye. This has caused vitreous haemorrhage requiring PPV. The fellow eye has inactive membranes which have remained stable over a 1-year period with 20/30 vision

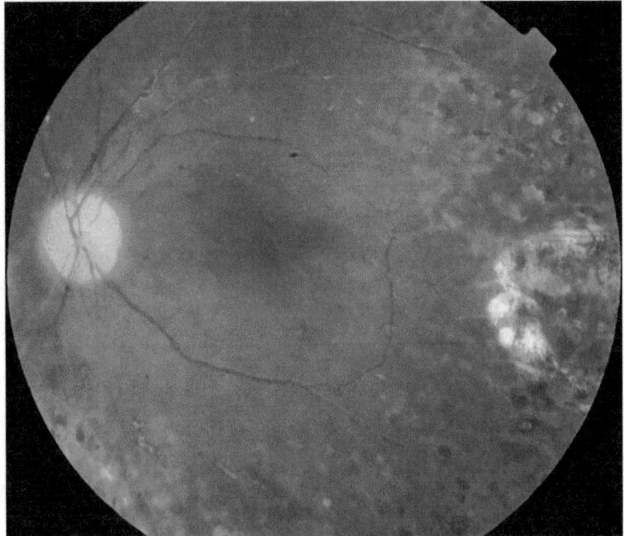

Fig. 14.20 The eye after vitrectomy

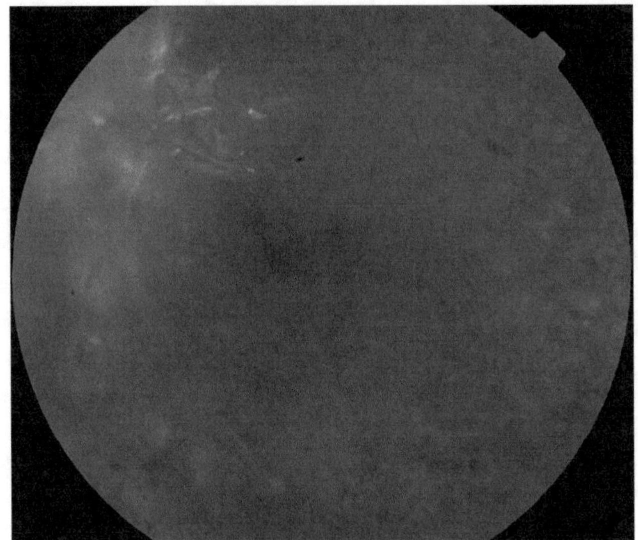

Fig. 14.19 Vitreous haemorrhage has occured Vitreous haemorrhage has occured

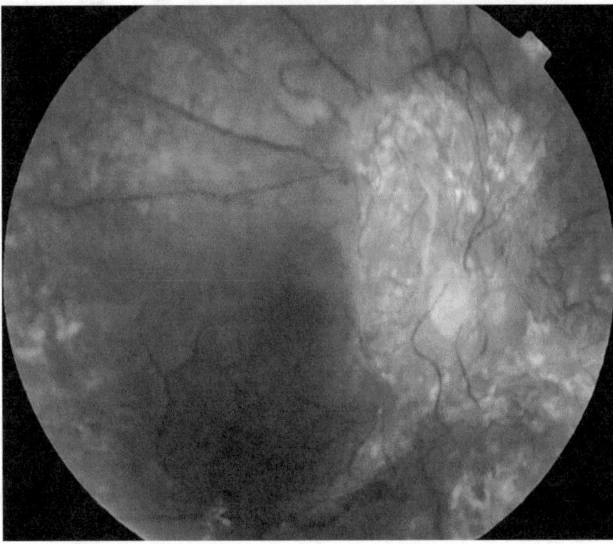

Fig. 14.21 Gliosed blood vessels in the other eye

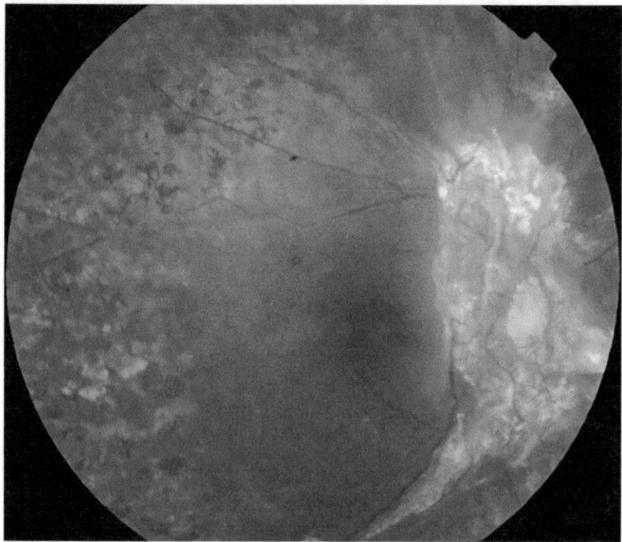

Fig. 14.22 These contracted further

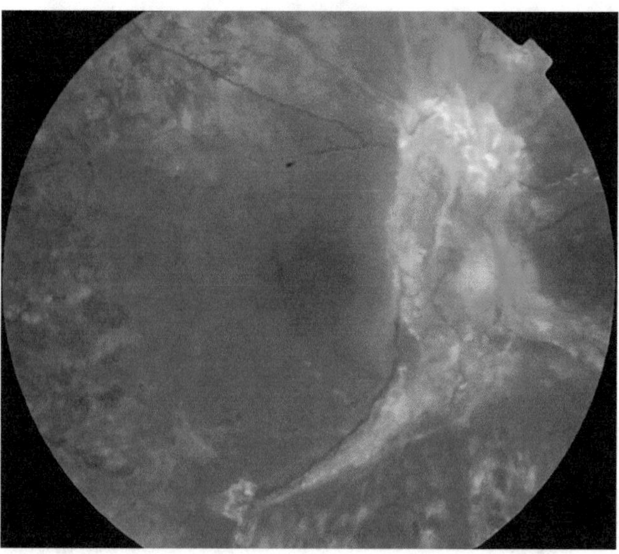

Fig. 14.23 The membranes were stable for some time but bled a few years later requiring vitrectomy

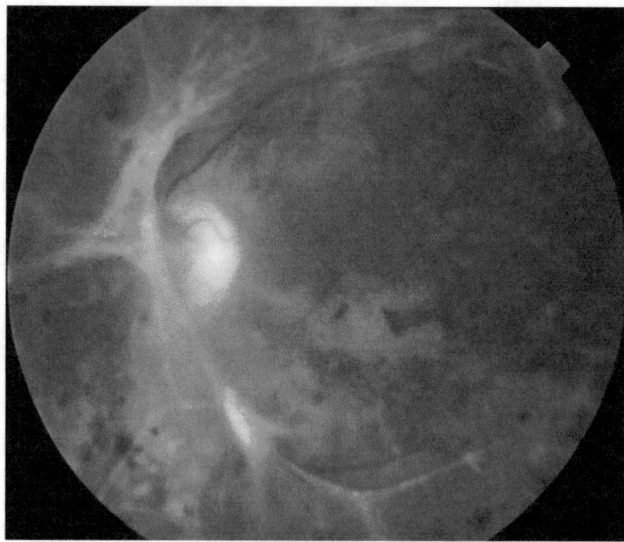

Fig. 14.24 This patient's neovascular membranes are stable 6 years after receiving a pancreatic transplant

References

1. Photocoagulation treatment of proliferative diabetic retinopathy: the second report of diabetic retinopathy study findings. Ophthalmology. 1978;85(1):82–106.
2. Photocoagulation treatment of proliferative diabetic retinopathy. Clinical application of diabetic retinopathy study (DRS) findings, DRS report number 8. The diabetic retinopathy study research group. Ophthalmology. 1981;88(7):583–600.
3. Early photocoagulation for diabetic retinopathy. ETDRS report number 9. Early treatment diabetic retinopathy study research group. Ophthalmology. 1991;98(5 Suppl):766–85.
4. Flynn HW Jr, Chew EY, Simons BD, Barton FB, Remaley NA, Ferris FL III. Pars plana vitrectomy in the early treatment diabetic retinopathy study. ETDRS report number 17. The early treatment diabetic retinopathy study research group. Ophthalmology. 1992;99(9):1351–7.
5. Ramulu PY, Do DV, Corcoran KJ, Corcoran SL, Robin AL. Use of retinal procedures in medicare beneficiaries from 1997 to 2007. Arch Ophthalmol. 128(10):1335–40. https://doi.org/10.1001/archophthalmol.2010.224.

6. Fajgenbaum MAP, Wong RS, Laidlaw DAH, Williamson TH. Vitreoretinal surgery on the fellow eye: a retrospective analysis of 18 years of surgical data from a tertiary center in England. Indian J Ophthalmol. 2018;66(5):681–6. https://doi.org/10.4103/ijo.IJO_1176_17.
7. Morse LS, Chapman CB, Eliott D, Benner JD, Blumenkranz MS, McCuen BW. Subretinal hemorrhages in proliferative diabetic retinopathy. Retina. 1997;17(2):87–93.
8. Early vitrectomy for severe vitreous hemorrhage in diabetic retinopathy. Two-year results of a randomized trial. Diabetic retinopathy vitrectomy study report 2. The diabetic retinopathy vitrectomy study research group. Arch Ophthalmol. 1985;103(11):1644–52.
9. Early vitrectomy for severe vitreous hemorrhage in diabetic retinopathy. Four-year results of a randomized trial: diabetic retinopathy vitrectomy study report 5. Arch Ophthalmol. 1990;108(7):958–64.
10. Genovesi-Ebert F, Rizzo S, Chiellini S, Di Bartolo E, Marabotti A, Nardi M. Reliability of standardized echography before vitreoretinal surgery for proliferative diabetic retinopathy. Ophthalmologica. 1998;212(Suppl 1):91–2.
11. Mandelcorn MS, Blankenship G, Machemer R. Pars plana vitrectomy for the management of sever diabetic retinopathy. Am J Ophthalmol. 1976;81(5):561–70.
12. Michels RG. Vitrectomy for complications of diabetic retinopathy. Arch Ophthalmol. 1978;96(2):237–46.
13. Aaberg TM. Clinical results in vitrectomy for diabetic traction retinal detachment. Am J Ophthalmol. 1979;88(2):246–53.
14. Huang YH, Yeh PT, Chen MS, Yang CH, Yang CM. Intravitreal bevacizumab and panretinal photocoagulation for proliferative diabetic retinopathy associated with vitreous hemorrhage. Retina. 2009;29(8):1134–40. https://doi.org/10.1097/IAE.0b013e3181b094b7.
15. Early vitrectomy for severe proliferative diabetic retinopathy in eyes with useful vision. Results of a randomized trial--diabetic retinopathy vitrectomy study report 3. The diabetic retinopathy vitrectomy study research group. Ophthalmology. 1988;95(10):1307–20.
16. Celebi S, Kukner AS. Photodisruptive Nd:YAG laser in the management of premacular subhyaloid hemorrhage. Eur J Ophthalmol. 2001;11(3):281–6.
17. Ulbig MW, Mangouritsas G, Rothbacher HH, Hamilton AM, McHugh JD. Long-term results after drainage of premacular subhyaloid hemorrhage into the vitreous with a pulsed Nd:YAG laser. Arch Ophthalmol. 1998;116(11):1465–9.
18. Rice TA, Michels RG, Rice EF. Vitrectomy for diabetic traction retinal detachment involving the macula. Am J Ophthalmol. 1983;95(1):22–33.
19. Blankenship GW. The lens influence on diabetic vitrectomy results. Report of a prospective randomized study. Arch Ophthalmol. 1980;98(12):2196–8.
20. Hu X, Pan Q, Zheng J, Song Z, Zhang Z. Reoperation following vitrectomy for diabetic vitreous hemorrhage with versus without preoperative intravitreal bevacizumab. BMC Ophthalmol. 2019;19(1):200. https://doi.org/10.1186/s12886-019-1179-x.
21. Khuthaila MK, Hsu J, Chiang A, DeCroos FC, Milder EA, Setlur V, et al. Postoperative vitreous hemorrhage after diabetic 23-gauge pars plana vitrectomy. Am J Ophthalmol. 2013;155(4):757–63., 63 e1-2. https://doi.org/10.1016/j.ajo.2012.11.004.

Diabetic Retinopathy 2

15

Contents

Diabetic Retinal Detachment

Clinical Features (Figs. 15.1, 15.2, and 15.3)

As in other epiretinal membranes, fibroblasts within the vascularised membranes contract and the tangential traction so produced is stabilised and consolidated by collagen synthesis. The tangential traction results initially in folding of the inner retinal layers (internal limiting membrane and nerve fibre layer) and can then progress to traction retinal detachment.

Contraction of the neovascular membranes both anteroposteriorly and tangentially combined with shrinkage of the vitreous gel pulls the retina at its points of adhesion into the centre of the eye. Without a retinal hole to allow accumulation of subretinal fluid the retina detaches with a concave configuration. Two forces are acting on the retina, one the action of the RPE to keep the retina flat and two the action of the shrinking vitreous and neovascular membranes pulling the retina centrally into the vitreous cavity.

During this process the vitreous cortex often splits leaving a thin layer on the retina that should be elevated during surgery to allow easier dissection of the fibrotic neovascular membranes [1, 2]. The vitreous detachment on the inner surface of the vitreoschisis is taught, stretches from the vitreous base to the neovascular membranes and between the membranes. The areas of detachment surround neovascularisation on the retinal arcades and are often multifocal. Eventually the macula detaches severely reducing the visual acuity, whilst the periphery remains flat. The extent of tractional

T. H. Williamson, *Vitreoretinal Surgery*, https://doi.org/10.1007/978-3-030-68769-4_15

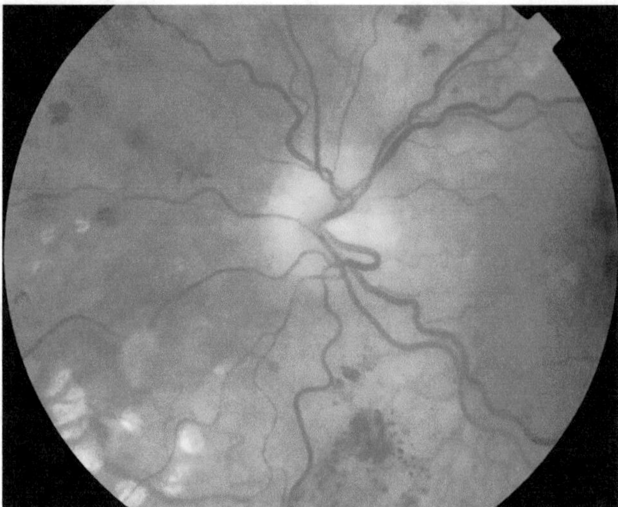

Fig. 15.1 Traction on the retina can create a retinal break as in this patient who has an avulsed blood vessel and an operculum on the nasal side of the disc overlying a retinal hole. Often as in this eye progression to RRD does not occur, this may be due to the stiff immobile vitreous in diabetes. The immobility of the vitreous prevents the creation of fluid currents thought to be necessary for SRF to accumulate

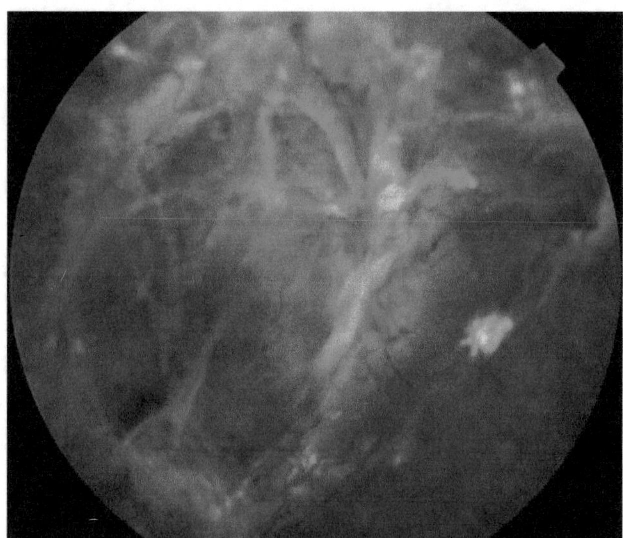

Fig. 15.2 Unfortunately, despite the advantages in screening and in treatment by pan retinal photocoagulation, patients still attend with very severe tractional retinal detachments as seen in this picture. The appearance can be deceptive with dissections easier than at first apparent. As with all diabetic tractional retinal detachments the key is determining the right layer and getting behind the posterior hyaloid, membrane, and cortex. Elevation of cortex remnants in a vitreoschisis aids removal of the vitreous gel and reattachment of the retina

retinal detachment (TRD) varies from a single focus to large areas of the retina. Similarly, and more important to the surgeon the areas of adhesion of the neovascular membrane to the retina vary, often being most pronounced on the vascular arcades and around the optic disc.

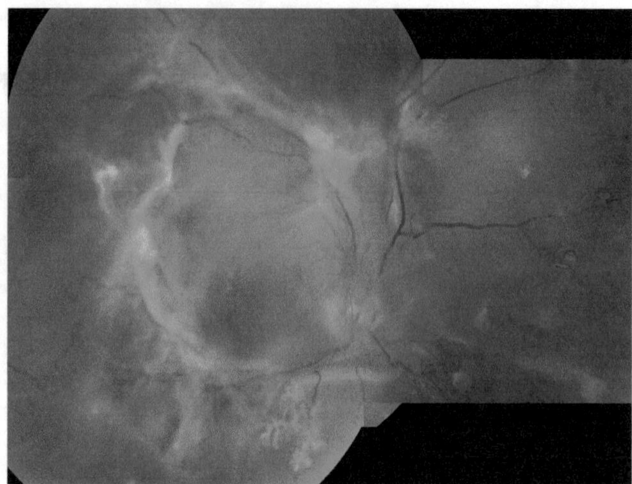

Fig. 15.3 The membranes in diabetic TRD usually form over the retinal vasculature, the optic disc and temporal to the macula encircling the macula. However, membranes can be seen anywhere in the retina

Traction on the disc can reduce vision by damaging the superficial nerve fibres [3] indeed axons are found in tissue removed from the disc surgically [4].

Traction on the retina may split the retina causing retinoschisis [4].

Occasionally a hole appears in the fragile ischemic retina allowing subretinal fluid accumulation. The retinal detachment then takes on a convex configuration and may extend further anteriorly in a bullous fashion. (Figs. 15.4, 15.5, and 15.6).

Application of panretinal photocoagulation to eyes with tractional retinal detachment can cause further contraction of the membranes and macular detachment [5]. Therefore, in patients with established TRDs but with no PRP it is often safer to proceed to PPV rather than try PRP alone (Figs. 15.7, 15.8, 15.9, 15.10 and 15.11).

Surgery

Tractional Retinal Detachment (Table 15.1)

Additional surgical steps.

Insert a chandelier light pipe.

Remove vitreous haemorrhage as above but retain any traction on the retina.

Create holes in the posterior hyaloid to allow easy access to the areas of retinal elevation and vitreoretinal adhesion.

Detect and elevate the posterior layer of any vitreoschisis.

Dissect the tractional membranes off the retina with a bimanual method.

Complete the removal of the vitreous.

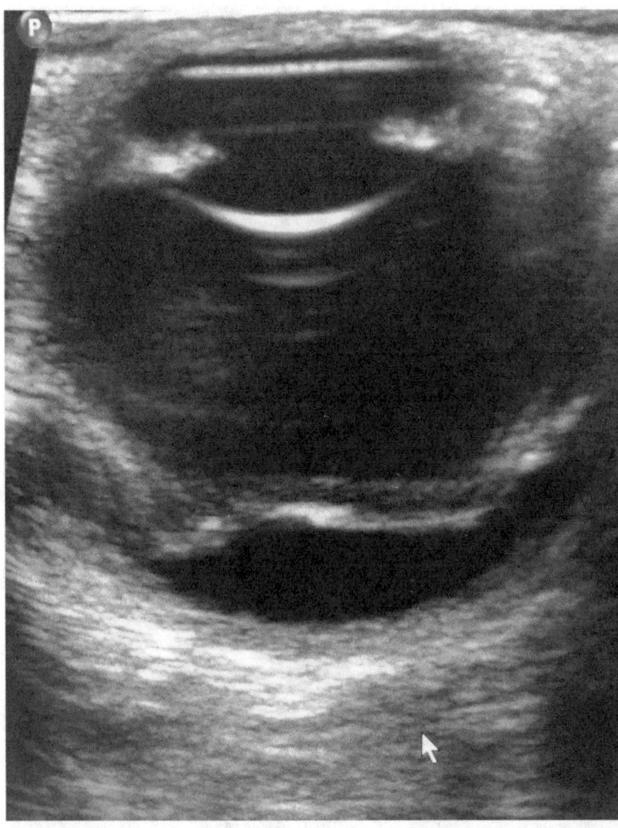

Fig. 15.4 A vitreous haemorrhage with attachment of the vitreous to an area of TRD

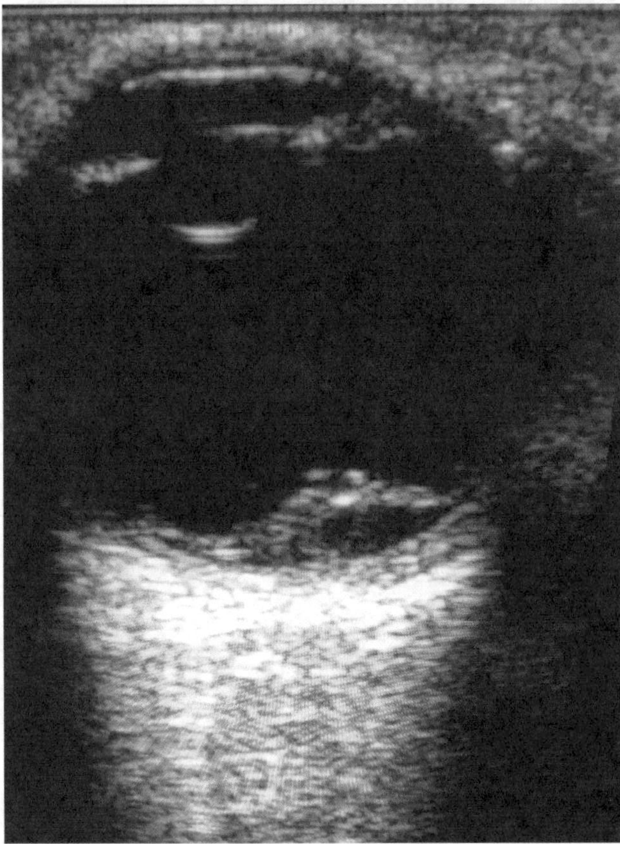

Fig. 15.5 A TRD on US

Fig. 15.6 A "tabletop" TRD. It is still worth operating to see if some vision can be recovered

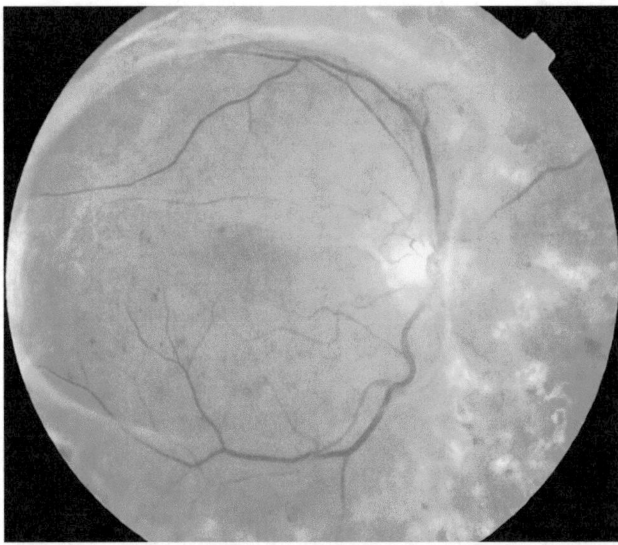

Fig. 15.7 The fovea is just being elevated by the TRD in this patient as shown by the OCT image

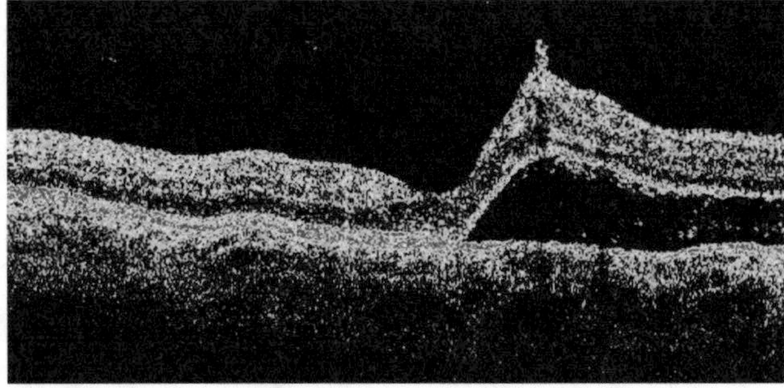

Fig. 15.8 SRF is encroaching the fovea as seen on OCT

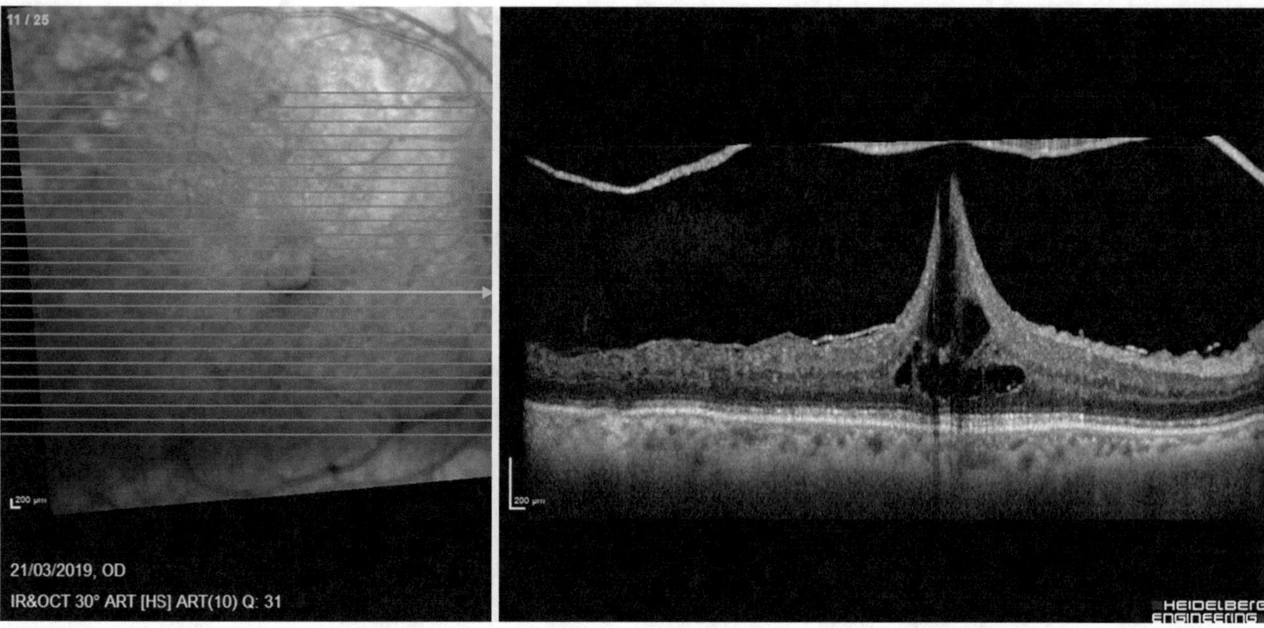

Fig. 15.9 Tractional retinal elevation in DMR can lead to schisis of the retina

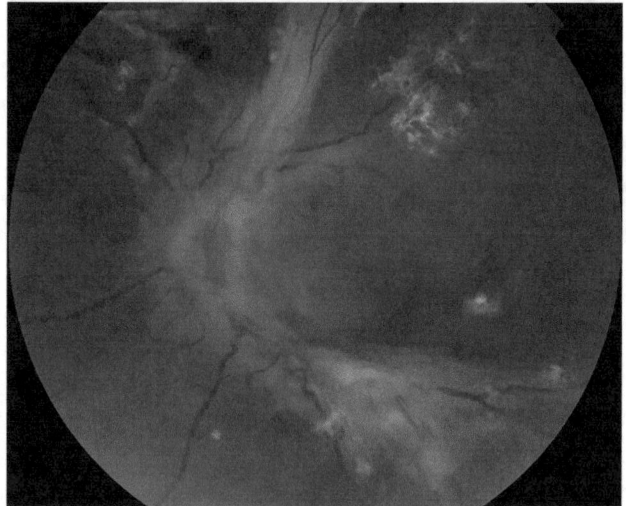

Fig. 15.10 If you see asymmetrical disease, check the eye with less retinopathy for a PVD or check the carotid arteries for stenosis (the worse stenosis is on the same side as the eye with less retinopathy)

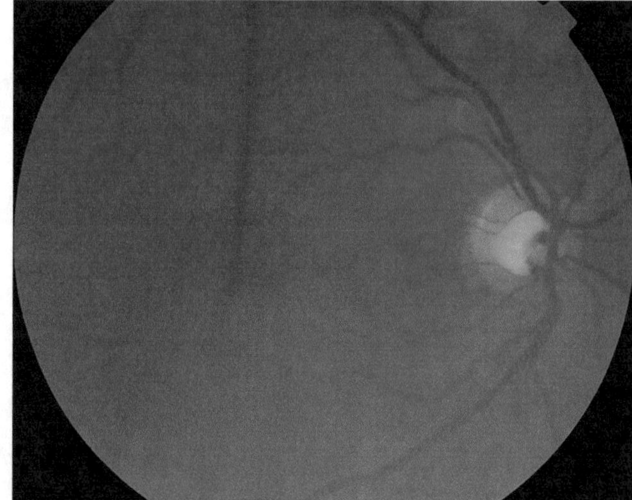

Fig. 15.11 The other eye has minimal retinopathy

Table 15.1 Difficulty rating for diabetic tractional retinal detachment

Difficulty rating	High
Success rates	Moderate
Complication rates	High
When to use in training	Late

Apply panretinal photocoagulation (Figs. 15.12, 15.13, and 15.14).

(Fig. 15.15) Where significant neovascular membranes exist or retinal detachment is present dissection by delamination of any membranes is required. The membranes are best removed in total ("en bloc") to prevent future reproliferation and subsequent detachment [6–8]. The core of the vitreous is removed whilst retaining the taught peripheral gel thereby maintaining traction upon the membrane. A hole is made in the cortical gel to allow access of instruments to the retinal surface. The outer portion of the vitreous cortex on the retinal surface is then elevated to find the plane of cleavage of the internal limiting membrane and posterior hyaloid membrane. The posterior hyaloid and the neovascular membranes are then dissected away from the retina to relieve traction and allow the retina to reattach. Modern small gauge cutters ((27 gauge is preferred) have orifices which are nearer the tip end of the cutter shaft [9] (Fig. 15.16). This allows the surgeon to get very close to the retina without engaging it. Membranes are easily nibbled off the surface of the retina. Using a bimanual technique allows the membranes to be elevated locally for dissection and cutting. This speeds up the dissection compared with the use of passive traction alone. In addition, it allows the surgeon to fold the membrane upon itself for controlled division of pegs (see ERM surgery). The

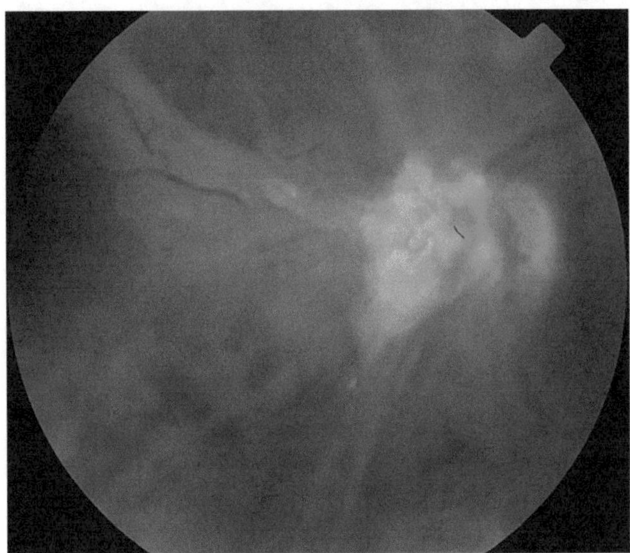

Fig. 15.12 The membranes can cause traction and damage on the optic nerve reducing visual recovery postoperatively

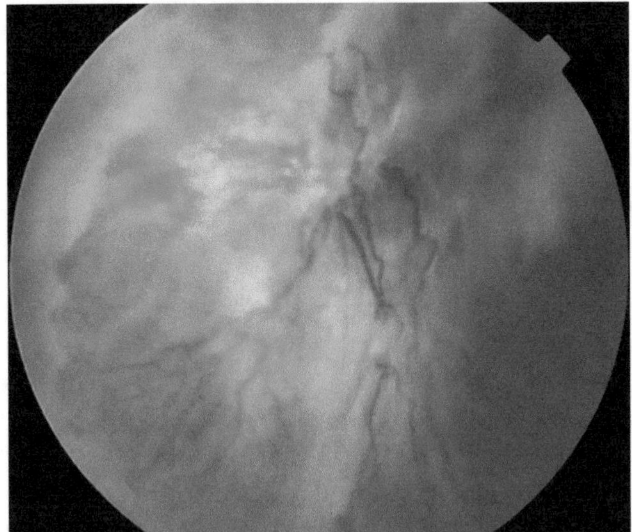

Fig. 15.13 A combination of rhegmatogenous and tractional retinal detachment may occur. Problems exist when the patient has a rhegmatogenous element in addition producing PVR. Other indicators of relatively poor prognosis are subretinal haemorrhage and iris neovascularisation

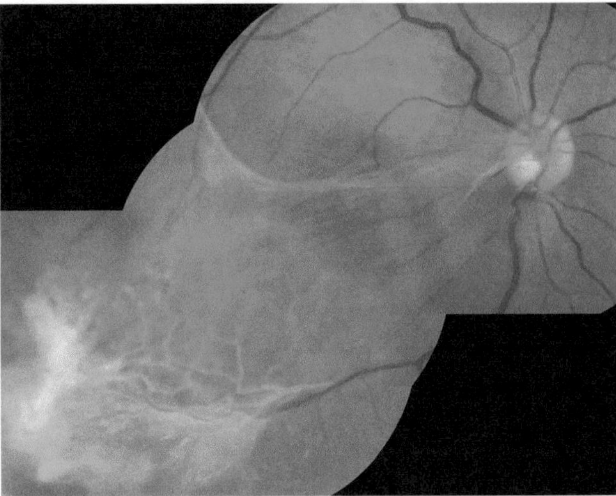

Fig. 15.14 Occasionally an eye in which neovascularisation has been stabilised by laser will have inactive membrane overlying the macula

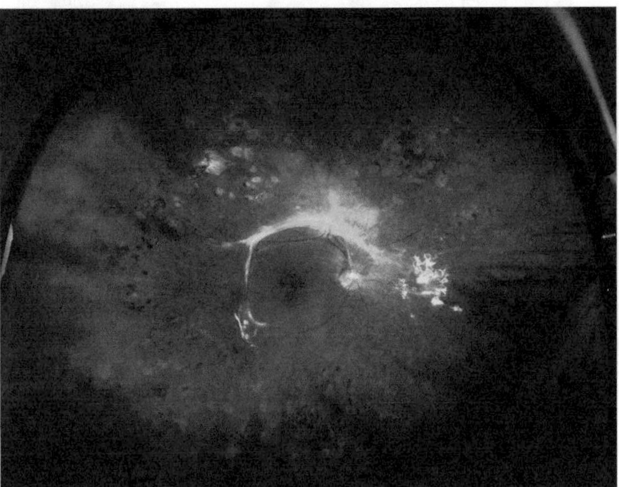

Fig. 15.15 Despite only minimal PRP these membranes are stable perhaps indicating a "burnt out" retinopathy

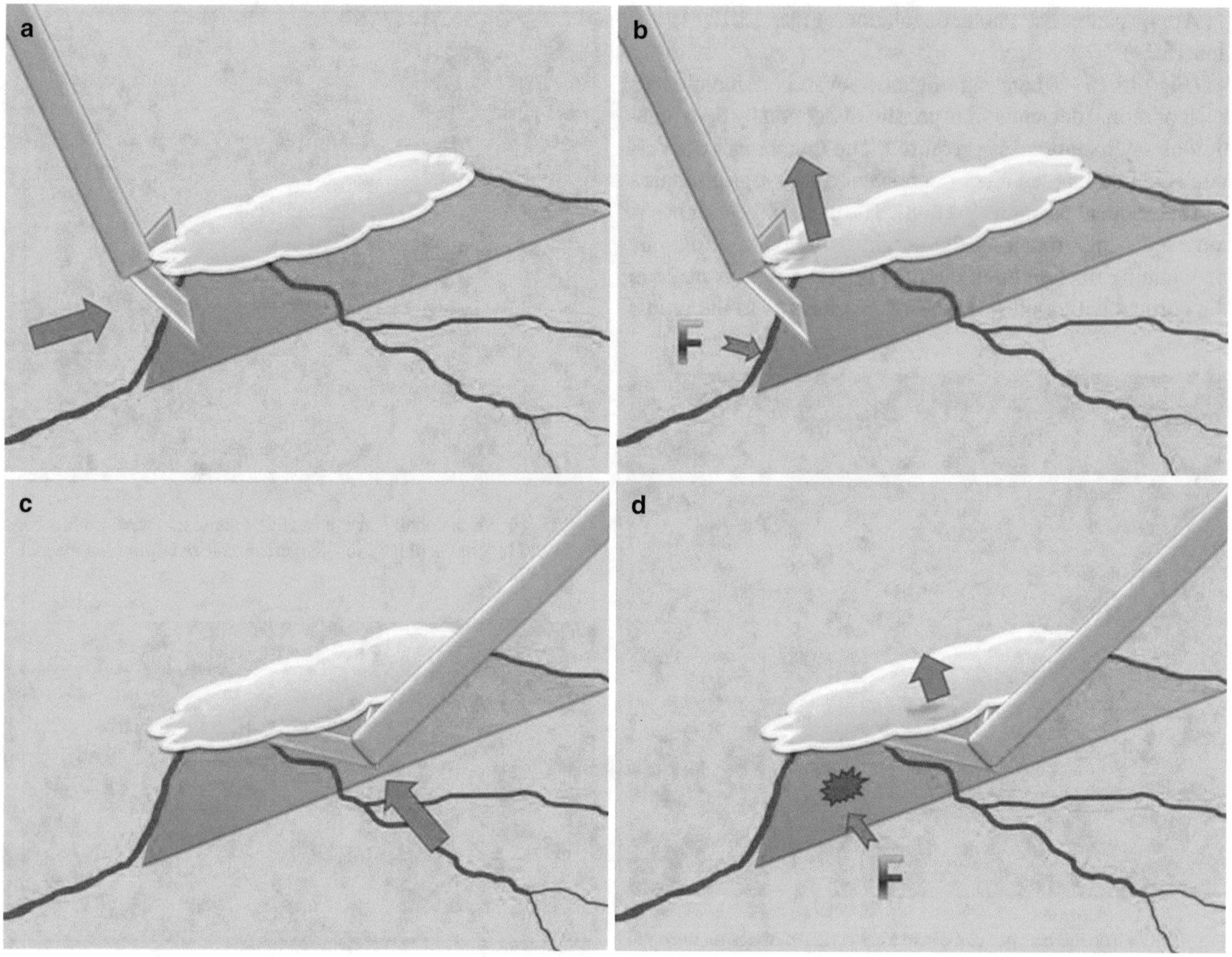

Fig. 15.16 Try to work along a ridge of adhesion (often along a large blood vessel) (**a** and **b**) rather than across it because the scissors can straddle the ridge and keep away from the retina and any forces (F) are applied to the relatively strong blood vessel. Going across the ridge (**c** and **d**) risks the tips of the scissors incising the retina and the forces are applied to the weak retina on the slope of the ridge

ability to lift membranes with serrated forceps reduces the need to maintain anterior–posterior traction which frees up the removal process of the vitreous (Fig. 15.17).

Note: In TRD the membranes can be trimmed down by these cutters effectively shaving down the membrane until the retina is cleared rather than using scissors to dissect off the membrane.

Elevating the cortical gel and posterior hyaloid which is still attached to the surface of the retina is the key manoeuvre of the operation. Having made the hole in the elevated vitreous cortex, use the edge of the scissors or the cutter to run along the slope of an area of TRD. Try to catch the posterior hyaloid and see it lifts both outwards towards the equator and towards the TRD. Elevate the PHM up to the edge of the TRD and then use the plane between this and the retina to elevate the membranes. Alternatively, the correct plane can sometimes be found by starting in the macular area and working outwards towards the arcades (Fig. 15.18).

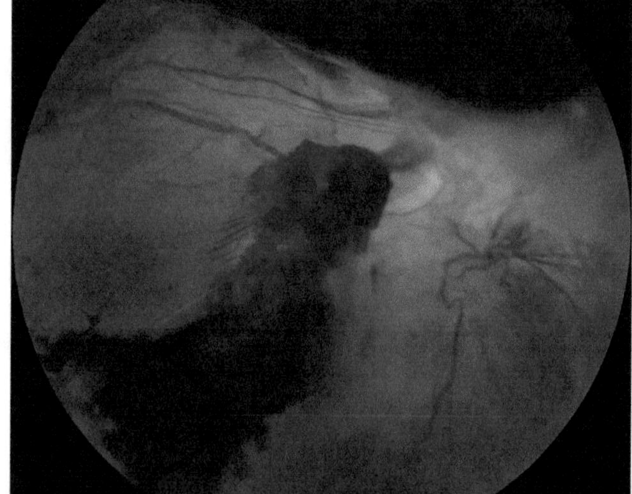

Fig. 15.17 A severe TRD with vitreous haemorrhages

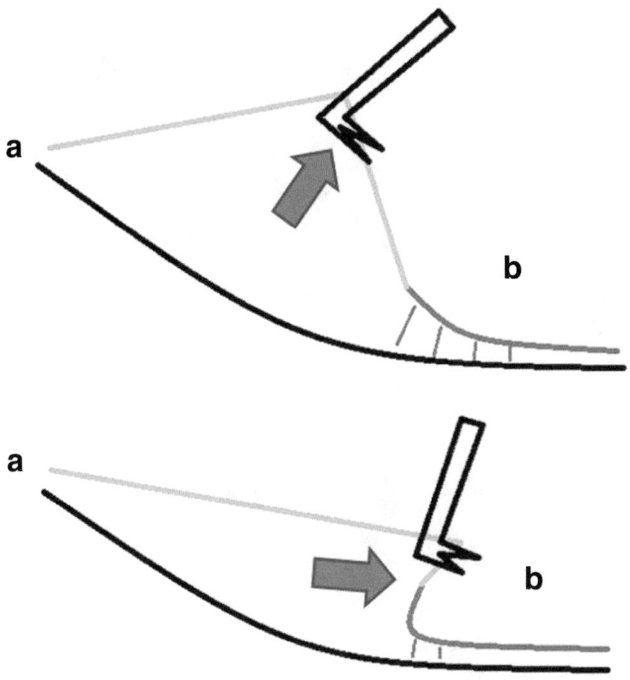

Fig. 15.18 When using the posterior hyaloid to lift a membrane (e.g. TRD membrane) to look for pegs at site (**b**) stay close to the edge of the membrane. Lifting further away from the membrane requires a vertical movement to avoid traction at point (**a**) to see the pegs. This will also put a force on pegs deeper under the membrane which you cannot see. If you stay close to the membrane edge, a tangential motion is possible without undue force at point (**a**) and only applying force to pegs at the edge of the membrane

Note:

The PHM very often ends in the peripheral retina and does not often extend to the vitreous base in severe TRD.

In this plane the membranes will separate much more easily. Cutting through cortical gel is much more difficult to achieve and will leave membrane on the retina allowing later reproliferation. Some of the membrane will lift off but sites of adhesion that will not lift must be cut. Keep your visualisation to a maximum by trimming any elevated membrane with the cutter whilst maintaining some antero-posterior traction on the TRD. As with any membrane, work around points of adhesion lifting the membrane around a difficult site before tackling it. Usually I will elevate and PHM around the TRD 360°, if I can, before dissecting the area of TRD itself. When lifting the PHM elevate close to the edge of the TRD and then move tangentially out to elevate the PHM in the periphery. If using the PHM to lift the edge of the TRD, stay close to the TRD to achieve a large angle on the edge of the TRD without applying forces on the vitreous base (Figs. 15.19 and 15.20).

Most TRDs are made up of peg attachments except:

- At the optic disc where a larger area of adhesion approximately ½ a disc area is seen. This will usually peel off the disc with scissors or the cutter surprisingly easily though be aware of the major blood vessels and vulnerability of the surface of the optic nerve head.
- Where there is schitic retina there can sometimes be a sheet of adhesion of the membrane to the retina.

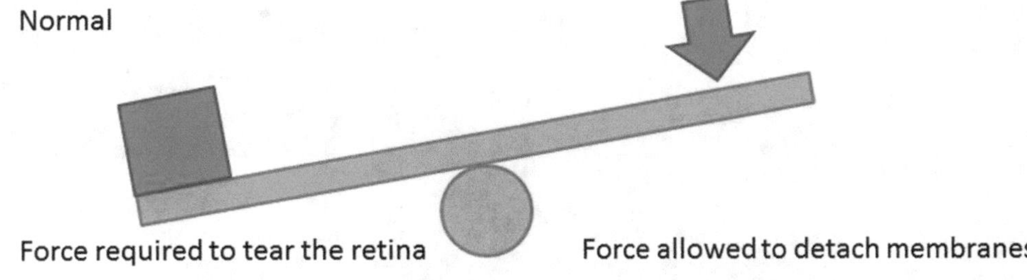

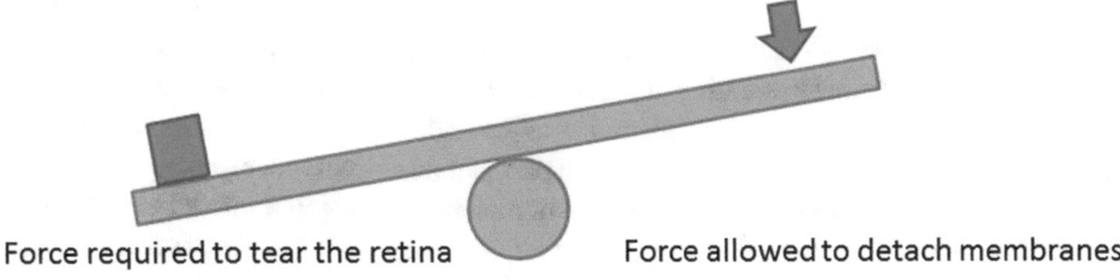

Fig. 15.19 The balancing act between pulling on an ERM and avoiding a retinal tear. In the normal eye a large force is required before the retina tears, so that a relatively large force can be applied to pull off an ERM. In the ischaemic diabetic retina, a small force may tear the retina therefore only a small force can be applied to ERM to remove it

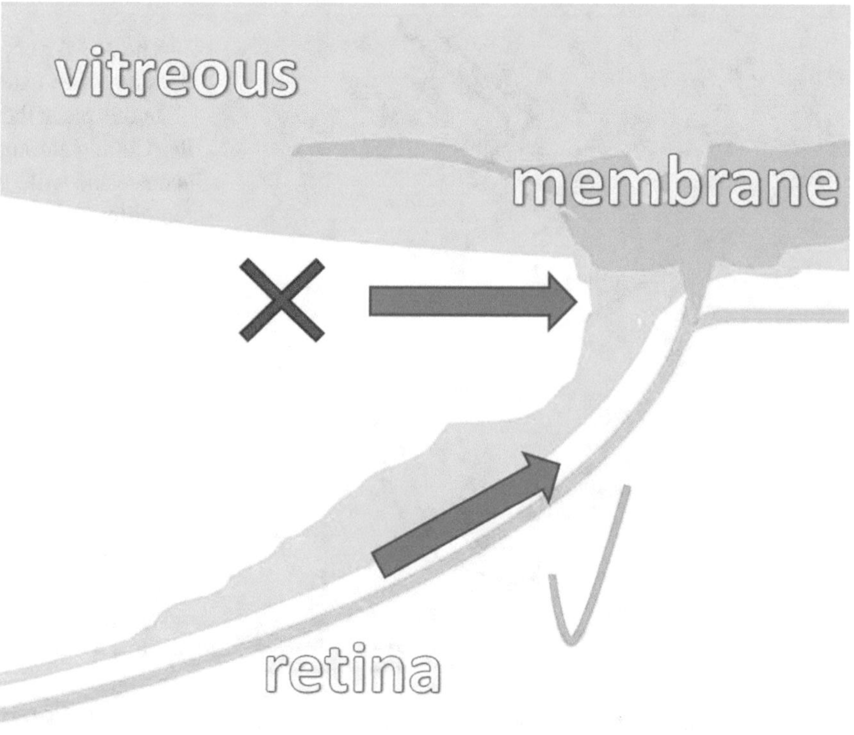

Fig. 15.20 It is important to dissect under the outer layer of a vitreoschisis which is easier than cutting through the vitreous to get to pegs of membranous attachment and avoids leaving vitreous on the retina

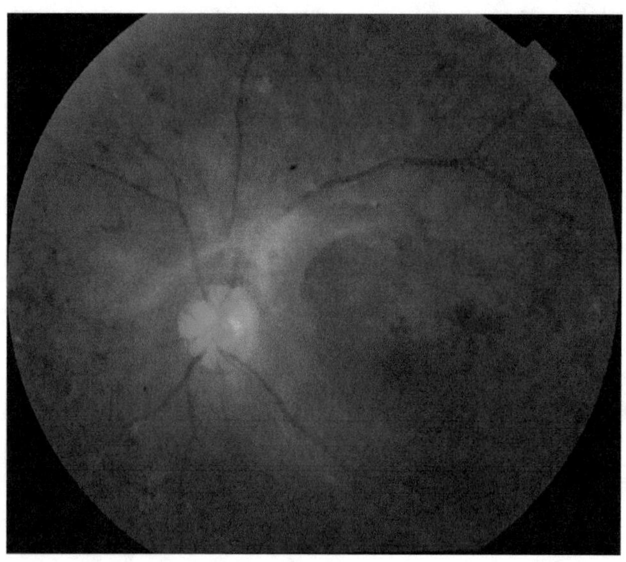

Fig. 15.21 The OCT of this patient shows the pegs of attachment between the membranes and the retina

- Retinoschisis is an occasional feature in retina in TRD and is presumably due to splitting of the retina from traction. It may prevent flattening of the retina at the end of the operation and application of laser. Often partial thickness inner retinal holes are seen. Dissection of membrane is often difficult from the surface of the schitic area (Figs. 15.21, 15.22, 15.23, 15.24, 15.25, 15.26, and 15.27).

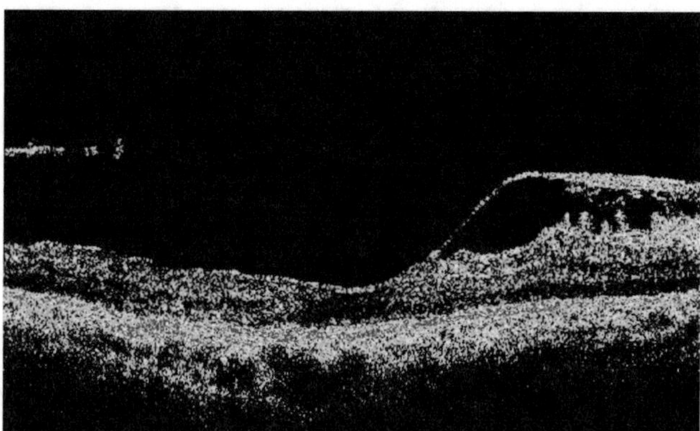

Fig. 15.22 An OCT shows the pegs of attachment under the membrane

Peroperative Panretinal Photocoagulation

Once the membranes have been dissected apply panretinal photocoagulation. Use a similar method as in the outpatients by first demarcating the edge of the macula on the temporal side with a row of laser. This stops you drifting into the macula. The blood vessels and optic nerve are you borders elsewhere. Then fill the peripheral retina with laser using a curved endolaser fibre optic. Some surgeons laser out to the ora serrata to reduce the chance of far peripheral ischaemia inducing neovascularisation at the vitreous base a suspected cause of late rebleeds. For this a chandelier is

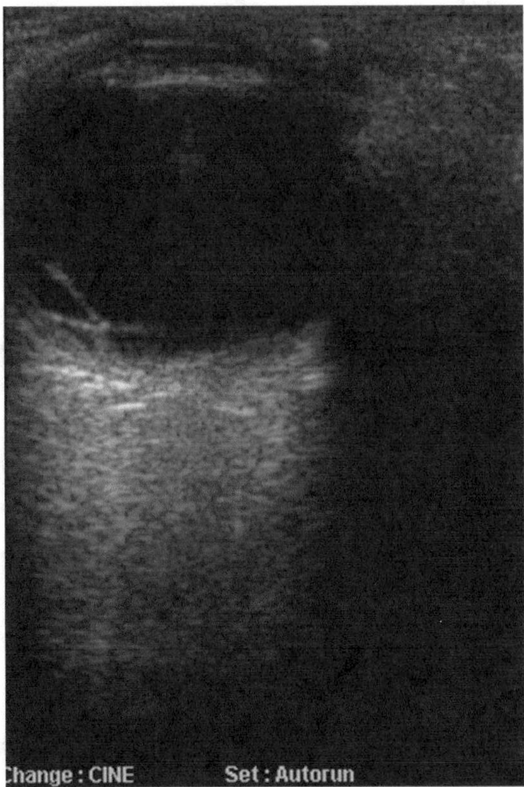

Fig. 15.23 TRDs are characterised by a triangular shaped elevation of the retina with attachment to the vitreous. The vitreous is usually immobile in these patients

helpful as you can indent the far periphery to apply the laser. If you are intending to insert a gas bubble, laser all the flat retina before you insert the gas. Gas insertion in a diabetic eye can induce a peroperative lens opacity which can reduce the view. Any elevated retina will need to be flattened under air and lasered. The wider view of the peripheral retina in an air filled can allow further anterior peripheral PRP. Be careful of the back of the lens (most of these patients are phakic) when applying laser to the anterior retina. Make sure you know where any breaks are and laser them. If there is retinal detachment, e.g. from TRD but no retinal break, the subretinal fluid can be left alone, however, you will not be able to laser that area. If you have made a hole in an area of TRD, you will need to drain the SRF and laser the hole.

Anti-VEGF Pre-Treatment

In patients with active neovascularisation, surgery on the eye can be greatly facilitated by preoperative injection of an Anti-VEGF therapy. Bevacizumab 1.25 mg injected into the vitreous cavity one week before the PPV surgery causes regression of the neovascular membrane, reduces peroperative bleeding [10–17] and may reduce postoperative rebleed rates [18]. It is recommended to use this routinely in these patients because surgery is greatly facilitated.

The timing of the injection is usually 1 week before. If there is a longer delay between Bevacizumab injection and PPV, there is a risk of TRD progression from contraction of membranes [19]. Risk of progression of TRD appears to be dose dependant [20] (Figs. 15.28, 15.29, and 15.30).

Bimanual Surgery

Chandelier illumination during PPV allows the surgeon the use of both hands for instrumentation. In complex dissection of membranes, the edge of membranes can be lifted by grasping with forceps whilst the other hand dissects with scissors. The membrane can be pulled over an area of attachment to reveal pegs which can be cut. Illumination is not directed at the site of interest therefore it is useful to experiment with different chandeliers till you find one that suits you. I place the chandelier at 12 o'clock and fix on the forehead. The chandelier should have a stiff but bendable shaft to allow direction of the light. Most now have a trochar through which the fibreoptic is inserted.

This method is particularly useful in combined TRD/RRD surgery where the retina is mobile and there is no natural traction on the membranes from the vitreous (the elevation of the retina relieves the traction) to allow easy dissection. It is also useful in more straightforward TRD and can speed the surgery. Usually the sclerotomies for the chandeliers can be made transconjunctivally and left unsutured after removal (Figs. 15.31 and 15.32).

Dealing with Bleeding Vessels

Elevate the infusion bottle.

Apply pressure to the bleeding site with a blunt instrument, e.g. flute needle tip. You will need to maintain the pressure for at least 60 seconds for the clot to form. This requires patience and a steady hand.

If there is a blood clot, trim this with a cutter so that a plug of thrombus remains at the bleeding point. Do not pull the thrombus off because this will recommence the bleeding.

Some argue that insertion of air will reduce the risk of further bleeding but this is not confirmed by studies [21].

Apply minimal endodiathermy, use diathermy only occasionally, the tips of the instruments are sharp and difficult to insert into valve trochars, in the meantime the bleed proceeds to reduce your vision once in the eye and it can be difficult to find the bleeding point. In addition, removal of the diathermy tips off the burn sometimes dislodges the clot again because the tip must touch the tissue. An alternative is to use an endolaser pointing at the bleed but not touching it, to heat the

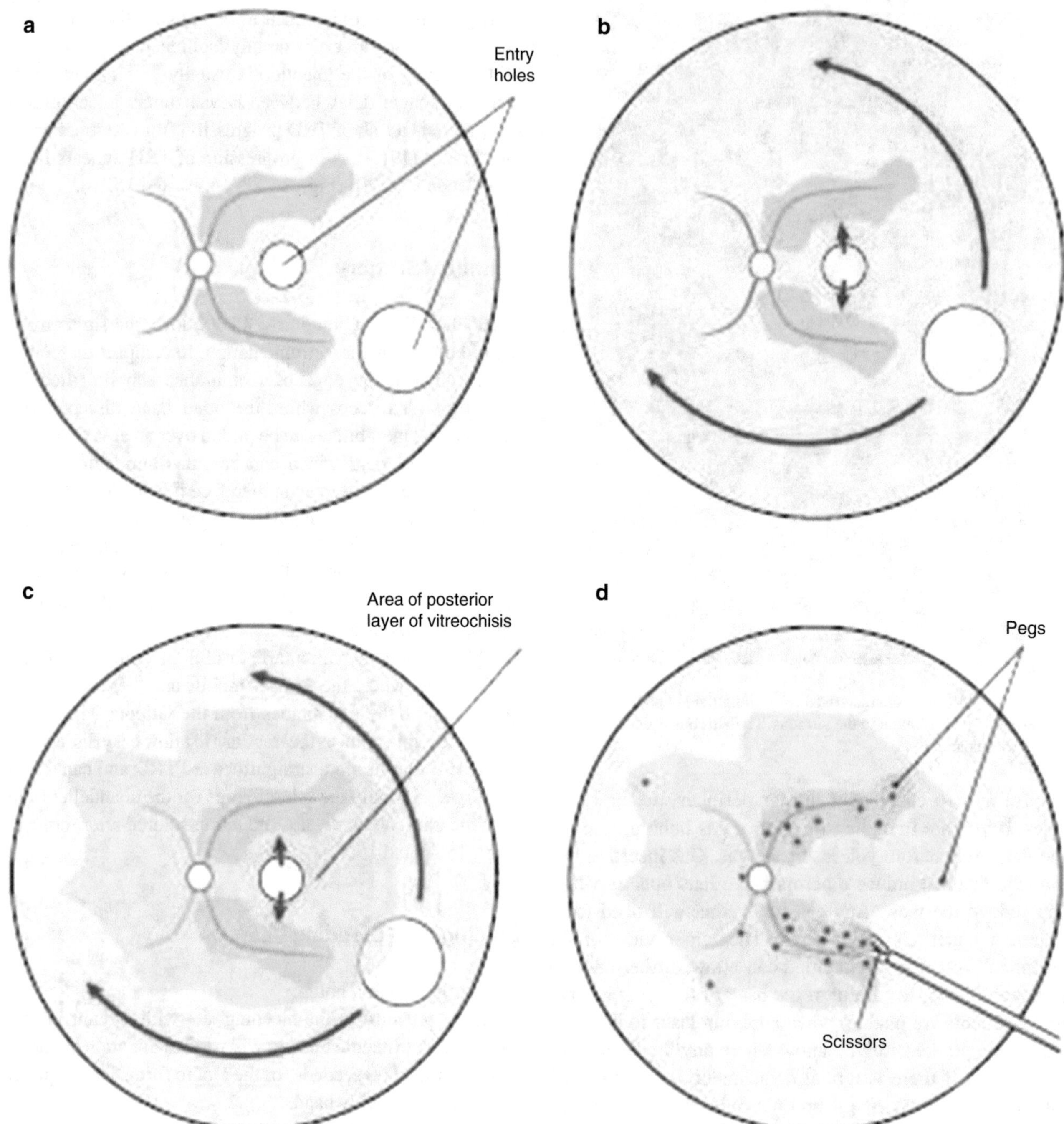

Fig. 15.24 Try to find a route through the posterior hyaloid membrane to allow easy dissection of the membranes and insertion of your scissors underneath the posterior hyaloid membrane to aid dissection (**a**). These can be found conveniently in locations such as superotemporally or superonasally, so that you have access with right or left hands to the membranes or over the macula itself where it is possible to start centrally and work peripherally through the membranes (**b**). Once you have found your appropriate layer (**c**), 45° angle scissors or the small gauge cutter are used to dissect off the membrane from the retina. You must cut pegs of attachment of the membrane to the retina (**d**). Cutting, rather than pulling these apart, reduces bleeding and improves your postoperative rebleed rate, whilst minimising any chance of iatrogenic tears. Once you have made your access incisions in the posterior vitreous, work around the most severe membranes which are often on the arcades and disc, lifting the hyaloid around these sites, so that you can determine the most adherent foci before working down onto the most severe membranes themselves. Often these are found concentrated around blood vessels and the optic disc, but also can be found sporadically around the retina

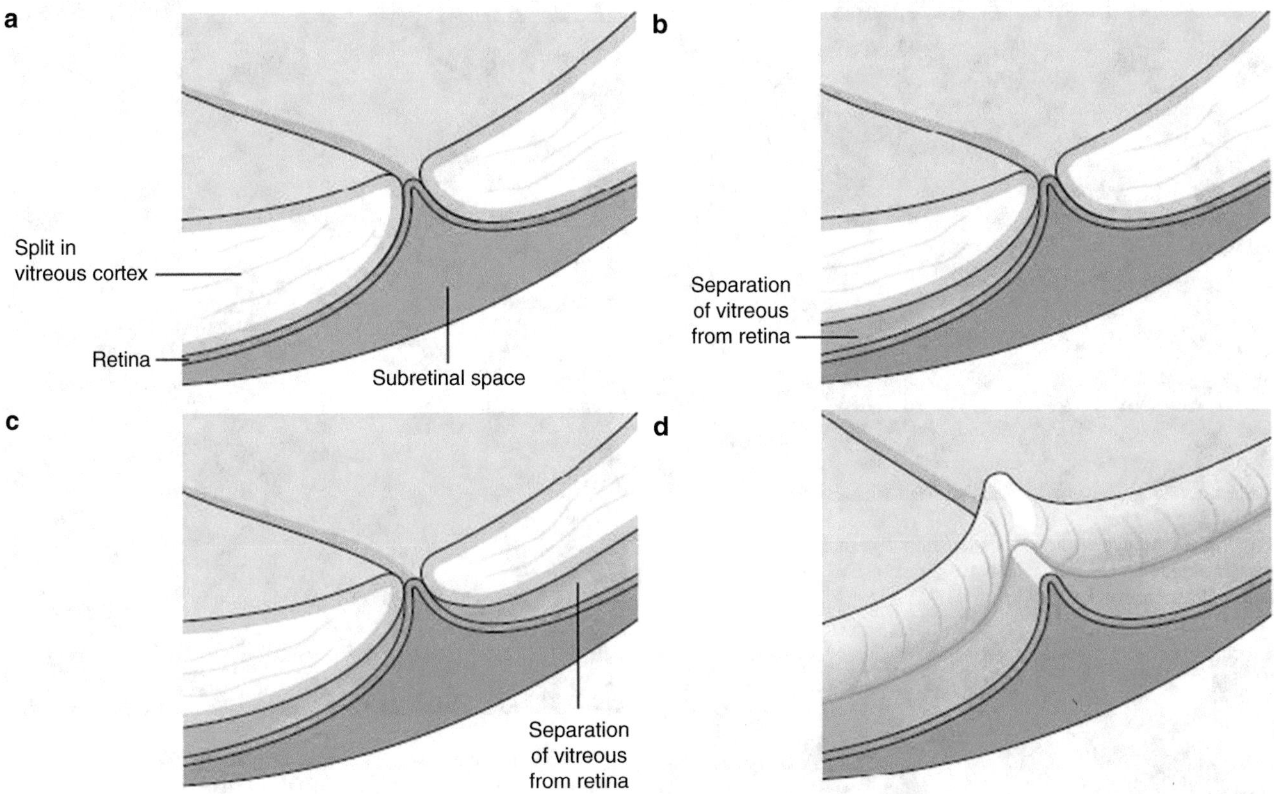

Fig. 15.25 Lift the vitreoschisis (**a**, **b** and **c**) on either side of the line of adhesion before working along the line of adhesion to detach the membrane (**d**)

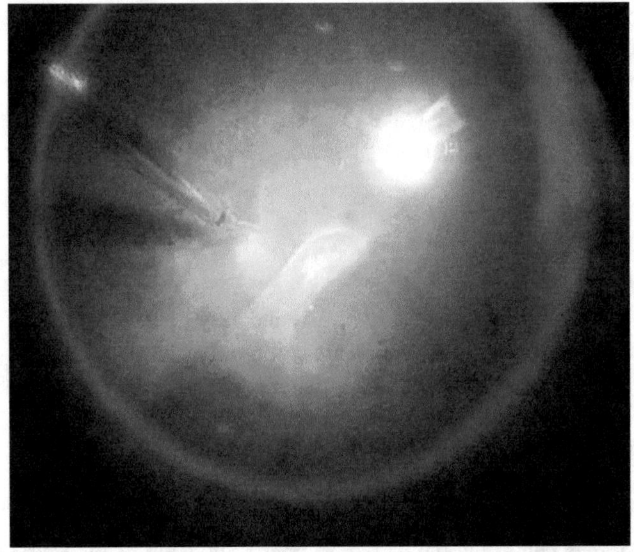

Fig. 15.26 A peroperative picture shows a membrane which may tempt the surgeon into performing a dissection off only the anterior layer, but in fact, re-examination of the eye shows another layer indicated by the position of the scissors; a more posterior layer which is attached to the retina. This is the posterior hyaloid membrane and cortical remnants that make up the posterior leaf of the vitreoschisis. These must be elevated to find the right plane for removal of the membranes

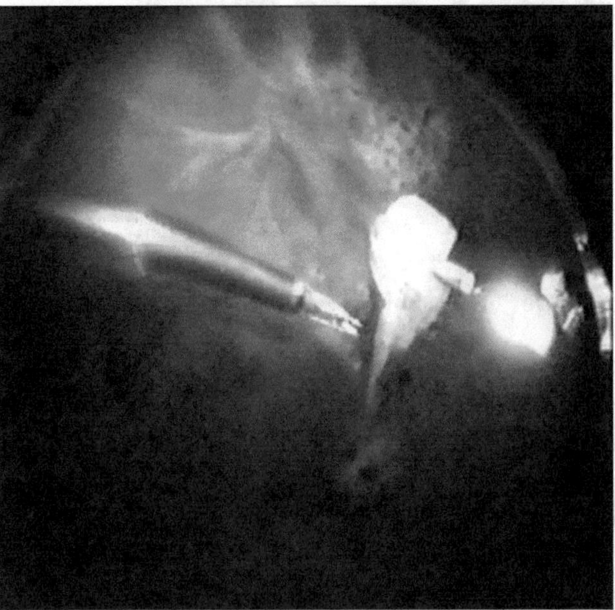

Fig. 15.27 When dissections are difficult use bimanual surgery (with illuminated forceps or insert a chandelier) to hold membranes so that pegs can be seen and cut with scissors

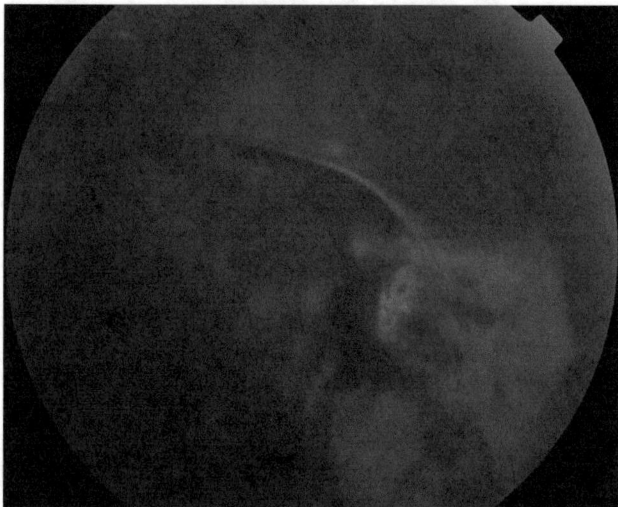

Fig. 15.28 An eye with vitreous haemorrhage and active membranes was injected with bevacizumab to shrink active neovascularisation before delamination surgery

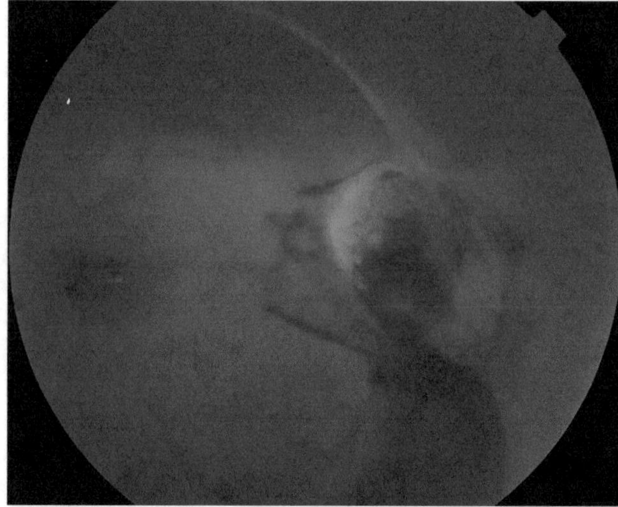

Fig. 15.29 The fundus after bevacizumab injection

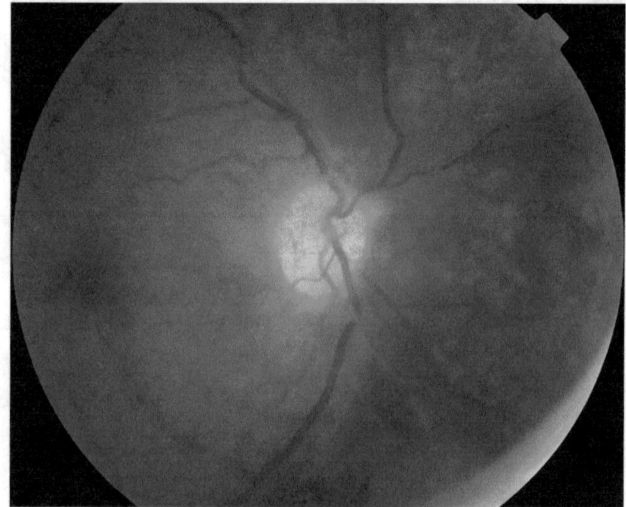

Fig. 15.30 The retina after PPV and delamination

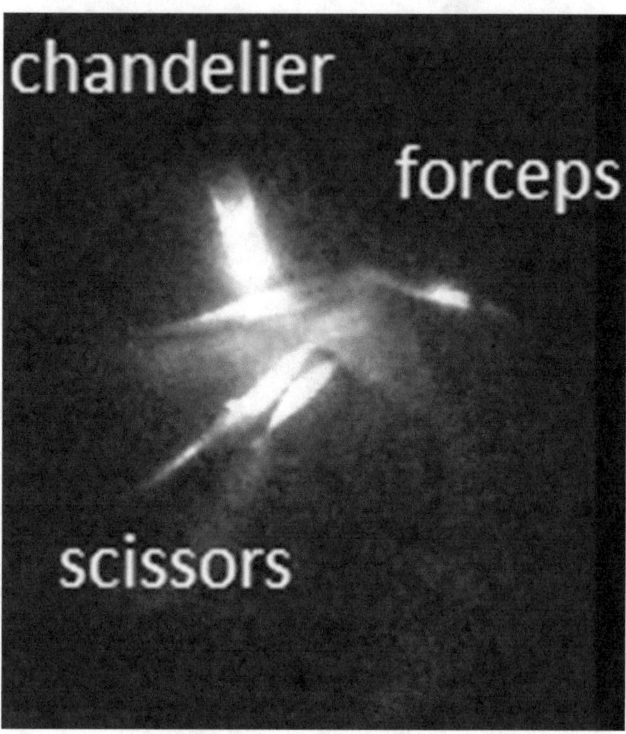

Fig. 15.31 Bimanual surgery is extremely useful for dissecting membranes off the retina in combined TRD/RRD and in complex TRD

thrombus and coagulate the tissue. This has the advantage that the tissue is not touched and therefore the clot is not pulled off (Fig. 15.33).

The retina can be flattened in 86% with better results in younger patients and those without iris neovascularisation [22, 23] (Figs. 15.34 and 15.35).

Apply panretinal photocoagulation (PRP) to the retina.

Iatrogenic Breaks

The diabetic retina is very fragile and easy to tear during dissection, breaks in the retina are commonly produced, 20% to 35% of eyes [8, 24, 25]. In general, creation of iatrogenic breaks is better than leaving membrane on the retina. If they occur flatten them, laser the edges, and provide tamponade with intraocular gas. Try to avoid leaving tractional membranes near breaks as postoperative contraction of the membranes can allow the breaks to open. Adhesion of the retina because of PRP makes it difficult for the break to accumulate SRF; however, tractional membranes will overcome this adhesion and lift the retina. Iatrogenic break formation increases the risk of postoperative retinal detachment by a factor of 3 [26] (Figs. 15.36, 15.37, 15.38, 15.39, 15.40 and 15.41).

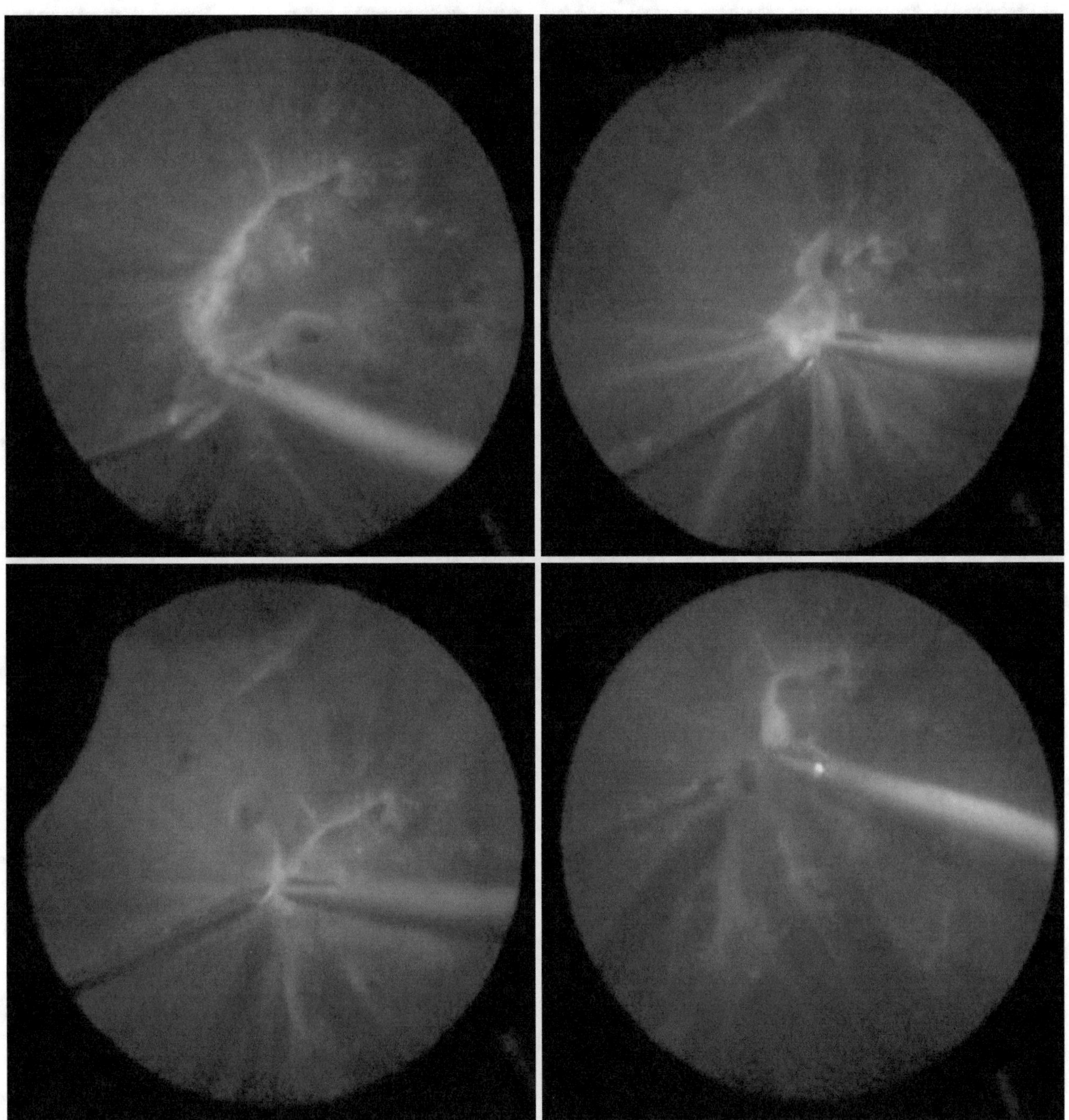

Fig. 15.32 When dissecting along an area of adhesion work your way along its long axis, using your unfavoured hand to cut (in this case the left hand) if needed, and using a bimanual method with forceps lifting up the membrane to reveal pegs of adhesion

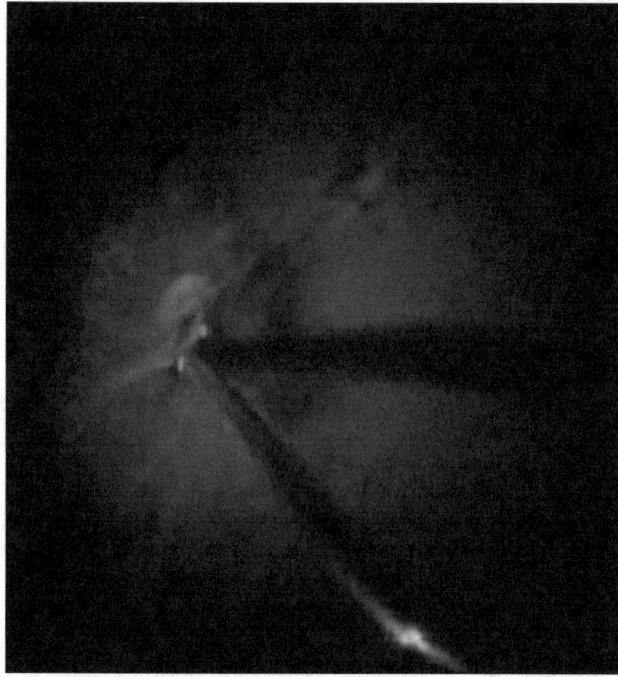

Fig. 15.33 Applying pressure to a bleeding vessel

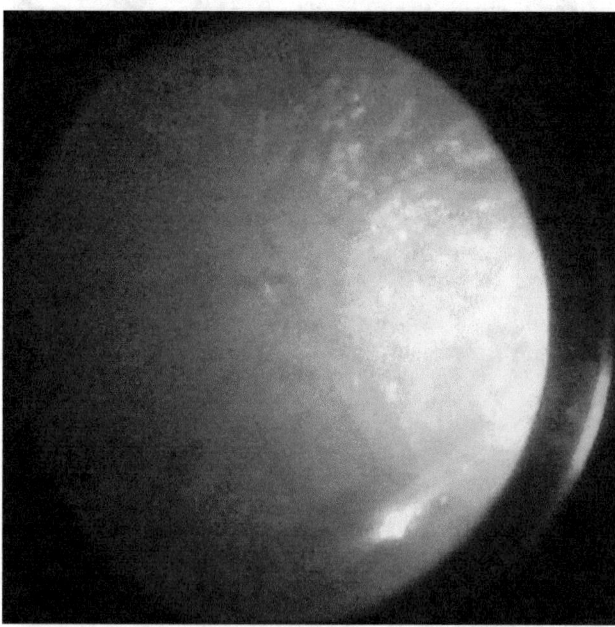

Fig. 15.34 Lasers are almost universally required in diabetic patients, even if laser has already been applied. This is to prevent iris neovascularisation and neovascular glaucoma, an uncommon, but devastating complication after diabetic tractional retinal detachment surgery, which is most common when the retina re-detaches postoperatively

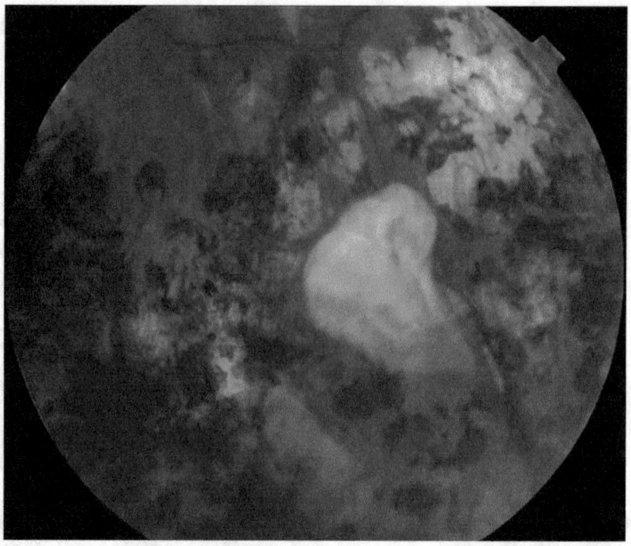

Fig. 15.35 Segmentation of membranes can be successful, but in general it is a riskier process and surgeons should be encouraged to remove as much membrane or all membrane if possible, even if small iatrogenic tears occur

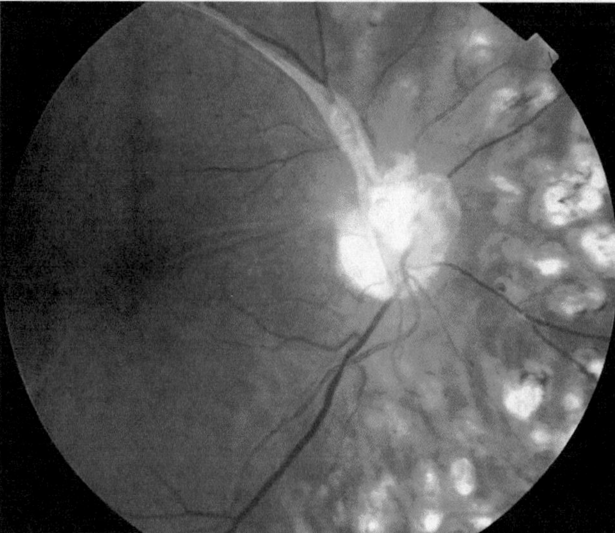

Fig. 15.36 Leaving membrane on the retina postoperatively encourages contraction of the membrane and striae of the retina

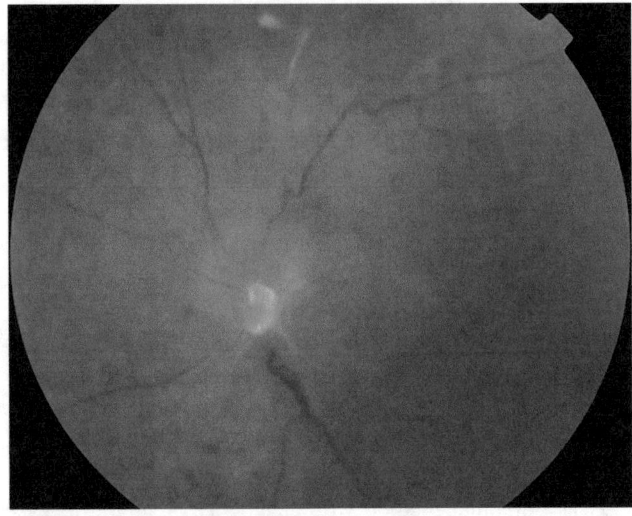

Fig. 15.37 Leaving a focus of membrane on the disc after TRD surgery can allow wrinkling of the macular retina as the membrane contracts postoperatively

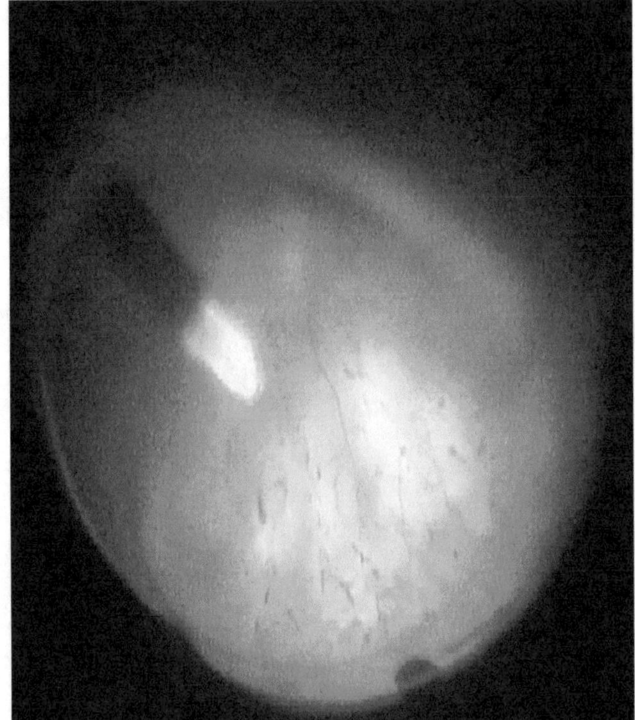

Fig. 15.38 Even pan retinal photocoagulation will not hold back a retinal detachment if it were to extend as in this eye

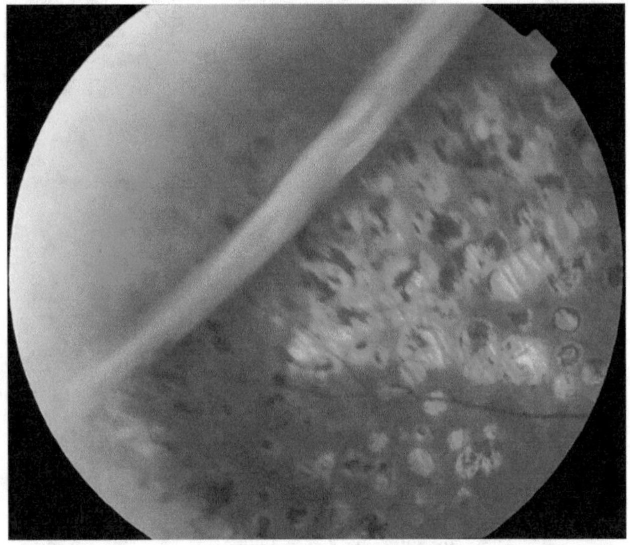

Fig. 15.39 This patient had a peripheral giant retinal tear causing retinal detachment after vitrectomy which remained peripheral due to preexisting PRP

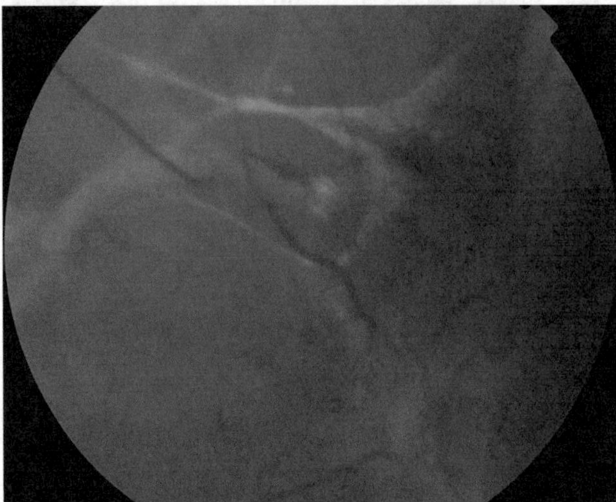

Fig. 15.40 PVR can occur in TRD patients as in this eye with subretinal bands. The risk is that the bands may hold up the retina postoperatively, and therefore the surgeon may need to consider inserting silicone oil to hold the retina in place leaving the bands to atrophy over time with later removal of the oil

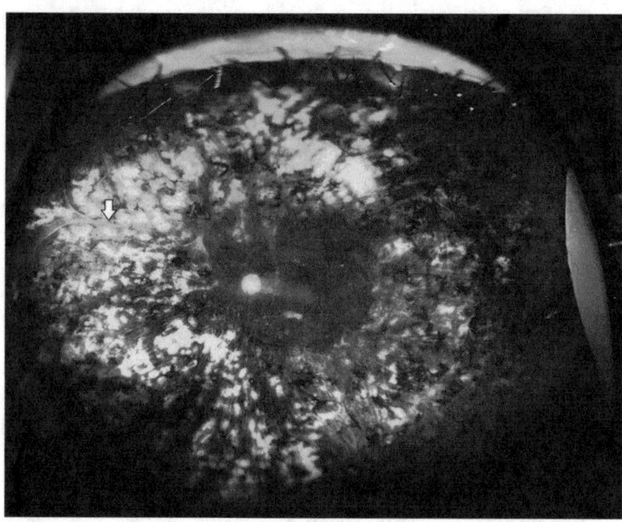

Fig. 15.41 There are subretinal bands under this retina which in this case have not prevented reattachment of the retina after PPV

Silicone Oil

Avoid silicone oil use if possible because this seems to adversely affect the outcome of surgery by stimulating membrane formation [27, 28], spontaneous break formation [29], and migration of subretinal oil postoperatively. The functional success rates are low [30, 31] and the capacity for silicone oil removal is restricted [32]. Silicone oil is impervious to oxygen and therefore may exacerbate the ischaemia of the eye [33]. It is used in only 5% of my patients at primary surgery [26].

Surgical Pearl

Operating on Tractional Retinal Detachment

- Do a thorough anterior indented vitrectomy ("Basal trim") in all cases especially around sclerostomies to reduce scaffold for entry site or anterior neovascularisation, and to allow rapid clearance of postoperative vitreous cavity haemorrhage.
- Doing an anterior chamber paracentesis in older phakic patients can significantly improve access to the anterior vitreous [34].
- Use preoperative anti-VEGFs 3–5 days preop and intermittent short bursts of raised IOP to control bleeding.
- Look after the corneal epithelium with corneal hydration agents throughout surgery.
- Vitreoschisis is near universal in severe PDR and diluted (1: 3) triamcinolone staining is especially useful in its detection and removal.
- The Finesse flex loop is a useful instrument to help elevate areas of tenuous vitreoschisis especially over the fovea.
- Laser the anterior retina up to the ora serrata especially behind the sclerostomies in severe diabetics to reduce the rate of entry site neovascularisation.

Professor David Steel, Sunderland Eye Hospital, Sunderland, UK

Combined TRD and RRD (Table 15.2).

This is a difficult problem because the retina will lift with the membranes during dissection. The patient needs to be operated on urgently because PVR can occur. Use of a small bubble of heavy liquid will stabilise the retina during surgery [35]. A bimanual method with chandelier or multiport system should be used to allow manipulation of the retina and membrane [36, 37]. Bimanual surgery allows dissection of membranes on a mobile retina. Find and treat the retinal break and tamponade with gas, apply PRP. The outcomes for this are reduced often because of PVR with only 50% achieving improved vision [38] (Fig. 15.42).

Table 15.2 difficulty rating for PPV for combined TRD and RRD

Difficulty rating	Very high
Success rates	Low
Complication rates	High
When to use in training	Late

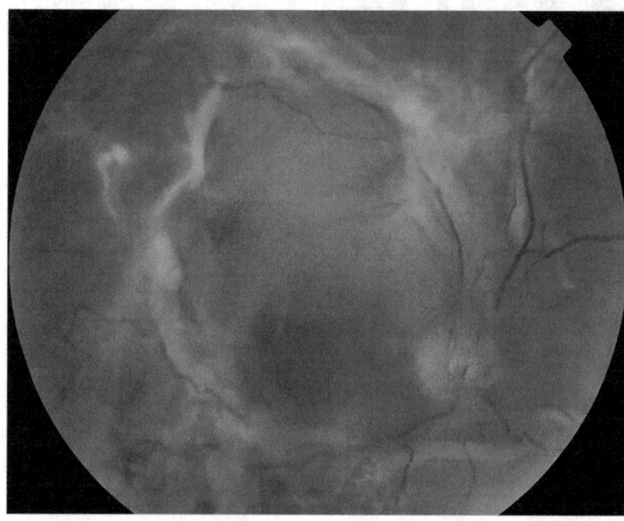

Fig. 15.42 This patient has active neovascularisation with a combined TRD and RRD. An appropriate surgical approach would be intravitreal injection of an anti-VEGF agent, followed a week later by PPV using a chandelier to allow bimanual dissection of the membranes, with PRP and postoperative tamponade with 14% perfluorocarbon in air if there are any retinal breaks

Note:

Make sure that all membranes are removed near breaks in the retina.

Postoperative Complications

Cataract

This is less common in eyes with diabetic retinopathy than other eyes treated with PPV. The reason for this is unclear but may be due to less oxidative stress on the lens in ischemic diabetic eyes [39]. Cataract formation in ischaemic conditions (diabetic retinopathy, retinal vein occlusion, sickle cell disease) is slower than in other eyes.

Vitreous Cavity Haemorrhage VCH

Postoperative VCH is present in up to 60% immediately after surgery [40]. In the immediate postoperative period, some VCH is common. Monitor with ultrasound. In general, in a vitrectomised eye with diffuse VCH, if some of the features of the fundus are visible such as the optic nerve head or blood vessels the VCH will clear in a few weeks. Check the IOP in case of erythroclastic glaucoma.

Persistent or recurrent haemorrhage occurs in 12 to 27% [40–44] with 5 to 10% requiring surgery [26, 40, 45, 46] to clear out the haemorrhage. Postoperative vitreous haemorrhage spontaneously clears more quickly in aphakes [46] and is reduced by peroperative endolaser [47]. Neovascular membranes at the vitreous base or adjacent to sclerotomy sites have been detected in 13% of postvitrectomy eyes and been blamed for postoperative haemorrhage [48–50]. These can be detected on ultrasound biomicroscopy and treated with cryotherapy [51].

Techniques involving exchange of the vitreous cavity fluid for air as office procedures have been described; however, further vitrectomy and panretinal photocoagulation by endolaser is recommended. The use of C3F8 gas may reduce the early postoperative vitreous haemorrhage rate [52] and Anti-VEGF pre-treatment therapy may reduce late bleeds.

Rhegmatogenous Retinal Detachment

This is described in 1 to 9% of eyes [43, 45] and is frequently associated with iris neovascularisation, 83% [53]. If a RRD subsequently occurs recourse to oil may be necessary, but treatment of postoperative RRD is associated with a poor outcome [54]. It is important to detect the RRD early and treat early for best results. TRD patients may need more frequent review in the postoperative period.

Iris Neovascularisation

This is described in 2 to 15% and is very common when postoperative RRD is present [55, 56]. Treatment of the RRD can induce regression of the INV [57] (Fig. 15.43).

Phthisis Bulbi

This is reported in 3 to 4% after surgery [45, 58].

Maculopathy

Slow reabsorption of subfoveal fluid on OCT after TRD surgery has been described in a few patients, taking 6 months to flatten [59, 60]. The macula is vulnerable to ischemia and thinning, cystoid macular oedema, and ERM in addition (Figs. 15.44, 15.45, and 15.46).

Survival after Surgery

Five year survival after surgery for the complications of diabetic retinopathy varies from 68% to 80% and is particularly poor for those with cardiac disease [61–63]. A recent study has shown median survival of 2 years post-surgery for TRD and 49% all-cause mortality at 10 years compared to 2% for diabetics without TRD [64].

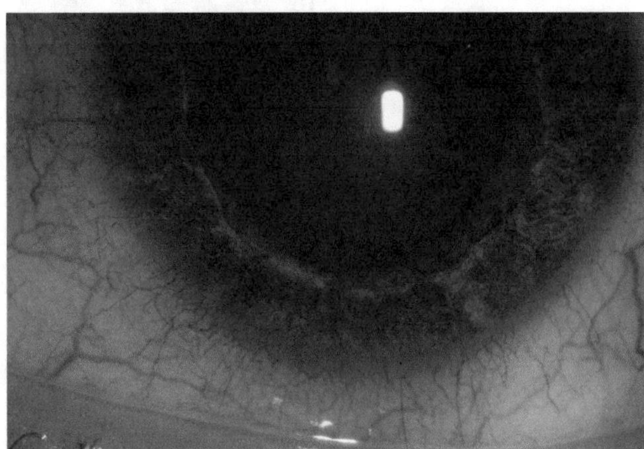

Fig. 15.43 An eye with neovascular glaucoma from diabetic retinopathy

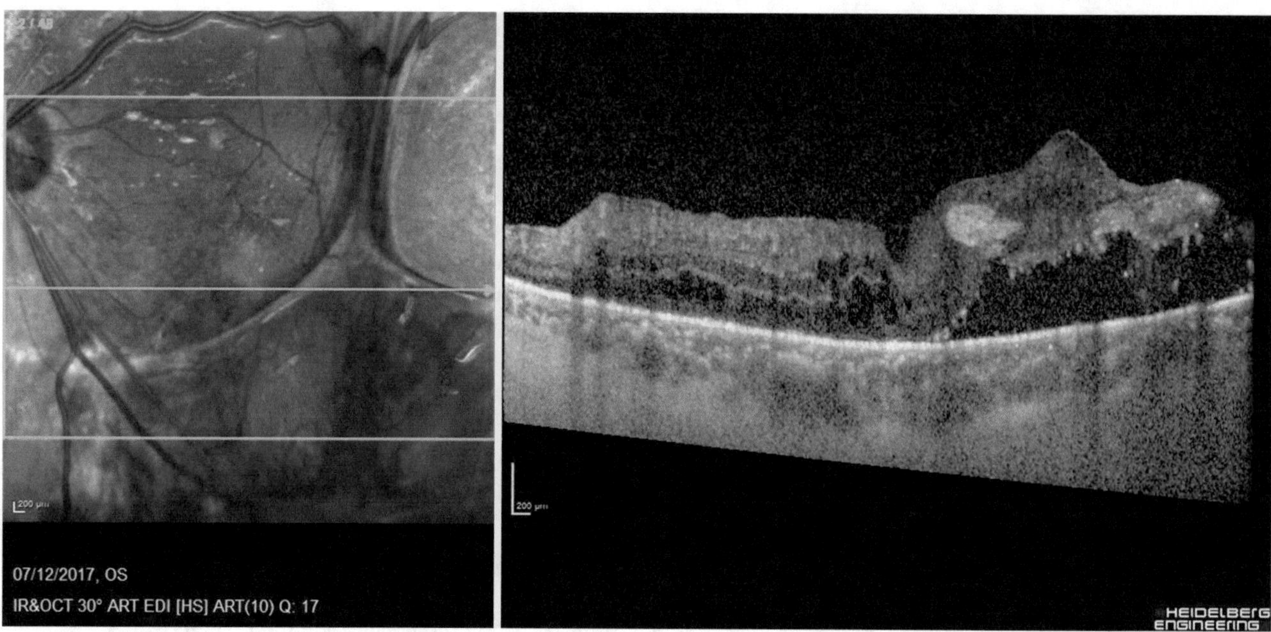

Fig. 15.44 A chronic TRD with persistent SRF postoperatively early on

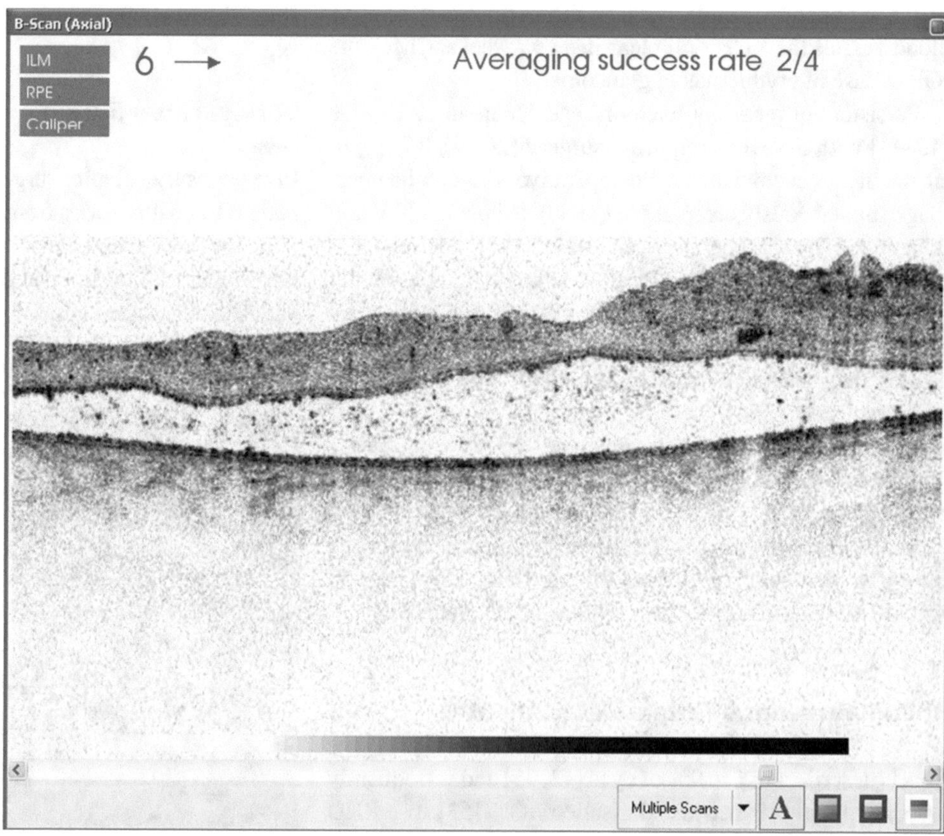

Fig. 15.45 Persistent SRF in a postoperative TRD

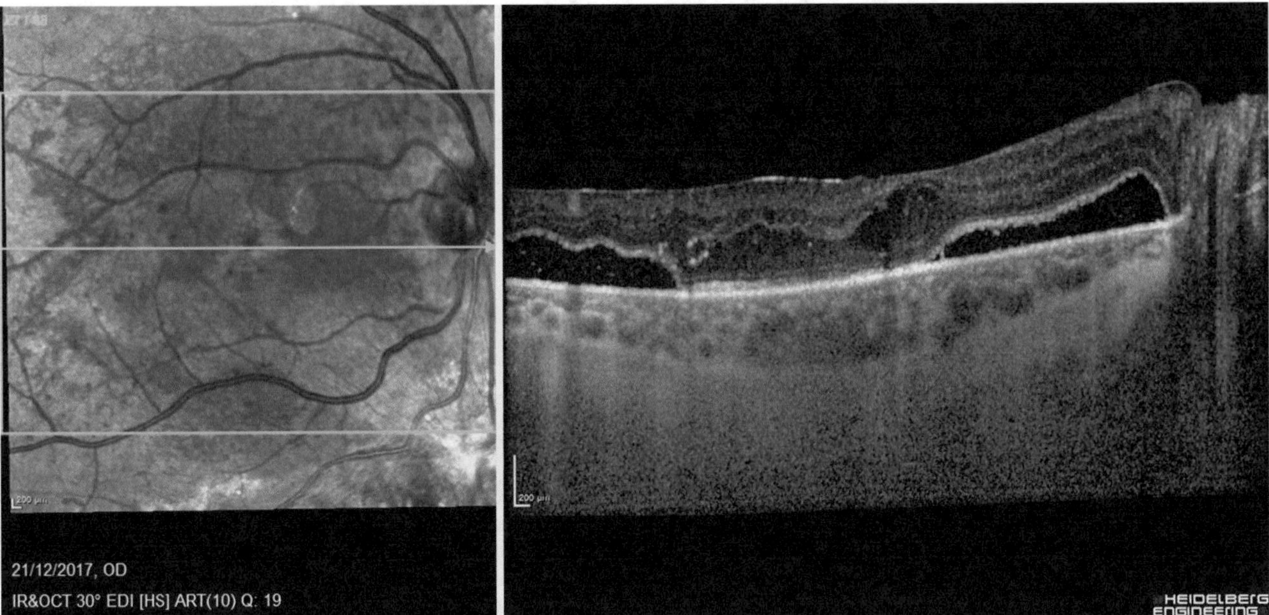

Fig. 15.46 SRF in a postoperative TRD operation. This should resolve after a duration of months

Success Rates

For visual improvement:

- Vitreous haemorrhage 90% chance of improvement of vision.
  - The DRVS from the 1980s included, in group 1, patients with recent severe vitreous haemorrhage (VA < = 5/200). Patients were randomised to PPV in 3 months or 1 year [65].
  - Chance of at least 10/20 was 25% in the early PPV patients 15% in late PPV.
  - Chance of NPL was 25% with the early PPV 19% in late PPV (not statistically significant).
  - Most benefit was found for early PPV in type 1 diabetics.
- TRD, 60% chance of improvement of vision.
  - 50% achieve 20/200 or better [22], 86% flat retina. Recurrent tractional retinal detachment has been described in 22% and rhegmatogenous retinal detachment in 7%.
  - DRVS group 2 included advanced proliferative diabetic retinopathy and vision at least 10/200 randomised to PPV or conventional management.
  - Chance of VA at least 10/20 was 44% in the PPV group compared to 28%.
- Combined TRD/RRD chance of improved vision is approximately 50%.

The risk of no perception of light after PPV for diabetic retinopathy is 7%, increased in those patients with peroperative iris neovascularisation, or postoperative haemorrhage, macular ischemia, or iris neovascularisation [66]. Overall, the reoperation rate is 16% [66].

Diabetic Maculopathy

The mainstay of treatment of diabetic macular oedema is intravitreal injection of Anti-VEGF agents (Figs. 15.47, 15.48, and 15.49).

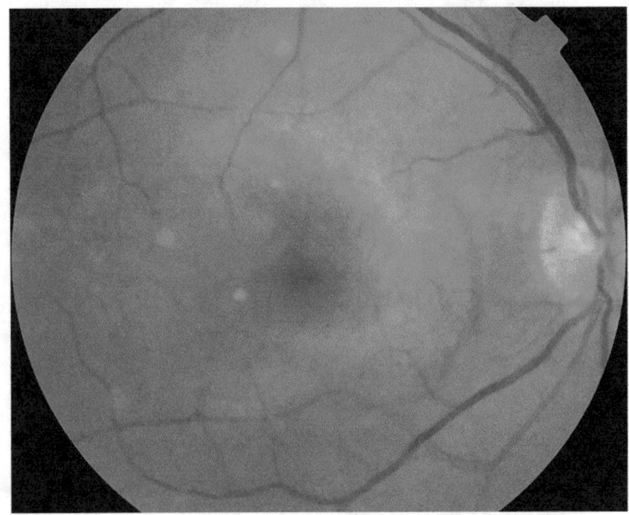

Fig. 15.47 Diabetic retinopathy may produce changes in the vitreous which stimulate shrinkage with traction on the retina. A specific form of traction is a taught thickened posterior hyaloid membrane seen as a "sheen" over the macula in an eye with an attached vitreous. An OCT shows a thickened sheet near the retina with pegs attached to the retinal surface. This may respond well to vitrectomy and peel. Whereas other ERMs associated with diabetic maculopathy may show disappointing visual recovery after surgery

This is the major cause of visual loss in Type 2 diabetes and is present in many patients undergoing vitrectomy [67]. A multitude of investigations have been performed to determine the role of vitrectomy in diabetic macular oedema [68–79]. Randomised controlled trials without the addition of cataract surgery have shown no benefit [80]. The PPV appears to normalise retinal microcirculation from its hyperdynamic preoperative state [81]. The specific presentation of taught thickened posterior hyaloid membrane where a contraction of the vitreous is seen as a diffuse area of traction on the macula appears to respond to surgery probably because the diabetic maculopathy associated with this condition is less [82] (Figs. 15.50 and 15.51).

Macular holes (foveal) can appear in the diabetic macula [5].

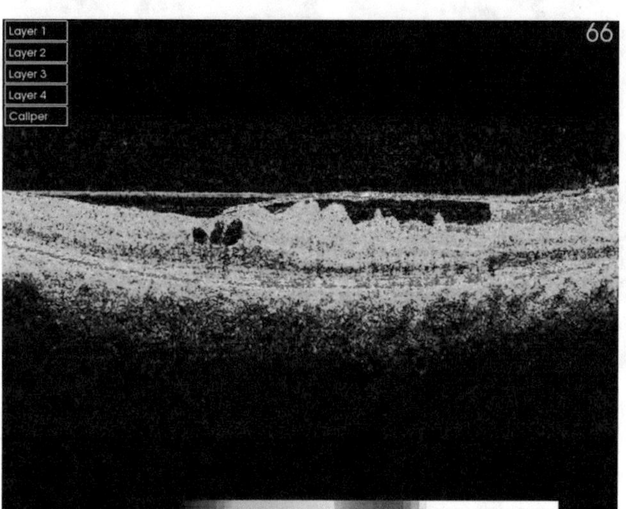

Fig. 15.48 An OCT shows the broad area of attachments to the macula

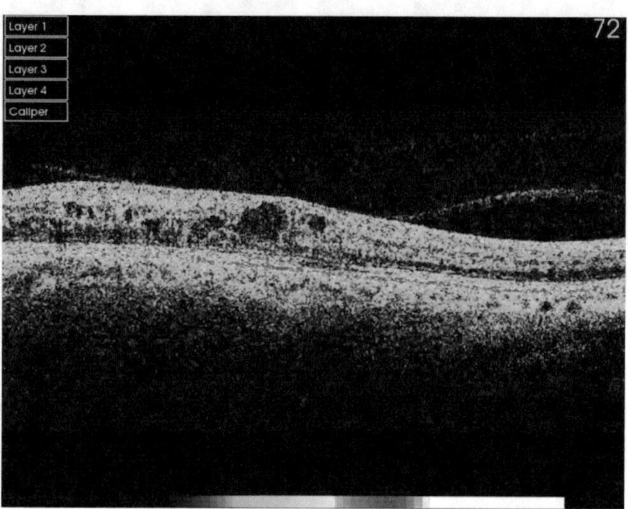

Fig. 15.49 OCT shows a partial detachment of the vitreous from the macula in diabetic macular oedema prompting some surgeons to perform vitrectomy in these eyes

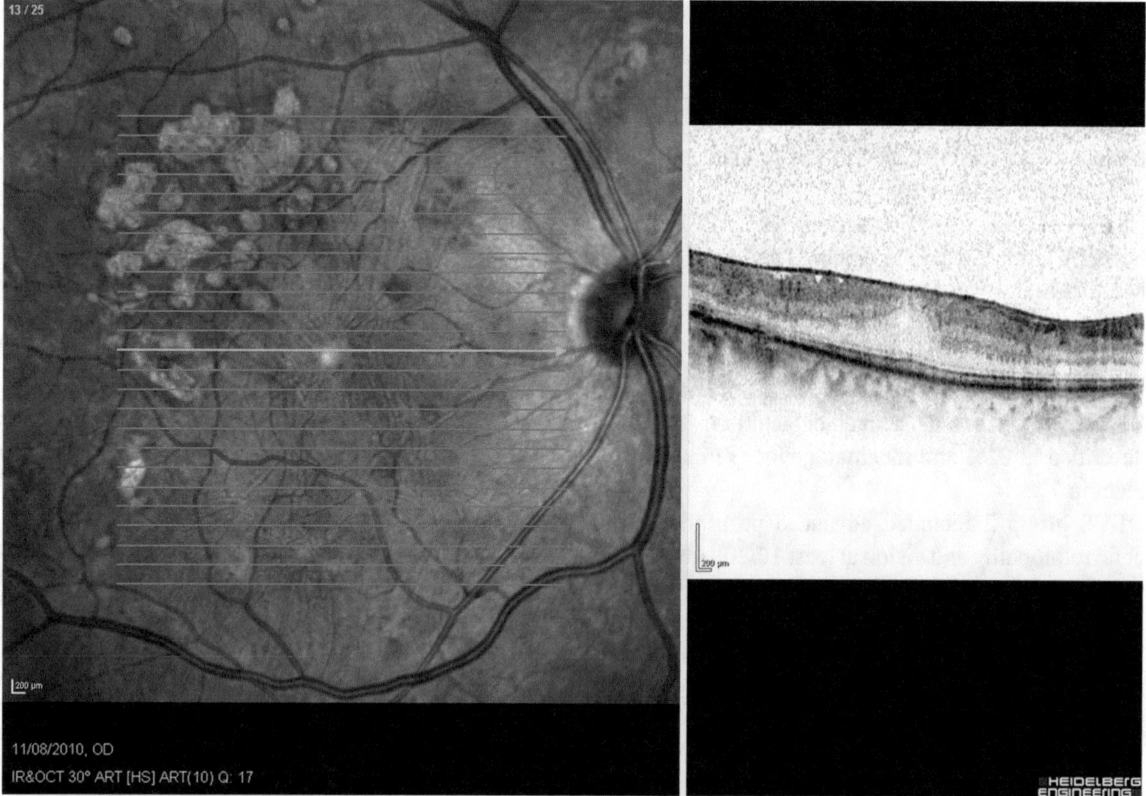

Fig. 15.50 ERM can be seen in DMR. Visual improvement after surgery can be disappointing perhaps because of underlying retinal damage and cystoid macular oedema

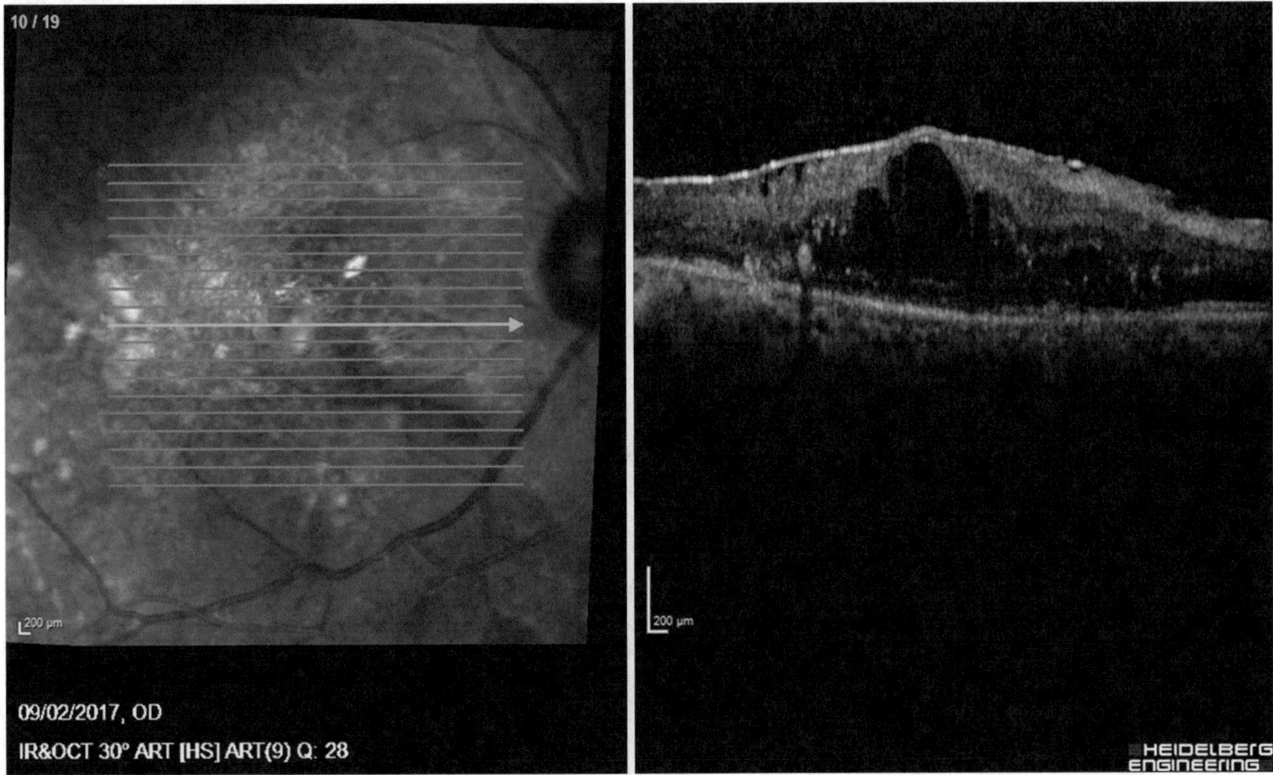

Fig. 15.51 An ERM in diabetic retinopathy. Surgical results are variable because the underlying retina is weak

Removal of massive subretinal exudation has been performed but is of uncertain worth [83–85] and drainage of fluid from cystoid spaces via retinal puncture has been attempted [86].

Surgical Pearl

Tangential Endo-Photocoagulation to Microaneurysms in Diabetic Macular Oedema

Direct laser photocoagulation (PC) of microaneurysms (MAs) is effective as a treatment for diabetic macula oedema (DME) even in the era of anti-VEGF. Endo-PC to MAs during surgery is recommended in cases with DME when vitrectomy is performed for retinal detachment, vitreous haemorrhage or epiretinal membrane associated with diabetic retinopathy.

Direct PC becomes more effective when MAs closer to the FAZ (foveal avascular zone) are coagulated. However, failing to accurately aim onto a MA causes a burn in the RPE (retinal pigment epithelium) and the photoreceptors resulting in a decrease of retinal sensitivity especially when closer to the fovea. To avoid this adverse effect, we apply tangential endo-PC to MAs.

A flexible, adjustable, angled or bent/curved tip endolaser probe is recently available, which enables irradiation of the laser beam tangentially to the retina surface when applying the curvature. In addition, making the direction of the aiming beam away from the fovea avoids undesirable burns near the fovea. Even there is failure to coagulate the MA, the burn will occur in a spot apart from the fovea (Fig. 15.52).

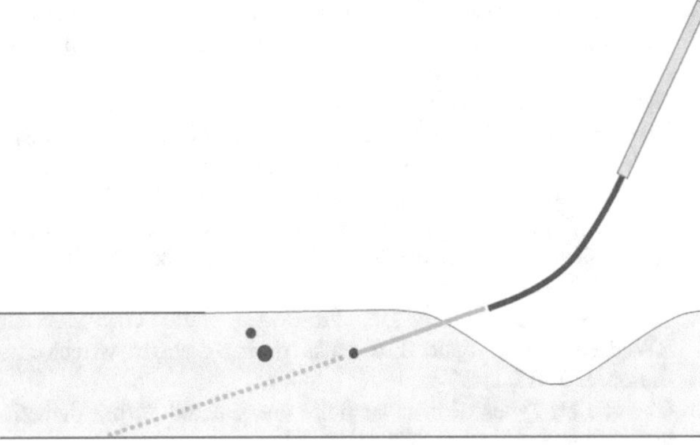

Fig. 15.52 Applying tangential laser to microaneurysms in DMR

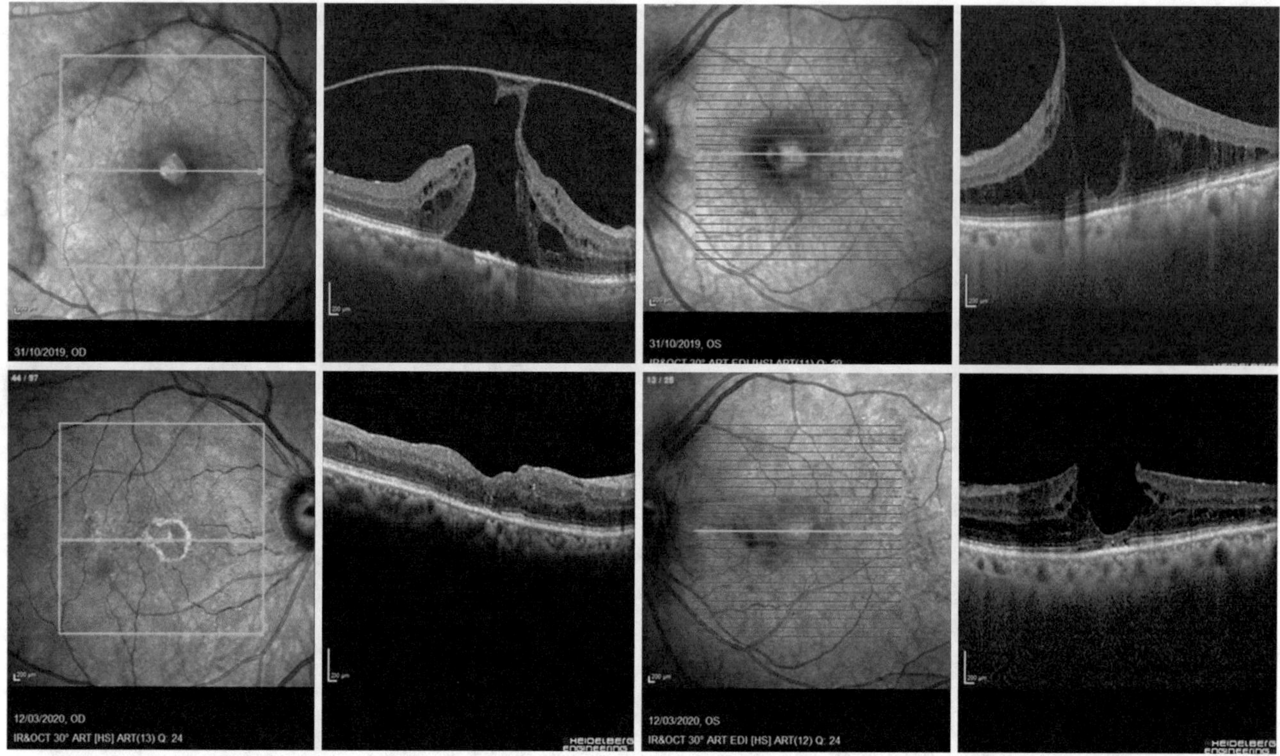

Fig. 15.53 A diabetic patient with a right macular hole and left severe VMT. The macular hole was closed with PPV, gas, and ILM flap. The VMT spontaneously separated

The followings are my setting of tangential endo-PC to MAs; 27G laser probe (rather than 25G), low power (no higher than 100 mW), short duration (no longer than 50 ms), a single irradiation with the probe close to the retina surface, even touching the retina.

Motohiro Kamei, Aichi Medical University, Nagakute, Japan (Fig. 15.53)

References

1. Schwatz SD, Alexander R, Hiscott P, Gregor ZJ. Recognition of vitreoschisis in proliferative diabetic retinopathy. A useful landmark in vitrectomy for diabetic traction retinal detachment. Ophthalmology. 1996;103(2):323–8.
2. Chu TG, Lopez PF, Cano MR, Freeman WR, Lean JS, Liggett PE, et al. Posterior vitreoschisis. An echographic finding in proliferative diabetic retinopathy. Ophthalmology. 1996;103(2):315–22.
3. Kroll P, Wiegand W, Schmidt J. Vitreopapillary traction in proliferative diabetic vitreoretinopathy [ssee comments]. Br J Ophthalmol. 1999;83(3):261–4.
4. Pendergast SD, Martin DF, Proia AD, Jaffe GJ, McCuen BW. Removal of optic disc stalks during diabetic vitrectomy. Retina. 1995;15(1):25–8.
5. Ghoraba H. Types of macular holes encountered during diabetic vitrectomy. Retina. 2002;22(2):176–82.
6. Kakehashi A. Total en bloc excision: a modified vitrectomy technique for proliferative diabetic retinopathy. Am J Ophthalmol. 2002;134(5):763–5.
7. Williams DF, Williams GA, Hartz A, Mieler WF, Abrams GW, Aaberg TM. Results of vitrectomy for diabetic traction retinal detachments using the en bloc excision technique. Ophthalmology. 1989;96(6):752–8.
8. Abrams GW, Williams GA. "En bloc" excision of diabetic membranes. Am J Ophthalmol. 1987;103(3 Pt 1):302–8.
9. Khan MA, Shahlaee A, Toussaint B, Hsu J, Sivalingam A, Dugel PU, et al. Outcomes of 27 gauge microincision vitrectomy surgery for posterior segment disease. Am J Ophthalmol. 2016;161:36–43. e1-2. https://doi.org/10.1016/j.ajo.2015.09.024.
10. Yang CM, Yeh PT, Yang CH, Chen MS. Bevacizumab pretreatment and long-acting gas infusion on vitreous clear-up after diabetic vitrectomy. Am J Ophthalmol. 2008;146(2):211–7. https://doi.org/10.1016/j.ajo.2008.04.028.
11. avastin 1.
12. Chen E, Park CH. Use of intravitreal bevacizumab as a preoperative adjunct for tractional retinal detachment repair in severe proliferative diabetic retinopathy. Retina. 2006;26(6):699–700. https://doi.org/10.1097/01.iae.0000225351.87205.
13. Gandhi JS, Tan LT, Pearce I, Charles SJ. Bevacizumab (Avastin) as a surgical adjunct in diabetic vitrectomy for fibrovascular disease. Eye. 2008; https://doi.org/10.1038/eye.2008.99.
14. Ishikawa K, Honda S, Tsukahara Y, Negi A. Preferable use of intravitreal bevacizumab as a pretreatment of vitrectomy for severe proliferative diabetic retinopathy. Eye. 2007; https://doi.org/10.1038/sj.eye.6702983.
15. Miki A, Oshima Y, Otori Y, Kamei M, Tano Y. Efficacy of intravitreal bevacizumab as adjunctive treatment with pars plana vitrectomy, endolaser photocoagulation, and trabeculectomy for neovascular glaucoma. Br J Ophthalmol. 2008;92(10):1431–3. https://doi.org/10.1136/bjo.2007.129833.
16. Romano MR, Gibran SK, Marticorena J, Wong D, Heimann H. Can a preoperative bevacizumab injection prevent recurrent postvit-

rectomy diabetic vitreous haemorrhage? Eye. 2008; https://doi.org/10.1038/eye.2008.354.

17. Ahmadieh H, Shoeibi N, Entezari M, Monshizadeh R. Intravitreal bevacizumab for prevention of early postvitrectomy hemorrhage in diabetic patients: a randomized clinical trial. Ophthalmology. 2009;116(10):1943–8. https://doi.org/10.1016/j.ophtha.2009.07.001.
18. Smith JM, Steel DH. Anti-vascular endothelial growth factor for prevention of postoperative vitreous cavity haemorrhage after vitrectomy for proliferative diabetic retinopathy. Cochrane Database Syst Rev. 2015;8:Cd008214. https://doi.org/10.1002/14651858.CD008214.pub3.
19. Arevalo JF, Maia M, Flynn HW Jr, Saravia M, Avery RL, Wu L, et al. Tractional retinal detachment following intravitreal bevacizumab (Avastin) in patients with severe proliferative diabetic retinopathy. Br J Ophthalmol. 2008;92(2):213–6. https://doi.org/10.1136/bjo.2007.127142.
20. Castillo Velazquez J, Aleman I, Rush SW, Rush RB. Bevacizumab before diabetic vitrectomy: a clinical trial assessing 3 dosing amounts. Ophthalmol Retina. 2018;2(10):1010–20. https://doi.org/10.1016/j.oret.2018.04.014.
21. Joondeph BC, Blankenship GW. Hemostatic effects of air versus fluid in diabetic vitrectomy. Ophthalmology. 1989;96(12):1701–6.
22. La Heij EC, Tecim S, Kessels AG, Liem AT, Japing WJ, Hendrikse F. Clinical variables and their relation to visual outcome after vitrectomy in eyes with diabetic retinal traction detachment. Graefes Arch Clin Exp Ophthalmol. 2004;242(3):210–7.
23. Sakamoto T, Fujisawa K, Kinukawa N, Ishibashi T, Inomata H. Re-worsening factor after successful vitrectomy for diabetic retinopathy: optic disc fibrovascular proliferation and macular disease. Ophthalmologica. 2002;216(2):101–7.
24. Carter JB, Michels RG, Glaser BM, de BS. Iatrogenic retinal breaks complicating pars plana vitrectomy. Ophthalmology. 1990;97(7):848–53.
25. Oyakawa RT, Schachat AP, Michels RG, Rice TA. Complications of vitreous surgery for diabetic retinopathy. I. Intraoperative complications. Ophthalmology. 1983;90(5):517–21.
26. Gupta B, Wong R, Sivaprasad S, Williamson TH. Surgical and visual outcome following 20-gauge vitrectomy in proliferative diabetic retinopathy over a 10-year period, evidence for change in practice. Eye (Lond). 2012; https://doi.org/10.1038/eye.2011.348.
27. Pearson RV, McLeod D, Gregor ZJ. Removal of silicone oil following diabetic vitrectomy. Br J Ophthalmol. 1993;77(4):204–7.
28. Heimann K, Dahl B, Dimopoulos S, Lemmen KD. Pars plana vitrectomy and silicone oil injection in proliferative diabetic retinopathy. Graefes Arch Clin Exp Ophthalmol. 1989;227(2):152–6.
29. Wilson-Holt N, Gregor Z. Spontaneous relieving retinotomies in diabetic silicone filled eyes. Eye. 1992;6(Pt 5):461–4.
30. Karel I, Kalvodova B. Long-term results of pars plana vitrectomy and silicone oil for complications of diabetic retinopathy. Eur J Ophthalmol. 1994;4(1):52–8.
31. Gonvers M. Temporary silicone oil tamponade in the treatment of complicated diabetic retinal detachments. Graefes Arch Clin Exp Ophthalmol. 1990;228(5):415–22.
32. Castellarin A, Grigorian R, Bhagat N, Del Priore L, Zarbin MA. Vitrectomy with silicone oil infusion in severe diabetic retinopathy. Br J Ophthalmol. 2003;87(3):318–21.
33. de Juan E, Jr., Hardy M, Hatchell DL, Hatchell MC. The effect of intraocular silicone oil on anterior chamber oxygen pressure in cats. Arch Ophthalmol. 1986;104(7):1063–4.
34. Mulder V, Veckeneer M, van Rooij J, Delaey C, van Meurs JC. Intentional continuous shallowing of the anterior chamber, a procedure to prevent lens touch during phakic vitrectomy. Acta Ophthalmol. 2016;94(2):e163–4. https://doi.org/10.1111/aos.12804.
35. Imamura Y, Minami M, Ueki M, Satoh B, Ikeda T. Use of perfluorocarbon liquid during vitrectomy for severe proliferative diabetic retinopathy. Br J Ophthalmol. 2003;87(5):563–6.
36. Steinmetz RL, Grizzard WS, Hammer ME. Vitrectomy for diabetic traction retinal detachment using the multiport illumination system. Ophthalmology. 2002;109(12):2303–7.
37. Han DP, Murphy ML, Mieler WF. A modified en bloc excision technique during vitrectomy for diabetic traction retinal detachment. Results and complications. Ophthalmology. 1994;101(5):803–8.
38. Rice TA, Michels RG, Rice EF. Vitrectomy for diabetic rhegmatogenous retinal detachment. Am J Ophthalmol. 1983;95(1):34–44.
39. Holekamp NM, Shui YB, Beebe D. Lower intraocular oxygen tension in diabetic patients: possible contribution to decreased incidence of nuclear sclerotic cataract. Am J Ophthalmol. 2006;141(6):1027–32.
40. Tolentino FI, Cajita VN, Gancayco T, Skates S. Vitreous hemorrhage after closed vitrectomy for proliferative diabetic retinopathy. Ophthalmology. 1989;96(10):1495–500.
41. Steel DH, Habib MS, Park S, Hildreth AJ, Owen RI. Entry site neovascularization and vitreous cavity hemorrhage after diabetic vitrectomy. The predictive value of inner sclerostomy site ultrasonography. Ophthalmology. 2008;115(3):525–32. https://doi.org/10.1016/j.ophtha.2007.08.034.
42. Laatikainen L, Summanen P, Immonen I. Effect of tranexamic acid on postvitrectomy haemorrhage in diabetic patients. Int Ophthalmol. 1987;10(3):153–5.
43. Virata SR, Kylstra JA. Postoperative complications following vitrectomy for proliferative diabetic retinopathy with sew-on and noncontact wide-angle viewing lenses. Ophthalmic Surg Lasers. 2001;32(3):193–7.
44. Koutsandrea CN, Apostolopoulos MN, Chatzoulis DZ, Parikakis EA, Theodossiadis GP. Hemostatic effects of SF6 after diabetic vitrectomy for vitreous hemorrhage. Acta Ophthalmol Scand. 2001;79(1):34–8.
45. Brown GC, Tasman WS, Benson WE, McNamara JA, Eagle RC Jr. Reoperation following diabetic vitrectomy. Arch Ophthalmol. 1992;110(4):506–10.
46. Novak MA, Rice TA, Michels RG, Auer C. Vitreous hemorrhage after vitrectomy for diabetic retinopathy. Ophthalmology. 1984;91(12):1485–9.
47. Liggett PE, Lean JS, Barlow WE, Ryan SJ. Intraoperative argon endophotocoagulation for recurrent vitreous hemorrhage after vitrectomy for diabetic retinopathy. Am J Ophthalmol. 1987;103(2):146–9.
48. West JF, Gregor ZJ. Fibrovascular ingrowth and recurrent haemorrhage following diabetic vitrectomy. Br J Ophthalmol. 2000;84(8):822–5.
49. Sawa H, Ikeda T, Matsumoto Y, Niiya A, Kinoshita S. Neovascularization from scleral wound as cause of vitreous rebleeding after vitrectomy for proliferative diabetic retinopathy. Jpn J Ophthalmol. 2000;44(2):154–60.
50. Lewis H, Abrams GW, Williams GA. Anterior hyaloidal fibrovascular proliferation after diabetic vitrectomy. Am J Ophthalmol. 1987;104(6):607–13.
51. Hershberger VS, Augsburger JJ, Hutchins RK, Raymond LA, Krug S. Fibrovascular ingrowth at sclerotomy sites in vitrectomized diabetic eyes with recurrent vitreous hemorrhage: ultrasound biomicroscopy findings. Ophthalmology. 2004;111(6):1215–21.
52. Yang CM, Yeh PT, Yang CH. Intravitreal long-acting gas in the prevention of early postoperative vitreous hemorrhage in diabetic vitrectomy. Ophthalmology. 2007;114(4):710–5. https://doi.org/10.1016/j.ophtha.2006.07.047.
53. Wand M, Madigan JC, Gaudio AR, Sorokanich S. Neovascular glaucoma following pars plana vitrectomy for complications of diabetic retinopathy. Ophthalmic Surg. 1990;21(2):113–8.

54. Rinkoff JS, De Juan E, Jr., McCuen BW. Silicone oil for retinal detachment with advanced proliferative vitreoretinopathy following failed vitrectomy for proliferative diabetic retinopathy. Am J Ophthalmol. 1986;101(2):181–6.
55. Kadonosono K, Matsumoto S, Uchio E, Sugita M, Akura J, Ohno S. Iris neovascularization after vitrectomy combined with phacoemulsification and intraocular lens implantation for proliferative diabetic retinopathy. Ophthalmic Surg Lasers. 2001;32(1):19–24.
56. Helbig H, Kellner U, Bornfeld N, Foerster MH. Rubeosis iridis after vitrectomy for diabetic retinopathy. Graefes Arch Clin Exp Ophthalmol. 1998;236(10):730–3.
57. Scuderi JJ, Blumenkranz MS, Blankenship G. Regression of diabetic rubeosis iridis following successful surgical reattachment of the retina by vitrectomy. Retina. 1982;2(4):193–6.
58. Oldendoerp J, Spitznas M. Factors influencing the results of vitreous surgery in diabetic retinopathy. I. Iris Rubeosis and/or active neovascularization at the fundus. Graefes Arch Clin Exp Ophthalmol. 1989;227(1):1–8.
59. Barzideh N, Johnson TM. Subfoveal fluid resolves slowly after pars plana vitrectomy for tractional retinal detachment secondary to proliferative diabetic retinopathy. Retina. 2007;27(6):740–3. https://doi.org/10.1097/IAE.0b013e318030c663.
60. Karimov MI, Gasymov EM, Aliyeva IJ, Akhundova LA, Rustambayova GR, Aliyev KD. An optical coherence tomography study of residual subfoveal fluid after successful pars plana vitrectomy in patients with diabetic tractional macular detachment. Eye (Lond). 2018;32(9):1472–7. https://doi.org/10.1038/s41433-018-0111-6.
61. Gollamudi SR, Smiddy WE, Schachat AP, Michels RG, Vitale S. Long-term survival rate after vitreous surgery for complications of diabetic retinopathy. Ophthalmology. 1991;98(1):18–22.
62. Summanen P, Karhunen U, Laatikainen L. Characteristics and survival of diabetic patients undergoing vitreous surgery. Acta Ophthalmol(Copenh). 1987;65(2):197–202.
63. Helbig H, Kellner U, Bornfeld N, Foerster MH. Life expectancy of diabetic patients undergoing vitreous surgery. Br J Ophthalmol. 1996;80(7):640–3.
64. Shukla SY, Hariprasad AS, Hariprasad SM. Long-term mortality in diabetic patients with Tractional retinal detachments. Ophthalmol Retina. 2017;1(1):8–11. https://doi.org/10.1016/j.oret.2016.09.002.
65. Two-year course of visual acuity in severe proliferative diabetic retinopathy with conventional management. Diabetic retinopathy vitrectomy study (DRVS) report #1. Ophthalmology. 1985;92(4):492–502.
66. Mason JO III, Colagross CT, Haleman T, Fuller JJ, White MF, Feist RM, et al. Visual outcome and risk factors for light perception and no light perception vision after vitrectomy for diabetic retinopathy. Am J Ophthalmol. 2005;140(2):231–5.
67. Tong L, Vernon SA, Kiel W, Sung V, Orr GM. Association of macular involvement with proliferative retinopathy in type 2 diabetes. Diabet Med. 2001;18(5):388–94.
68. Kuhn F, Kiss G, Mester V, Szijarto Z, Kovacs B. Vitrectomy with internal limiting membrane removal for clinically significant macular oedema. Graefes Arch Clin Exp Ophthalmol. 2004;
69. Micelli FT, Cardascia N, Durante G, Vetrugno M, Cardia L. Pars plana vitrectomy in diabetic macular edema. Doc Ophthalmol. 1999;97(3–4):471–4.
70. Ikeda T, Sato K, Katano T, Hayashi Y. Vitrectomy for cystoid macular oedema with attached posterior hyaloid membrane in patients with diabetes. Br J Ophthalmol. 1999;83(1):12–4.
71. Ikeda T, Sato K, Katano T, Hayashi Y. Attached posterior hyaloid membrane and the pathogenesis of honeycombed cystoid macular edema in patients with diabetes. Am J Ophthalmol. 1999;127(4):478–9.
72. Tachi N, Ogino N. Vitrectomy for diffuse macular edema in cases of diabetic retinopathy. Am J Ophthalmol. 1996;122(2):258–60.
73. Yamamoto T, Hitani K, Tsukahara I, Yamamoto S, Kawasaki R, Yamashita H, et al. Early postoperative retinal thickness changes and complications after vitrectomy for diabetic macular edema. Am J Ophthalmol. 2003;135(1):14–9.
74. Harbour JW, Smiddy WE, Flynn HW Jr, Rubsamen PE. Vitrectomy for diabetic macular edema associated with a thickened and taut posterior hyaloid membrane. Am J Ophthalmol. 1996;121(4):405–13.
75. Pendergast SD, Hassan TS, Williams GA, Cox MS, Margherio RR, Ferrone PJ, et al. Vitrectomy for diffuse diabetic macular edema associated with a taut premacular posterior hyaloid. Am J Ophthalmol. 2000;130(2):178–86.
76. La Heij EC, Hendrikse F, Kessels AG, Derhaag PJ. Vitrectomy results in diabetic macular oedema without evident vitreomacular traction. Graefes Arch Clin Exp Ophthalmol. 2001;239(4):264–70.
77. Sato Y, Lee Z, Shimada H. Vitrectomy for diabetic cystoid macular edema. Jpn J Ophthalmol. 2002;46(3):315–22.
78. Otani T, Kishi S. A controlled study of vitrectomy for diabetic macular edema. Am J Ophthalmol. 2002;134(2):214–9.
79. Lewis H, Abrams GW, Blumenkranz MS, Campo RV. Vitrectomy for diabetic macular traction and edema associated with posterior hyaloidal traction. Ophthalmology. 1992;99(5):753–9.
80. Thomas D, Bunce C, Moorman C, Laidlaw DA. A randomised controlled feasibility trial of vitrectomy versus laser for diabetic macular oedema. Br J Ophthalmol. 2005;89(1):81–6. https://doi.org/10.1136/bjo.2004.044966.
81. Park JH, Woo SJ, Ha YJ, Yu HG. Effect of vitrectomy on macular microcirculation in patients with diffuse diabetic macular edema. Graefes Arch Clin Exp Ophthalmol. 2009;247(8):1009–17. https://doi.org/10.1007/s00417-009-1062-1.
82. Laidlaw DA. Vitrectomy for diabetic macular oedema. Eye. 2008;22(10):1337–41. https://doi.org/10.1038/eye.2008.84.
83. Yang CM. Surgical treatment for severe diabetic macular edema with massive hard exudates. Retina. 2000;20(2):121–5.
84. Sakuraba T, Suzuki Y, Mizutani H, Nakazawa M. Visual improvement after removal of submacular exudates in patients with diabetic maculopathy. Ophthalmic Surg Lasers. 2000;31(4):287–91.
85. Takagi H, Otani A, Kiryu J, Ogura Y. New surgical approach for removing massive foveal hard exudates in diabetic macular edema. Ophthalmology. 1999;106(2):249–56.
86. Singh RP, Margolis R, Kaiser PK. Cystoid puncture for chronic cystoid macular oedema. Br J Ophthalmol. 2007;91(8):1062–4. https://doi.org/10.1136/bjo.2006.101790.

16 Other Vascular Disorders

Contents

Introduction

There are several conditions that stimulate neovascularisation of the retina with subsequent complications such as vitreous haemorrhage and tractional retinal detachment from the pathological separation of the vitreous. The most common is severe diabetic retinopathy but also retinal vein occlusion, sickle cell retinopathy and retinal vasculitis (Fig. 16.1).

Retinal Vein Occlusion

Retinal vein occlusions (RVO) are the second commonest vascular events in the eye after diabetic retinopathy. The eye is unusual in suffering from occlusion of the veins more often than arteries. Retinal vein occlusion can be divided into two groups, branch retinal vein occlusion, BRVO, and central retinal vein occlusion, CRVO (which includes hemi retinal vein occlusion). BRVO occurs most commonly

T. H. Williamson, *Vitreoretinal Surgery*, https://doi.org/10.1007/978-3-030-68769-4_16

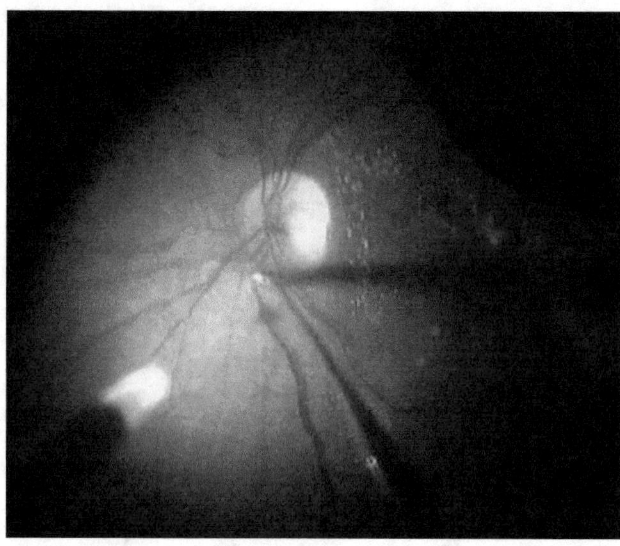

Fig. 16.1 It is possible to dissect the overlying artery off the underlying occluded retinal vein in a branch retinal vein occlusion to try to relieve the blockage

where a retinal arteriole crosses over a venule. Sharing an adventitial sheath in the presence of the thickened arteriolar wall may compress the thinner walled venule resulting in occlusion. In CRVO, pathological evidence suggests the site of obstruction is situated at the lamina cribrosa [1]. Several innovations have been designed but none are of proven benefit.

New methods:

Chorioretinal Anastomosis	CRVO
Intravitreal Steroid Injection	CRVO and BRVO
Pars Plana Vitrectomy	CRVO and BRVO
Arteriovenous Decompression	BRVO
Radial Optic Neurotomy	CRVO
Tissue Plasminogen Activator	CRVO

These methods have been superseded by intravitreal Anti-VEGF injections [2, 3]. However, Anti-VEGF does not, in general reverse the ischaemic variants of RVO.

Chorioretinal Anastomosis

Chorioretinal anastomosis using argon laser has been successful in improving vision in one-third of eyes in the nonischemic variant of the disorder in selected patients but has been associated with frequent complications [4–6]. This therapy is not generally used in ischemic CRVO because of a high complication rate of choroidal neovascularisation.

Table 16.1 Difficulty rating for arteriovenous decompression

Difficulty Rating	High
Success rates	Unknown
Complication rates	Low
When to use in training	Late

Arteriovenous Decompression (Table 16.1)

Grid macular laser therapy in BRVO can control macular oedema, with 60% of treated cases retaining 20/40 vision or better at 3 years [7] and reduce the incidence of vitreous haemorrhage by half [7, 8]. In BRVO, the site of occlusion can easily be visualised and is thought to occur because of arteriosclerosis in the media of the artery giving rise to a compressive effect on the adjacent vein. At the arteriovenous crossing, the artery is generally located anterior to the occluded vein, within a common adventitial sheath. Charles attempted to relieve the blockage by dissecting the arteriole off the venule at the arteriovenous crossing in one patient [9]. The technique was revisited with reported success in 10 out of 15 patients, with an average gain of four lines of vision [10]. In a non-randomised comparative study, patients receiving intervention performed better, with 75% doubling their visual angles compared to 40% with conventional treatment [11]. Opremcak has designed an instrument for the blunt dissection of the arteriole from the venule by inserting a spatulated knife between the blood vessels. Potential complications include retinal tear or detachment, vitreous haemorrhage, retinal gliosis at the incision site, arcuate scotoma, and cataract. Resolution of macular oedema following sheathotomy has been confirmed using optical coherence tomography (OCT) [12]. There are also theoretical reasons whereby the localised ischemia of the retina in BRVO might be improved by the PPV procedure because removal of the vitreous gel may allow oxygenation of the retina from other sites in the eye with good blood flow [13]. Indeed, some investigators have tried PPV and gas alone [14] (Figs. 16.2, 16.3 and 16.4).

Radial Optic Neurotomy (Table 16.2 and Fig. 16.5)

Usually, CRVO is associated with severe irreversible visual loss and with the improvement of vision in only 20% [15]. Incision of the optic nerve on the nasal side (radial optic neurotomy) has been described [16–18] but is of unproven benefit as yet despite large case series [16, 19]. It is thought that the neurotomy may help blood flow in the central retinal vein by relieving pressure on the vein as it exits the lamina cribrosa, assuming that CRVO is a "neurovascular compres-

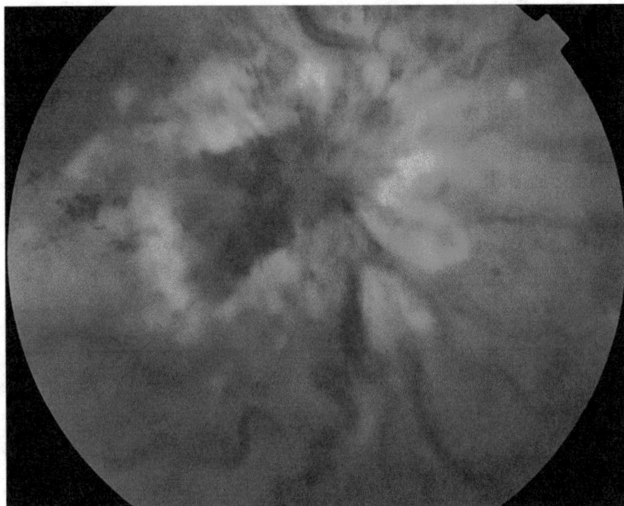

Fig. 16.2 CRVO can be excessively severe, as in this patient

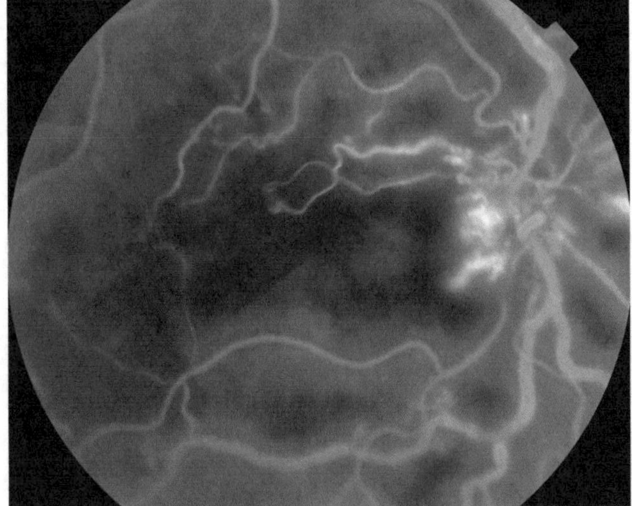

Fig. 16.3 Severe ischaemia on FFA

sion syndrome," resulting from increased pressure within the confined space of the scleral outlet. Intravitreal pO2 is severely reduced in CRVO and may be increased by vitrectomy [20].

Intravitreal Steroid and Anti-VEGF Agents (Table 16.3)

Cystoid macular oedema (CMO) is a major cause of visual loss in RVO. Injections of varying doses of Triamcinolone into the vitreous cavity (1–21 mg) have been investigated for reversing CMO in uveitis, post-cataract surgery, retinal vein occlusion, telangiectasia, and diabetes [21–37].

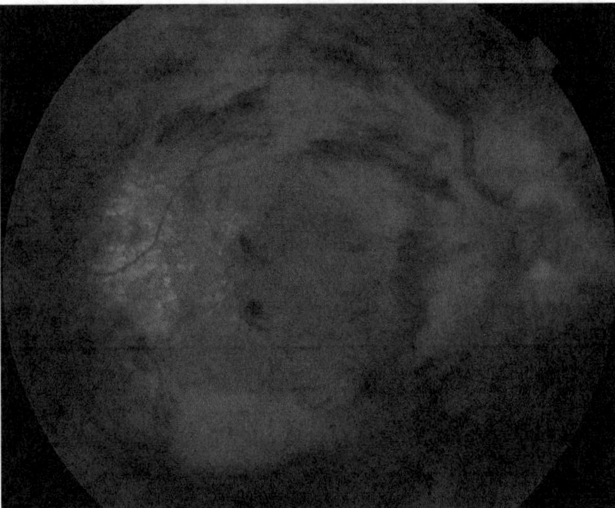

Fig. 16.4 A 13-year-old girl with CRVO in whom the onset was associated with a bout of diarrhoea on ski trip and a short-haul plane journey. She had a familial cholesterolaemia

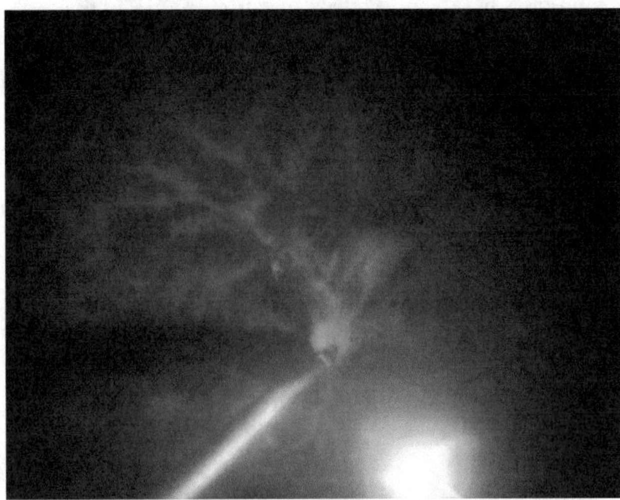

Fig. 16.5 Incising the optic nerve in radial optic neurotomy is of uncertain worth in the treatment of central retinal vein occlusion

Table 16.2 Difficulty rating for RON

Difficulty rating	Low
Success rates	Unknown
Complication rates	Low
When to use in training	Late

Table 16.3 Difficulty rating for intravitreal steroid injection

Difficulty Rating	Low
Success rates	Slight
Complication rates	Low
When to use in training	Early

Dexamethasone pellets can be inserted into the vitreous and have shown some efficacy for improved vision over 6 and 12 months [38] but as with triamcinolone repeated injections are required.

The steroid stabilises the leaky vascular endothelium reducing the extracellular fluid accumulation perhaps by downregulating vascular endothelial growth factor (VEGF) [39]. In many cases, the feasibility of steroid is lessened because the duration of action is only a few months, requiring the administration of repeated injections in chronic conditions. Unfortunately, those repeat injections are associated with a reduced or absent response with time [36]. Dexamethasone has, however, been associated with less frequent IOP elevation than triamcinolone injection, which in the later can be severe and require surgery for IOP control. Ozurdex is a slow-release implant of dexamethasone for the treatment of macular oedema.

Anti-VEGF agents have been used widely for cystoid macular oedema for many causes, including RVO. Anti-VEGF reduces CMO and improves vision with low complication rates but requires repeat injection. Anti-VEGF agents are also useful for controlling neovascular glaucoma (Figs. 16.6 and 16.7).

Tissue Plasminogen Activator

TPA may not cross the vasculature to enter the central retinal vein, therefore investigators have attempted to insert TPA directly into the vein [40] using a 33-G cannula. The technique does not seem to have had a major effect on visual acuity and vitreous haemorrhage is common [41]. More recently, Weiss has added intravitreal steroid injections to try to improve success rates [28].

Sickle Cell Disease

Introduction

The sickle cell haemoglobinopathies result from an abnormality in the beta chain of the haemoglobin molecule. They are hereditary disorders that cause red blood cells to take on a sickle shape. These blood cells are rigid and pass with more difficulty through blood vessels causing vascular occlusion in multiple organs, including the retina. There is chronic haemolytic anaemia and vaso-occlusive crises and a number of clinical features in the eye [42]. Sickling occurs more in hypoxic or acidotic conditions (Fig. 16.8).

Types of Sickle Cell Disease

- Sickle cell trait (Hb AS)
- Sickle cell anaemia, Homozygous sickle cell disease (SS disease)
- Sickle cell disease, Heterozygous sickle cell C disease (SC disease)
- Sickle cell thalassaemia disease (S-thal disease)
- Systemic investigations

Systemic Investigation

Ask for a history of systemic crisis, medications, racial and family history and check haemoglobin electrophoresis and full blood count.

Inheritance and Race

It is an autosomal incomplete dominant condition (inheritance is like recessive inheritance, e.g. 1 in 4 chance of SS if both parents AS), but the S gene can have effects if combined with the C gene or thalassaemia gene.

The sickle gene is present in approximately 8% of the black population in the USA but can be higher or lower depending on geographical location. The gene is thought to have originated in West Africa and become more prevalent because of its protective effect in falciparum malaria (shorter living red blood cells and relative hypoxia may be detrimental to the infection). The gene is also seen in eastern Mediterranean and Middle Eastern patients.SC disease is traditionally thought to develop more retinal complications; however, the complications are also seen in SS disease. Most cases of retinopathy seem to appear between 20 and 40 years and stabilise or regress thereafter.

Systemic Manifestations

- Painful vaso-occlusive crisis
- Acute chest crisis
- Anaemia
- Leg ulcers
- Bacterial infections
- Arthritis and swelling in the hands and feet
- Bone necrosis
- Splenomegaly
- Hepatomegaly
- Heart and lung damage

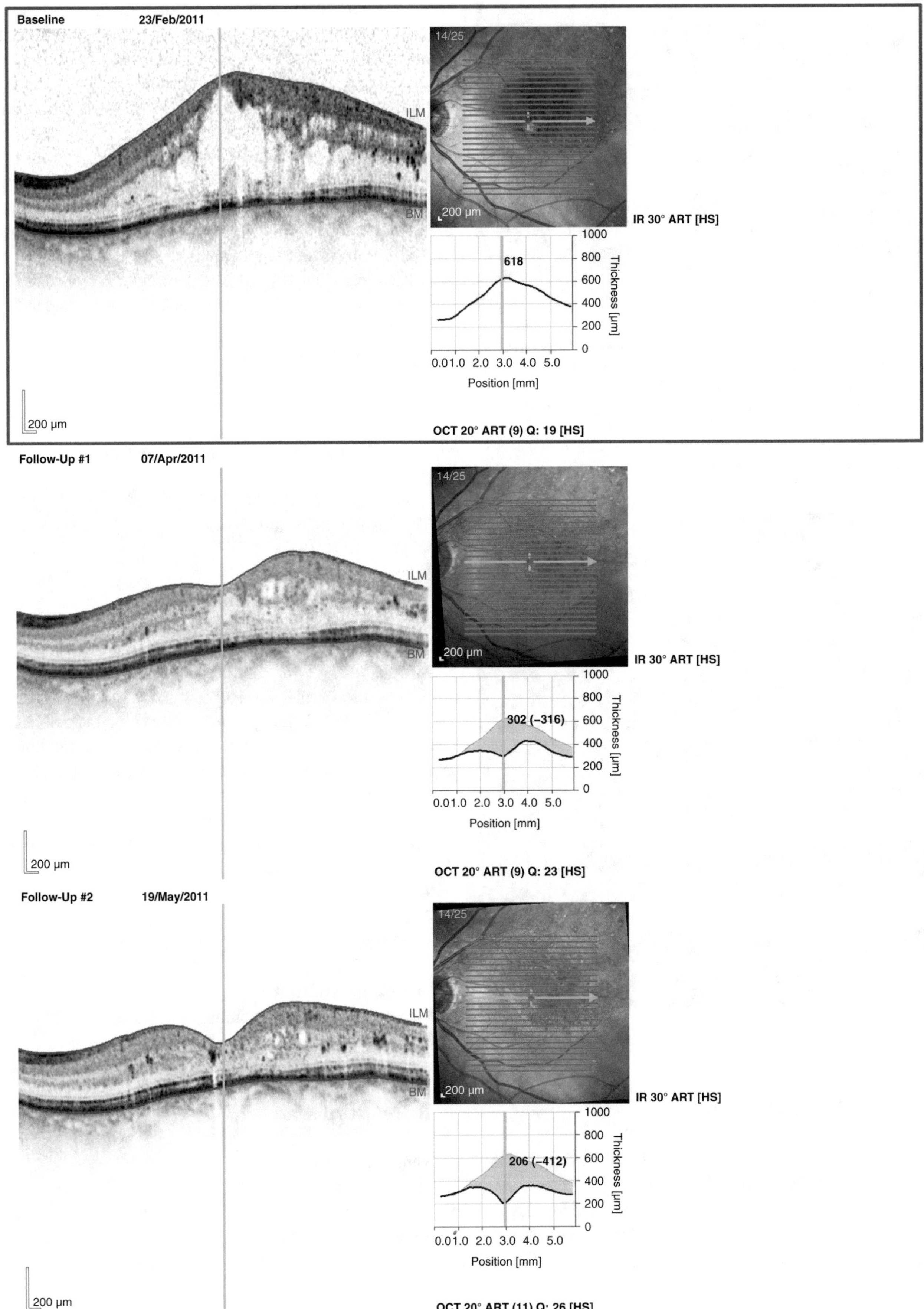

Fig. 16.6 CMO of the retina from BRVO, reduced by the intravitreal injection of bevacizumab

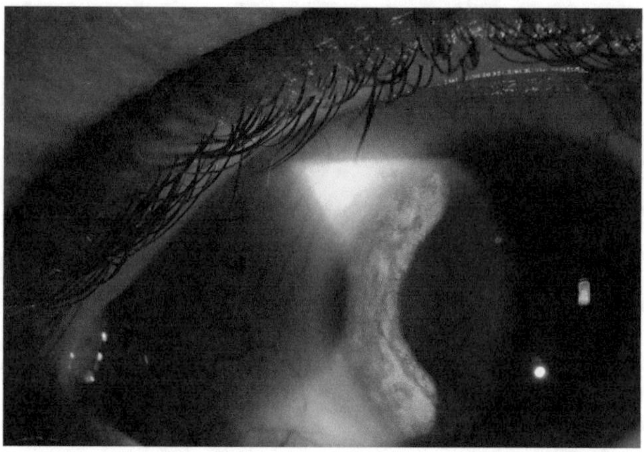

Fig. 16.7 Iris neovascularisation after CRVO. The neovascularisation can be reversed by injection of anti-VEGF into the vitreous. This may temporarily reduce the IOP to allow PRP or other measures such as PPV to reverse the ischaemia. Repeated injections can be used to prolong the duration of residual vision in the eye (for up to 2 years), although these patients will usually eventually suffer further loss of vision from retinal ischaemia and CMO

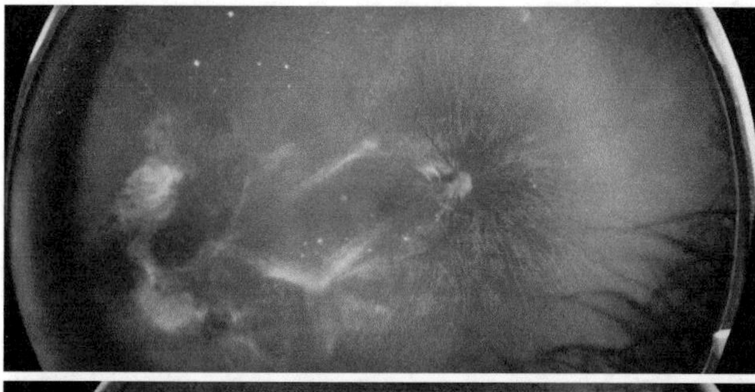

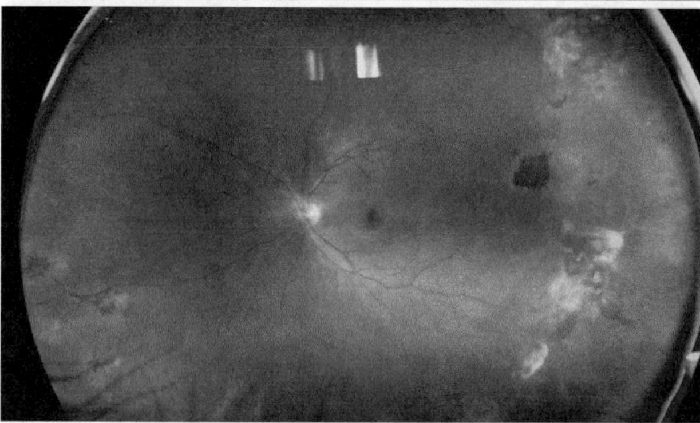

Fig. 16.8 Sickle cell retinopathy with TRD on the right and sea fans and black sunbursts on the left

Ophthalmic Presentation

The blood cells occlude the retinal blood vessel causing hypoxia stimulating neovascularisation [43]. These may bleed or produce traction on the retina, which may be implicated in retinal break formation and retinal detachment. The process also causes secondary changes in the vitreous, which stimulates epiretinal membrane formation and macular holes. Retinal complications are seen in 43% of patients aged between 20 and 30 years with sickle cell [44]. In one study, blindness in patients with proliferative vitreoretinopathy was seen in 12% [45]. However, in a large study of young patients in Jamaica (307 patients with SS and 166 with SC), followed for 20 years up to the age of 26 years, only two patients had sight-threatening disease, one patient suffering irreversible sight loss in one eye and one patient with a successfully treated RRD [44]. A description of the natural history of the condition has demonstrated a moderate risk of vitreous haemorrhage (5.3%) and macular lesions (4.6%), and a low risk of retinal detachment (2%) over a mean follow up of 6.3 years [42].

The asymptomatic patient:

- Black sunburst spots
- Iridescent spots
- Retinal haemorrhages (salmon patches) and
- Sea fan neovascular proliferation

The symptomatic patient [46]:

- Vitreous haemorrhage
- Tractional retinal detachment (TRD)
- Rhegmatogenous retinal detachment (RRD)
- Macular epiretinal membrane (ERM)
- Macular hole

The conjunctival and optic nerve head blood vessels show characteristic segmentation of blood columns in the homozygous sickle cell disease (SS). There may be comma-shaped vessels on the bulbar conjunctiva and iris atrophy. Spontaneous hyphaema can occur and cause raised intraocular pressure and has a risk of rebleeding. Surgical intervention is sometimes required.

The optic nerve may show dark red spots or clumps on the surface.

The Macula

- Chronic retinal ischaemia.
- Macular epiretinal membrane.
- Macular hole.
- An association with angioid streaks has been described.

The peripheral retina

- Nonproliferative changes.
- Venous tortuosity.
- Salmon patch haemorrhage, round or oval intraretinal haemorrhages in the mid periphery initially bright red then fading to the colour of salmon flesh.

- Black sunburst, hypertrophy of the retinal pigment epithelium with spiky border.
- Iridescent white spots.
- Proliferative changes, Goldberg classification [47].
- Peripheral arteriolar occlusion in the far periphery.
- Arteriolar venular anastomosis is seen at the junction of the perfused and non-perfused retina. Best seen on angiography, flat on the retina and non-leaking.
- Neovascular proliferation in the far periphery giving a "sea fan" appearance. These often auto infarct and are commonest in SC disease.
- Vitreous haemorrhage.
- Retinal detachment either tractional or rhegmatogenous (Figs. 16.9 and 16.10).

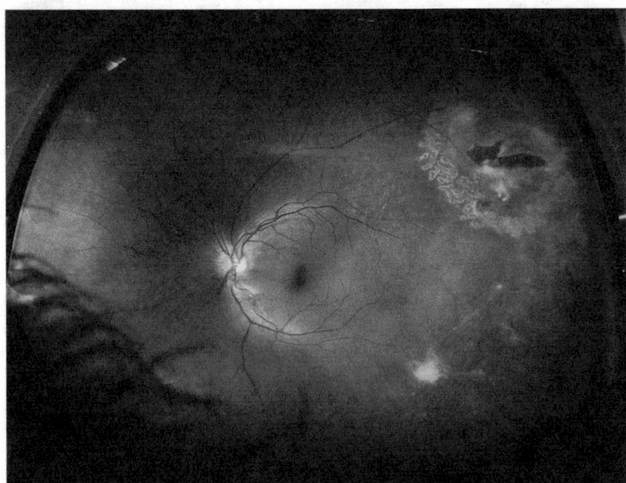

Fig. 16.9 A large retinal tear in a patient with a sickle was found 6 months after PVD symptoms and was treated with laser

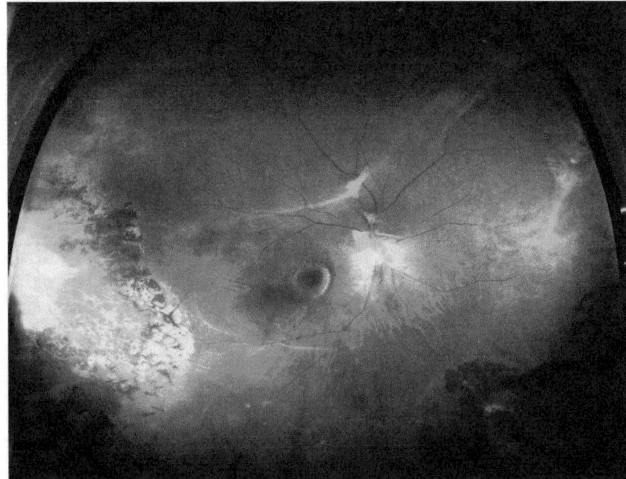

Fig. 16.10 A longstanding atrophic macular hole in a patient with sickle retinopathy

Laser Therapy

The use of scatter laser as a means of regressing neovascularization is controversial because of the high incidence of auto infarction of the retinal proliferation in 30% [48]. Occlusion of the feeder vessels supplying sea fans has been employed, feeder vessel laser has been associated with retinal break formation and choroidal neovascularization but has been shown in a small randomised study to reduce the risk of vitreous haemorrhage [45]. It has been used to treat a patient with exudative retinal detachment apparently from sickle cell retinopathy (Figs. 16.11, 16.12, 16.13, 16.14, 16.15, 16.16, 16.17, 16.18 and 16.19).

Surgery

Patients with vitreous haemorrhage, TRD, RRD, and macular disorders such as ERM and macular holes can be treated with pars plana vitrectomy [49]. Peroperative complications are frequent; in particular, a high incidence of iatrogenic tears formation during PPV, especially around sea fan complexes, if you attempt to delaminate. Sea fans are better left in situ and a segmentation technique used to remove vitreal attachments. There is no need to try to induce regression of the sea fans with scatter laser or feeder vessel laser. Cataract formation after surgery is uncommon, perhaps relating to the young age of many of the patients or to the relative ischemia of these eyes, which may protect against cataractogenesis as has been suggested in diabetic retinopathy.

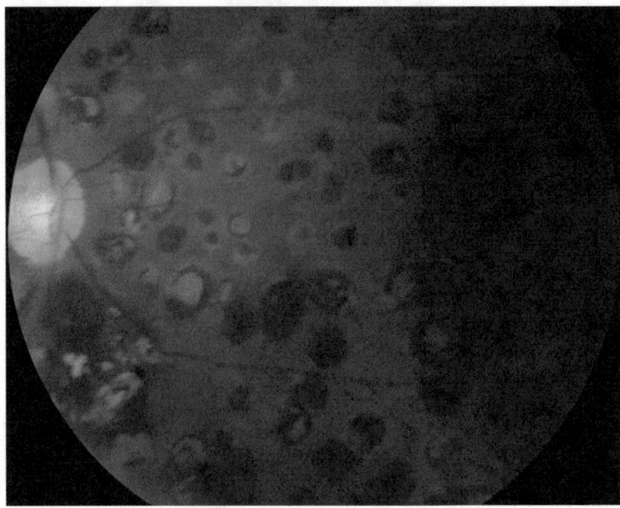

Fig. 16.11 It would appear the panretinal photocoagulation is not necessary in sickle cell retinopathy

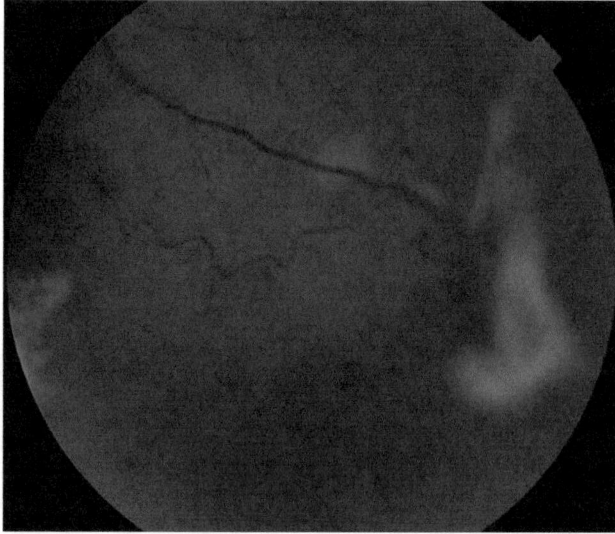

Fig. 16.12 Patients with sea fans in the periphery can present with vitreous haemorrhage or retinal detachment. Although these patients are difficult to operate on, success rates tend to be high. The sea fans are very adherent to overlying vitreous and cannot be dissected and must be segmented, but the neovascular process is inactive, so the eyes tend to respond to surgery well without laser photocoagulation

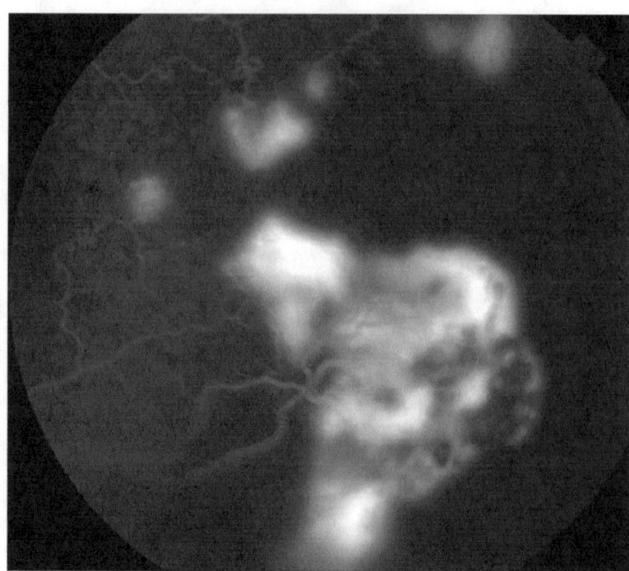

Fig. 16.14 A fluorescein angiogram of a sea fan complex showing leakage from the neovascularisation and far peripheral capillary drop out

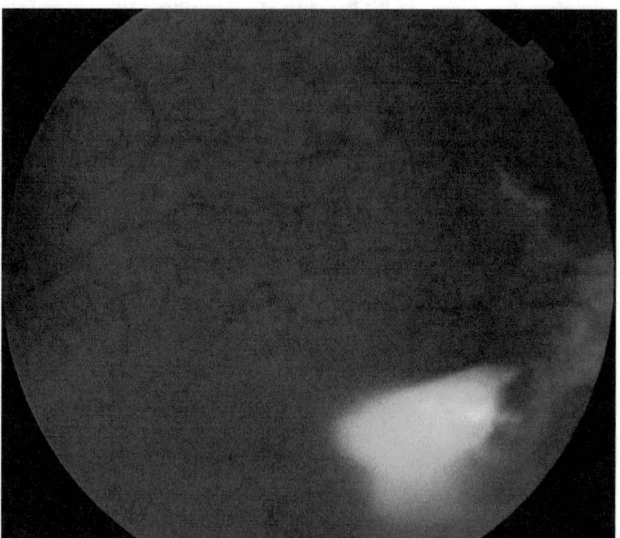

Fig. 16.13 A sea fan complex with thick membrane and blood, with leakage seen on FFA. These do not dissect off the retina and should be segmented

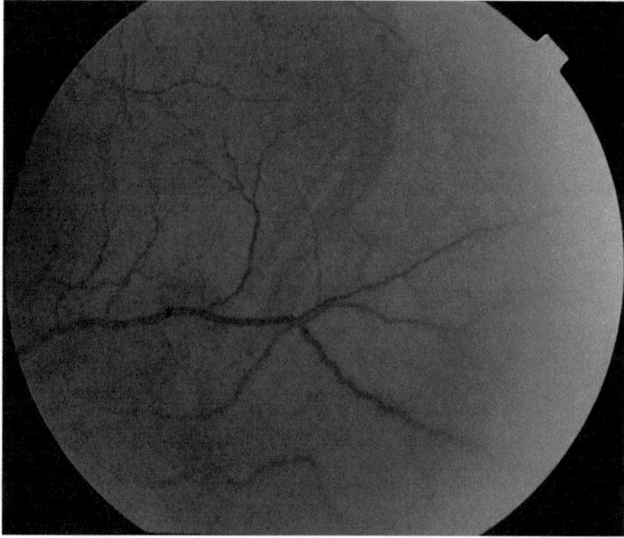

Fig. 16.15 Because the vitreous is often attached to sickle cell patients, not all retinal detachments will proceed or progress and these can be watched on occasion carefully. Such retinal detachments may spontaneously regress

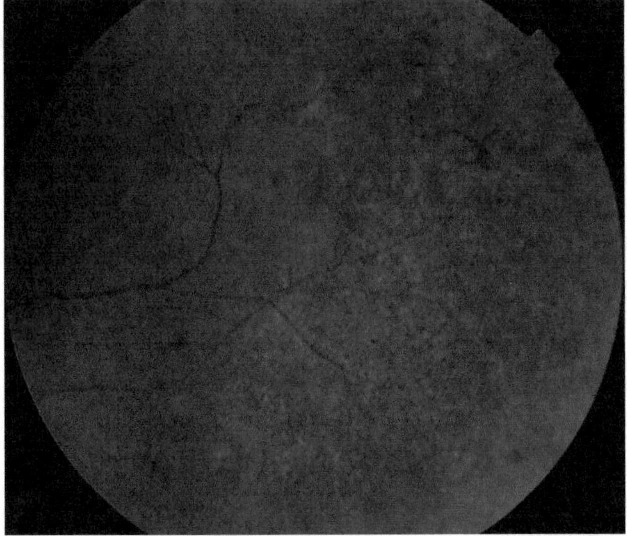

Fig. 16.16 The retina flattened without surgery

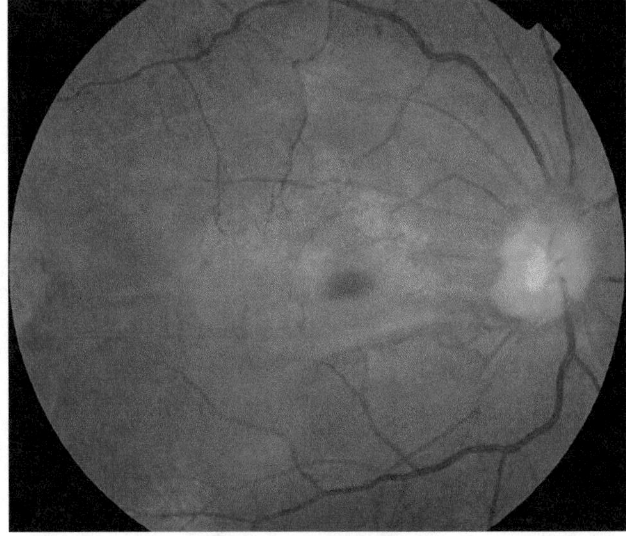

Fig. 16.18 The sickle retinopathy may cause ERM

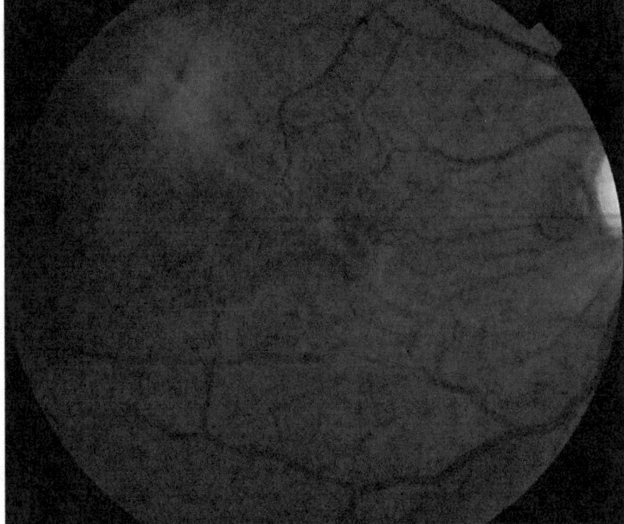

Fig. 16.17 Macular ERM can appear in sickle cell retinopathy, usually with an attached vitreous gel presumably because of changes in vitreal structure secondary to the peripheral retinopathy

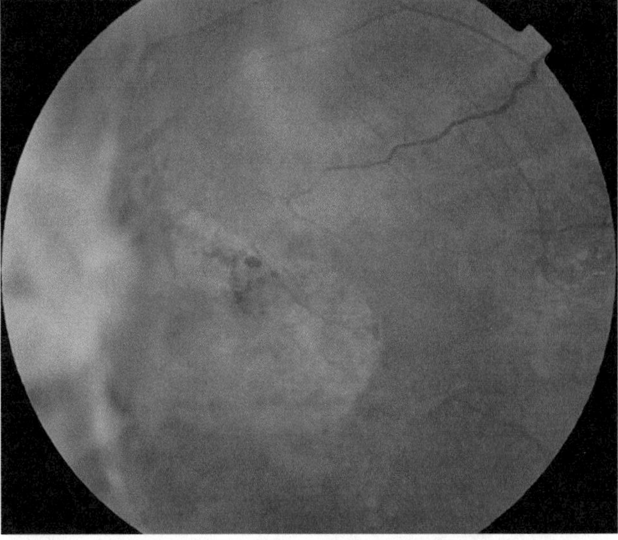

Fig. 16.19 Tractional retinal detachments can occur with sickle cell. Any membrane that can be, should be dissected and removed, but often membrane is adherent to sea fans and must be left behind

There is less use of scleral buckling or scatter photocoagulation (which has been used both preoperatively and peroperatively). Both interventions are associated with the development of anterior segment ischemia in these patients [50], a complication rarely seen today[7].

Not all patients with vitreoretinal complications from sickle cell retinopathy require surgery. Vitreous haemorrhage can be allowed to clear without detriment, and TRD observed without a progression in some patients. Indeed, patients may show spontaneous improvement.

Exchange transfusion once used before surgery is no longer considered necessary and has been abandoned.

Note; Avoid carbonic anhydrase inhibitors (e.g. Acetazolamide) in case of the induction of acidosis.

Some suggest avoiding topical epinephrine and related drugs in case of exacerbating local ischaemia.

Avoid scleral buckling in case of inducing anterior segment ischaemia.

Visual Outcome

In general, the risk to vision is low, and most complications are responsive to surgery. After the age of 40 years the condition usually stabilises. In one study, outcomes for visions were good, with 10 of 18 eyes achieving 6/12 vision or better and 15 eyes (83%) with improved vision postoperatively.

Screening

The need for surveillance is doubtful because:

- There is doubt over the effectiveness of prophylactic therapy, e.g. scatter laser (in contrast to diabetic retinopathy where it is of proven benefit).
- The relatively low prevalence of sight-threatening complications.
- That sight-threatening complications present symptomatically and usually progress slowly.
- That sight-threatening complications respond well to surgery if necessary.

Survival

- Sickle cell anaemia (homozygous SS), the median age at death is 42 years for males and 48 years for females [51].
- Sickle cell haemoglobin SC disease, the median age at death is 60 years for males and 68 years for females.
- Eighteen percent of the deaths occur in patients with the presence of organ failure usually renal.
- Thirty-three percent die during an acute sickle crisis (78% had pain, chest syndrome, or both; 22% had stroke).

Retinal Vasculitis

Retinal neovascularisation can occur and cause vitreous haemorrhage or tractional retinal detachment. The former may be surgically removed, but care is required because of accentuated vitreoretinal adhesions and usually an attached vitreous gel. PRP is usually not required but an increase in immune suppressive cover may help the new vessels to regress. Traction retinal detachment tends to be associated with severe subretinal exudation and cholesterol crystal formation. Dissection of traction membranes is difficult and visual recovery is frequently poor.

Central Retinal Artery Occlusion

In experimental surgery, the embolus in central retinal artery occlusion (CRAO) has been surgically removed by incising the wall of the artery over the embolus [52]. The embolus exits the artery spontaneously or by grasping the embolus with forceps. Only a few patients have been described. Massage of the embolus away from the optic nerve has been reported [53] (Fig. 16.20).

Summary

Vitrectomy methods are established to treat the ocular complications of diabetic retinopathy. The methods of membrane dissection require new skills for delamination of the membranes off the fragile retina. The same skills can be applied to other similar conditions.

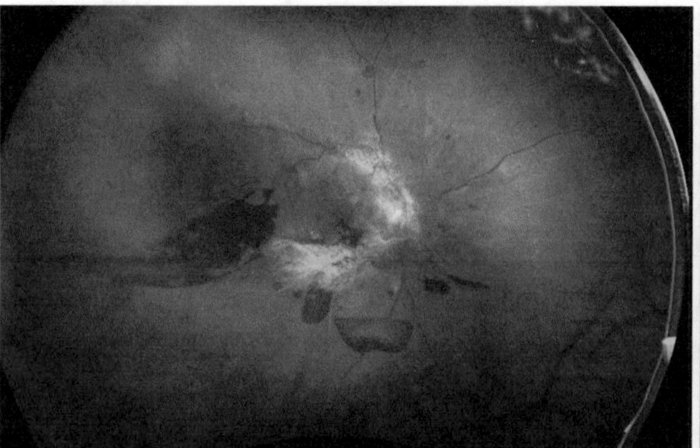

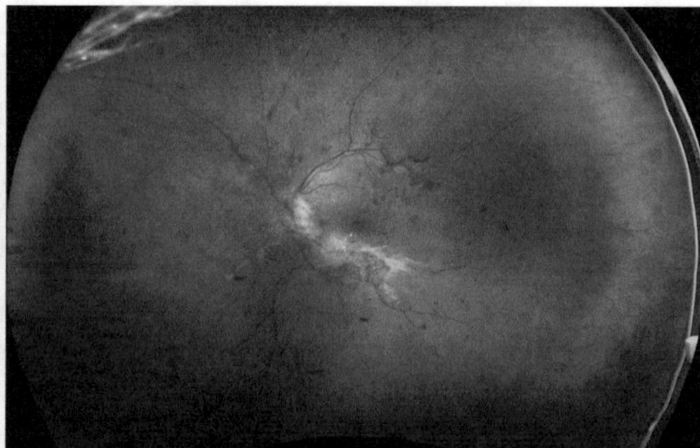

Fig. 16.20 Preretinal neovascular membranes after ischaemia from malignant hypertension

References

1. Green WR, Chan CC, Hutchins GM, Terry JM. Central retinal vein occlusion: a prospective histopathologic study of 29 eyes in 28 cases. Trans Am Ophthalmol Soc. 1981;79:371–422.
2. Thach AB, Yau L, Hoang C, Tuomi L. Time to clinically significant visual acuity gains after ranibizumab treatment for retinal vein occlusion: BRAVO and CRUISE trials. Ophthalmology. 2014;121(5):1059–66. https://doi.org/10.1016/j.ophtha.2013.11.022.
3. Varma R, Bressler NM, Suner I, Lee P, Dolan CM, Ward J, et al. Improved vision-related function after ranibizumab for macular edema after retinal vein occlusion: results from the BRAVO and CRUISE trials. Ophthalmology. 2012;119(10):2108–18. https://doi.org/10.1016/j.ophtha.2012.05.017.
4. Browning DJ, Antoszyk AN. Laser chorioretinal venous anastomosis for nonischemic central retinal vein occlusion. Ophthalmology. 1998;105(4):670–7.
5. McAllister IL, Douglas JP, Constable IJ, Yu DY. Laser-induced chorioretinal venous anastomosis for nonischemic central retinal vein occlusion: evaluation of the complications and their risk factors. Am J Ophthalmol. 1998;126(2):219–29.
6. McAllister IL, Constable IJ. Laser-induced chorioretinal venous anastomosis for treatment of nonischemic central retinal vein occlusion. Arch Ophthalmol. 1995;113(4):456–62.
7. Branch Vein Occlusion Study Group. Argon laser photocoagulation for macular oedema in branch vein occlusion. Am J Ophthalmol. 1984;98:271–82.
8. Branch Vein Occlusion Study Group. Argon laser scatter photocoagulation for prevention of neovascularisation and vitreous haemorrhage in branch vein occlusion. A randomized clinical trial. Arch Ophthalmol. 1986;104:34–41.
9. Osterloh MD, Charles S. Surgical decompression of branch retinal vein occlusions. Arch Ophthalmol. 1988;106:1469–71.
10. Opremcak EM, Bruce RA. Surgical decompression of branch retinal vein occlusion via arteriovenous crossing sheathotomy: a prospective review of 15 cases. Retina. 1999;19(1):1–5.
11. Mason J III, Feist R, White M Jr, Swanner J, McGwin G Jr, Emond T. Sheathotomy to decompress branch retinal vein occlusion: a matched control study. Ophthalmology. 2004;111(3):540–5.
12. Fujii GY, De Juan E Jr, Humayan MS. Improvements after sheathotomy for branch retinal vein occlusion documented by optical coherence tomography and scanning laser ophthalmoscope. Opthalmic Surg Lasers Imaging. 2003;34:49–52.
13. Cringle SJ, Yu DY, Alder VA. Intravitreal and intraretinal oxygen tension in the rat eye. Afv Exp Med Biol. 1992;316:113–7.
14. Saika S, Tanaka T, Miyamoto T, Ohnishi Y. Surgical posterior vitreous detachment combined with gas/air tamponade for treating macular edema associated with branch retinal vein occlusion: retinal tomography and visual outcome. Graefes Arch Clin Exp Ophthalmol. 2001;239(10):729–32.
15. Vein T. Natural history and clinical management of central retinal vein occlusion. The central vein occlusion study group. Arch Ophthalmol. 1997;115(4):486–91.
16. Opremcak EM, Bruce RA, Lomeo MD, Ridenour CD, Letson AD, Rehmar AJ. Radial optic neurotomy for central retinal vein occlusion: a retrospective pilot study of 11 consecutive cases. Retina. 2001;21(5):408–15.
17. Williamson TH, Poon W, Whitefield L, Strothidis N, Jaycock P. A pilot study of pars plana vitrectomy, intraocular gas, and radial neurotomy in ischaemic central retinal vein occlusion. Br J Ophthalmol. 2003;87(9):1126–9.
18. Garcia-Arumi J, Boixadera A, Martinez-Castillo V, Castillo R, Dou A, Corcostegui B. Chorioretinal anastomosis after radial optic neurotomy for central retinal vein occlusion. Arch Ophthalmol. 2003;121(10):1385–91.
19. Opremcak EM, Rehmar AJ, Ridenour CD, Kurz DE, Borkowski LM. Radial optic neurotomy with adjunctive intraocular triamcinolone for central retinal vein occlusion: 63 consecutive cases. Retina. 2006;26(3):306–13.
20. Williamson TH, Grewal J, Gupta B, Mokete B, Lim M, Fry CH. Measurement of PO2 during vitrectomy for central retinal vein occlusion, a pilot study. Graefes Arch Clin Exp Ophthalmol. 2009;247(8):1019–23. https://doi.org/10.1007/s00417-009-1072-z.
21. Jonas JB, Akkoyun I, Kamppeter B, Kreissig I, Degenring RF. Branch retinal vein occlusion treated by intravitreal triamcinolone acetonide. Eye. 2005;19(1):65–71.
22. Jonas JB, Akkoyun I, Kreissig I, Degenring RF. Diffuse diabetic macular oedema treated by intravitreal triamcinolone acetonide: a comparative, non-randomised study. Br J Ophthalmol. 2005;89(3):321–6.
23. Jonas JB, Harder B, Kamppeter BA. Inter-eye difference in diabetic macular edema after unilateral intravitreal injection of triamcinolone acetonide. Am J Ophthalmol. 2004;138(6):970–7.
24. Spandau UH, Derse M, Schmitz-Valckenberg P, Papoulis C, Jonas JB. Dosage dependency of intravitreal triamcinolone acetonide as treatment for diabetic macular oedema. Br J Ophthalmol. 2005;89(8):999–1003.
25. Alldredge CD, Garretson BR. Intravitreal triamcinolone for the treatment of idiopathic juxtafoveal telangiectasis. Retina. 2003;23(1):113–6.
26. Antcliff RJ, Spalton DJ, Stanford MR, Graham EM, Ffytche TJ, Marshall J. Intravitreal triamcinolone for uveitic cystoid macular edema: an optical coherence tomography study. Ophthalmology. 2001;108(4):765–72.
27. Benhamou N, Massin P, Haouchine B, Audren F, Tadayoni R, Gaudric A. Intravitreal triamcinolone for refractory pseudophakic macular edema. Am J Ophthalmol. 2003;135(2):246–9.
28. Bynoe LA, Weiss JN. Retinal endovascular surgery and intravitreal triamcinolone acetonide for central vein occlusion in young adults. Am J Ophthalmol. 2003;135(3):382–4.
29. Conway MD, Canakis C, Livir-Rallatos C, Peyman GA. Intravitreal triamcinolone acetonide for refractory chronic pseudophakic cystoid macular edema. J Cataract Refract Surg. 2003;29(1):27–33.
30. Martidis A, Duker JS, Puliafito CA. Intravitreal triamcinolone for refractory cystoid macular edema secondary to birdshot retinochoroidopathy. Arch Ophthalmol. 2001;119(9):1380–3.
31. Greenberg PB, Martidis A, Rogers AH, Duker JS, Reichel E. Intravitreal triamcinolone acetonide for macular oedema due to central retinal vein occlusion. Br J Ophthalmol. 2002;86(2):247–8.
32. Martidis A, Duker JS, Greenberg PB, Rogers AH, Puliafito CA, Reichel E, et al. Intravitreal triamcinolone for refractory diabetic macular edema. Ophthalmology. 2002;109(5):920–7.
33. Degenring RF, Jonas JB. Intravitreal injection of triamcinolone acetonide as treatment for chronic uveitis. Br J Ophthalmol. 2003;87(3):361.
34. Degenring RF, Kamppeter B, Kreissig I, Jonas JB. Morphological and functional changes after intravitreal triamcinolone acetonide for retinal vein occlusion. Acta Ophthalmol Scand. 2003;81(4):399–401.
35. Jonas JB, Kreissig I, Degenring RF. Intravitreal triamcinolone acetonide for pseudophakic cystoid macular edema. Am J Ophthalmol. 2003;136(2):384–6.
36. Williamson TH, O'Donnell A. Intravitreal triamcinolone acetonide for cystoid macular edema in nonischemic central retinal vein occlusion. Am J Ophthalmol. 2005;139(5):860–6.

37. Jonas JB, Kreissig I, Degenring RF. Intravitreal triamcinolone acetonide as treatment of macular edema in central retinal vein occlusion. Graefes Arch Clin Exp Ophthalmol. 2002;240(9):782–3.
38. Haller JA, Bandello F, Belfort R Jr, Blumenkranz MS, Gillies M, Heier J, et al. Randomized, sham-controlled trial of dexamethasone intravitreal implant in patients with macular edema due to retinal vein occlusion. Ophthalmology. 2010;117(6):1134–46.e3. doi: S0161-6420(10)00311-8 [pii]. https://doi.org/10.1016/j.ophtha.2010.03.032.
39. Jonas JB, Sofker A. Intraocular injection of crystalline cortisone as adjunctive treatment of diabetic macular edema. Am J Ophthalmol. 2001;132(3):425–7.
40. Weiss JN. Treatment of central retinal vein occlusion by injection of tissue plasminogen activator into a retinal vein. Am J Ophthalmol. 1998;126(1):142–4.
41. Weiss JN, Bynoe LA. Injection of tissue plasminogen activator into a branch retinal vein in eyes with central retinal vein occlusion. Ophthalmology. 2001;108(12):2249–57.
42. Clarkson JG. The ocular manifestations of sickle-cell disease: a prevalence and natural history study. Trans Am Ophthalmol Soc. 1992;90:481–504.
43. Saidkasimova S, Shalchi Z, Mahroo OA, Shunmugam M, Laidlaw DA, Williamson TH, et al. Risk factors for visual impairment in patients with sickle cell disease in London. Eur J Ophthalmol. 2016;26(5):431–5. https://doi.org/10.5301/ejo.5000767.
44. Downes SM, Hambleton IR, Chuang EL, Lois N, Serjeant GR, Bird AC. Incidence and natural history of proliferative sickle cell retinopathy: observations from a cohort study. Ophthalmology. 2005;112(11):1869–75.
45. Condon P, Jampol LM, Farber MD, Rabb M, Serjeant G. A randomized clinical trial of feeder vessel photocoagulation of proliferative sickle cell retinopathy. II. Update and analysis of risk factors. Ophthalmology. 1984;91(12):1496–8.
46. Brazier DJ, Gregor ZJ, Blach RK, Porter JB, Huehns ER. Retinal detachment in patients with proliferative sickle cell retinopathy. Trans Ophthalmol Soc UK. 1986;105(Pt 1):100–5.
47. Goldberg MF. Classification and pathogenesis of proliferative sickle retinopathy. Am J Ophthalmol. 1971;71(3):649–65.
48. Fox PD, Minninger K, Forshaw ML, Vessey SJ, Morris JS, Serjeant GR. Laser photocoagulation for proliferative retinopathy in sickle haemoglobin C disease. Eye. 1993;7(Pt 5):703–6.
49. Williamson TH, Rajput R, Laidlaw DA, Mokete B. Vitreoretinal management of the complications of sickle cell retinopathy by observation or pars plana vitrectomy. Eye. 2009;23(6):1314–20. doi: eye2008296 [pii]. https://doi.org/10.1038/eye.2008.296.
50. Cohen SB, Fletcher ME, Goldberg MF, Jednock NJ. Diagnosis and management of ocular complications of sickle hemoglobinopathies: part V. Ophthalmic Surg. 1986;17(6):369–74.
51. Platt OS, Brambilla DJ, Rosse WF, Milner PF, Castro O, Steinberg MH, et al. Mortality in sickle cell disease. Life expectancy and risk factors for early death. N Engl J Med. 1994;330(23):1639–44.
52. Garcia-Arumi J, Martinez-Castillo V, Boixadera A, Fonollosa A, Corcostegui B. Surgical embolus removal in retinal artery occlusion. Br J Ophthalmol. 2006;90(10):1252–5. doi: bjo.2006.097642 [pii]. https://doi.org/10.1136/bjo.2006.097642.
53. Lu N, Wang NL, Wang GL, Li XW, Wang Y. Vitreous surgery with direct central retinal artery massage for central retinal artery occlusion. Eye (Lond). 2009;23(4):867–72. doi: eye2008126 [pii]. https://doi.org/10.1038/eye.2008.126.

Complications of Anterior Segment Surgery

17

Contents

T. H. Williamson, *Vitreoretinal Surgery*, https://doi.org/10.1007/978-3-030-68769-4_17

Introduction

Cataract Surgery in the modern setting means phacoemulsification with a small incision and a sutureless wound. This is a rapid procedure with a high rate of success, approximately 95%. There remains a small complication rate of approximately 2%.

Some of these are serious complications and will often involve the vitreoretinal surgeon in remedying the situation (Fig. 17.1).

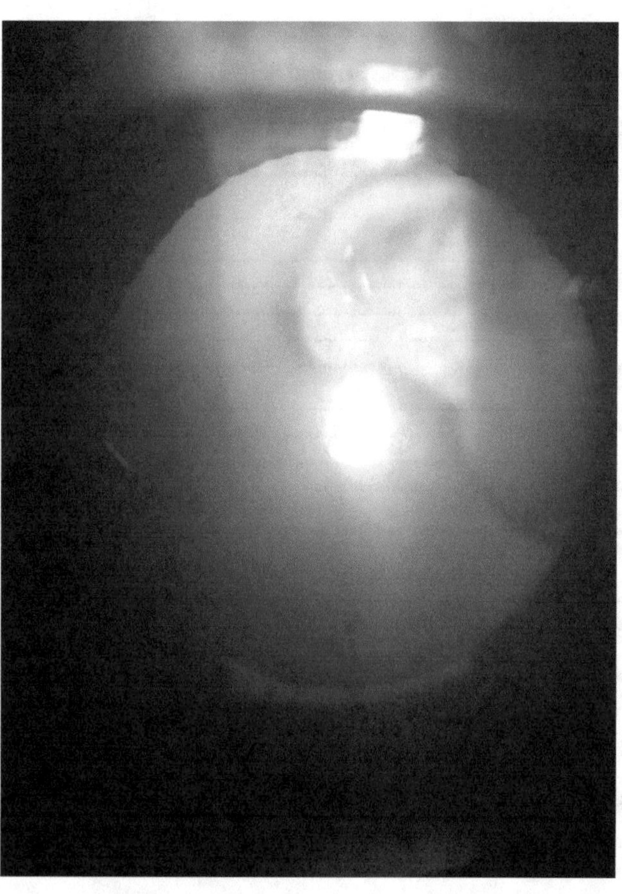

Fig. 17.1 Shrunken contracted capsule

Dropped Nucleus

Clinical Features

Dropped Nucleus Incidence	0.09–0.8% [1–4]

The phrase "dropped nucleus" has been used to describe the dislocation of the nucleus (or part of the nucleus) of a cataract during phacoemulsification into the vitreous cavity. A dropped nucleus may happen to any case with an increased risk of capsular rupture or zonular dehiscences such as trauma, pseudo exfoliation or hard nuclei, or because of the inexperience of the surgeon [1]. The positive pressure applied by the infusion fluid during phacoemulsification means that a tear in the posterior capsule of the lens will result in the dislocation of the contents of the anterior chamber (most often the lens) into the vitreous cavity. The higher density of the lens compared to the vitreous also encourages its dislocation into the posterior segment. The nucleus can be seen in the inferior vitreous accompanied by fluffy white soft cortical lens material. This results in the following:

- Uveitis. The lens material stimulates uveitis which in the short term can be controlled, if the nucleus remains in the posterior segment for months chronic uveitis is stimulated, which may persist after surgery.
- Glaucoma, a severe rise in intraocular pressure can usually be controlled by topical medication in the short term till the removal of the nucleus is performed. However, if the nucleus remains in the eye for a prolonged period, glaucoma may not reverse after lens removal.
- Retinal detachment. The disruption to the vitreous may produce retinal detachment by tearing the retina, 4–8% of patients [5, 6]. There is an increased risk of RRD approximately 4% before PPV and 4% after PPV with retinal tears also requiring treatment during PPV in a few patients [7]. RRD is reported earlier in these patients (mean 4 months) than after routine cataract extraction (mean 16 months) [8].

The patient is understandably disappointed having expected a straightforward operation and improved vision. Instead, they often have reduced vision and discomfort from uveitis (56%), raised IOP (52%) and corneal oedema (46%) [9]. Pars plana vitrectomy and removal of the nucleus are required within 1 or 2 weeks to avoid glaucomatous damage or chronic uveitis or cystoid macular oedema [10]. Most patients if treated promptly will achieve good vision. However, occasionally an eye will end up blind from associated choroidal haemorrhage or retinal detachment. Rarely dropped nucleus will present with endophthalmitis [11]. The risk of endophthalmitis seems to be doubled over other surgery [12].

Note: Rapid referral for vitrectomy is required.

Surgery (Table 17.1)

Additional surgical steps

1. Sew up the cataract wound.
2. Clear the anterior segment and capsule of soft lens material.
3. Use the vitreous cutter to remove the soft lens material in the vitreous cavity.
4. Use the fragmatome to remove the nucleus if the cutter is not enough.
5. Detach the posterior hyaloid if required.
6. Insert an intraocular lens implant.

"Fishing" for the nucleus via the anterior segment by the phacoemulsification surgeon is not advisable as this can cause giant retinal tears from traction on the vitreous even after anterior vitrectomy [13]. The timing of surgery by PPV has created controversy in the past [7, 14–20] but it is now recommended that a patient who has suffered a dropped nucleus during phacoemulsification cataract extraction be operated on within 2 weeks from the onset of the complication. This minimises the risk of secondary complications such as intractable glaucoma and cystoid macula oedema from the uveitis [10, 21]. Patients presenting with these complications in the short term usually have these reversed after PPV [22] (Figs. 17.2 and 17.3).

Table 17.1 Difficulty rating for PPV for dropped nucleus

Difficulty rating	Moderate
Success rates	Moderate
Complication rates	Low
When to use in training	Middle

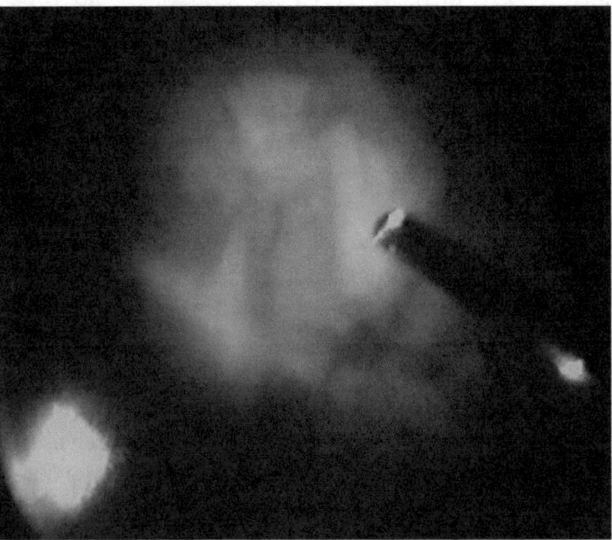

Fig. 17.2 Soft lens material can be removed easily by the vitreous cutter as can moderate amounts of the lens nucleus

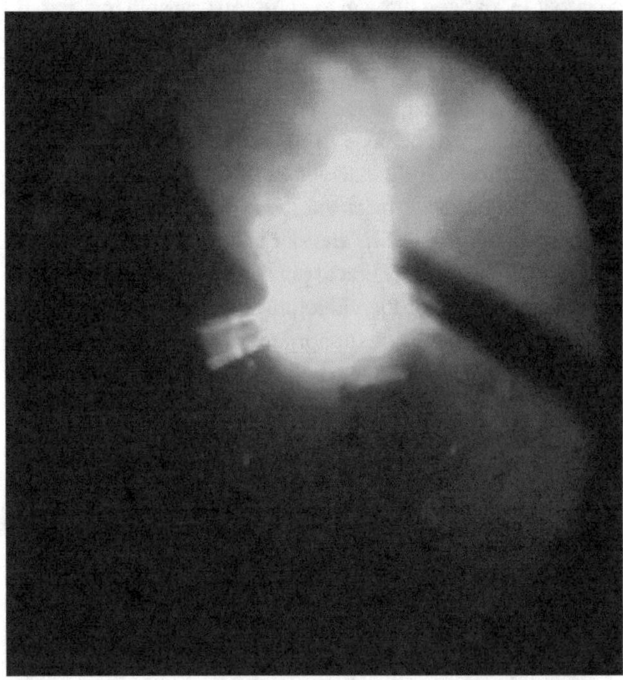

Fig. 17.3 The hard nuclear material is removed with a Fragmatome whilst supporting the lens with the light pipe. Whiter and fluffier softer lens material can be removed with the cutter

Primary Management

If the surgeon who has dropped the nucleus has the capability to perform a vitrectomy and removal of the fragments, then this can be performed immediately. However, unless this facility is available, it is best to close the eye, tidy up the vitreous, leave lens implantation until the next surgery and ensure closure of the cataract wound. By delaying the surgery for 1 or 2 weeks allows the use of elective surgical time and provides time to discuss the problem with the patient and allows them a chance to gather their thoughts before proceeding to another operation. Uveitis during this period readily responds to topical steroid therapy and raised IOP responds to topical antihypertensive therapy with temporary use of acetazolamide orally if required.

Vitrectomy Surgery

At PPV surgery, the first thing to do is to secure the anterior chamber. Most wounds are now so small that they can usually be left without a suture but check the wound and rehydrate if necessary, the wound has not usually been sealed by the time of the PPV. If the wound remains unstable use a 10/0 absorbable suture to close the wound, any pressure on the posterior edge of the wound will open it during the vitrectomy. Create sclerotomies as usual and excise any vitreous from the anterior chamber by passing through the posterior capsule into the AC (do not use old wounds if you want to go from the front create a new paracentesis for the cutter to enter). Remove any soft lens material from within the capsule using the cutter on aspirate only. This can be done in the same fashion as a normal SLM aspiration during cataract extraction but by accessing from the posterior segment via the posterior capsular break. Preserve as much capsule, anterior and posterior, as is possible, as it will be the intention to put in a posterior chamber lens implant at the end of the vitrectomy, and this capability will depend on the amount of supporting capsule. Then perform a PPV, taking note of whether the vitreous has detached or not. Gain access to the nucleus, remove any SLM from around the nucleus and then assess the size of the nucleus to be removed.

If there is less than a quarter of the nucleus in the posterior segment a chop and cut procedure will be adequate, whereby the nucleus is delaminated against the cutter, and small fragments of the nucleus are chopped by the cutter. If there is more than a quarter of the nucleus in the back of the eye, then a fragmatome is required to phaco-emulsify the nucleus to speed its extraction. In this case, it is prudent to apply a small protective bubble of heavy liquid to the posterior pole, as it is likely that the nucleus will occasionally fall from the fragmatome tip, and may strike the macula or the optic disc [23]. If the fragmatome is still 20 gauge, create a self-sealing sclerotomy near the trochar for your dominant hand. This should be transconjunctival and can be closed without a suture after the fragmatome has been used.

Set the power of the fragmatome to low, 20% of normal and use a pulse mode of 8 pulses per second. This makes it easier to hold onto the lens nucleus during phacoemulsification. The nucleus tends to shoot away from the fragmatome tip when using the ultrasound continuously. It should be possible to manipulate the nucleus in a cartwheel fashion, using the light pipe and fragmatome, remove as much of the nucleus as possible in one sweep (Fig. 17.4).

Use the on-demand system for the fragmatome to avoid ultrasound near the retina causing any damage to the retinal surface:

- For linear aspiration use the foot pedal on direct depression.
- When the nucleus has been engaged by aspiration only, lift the nucleus away from the retina into the mid-vitreous.
- Once safely away from the retina kick the foot pedal to the side to engage ultrasound on maximum to commence the phacoemulsification (fragmatome).

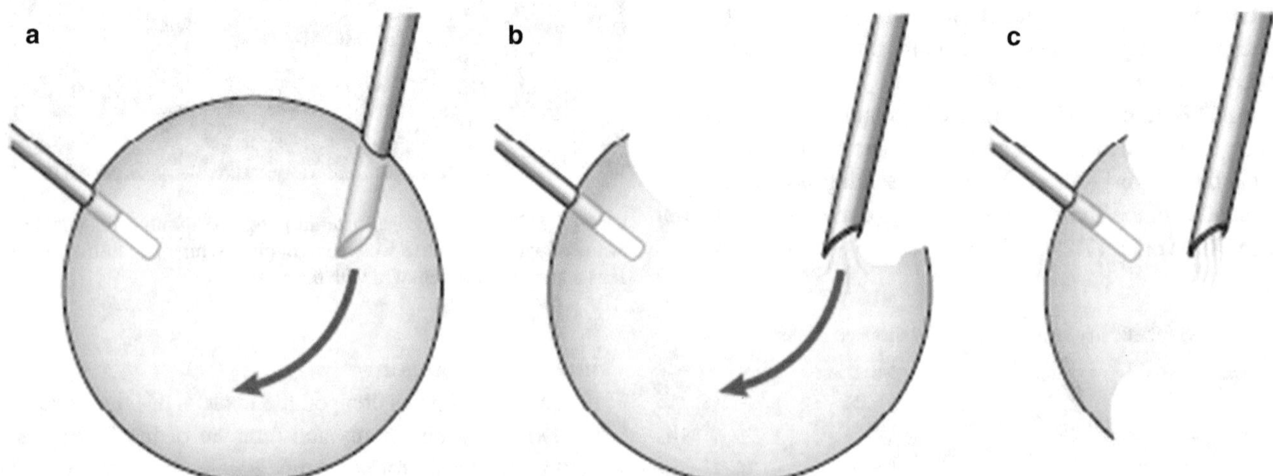

Fig. 17.4 Spike the lens or nucleus with the light pipe and, in a rotating manner, use the Fragmatome to emulsify and aspirate the nuclear fragments. Try to work towards the light pipe without dislodging the light pipe, so that there is minimal need for re-engaging the nucleus, thereby reducing manipulation and time spent near the retina

- If the nucleus disengages and drops cease aspiration (lift your foot) and start again.

Note the aspiration is high even at 150 mmHg (the bore of the fragmatome port is larger than a cutter) for a fluid-filled eye; therefore, rapid cessation of aspiration is required to prevent globe collapse, even if the infusion bottle height has been increased.

Eventually, the nucleus can be completely removed. If there is no posterior vitreous detachment, detach the posterior vitreous at this stage. This is difficult before fragmentation because the nucleus is resting on the vitreous cortex. Perform an internal search to detect retinal tears or retinal detachment, and treat these as they arise, do not put gas in yet, because insertion of intraocular gas may be problematic depending on the stability of the IOL (Fig. 17.5).

Thereafter, perform secondary lens implantation. It is prudent to stabilise the posterior segment by inserting heavy liquid. Leaving the infusion on, incise a corneal wound with the keratome. Switch off the infusion and fill the anterior chamber with viscoelastic which acts as a plug, preventing the egress of fluid through the corneal wound. Assess the state of the capsule. If there is plenty of capsule available (i.e. enough to encapsulate securely the IOL) insert the lens implant into the bag. If not, place the lens implant into the ciliary sulcus (requiring at least two-third of the capsule remaining). If possible, posteriorly dislocate the optic behind the capsule and the haptics in front of the sulcus. This keeps the optic away from the posterior iris. If there are less than two-thirds of the capsule, insert an anterior chamber lens implant. A few surgeons recommend sulcus sutured lenses but these have a chance of dislocation in 6 years, approximately 25% [24] (Fig. 17.6).

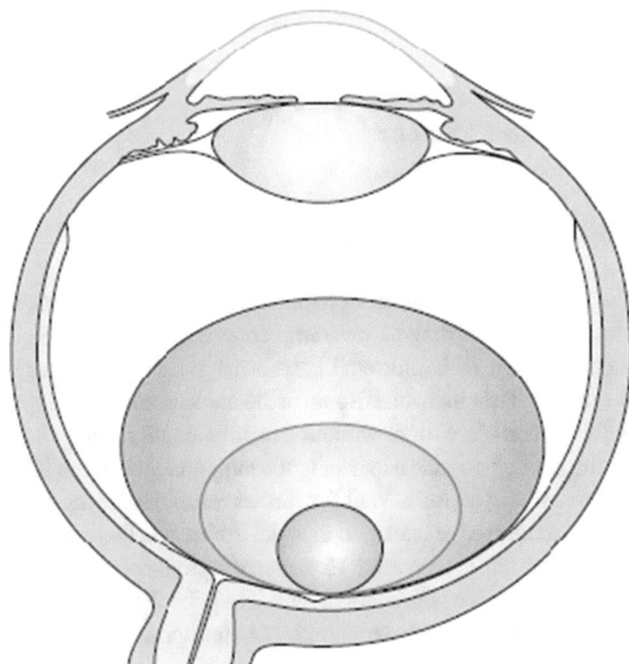

Fig. 17.5 Heavy liquids can be placed onto the posterior pole of the eye during the removal of dropped nucleus. A small bubble has a very convex surface upon which the fragments will slip back down onto the retina. Increasing the size of the bubble flattens the surface of the heavy liquids, facilitating the maintenance of fragments in the mid-vitreous cavity. However, if the bubble becomes too large, then there is reduced space for working between the bubble and the anterior segment. An ideal size is indicated by the blue circle

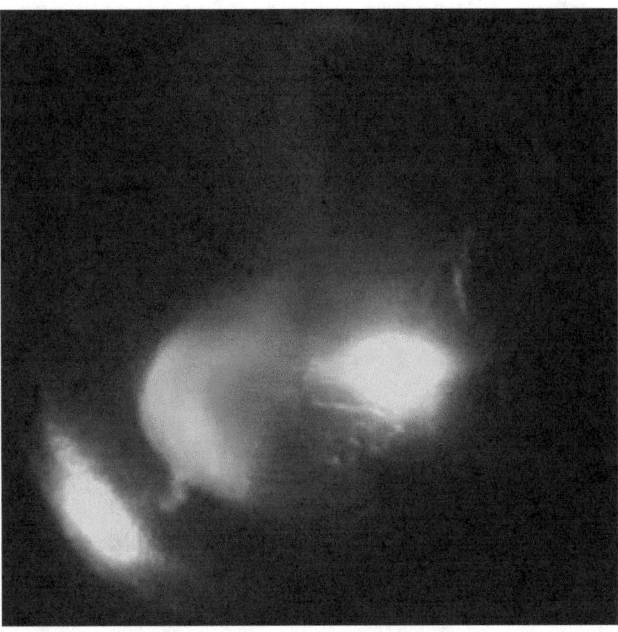

Fig. 17.6 This nucleus is blood stained because the eye has also suffered a choroidal haemorrhage

Difficult Situations

Concurrent Retinal Detachment and Dropped Nucleus

A mobile retina may cause problems whilst trying to perform fragmatome extraction. In this case, the heavy liquid will need to be inserted to stabilise the retina before removing the nucleus. Insert the IOL before the air exchange if you judge that it will allow a stable barrier between the anterior and posterior segments of the eye (with the posterior segment filled with heavy liquid) using viscoelastic in the anterior chamber as above. Remove the viscoelastic (it is difficult to do this after the air has been inserted), then perform an air/heavy liquid exchange; you may need to wipe the posterior lens surface to avoid condensation (see Chap. 3). Treat any retinal breaks (Figs. 17.7 and 17.8).

Air may get into the anterior chamber in the presence of a large posterior capsule rent or zonule dehiscence and particularly if an anterior chamber lens implant is present.

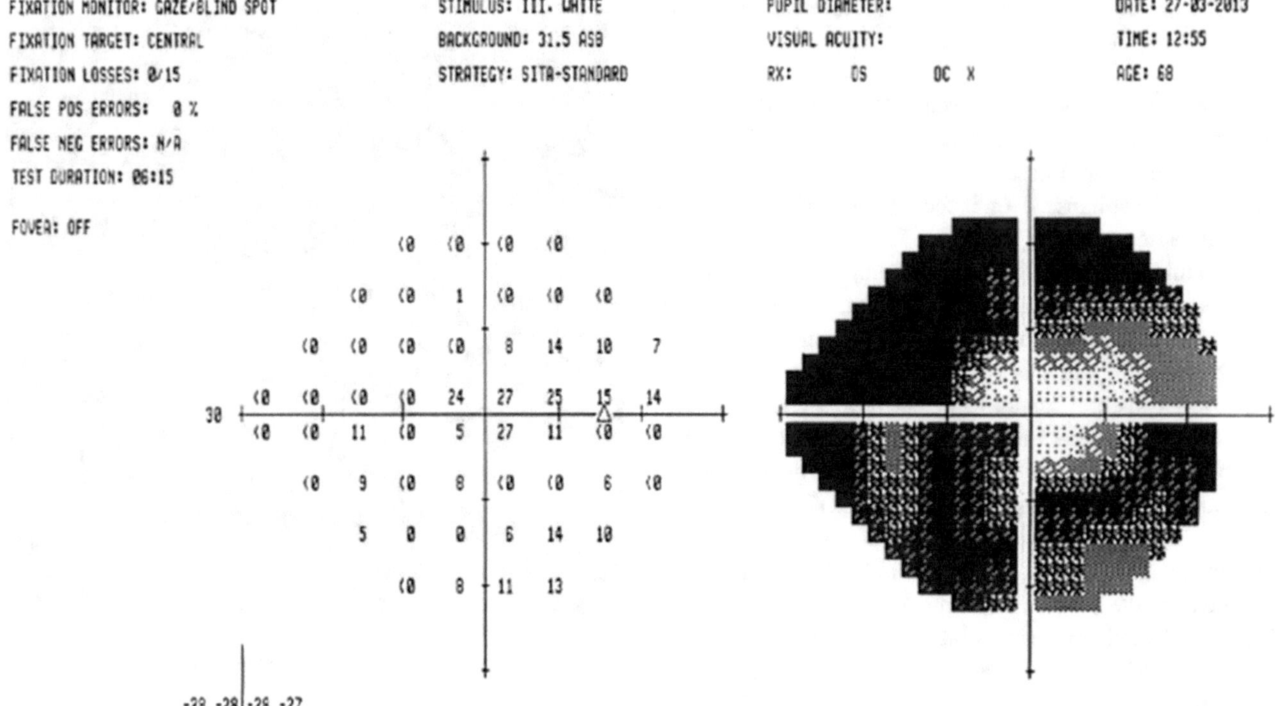

Fig. 17.7 Visual field loss from pressure problems from a dropped nucleus

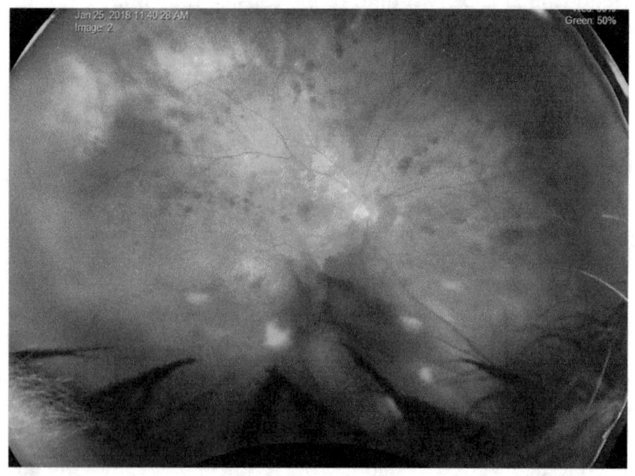

Fig. 17.8 Fragments of the dropped nucleus in a patient with DMR

Remove the IOL if gas tamponade is being used and:

- There is an ACIOL.
- Air is entering the anterior chamber repeatedly.

If there is no support for the IOL and you anticipate needing an ACIOL, sutured, haptic capture or iris clip IOL do this at a second operation once the gas bubble has dispersed. These lenses could be problematic in the presence of gas with the possibility of:

- Dislocation
- Corneal touch
- Displacement from the visual axis
- Pupil block glaucoma

Choroidal Haemorrhage

Very occasionally the dropped nucleus is associated with a choroidal haemorrhage. Consider preoperative suprachoroidal TPA injection with choroidal haemorrhage drainage through posterior scleral incisions. Remove the nucleus and fill the eye with silicone oil, with or without lens implantation depending on the ability to create a barrier to the tamponade with the IOL and remaining capsule. Wait for further resolution of the choroidal haemorrhage later, and then determine whether implantation is possible if required. However, the prognosis for vision in an eye like this is often poor, and it may be that vision will be limited and lens implantation is not appropriate.

Success Rates

The visual outcome is approximately a 60% chance of 20/40 vision or better, i.e. at least 20% less than after routine cataract extraction [7, 18, 25]. There seems to be little difference in outcome between surgery on the same day as the cataract operation and within 1 week or later [26, 27].

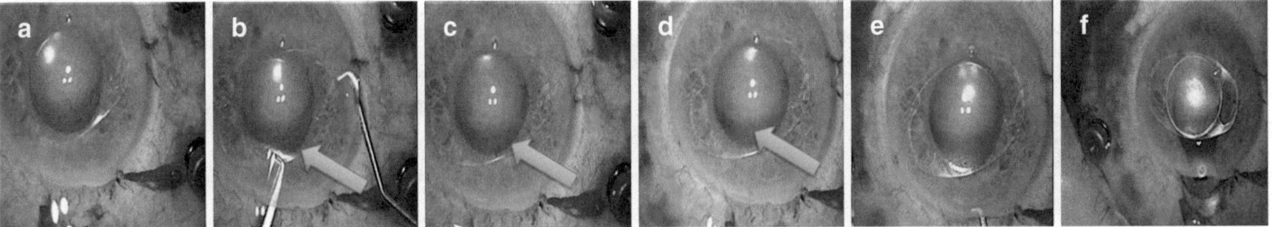

Fig. 17.9 Suprachoroidal haemorrhage developing over 1 minute during iris clip IOL insertion, (**a**): IOL in place, due to enclave final haptic, (**b**): Early SCH noted (arrow), (**c** and **d**): SCH growing (arrow), (**e**): No Red reflex, (**f**): Prolapse of iris, courtesy of Aman Chandra

Suprachoroidal Haemorrhage

Massive SCH occurs as a rare risk factor from anterior segment surgery often seen late as an expulsive haemorrhage [28–33]. An incidence of 0.04% has been described in the UK [34, 35]. The delay in detection peroperatively results in a large and often catastrophic haemorrhage (Fig. 17.9). This is a rare risk during surgery such as cataract extraction [34], trabeculectomy [36, 37] (glaucoma drainage implants [38]) and corneal grafting [29, 31, 39–42]. Wound leakage or insufficient infusion result in hypotony which allows vessel rupture in at-risk individuals with arteriopathy, high myopia or hypertension. Bleeds are made worse by delayed thrombus formation in those on anti-thrombotic or anti-platelet agents. The haemorrhage may occur intraoperatively or be delayed and occur after surgery [37, 38, 43–49] (Fig. 17.10).

- A late SCH can be seen in glaucoma for example when needling of a trabecular flap is performed [50].

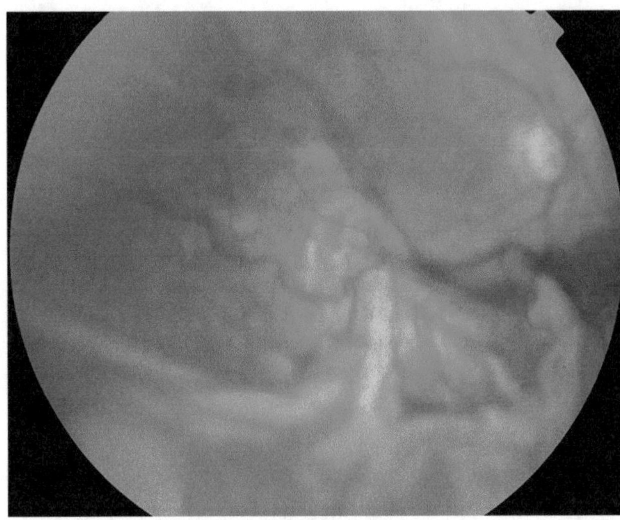

Fig. 17.10 A choroidal haemorrhage is settling after a complicated cataract operation. Secondary retinal detachment can occur with PVR. Close observation is required

What to Do if Choroidal Haemorrhage Occurs During Anterior Segment Surgery

- Early recognition: If there is a sudden change in intraocular pressure consider whether SCH has developed. Sudden changes can occur during any moment, but particularly if a complication such as PCR develops. Subsequent hardening/increase in intraocular pressure must alert the surgeon to the possibility of SCH.
- When recognised, close the main wound as efficiently as possible. Replace any expelled intraocular tissue if possible, but not at the expense of closing the wound.

Intraocular Lens Dislocations

Clinical Presentation

Prosthetic intraocular lens implants can also dislocate into the posterior segment, especially silicone plate IOLs after Yag capsulotomy (typically at 2 months after the laser procedure) [51, 52]. In some patients with weak zonular fibres (high myopes, trauma, exfoliation, Marfan's syndrome and Ehlers–Danlos syndrome) the whole lens and capsule may dislocate. This may occur after minor trauma to the eye. Patients with prior vitrectomy appear to be at more risk and the numbers of cases may be increasing [53].

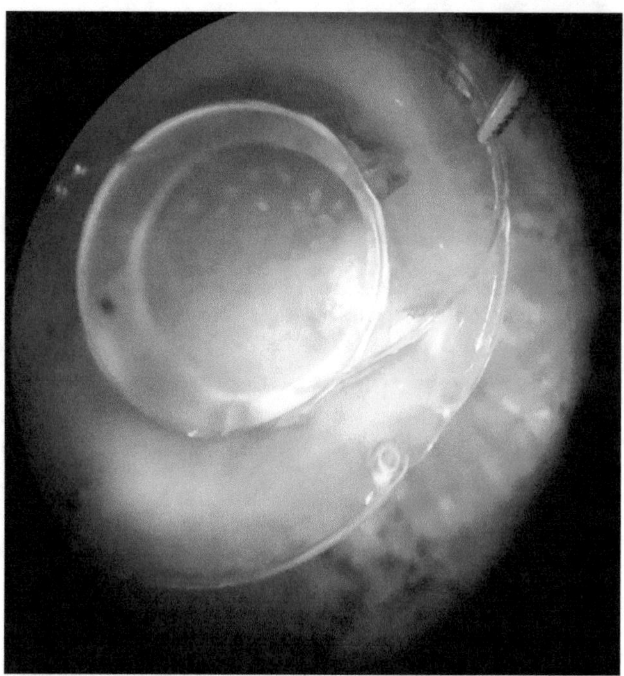

Fig. 17.11 Dislocations of IOLs from zonule breakdown many years after surgery seem to be on the increase. It is useful to remove the capsule and Sommerung's ring before trying to remove it from the eye

There are several options for surgery:

- Mild subluxation. Perform scleral suturing with Hoffman Pockets.
- Dislocation of a three-piece IOL. Perform haptic capture fixation.
- Dislocation of a one-piece IOL. Remove the IOL and perform haptic capture fixation with a three-piece IOL.
- Dislocation in an elderly patient. Consider removal of the IOL and an ACIOL replacement (Fig. 17.11).

Surgery

Usually, there is not enough capsular support to allow the implant to be inserted into the sulcus and the IOL must either be removed or sutured into place.

Removal of the IOL

- Insert a chandelier illumination.
- Perform the vitrectomy (it may or may not be detached) and make sure the vitreous is cleared away from the IOL. It is possible to elevate the IOL off the retina with the negative pressure of the orifice of the end of a flute needle, placed perpendicular to the surface of the optic. The IOL can then be lifted into the vitreous cavity and transferred to forceps. If the flute will not hold the IOL use forceps to grasp the edge of the optic or one of the haptics. Always keep a watch on the haptics making sure they do not scrape the retina or pull on the vitreous.
- If the IOL is still within the capsule, remove the capsule with the cutter.
- Dislocate the IOL into the anterior chamber but always be careful with the position of the IOL especially the haptics when under the iris and therefore unseen. There is the potential to engage the haptic into the vitreous base causing traction and giant retinal tears.
- If it is a three-piece IOL consider using the IOL for haptic capture fixation.
- Once in the anterior chamber; if the optic is of a soft material, it is worth cutting 75% of the way through the optic (lens cutting scissors are available) so that it can be removed through a smaller wound in the corneal periphery. Note it is not necessary to cut the optic in two and risk posterior dislocation of one half, with a cut through the optic the IOL can distort and therefore exit through a 3-mm wound (Fig. 17.12).

- An alternative method is to fold the IOL in the AC. Make a paracentesis at 6 o'clock and insert a dialler needle under the optic centrally. Through the superior 3 mm wound insert lens folding forceps, push these down onto the optic whilst the dialler needle remains stationery this folds the IOL over the needle. Remove the needle and then remove the folded IOL through the wound (Fig. 17.13).

Removal of an "In the Bag IOL" from the Anterior Segment

Use of the wrong IOL requires early recognition and remediation. Removal of a recently inserted IOL less than 6 weeks from surgery can be performed in the anterior segment by filling the bag with viscoelastic and dislocating the IOL into the anterior chamber before extraction.

Faulty lenses can cloud over reducing vision over time. If the IOL has been in the eye long enough for the capsule to scar and fuse, the IOL may need to be removed by first dislocating it into the posterior segment. Perform PPV and remove the posterior capsule whilst maintaining the anterior capsule. Allow the IOL to drop into the posterior segment and then lift it as above through the capsulorhexis in the anterior capsule. Extract as shown above. Insert a sulcus IOL and perform optic capture using the anterior capsule (Fig. 17.14).

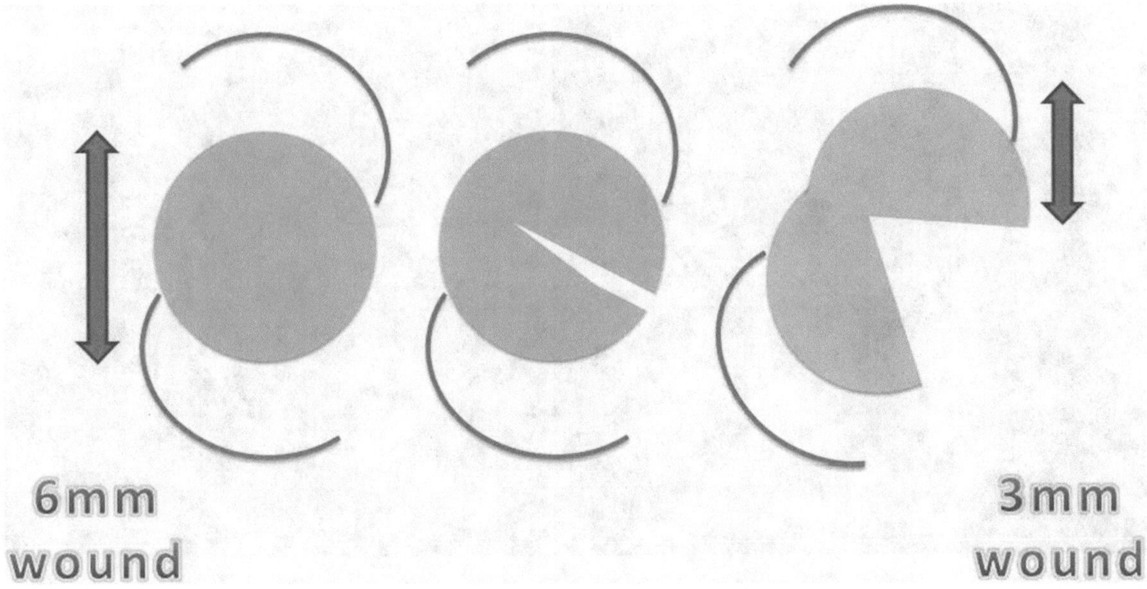

Fig. 17.12 To remove a flexible IOL from the AC through a small wound first cut 75% of the way across the optic, the IOL can then be removed through a smaller wound in one piece by pulling one half through the wound and the other attached half follows behind

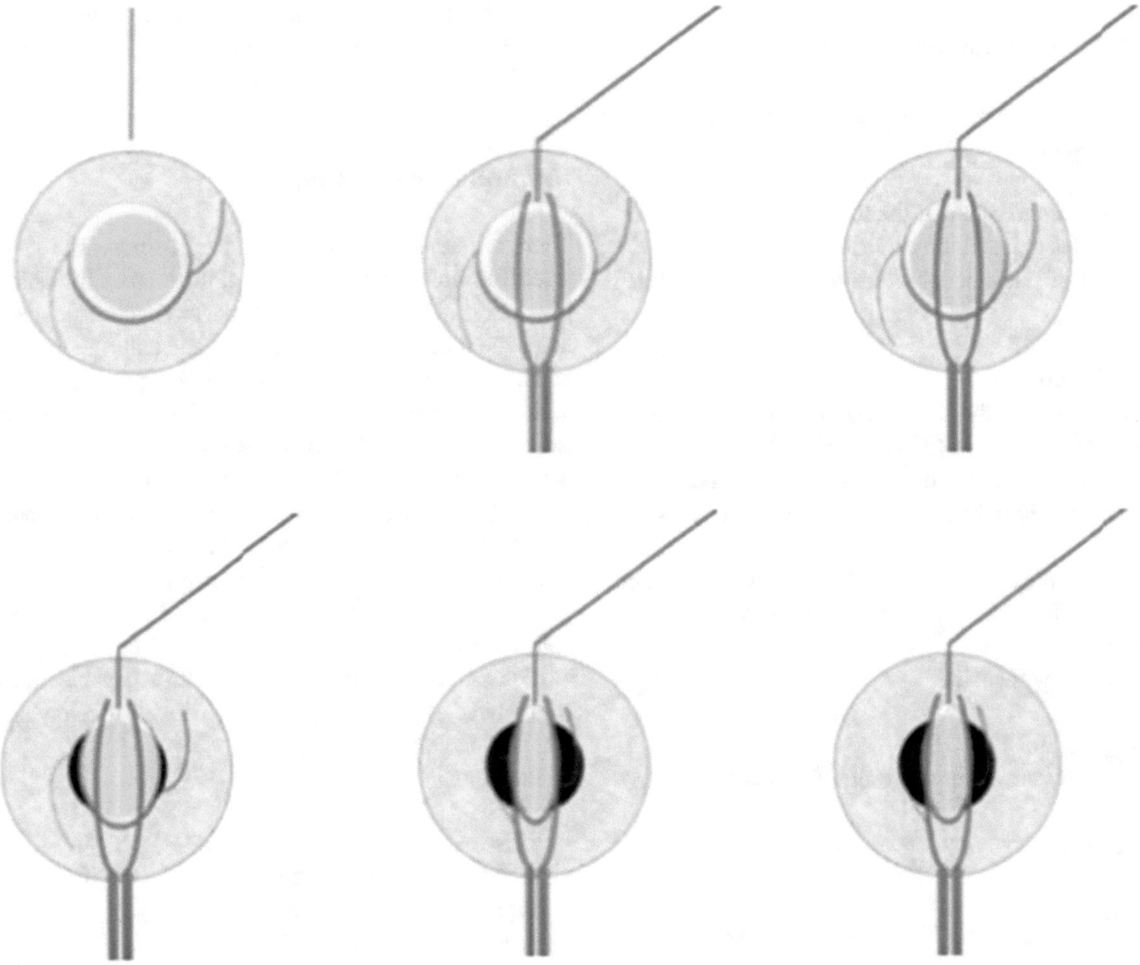

Fig. 17.13 To remove an IOL from the eye, a successful method is to fold the IOL inside the eye. Dislocate the IOL into the anterior chamber (AC). Insert an iris hook through a paracentesis at 6 o'clock and under the IOL. Create a 3 mm wound at 12 o'clock and insert folding forceps over the IOL. Push down on the IOL and iris hook to fold the IOL. Remove the iris hook. Once folded remove the IOL from the AC

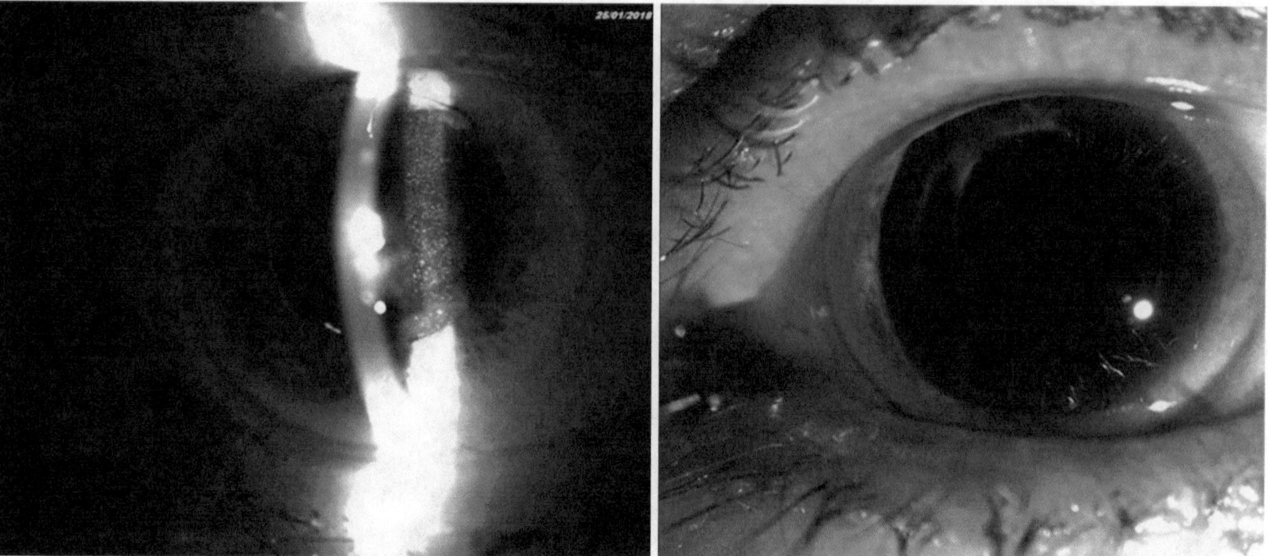

Fig. 17.14 A sulcus lens is secured away from the iris by optic capture

Surgical Options for the Aphakic Eye

Sutured Posterior Chamber IOLs

PC IOLs can be sutured into the ciliary sulcus using a variety of methods but employing:

- Suture tied to the haptic of the IOL
- Long needles to insert the Prolene suture
- Trap doors of sclera under which the knot of the suture is buried

A Simple Method

- Tie the suture to the haptic and insert a 27 g needle through the sclera opposite and behind the iris, insert the long needle through the orifice of the 27 g needle. Draw out the 27 g needle which pulls the long needle and suture with it.
- The long needle is passed partially through the sclera circumferentially a few times and will then stay tight without suturing.
- Repeat for the other side.

Hoffman Pocket

Hoffman pockets are extremely useful for this (Fig. 17.15).

Complications

- Suture erosion
- Lens tilt
- Lens dislocation
- Vitreous haemorrhage

Suturing of the IOL has a dislocation rate of 25% [54] in 5 years but is easy to do and safe if you are reusing the dislocated IOL. If 75% have a stable IOL at 5 years, then it is still an option if perhaps an interim one.

McCannell Iris Sutured IOL

There are several variations for this method. The key is to insert (or relocate) a PC IOL (e.g. three-piece foldable) with the optic in front of the pupil and the haptics behind. This holds the IOL in the pupillary plane and tents the iris over the haptics so that they can be seen. A long needle 10/0 non-absorbable suture is inserted through the peripheral cornea and is then passed through the mid iris under the haptic and through the iris again and out through the peripheral cornea opposite. The suture is retrieved by inserting a hook through a paracentesis adjacent to the haptic and using the hook to retrieve the suture both near and distal to the haptic. The suture is now available to tie over the iris. Once done on both haptics the optic can be reinserted into the posterior chamber (Fig. 17.16).

Note: if repositioning a lens with a capsule the optic would need to be freed up from the capsule to allow anterior displacement through the pupil.

Problems

- Iritis
- Secondary cystoid macular oedema
- Suture lysis and dislocation
- Haemorrhage from the iris
- Pigment dispersion (Fig. 17.17)

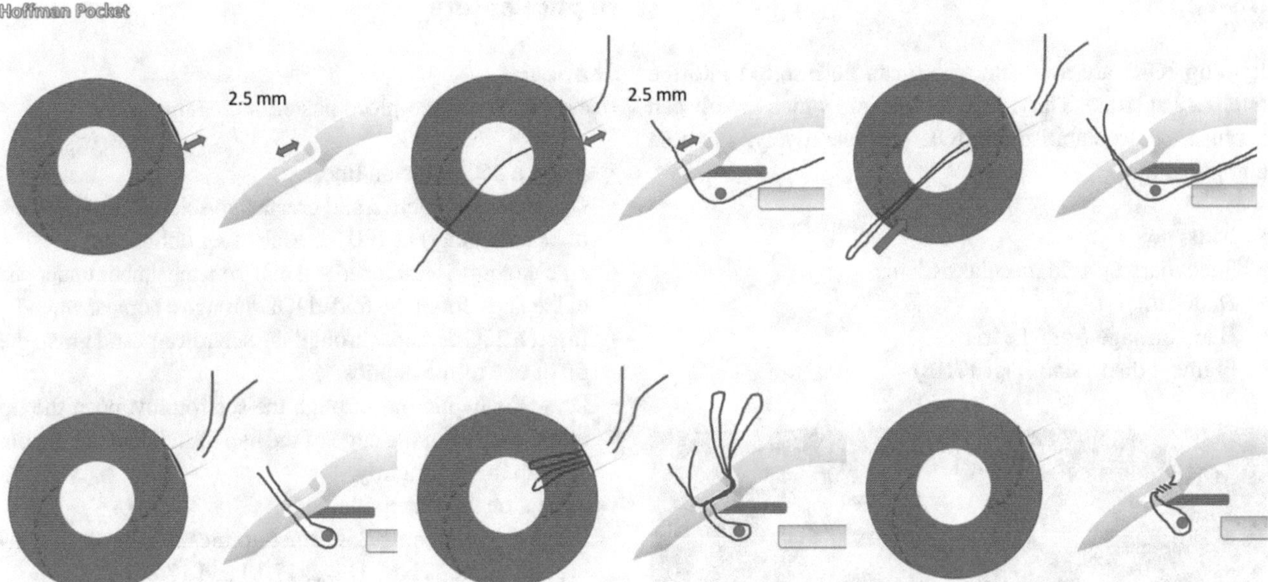

Fig. 17.15 The sequence for creating a Hoffman pocket and using this to secure a haptic of an IOL. From the cornea create a scleral tunnel to 2.5 mm. Pass a suture through the tunnel under the haptic. This goes out through a paracentesis opposite to the pocket. Re-enter the suture back through the same paracentesis and over the haptic and back across the tunnel. Pull loops of the sutures from the tunnel and cut. Tie the knot down into the tunnel to secure

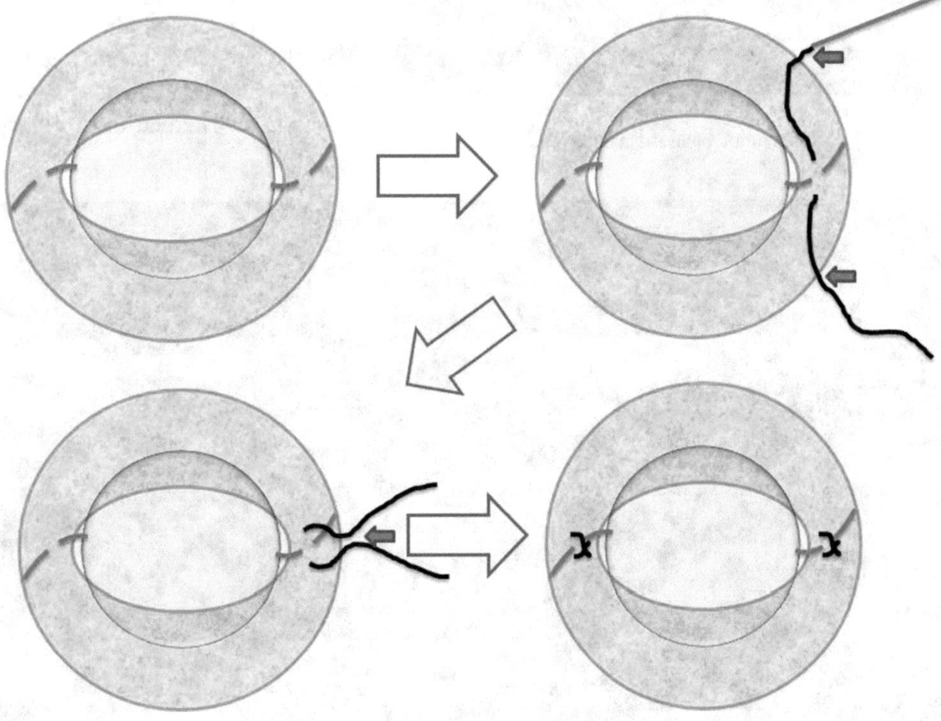

Fig. 17.16 For a McCannell suture (1), dislocate the optic through the pupil leaving the haptics posteriorly, (2), insert a suture using a long needle through the limbus (solid arrow) through the iris under the haptic and out through the limbus again (solid arrow), cut off the needle, (3), create a paracentesis (solid arrow) and hook and draw out the loops of suture then tie over the haptic, (4), repeat on other side and then push the optic through the pupil

Iris-Clip IOL

Iris-clip IOLs are available which can be inserted into the pupillary aperture. These have flanges into which the iris can be inserted to stabilise the IOL postoperatively. Possible complications:

- Iritis
- Secondary cystoid macular oedema
- Dislocation
- Haemorrhage from the iris
- Pigment dispersion (Fig. 17.18)

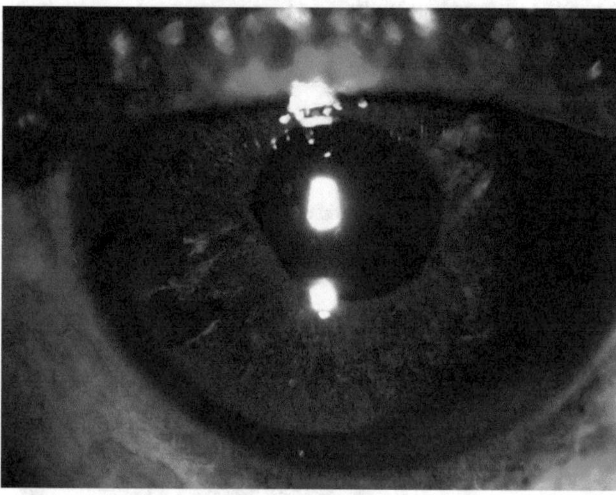

Fig. 17.17 A subluxation of an iris fixated IOL

Haptic Capture

Sharioch

Use a standard three-piece posterior chamber IOL.

- Insert a 25G infusion line.
- Open the conjunctiva and create two scleral flaps (as for a trabeculectomy) at 180° to each other obliquely.
- A sclerotomy is fashioned at 2 mm from the limbus under one of the flaps. Insert the folded IOL through a corneal wound.
- Insert a 25G forceps through the sclerotomy and grasp the tip of one of the haptics.
- Draw the haptic out through the sclerotomy, push the tip into the sclera at the edge of the flap to stabilise the haptic. Sew up the flap tightly.
- Repeat on the other side.
- Insert the remaining 25G sclerotomies to inspect the retina and vitreous base (Figs. 17.19 and 17.20).

Trochar

Set up for vitrectomy but insert two extra trochars transconjunctivally at the sites from which you wish to extract the haptics. When you are ready with micro-forceps inserted through the extra trochar grasp the end of the haptic. Whilst holding the haptic, advance the trochar up the shaft of the instrument. Pull the haptic out of the sclerotomy. Diathermy the end of the haptic to create a ball at the end. This can be done with handheld diathermy held close to the end of the haptic. The end must be dry and in the air for the heat to

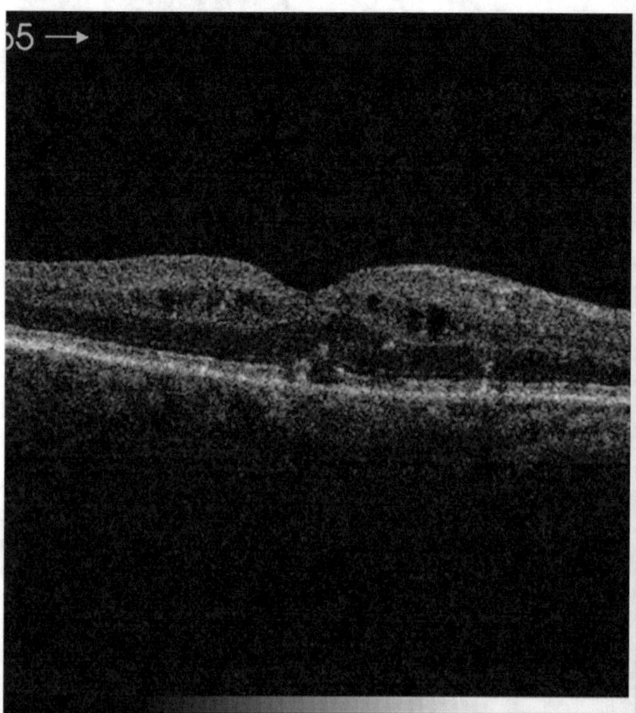

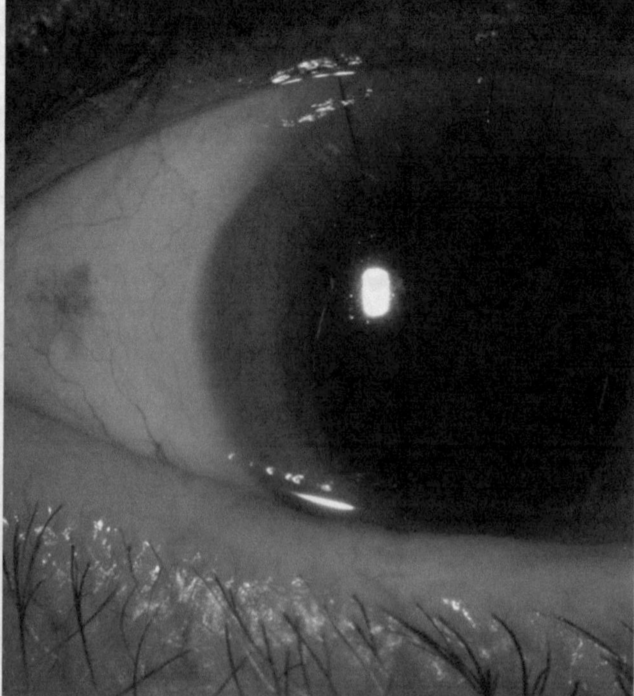

Fig. 17.18 An iris fixed IOL causing CMO

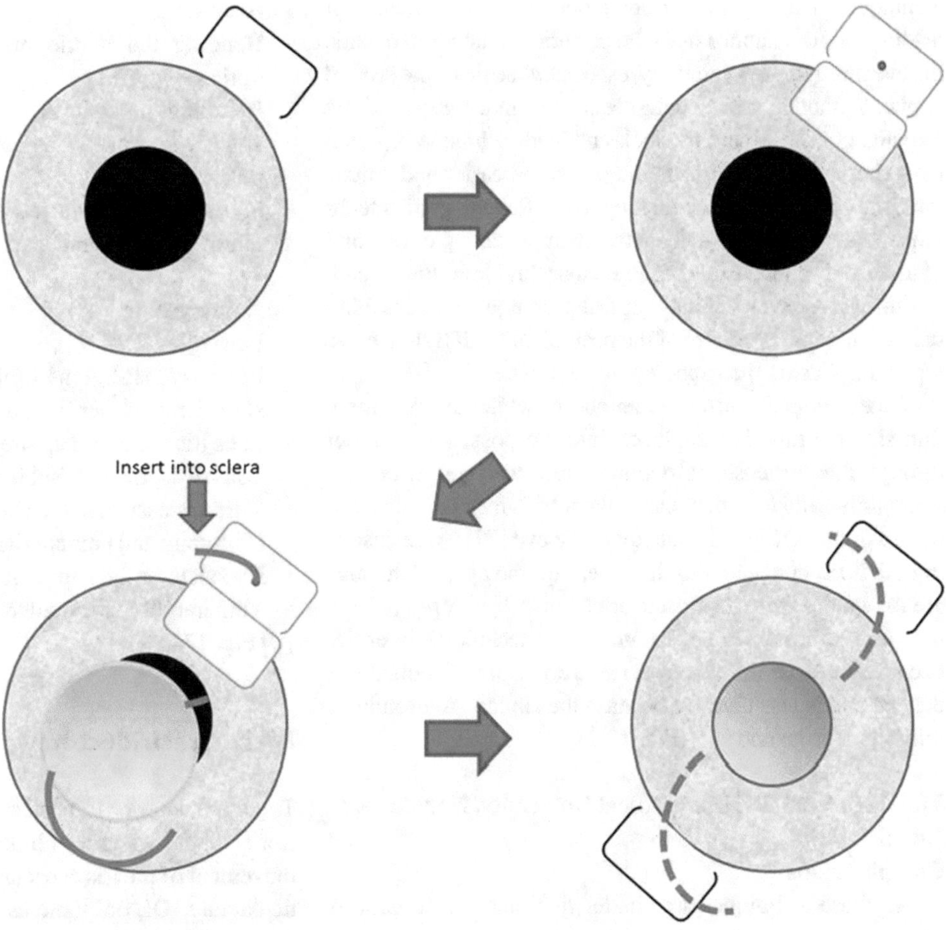

Fig. 17.19 The haptic capture technique can be used to place a standard three-piece foldable lens behind the iris in an aphakic eye. Create a scleral flap, then a sclerotomy in the bed of the flap, pull the end of the haptic through the sclerotomy and insert the end into the sclera at the edge of the flap incision, sew down the flap and repeat on the other side

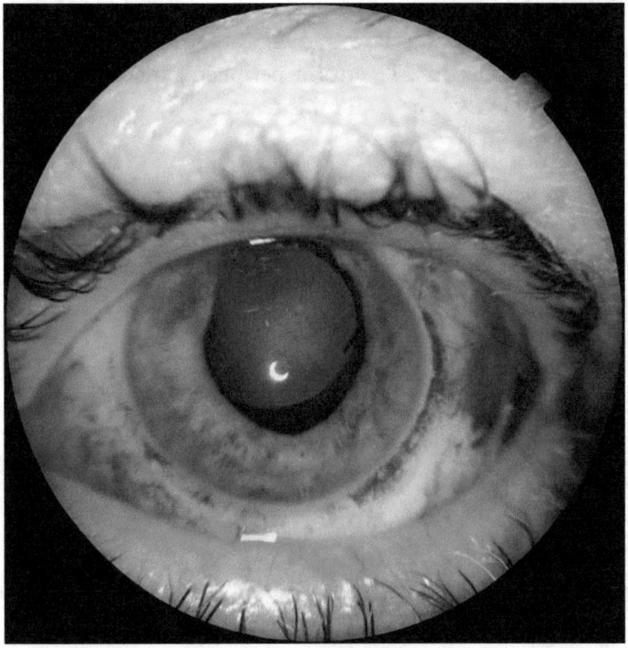

Fig. 17.20 An eye with a haptic capture IOL in situ 1 week after surgery

work. This is used to secure the haptic. The ball at the end can be inserted gently into the scleral tunnel created when inserting the trochar. Repeat on the other side.

Yamane

Instead of using trochars as above, the ends of the haptics can be inserted into the lumen of a needle. Bend a 26 G needle (or 30 G if you can get one with a large enough lumen) and insert transconjunctivally with a scleral tunnel at the site you wish to use to exit the haptic. Feed the end of the haptic into the lumen of the needle and remove the needle taking the haptic with it. The haptic is now externalised and you can diathermy as above for securing [55].

Surgical Pearl

Silicone Microtube Assisted Intrascleral IOL Fixation

Intrascleral fixation of a posterior chamber intraocular lens (IOL) has been getting popular compared with the suturing techniques. However, a current problem is the difficulty of leading the IOL haptics from the posterior chamber to outside the eye through the sclerotomy, especially the tip of the second haptic. Although the double-needle technique reported by Yamane et al. [55] and the lock-and-lead technique reported by Akimoto et al. [56] made the procedure easier and reduce the risks of complications relating to the forceps-guided technique including ciliary body detachment, breaking or bending of the haptic, and leakage of intraocular fluid from the wound, the difficulty level of this surgical technique remains high because it requires control of the position of the IOL in the eye while introducing the haptic tip into a thin needle.

We developed a novel technique in which an extremely thin silicone tube is introduced into the posterior chamber through the corneoscleral wound and drawn out through a sclerotomy, and the other end of the tube is then connected to the tip of the IOL haptic outside of the eye [57]. After inserting the IOL, connected to the tube, into the eye, the haptics are drawn out from the posterior chamber by simply pulling the tubing through a sclerotomy. This technique is easier because most of the manoeuvres are performed outside of the eye and is less invasive because the silicone microtube is thin, thread-like and soft (Fig. 17.21).

Motohiro Kamei, Aichi Medical University, Nagakute, Japan
Complications

All these techniques are challenging, and the surgeon is using a lens implant not designed for this purpose. Complications preoperatively and postoperatively are relatively common.

The second haptic is the most difficult to fix. Therefore, perform the nasal haptic first because the nose can make angulation of the forceps difficult.

Peroperative

- Bending the haptic may cause misalignment of the optic.
- Breaking the haptic, if the haptic is shortened only slightly it may still be able to be fixed with a good optic position.
- Separation of the haptic from the optic, you will need to remove the IOL and start again.

Postoperative

- Lens tilt
- Refractive shift, lens further forward leads to amblyopic shift. Lens further back a hypermetropic shift.
- Lens iris touch or capture
- Lens dislocation or subluxation
- Vitreous base damage and giant retinal tear
- Hypotony and conjunctival bleb formation
- Exposure of the haptic through the conjunctiva
- Vulnerability to ocular trauma and lens dislocation (Fig. 17.22)

Peripheral Iridectomy

There are anterior to posterior flows of aqueous in the anterior chamber when we blink or rub our eyes. This can cause movement of the iris especially if it is unsupported as in haptic capture IOL or atonic as it may become with rubbing of the iris. Therefore, the capture of the iris sphincter in this type of IOL insertion is common. A peripheral iridectomy allows the aqueous to flow into the posterior chamber without moving the iris. I perform peripheral iridectomy routinely now in these cases for this reason.

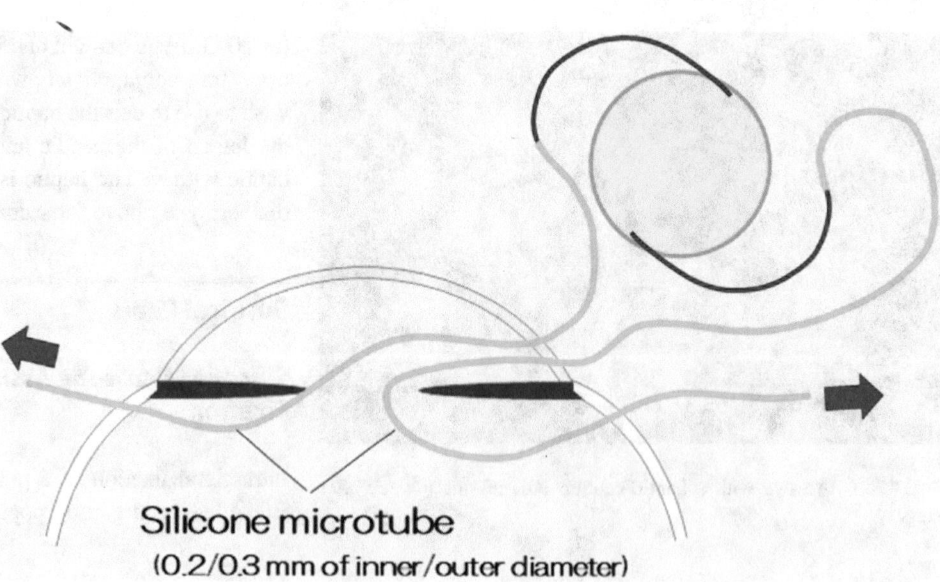

Fig. 17.21 Using a silicone tube to guide the haptic of an IOL during scleral fixation of the IOL

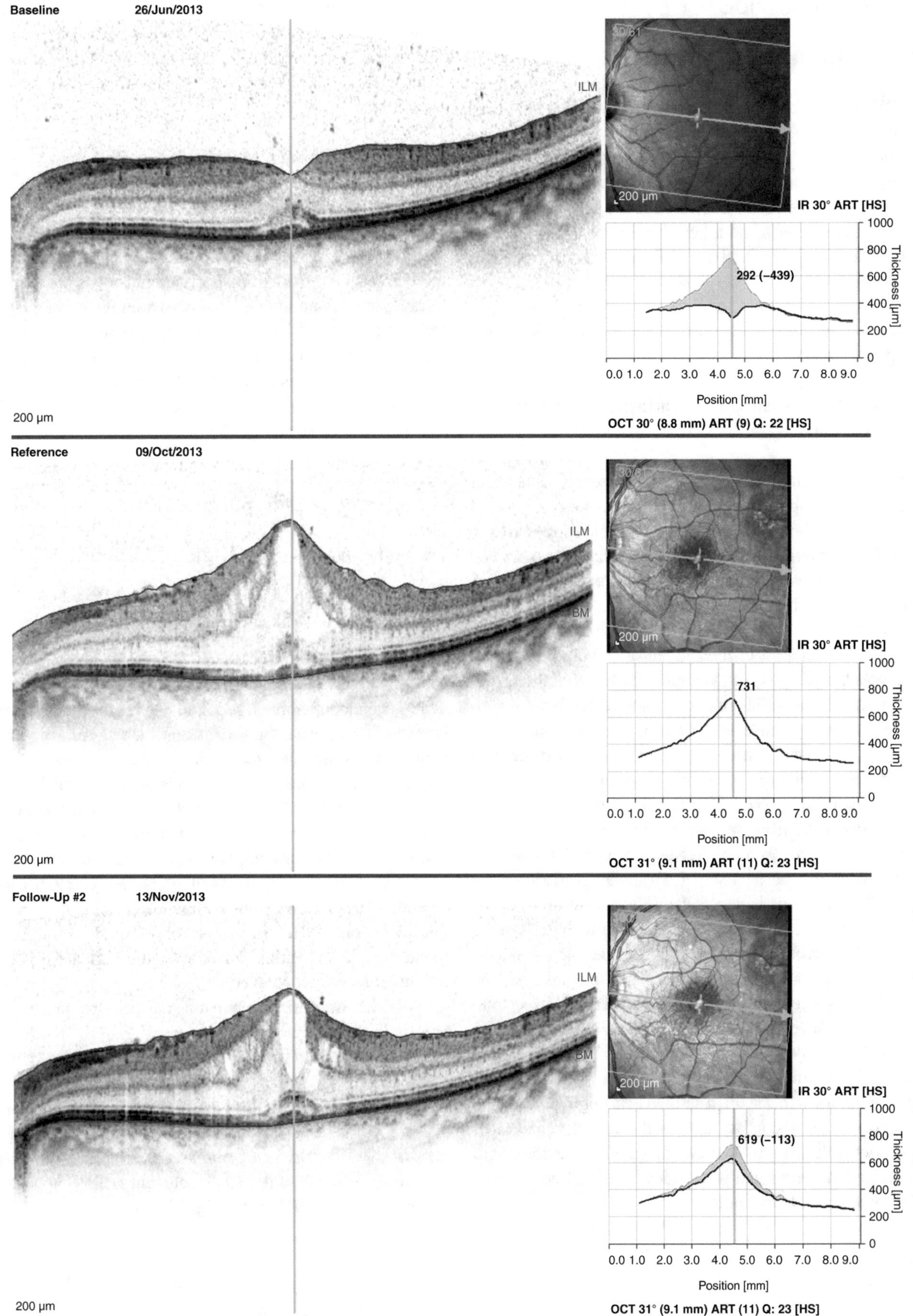

Fig. 17.22 CMO stimulated by the rub of the iris by haptic capture IOL

Anterior Chamber IOL

The modern design of open-loop AC IOL is less likely to cause corneal decompensation than older closed-loop models. This may be because the open loop allows the haptics to flex on rubbing the eye rather than vaulting the optic forward as with the closed-loop systems. They require a large 6 mm wound to insert and will require 10/0 nonabsorbable suture to the wound. The suture can be removed 3–4 months after surgery. Remember to do a peripheral iridectomy to avoid pupil block. Postoperative IOP rise is a possible complication.

Surgical Pearl

Secondary IOL Insertion Techniques, Choosing the Right Lens

Insertion of an intraocular lens in the absence of capsular support is developing into an area of expertise. A myriad of lens options is available to the VR surgeon and can be broadly divided into anterior chamber lenses, iris fixated lenses and scleral fixated lenses. Although most patients present for secondary IOL insertion following complex cataract surgery or trauma, there are a number of other conditions that can predispose to unstable or dislocated lenses in both phakic and pseudophakic patients for example pseudo-exfoliation, previous retinal surgery, inherited conditions e.g. Marfan's syndrome and peroperative lens trauma, e.g. tube surgery in glaucoma. Unstable lenses may also require replacement even if they are not displaced due to complications such as iris chafing, raised intraocular pressure, recurrent uveitis and macular oedema and corneal endothelial decompensation.

None of the lens fixation methods currently described are perfect; each has its own set of advantages and disadvantages. The ideal lens is very patient dependent and will be influenced by age, hobbies, occupation, refractive expectations, and systemic and ocular comorbidities. In an elderly patient with no previous history of glaucoma and systemic comorbidities where the priority is having a single procedure with little chance of future lens dislocation, an anterior chamber lens may be the most appropriate lens choice. In a young patient with a history of uveitis and with a hobby of rugby or other contact sport, a sutured lens might provide the best form of the secondary lens as there is less chance of dislocation following trauma compared with that seen with scleral capture lenses and where lens tilt would be undesirable due to possible iris touch.

VR surgeons should therefore familiarise themselves with more than one method of secondary IOL insertion to ensure that they are able to choose a lens based on patient characteristics rather than being limited by one lens type or technique.

Ms. Louisa Wickham, Moorfields Eye Hospital, London, UK

The Aphakic and Aniridic Eye

Occasionally you will be presented with an aphakic eye that has also lost its iris, e.g. aniridia or post-traumatic. In these cases, the use of silicone oil tamponade is problematic because there is no iris diaphragm to hold the oil in the posterior chamber and the oil will fill the anterior chamber risking glaucoma and corneal touch and decompensation. A clever technique has been described whereby sutures are inserted to hold the oil away from the cornea [58] (Figs. 17.23, 17.24, 17.25, 17.26 and 17.27).

Postoperative Endophthalmitis

Clinical Features (Figs. 17.28, 17.29, and 17.30)

Incidence of endophthalmitis in cataract surgery	0.028–0.14% [59–62]

If a patient experiences severe pain in the first week after cataract surgery the eye must be examined as quickly as possible for endophthalmitis. A high degree of urgency should be exercised because the sooner that the eye receives intraocular antibiotics the greater the chance of recovery. The patient often experiences a drop in vision with an aching pain in the eye. The eye is inflamed with signs of anterior uveitis followed by the formation of a hypopyon. Fibrin may be deposited on the lens implant and the iris blood vessels engorged. A view of the retina may not be possible because of infiltration of the vitreous with white cells but a red reflex may be visible. If the retina can be observed sheathing of the blood vessels and retinal haemorrhaging indicate a poorer prognosis for visual recovery.

Note: be aware that hypopyon and pain are not always present [63].

The priority is to inject intravitreal antibiotics as soon as possible.

Blebitis in patients with trabeculectomy may also lead to late endophthalmitis. In contrast to early postoperative infection, *Staphylococcus epidermidis* is less common in these cases [64]. The risk of retinal detachment is 8.3% in postoperative endophthalmitis [65] (Fig. 17.31).

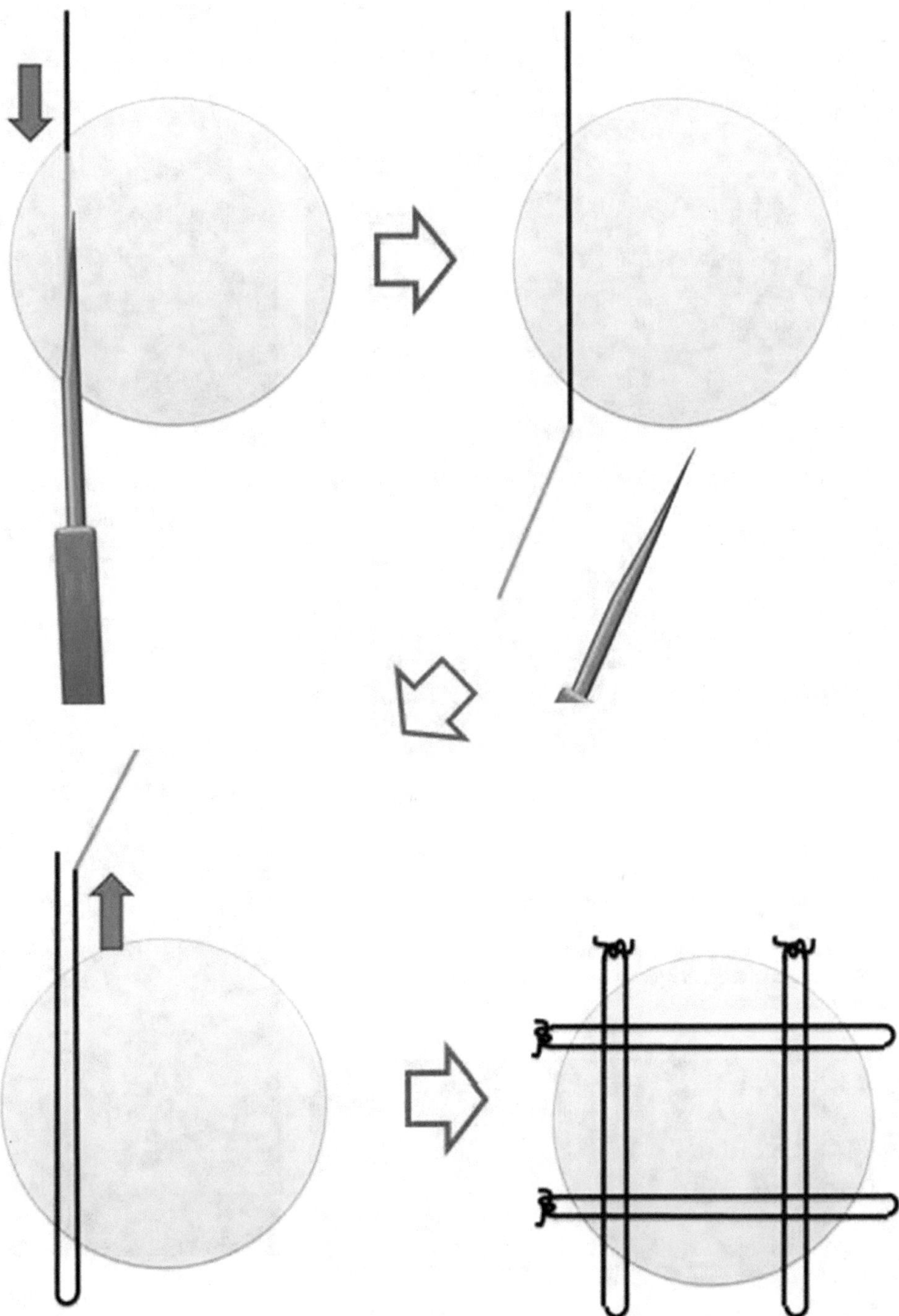

Fig. 17.23 In an aphakic aniridic eye a mesh of sutures can be used to prevent forward prolapse of silicone oil. First, pass a 10/0 Prolene with a straight needle through the sclera 1 mm posterior to the limbus. Draw the needle out of the eye by engaging the suture needle into the lumen of a hypodermic needle, e.g. 28 gauge. Pass the needle back in a similar fashion and then tie and bury the knot. Do this for two vertical and two horizontal sutures. The square mesh created will keep the oil in the posterior segment

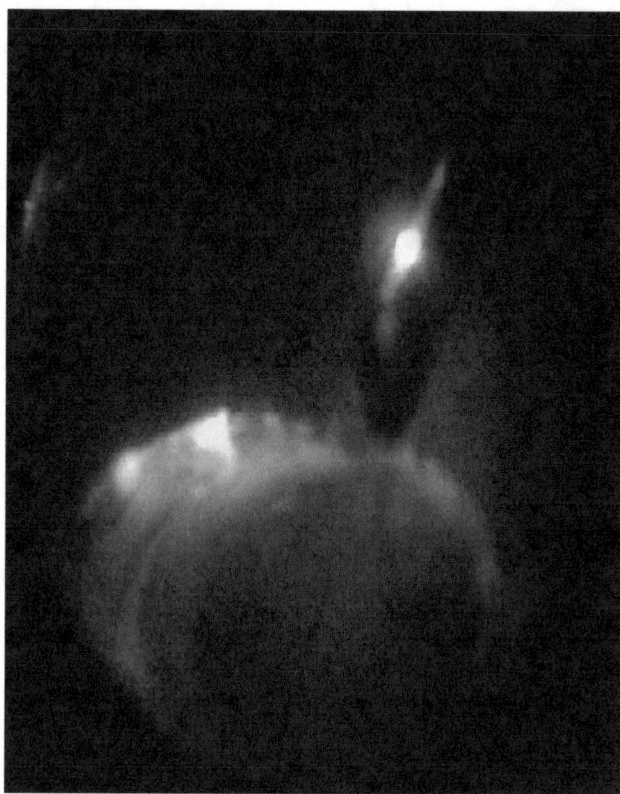

Fig. 17.24 Removal of dislocated intraocular lens implants provides several challenges. In this patient, the capsule and lens have fallen backward, but it remains hinged by the zonules at the 6 o'clock position. Many techniques exist to reposition such lenses including suturing of the lens to the sulcus, thereby avoiding complete removal of the lens. However, this runs the problems of suture erosion and breakage later. Modern anterior chamber lenses are useful in the elderly if you wish to remove the lens in total, in which case this will need to be done through the anterior segment

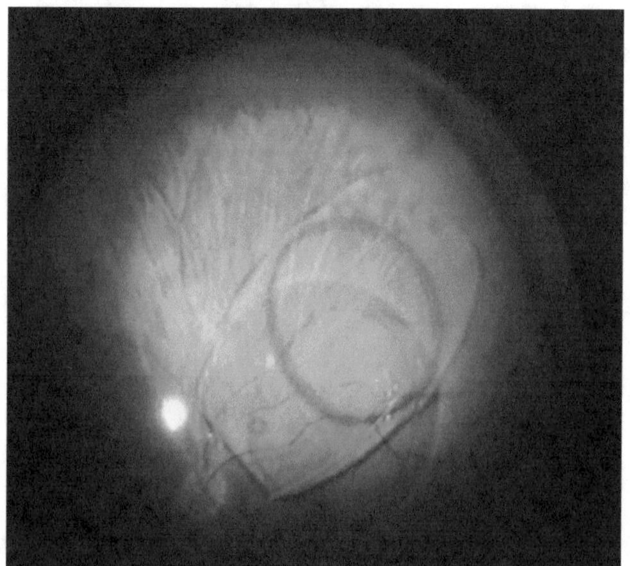

Fig. 17.25 Silicone plate haptic lens implants may dislocate posteriorly after Yag capsulotomy. These can be removed through the anterior segment and cut inside the eye to allow a smaller exit wound for the implant

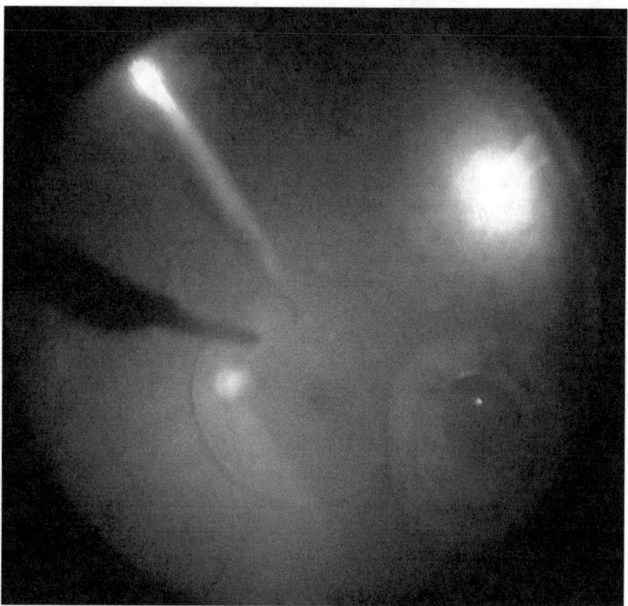

Fig. 17.26 If the zonular fibres give way the whole lens and capsule can dislocate posteriorly. This can be seen years after PPV

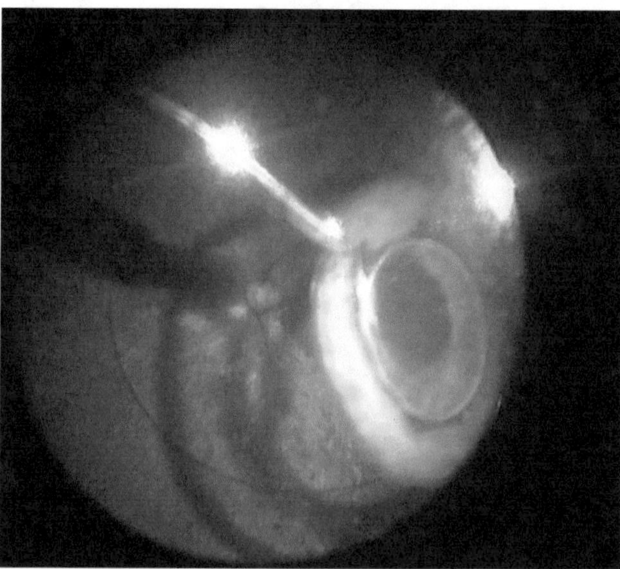

Fig. 17.27 The IOL can be lifted into the AC for removal

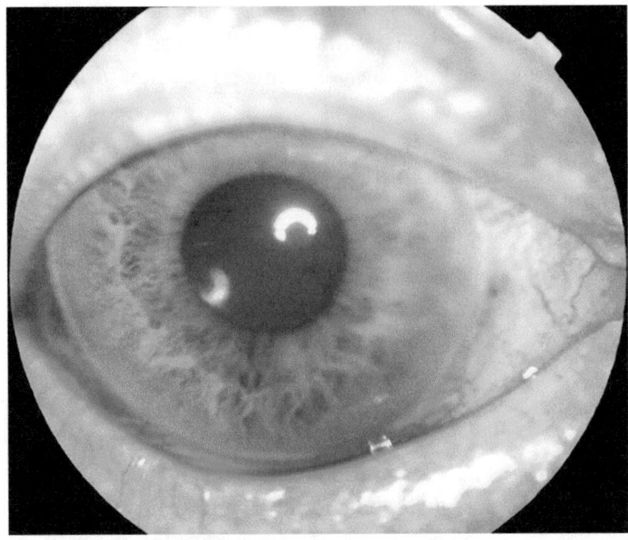

Fig. 17.28 A small hypopyon from postoperative endophthalmitis from *staphylococcus epidermidis*

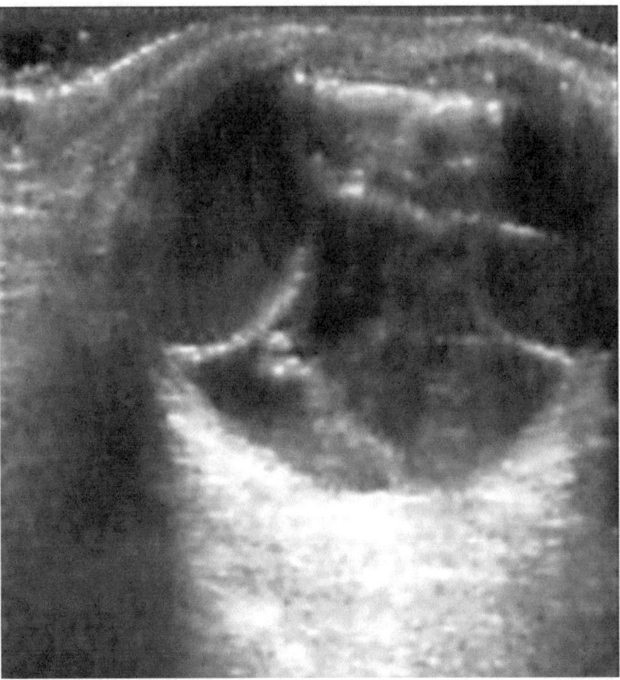

Fig. 17.30 Mixed disruption after pseudomonas corneal abscess and endophthalmitis with vitreous infiltrates, RD and choroidal effusions. Pseudomonas seems to be relatively less toxic to the retina than other severe infections

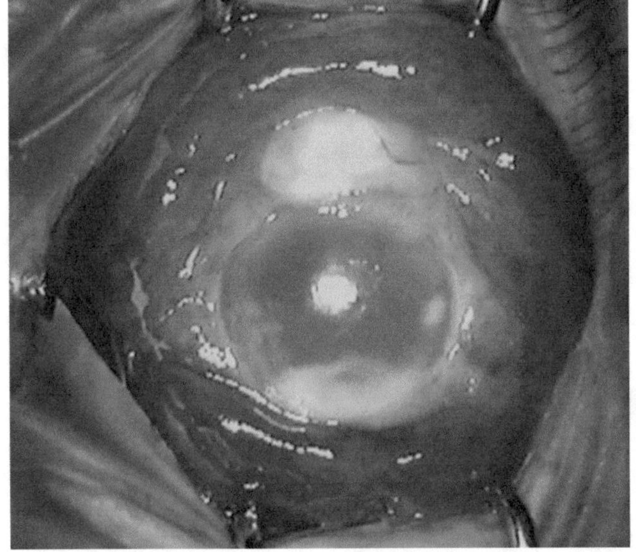

Fig. 17.29 This eye has suffered late postoperative endophthalmitis after trabeculectomy. There is a bleb abscess and a hypopyon

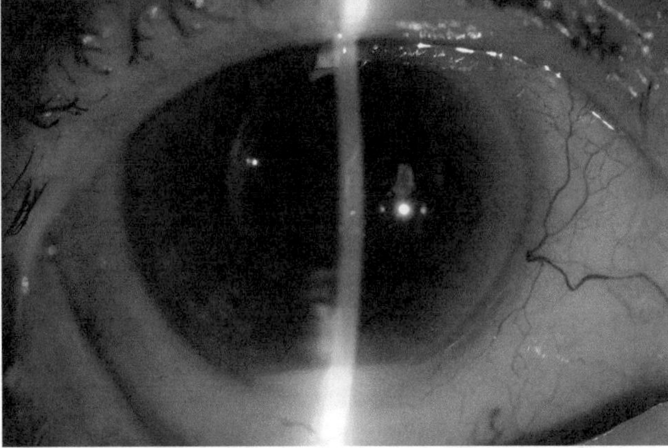

Fig. 17.31 Chronic postoperative endophthalmitis shows a hypopyon in a relatively quiet eye

Table 17.2 Difficulty rating for vitreous biopsy for endophthalmitis

Difficulty rating	Low
Success rates	Moderate
Complication rates	Low
When to use in training	Early

Surgery (Table 17.2)

Intervention should be performed as soon as possible after the infection is suspected because a delay will lead to further risk of visual loss.

Note. It is better to insert antibiotics occasionally inappropriately than to miss a case of endophthalmitis

Vitreous Tap

A fine needle is inserted transconjunctivally through the pars plana 3.5 mm from the limbus, topical anaesthesia can be used although the patient may feel the insertion of the needle in the inflamed eye. In endophthalmitis in an elderly patient, the vitreous is often liquefied and the tap procedure successful in obtaining a specimen for microbiological examination. Remove 0.1 ml of fluid vitreous. Leave the needle in situ and detach the syringe to send the sample to the laboratory, attach the antibiotics for insertion. The antibiotics should be drawn up in a 1 ml syringe. There is a dead space of 0.04 mls in the needle therefore you will need 0.14 mls in the syringe to inject 0.1 mls and prime the needle. Your pharmacy should make double the volume of the dose to allow you to prime the needle. Some antibiotics crystallise when inserted through the same needle; therefore, you may need two injection sites. The space created by the removal of the fluid vitreous will be filled by the antibiotics (for suggested drug dosages see Chap. 15).

Vitreous Biopsy

In most cases of endophthalmitis, a needle tap will obtain a sample; however, occasionally a dry tap is encountered. A vitreous cutter will provide a sample of whether the vitreous is liquefied or not. The increased reliability of the technique however may be outweighed by any delay in getting access to the vitrector and setting up any machinery. Small gauge instruments are ideal because there is no need for suturing or opening the conjunctiva. Place a three-way tap in the vitrector aspiration line and use this to extract the sample into a 1 m syringe. Cap the syringe and send it to the laboratory. As you remove the sample maintain pressure in the eye by pressing on the globe away from the biopsy site. Inject the antibiotics and gradually release the pressure.

If safe to do so a sample can be taken from the anterior chamber in addition.

No significant difference in complication rates or culture-positive rates has been demonstrated between vitreous needle taps and vitreous biopsy by vitrectomy cutter [66].

Infective Organisms

Only 56% to 69% of samples are culture positive [60, 67]. The bacteria involved vary from the virulent *Staphylococcus Aureus*, *Streptococcus pyogenes*, Hemophilus influenza [68], coliforms, *Pseudomonas aeruginosa* [69] and Klebsiella [70] to the less virulent *Staphylococcus epidermidis* (coagulase-negative staphylococci) and *Propionibacterium acnes* [71]. The less virulent organisms have a much better visual prognosis. Coagulase-negative staphylococci are the commonest pathogens and appear to come from the patient's eyelids or conjunctiva [72]. More recently methicillin-resistant *Staphylococcus aureus* has been implicated in postoperative endophthalmitis (18% of culture-positive endophthalmitis in one publication), with in vitro sensitivity to Gentamycin and Vancomycin [73]. Occasionally fungal postoperative infections are seen [74] (Fig. 17.32).

Frequency of isolation of organisms in positive biopsies (94% are Gram-positive) [67] (Fig. 17.33).

Coagulase-negative staphylococci	70%
Staphylococcus aureus	10%
Streptococci	9%
Gram-negative	6%
Enterococci	2%
Other Gram-positive	3%

Antibiotics

Intravitreal antibiotics are injected and provide a high concentration of drugs to treat the infection. For this reason, sys-

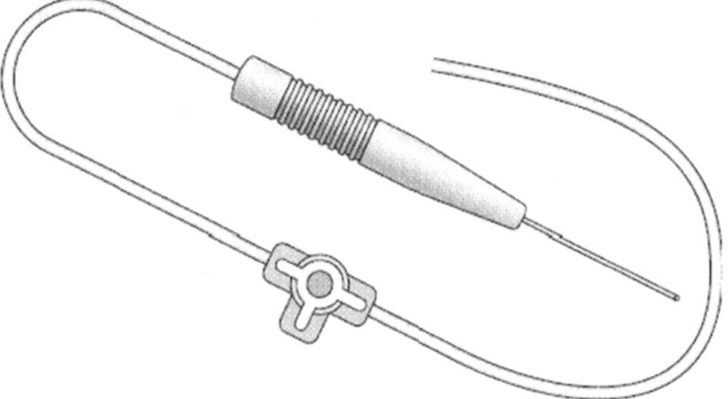

Fig. 17.32 When taking a sample, attach a three-way tap to the cutter to allow aspiration of fluids from the tubing

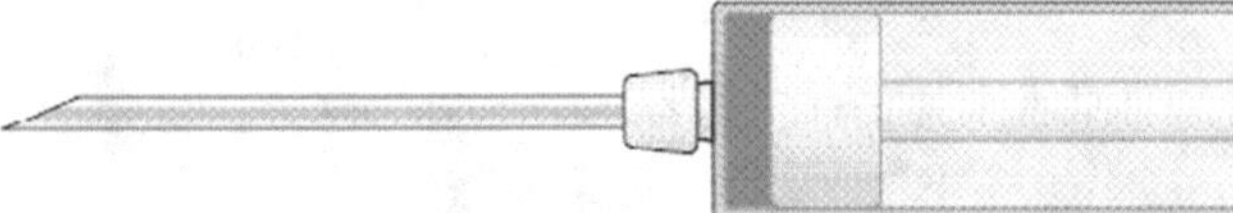

Fig. 17.33 There is a dead space of approximately 0.04 mls in the needle which must be accounted for during intravitreal injections

temic antibiotics appear to add little to the therapeutic effect [75]. Likewise, topical antibiotics will provide additional dosage to the anterior chamber but not to the vitreous and are only required in a moderate application unless there is an anterior abscess. Third-generation Cephalosporins are useful in combination with Vancomycin. Both persist in the eye for a week at therapeutic doses [76, 77]. Vancomycin is useful for Gram-positive organisms and Cephalosporins for Gram-negative organisms. In the latter, resistance has been described in 11% of Gram-negative organisms [67].

Aminoglycosides (gentamicin and amikacin) have been used in the past but are associated with retinal vascular occlusion in some patients which causes profound irreversible loss of vision [78–82].

Cephalosporins can also cause retinal toxicity in high doses and therefore it is preferable that the drug is made up in a controlled pharmaceutical environment.

The intravitreal steroid has been used as an adjunctive treatment but may be associated with a poorer visual outcome [83].

A repeat biopsy may be required in 10% for worsening inflammation, in which case the repeat biopsy has been associated with a positive culture in 42%. Repeat biopsy is often associated with a poor visual outcome [84].

The Role of Vitrectomy (Table 17.3 and Figs. 17.34, 17.35, 17.36 and 17.37)

Immediate PPV at presentation has been suggested from subgroup analysis in the Endophthalmitis Vitrectomy Study for those patients who present with light perception vision [75]. However, only patients whose irises were visible were included in this study, thus excluding those with severe hypopyon and corneal changes. Furthermore, those who were randomised to not receive PPV were not offered a PPV in follow-up to clear vitreous debris. This group may have had a reversible loss of vision from vitreous debris. For these reasons, immediate PPV should only be performed rarely. However, early intervention by vitrectomy at 48 hours may be justified in some cases [85, 86]. The fluid in the cassette from the vitrectomy machinery (containing BSS and diluted vitreous) can also be sent for culturing of bacteria with yields of 76% [87]. Polymerase chain reaction (PCR) to detect bacterial DNA can be useful especially if the patients have received prior antibiotic therapy. PPV may be required at a later stage to clear vitreous debris if there is visual potential (Fig. 17.38).

Table 17.3 Difficulty rating for PPV for endophthalmitis

Difficulty rating	Moderate
Success rates	Very low
Complication rates	High
When to use in training	Late

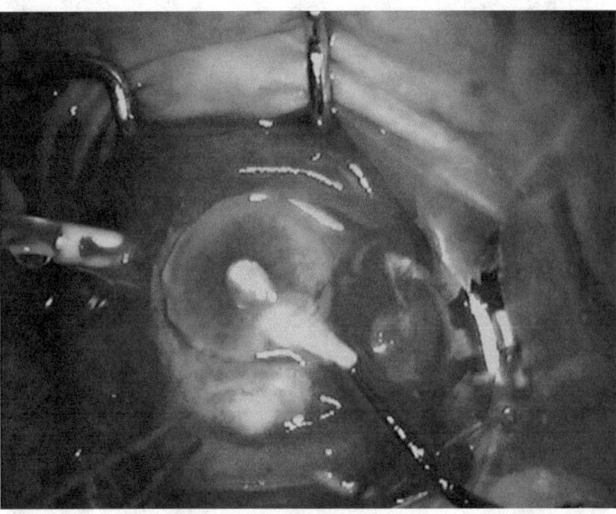

Fig. 17.34 When operating on endophthalmitis it will be necessary to clear the anterior segment. The hypopyon may be removed and have a fibrinous quality. The vitreous may be very murky and there may be pus on the retina and the retina may show vasculitis

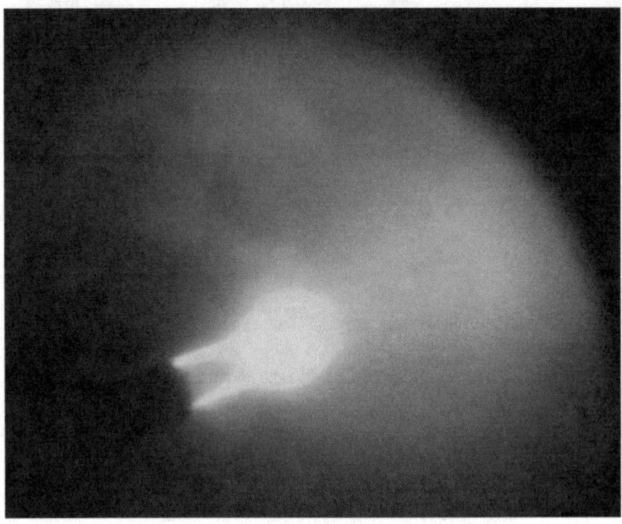

Fig. 17.35 The vitreous cavity is opaque

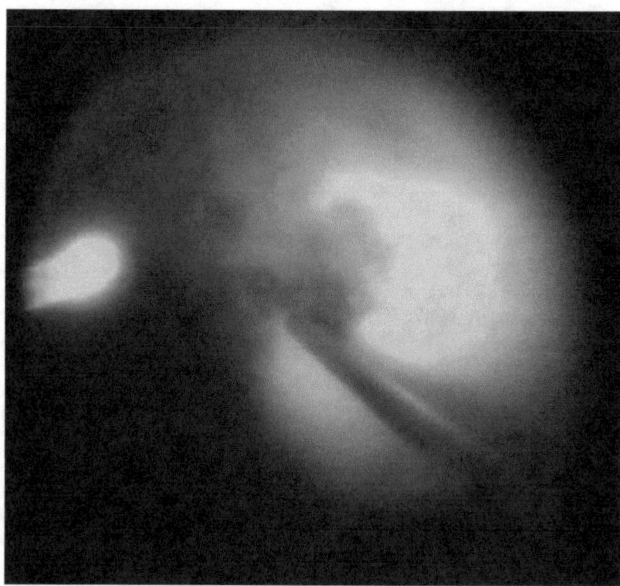

Fig. 17.36 There is pus on the retina

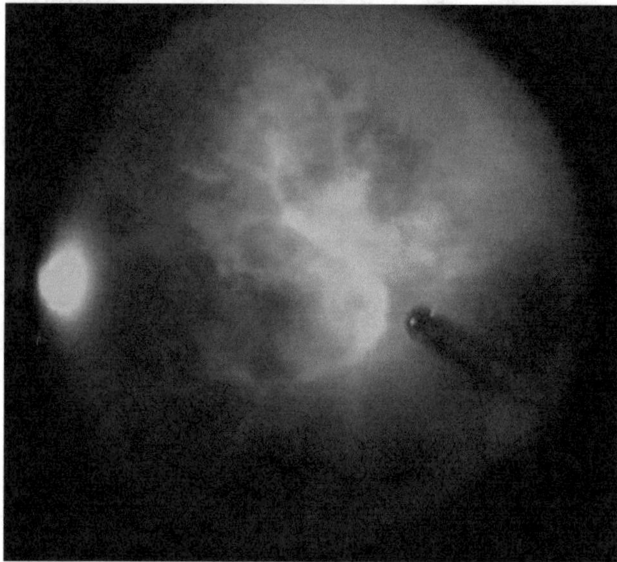

Fig. 17.37 There is vasculitis, a bad sign in infection

Success Rates

There is a 50% chance of moderate vision and 13% of NPL [60]. Only one-third achieve 20/40 or better [88, 89]. The best results are obtained by those patients with coagulase-negative staphylococci.

Visual Results by Organism [90].
(Rates of 20/100 or better)

• Coagulase-negative Staphylococci	84%
• Gram-negative	56%
• *Staphylococcus aureus*	50%
• Streptococci	30%
• Enterococci	14%

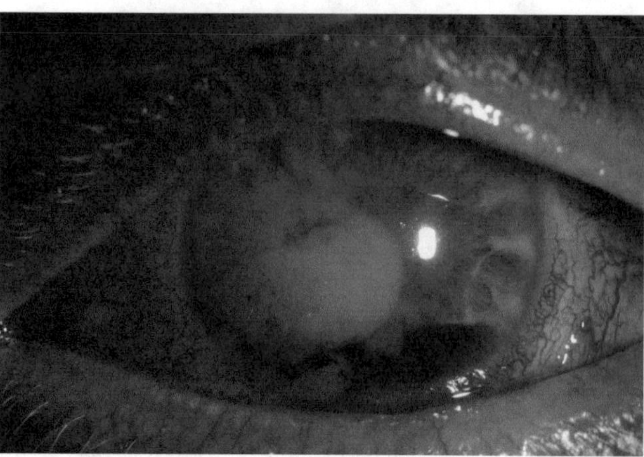

Fig. 17.38 A patient with endophthalmitis after placement of a radiotherapy plaque to treat a ciliary body malignant melanoma. The patient had raised IOP treated with Yag peripheral iridectomy, this caused an egress of pus into the anterior chamber. Vitreous biopsy and aqueous tap revealed staphylococcus coagulase negative. Intravitreal antibiotics with systemic ciprofloxacin allowed the resolution of the infection

Chronic Postoperative Endophthalmitis

This often masquerades as a panuveitis postoperatively; consequently, months may pass before the infection is considered. These eyes may have a white capsular plaque indicating the foci of infection around the IOL. Chronic endophthalmitis is caused by low virulence bacteria, classically *Propionibacterium acnes* or *staphylococcus epidermidis* but also from other organisms [91, 92] or even mixed colonies [93–96]. In chronic endophthalmitis the surgical approach can be separated into three stages:

1. Vitreous biopsy and intravitreal antibiotics with surgical capsulectomy, if this fails move on to,
2. PPV and then,
3. Removal of the IOL.

The best results are often obtained by PPV and removal of the IOL and capsule, but these have visual consequences. Electron microscopy can be used to identify the bacteria. Despite the eradication of the infection, the patient may still require medical therapy for chronic uveitis and CMO [71].

Consider the possibility that a retained nuclear fragment has been missed in chronic postoperative uveitis, see later in the chapter.

Needle-Stick Injury

Clinical Features (Figs. 17.39, 17.40, 17.41, 17.42, and 17.43)

- Incidence Globe penetration from the local anaesthetic needle in all patients is 0.014% and in patients with axial

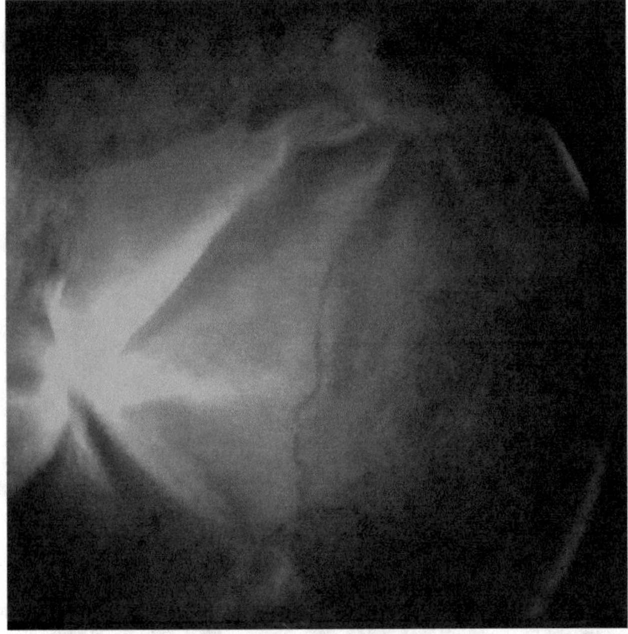

Fig. 17.39 An incarceration site has been created at the point of penetration of the back of the eye by a local anaesthetic needle. This has caused a retinal detachment like the types seen in perforating injury in trauma

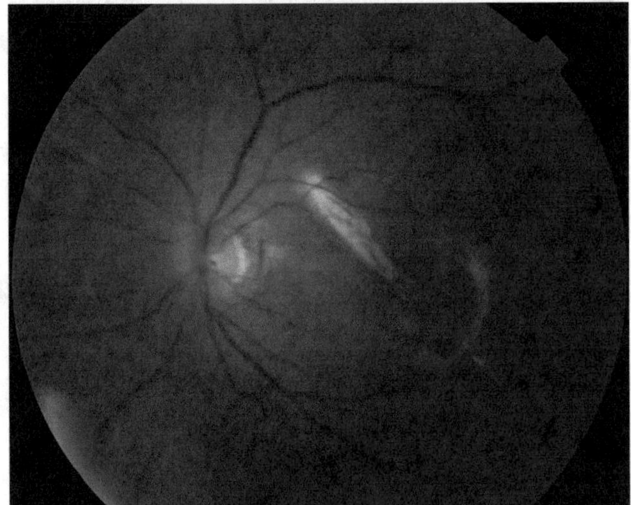

Fig. 17.40 The perils of orbital needle injections are illustrated in this patient who has a choroidal needle track clearly visible transecting the fovea (courtesy of Alistair Laidlaw)

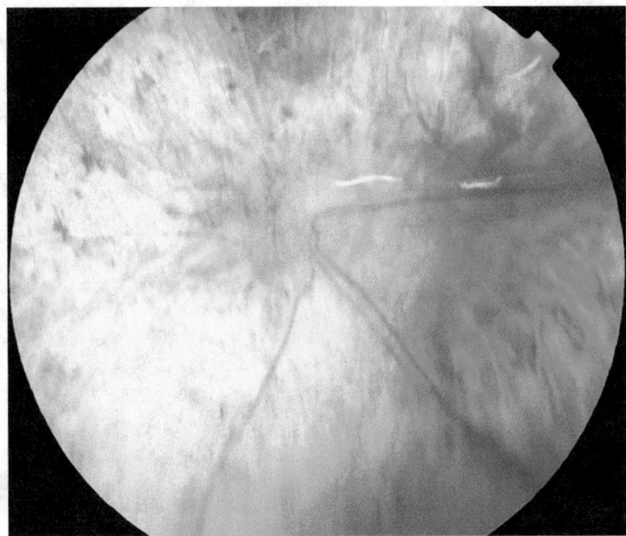

Fig. 17.41 Ten years after the injection of local anaesthesia into the eye the choroid and RPE are atrophic, the retinal is flat with oil in situ and vision is poor at hand movements

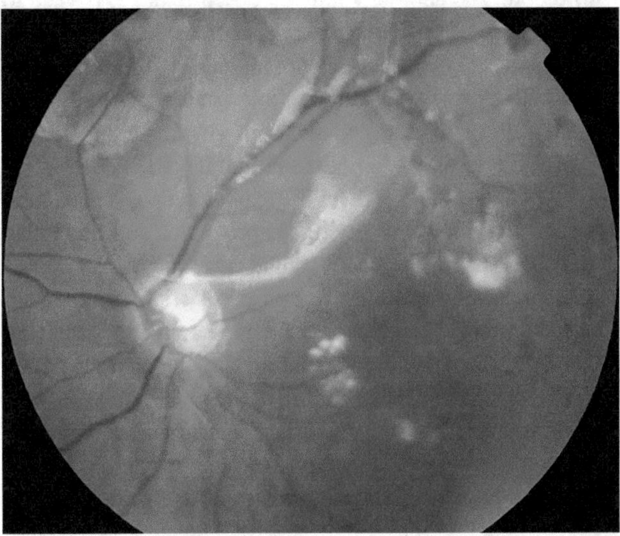

Fig. 17.42 This patient had undiagnosed posterior scleritis which had led to scleromalacia. In preparation for vitrectomy for vitreous haemorrhage (secondary to retinal vein occlusion and glaucoma), during sub tenons injection of local anaesthesia the cannula ruptured the thinned area of sclera and entered the eye causing a large area of scleral rupture and choroidal haemorrhage. The sclera was repaired with difficulty and the eye tamponaded with intraocular silicone oil. An early postoperative picture is shown with residual haemorrhage superiorly and an oil reflex. Eventually, the oil was removed with 6/60 vision from the retinal vein occlusion

length more than 26 mm is 0.7% [97], and posterior staphyloma is 0.13% [98].

- 53% of cases of globe perforation are myopic [99]
- 55% of cases are in eyes with normal axial lengths [97].

The needle used in local anaesthesia for ophthalmic surgery may penetrate the walls of the eye. The risk has been described in retrobulbar, peribulbar, sub-Tenon [100, 101] and even subconjunctival injections [99] but is less common now as topical anaesthesia is used for cataract surgery. Care must be exercised in eyes that are 25 mm or longer. These myopic eyes have thin sclera and are vulnerable to injury. Penetration of the coats of the eye may cause haemorrhage in the choroid, subretinal space or into the vitreous. Tears in the

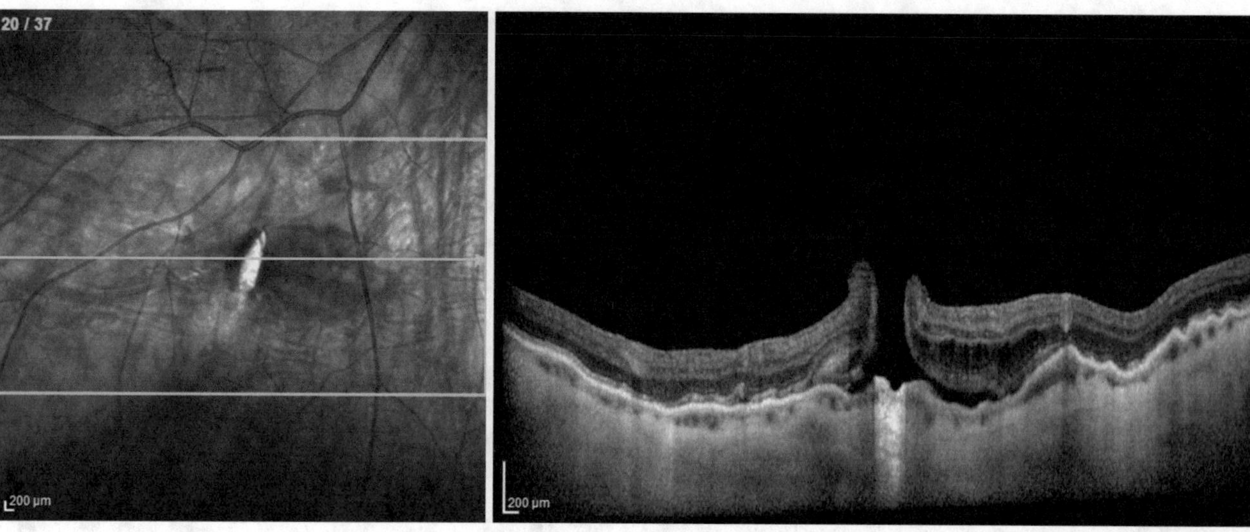

Fig. 17.43 OCT of a needlestick injury showing a hole in the retina

retina can result in retinal detachment. The cataract surgeon may present a postoperative patient who has an eye filled with blood. The aetiology may be obscure, but it is wise to have an index of suspicion that the eye has been injured during the anaesthesia. Although not all tears of the retina produced in this way will result in retinal detachment, it is worth considering a vitrectomy to clear out vitreous haemorrhage and to allow visualisation of the retina. If RRD occurs there is a 40% chance of PVR [97, 98]. Tears or retinal detachment can be dealt with by employing the principles outlined in the treatment of rhegmatogenous retinal detachment.

The incarceration sites from needle stick injuries are small but may be multiple as the person anaesthetising repeatedly inserts the needle whilst trying to reach the posterior orbit. Despite the penetration of the globe, most injuries do not produce the tractional retinal detachment that is associated with larger incarceration sites seen in trauma. PPV is required in 40–80% [102, 103] with a 50% chance of 20/40 vision or better. In rare circumstances, if an attempt has been made to inject the local anaesthesia whilst the needle tip is in the eye, the pressure rise can induce a scleral rupture similar to a blunt trauma [104, 105]. The need for vitrectomy depends on the presence of vitreous haemorrhage or retinal detachment (Fig. 17.44).

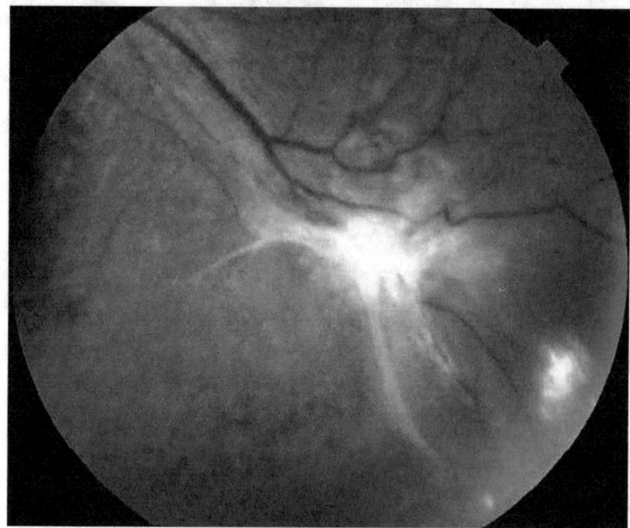

Fig. 17.44 An old incarceration site from a needle stick injury is seen with fibrous membranes tracking into the site of injury but without retinal detachment

Surgery (Table 17.4)

Laser around the needle sites can be used to prevent accumulation of subretinal fluid but these sites only uncommonly cause RD. The eye is more often operated upon for vitreous haemorrhage. Depending on the presentation, follow the principles outlined in the preceding chapters.

Table 17.4 Difficulty rating for surgery for needle stick injury

Difficulty rating	Moderate
Success rates	High
Complication rates	Low
When to use in training	Middle

Intraocular Haemorrhage

Incidence of choroidal haemorrhage	0.04–0.16% [31, 34] (Figs. 17.45, 17.46 and 17.47)

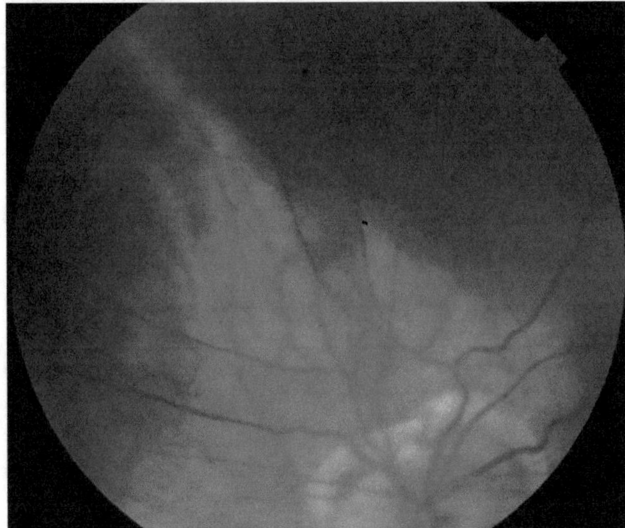

Fig. 17.45 A diffuse area of choroidal haemorrhage is shown superiorly in a high myope. These haemorrhages although occurring more commonly in high myopes often clear quickly in these eyes

Spontaneous choroidal haemorrhage occurs because of the sudden drop in intraocular pressure when the eye is opened during surgery. Any fragile blood vessels in the choroid may fracture and bleed causing the catastrophic "expulsive haemorrhage". The eyes of patients with high myopia, arteriopathy or old age are particularly at risk. Management of the condition is like the treatment of choroidal haemorrhage in trauma. Presentations tend to be severe if these occur because the anterior surgeon does not see the haemorrhage until late. In contrast, during retinal surgery, the haemorrhage is seen early and can often be controlled (Fig. 17.48).

A key sign indicating poorer visual outcome is if the macula is detached by the haemorrhage. In contrast, if the macula is flat between the choroidal elevations, there is more chance of visual recovery. Observe the choroidals carefully over weeks to watch for spontaneous resolution. If complications such as severe hyphaema (risking glaucoma and corneal staining), vitreous haemorrhage or retinal detachment occur intervene with surgery. a recent promising intervention is the injection of suprachoroidal tPA 50 micrograms/0.01 mls 24 h before the vitrectomy to help liquefy the haemorrhage (Fig. 17.49).

Retinal Detachment

4 year incidence [59].

All cataract extractions	1.17%
With vitreous loss at the cataract extraction	4.9%
Phacoemulsification	0.4%

(Increased in the white race, the young, male and those with YAG capsulotomy)

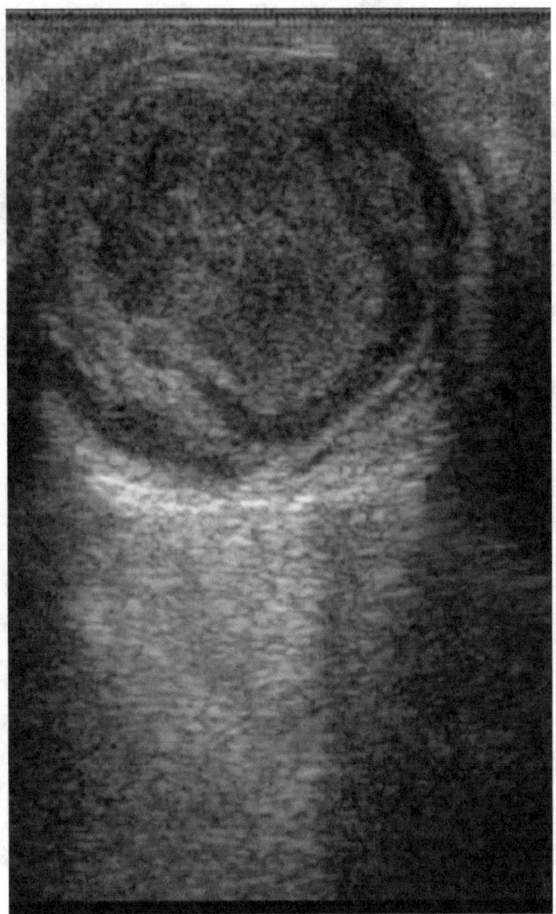

Fig. 17.46 A choroidal haemorrhage develops into a catastrophic expulsive haemorrhage because the cataract surgeon does not see anything happening until it is too late. The surgeon performing a vitrectomy usually notices something occurring because the retina is being continually visualised. Therefore, the surgeon can react more quickly to limit the size of the haemorrhage. In this patient, an expulsive occurred during extracapsular cataract extraction. At 3 weeks there was some resolution of the haemorrhage allowing space to perform surgery. Using an AC maintainer, the vitreous haemorrhage was removed and liquified choroidal haemorrhage expelled. The eye was filled with silicone oil to await further choroidal haemorrhage resolution and repeat surgery. The eye achieved CF vision

An increased risk of retinal detachment is associated with previous a cataract extraction. Approximately, 30% of rhegmatogenous retinal detachments are pseudophakic. This is easy to explain when the cataract surgery has been complicated by a vitreous loss where the vitreous disruption results in a posterior vitreous detachment or in further shrinkage of the vitreous and retinal tear formation. However, even uncomplicated cataract surgery seems to induce a doubling of the risk of retinal detachment compared with the phakic population. It may be that the loss of the larger volume of the crystalline lens, which is replaced, by the lower volume of the intraocular lens implant induces a structural change in the vitreous that must fill the gap. This may induce vitreous detachment or shrinkage. The retinal detachment risk appears

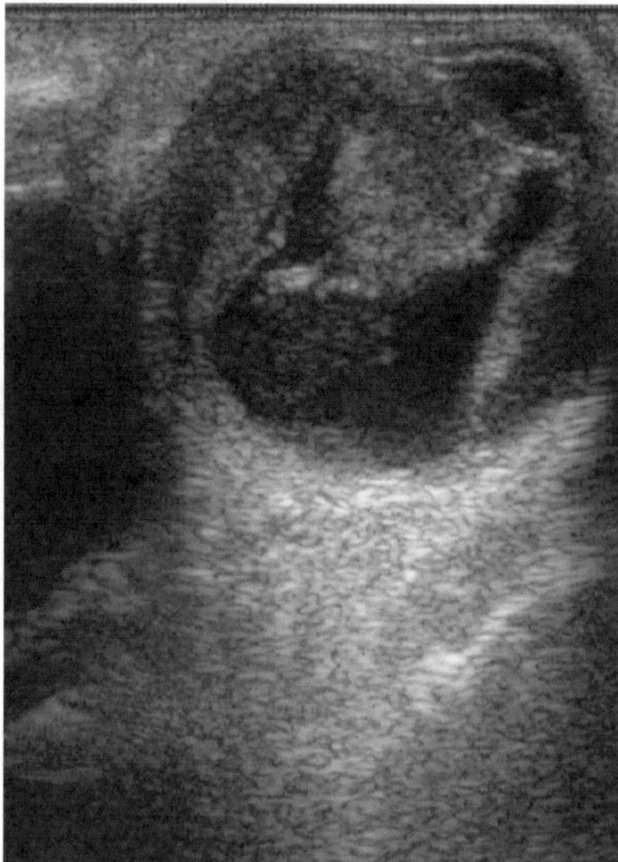

Fig. 17.47 An ultrasound of an expulsive choroidal haemorrhage

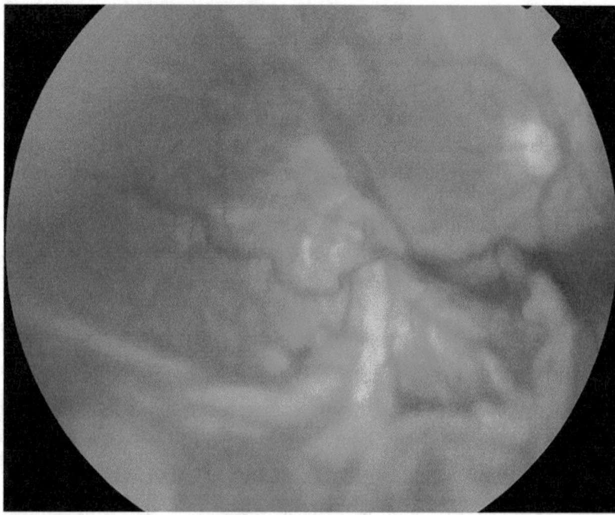

Fig. 17.48 A choroidal haemorrhage is settling after a complicated cataract operation. Secondary retinal detachment can occur with PVR. Close observation is required

at a mean of 15 months after the surgery and lasts 4 years. These patients may experience floaters and flashes but often present late with their macula detached. Therefore, it is important that the cataract surgeon is aware of the risk and that the retina is examined postoperatively. Pseudophakic RRD can be treated by the usual modalities although posterior capsule opacification would tend to steer the surgeon towards PPV. See also Chap. 7 (Fig. 17.50).

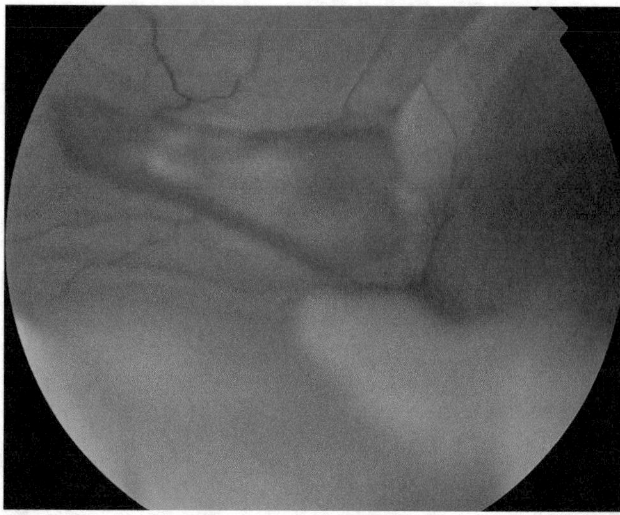

Fig. 17.49 A choroidal haemorrhage after needling of a trabeculectomy

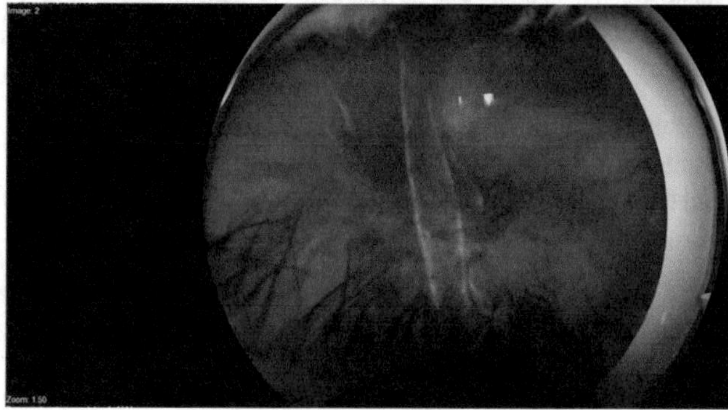

Fig. 17.50 A GRT folded over the macula and occurring 6 weeks after a phaco and IOL with vitreous loss

Chronic Uveitis

(Fig. 17.51) Some patients may develop chronic uveitis after cataract extraction. Check the operation notes in case a complicated operation has been described which may indicate a missed or ignored dropped nuclear fragment. With anterior uveitis check the angle with a gonioscope for a piece of nucleus inferiorly. Examination of the eye sometime after the cataract extraction reveals chronic vitritis often with raised intraocular pressure. The nuclear fragment may have been absorbed. Removal of the vitreous by PPV may improve but not cure the uveitis.

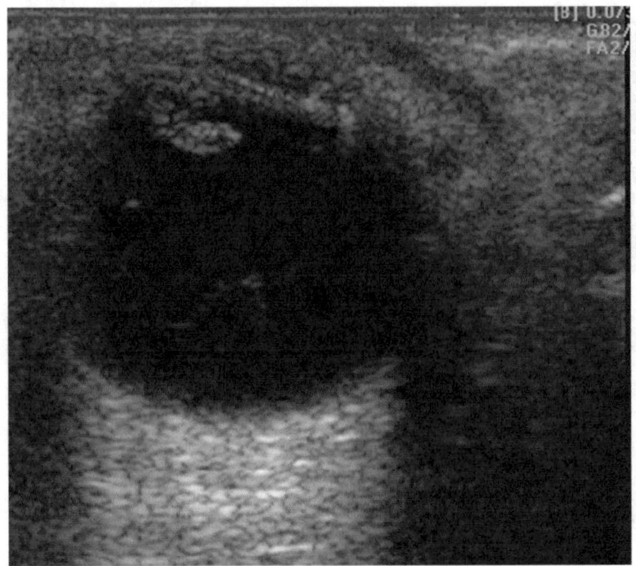

Fig. 17.51 An ultrasound of a patient with chronic uveitis after cataract extraction reveals lens material trapped in the capsule stimulating the uveitis

Another cause is low-grade endophthalmitis, see above. Vision is often permanently reduced due to cystoid macular oedema.

Postoperative Cystoid Macular Oedema (Figs. 17.52, 17.53 and 17.54)

The vitreoretinal surgeon may be asked to insert an intravitreal steroid for postoperative CMO but although efficacious in the short term the effect of the steroid is not lasting in improving the vision [106]. Thankfully, most are self-limiting. Alternatively, an intravitreal anti-VEGF agent can be used, thereby avoiding the IOP problems of IV steroid.

Special Notes

- Beware of the pain in the first week after cataract extraction indicating endophthalmitis.
- Beware floaters in the first year after cataract extraction in case of retinal detachment.
- Check if chronic uveitis in a pseudophakic eye started after the cataract extraction indicating an ignored dropped nucleus or *Propionibacterium acnes* infection.

Postoperative Vitreomacular Traction

Sudden onset vitreomacular traction can be seen rarely after cataract extraction [107]. This presents in the few weeks after surgery and usually spontaneously resolves if you wait

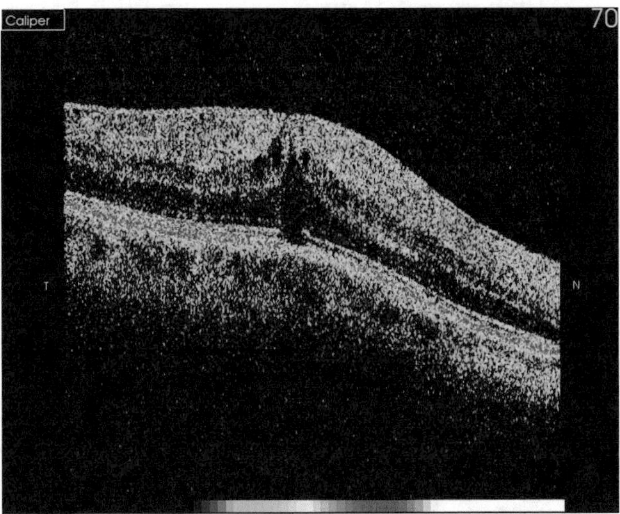

Fig. 17.52 Cystoid macular oedema can appear in vitrectomised eyes which subsequently have phacoemulsification cataract extraction. It is possible that the prostaglandins reach the macula more easily because the physical barrier of the vitreous has been removed

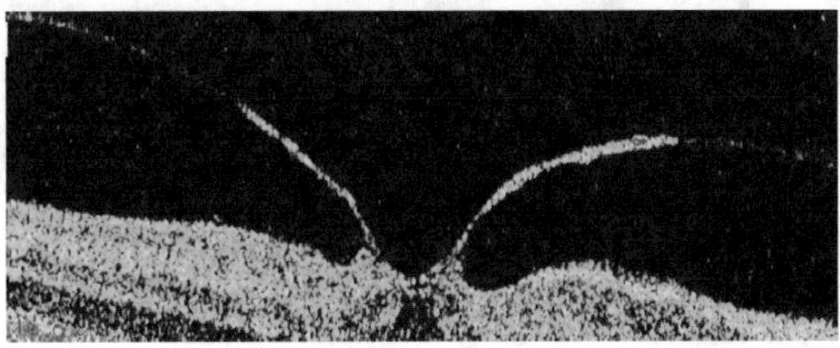

Fig. 17.53 Occasionally patients will experience distortion a few weeks after cataract extraction, this may be due to rapid onset vitreal traction which usually spontaneously separates

for a few months. If not, PPV can be used. The eye is at risk of residual metamorphopsia.

Postoperative Choroidal Effusion

Note: do not confuse postoperative choroidal effusions with RRD. These have a deep green colour and an appearance of a thicker consistency than RRD. They are more likely to occur with glaucoma drainage procedures. Most will resolve spontaneously. If not, perform PPV with a long infusion cannula (6 mm) or an anterior chamber placement of the infusion. Usually, the suprachoroidal fluid will leak from the superior sclerotomies as straw coloured or green fluid, when the infusion is switched on. Be careful when inserting small gauge trochars to make sure that the trochar has penetrated the vitreous cavity. Drainage from the sclerotomy with trochars is less good. Once in the eye, a 30G needle attached to

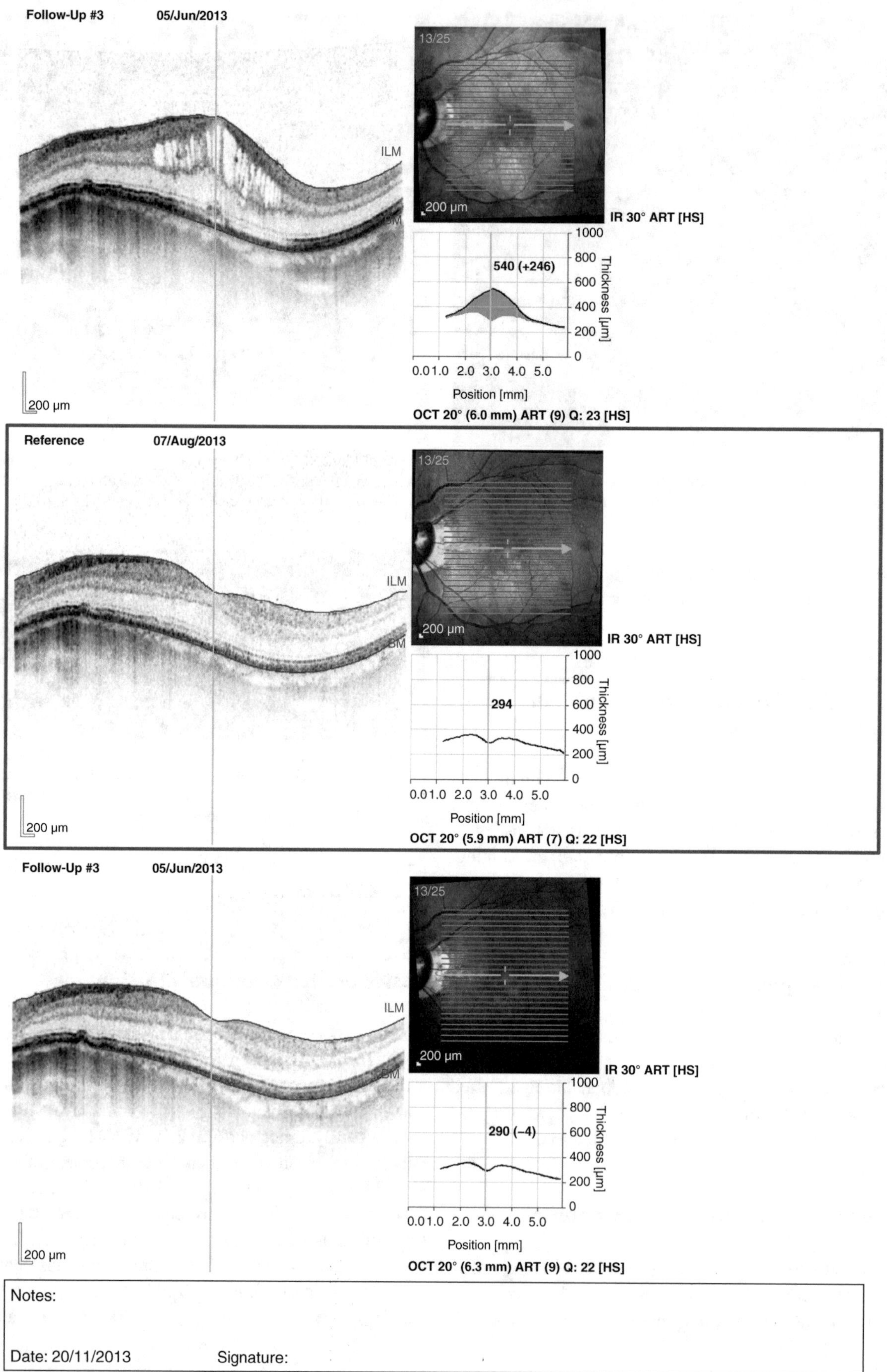

Fig. 17.54 CMO secondary to topical prostaglandin agonist, and after stopping the drops

a 1 ml syringe with the plunger out can be inserted transconjunctivally through the sclera and into the suprachoroidal space.

External Drainage

- Perform the PPV.
- With the syringe press the needle onto the sclera and watch for the indentation internally.
- Once you are happy that the indent of the needle is under elevated choroid and retina, insert the tip of the needle into the suprachoroidal space.
- Allow passive fluid drainage (PPV infusion on).

There is a worry that the needle will penetrate the retina; however, this is unlikely. Indeed, the retina can settle onto the needle tip whilst flattening without being penetrated.

You can insert heavy liquids to encourage the drainage of any residual fluid. No internal tamponade is required. Note this method of external drainage can be used for exudative RD with the needle inserted into the subretinal space thereby avoiding a retinotomy. The use of a 25-gauge trochar to drain the suprachoroidal space is an alternative option (Figs. 17.55, 17.56, 17.57 and 17.58).

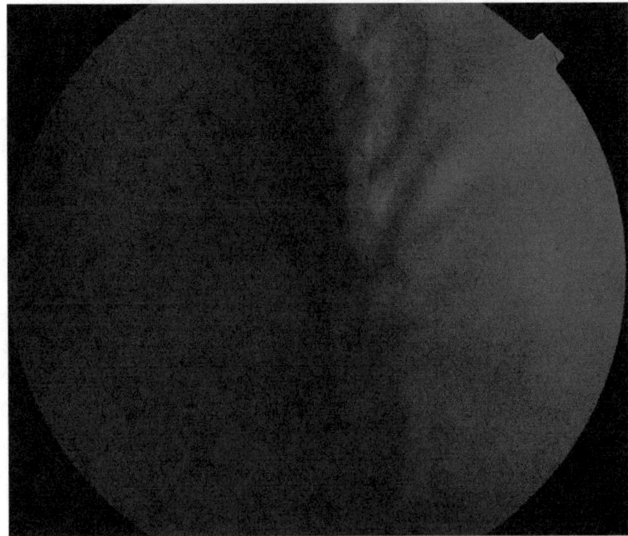

Fig. 17.55 Loss of intraocular pressure has caused the development of extensive choroidal effusions, which have a dark green colour. The disc can just be seen between the two edges of the choroidal effusions. In some instances, these may meet each other. Drainage of choroidal effusions may be necessary to restore vision. If the effusions are recurrent, examine the eye with ultrasound biomicroscopy for a cyclodialysis cleft

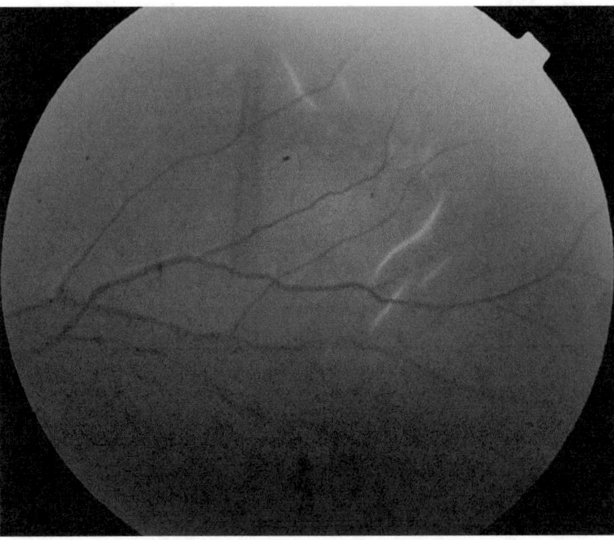

Fig. 17.56 A resolved effusion may leave some folds in the choroid in the early stages

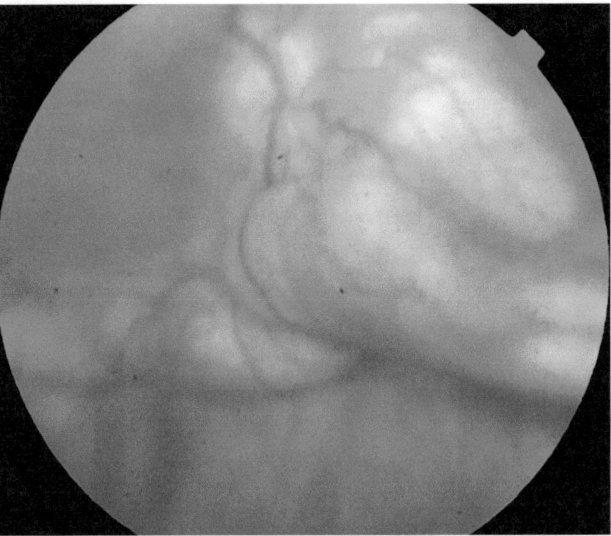

Fig. 17.57 Do not leave unstable anterior segment wounds in vitrectomised eyes. Any wound leak can cause severe hypotony with globe collapse as in this eye. The sclera is infolded

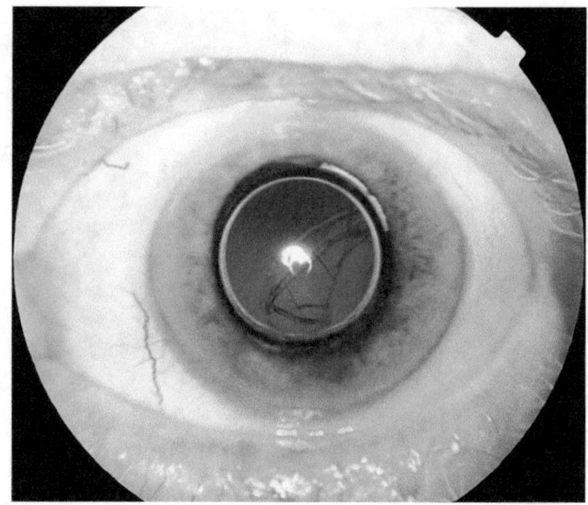

Fig. 17.58 The capsule of this patient has rolled up behind the lens implant reducing vision this can be removed by surgical capsulectomy with the vitreous cutter but the support for the IOL may be compromised by the removal of the anterior hyaloid. Therefore, the patient must be warned about the possibility of dislocation of the IOL postoperatively

Summary

Vitreoretinal procedures are used to correct the various complications of intraocular surgery. The vitreoretinal surgeon requires anterior segment surgical skills because cataract extraction is often required during vitrectomy to maximise visualisation of the retina and because vitreoretinal surgery may require anterior segment intervention in addition (Figs. 17.59, 17.60 and 17.61).

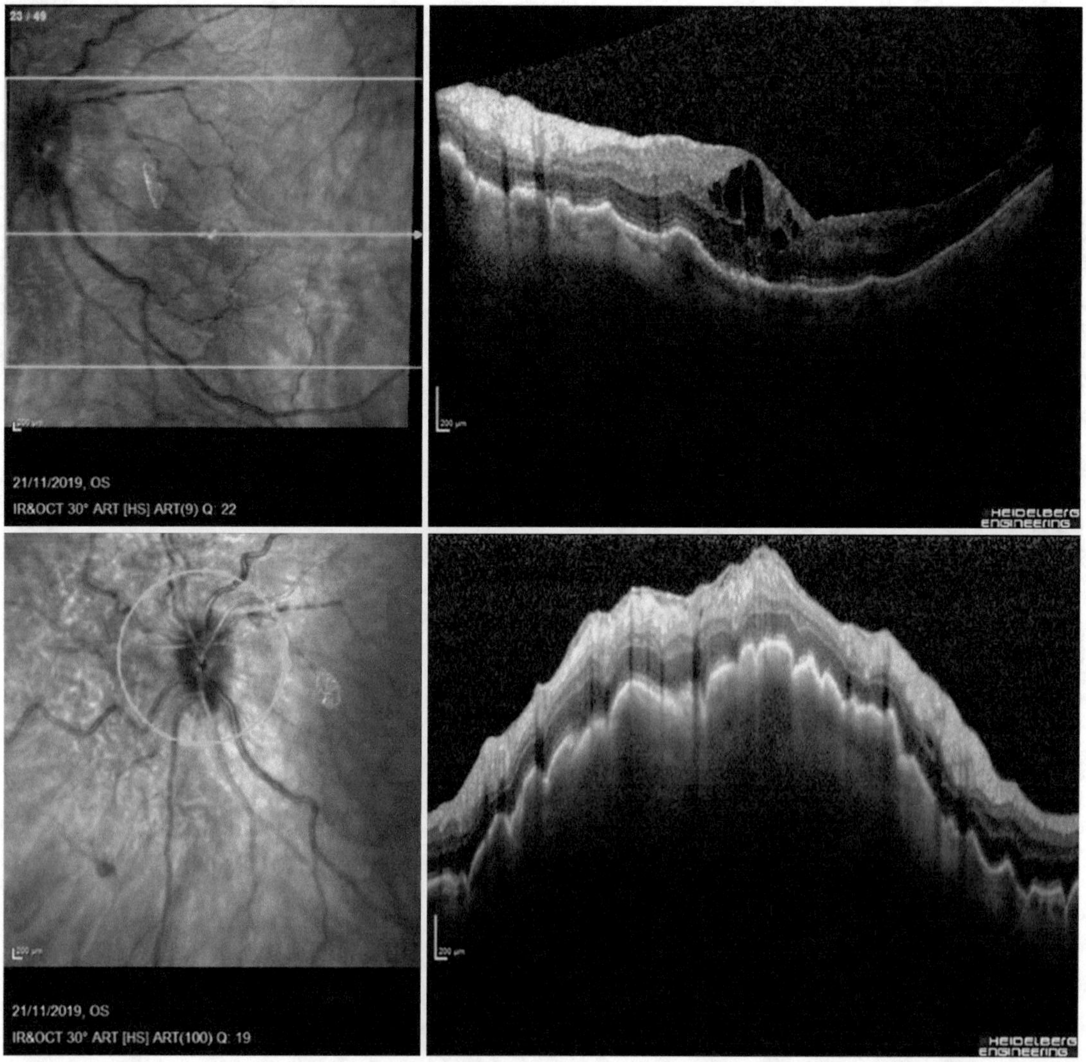

Fig. 17.59 A hypotonous eye from cycloablation for ocular hypertension, shows wrinkling of the posterior layers of the eye

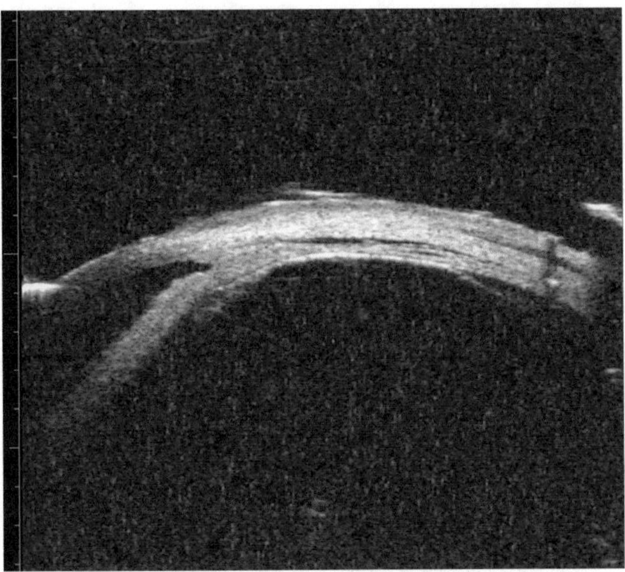

Fig. 17.60 A cyclodialysis cleft creating hypotony may occur after anterior segment surgery

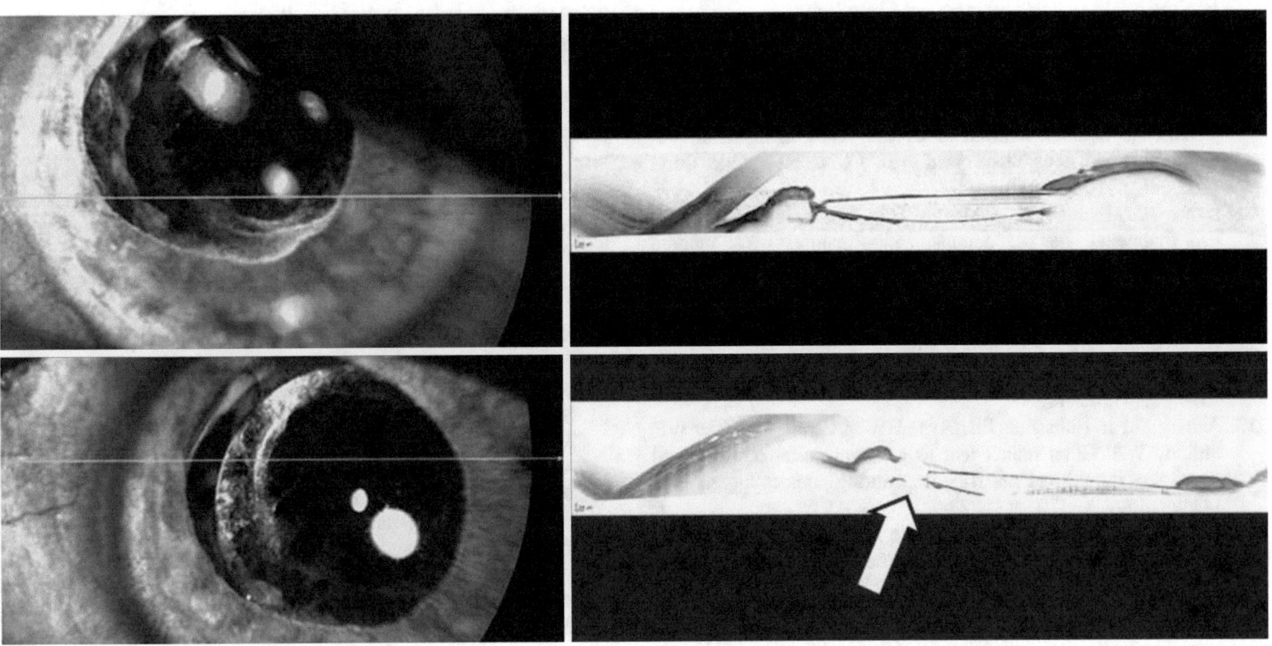

Fig. 17.61 Creating a hole in the capsule next to the IOL reversed aqueous misdirection. Some patients will need a vitrectomy

References

1. Aasuri MK, Kompella VB, Majji AB. Risk factors for and management of dropped nucleus during phacoemulsification. J Cataract Refract Surg. 2001;27(9):1428–32.
2. Kageyama T, Ayaki M, Ogasawara M, Asahiro C, Yaguchi S. Results of vitrectomy performed at the time of phacoemulsification complicated by intravitreal lens fragments. Br J Ophthalmol. 2001;85(9):1038–40.
3. Mathai A, Thomas R. Incidence and management of posteriorly dislocated nuclear fragments following phacoemulsification. Indian J Ophthalmol. 1999;47(3):173–6.
4. Stilma JS, van der Sluijs FA, van Meurs JC, Mertens DA. Occurrence of retained lens fragments after phacoemulsification in the Netherlands. J Cataract Refract Surg. 1997;23(8):1177–82.
5. Ross WH. Management of dislocated lens fragments after phacoemulsification surgery. Can J Ophthalmol. 1996;31(5):234–40.
6. Oruc S, Kaplan HJ. Outcome of vitrectomy for retained lens fragments after phacoemulsification. Ocul Immunol Inflamm. 2001;9(1):41–7.
7. Hansson LJ, Larsson J. Vitrectomy for retained lens fragments in the vitreous after phacoemulsification. J Cataract Refract Surg. 2002;28(6):1007–11.
8. Haddad WM, Monin C, Morel C, Larricart P, Quesnot S, Ameline B, et al. Retinal detachment after phacoemulsification: a study of 114 cases. Am J Ophthalmol. 2002;133(5):630–8.
9. Gilliland GD, Hutton WL, Fuller DG. Retained intravitreal lens fragments after cataract surgery. Ophthalmology. 1992;99(8):1263–7.
10. Rossetti A, Doro D. Retained intravitreal lens fragments after phacoemulsification: complications and visual outcome in vitrectomized and nonvitrectomized eyes. J Cataract Refract Surg. 2002;28(2):310–5.
11. Irvine WD, Flynn HW Jr, Murray TG, Rubsamen PE. Retained lens fragments after phacoemulsification manifesting as marked intraocular inflammation with hypopyon. Am J Ophthalmol. 1992;114(5):610–4.
12. Kim JE, Flynn HW Jr, Rubsamen PE, Murray TG, Davis JL, Smiddy WE. Endophthalmitis in patients with retained lens fragments after phacoemulsification. Ophthalmology. 1996;103(4):575–8.
13. Aaberg TM Jr, Rubsamen PE, Flynn HW Jr, Chang S, Mieler WF, Smiddy WE. Giant retinal tear as a complication of attempted removal of intravitreal lens fragments during cataract surgery. Am J Ophthalmol. 1997;124(2):222–6.
14. Al-Khaier A, Wong D, Lois N, Cota N, Yang YC, Groenewald C. Determinants of visual outcome after pars plana vitrectomy for posteriorly dislocated lens fragments in phacoemulsification. J Cataract Refract Surg. 2001;27(8):1199–206.
15. Bessant DA, Sullivan PM, Aylward GW. The management of dislocated lens material after phacoemulsification. Eye. 1998;12(Pt 4):641–5.
16. Borne MJ, Tasman W, Regillo C, Malecha M, Sarin L. Outcomes of vitrectomy for retained lens fragments. Ophthalmology. 1996;103(6):971–6.
17. Hutton WL, Snyder WB, Vaiser A. Management of surgically dislocated intravitreal lens fragments by pars plana vitrectomy. Ophthalmology. 1978;85(2):176–89.
18. Kim JE, Flynn HW Jr, Smiddy WE, Murray TG, Rubsamen PE, Davis JL, et al. Retained lens fragments after phacoemulsification. Ophthalmology. 1994;101(11):1827–32.
19. Margherio RR, Margherio AR, Pendergast SD, Williams GA, Garretson BR, Strong LE, et al. Vitrectomy for retained lens fragments after phacoemulsification. Ophthalmology. 1997;104(9):1426–32.
20. Stefaniotou M, Aspiotis M, Pappa C, Eftaxias V, Psilas K. Timing of dislocated nuclear fragment management after cataract surgery. J Cataract Refract Surg. 2003;29(10):1985–8.
21. Yeo LM, Charteris DG, Bunce C, Luthert PJ, Gregor ZJ. Retained intravitreal lens fragments after phacoemulsification: a clinicopathological correlation. Br J Ophthalmol. 1999;83(10):1135–8.
22. Vilar NF, Flynn HW Jr, Smiddy WE, Murray TG, Davis JL, Rubsamen PE. Removal of retained lens fragments after phacoemulsification reverses secondary glaucoma and restores visual acuity. Ophthalmology. 1997;104(5):787–91.
23. Wallace RT, McNamara JA, Brown G, Benson W, Belmont J, Goldberg R, et al. The use of perfluorophenanthrene in the removal of intravitreal lens fragments. Am J Ophthalmol. 1993;116(2):196–200.
24. Vote BJ, Tranos P, Bunce C, Charteris DG, Da CL. Long-term outcome of combined pars plana vitrectomy and scleral fixated sutured posterior chamber intraocular lens implantation. Am J Ophthalmol. 2006;141(2):308–12.
25. Smiddy WE, Guererro JL, Pinto R, Feuer W. Retinal detachment rate after vitrectomy for retained lens material after phacoemulsification. Am J Ophthalmol. 2003;135(2):183–7.
26. Modi YS, Epstein A, Smiddy WE, Murray TG, Feuer W, Flynn HW Jr. Retained lens fragments after cataract surgery: outcomes of same-day versus later pars plana vitrectomy. Am J Ophthalmol. 2013;156(3):454–9e1. https://doi.org/10.1016/j.ajo.2013.04.038.
27. Peck T, Park J, Bajwa A, Shildkrot Y. Timing of vitrectomy for retained lens fragments after cataract surgery. Int Ophthalmol. 2018;38(6):2699–707. https://doi.org/10.1007/s10792-017-0719-8.
28. Obuchowska I, Mariak Z. Risk factors of massive suprachoroidal hemorrhage during extracapsular cataract extraction surgery. Eur J Ophthalmol. 2005;15(6):712–7. https://doi.org/10.1177/112067210501500609.
29. Reynolds MG, Haimovici R, Flynn HW Jr, DiBernardo C, Byrne SF, Feuer W. Suprachoroidal hemorrhage. Clinical features and results of secondary surgical management. Ophthalmology. 1993;100(4):460–5.
30. Sharma T, Virdi DS, Parikh S, Gopal L, Badrinath SS, Mukesh BN. A case-control study of suprachoroidal hemorrhage during pars plana vitrectomy. Ophthalmic Surg Lasers. 1997;28(8):640–4.
31. Speaker MG, Guerriero PN, Met JA, Coad CT, Berger A, Marmor M. A case-control study of risk factors for intraoperative suprachoroidal expulsive hemorrhage. Ophthalmology. 1991;98(2):202–9.
32. Welch JC, Spaeth GL, Benson WE. Massive suprachoroidal hemorrhage. Follow-up and outcome of 30 cases. Ophthalmology. 1988;95(9):1202–6.
33. Wong KK, Saleh TA, Gray RH. Suprachoroidal hemorrhage during cataract surgery in a vitrectomized eye. J Cataract Refract Surg. 2005;31(6):1242–3. https://doi.org/10.1016/j.jcrs.2004.10.073.
34. Ling R, Cole M, James C, Kamalarajah S, Foot B, Shaw S. Suprachoroidal haemorrhage complicating cataract surgery in the UK: epidemiology, clinical features, management, and outcomes. Br J Ophthalmol. 2004;88(4):478–80.
35. Ling R, Kamalarajah S, Cole M, James C, Shaw S. Suprachoroidal haemorrhage complicating cataract surgery in the UK: a case control study of risk factors. Br J Ophthalmol. 2004;88(4):474–7. https://doi.org/10.1136/bjo.2003.026179.
36. Hussain N, Hussain A, Khan NA. Favorable outcome after choroidal drainage for postoperative kissing suprachoroidal hemorrhage following trabeculectomy in a high myopic vitrectomised eye. Saudi J Ophthalmol. 2018;32(2):146–50. https://doi.org/10.1016/j.sjopt.2017.10.002.

37. Lin HZ, Huang CT, Lee YC. A blood clot hanging in the anterior chamber due to delayed suprachoroidal hemorrhage after trabeculectomy. Ci Ji Yi Xue Za Zhi. 2016;28(2):73–5. https://doi.org/10.1016/j.tcmj.2015.06.003.
38. Balekudaru S, Basu T, Sen P, Bhende P, Lingam V, George R. Risk factors and outcomes of management of delayed suprachoroidal haemorrhage following Ahmed glaucoma valve implantation in children. Br J Ophthalmol. 2020;104(1):115–20. https://doi.org/10.1136/bjophthalmol-2018-313804.
39. Bandivadekar P, Gupta S, Sharma N. Intraoperative Suprachoroidal hemorrhage after penetrating Keratoplasty: case series and review of literature. Eye Contact Lens. 2016;42(3):206–10. https://doi.org/10.1097/ICL.0000000000000164.
40. Dockery PW, Joubert K, Parker JS, Parker JS. Suprachoroidal hemorrhage during Descemet membrane endothelial Keratoplasty. Cornea. 2020;39(3):376–8. https://doi.org/10.1097/ICO.0000000000002199.
41. Ingraham HJ, Donnenfeld ED, Perry HD. Massive suprachoroidal hemorrhage in penetrating keratoplasty. Am J Ophthalmol. 1989;108(6):670–5. https://doi.org/10.1016/0002-9394(89)90859-3.
42. Price FW Jr, Whitson WE, Ahad KA, Tavakkoli H. Suprachoroidal hemorrhage in penetrating keratoplasty. Ophthalmic Surg. 1994;25(8):521–5.
43. Ariano ML, Ball SF. Delayed nonexpulsive suprachoroidal hemorrhage after trabeculectomy. Ophthalmic Surg. 1987;18(9):661–6.
44. Becquet F, Caputo G, Mashhour B, Chauvaud D, Pouliquen Y. Management of delayed massive suprachoroidal hemorrhage: a clinical retrospective study. Eur J Ophthalmol. 1996;6(4):393–7.
45. Duncker GI, Rochels R. Delayed suprachoroidal hemorrhage after penetrating keratoplasty. Int Ophthalmol. 1995;19(3):173–6. https://doi.org/10.1007/BF00133734.
46. Ghorayeb G, Khan A, Godley BF. Delayed suprachoroidal hemorrhage after cataract surgery. Retin Cases Brief Rep. 2012;6(4):390–2. https://doi.org/10.1097/ICB.0b013e3182437da2.
47. Jin W, Xing Y, Xu Y, Wang W, Yang A. Management of delayed suprachoriodal haemorrhage after intraocular surgery and trauma. Graefes Arch Clin Exp Ophthalmol. 2014;252(8):1189–93. https://doi.org/10.1007/s00417-013-2550-x.
48. Song W, Zhang Y, Chen H, Du C. Delayed suprachoroidal hemorrhage after cataract surgery: a case report and brief review of literature. Medicine (Baltimore). 2018;97(2):e8697. https://doi.org/10.1097/MD.0000000000008697.
49. Syam PP, Hussain B, Anand N. Delayed suprachoroidal hemorrhage after needle revision of trabeculectomy bleb in a patient with hairy cell leukemia. Am J Ophthalmol. 2003;136(6):1155–7. https://doi.org/10.1016/s0002-9394(03)00574-9.
50. Howe LJ, Bloom P. Delayed suprachoroidal haemorrhage following trabeculectomy bleb needling. Br J Ophthalmol. 1999;83(6):757. https://doi.org/10.1136/bjo.83.6.753f.
51. Agustin AL, Miller KM. Posterior dislocation of a plate-haptic silicone intraocular lens with large fixation holes. J Cataract Refract Surg. 2000;26(9):1428–9.
52. Schneiderman TE, Vine AK. Retained lens fragment after phacoemulsification. Ophthalmology. 1995;102(12):1735–6.
53. Stuart AJ, Kontos A, Williamson TH. Managing cases of dislocated intraocular lenses; a retrospective review of cases over a 13 year period. Adv Ophthalmol Vis Syst. 2015;3(3):1–4.
54. Johnston RL, Charteris DG, Horgan SE, Cooling RJ. Combined pars plana vitrectomy and sutured posterior chamber implant. Arch Ophthalmol. 2000;118(7):905–10.
55. Yamane S, Inoue M, Arakawa A, Kadonosono K. Sutureless 27-gauge needle-guided intrascleral intraocular lens implantation with lamellar scleral dissection. Ophthalmology. 2014;121(1):61–6. https://doi.org/10.1016/j.ophtha.2013.08.043.
56. Takayama K, Akimoto M, Taguchi H, Nakagawa S, Hiroi K. Transconjunctival sutureless intrascleral intraocular lens fixation using intrascleral tunnels guided with catheter and 30-gauge needles. Br J Ophthalmol. 2015;99(11):1457–9. https://doi.org/10.1136/bjophthalmol-2014-306579.
57. Kataoka T, Kamei M. Silicone microtube-assisted scleral fixation of a posterior chamber intraocular Lens. Retina. 2018;38(Suppl 1):S146–S53. https://doi.org/10.1097/IAE.0000000000002143.
58. Gentile RC, Eliott D. Silicone oil retention sutures in aphakic eyes with iris loss. Arch Ophthalmol. 128(12):1596–9. 28/12/1596 [pii]. https://doi.org/10.1001/archophthalmol.2010.300.
59. Javitt JC, Vitale S, Canner JK, Street DA, Krakauer H, McBean AM, et al. National outcomes of cataract extraction. Endophthalmitis following inpatient surgery. Arch Ophthalmol. 1991;109(8):1085–9.
60. Kamalarajah S, Silvestri G, Sharma N, Khan A, Foot B, Ling R, et al. Surveillance of endophthalmitis following cataract surgery in the UK. Eye. 2004;18(6):580–7.
61. Wykoff CC, Parrott MB, Flynn HW Jr, Shi W, Miller D, Alfonso EC. Nosocomial acute-onset postoperative endophthalmitis at a university teaching hospital (2002–2009). Am J Ophthalmol. 150(3):392–8e2. doi: S0002-9394(10)00266-7 [pii]. https://doi.org/10.1016/j.ajo.2010.04.010.
62. Pershing S, Lum F, Hsu S, Kelly S, Chiang MF, Rich WL 3rd, et al. Endophthalmitis after cataract surgery in the United States: a report from the intelligent research in sight registry, 2013–2017. Ophthalmology. 2020;127(2):151–8. https://doi.org/10.1016/j.ophtha.2019.08.026.
63. Wisniewski SR, Capone A, Kelsey SF, Groer-Fitzgerald S, Lambert HM, Doft BH. Characteristics after cataract extraction or secondary lens implantation among patients screened for the Endophthalmitis vitrectomy study. Ophthalmology. 2000;107(7):1274–82.
64. Ciulla TA, Beck AD, Topping TM, Baker AS. Blebitis, early endophthalmitis, and late endophthalmitis after glaucoma-filtering surgery. Ophthalmology. 1997;104(6):986–95.
65. Doft BM, Kelsey SF, Wisniewski SR. Retinal detachment in the endophthalmitis vitrectomy study. Arch Ophthalmol. 2000;118(12):1661–5.
66. Han DP, Wisniewski SR, Kelsey SF, Doft BH, Barza M, Pavan PR. Microbiologic yields and complication rates of vitreous needle aspiration versus mechanized vitreous biopsy in the Endophthalmitis vitrectomy study. Retina. 1999;19(2):98–102.
67. Han DP, Wisniewski SR, Wilson LA, Barza M, Vine AK, Doft BH, et al. Spectrum and susceptibilities of microbiologic isolates in the Endophthalmitis vitrectomy study. Am J Ophthalmol. 1996;122(1):1–17.
68. Yoder DM, Scott IU, Flynn HW Jr, Miller D. Endophthalmitis caused by *Haemophilus influenzae*. Ophthalmology. 2004;111(11):2023–6.
69. Eifrig CW, Scott IU, Flynn HW Jr, Miller D. Endophthalmitis caused by *Pseudomonas aeruginosa*. Ophthalmology. 2003;110(9):1714–7.
70. Scott IU, Matharoo N, Flynn HW Jr, Miller D. Endophthalmitis caused by Klebsiella species. Am J Ophthalmol. 2004;138(4):662–3.
71. Meisler DM, Mandelbaum S. Propionibacterium-associated endophthalmitis after extracapsular cataract extraction. Review of reported cases. Ophthalmology. 1989;96(1):54–61.
72. Bannerman TL, Rhoden DL, McAllister SK, Miller JM, Wilson LA. The source of coagulase-negative staphylococci in the Endophthalmitis vitrectomy study. A comparison of eyelid and intraocular isolates using pulsed-field gel electrophoresis. Arch Ophthalmol. 1997;115(3):357–61.

73. Deramo VA, Lai JC, Winokur J, Luchs J, Udell IJ. Visual outcome and bacterial sensitivity after methicillin-resistant *Staphylococcus aureus*-associated acute endophthalmitis. Am J Ophthalmol. 2008;145(3):413–7. doi: S0002-9394(07)00927-0 [pii]. https://doi.org/10.1016/j.ajo.2007.10.020.
74. Narang S, Gupta A, Gupta V, Dogra MR, Ram J, Pandav SS, et al. Fungal endophthalmitis following cataract surgery: clinical presentation, microbiological spectrum, and outcome. Am J Ophthalmol. 2001;132(5):609–17.
75. Results of the Endophthalmitis Vitrectomy Study. A randomized trial of immediate vitrectomy and of intravenous antibiotics for the treatment of postoperative bacterial endophthalmitis. Endophthalmitis vitrectomy study group. Arch Ophthalmol. 1995;113(12):1479–96.
76. Ferencz JR, Assia EI, Diamantstein L, Rubinstein E. Vancomycin concentration in the vitreous after intravenous and intravitreal administration for postoperative endophthalmitis. Arch Ophthalmol. 1999;117(8):1023–7.
77. Gan IM, van Dissel JT, Beekhuis WH, Swart W, van Meurs JC. Intravitreal vancomycin and gentamicin concentrations in patients with postoperative endophthalmitis. Br J Ophthalmol. 2001;85(11):1289–93.
78. Campochiaro PA, Conway BP. Aminoglycoside toxicity--a survey of retinal specialists. Implications for ocular use. Arch Ophthalmol. 1991;109(7):946–50.
79. Waltz K, Margo CE. Intraocular gentamicin toxicity. Arch Ophthalmol. 1991;109(7):911.
80. Jackson TL, Williamson TH. Amikacin retinal toxicity. Br J Ophthalmol. 1999;83(10):1199–200.
81. Campochiaro PA, Lim JI. Aminoglycoside toxicity in the treatment of endophthalmitis. The aminoglycoside toxicity study group. Arch Ophthalmol. 1994;112(1):48–53.
82. Seawright AA, Bourke RD, Cooling RJ. Macula toxicity after intravitreal amikacin. Aust N Z J Ophthalmol. 1996;24(2):143–6.
83. Shah GK, Stein JD, Sharma S, Sivalingam A, Benson WE, Regillo CD, et al. Visual outcomes following the use of intravitreal steroids in the treatment of postoperative endophthalmitis. Ophthalmology. 2000;107(3):486–9.
84. Doft BH, Kelsey SF, Wisniewski SR. Additional procedures after the initial vitrectomy or tap-biopsy in the Endophthalmitis vitrectomy study. Ophthalmology. 1998;105(4):707–16.
85. Soliman MK, Gini G, Kuhn F, Iros M, Parolini B, Ozdek S, et al. International practice patterns for the management of acute postsurgical and postintravitreal injection endophthalmitis: European vitreo-retinal society endophthalmitis study report 1. Ophthalmol Retina. 2019;3(6):461–7. https://doi.org/10.1016/j.oret.2019.03.009.
86. Clarke B, Williamson TH, Gini G, Gupta B. Management of bacterial postoperative endophthalmitis and the role of vitrectomy. Surv Ophthalmol. 2018;63(5):677–93. https://doi.org/10.1016/j.survophthal.2018.02.003.
87. Chiquet C, Maurin M, Thuret G, Benito Y, Cornut PL, Creuzot-Garcher C, et al. Analysis of diluted vitreous samples from vitrectomy is useful in eyes with severe acute postoperative endophthalmitis. Ophthalmology. 2009;116(12):2437–41e1. doi: S0161-6420(09)00609-5 [pii]. https://doi.org/10.1016/j.ophtha.2009.06.007.
88. Ng JQ, Morlet N, Pearman JW, Constable IJ, McAllister IL, Kennedy CJ, et al. Management and outcomes of postoperative Endophthalmitis since the Endophthalmitis vitrectomy study the Endophthalmitis population study of Western Australia (EPSWA)'s fifth report. Ophthalmology. 2005;
89. Doft BH, Kelsey SF, Wisniewski S, Metz DJ, Lobes L, Rinkoff J, et al. Treatment of endophthalmitis after cataract extraction. Retina. 1994;14(4):297–304.
90. Endophthalmitis Vitrectomy Study Group. Microbiologic factors and visual outcome in the endophthalmitis vitrectomy study. Am J Ophthalmol. 1996;122(6):830–46.
91. Chien AM, Raber IM, Fischer DH, Eagle RC Jr, Naidoff MA. *Propionibacterium acnes* endophthalmitis after intracapsular cataract extraction. Ophthalmology. 1992;99(4):487–90.
92. Chen JC, Roy M. Epidemic Bacillus endophthalmitis after cataract surgery II: chronic and recurrent presentation and outcome. Ophthalmology. 2000;107(6):1038–41.
93. Adan A, Casaroli-Marano RP, Gris O, Navarro R, Bitrian E, Pelegrin L, et al. Pathological findings in the lens capsules and intraocular lens in chronic pseudophakic endophthalmitis: an electron microscopy study. Eye. 2008;22(1):113–9. doi: 6702615 [pii]. https://doi.org/10.1038/sj.eye.6702615.
94. Modi D, Pyatetsky D, Edward DP, Ulanski LJ, Pursell KJ, Tessler HH, et al. *Mycobacterium haemophilum*: a rare cause of endophthalmitis. Retina. 2007;27(8):1148–51. https://doi.org/10.1097/IAE.0b013e318030e622. 00006982-200710000-00028 [pii]
95. Nehemy MB, Vasconcelos-Santos DV, Torqueti-Costa L, Magalhaes EP. Chronic endophthalmitis due to verticillium species after cataract surgery treated (or managed) with pars plana vitrectomy and oral and intravitreal voriconazole. Retina. 2006;26(2):225–7. doi: 00006982-200602000-00019 [pii]
96. Newell CK, Steinmetz RL, Brooks HL Jr. Chronic postoperative endophthalmitis caused by Bipolaris australiensis. Retina. 2006;26(1):109–10. doi: 00006982-200601000-00020 [pii]
97. Duker JS, Belmont JB, Benson WE, Brooks HL Jr, Brown GC, Federman JL, et al. Inadvertent globe perforation during retrobulbar and peribulbar anesthesia. Patient characteristics, surgical management, and visual outcome. Ophthalmology. 1991;98(4):519–26.
98. Edge R, Navon S. Scleral perforation during retrobulbar and peribulbar anesthesia: risk factors and outcome in 50,000 consecutive injections. J Cataract Refract Surg. 1999;25(9):1237–44.
99. Gadkari SS. Evaluation of 19 cases of inadvertent globe perforation due to periocular injections. Indian J Ophthalmol. 2007;55(2):103–7.
100. Frieman BJ, Friedberg MA. Globe perforation associated with subtenon's anesthesia. Am J Ophthalmol. 2001;131(4):520–1.
101. Faure C, Faure L, Billotte C. Globe perforation following no-needle sub-Tenon anesthesia. J Cataract Refract Surg. 2009;35(8):1471–2. doi: S0886-3350(09)00403-9 [pii]. https://doi.org/10.1016/j.jcrs.2009.03.024.
102. Puri P, Verma D, McKibbin M. Management of ocular perforations resulting from peribulbar anaesthesia. Indian J Ophthalmol. 1999;47(3):181–3.
103. McCombe M, Heriot W. Penetrating ocular injury following local anaesthesia. Aust N Z J Ophthalmol. 1995;23(1):33–6.
104. Wadood AC, Dhillon B, Singh J. Inadvertent ocular perforation and intravitreal injection of an anesthetic agent during retrobulbar injection. J Cataract Refract Surg. 2002;28(3):562–5.
105. Minihan M, Williamson TH. Ocular explosions from periocular anesthetic injections. Ophthalmology. 2000;107(11):1965.
106. Benhamou N, Massin P, Haouchine B, Audren F, Tadayoni R, Gaudric A. Intravitreal triamcinolone for refractory pseudophakic macular edema. Am J Ophthalmol. 2003;135(2):246–9.
107. Costen MT, Williams CP, Asteriades S, Luff AJ. An unusual maculopathy after routine cataract surgery. Eye (Lond). 2007;21(11):1416–8. doi: 6702587 [pii]. https://doi.org/10.1038/sj.eye.6702587.

Trauma

18

Contents

T. H. Williamson, *Vitreoretinal Surgery*, https://doi.org/10.1007/978-3-030-68769-4_18

Introduction

Ocular trauma remains a leading cause of visual loss, most often affecting men (on average five males are affected to one female). Patients are usually aged less than 30 years, and trauma is often associated with alcohol and illicit drug usage [1]. In the elderly, males and females are equally involved [2]. Incidence has been estimated as 3:10000 of the population [3, 4]. Severe injuries account for 5% of all eye injuries [5]. Aetiology is variable but certain associations are common, e.g. assault, sport, children at play, road traffic accidents, industrial, domestic and war injuries [6–9].

The patterns of ocular trauma are constantly changing depending on social, demographic and geographical variations. The clinical characteristics vary widely. Intraocular foreign bodies are common in war [9] and road traffic accidents especially when car seat belts are not worn [10]. In children, sharp objects are commonly implicated and the complication of amblyopia limits visual recovery [11]. The wearing of spectacles has been found to be protective [12].

Classification (Fig. 18.1)

The Birmingham Eye Trauma Classification (BETT) is a useful system to allow the organisation of the clinical presentation of these patients and aid communication of findings between clinicians [13].

It is worth learning and using the terminology from BETT.

1. Eyewall Sclera and cornea
2. Closed globe injury No full-thickness wound of the eyewall
3. Open globe injury Full-thickness wound of the eyewall
4. Contusion There is no (full-thickness) wound.
5. Lamellar laceration Partial-thickness wound of the eyewall
6. Rupture Full-thickness wound of the eyewall, caused by a blunt object
7. Laceration Full-thickness wound of the eyewall, caused by a sharp object
8. Penetrating injury Entrance wound or wounds from object or objects
9. IOFB Intraocular foreign body in the eye
10. Perforating injury Entrance and exit wounds from the same object

The BETT however is less good for describing the mode of injury which can be from blunt objects as in assaults from fists, feet, wooden bats or other causes, e.g. balls in sport, airbags [14–16], paintballs [17] and bungee elastic cords [18], from sharp instruments such as broken glass, knives or fragments of metal.

Trauma was a very early indication for the use of vitrectomy [19–25] with increased experience and availability of techniques leading to improved success rates [26] (Figs. 18.2 and 18.3)

Contusion Injuries (Figs. 18.4, 18.5, 18.6, 18.7, 18.8, 18.9, 18.10, 18.11, 18.12, 18.2)

Clinical Presentation

Presentations of Contusion Injury

- Subluxated or dislocated lens
- Vitreous haemorrhage
- Macular oedema and commotio retinae
- Retinal detachment

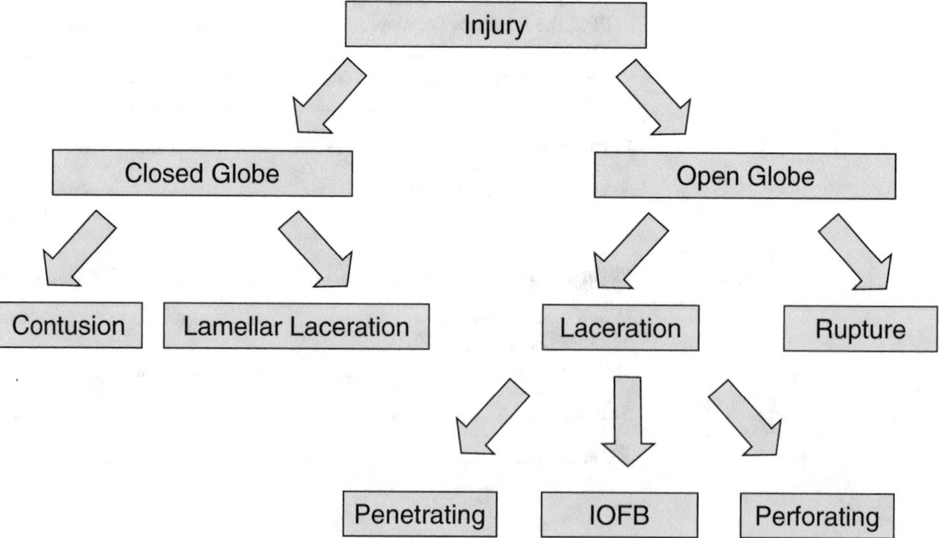

Fig. 18.1 The Birmingham Eye Trauma Terminology is a useful method for classifying trauma and allows adequate communication between surgeons

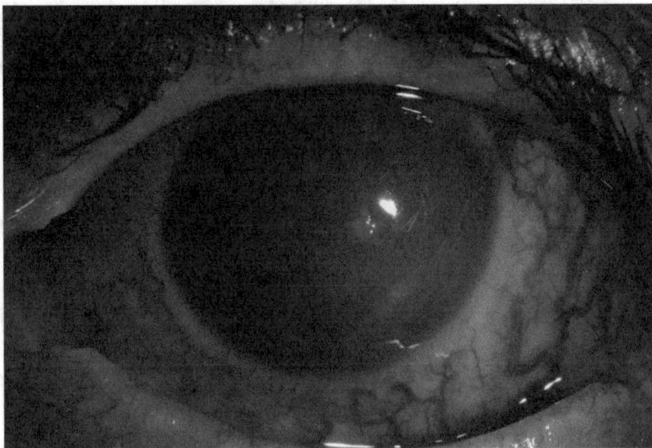

Fig. 18.2 This patient's cornea shows severe staining of the corneal stroma after hyphaema from a severe injury to the eye from an assault. This can make visualisation of the posterior segment difficult during PPV. Usually, with corneal opacities, it remains possible to visualise through a segment of clear cornea, in rare cases a keratoprosthesis (e.g. Ekhart) is required

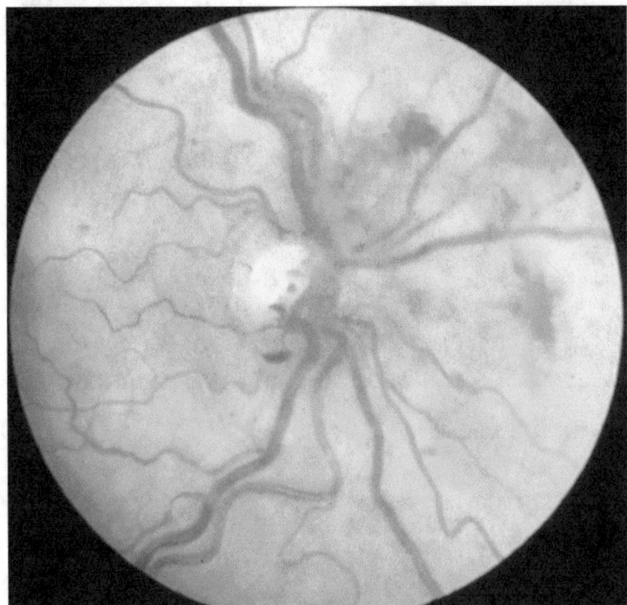

Fig. 18.3 The shock wave from a high-velocity projectile is enough to disrupt the structure of the retina

  - Dialysis usually with a "bucket handle" vitreous base avulsion
  - Giant retinal tear
  - Ragged retinal tear in an area of commotion retinae
  - Pars ciliaris tear
  - U tears from induced PVD
- Late retinal pigment epithelial changes
- Macular hole
- Choroidal rupture, haemorrhage
- Submacular haemorrhage

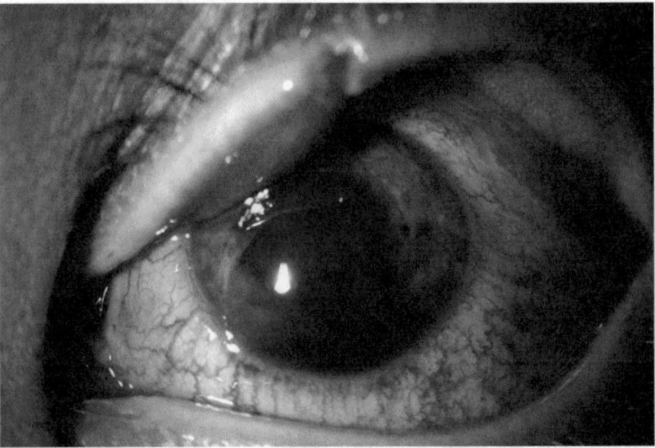

Fig. 18.4 This patient was struck by weight from a fishing line and has suffered a blunt injury that damaged the upper lid. It caused a hyphaema and an optic nerve avulsion

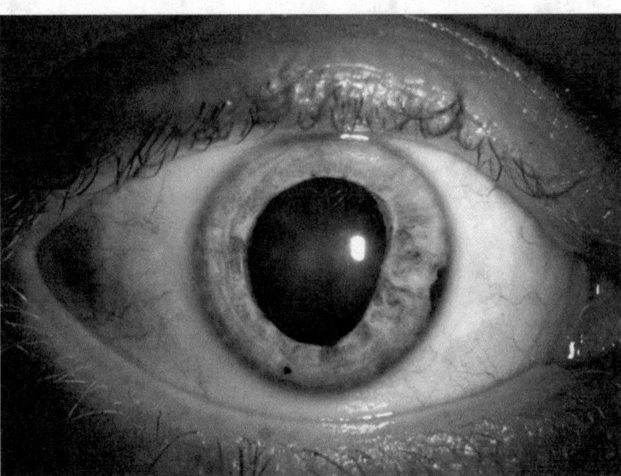

Fig. 18.5 This patient has suffered an iris root dialysis from a blast injury during a terrorist bomb attack. The eye was hypotonous for many weeks post injury but finally recovered to 20/20 after cataract extraction

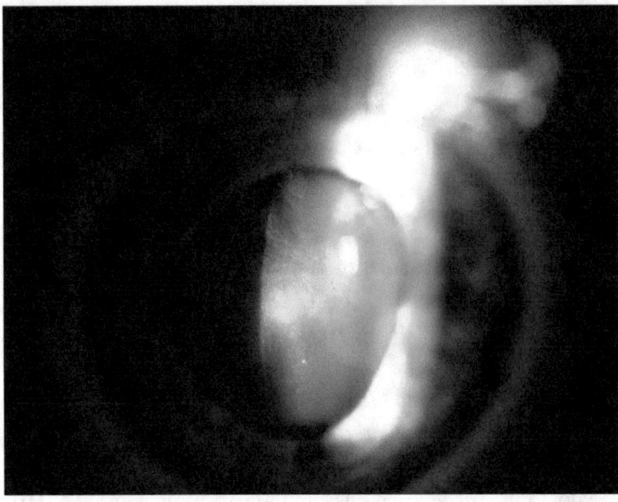

Fig. 18.6 The patient suffered a typical traumatic sunflower cataract

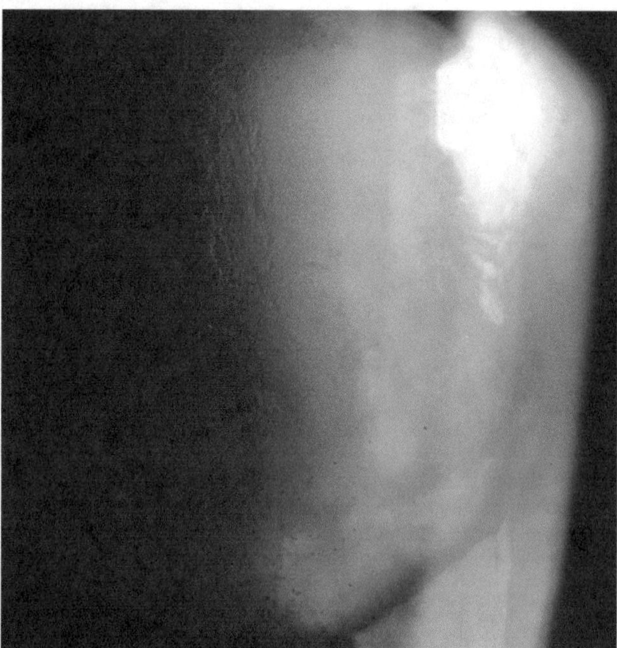

Fig. 18.7 The vitreous in the AC in this patient with contusion injury indicates zonular dehiscence. The patient had lenticulodonesis which was too unstable for routine phacoemulsification cataract extraction and required PPV and cataract extraction with anterior chamber lens insertion

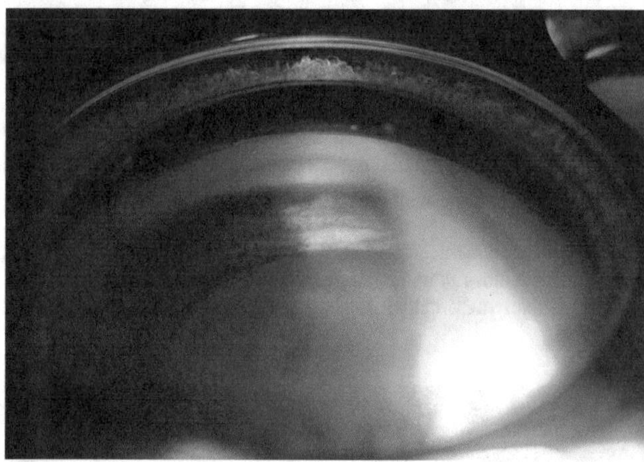

Fig. 18.8 Angle recession is visible in a patient who suffered a blunt injury whilst shaking out wet clothing when the metal zip of a shirt hit her eye

- Choroidal neovascular membrane
- Optic nerve avulsion (Figs. 18.13, 18.14, 18.15, 18.16, 18.17, 18.18, 18.19, 18.20, 18.21, 18.22 and 18.23)

Contusion injuries occur when the eye is struck by an object, but the eyewall remains intact. This is common in assaults from the use of fists or feet or from injury from balls in sport but can also be encountered from airbags [14–16], paintballs [17], and bungee elastic cords [18]. In mild injury,

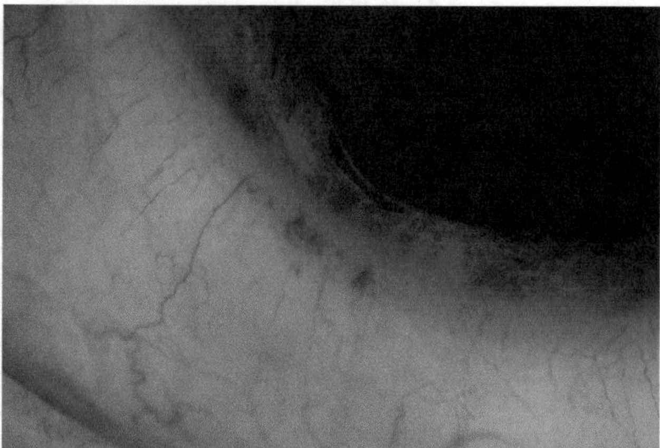

Fig. 18.9 Paintball gaming is associated with blunt injuries to the eye when the participants remove their googles to clear them of condensation and are struck in the eye by a paint pellet. This patient suffered an iridodialysis and rupture in the posterior lens capsule which caused a rapid onset cataract

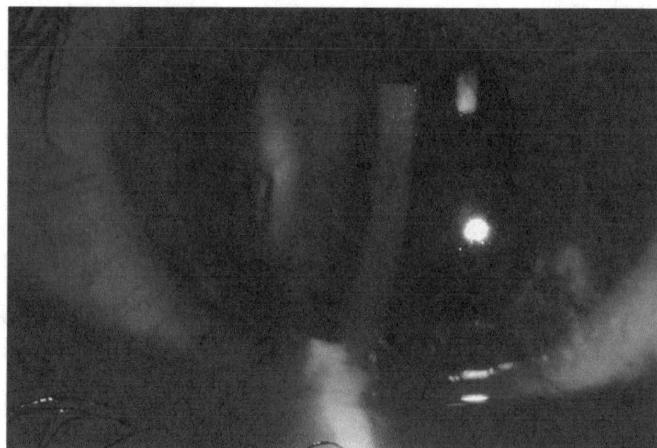

Fig. 18.10 Traumatic lens injury

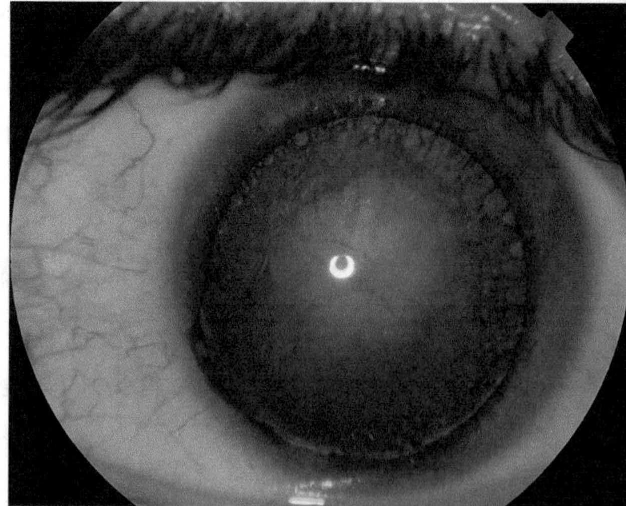

Fig. 18.11 Two months after the injury with the paintball, an extensive posterior subcapsular cataract has developed

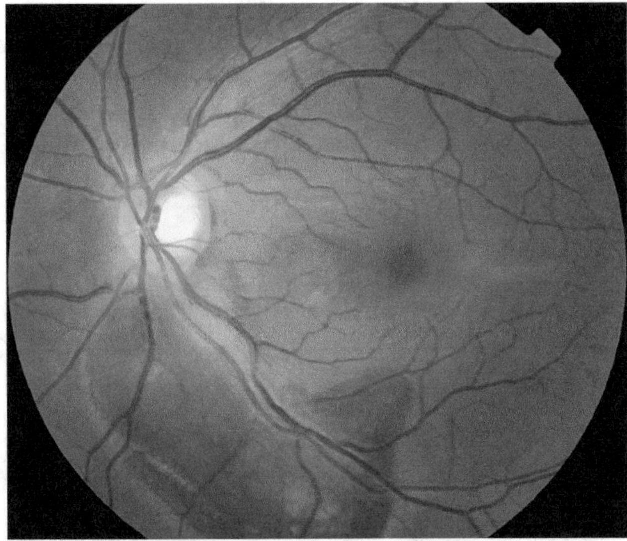

Fig. 18.12 This patient was punched in the eye causing a subretinal haemorrhage which is likely to have an underlying choroidal haemorrhage, vision was 20/20

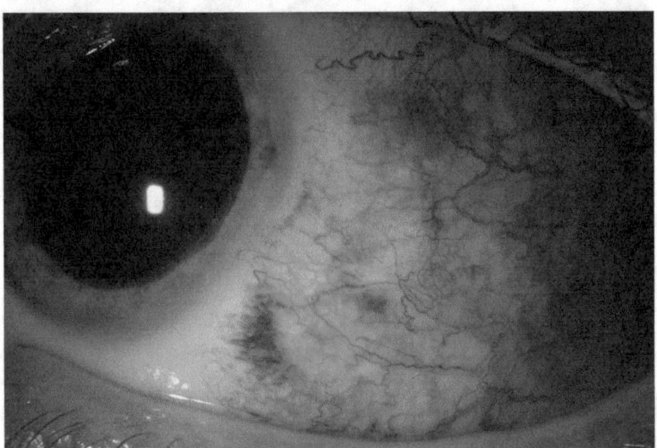

Fig. 18.13 This eye was struck by a squash ball. There are minimal signs on the exterior of the eye

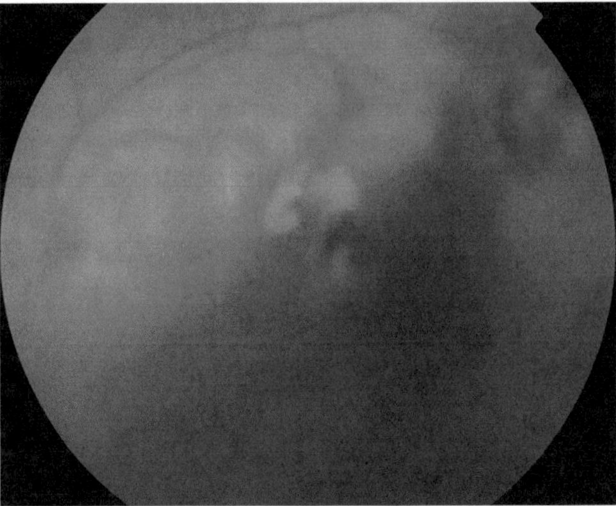

Fig. 18.14 The eye was filled with vitreous haemorrhage and rolled up retina could be seen near the macula

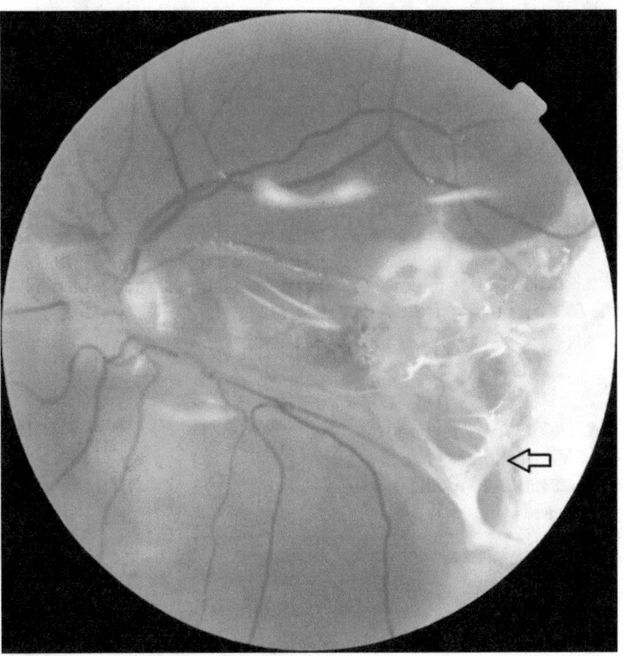

Fig. 18.15 After removal of the vitreous haemorrhage a large area of severe chorioretinal damage was found. PVR developed postoperatively causing the folding of the retina over the disc and transretinal fibrosis at the edge of the scar

the retina shows commotio (whitening) which clears after a few days, sometimes accompanied by macular oedema (Berlin's oedema).

Vision can be lost from macular oedema, commotio retinae, choroidal rupture, lens dislocation, glaucoma, hyphaema, retinal detachment, choroidal haemorrhage, and vitreous haemorrhage.

Corneal staining may result from hyphaema and choroidal neovascular membrane from choroidal rupture. The retina may show late retinal pigment epithelial changes from diffuse retinal damage.

Lens dislocation may occur in patients with pseudoexfoliation, or pseudophakia or in highly myopic eyes.

Ultrasound is helpful to assess the type of haemorrhage in patients with medial opacities to determine a prognosis for vision and surgical options. Traumatic macular hole formation may occur (Figs. 18.24, 18.25 and 18.26).

Types of Retinal Break

Dialysis (Fig. 18.27)

In blunt trauma the commonest break is inferotemporal dialysis then superonasal (see Chap. 6). The slow onset detachment may not become symptomatic until months or years after the injury when the macula detaches. Occasionally, an avulsion of the vitreous base is seen comprising a strip of ciliary epithelium, ora serrata, and immediately post-oral retina into which the basal vitreous gel remains inserted. This "bucket handle" often in the superonasal quadrant hangs down in the vitreous cavity. The free posterior edge of the torn retina becomes detached. Beware that some patients can present with giant dialysis (90–360°) in contusion injuries. If the dialysis detaches early the retina is mobile. If it appears late, the retina and break are usually stiff and immobile.

Fig. 18.16 Notice removal of the transretinal fibrosis and flattening of the fold over the optic disc after surgery

Par Ciliaris Tears

In a few cases, retinal tears may be found in the non-pigmented epithelium of the pars ciliaris. These are difficult

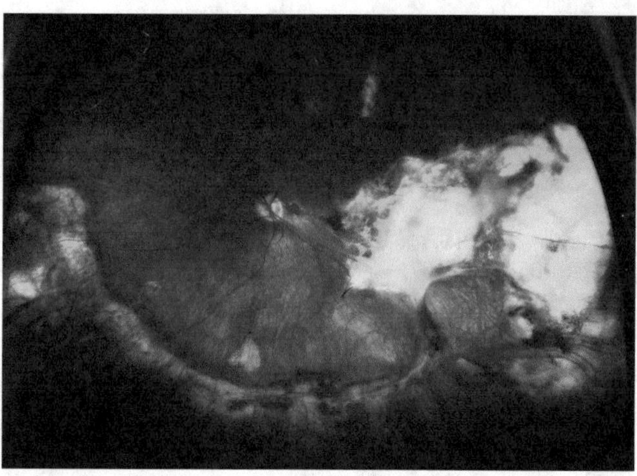

Fig. 18.18 Squash ball injury, 10 months after the removal of the silicone oil the retina remains stable, the traumatic scar in the macular and temporal retina can be seen. Note the retinectomy edge inferiorly and nasally

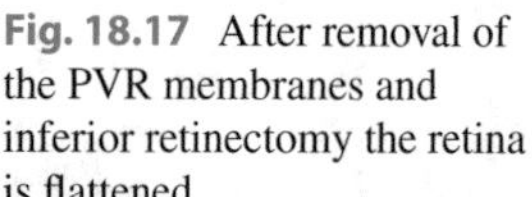

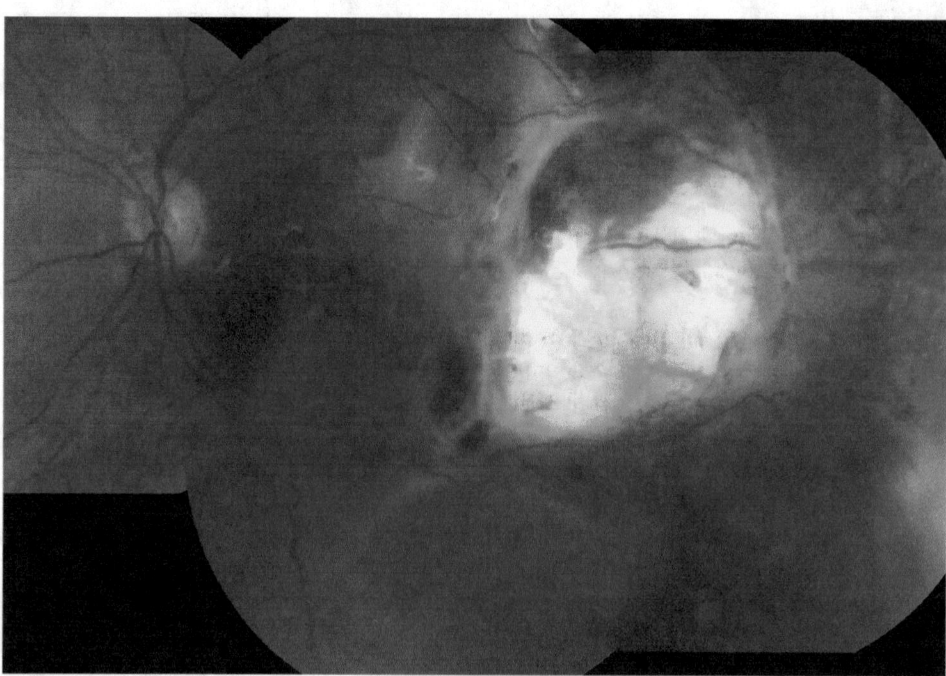

Fig. 18.17 After removal of the PVR membranes and inferior retinectomy the retina is flattened

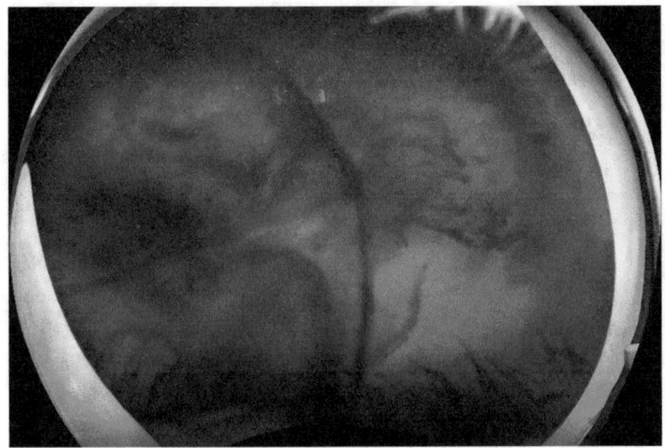

Fig. 18.19 A vitreous haemorrhage from the eye being struck by a rebounding nail from a nail gun

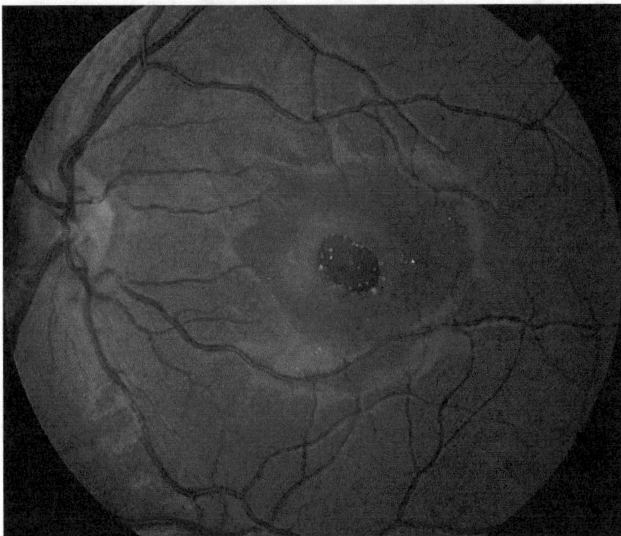

Fig. 18.20 A traumatic macular hole

to detect, typically causing a slow onset shallow retinal detachment [27]. This should be considered in children with a poor history and a chronic RRD.

Ragged Tear in Commotion Retinae

In severe injury, the choroid and retina have an ischemic and haemorrhagic appearance (scloptera) and can produce a ragged degenerative break that may be large. This should be treated by observation at first. The attached vitreous creates a slow onset RRD. Once retinal detachment appears, intervention is indicated [28].

Giant Retinal Tears

Occasionally, posterior vitreous detachment related tears can be seen most classically giant retinal tears but occasionally U tears.

Note: In contusion injury it is often possible to wait and see what develops (Figs. 18.28, 18.29, 18.30, 18.31, 18.32, 18.33, 18.34, 18.35, 18.36, 18.37, 18.38, 18.39 and 18.40).

Surgery (Table 18.1)

Posterior segment surgery may be necessary for:

- Dislocation or subluxation of the lens
- Vitreous haemorrhage
- Choroidal haemorrhage
- Retinal detachment
- Macular hole
- Macular subretinal haemorrhage

Note: when the view is extremely poor it may be useful to put the infusion (with small gauge instrumentation insert the cannula without using the stent) in through the limbus into the AC. Once some of the anterior vitreous haemorrhages have been cleared with the cutter, the infusion can be moved to its usual position and be checked visually before switching on.

Surgery for RRD depends on the type of break and the principles outlined in the previous chapters.

Choroidal Haemorrhage

Switch on the infusion. When fashioning the superior sclerotomies green liquefied blood will exit via the sclerotomies if choroidal haemorrhage. Usually, a considerable residual clot remains in the suprachoroidal space. It is not usually possible to remove this. Excise the vitreous cavity haemorrhage whilst being aware of the chorioretinal elevation. Silicone oil is inserted to prevent further vitreous cavity opacity. As the choroidal haemorrhage resolves over weeks or months, under fill of the silicone oil will become apparent causing the refractive visual disturbance. Rarely, a suprachoroidal cystic space remains, permanently elevating the retina and choroid.

A recent innovation is to insert 0.05 mls of 50 micrograms of Tissue Plasminogen Activator (TPA) a few hours prior to the vitrectomy. This may help liquify any choroidal haemorrhage.

Other Presentations

Dislocation of the lens is a common complication and managed as per the principles described elsewhere (see Chap. 16).

Vitreous haemorrhage can be dealt with by PPV but be aware that there is likely to be other intraocular injuries. The haemorrhage can be very thick, and the cutter may not be as efficient in its removal. There may or may not be a PVD.

Choroidal haemorrhage will usually breakthrough into the vitreous cavity sometimes causing hyphaema (in severe

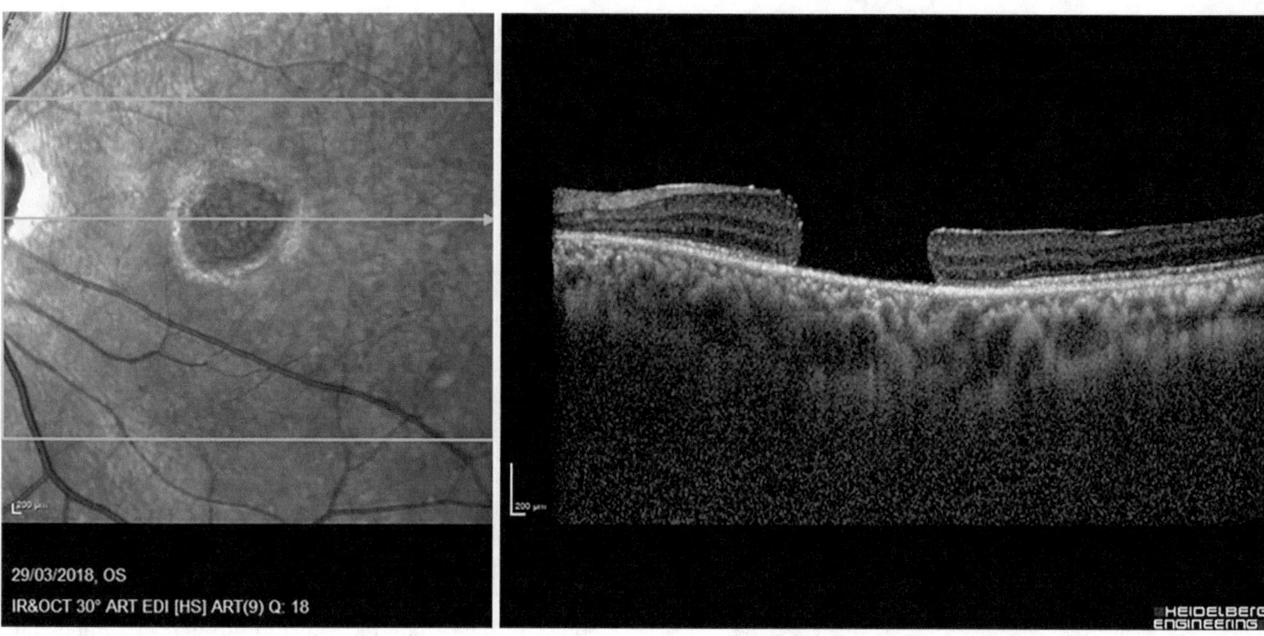

Fig. 18.21 A traumatic MH

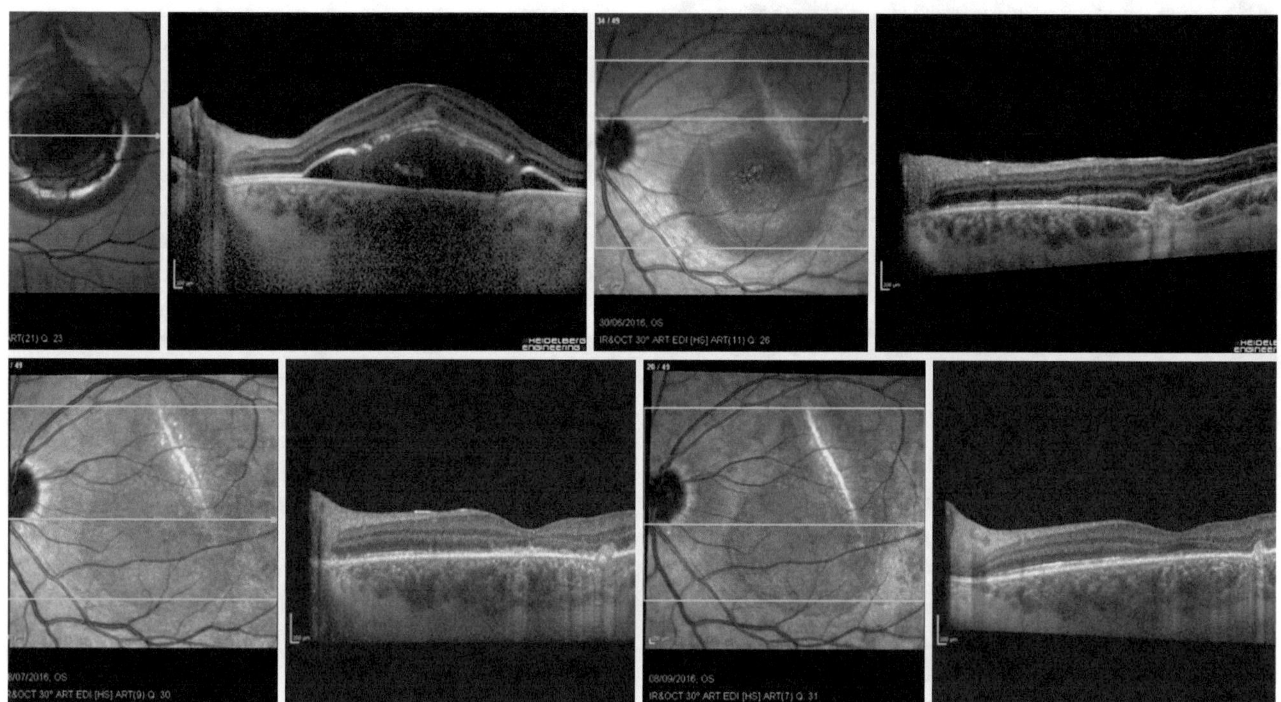

Fig. 18.22 Squash ball injury with subretinal haemorrhage with a pneumatic displacement of the blood. The final vision was 6/36

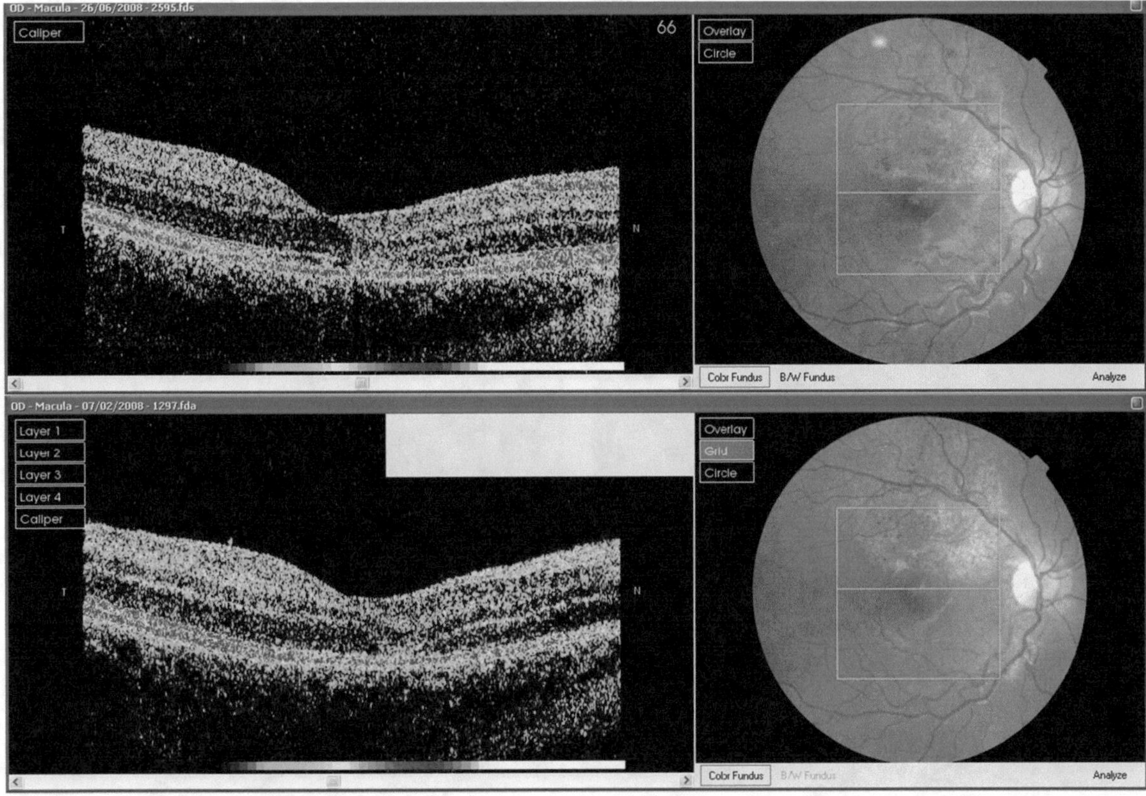

Fig. 18.23 These images show the evolution of pigmentary changes and OCT findings in the retina over 6 months from a contusion injury from a football hitting the eye, early scan on the bottom and late on top

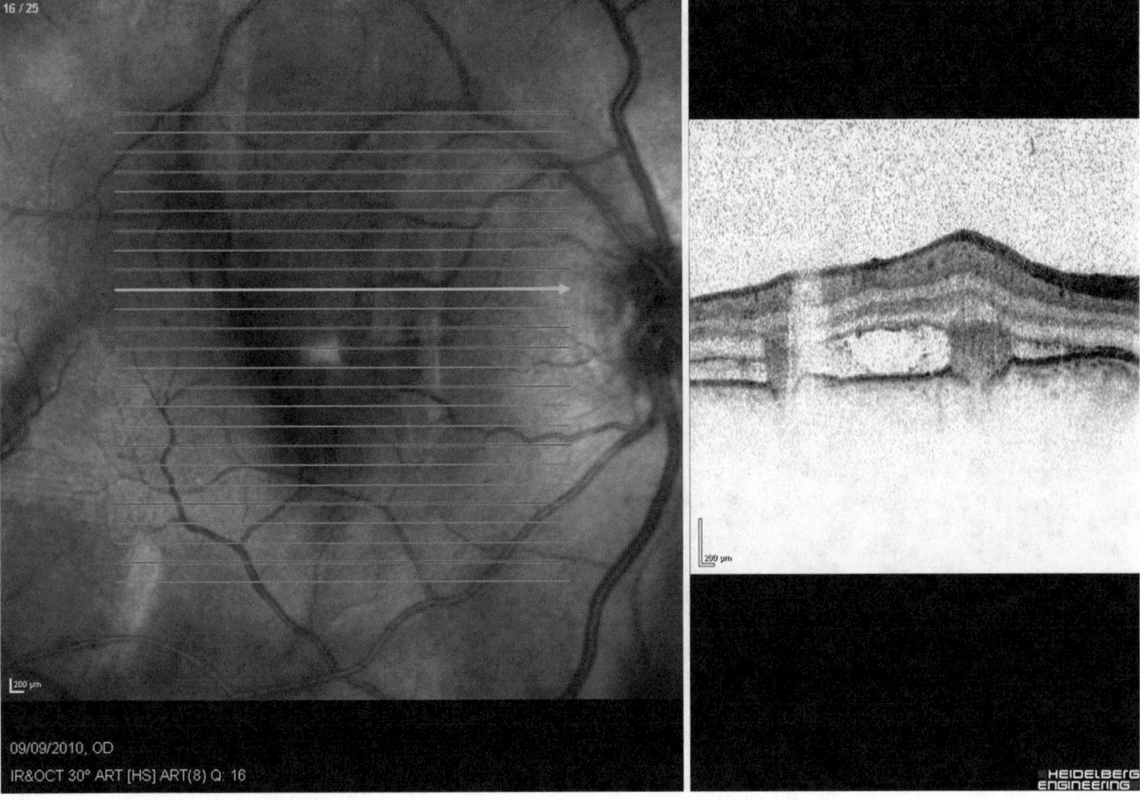

Fig. 18.24 This eye was struck by an elasticated cord used for holding luggage on a roof rack. This has caused choroidal ruptures seen on an OCT lifting the retina

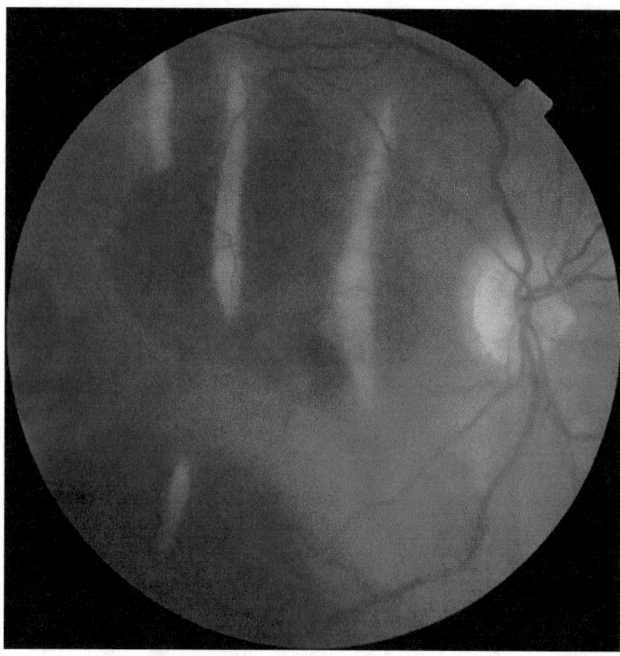

Fig. 18.25 Choroidal ruptures

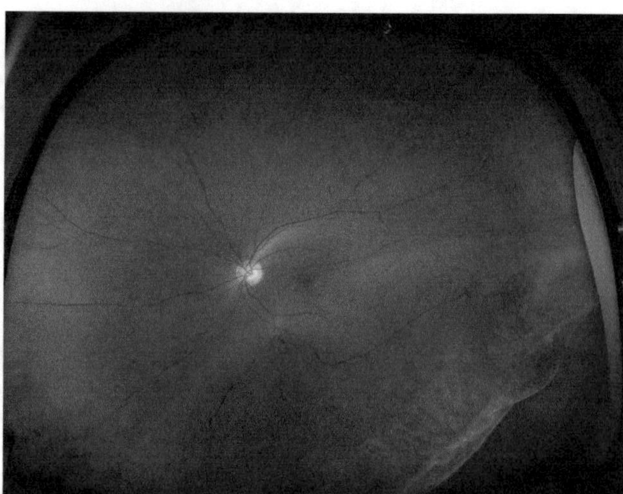

Fig. 18.27 This patient had been struck in the eye by a tennis ball 9 months previously. There is now an RRD with inferotemporal dialysis

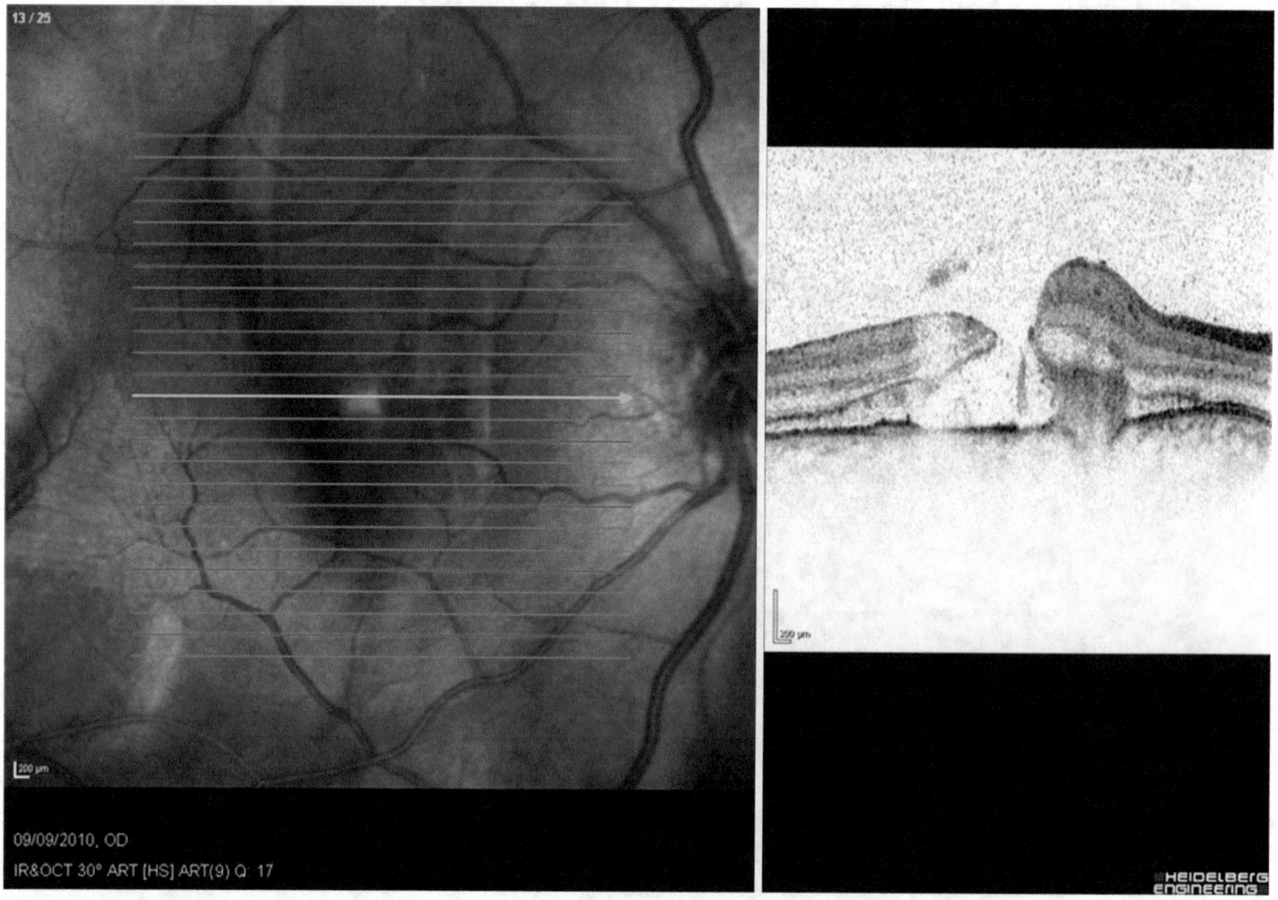

Fig. 18.26 In the fovea, there is evidence of a macular hole

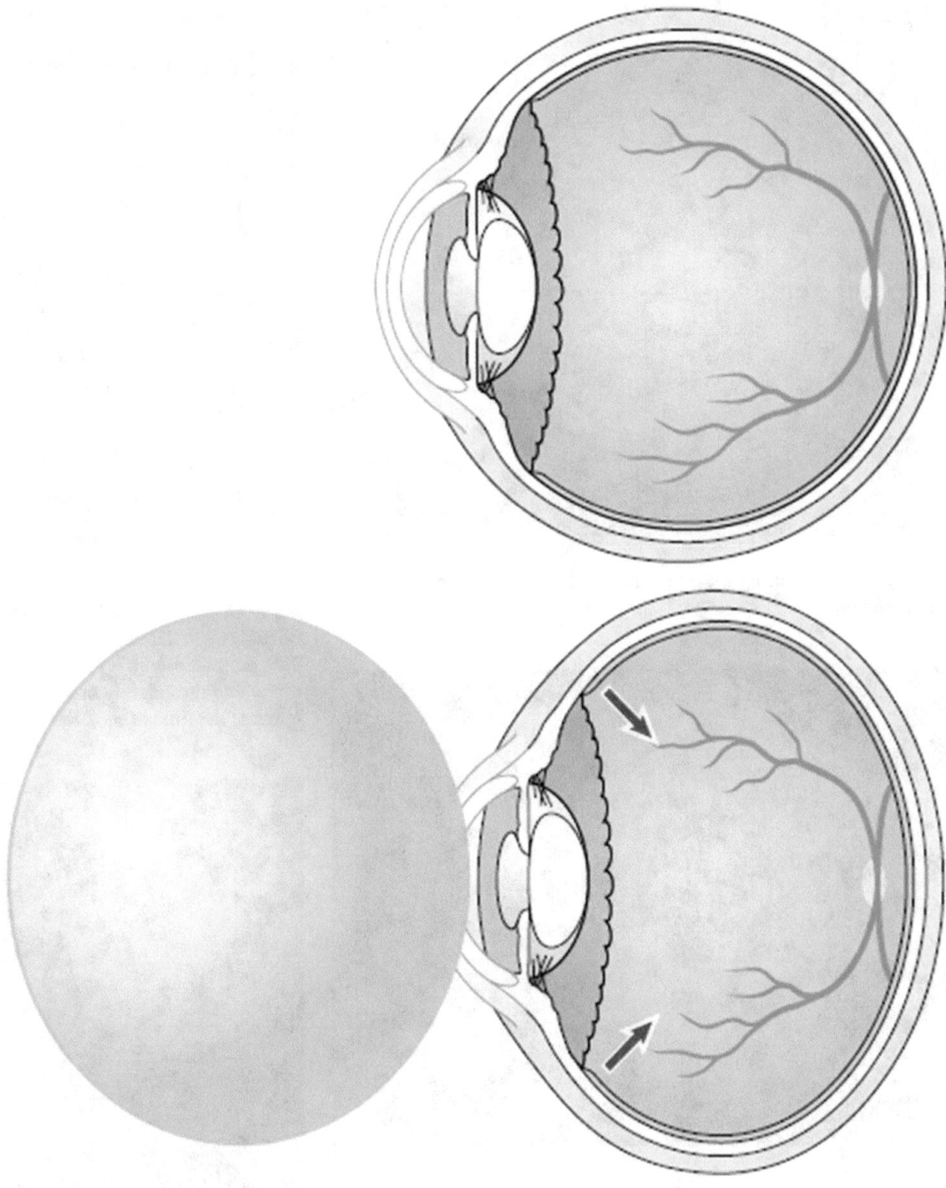

Fig. 18.28 A squash ball is ideally sized to transfer all its energy to the same sized globe. The impact causes distortion of the globe which allows the vitreous base to move inwards relative to the adjacent sclera, the probable mechanism for retinal dialysis formation

cases eight ball hyphaema, i.e. completely filling the anterior chamber, with a risk of corneal staining) and erythroclastic glaucoma. On insertion of the infusion cannula (use a 6 mm cannula if necessary), take extra care not to infuse suprachoroidal fluid by checking the cannula is through all layers. If in doubt insert an AC maintainer till your view improves.

The macula can be operated upon as per the diagnosis with PPV, ILM and gas for macular holes and pneumatic displacement for subretinal haemorrhage (Figs. 18.41, 18.42, 18.43, 18.44, 18.45, 18.46 and 18.47).

Visual Outcome

The visual outcome is dependent on the mechanism of injury, but contusion injury severe enough to require vitreoretinal intervention is associated with only a 50% chance of better than 20/200 vision (Figs. 18.48, 18.49, and 18.50).

Rupture

Clinical Presentation (Figs. 18.51, 18.52, and 18.53) [29]

Blunt trauma may rupture the eyewall, most commonly the sclera at the limbus or posterior to the extraocular muscle insertions, often with immediate loss of the crystalline lens and prolapse of the choroid and retina. Old surgical wounds are also prone to opening, e.g. corneal grafts and extracapsular cataract extraction wounds. Rupture may be commoner than anticipated. In one study, 72% of eyes with severe blunt

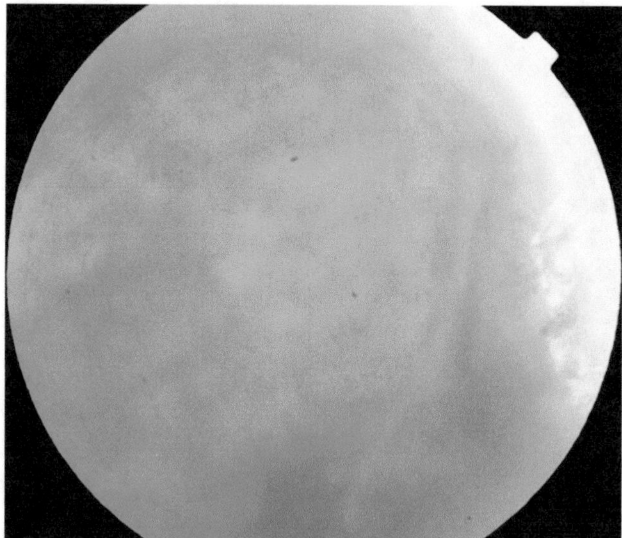

Fig. 18.29 In blunt injuries, the vitreous base can become separated from the retina

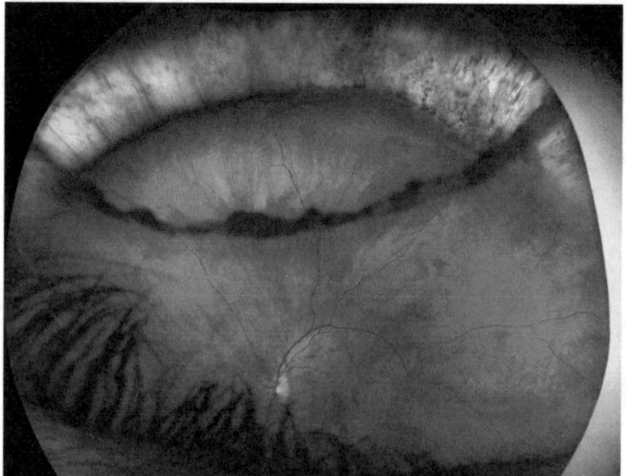

Fig. 18.30 A buckle was applied to treat this traumatic retinal dialysis. The bucket handle dehiscence of the vitreous base can still be seen

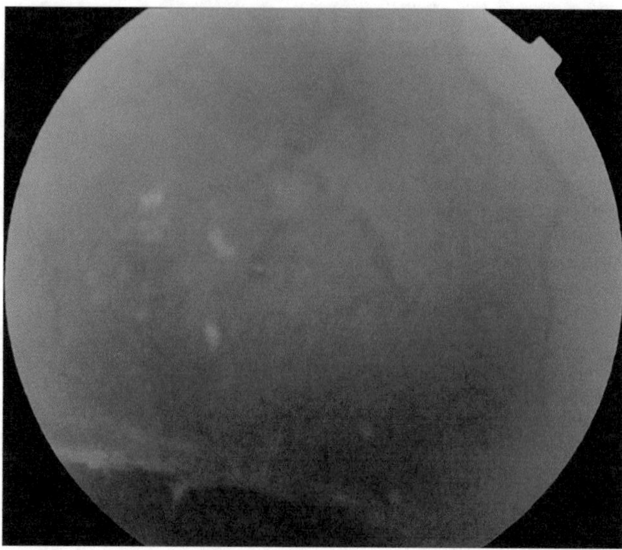

Fig. 18.31 The retinas are shown from a 13-year-old who was suffering from domestic violence. She presented with bilateral inferotemporal dialyses and whilst awaiting operation was struck in the left eye. She then presented with a tear at the posterior edge of the RRD in the left eye which presumably occurred from a shock wave of SRF ripping the retina at the time of the blow

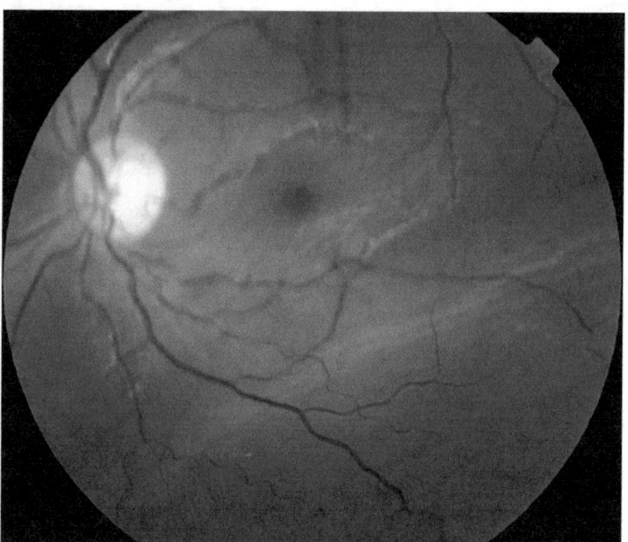

Fig. 18.32 Macula was detached

trauma had scleral ruptures, 47% of these were undetected preoperatively [30]. Computed tomography (CT) cannot be relied upon to detect globe rupture [31].

The severe fibrotic response that trauma induces [32] leads to a high incidence of retinal detachment which may progress rapidly to closed funnel detachments within weeks. Surgical exploration of the globe is advised. Incarceration of vitreous, choroid and retina into scleral ruptures cause traction on these structures.

In practice, if rupture is present, the posterior segment is often disrupted with choroidal and vitreous haemorrhage and there is a deepened anterior chamber. Take care not to exacerbate extrusion of intraocular contents by applying pressure to the globe during examination or surgery.

Note: the IOP may be normal or even high because the scleral rupture may block off with intraocular tissue.

Ultrasound can be employed but with copious contact jelly to avoid direct pressure on the damaged globe.

Note: In eyes with rupture of the globe, primary closure with vitreoretinal intervention at 2 weeks, if necessary, is advised (Figs. 18.54, 18.55, 18.56, 18.57 and 18.58).

Surgery (Table 18.2, Figs. 18.59 and 18.60)

In more severe blunt injury in which the globe cannot be examined clinically to exclude rupture, a surgical explora-

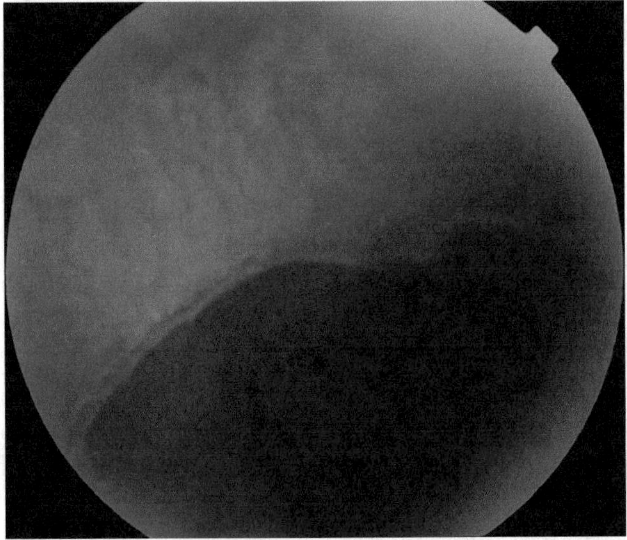

Fig. 18.33 Peripheral dialysis

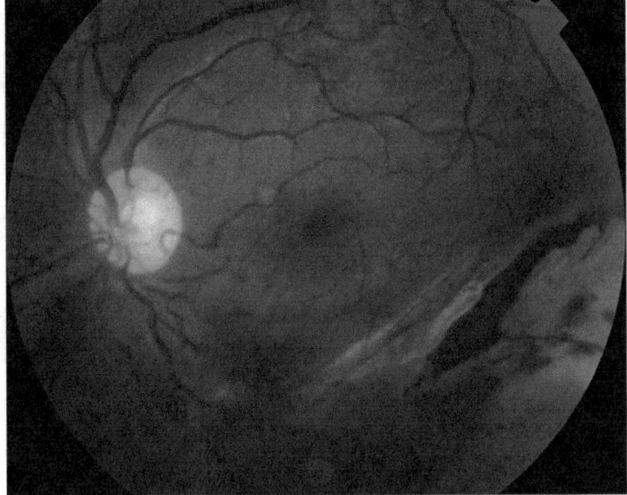

Fig. 18.34 Further blunt trauma caused a posterior rip in the retina

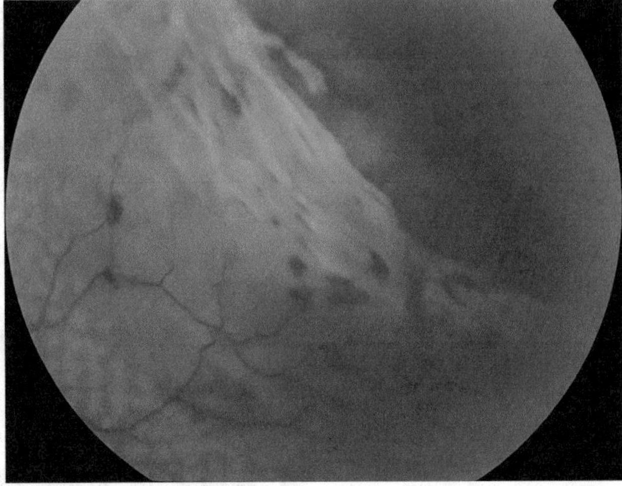

Fig. 18.35 This eye was struck by a soccer football and suffered a contusion injury with a ragged tear from the disintegration of the retina in an eye with vitreous attached. The edge was lasered and the retina monitored for extension of the SRF

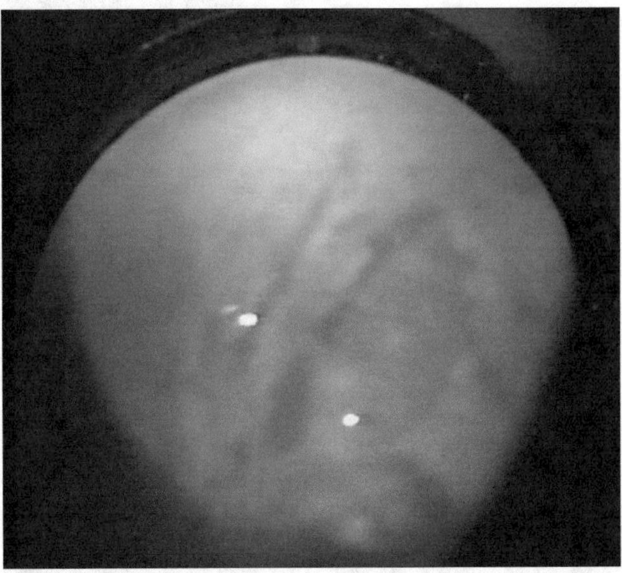

Fig. 18.36 This patient was struck in the eye with a champagne cork. This caused a localised retinal detachment with a typical traumatic ragged break which was treated by plombage

tion of the globe should be considered. A primary repair of any scleral laceration should be performed with the abscission of any extruding intraocular tissues to allow a clean closure of the sclera. Some surgeons advocate the use of 7/0 nylon for posterior ruptures; however, I have found adequate closure with 7/0 Vicryl.

The timing of the vitrectomy to clear vitreous haemorrhage is a balance between allowing some settling of immediate inflammation and engorgement of the eye and the risk of development of a closed funnel retinal detachment from PVR. A PPV at 2–3 weeks is suggested. The lens is frequently lost through the wound so that the use of a 6-mm long infusion cannula to avoid suprachoroidal infusion of fluid is safe and often recommended. Once the view of the retina has been obtained by careful vitrectomy, the incarceration site should be examined. If the rupture is at the corneoscleral limbus retinal involvement may be minimal and if the vitreous haemorrhage is not too severe PPV can be avoided allowing spontaneous clearance. If the retina is incarcerated, a retinectomy may be necessary to avoid dragging of the retina and tractional or secondary rhegmatogenous retinal detachment.

Some have advocated the removal of the choroid around the wound to leave a colobomatous area. This can be sealed off by a laser. Hopefully, removal of the tissue around the wound reduces the risk of progressive incarceration.

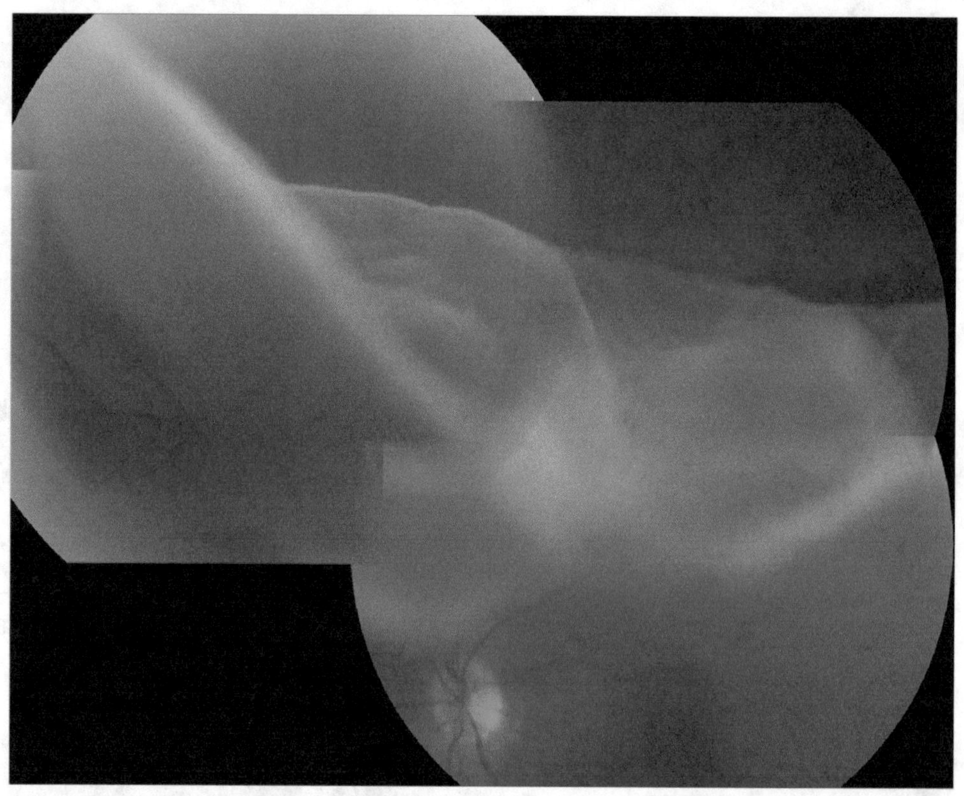

Fig. 18.37 This patient was struck in the eye accidentally resulting in the development of a giant retinal tear

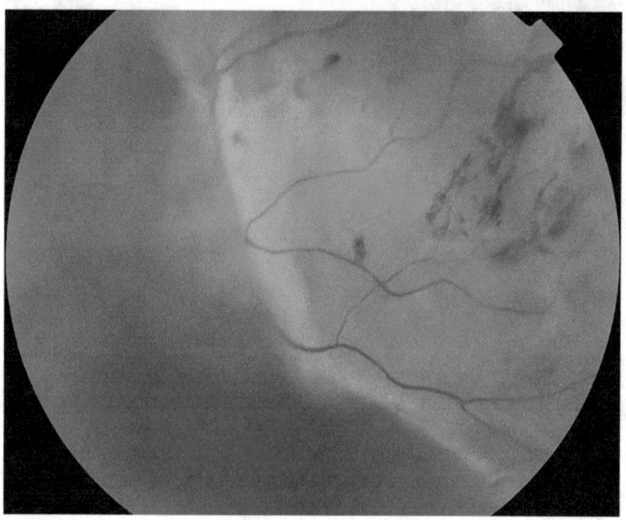

Fig. 18.38 A retinal break in retinal detachment with commotio retinae

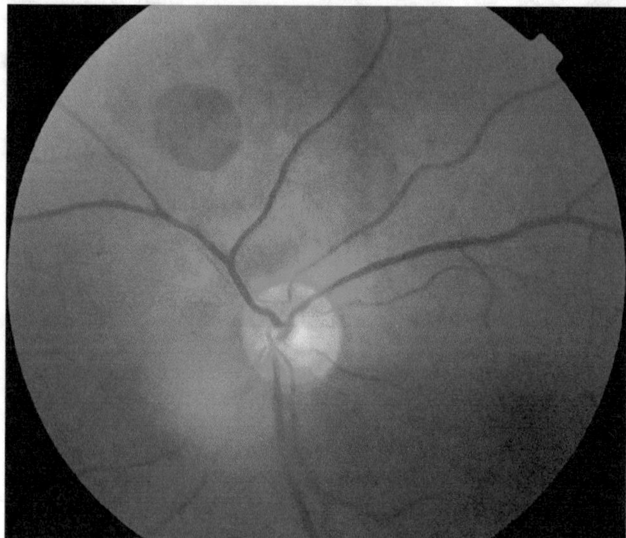

Fig. 18.39 This patient noticed a floater after being struck in the eye. He had an operculated retinal break above the disc which was lasered but was very unlikely to progress

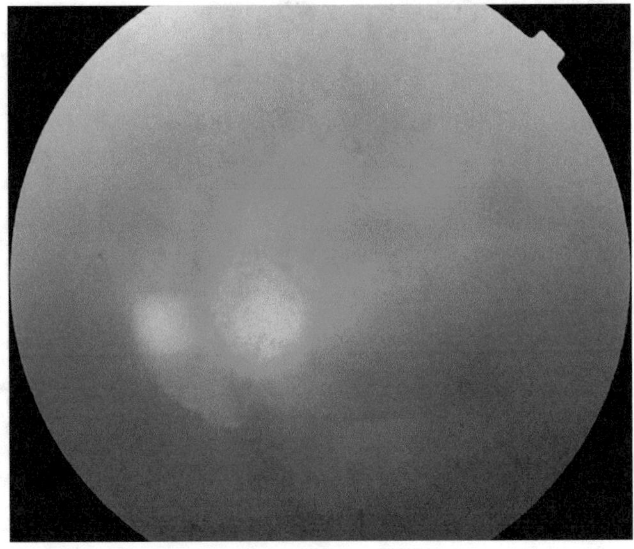

Fig. 18.40 The operculum from the hole

Table 18.1 Difficulty rating for surgery for contusion injury

Difficulty rating	Moderate
Success rates	Moderate
Complication rates	Low
When to use in training	Late

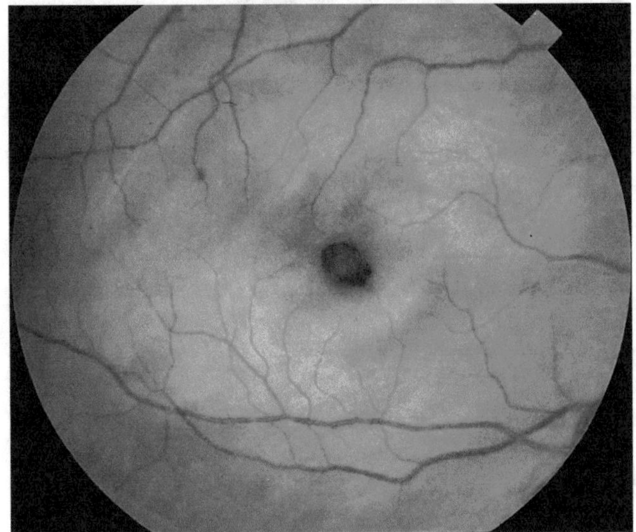

Fig. 18.41 This patient who suffered macular oedema from a severe blunt trauma also produced a macular hole

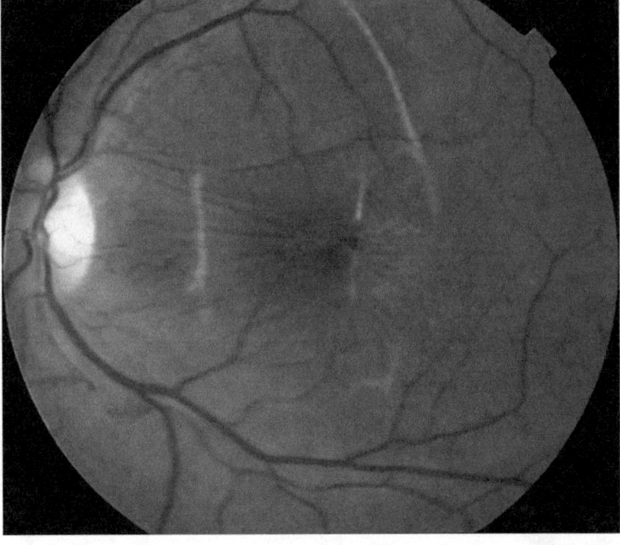

Fig. 18.42 Choroidal ruptures occur in blunt trauma and are circumferential white lines. In this case, one is close to the fovea. These patients can produce Type II choroidal neovascular membranes from these defects

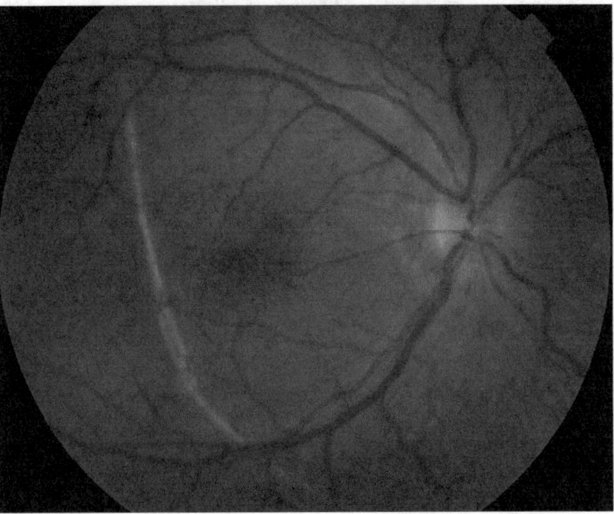

Fig. 18.43 A long choroidal rupture from contusion injury caused by a fist hitting the eye during an assault. Notice associated macular wrinkling

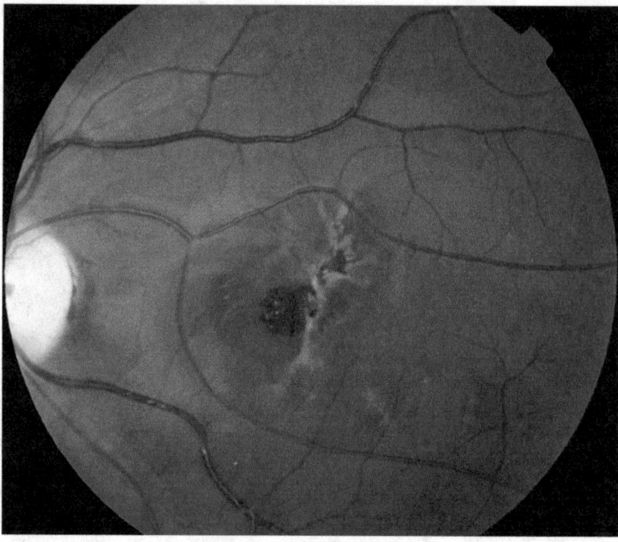

Fig. 18.44 A traumatic macular hole adjacent to a choroidal rupture. The surgery did not close the hole perhaps because of adhesion to the rupture site

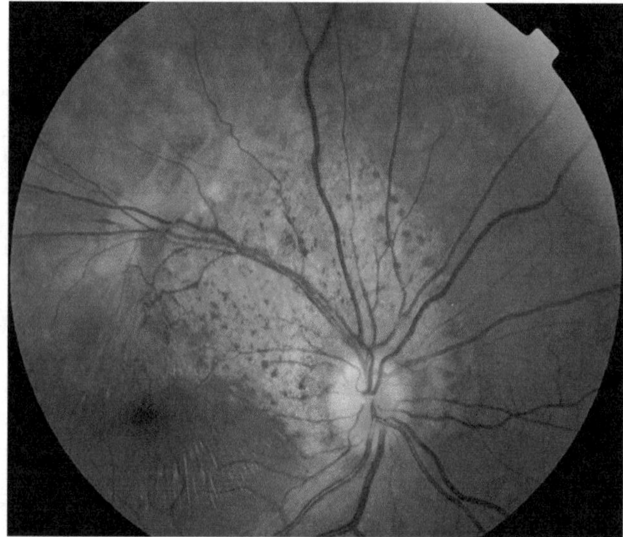

Fig. 18.45 This patient has suffered trauma diffusely to the eye from a football injury resulting in retinal pigment epithelial changes which come close to the fovea and reduce the central vision

Not all incarcerations will progress, and some can be observed to watch for progression. Silicone oil insertion is recommended if an intervention has been performed because of the risk of ongoing PVR formation. Unfortunately, these eyes are prone to late PVR even with silicone oil in, or weeks after silicone oil removal.

Visual Outcome

Studies have reported 40% with no light perception [33–35]. In addition, there may be cosmetic morbidity with a high risk of phthisis bulbi, occurring in up to two-third of the patients [35] (Fig. 18.61).

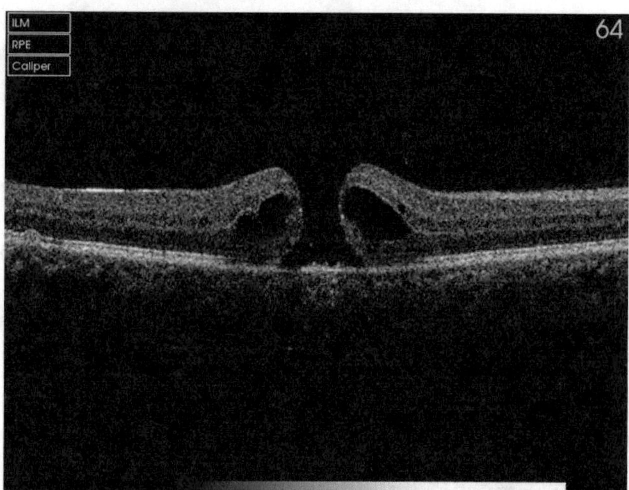

Fig. 18.46 A traumatic macular hole closed postoperatively

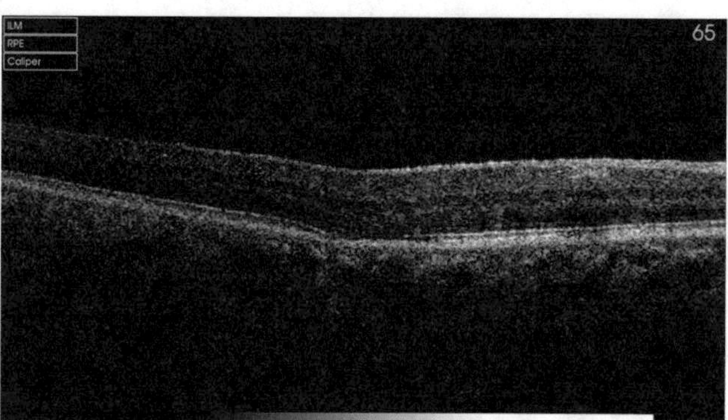

Fig. 18.47 The hole was closed by surgery

Penetrating Injury (Figs. 18.62 and 18.63)

Clinical Presentation

Sharp instruments may penetrate the sclera commonly in the assault with glass bottles or knifes, but also other situations such as working with a screwdriver or other tool usually being used to loosen objects and being drawn back into the eye, or even eating utensils [36]. Projectiles such as pellets from air guns cause severe injury with the pellets often stopping at the orbital apex where additional damage is suffered by the optic nerve [37–39]. The tissues damaged depend on the site of entry, depth of penetration and the size of the object. As a result, any intraocular structure may be disrupted. Incarceration sites are problematic when the site of entry involves the sclera rather than the cornea, resulting in later retinal detachment and phthisis. The injury can cause giant retinal tears [40] or introduce material into the eye such as cilia [41, 42] or fly larvae [43].

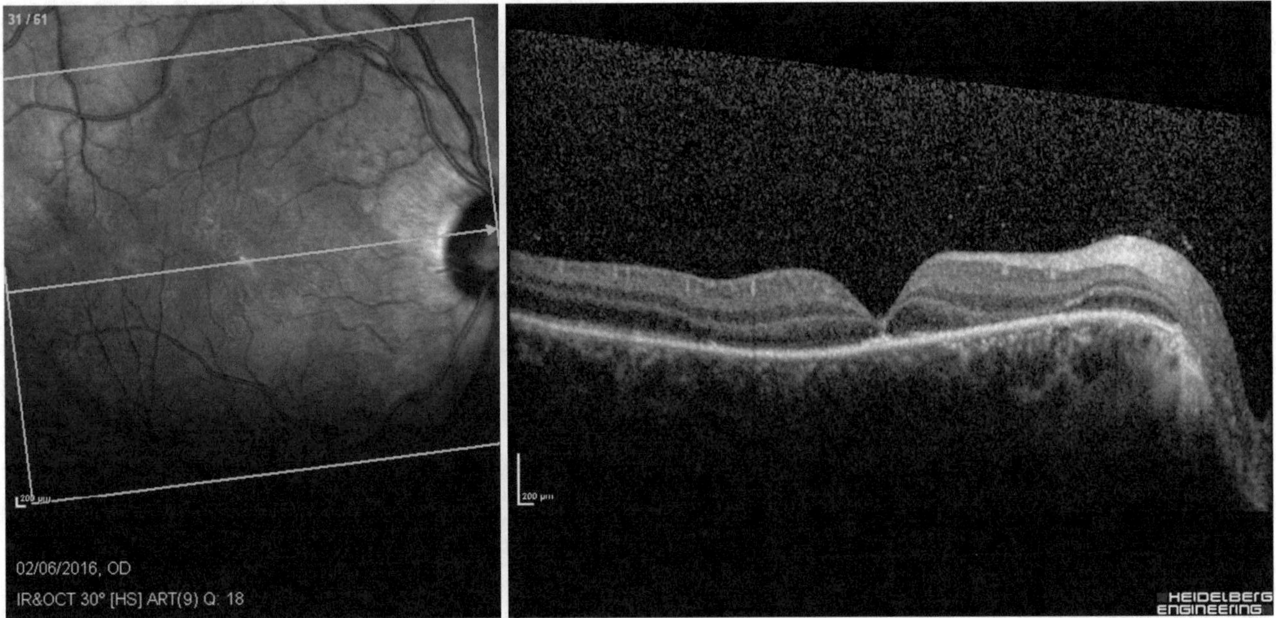

Fig. 18.48 A contusion injury has led to the loss of receptors and a thin fovea

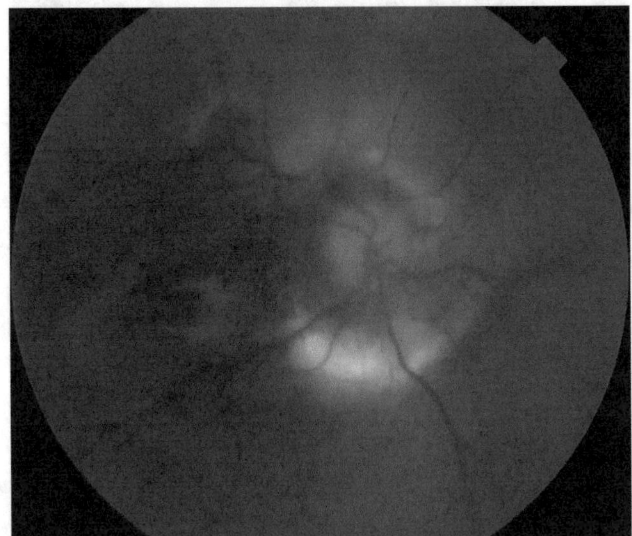

Fig. 18.49 This patient has suffered an avulsed optic nerve from trauma. This is evidenced by choroidal ruptures and subretinal haemorrhage around the optic nerve

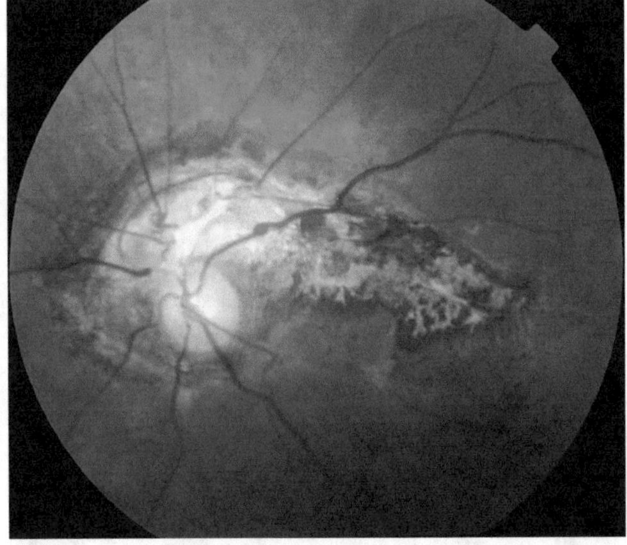

Fig. 18.50 The late sequelae from optic nerve avulsion are seen with widespread chorioretinal damage around the nerve head and extending into the macula

Endophthalmitis

Endophthalmitis may complicate any penetrating injury encountered in approximately 7% [44] with approximately 20% having virulent organisms [45]. Species of streptococcus, staphylococcus and bacillus are common in adults, with streptococcus commonest in children [46–48]. *Bacillus cereus* is highly virulent and only a very rare cause of endophthalmitis without trauma [49, 50]. In trauma, unusual organisms can be detected [51]. Prophylactic intravitreal antibiotics have been reported to reduce endophthalmitis rates from 18% to 6% in a study from India [52].

Retinal Detachment (Fig. 18.64)

Many types of retinal break are found in these traumatised eyes; they may develop at the time of impact or penetration, or subsequently from the incarceration of the retina.

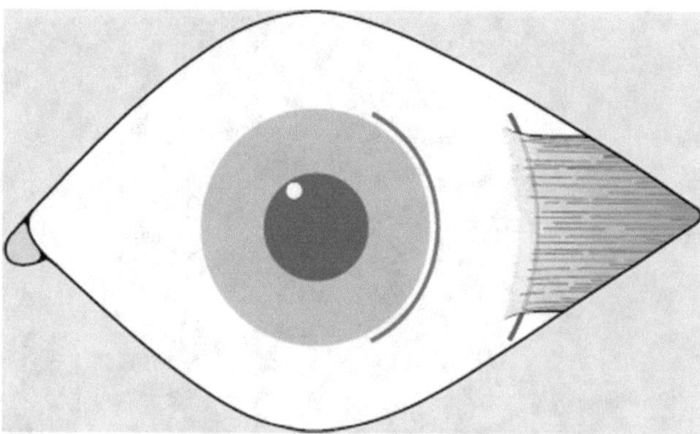

Fig. 18.51 The common sites of globe rupture from blunt trauma are at the limbus and just behind the extraocular muscles where the coats of the eye are at their weakest

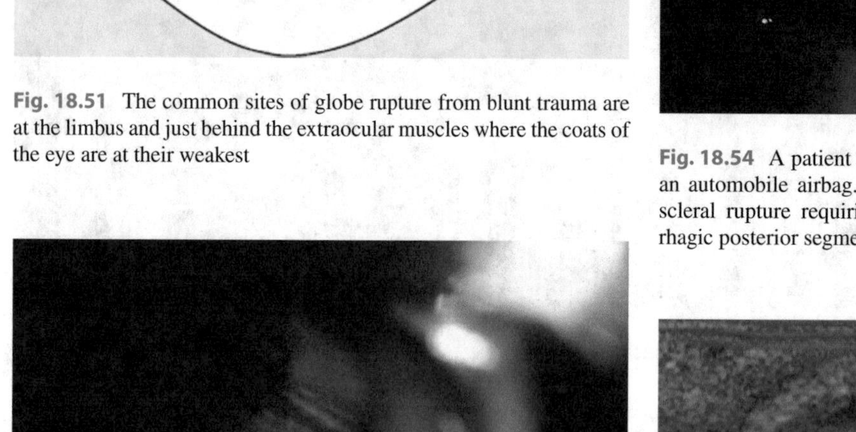

Fig. 18.52 An anterior incarceration site from a scleral rupture is present with vitreous and haemorrhage being dragged into the wound

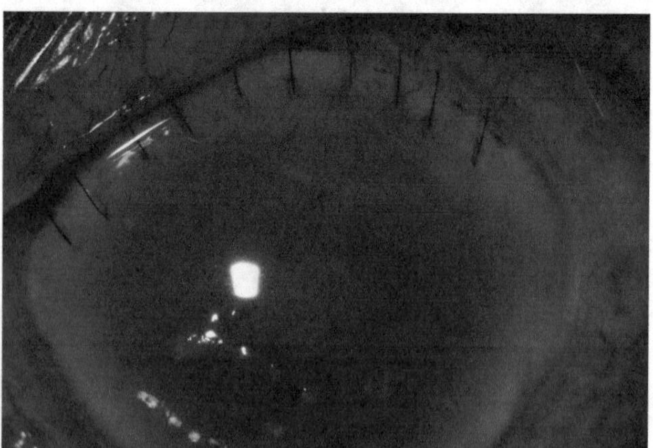

Fig. 18.53 Patients with pre-existing wounds are prone to rupture of the wound site in trauma. This patient suffered a rupture of her wound site (from previous extracapsular cataract extraction) after falling and hitting the eye on the corner of some furniture

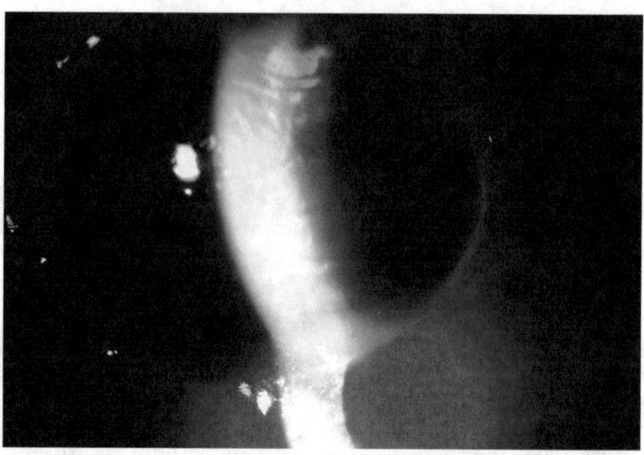

Fig. 18.54 A patient received a blow to the eye from an expansion of an automobile airbag. Initially, there was an eight ball hyphaema, a scleral rupture requiring immediate repair and a disrupted haemorrhagic posterior segment on ultrasound

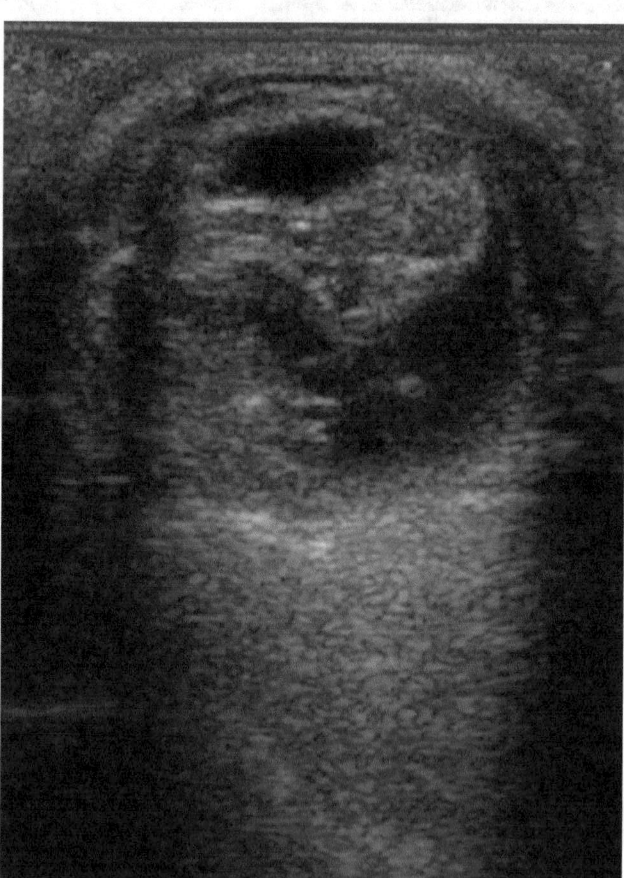

Fig. 18.55 An ultrasound at presentation

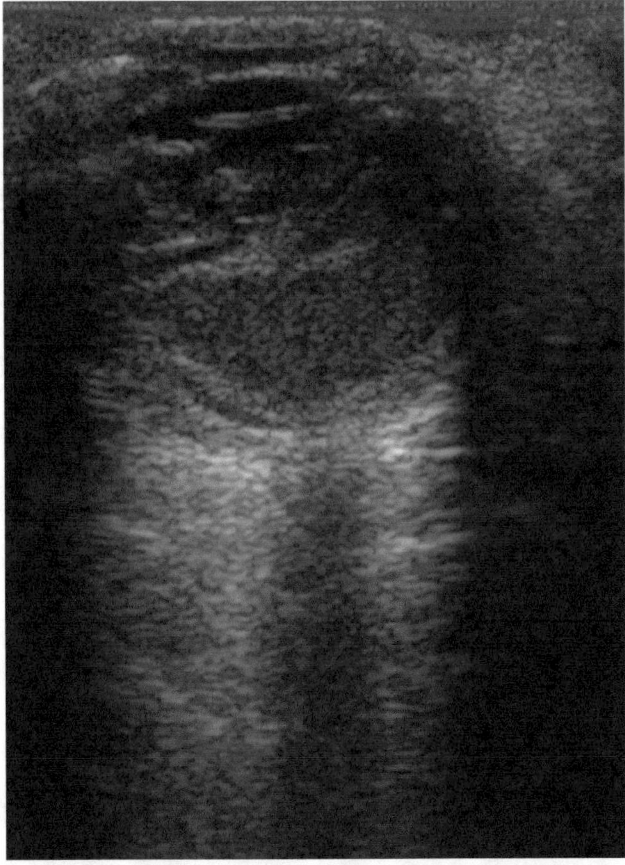

Fig. 18.56 By waiting 2 weeks, the interpretation of the structures of the posterior segment on ultrasound was improved allowing identification of surgical landmarks. The vitreous gel was incarcerated into the scleral wound causing it to detach leaving a subhyaloid haemorrhage and an area of tractional RD from the disc to the incarceration

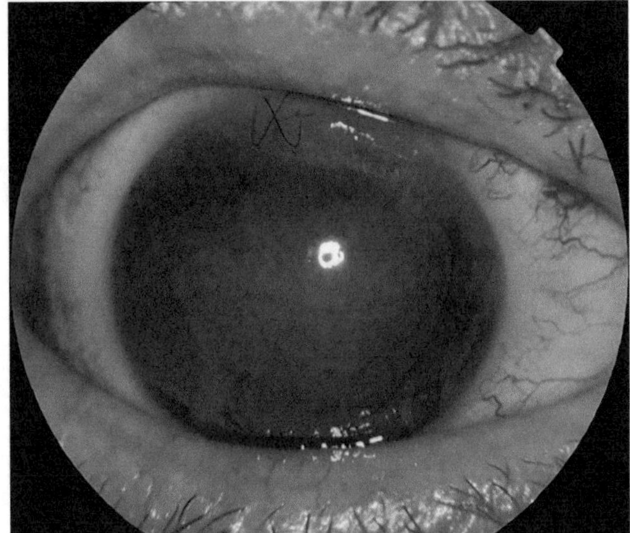

Fig. 18.57 In the early postoperative period after PPV, the anterior segment was much improved, and the retina could be viewed

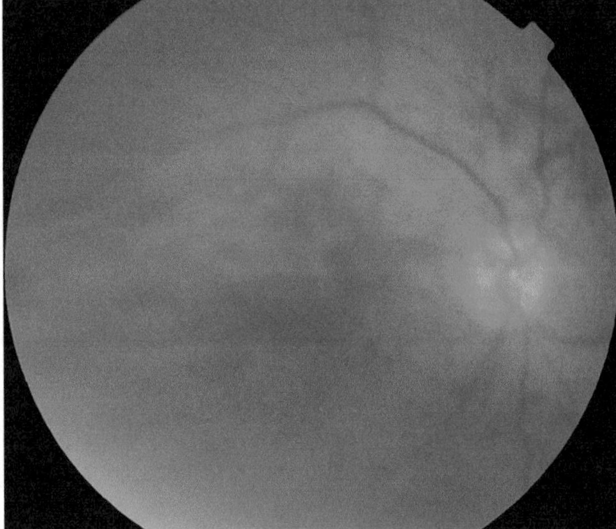

Fig. 18.58 The retina was relatively healthy

Table 18.2 Difficulty rating for surgery for rupture

Difficulty rating	High
Success rates	Low
Complication rates	High
When to use in training	Late

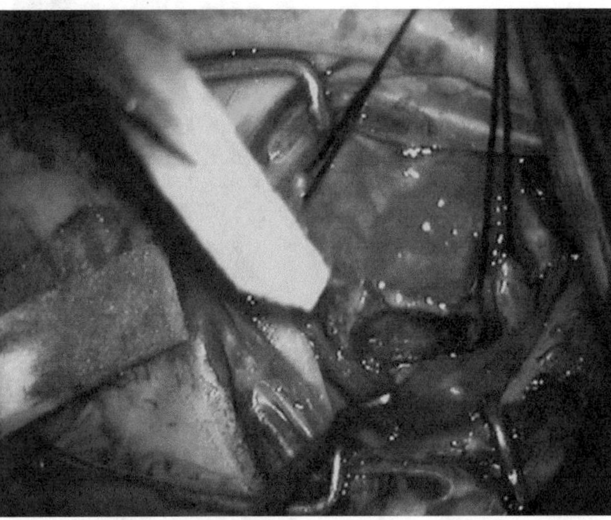

Fig. 18.59 This patient suffered blunt trauma with a haemorrhagic globe. The eye is being explored. A scleral rupture was discovered at 12 o'clock where the lens has been extruded from the eye and was found encapsulated underneath the superior rectus

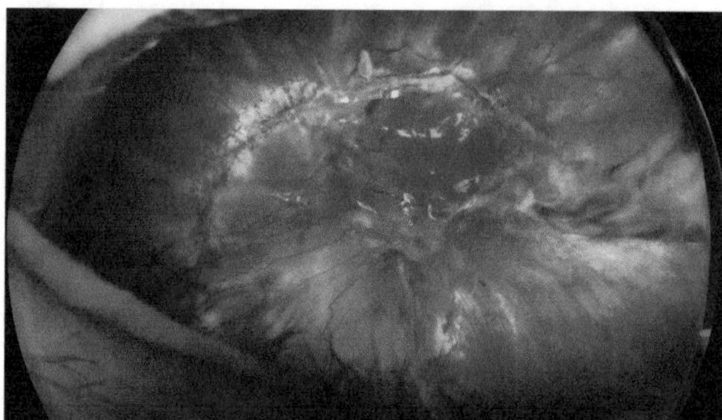

Fig. 18.60 This patient was struck in the eye by a golf ball, rupturing the eye. At this point, with 360-degree retinectomy and SRF, a discussion was held with the patient whether to proceed with further surgery. Eventually, the retina was flattened with further membrane peel, with minimal vision

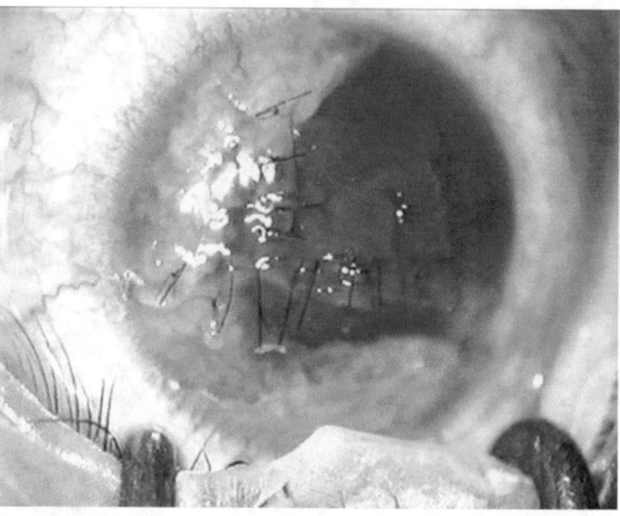

Fig. 18.62 This child was struck by a toy sword during play causing a penetrating injury and a haemorrhagic retinal detachment

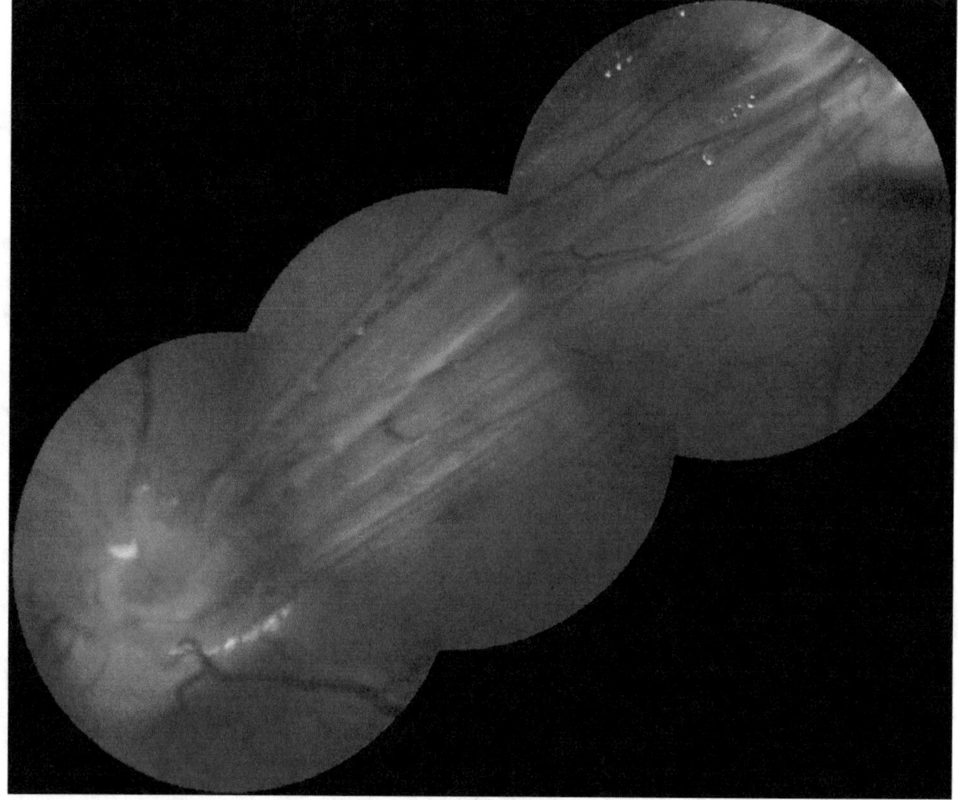

Fig. 18.61 This composite photograph shows the effects of incarceration site superonasally which is dragging the retina into the incarceration causing tractional retinal detachment, despite silicone oil insertion

Penetrating trauma can tear the retina at the site of injury or may produce incarceration of the vitreous, retina and choroid. The latter progressively scars, shortening the vitreous and retina, which can produce tears often in the incarceration site (Figs. 18.65, 18.66, 18.67 and 18.68).

Note: In penetrating injury perform primary closure and watch for traction.

Surgery (Table 18.3, Figs. 18.69, 18.70, 18.71, 18.72, and 18.73)

The surgical management is like blunt injury with rupture except that there may be damaged or undamaged crystalline lens in situ and visualisation through the anterior segment may be poorer because of corneal lacerations, hyphaema or cataract. Corneal or

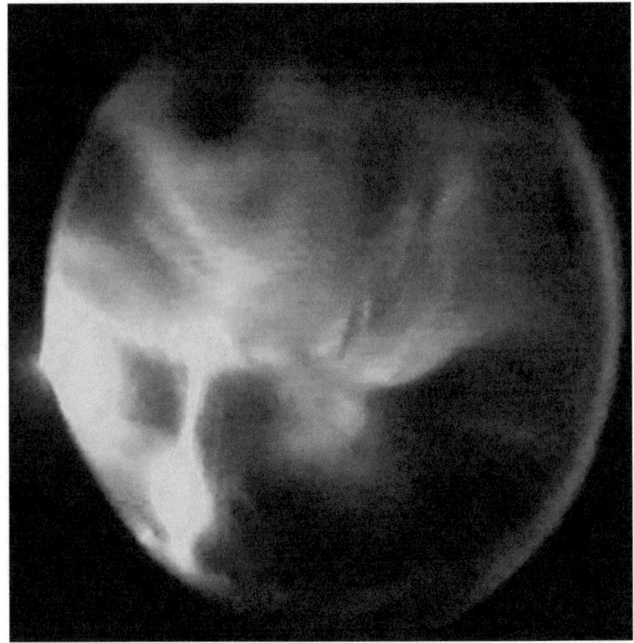

Fig. 18.63 The fundus was severely damaged with retinal detachment and choroidal haemorrhage

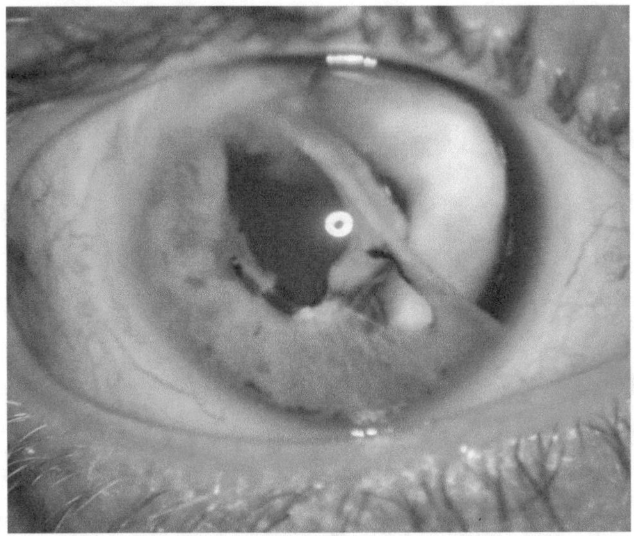

Fig. 18.64 Iridodialysis and a Sommerung's ring (ring of calcified lens material) from a penetrating injury from a road traffic accident many years ago. These eyes can develop late-onset RRD

scleral lacerations require primary repair immediately. If the penetrating object is likely to be infective intravitreal antibiotics may be necessary, but this is less indicated than in IOFB. An intravitreal injection may be hazardous in penetrating injury because of the more disrupted posterior segment and the possibility of retinal or choroidal elevation. With wide-angle viewing systems a small area of clear cornea is sufficient to allow surgery, only very rarely is recourse to keratoprosthesis required.

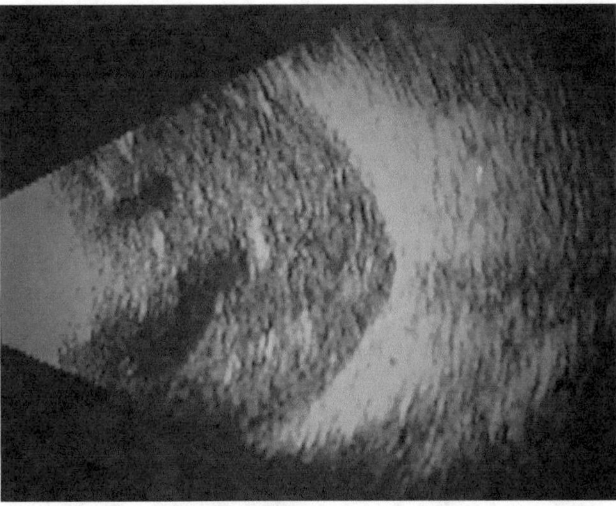

Fig. 18.65 An ultrasound of an eye with choroidal haemorrhage from trauma

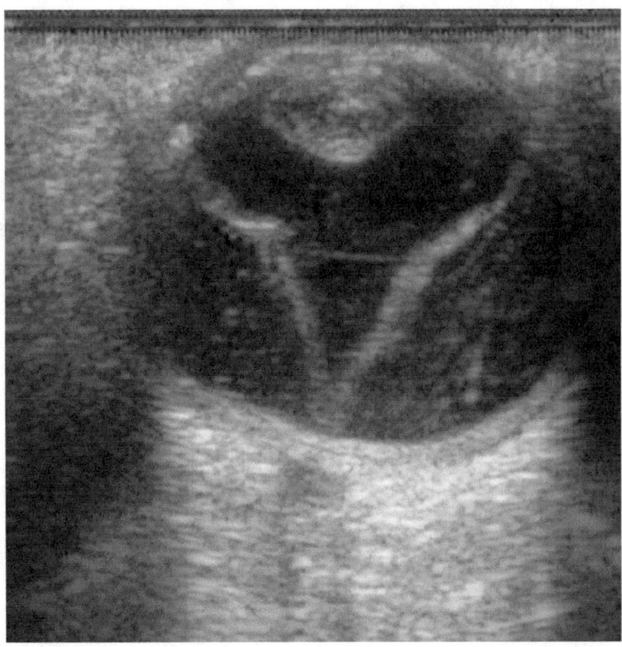

Fig. 18.66 A closed "funnel" RRD from PVR on ultrasound, CP12 and CA12

Surgical Pearl

Corneal Suturing

A few brief tips to achieve optimal wound healing, which is aimed at minimising the oedema (an immediate goal so that corneal opacity does not prevent concurrent or early posterior segment surgery) and at minimising the effects of scar formation.

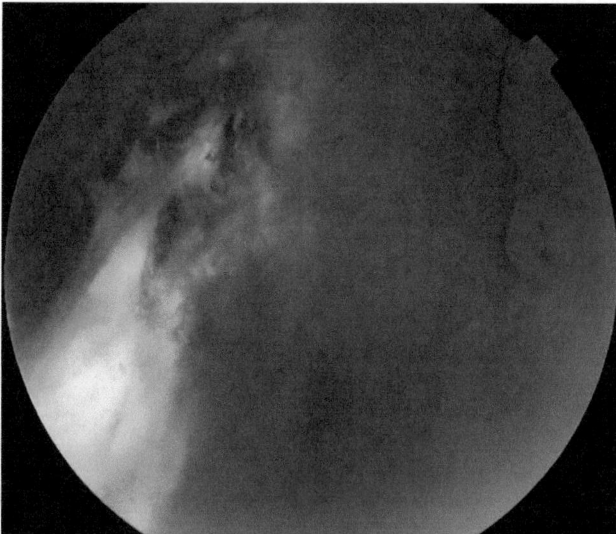

Fig. 18.67 This patient was shot bilaterally with pellets from his shotgun. This caused a glancing blow to his right eye as evidenced in this picture. The eye retained 20/60 vision with a flat retina without silicone oil

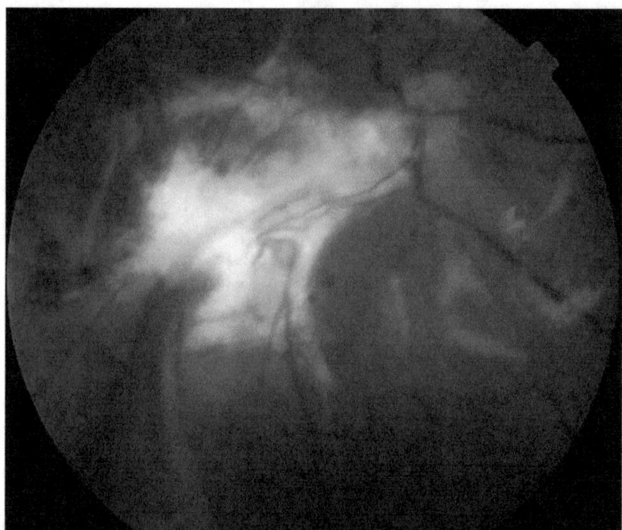

Fig. 18.68 A pellet caused a perforating injury in the other eye. This eye went phthisical

Table 18.3 Difficulty rating for surgery for penetrating injury

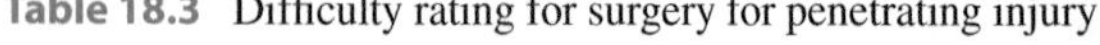

Difficulty rating	High
Success rates	Low
Complication rates	High
When to use in training	Late

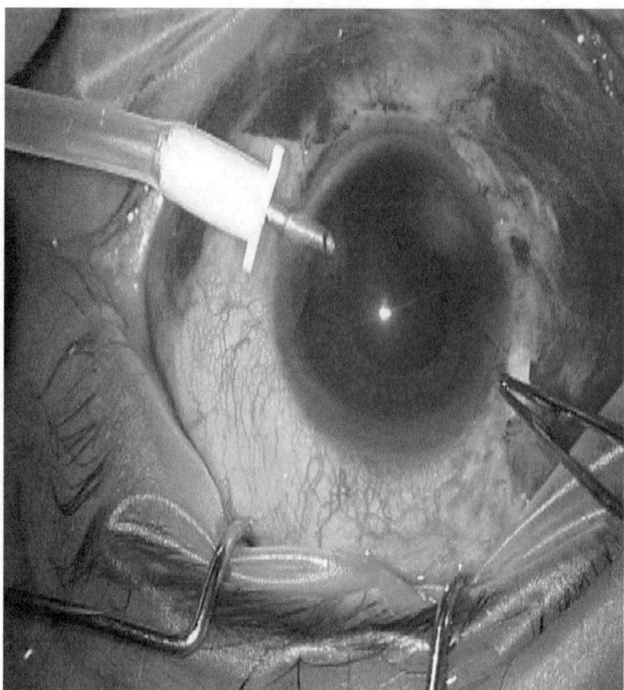

Fig. 18.69 When commencing the operation on a severely traumatised eye the infusion should be placed into the anterior chamber until this has been cleared to allow visualisation of a pars plana infusion

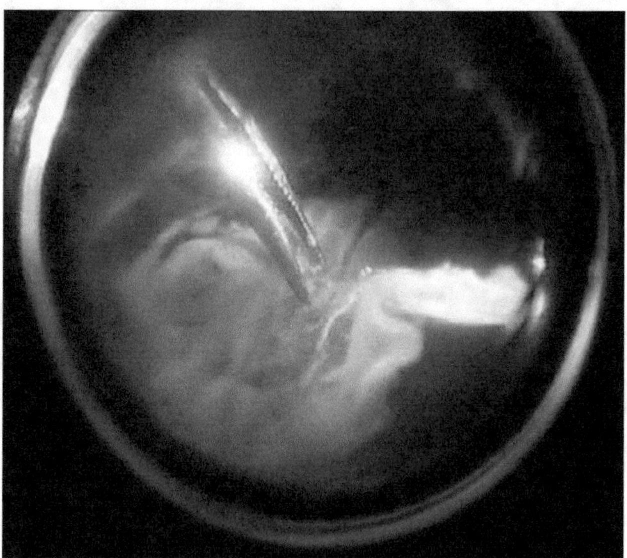

Fig. 18.70 This patient has had a 360° retinotomy and has a purse-string subretinal proliferative vitreoretinopathy which is being removed from the back surface of the retina

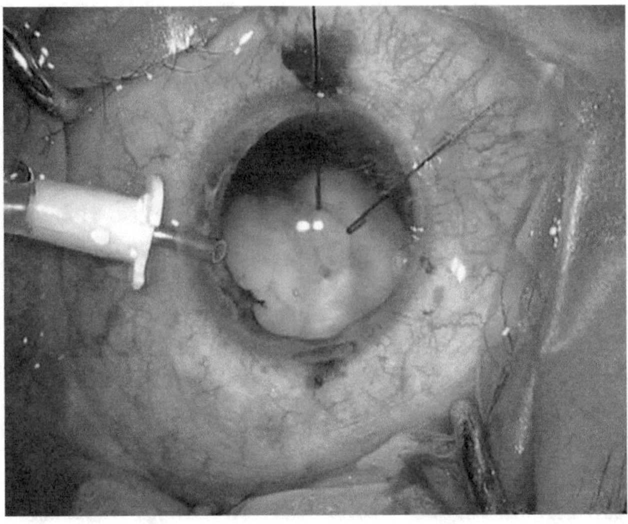

Fig. 18.71 In a patient with dislocated lens from trauma or other causes, iris hooks can be used to stabilise the capsule whilst the lens is aspirated. If possible, the capsule should be retained for insertion of a posterior chamber lens often with a capsular tension ring to maintain the shape of the capsule

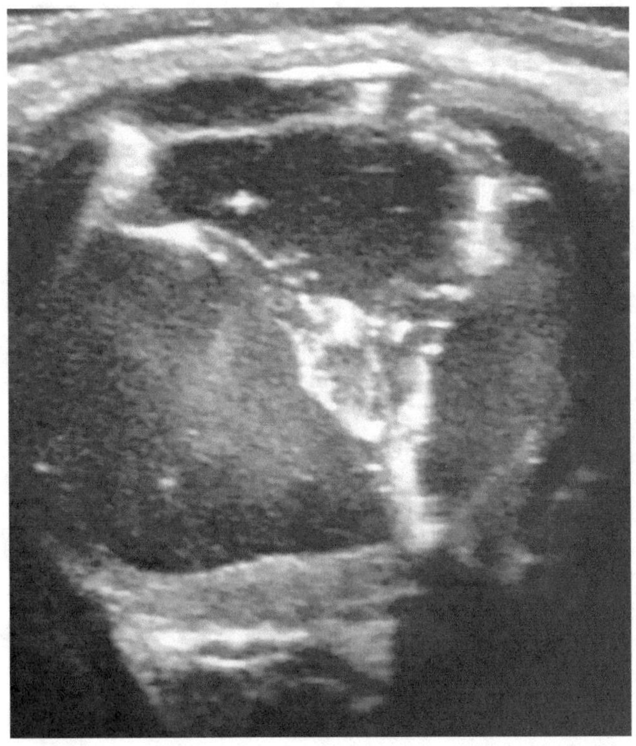

Fig. 18.72 A late presentation of a total retinal detachment after severe trauma. There is a closed funnel RRD and hypotony, choroidal thickening, shortening of the eye by 20% compared with the other eye. A decision needs to be made on the chances of reattaching the retina after 360-degree retinectomy (50–60% chance) and reconstruction of the anterior segment where the cornea is totally opaque. The low risk of sympathetic ophthalmia needs to be discussed

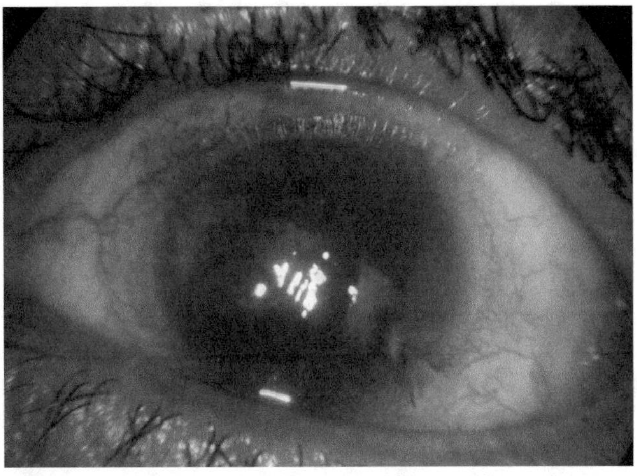

Fig. 18.73 The same patient as above, who will need restorative surgery on the anterior segment to allow visualisation of the RRD and restoration of vision

- Plan every step of the suturing process before the first suture is placed.
- Use 10–0 nylon.
- Always use interrupted sutures except at, or close to, the limbus.
- If the wound is trans-corneal, start from the two wound ends with large suture bites and alternatively advance from the end towards the centre with progressively shorter bites.
- Avoid placing sutures in the corneal apex.
- Except in the limbus, the sutures should be of 100% depth (the back of the suture rests in the anterior chamber).
- The length of the bites should be identical on the two sides, except if the wound is oblique; in this case, to prevent override, the bite on the surface should be of the same length on one side as it is in the anterior chamber on the other side.
- As a rule, use rather long bites to reduce the number of sutures and thus scarring.
- Do not overtighten the sutures.
- Make sure the knot is not too large since this makes both burying the knot (an absolute must) and removing it difficult.
- When removing the suture, sterilise the eye surface the same way as done for intravitreal injection.

Ferenc Kuhn, Retina Specialists of Alabama, Birmingham, Alabama, USA

Visual Outcome

These types of injury are associated with a poor visual outcome with 77.8% with 20/200 or worse vision and 27.8% with phthisis bulbi, and 50% redetachment rate, with only

60–80% achieving a flat retina [53, 54]. Poor starting vision, the presence of an RAPD, a large or posterior wound are reported to result in poorer prognosis [55, 56].

Trauma Scores

There are two models for the prediction of visual outcome in open globe injury, the ocular trauma score (OTS) and the classification and regression tree (CART) [57, 58] both have been found to be predictive of outcome [59] (Table 18.4).

Ocular Trauma Score [57]. Calculate the score for the traumatised eye (Table 18.5).

Ocular Trauma Score. Probability of achieving a visual acuity depending on the score attained (Fig. 18.74).

Intraocular Foreign Bodies

Clinical Presentation (Figs. 18.75, 18.76, 18.77, 18.78, 18.79, 18.80, 18.81, 18.82, 18.83, 18.84, 18.85 and 18.86)

IOFBs are typically caused by striking metal on metal such as hammering on a chisel. IOFBs have been described from glass from car windscreens [10], plastic fireworks and strimmers [60], organic material in rural settings, shotgun pellets [61, 62], graphite pencil lead [63] and fragments from lawnmower blades [64]. Diagnosis of ocular retention of a small foreign body depends on careful attention to the details and the circumstances of the injury, and scrutiny for evidence of ocular penetration, such as a small entry site in the anterior sclera and signs of vitreous disturbance. Immediate posterior segment damage after foreign body penetration is generally restricted to the site of ultimate impaction. Initially, local tissue whitening may be visible together with bleeding into the cortical gel in the vicinity of the impact site and along the "track" or path of the foreign body's penetration through the gel. The integrity of the retina is usually secured by chorioretinal scarring around the foreign body, but a small retinal break, subsequently causing retinal detachment may develop if the foreign body ricochets off the retina rather than impacting within it.

If the retina is damaged, RRD is reported in 25% [65]. IOFBs often sit in the vitreous cavity without causing a retinal tear. Subsequently, fibroblast proliferation may occur either locally at the impact site (encapsulating the foreign body or puckering and distorting the underlying and adjacent retina) or along the haemorrhagic track to form a trans gel traction band. The visual loss depends on the site of impaction (macular, papillary or peripheral), on opacities in the media (cataract or vitreous haemorrhage), or retinal detachment.

Table 18.4 OTS scoring

Initial visual acuity	Raw points
1. Initial visual acuity	NLP = 60 LP to HM = 70 1/200 to 19/200 = 80 20/200 to 20/50 = 90 >= 20/40 = 100
2. Globe rupture	−23
3. Endophthalmitis	−17
4. Perforating injury	−14
5. Retinal detachment	−11
6. Afferent pupillary defect	−10
Raw score = sum of raw points	

Table 18.5 OTS scoring

Raw sum score	OTS score	NLP	LP/ HM	1/200–19/200	20/2000–20/50	>= 20/40
0–44	1	73%	17%	7%	2%	1%
45–65	2	28%	26%	18%	13%	15%
66–80	3	2%	11%	15%	28%	44%
81–91	4	1%	2%	2%	21%	74%
92–100	5	0%	1%	2%	5%	92%

Diagnostic Imaging

1. CT scanning, with thin sections, is the investigation of choice if the IOFB cannot be seen on fundoscopy.
2. X-ray. Screening for a suspected foreign body can be performed by plain X-ray.
3. Ultrasound examination may be valuable for detecting non-radiolucent foreign bodies but is a relatively inefficient method for detecting small metallic foreign bodies, especially if they are embedded in the ocular coats. Foreign bodies can give rise to high amplitude echoes provided they are appropriately orientated to the sound beam; a variety of artefacts arising from metallic particles aid in their identification and localisation, but the main value of ultrasound is in determining the vitreoretinal complications of foreign body impaction.

An intraocular foreign body is an absolute contraindication to MRI scanning in case a ferromagnetic particle rotates or moves in the magnetic field (Fig. 18.87).

IOFB Materials

Surgical removal of the foreign body is indicated because of the risk of generalised posterior segment complications such as severe vitritis and endophthalmitis (from bacterial or toxic chemical penetration along with the foreign body, or acute chalcosis). Copper containing IOFBs cause chalcosis which

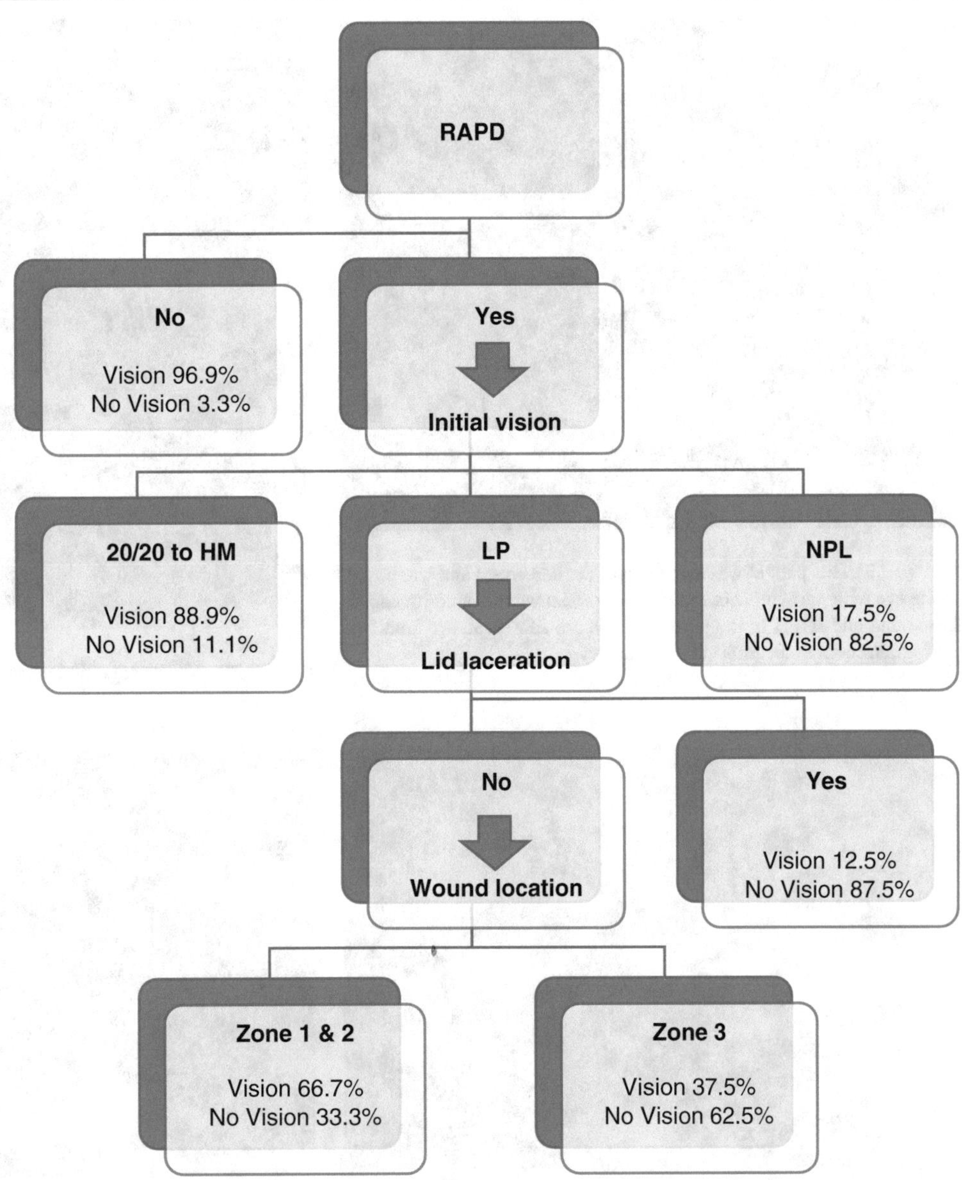

Fig. 18.74 The CART predictive model for visual outcome after open globe injury is shown for visual survival (light perception, LP or better) and no vision (no perception of light, NLP). Zone 1 = full-thickness wound confined to the cornea, zone 2 = involved the anterior 5 mm of the sclera and zone 3 more posterior than 5 mm from the limbus

can be rapidly damaging to the eye if the copper content is 85% or more [66].

Siderosis results from the chemical destruction and ocular absorption of retained ferrous material. Ferrous IOFBs cause siderosis which is slow in onset over weeks and months and can minimally affect vision. Features are tonic pupil, greenish tinge to the iris and late-onset cataract formation [67, 68]. Retinal damage from this is slow to occur and some patients may have only mild loss of vision over years. Electroretinography demonstrates a reduction in retinal function with reduced amplitudes. The IOFB may dissolve over years making it undetectable on ophthalmoscopy or CT scan.

Endophthalmitis occurs in 5–8% of cases [69, 70].

Note: Insert intravitreal antibiotics and repair any globe lacerations immediately at presentation followed by later surgery for removal of the IOFB within a few days (Figs. 18.88, 18.89, 18.90, 18.91, 18.92, 18.93, 18.94, 18.95 and 18.96).

Surgery (Table 18.6)

Perform a primary closure with intravitreal antibiotics.

Perform a PPV with additional surgical steps:

1. Deal with medial opacities.
2. Loosen the IOFB if incarcerated.
3. Create a large sclerotomy.
4. Grasp the IOFB with foreign body forceps.
5. Extract the IOFB.
6. Sew up the extra sclerotomy.

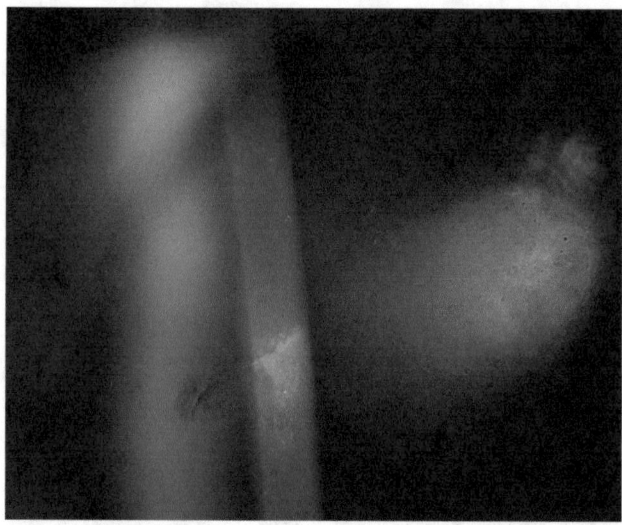

Fig. 18.75 This patient was using a hammer and chisel and was struck in the eye with a fragment of metal. The corneal wound, anterior capsular wound and IOFB in the posterior lens are shown. It was removed during phacoemulsification cataract surgery

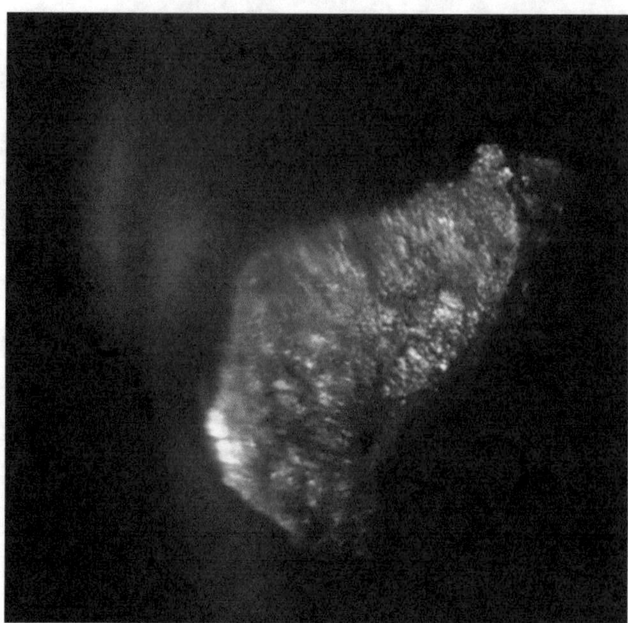

Fig. 18.78 IOFB magnified

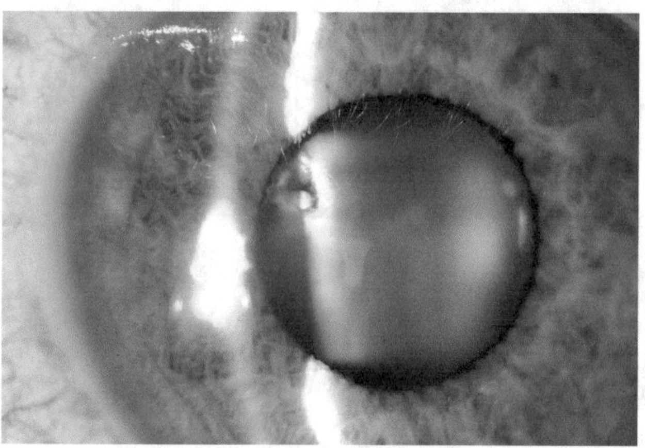

Fig. 18.76 Anterior capsular wound

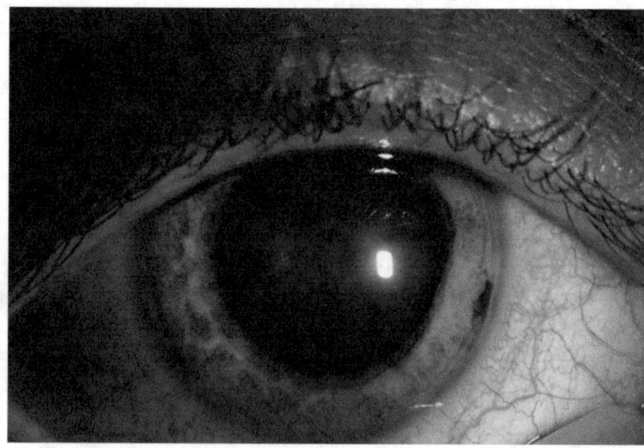

Fig. 18.79 A defect in the iris where an IOFB has entered, shown on diffuse illumination and transillumination

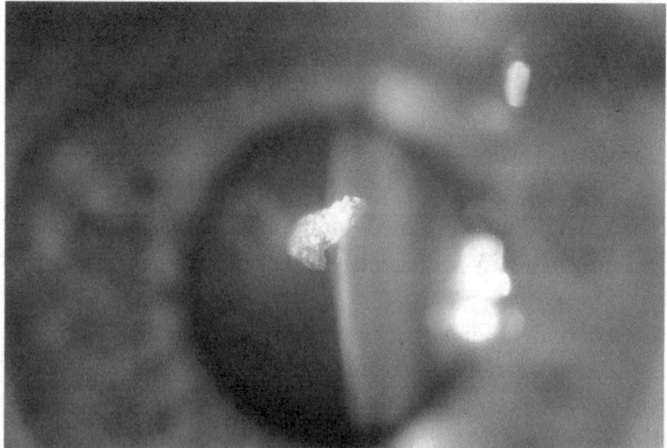

Fig. 18.77 IOFB in the lens

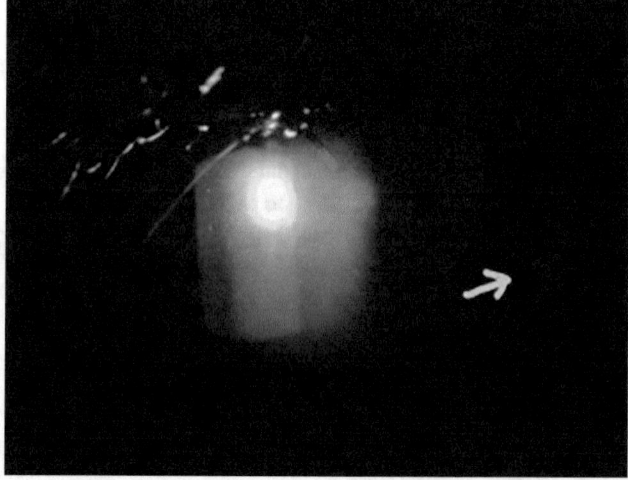

Fig. 18.80 Transillumination can be used to show the defect

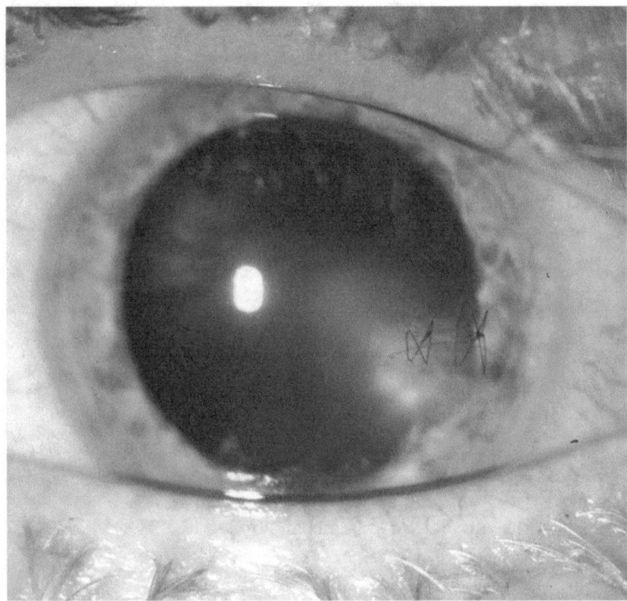

Fig. 18.81 In this patient with IOFB, the entry can be seen through the cornea, iris and lens

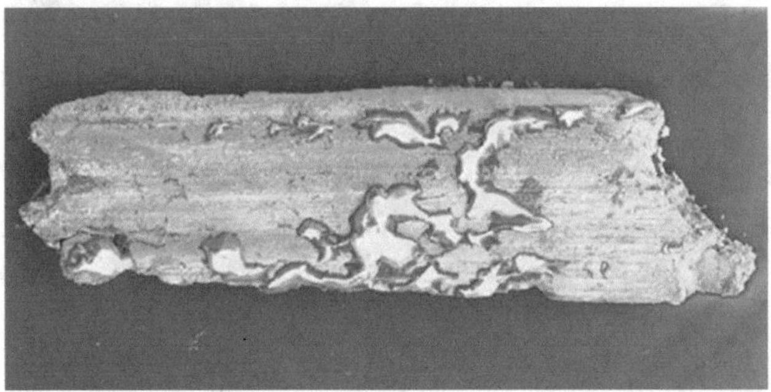

Fig. 18.82 An example of a fragment of metal removed from an eye. Often the foreign bodies are made of alloy metals. Foreign bodies vary in size from 1 mm to a few millimetres. They are commonly metallic but may be of other substances also

7. Peel the posterior hyaloid off the retina.
8. Insert intravitreal antibiotics.

The Primary Procedure

Identify and repair the entry site wound as soon as possible after the injury. At this time a vitreous sample should be taken, and intravitreal antibiotics inserted with later PPV [71]. Most foreign bodies are ferrous, steel or alloy and therefore can remain in the eye for a few days without toxicity to the eye. The risk of endophthalmitis (8%) justifies the insertion of antibiotics at an early stage. It is not uncommon to encounter a patient who has had a primary closure in a referring hospital but has endophthalmitis by the time they reach the tertiary referral centre. Once the biopsy has been performed the surgical removal of the IOFB can be scheduled. One exception is if the foreign body contains a high concentration of copper (more than 85%), in which case the removal must be performed as soon after the injury as possible (Figs. 18.97 and 18.98)

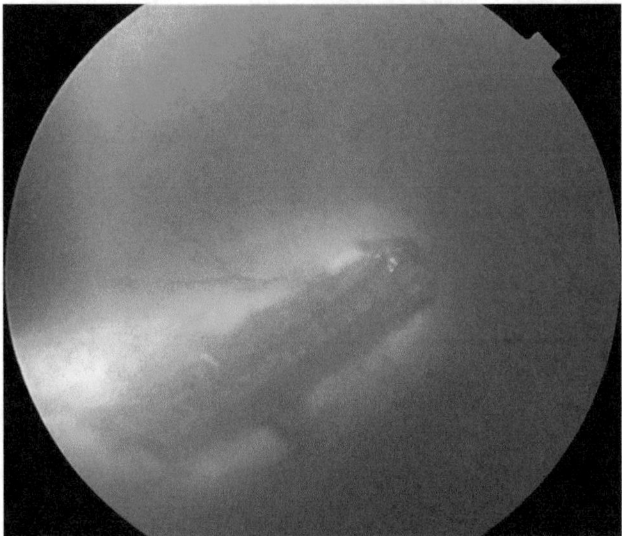

Fig. 18.83 A large intraocular foreign body is seen in the retina producing a whitened reaction around the foreign body

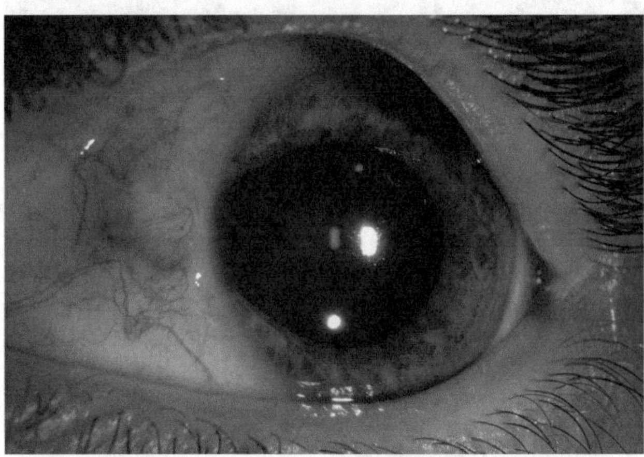

Fig. 18.84 In trauma, history is an important means of determining the likely type of injury. This patient presented late with IOFB after initially describing to the referring doctor a blunt injury from an iron bar for which a rupture or laceration was repaired. During an examination for a vitreoretinal opinion 3 weeks later the wound was felt to be suspicious of IOFB and the patient questioned again. He provided a prior history of possible IOFB from hammering concrete. The IOFB was seen on ultrasound and removed via PPV

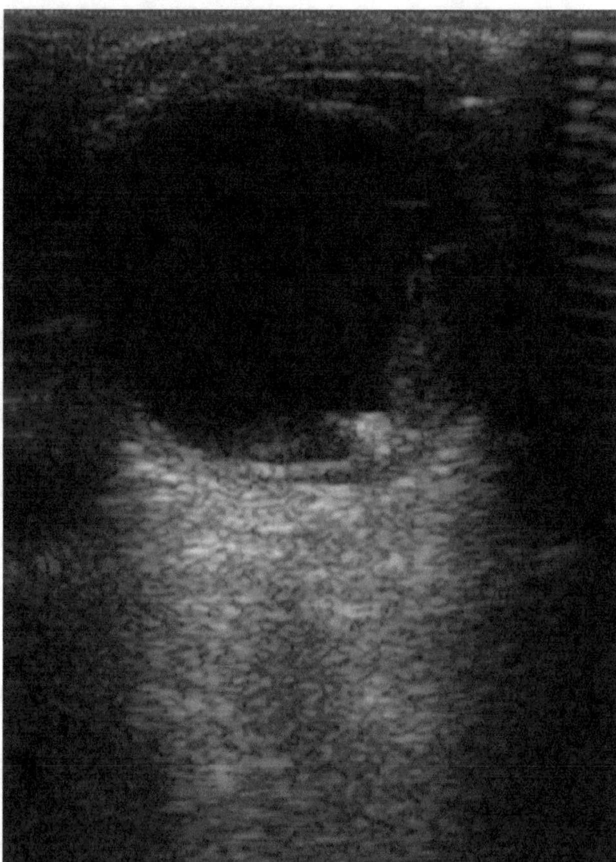

Fig. 18.85 Ultrasound shows the IOFB

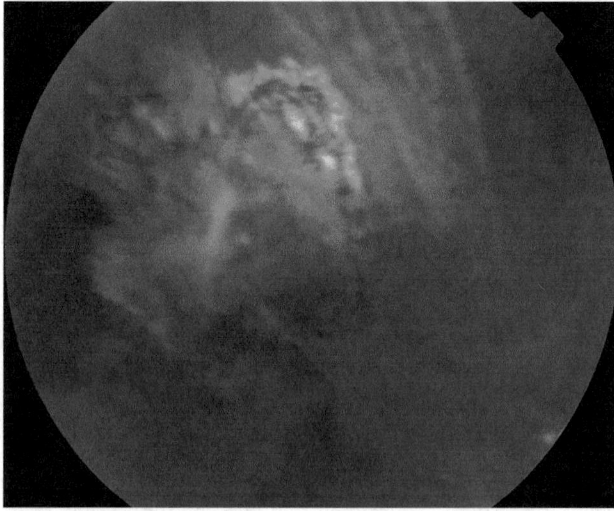

Fig. 18.86 The IOFB impact site

PPV, the Anterior Segment

Deal with any problems with the anterior segment first.

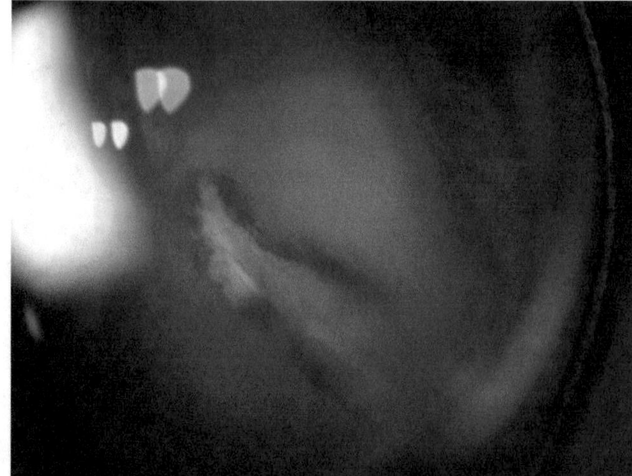

Fig. 18.87 A vitreoretinal traction band from an IOFB

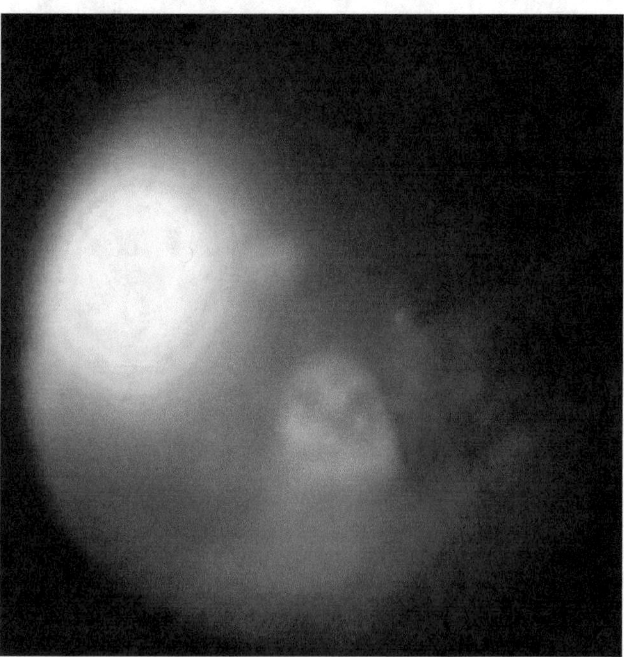

Fig. 18.88 This patient was shot in the eye with a shotgun pellet which caused endophthalmitis. The shotgun pellet was removed, and intravitreal antibiotics inserted with a visual recovery of 20/120

The Lens

Small capsular tears may self-seal with only the development of localised cataract so that some crystalline lenses can be preserved [72]. Phacoemulsification the lens if it is going cataractous but be aware there may be damage to the anterior or posterior capsules, or to the zonular fibres [73]. The patients are usually young and therefore the lens is often soft, requiring only phaco-assisted aspiration. Dropping the lens into the vitreous is not high risk because the lens is soft. In

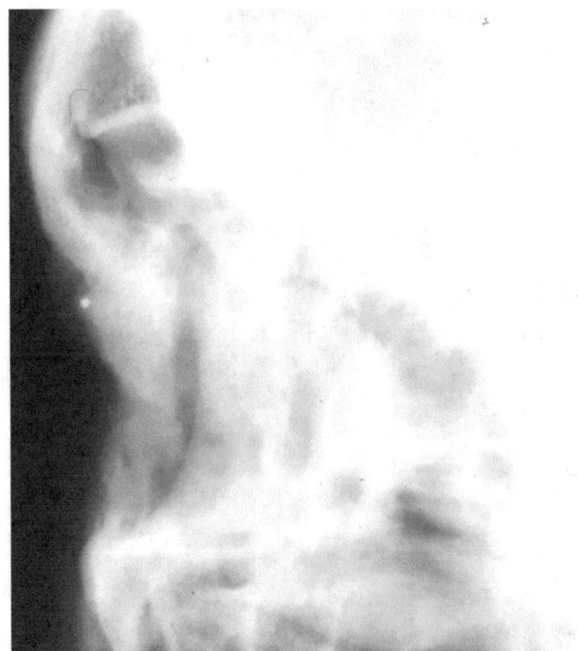

Fig. 18.89 A metallic IOFB seen on plain X-ray

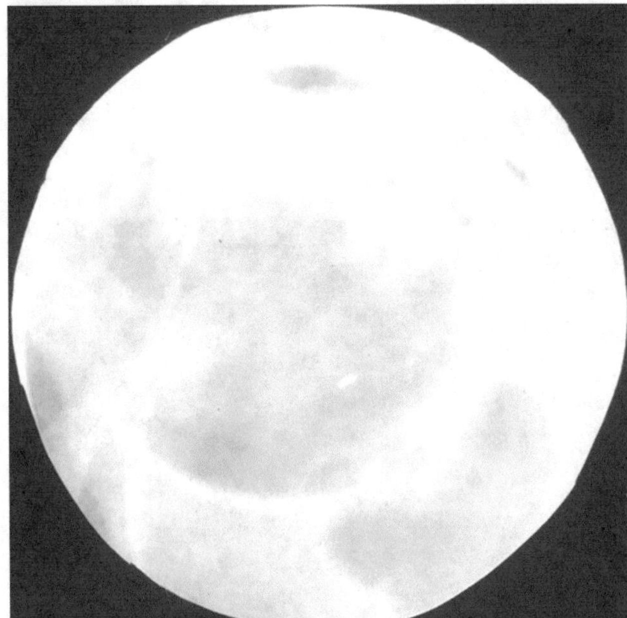

Fig. 18.90 IOFB on Xray

any case, if some lens material dislocates this can be dealt with during the PPV. If the IOFB is large and the intention is to remove it through the anterior chamber delay the IOL implantation until the end of the operation. If the capsular damage is severe and the nucleus hard, dislocate the lens into the anterior chamber to phaco it there, alternatively dislocate the nucleus into the posterior chamber and fragmatome from there. Try to preserve the capsule to allow support for the IOL. If removing the nucleus by fragmatome from the

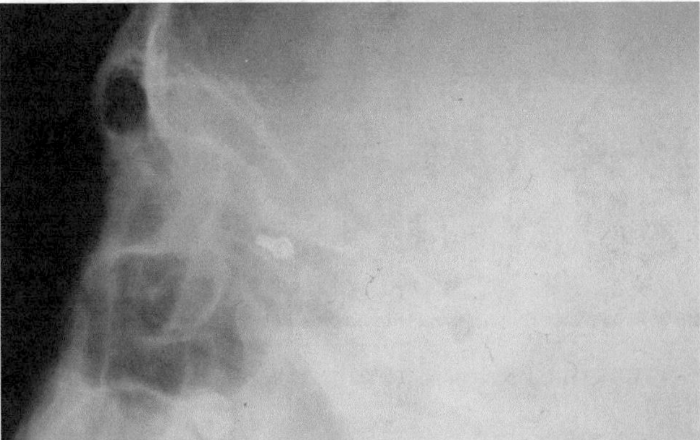

Fig. 18.91 An orbital air gun pellet seen on X-ray and on CT scan

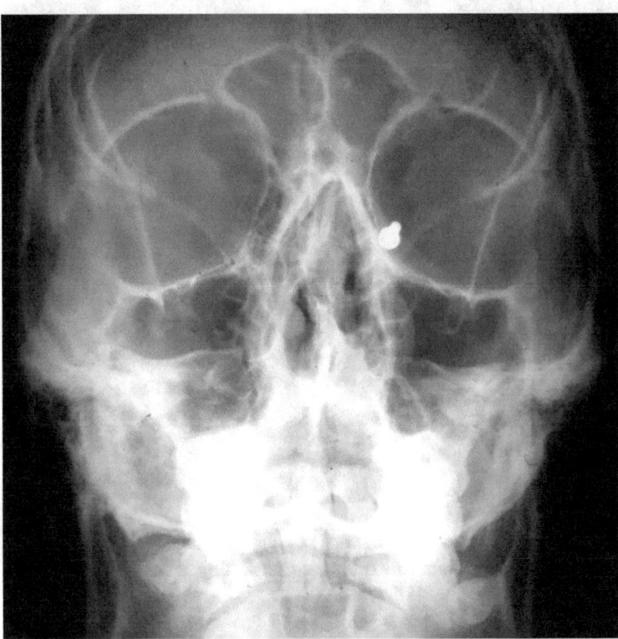

Fig. 18.92 Air gun pellet on Xray

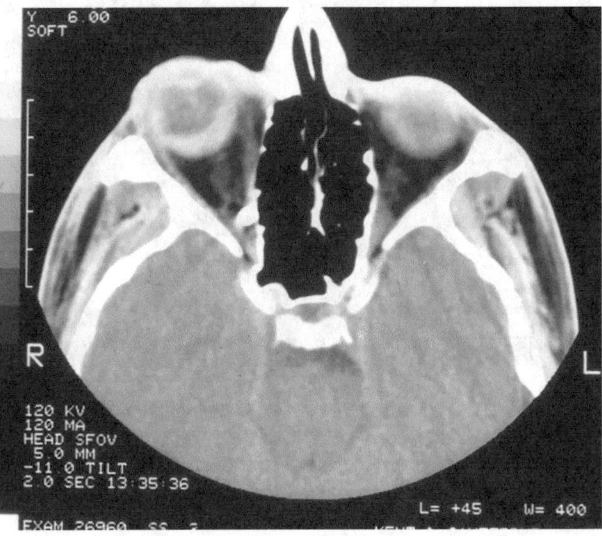

Fig. 18.93 Air gun pellet on CT scan

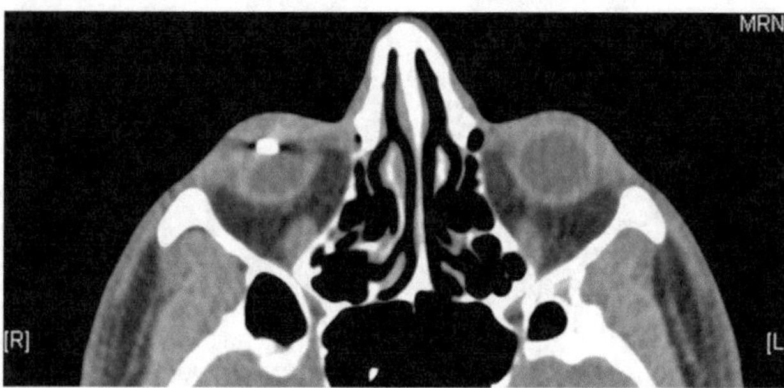

Fig. 18.94 A CT scan of an IOFB, the scan exaggerates the size of the IOFB

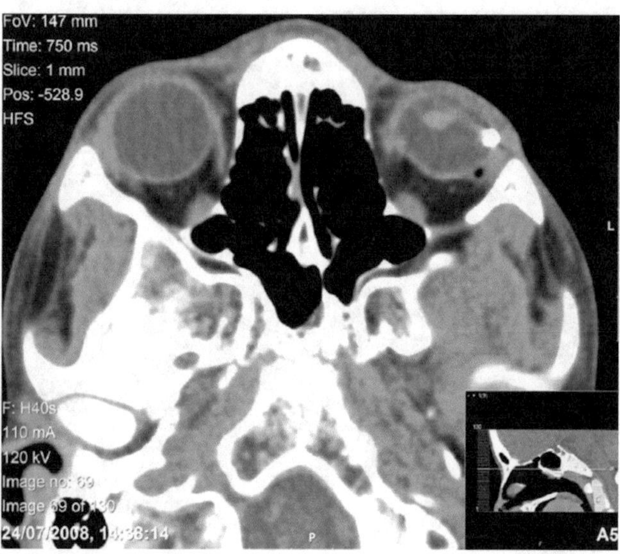

Fig. 18.95 This 13-year-old boy was hitting nail gun pellets with a hammer causing them to explode unfortunately a fragment lacerated and entered the eye

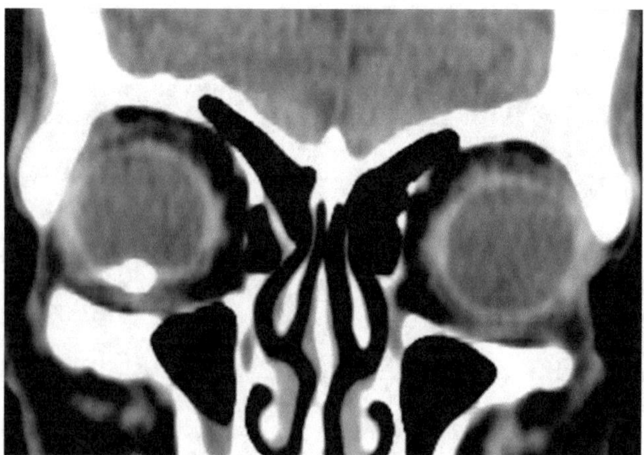

Fig. 18.96 An IOFB entered the eye of this patient during work on the London underground. He had taken off his goggles whilst an adjacent worker was breaking concrete with a powered hammer

Table 18.6 Difficulty rating for surgery for IOFB

Difficulty rating	Moderate
Success rates	High
Complication rates	Moderate
When to use in training	Middle

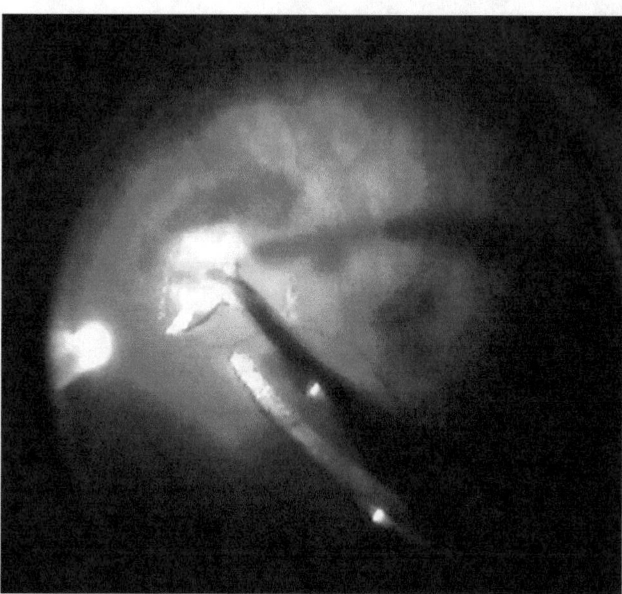

Fig. 18.97 Foreign body forceps are used in this patient with diamond-dusted tips to allow secure grasping of foreign bodies and manipulation of any incarceration sites

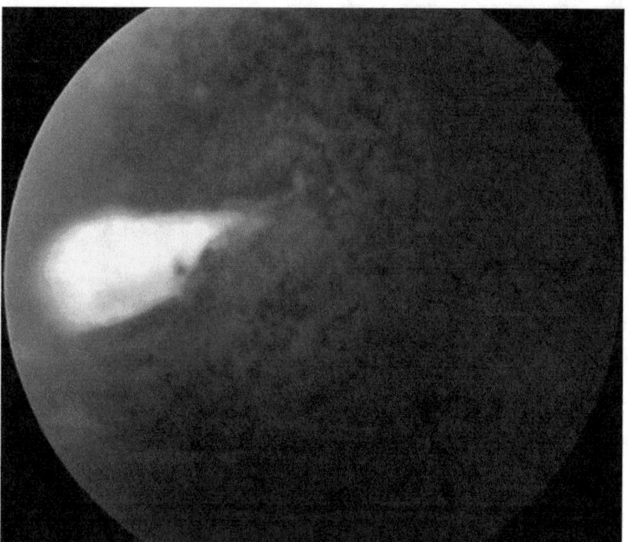

Fig. 18.98 A patient is shown after removal of an IOFB with a laser around the impact site. There is a defect in the retina and choroid. The scleral is visible and the retinal remains flat without the need for tamponade

posterior approach, maintain anterior capsule for a sulcus fixated IOL with optic capture.

PPV, the Posterior Segment

Perform the PPV and clear the vitreous away from the IOFB so that it is loosened and so as not incarcerate vitreous into the forceps during extraction. If the IOFB is small enough remove it through a sclerotomy. Judge the size of the IOFB in cross section remembering that a square end requires an even larger slit for removal. Add the size of the forceps tips (most are larger than 20 gauge) into the estimation of the size of sclerotomy. Enlarge the sclerotomy, which is furthest from the IOFB. By using this sclerotomy the IOFB can be removed in a perpendicular fashion from the retina whilst avoiding any scraping the retina or choroid. Insert diamond-dusted IOFB forceps through this sclerotomy. Grasp the free end of the IOFB. Take care that you do not grab either retina or vitreous. If you do, disengage and clear more vitreous from the IOFB, or using one leg of the forceps, tip the IOFB gently away from the retina and try again.

Bring the IOFB into the vitreous cavity and without releasing the forceps draw it to the sclerotomy and remove it through the sclerotomy. Sew over this sclerotomy. You will most likely have to induce a posterior vitreous detachment and then remove the remaining vitreous. Removing the posterior hyaloid will reduce the chance of tractional bands causing later tractional retinal detachment.

Inspect the impact site.

Several situations arise:

1. Local whitening of the retina without tear. Take no action and close.
2. Tear to the retina. Apply laser around the tear and fill the eye with the appropriate gas.
3. Tear to the retina and choroid. Laser the retina and insert silicone oil.
4. Tear to the retina and choroid and perforation of the sclera, i.e. a perforating injury. Prognosis is poorer. Laser around the impact site and insert silicone oil if possible.

Publications describing patients who have not received retinopexy or PVD peel during surgery but these procedures now have low morbidity and their avoidance is not recommended [74].

Occasionally the IOFB is so large that to remove it through a sclerotomy would require a wound so big that it would destabilise the globe during the operation. A large IOFB usually injures the lens, often with pre-existing disruption of the integrity of the capsule. Therefore, a cataract extraction has been necessary. This provides the surgeon with two features which are useful.

1. A pre-existing wound used for the cataract extraction.
2. Access to the anterior chamber from the posterior chamber.

In this circumstance, fill the anterior chamber with viscoelastic. Grasp the IOFB with the forceps and pass the IOFB through the pupil into the anterior chamber. With the free hand, cut the sutures, open the cataract wound, insert forceps into the anterior chamber, take hold of the IOFB and remove it through the wound (Figs. 18.99 and 18.100)

The Magnet

This is used less often now because of a reported higher incidence of postoperative retinal detachment at 15% and phthisis at 5% [75–77].

Coexisting problems may occur and can be dealt with using the principles described elsewhere in this book.

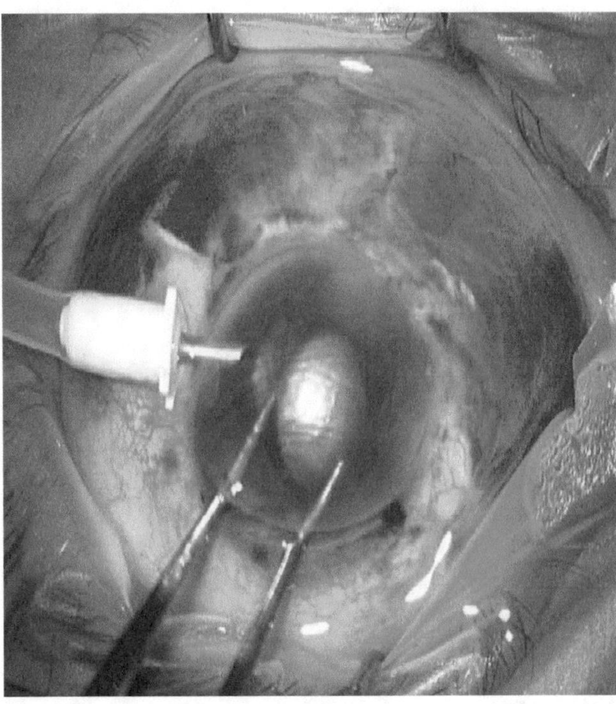

Fig. 18.99 An airgun pellet has been removed via a corneal section. This pellet was lodged at 6 o'clock damaging the lens and the posterior segment

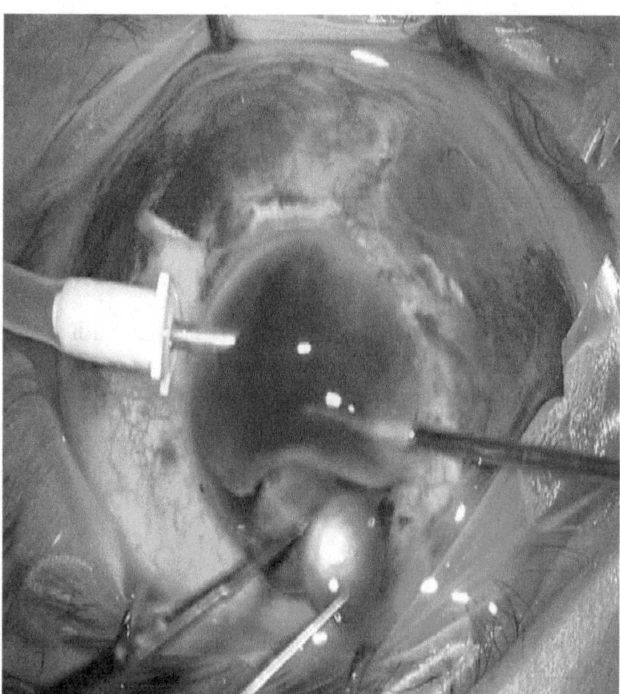

Fig. 18.100 A large wound was required to remove the pellet

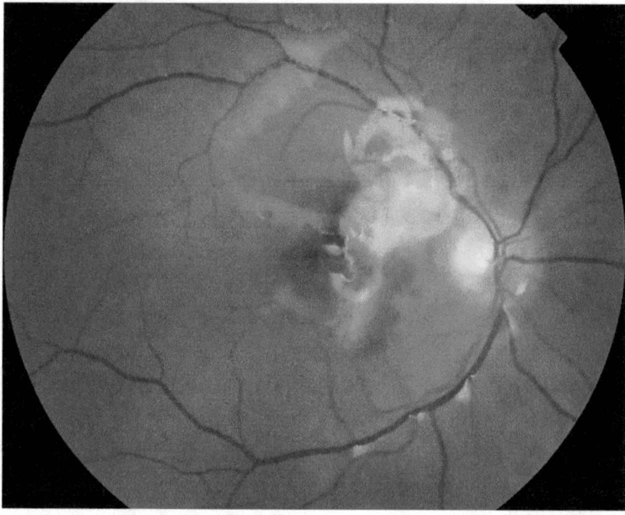

Fig. 18.101 An IOFB impact site on the macula which was complicated postoperatively with the development of a secondary CNV at 9 months, as seen on the FFA. Vision was counting fingers throughout

1. Retinal Detachment
2. Vitreous haemorrhage
3. Choroidal haemorrhage
4. Endophthalmitis

Unusual Problems

1.	Wooden IOFB	Risk of infection is high.
2.	Plastic IOFB	Will not appear on X-ray
3.	Multiple IOFBs	Must be considered, detected and removed

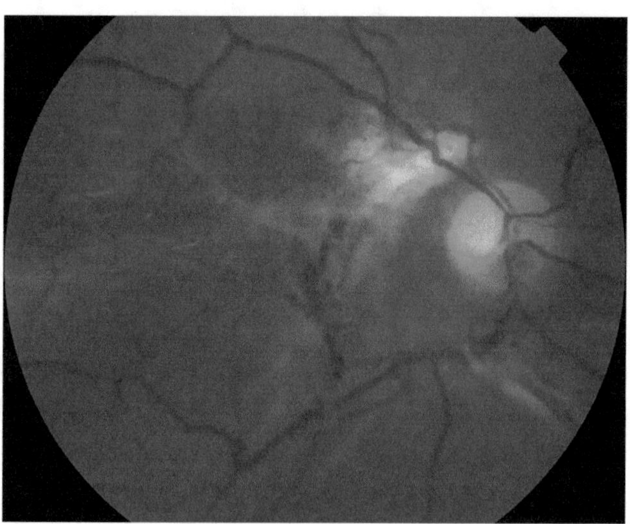

Fig. 18.102 Healing of the impact site

Visual Outcome (Figs. 18.101, 18.102, 18.103, 18.104)

IOFBs tend to demonstrate a less severe outcome than other severe ocular trauma with only 27% retaining 20/200 or worse vision and 50% attaining 20/40 vision or better [78]. The visual outcome is worse when there is retinal detachment, a large IOFB or additional anterior segment injury [70].

Siderosis

This is a late complication of retained iron. It takes weeks and months to affect the retina. The IOFB may dissolve and no longer be detectable. Features are tonic pupil, greenish tinge to the iris and late-onset cataract formation [67, 68]. Retinal damage from this is slow to occur and some patients may have only mild loss of vision over years. Electroretinography demonstrates reduction in retinal function with reduced amplitudes (Figs. 18.105, 18.106, 18.107, 18.108, and 18.109).

Perforating Injury

Perforating injury, where the projectile enters and exits the eye, has a very high retinal detachment rate and only one third achieve moderate vision [55, 79].

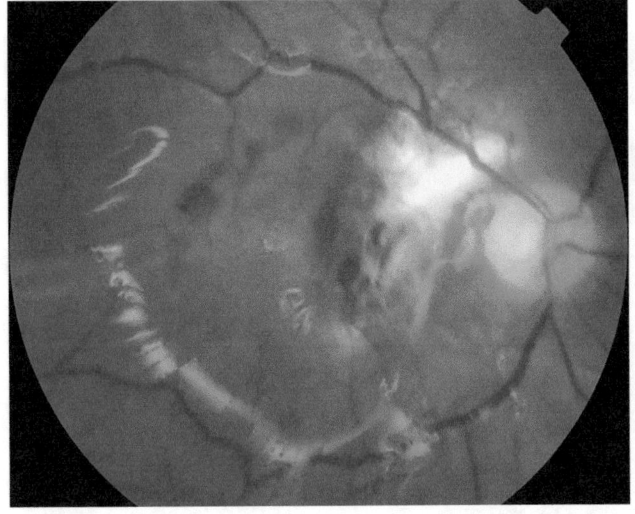

Fig. 18.103 A CNV appeared

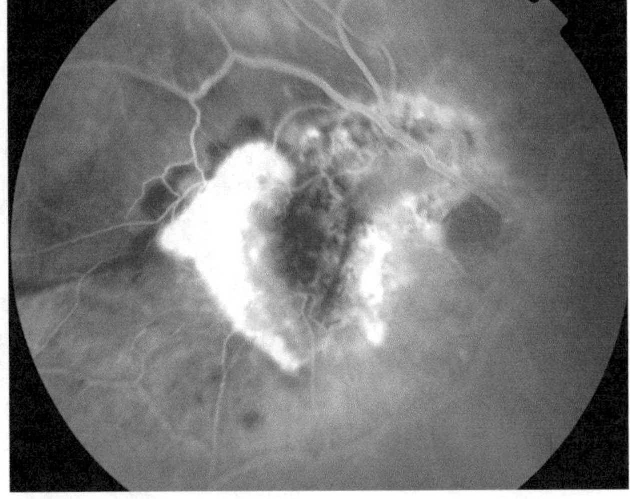

Fig. 18.104 FFA of the CNV

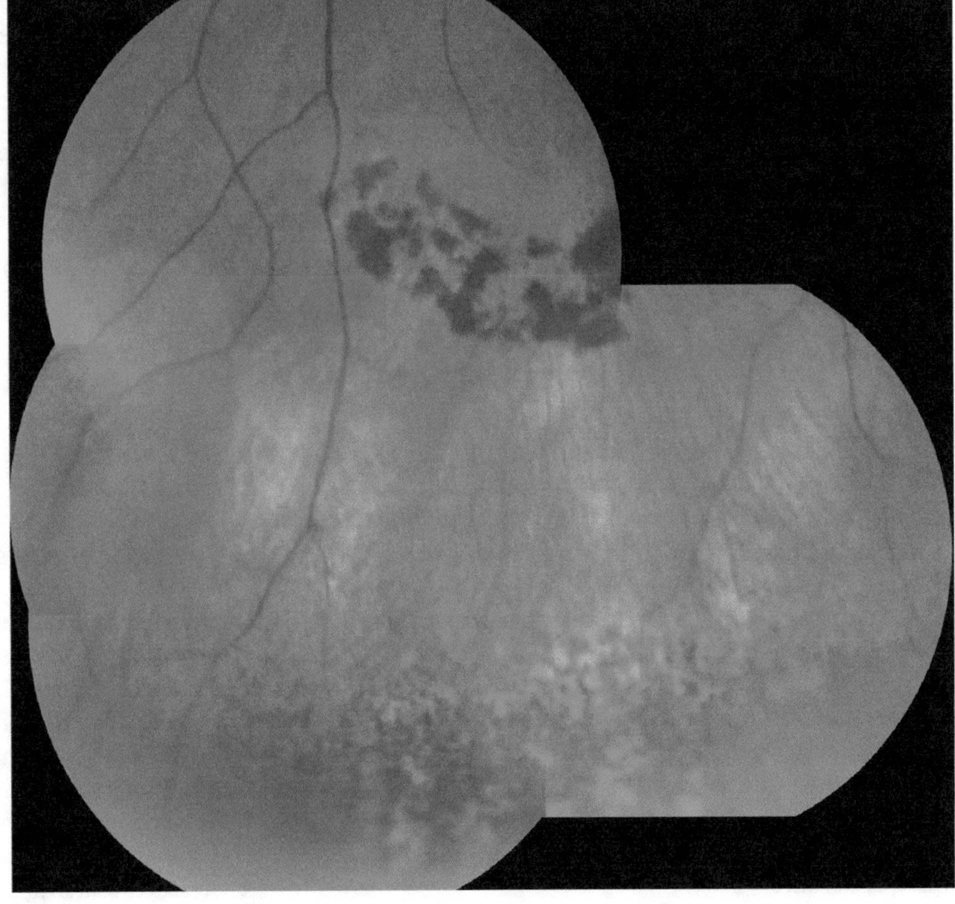

Fig. 18.105 An IOFB was removed after a delay of 6 weeks, damage of the retina can be seen from siderosis near the site of the IOFB

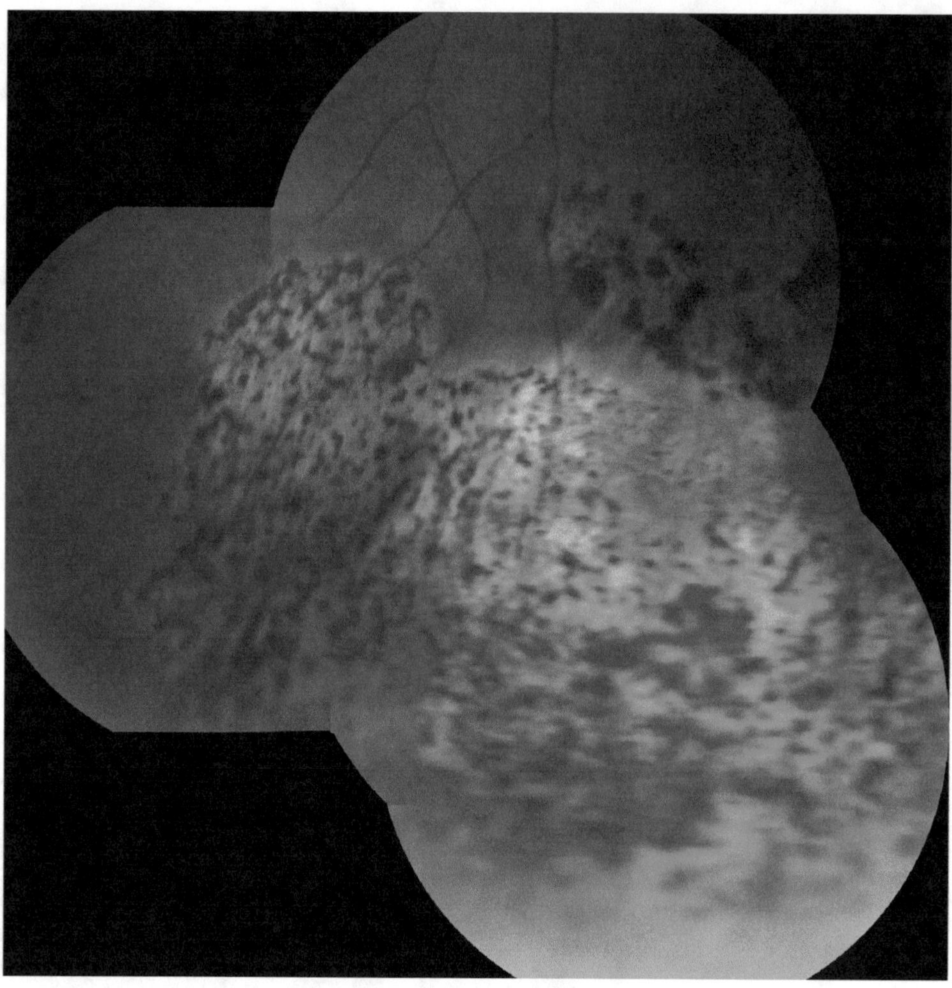

Fig. 18.106 Two months later the changes in the RPE are more extensive from siderosis

This may occur from:

1. An FB entering and exiting the eye and remaining in the orbit, e.g. shot gum pellet, air rifle pellet. Repair of the eye is required but the FB can be left in the orbit.
2. An IOFB entering the eye perforating the scleral posteriorly but remaining in situ in the posterior sclera, e.g. fragment of metal from hammer and chisel.
3. An injury with a long sharp instrument entering the eye deep enough to injure the posterior sclera.

Sometimes, the exit wound at the posterior of the eye is found unexpectedly during surgery. Often there is the incarceration of tissue that self-seals the exit allowing the internal filling of the eye with silicone oil. IOP during silicone oil insertion should be kept to a minimum to avoid posterior egress of the oil.

There is a high risk of traction from the incarceration site postoperatively but surprisingly a stable eye with some vision can be obtained and if the retina is stable or can be stabilised by further surgery silicone oil can be removed later. Theoretically, an increased risk of sympathetic ophthalmia could occur but as these cases are rare an assessment of this risk is not available (Figs. 18.110, 18.111, and 18.112).

Sympathetic Ophthalmia

This is a panuveitis of both the affected and fellow eye stimulated by the exposure of intraocular antigens to the immune system. Look for deep white spots in the retina, Dalen Fuchs's nodules. The risk after trauma appears to be low (0.1–0.3%) [80–82]. It may indeed be commoner after posterior segment surgery, i.e. PPV, than after trauma [83]. Improved control of the condition with immune suppression and better visual outcome has caused a shift away from primary enucleation (removal of the eye at presentation) as a method to prevent uveitis. In severe ocular trauma the eye can be repaired with, on occasion, surprising visual recovery, or maintenance of a cosmetically acceptable eye; therefore,

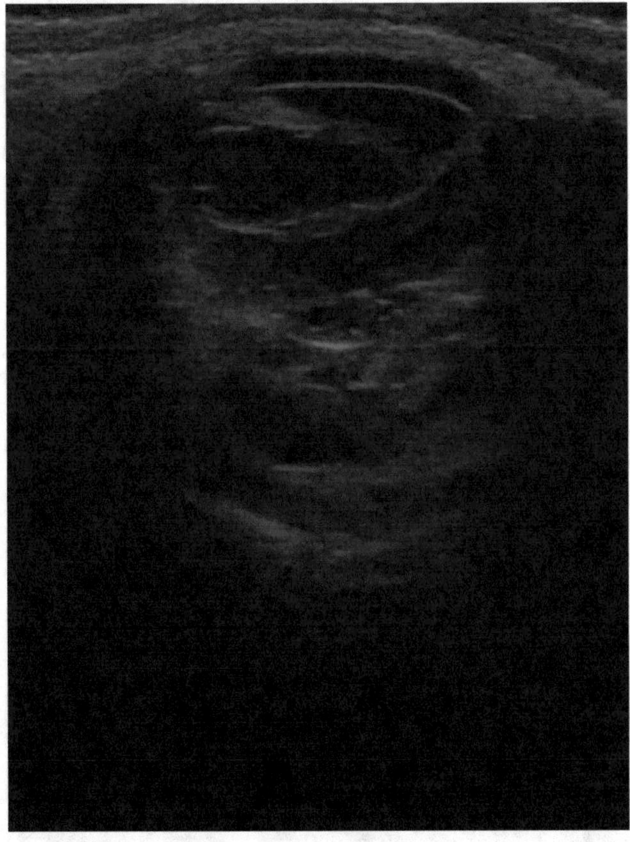

Fig. 18.107 A patient shot in the face by a shotgun blast and likely to have a perforating injury in this eye. There is disruption of the anterior segment, vitreous haemorrhage, PVR retinal detachment, choroidal thickening, shortening of the eye and hypotony. The eye is going into a phthisis bulbi

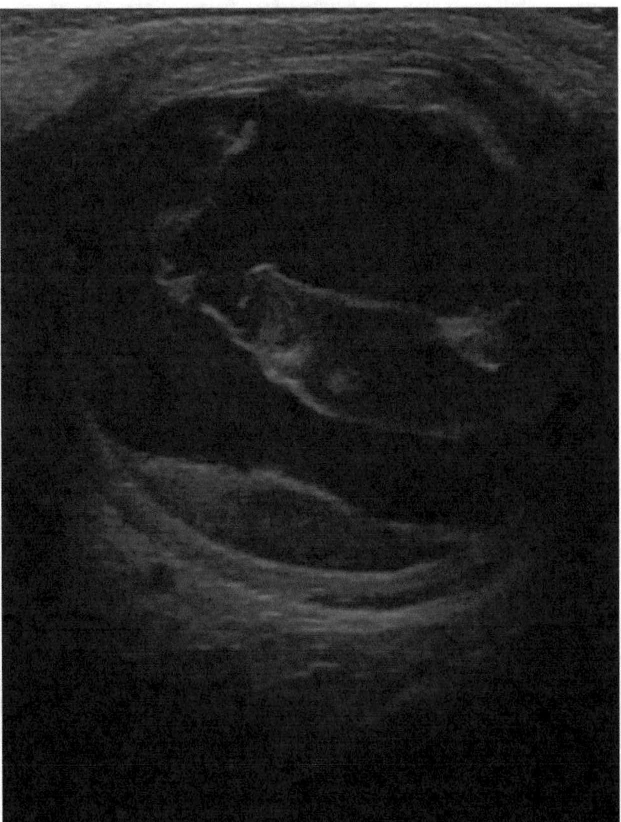

Fig. 18.108 The other eye of the patient shot in the face by a shotgun. This eye has a severe central corneal wound, is aphakic. On ultrasound, the posterior segment shows an incarcerated vitreous with haemorrhage and an inferior retinal elevation which may be serous from a resolution of subretinal haemorrhage. Elsewhere the retina is in place and visual recovery is possible depending on the status of the macula and success of anterior segment reconstruction

enucleation is not favoured. I am yet to see a proven case of sympathetic ophthalmia in my practice of more than 10,000 vitreoretinal operations, including patients with severe ocular trauma, and I have not performed enucleation or evisceration on any of my patients.

Proliferative Vitreoretinopathy

The incidence of PVR with different presentation patterns is shown in Table 18.7 [84], with vitreous haemorrhage the strongest predictor of its development. The complication is associated with a poorer visual outcome and is the reason for the urgency of operation after the presentation, frequent use of silicone oil insertion and careful follow up.

Phthisis bulbi (Fig. 18.113)

If a hypotonous eye is going phthisical, urgent insertion of silicone oil to allow preservation of the size of the globe is advised. If cyclitic membranes are present these can be dissected and segmented in an attempt to regain some function of the ciliary body [85, 86]. This may allow adequate cosmesis with a slight reduction in the size of the eye seen as mild ptosis by the patient or allow cornea scleral shell application if the shrinkage is noticeable or the anterior segment is unsightly. This is preferable to evisceration or enucleation (and its attendant orbital fat atrophy) if the eye is not painful. Band keratopathy may eventually occur if the eye remains formed. This may cause intermittent epithelial breakdown causing pain, usually a severe sudden onset pain lasting a few hours at a time. It can be treated with Excimer laser ablation.

Note: Hypotony is a key surrogate marker for the health of the eye; if the IOP is in the normal range then you can perform further surgery to maximise the vision. If the IOP is low with silicone oil in the eye and there is no other reason such as persistent RD, then the eye is unlikely to tolerate repeat operations. In this case, it may be best to leave the silicone oil in situ to maintain the cosmetic appearance of the eye. Cosmesis is important in these patients who are often relatively young.

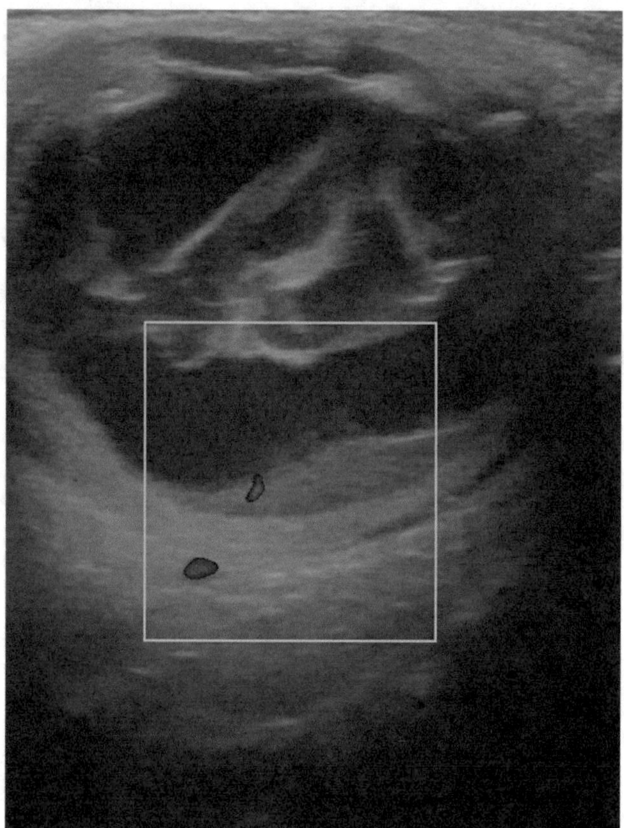

Fig. 18.109 Colour Doppler ultrasound shows a retinal blood vessel in the elevation

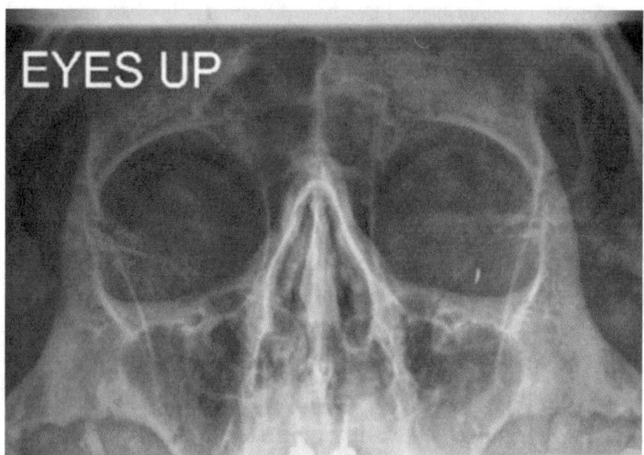

Fig. 18.110 X-rays showing an IOFB which has perforated the globe (entry and exit wound)

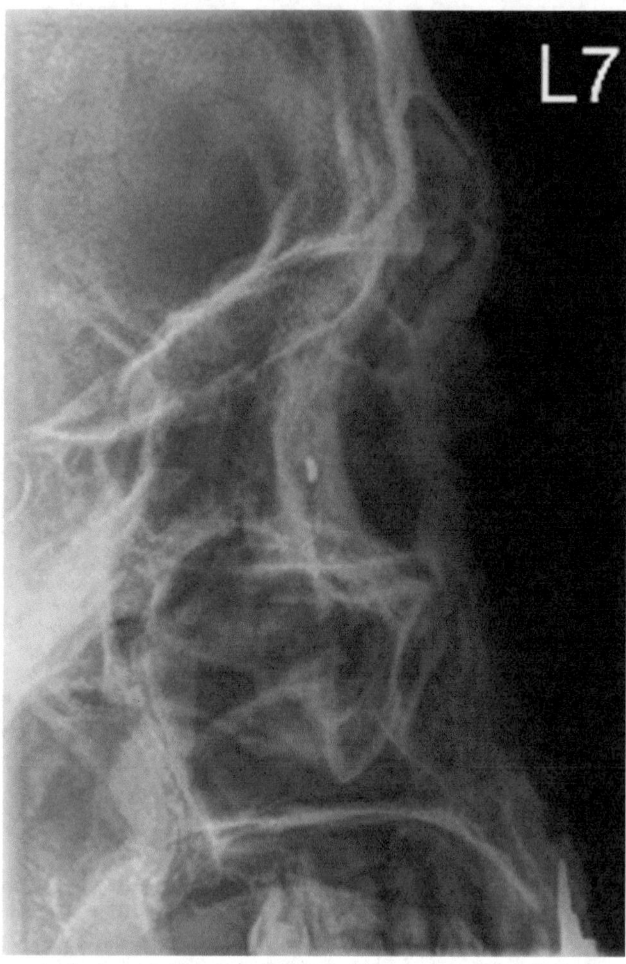

Fig. 18.111 Xray of the IOFB

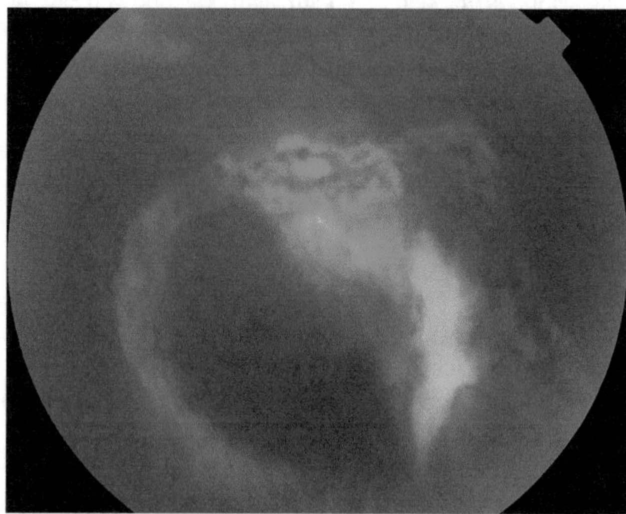

Fig. 18.112 The posterior wound with the surrounding laser is stable in this eye after repair of the perforation and removal of the IOFB

When Not to Operate

At Presentation

There are circumstances in severe trauma in which the chance of success from surgery is so low that to put the patient through surgery may not be the best approach. Surgery on a severely damaged eye may turn a blind comfortable eye into a blind painful eye. For example, severe trauma with a closed CA12 CP12 funnel RRD is unlikely to

Table 18.7 PVR and trauma

	Frequency of PVR %	Median duration till PVR develops (months)
Perforation	43	1.3
Rupture	21	2.1
Penetration	15	3.2
IOFB	11	3.1
Contusion	1	5.7

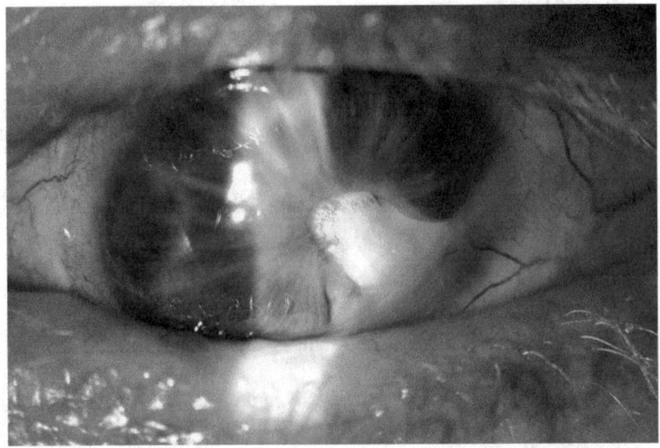

Fig. 18.113 This patient has suffered a phthisis of his eye after receiving a blunt trauma from a rubber surround for a car window screen which burst during the fitting of the screen

obtain any useful vision even if a small island of the retina is attached. The surgery is fraught with difficulty such as bleeding and there may be choroidal haemorrhage in addition. Evacuation of solid choroidal haemorrhage by surgical aspiration is rarely effective. By operating the discomfort of the eye is increased and may take months to subside. Patients with severe trauma and choroidal haemorrhage often have an ache which improves slowly over many weeks after the injury, surgery increases the pain again and slows the recovery. Visual acuity of no perception of light is not a reason to avoid surgery as 26% of patients who had NPL at presentation or on day one postoperatively have been shown to recover some vision [87].

Postoperatively

Be careful of repeated operations in an eye with a low IOP as each operation may exacerbate the risk of phthisis bulbi. Make sure you have a good reason to operate and a plan for improving the situation, otherwise "cut your losses". Be aware that patients do not want their cosmetic appearance affected for no visual gain or to continue their period of pain and discomfort.

Summary

1. Contusion injury should be treated conservatively with complications such as vitreous haemorrhage and retinal detachment operated upon as indicated. Retinal dialysis the commonest cause of a late-onset retinal detachment is easily treated by cryotherapy and explant. Giant retinal tears require vitrectomy and endotamponade often with silicone oil insertion. If a ragged tear of the retina occurs in traumatised retina, often these can be observed and only treated if an extension of a retinal detachment occurs. Macular holes can spontaneously close or be closed by vitrectomy and gas [88].
2. Rupture requires immediate repair requiring surgical exploration of the globe at presentation. Thereafter, the eye can be operated upon at 1–2 weeks for complications. If the rupture has involved the choroid and retina often surgery will be required to relieve traction on the retina by surgical relieving retinectomy.
3. The entry wound should be closed in the first instance with intravitreal antibiotics inserted. It is increasingly rare to use the surgical magnet for IOFB. Most can be removed on the next day using vitrectomy, diamond-dusted intraocular forceps and extraction through a sclerotomy. An IOFB is visible during vitrectomy in this figure.
4. Penetrating injury requires immediate repair and perhaps intravitreal antibiotics because of a risk of bacterial endophthalmitis. If the injury has involved the choroid and retina often surgery will be required to relieve traction on the retina by relieving retinectomy.

References

1. Parver LM, Dannenberg AL, Blacklow B, Fowler CJ, Brechner RJ, Tielsch JM. Characteristics and causes of penetrating eye injuries reported to the National eye Trauma System Registry, 1985–91. Public Health Rep. 1993;108(5):625–32.
2. Tielsch JM, Parver L, Shankar B. Time trends in the incidence of hospitalized ocular trauma. Arch Ophthalmol. 1989;107(4): 519–23.
3. Tielsch JM, Parver LM. Determinants of hospital charges and length of stay for ocular trauma. Ophthalmology. 1990;97(2):231–7.
4. Canavan YM, O'Flaherty MJ, Archer DB, Elwood JH. A 10-year survey of eye injuries in Northern Ireland, 1967–76. Br J Ophthalmol. 1980;64(8):618–25.
5. Schein OD, Hibberd PL, Shingleton BJ, Kunzweiler T, Frambach DA, Seddon JM, et al. The spectrum and burden of ocular injury. Ophthalmology. 1988;95(3):300–5.
6. Liggett PE, Pince KJ, Barlow W, Ragen M, Ryan SJ. Ocular trauma in an urban population. Review of 1132 cases. Ophthalmology. 1990;97(5):581–4.

7. Khatry SK, Lewis AE, Schein OD, Thapa MD, Pradhan EK, Katz J. The epidemiology of ocular trauma in rural Nepal. Br J Ophthalmol. 2004;88(4):456–60.
8. Appiah AP. The nature, causes, and visual outcome of ocular trauma requiring posterior segment surgery at a county hospital. Ann Ophthalmol. 1991;23(11):430–3.
9. Ahmadieh H, Soheilian M, Sajjadi H, Azarmina M, Abrishami M. Vitrectomy in ocular trauma. Factors influencing final visual outcome. Retina. 1993;13(2):107–13.
10. Ghoraba H. Posterior segment glass intraocular foreign bodies following car accident or explosion. Graefes Arch Clin Exp Ophthalmol. 2002;240(7):524–8.
11. Alfaro DV, Chaudhry NA, Walonker AF, Runyan T, Saito Y, Liggett PE. Penetrating eye injuries in young children. Retina. 1994;14(3):201–5.
12. May DR, Kuhn FP, Morris RE, Witherspoon CD, Danis RP, Matthews GP, et al. The epidemiology of serious eye injuries from the United States eye injury registry. Graefes Arch Clin Exp Ophthalmol. 2000;238(2):153–7.
13. Kuhn F, Morris R, Witherspoon CD, Heimann K, Jeffers JB, Treister G. A standardized classification of ocular trauma. Ophthalmology. 1996;103(2):240–3.
14. Han DP. Retinal detachment caused by air bag injury. Arch Ophthalmol. 1993;111(10):1317–8.
15. Pieramici DJ, Kuhn F. Frontal air bags and eye injury patterns in automobile crashes. Arch Ophthalmol. 2003;121(12):1807–8.
16. Pearlman JA, Au Eong KG, Kuhn F, Pieramici DJ. Airbags and eye injuries: epidemiology, spectrum of injury, and analysis of risk factors. Surv Ophthalmol. 2001;46(3):234–42.
17. Mason JO III, Feist RM, White MF Jr. Ocular trauma from paintball-pellet war games. South Med J. 2002;95(2):218–22.
18. Cooney MJ, Pieramici DJ. Eye injuries caused by bungee cords. Ophthalmology. 1997;104(10):1644–7.
19. Peyman GA, Raichand M, Goldberg MF, Brown S. Vitrectomy in the management of intraocular foreign bodies and their complications. Br J Ophthalmol. 1980;64(7):476–82.
20. Coleman DJ. Early vitrectomy in the management of the severely traumatized eye. Am J Ophthalmol. 1982;93(5):543–51.
21. Conway BP, Michels RG. Vitrectomy techniques in the management of selected penetrating ocular injuries. Ophthalmology. 1978;85(6):560–83.
22. Ryan SJ. Results of pars plana vitrectomy in penetrating ocular trauma. Int Ophthalmol. 1978;1(1):5–8.
23. Mody KV, Blach RK, Leaver PK, McLeod D. Closed vitrectomy after trauma. Trans Ophthalmol Soc UK. 1978;98(1):55–8.
24. Mandelcorn MS. Results after vitrectomy in trauma. Can J Ophthalmol. 1977;12(1):34–7.
25. Hutton WL, Snyder WB, Vaiser A. Vitrectomy in the treatment of ocular perforating injuries. Am J Ophthalmol. 1976;81(6):733–9.
26. Pieramici DJ, MacCumber MW, Humayun MU, Marsh MJ, De Juan E Jr. Open-globe injury. Update on types of injuries and visual results. Ophthalmology. 1996;103(11):1798–803.
27. Alappatt JJ, Hutchins RK. Retinal detachments due to traumatic tears in the pars plana ciliaris. Retina. 1998;18(6):506–9.
28. Martin DF, Awh CC, McCuen BW, Jaffe GJ, Slott JH, Machemer R. Treatment and pathogenesis of traumatic chorioretinal rupture (sclopetaria). Am J Ophthalmol. 1994;117(2):190–200.
29. trauma.
30. Russell SR, Olsen KR, Folk JC. Predictors of scleral rupture and the role of vitrectomy in severe blunt ocular trauma. Am J Ophthalmol. 1988;105(3):253–7.
31. Joseph DP, Pieramici DJ, Beauchamp NJ Jr. Computed tomography in the diagnosis and prognosis of open-globe injuries. Ophthalmology. 2000;107(10):1899–906.
32. Winthrop SR, Cleary PE, Minckler DS, Ryan SJ. Penetrating eye injuries: a histopathological review. Br J Ophthalmol. 1980;64(11):809–17.
33. Morris RE, Witherspoon CD, Helms HA Jr, Feist RM, Byrne JB Jr. Eye injury registry of Alabama (preliminary report): demographics and prognosis of severe eye injury. South Med J. 1987;80(7):810–6.
34. Soheilian M, Peyman GA, Wafapoor H, Navarro GC, Thompson H. Surgical management of traumatic retinal detachment with perfluorocarbon liquid. Vitreon Study Group. Int Ophthalmol. 1996;20(5):241–9.
35. Liggett PE, Gauderman WJ, Moreira CM, Barlow W, Green RL, Ryan SJ. Pars plana vitrectomy for acute retinal detachment in penetrating ocular injuries. Arch Ophthalmol. 1990;108(12):1724–8.
36. Feist RM, Lim JI, Joondeph BC, Pflugfelder SC, Mieler WF, Ticho BH, et al. Penetrating ocular injury from contaminated eating utensils. Arch Ophthalmol. 1991;109(1):63–6.
37. Pulido JS, Gupta S, Folk JC, Ossoiny KC. Perforating BB gun injuries of the globe. Ophthalmic Surg Lasers. 1997;28(8):625–32.
38. Enger C, Schein OD, Tielsch JM. Risk factors for ocular injuries caused by air guns. Arch Ophthalmol. 1996;114(4):469–74.
39. Schein OD, Enger C, Tielsch JM. The context and consequences of ocular injuries from air guns. Am J Ophthalmol. 1994;117(4):501–6.
40. Aylward GW, Cooling RJ, Leaver PK. Trauma-induced retinal detachment associated with giant retinal tears. Retina. 1993;13(2):136–41.
41. Gupta AK, Ghosh B, Mazumdar S, Gupta A. An unusual intraocular foreign body. Acta Ophthalmol Scand. 1996;74(2):200–1.
42. Fortuin ME, Blanksma LJ. An unusual complication of perforating wounds of the eye. Doc Ophthalmol. 1986;61(3–4):197–203.
43. Gozum N, Kir N, Ovali T. Internal ophthalmomyiasis presenting as endophthalmitis associated with an intraocular foreign body. Ophthalmic Surg Lasers Imaging. 2003;34(6):472–4.
44. Essex RW, Yi Q, Charles PG, Allen PJ. Post-traumatic endophthalmitis. Ophthalmology. 2004;111(11):2015–22. doi: S0161-6420(04)00126-5 [pii]. https://doi.org/10.1016/j.ophtha.2003.09.041.
45. Lieb DF, Scott IU, Flynn HW Jr, Miller D, Feuer WJ. Open globe injuries with positive intraocular cultures: factors influencing final visual acuity outcomes. Ophthalmology. 2003;110(8):1560–6.
46. Miller JJ, Scott IU, Flynn HW Jr, Smiddy WE, Murray TG, Berrocal A, et al. Endophthalmitis caused by Bacillus species. Am J Ophthalmol. 2008;145(5):883–8. doi: S0002-9394(08)00005-6 [pii]. https://doi.org/10.1016/j.ajo.2007.12.026.
47. Alfaro DV, Roth D, Liggett PE. Posttraumatic endophthalmitis. Causative organisms, treatment, and prevention. Retina. 1994;14(3):206–11.
48. Alfaro DV, Roth DB, Laughlin RM, Goyal M, Liggett PE. Paediatric post-traumatic endophthalmitis. Br J Ophthalmol. 1995;79(10):888–91.
49. Reynolds DS, Flynn HW Jr. Endophthalmitis after penetrating ocular trauma. Curr Opin Ophthalmol. 1997;8(3):32–8.
50. Foster RE, Martinez JA, Murray TG, Rubsamen PE, Flynn HW Jr, Forster RK. Useful visual outcomes after treatment of *Bacillus cereus* endophthalmitis. Ophthalmology. 1996;103(3):390–7.
51. Essex RW, Charles PG, Allen PJ. Three cases of post-traumatic endophthalmitis caused by unusual bacteria. Clin Exp Ophthalmol. 2004;32(4):445–7. https://doi.org/10.1111/j.1442--9071.2004.00855.x. CEO855 [pii]
52. Narang S, Gupta V, Gupta A, Dogra MR, Pandav SS, Das S. Role of prophylactic intravitreal antibiotics in open globe injuries. Indian J Ophthalmol. 2003;51(1):39–44.
53. Meredith TA, Gordon PA. Pars plana vitrectomy for severe penetrating injury with posterior segment involvement. Am J Ophthalmol. 1987;103(4):549–54.

54. Ung C, Stryjewski TP, Eliott D. Indications, findings, and outcomes of pars Plana Vitrectomy after open globe injury. Ophthalmol Retina. 2019; https://doi.org/10.1016/j.oret.2019.09.003.
55. Pieramici DJ, Eong KG, Sternberg P Jr, Marsh MJ. The prognostic significance of a system for classifying mechanical injuries of the eye (globe) in open-globe injuries. J Trauma. 2003;54(4):750–4.
56. Esmaeli B, Elner SG, Schork MA, Elner VM. Visual outcome and ocular survival after penetrating trauma. A clinicopathologic study. Ophthalmology. 1995;102(3):393–400.
57. Kuhn F, Maisiak R, Mann L, Mester V, Morris R, Witherspoon CD. The ocular trauma score (OTS). Ophthalmol Clin N Am. 2002;15(2):163–5. vi
58. Schmidt GW, Broman AT, Hindman HB, Grant MP. Vision survival after open globe injury predicted by classification and regression tree analysis. Ophthalmology. 2008;115(1):202–9. doi: S0161-6420(07)00380-6 [pii]. https://doi.org/10.1016/j.ophtha.2007.04.008.
59. Man CY, Steel D. Visual outcome after open globe injury: a comparison of two prognostic models--the ocular trauma score and the classification and regression tree. Eye (Lond). 24(1):84–9. doi: eye200916 [pii]. https://doi.org/10.1038/eye.2009.16.
60. Lambert HM, Sipperley JO. Intraocular foreign body from a nylon line grass trimmer. Ann Ophthalmol. 1983;15(10):936–7.
61. Alfaro DV, Tran VT, Runyan T, Chong LP, Ryan SJ, Liggett PE. Vitrectomy for perforating eye injuries from shotgun pellets. Am J Ophthalmol. 1992;114(1):81–5.
62. Morris RE, Witherspoon CD, Feist RM, Byrne JB Jr, Ottemiller DE. Bilateral ocular shotgun injury. Am J Ophthalmol. 1987;103(5):695–700.
63. Hamanaka N, Ikeda T, Inokuchi N, Shirai S, Uchihori Y. A case of an intraocular foreign body due to graphite pencil lead complicated by endophthalmitis. Ophthalmic Surg Lasers. 1999;30(3):229–31.
64. John G, Witherspoon CD, Feist RM, Morris R. Ocular lawnmower injuries. Ophthalmology. 1988;95(10):1367–70.
65. Ahmadieh H, Sajjadi H, Azarmina M, Soheilian M, Baharivand N. Surgical management of intraretinal foreign bodies. Retina. 1994;14(5):397–403.
66. Billi B, Lesnoni G, Scassa C, Giuliano MA, Coppe AM, Rossi T. Copper intraocular foreign body: diagnosis and treatment. Eur J Ophthalmol. 1995;5(4):235–9.
67. Weiss MJ, Hofeldt AJ, Behrens M, Fisher K. Ocular siderosis. Diagnosis Manage Retina. 1997;17(2):105–8.
68. Sneed SR, Weingeist TA. Management of siderosis bulbi due to a retained iron-containing intraocular foreign body. Ophthalmology. 1990;97(3):375–9.
69. Thompson JT, Parver LM, Enger CL, Mieler WF, Liggett PE. Infectious endophthalmitis after penetrating injuries with retained intraocular foreign bodies. National Eye Trauma Syst Ophthalmol. 1993;100(10):1468–74.
70. Jonas JB, Knorr HL, Budde WM. Prognostic factors in ocular injuries caused by intraocular or retrobulbar foreign bodies. Ophthalmology. 2000;107(5):823–8.
71. Knox FA, Best RM, Kinsella F, Mirza K, Sharkey JA, Mulholland D, et al. Management of endophthalmitis with retained intraocular foreign body. Eye. 2004;18(2):179–82.
72. Pieramici DJ, Capone A Jr, Rubsamen PE, Roseman RL. Lens preservation after intraocular foreign body injuries. Ophthalmology. 1996;103(10):1563–7.
73. Tyagi AK, Kheterpal S, Callear AB, Kirkby GR, Price NJ. Simultaneous posterior chamber intraocular lens implant combined with vitreoretinal surgery for intraocular foreign body injuries. Eye. 1998;12(Pt 2):230–3.
74. Ambler JS, Meyers SM. Management of intraretinal metallic foreign bodies without retinopexy in the absence of retinal detachment. Ophthalmology. 1991;98(3):391–4.
75. Chiquet C, Zech JC, Gain P, Adeleine P, Trepsat C. Visual outcome and prognostic factors after magnetic extraction of posterior segment foreign bodies in 40 cases. Br J Ophthalmol. 1998;82(7):801–6.
76. Karel I, Diblik P. Management of posterior segment foreign bodies and long-term results. Eur J Ophthalmol. 1995;5(2):113–8.
77. Chow DR, Garretson BR, Kuczynski B, Williams GA, Margherio R, Cox MS, et al. External versus internal approach to the removal of metallic intraocular foreign bodies. Retina. 2000;20(4):364–9.
78. Wani VB, Al Ajmi M, Thalib L, Azad RV, Abul M, Al Ghanim M, et al. Vitrectomy for posterior segment intraocular foreign bodies: visual results and prognostic factors. Retina. 2003;23(5):654–60.
79. Ramsay RC, Cantrill HL, Knobloch WH. Vitrectomy for double penetrating ocular injuries. Am J Ophthalmol. 1985;100(4):586–9.
80. Allen JC. Sympathetic ophthalmia, a disappearing disease. JAMA. 1969;209(7):1090.
81. Kraus-Mackiw E. Prevention of sympathetic ophthalmia. State of the art 1989. Int Ophthalmol. 1990;14(5–6):391–4.
82. Liddy L, Stuart J. Sympathetic ophthalmia in Canada. Can J Ophthalmol. 1972;7(2):157–9.
83. Kilmartin DJ, Dick AD, Forrester JV. Prospective surveillance of sympathetic ophthalmia in the UK and Republic of Ireland. Br J Ophthalmol. 2000;84(3):259–63.
84. Cardillo JA, Stout JT, LaBree L, Azen SP, Omphroy L, Cui JZ, et al. Post-traumatic proliferative vitreoretinopathy. The epidemiologic profile, onset, risk factors, and visual outcome. Ophthalmology. 1997;104(7):1166–73.
85. Essex RW, Tufail A, Bunce C, Aylward GW. Two-year results of surgical removal of choroidal neovascular membranes related to non-age-related macular degeneration. Br J Ophthalmol. 2007;91(5):649–54. doi: 91/5/649 [pii]. https://doi.org/10.1136/bjo.2005.089458.
86. Banaee T, Ahmadieh H, Abrishami M, Moosavi M. Removal of traumatic cyclitic membranes: surgical technique and results. Graefes Arch Clin Exp Ophthalmol. 2007;245(3):443–7. https://doi.org/10.1007/s00417-006-0337-z.
87. Salehi-Had H, Andreoli CM, Andreoli MT, Kloek CE, Mukai S. Visual outcomes of vitreoretinal surgery in eyes with severe open-globe injury presenting with no-light-perception vision. Graefes Arch Clin Exp Ophthalmol. 2009;247(4):477–83. https://doi.org/10.1007/s00417-009-1035-4.
88. Kuhn F, Morris R, Mester V, Witherspoon CD. Internal limiting membrane removal for traumatic macular holes. Ophthalmic Surg Lasers. 2001;32(4):308–15.

Uveitis and Allied Disorders

19

Contents

Introduction

Non-infectious Uveitis of the Posterior Segment (Fig. 19.1)

The variety of possible presentations of uveitis of the posterior segment makes it difficult to generalise on the surgical approach [1–3]. Bilateral surgery over 10 years in vitritis is 10% {Fajgenbaum, 2018 #11883}. The conditions that the surgeon may encounter, depending on the racial mix and geographical location, include:

- Intermediate uveitis
- Sarcoidosis
- Uveitis of juvenile chronic arthritis
- Behcet's disease
- Idiopathic vasculitis including Eales' disease
- Birdshot chorioretinopathy

T. H. Williamson, *Vitreoretinal Surgery*, https://doi.org/10.1007/978-3-030-68769-4_19

- Vogt–Koyanagi–Harada syndrome
- Sympathetic uveitis
- Takayasu's arteritis (Figs. 19.2, 19.3, 19.4, 19.5, 19.6 and 19.7)

In the western population, the commonest presentations are likely to be intermediate uveitis, sarcoidosis and juvenile chronic arthritis. Although often relatively controllable with systemic therapy, those patients with more severe disease may require vitreoretinal intervention for the following reasons (Fig. 19.8):

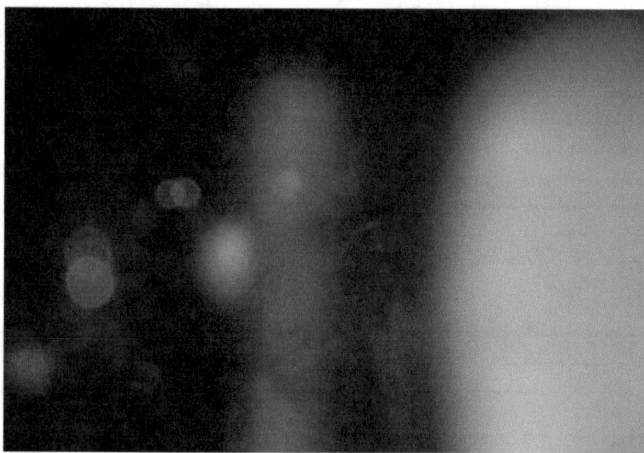

Fig. 19.1 Use the slit lamp beam to detect cells in the vitreous in inflammatory conditions. Check for cells in any odd presentation of macular ERM or retinal detachment in case there is an underlying inflammatory cause

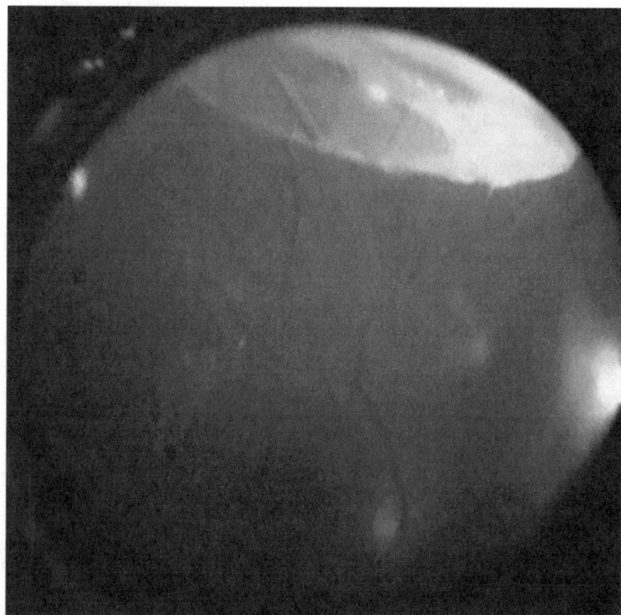

Fig. 19.2 Indentation reveals snow banking in this patient with intermediate uveitis

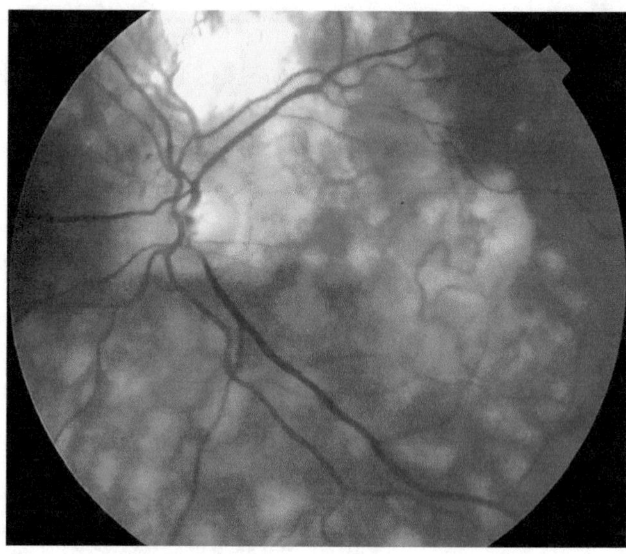

Fig. 19.3 Sarcoidosis is a common cause of posterior uveitis

- Diagnostic confirmation
- Vitreous opacification
- Rhegmatogenous retinal detachment (RRD)
- Tractional retinal detachment (TRD)
- Exudative retinal detachment
- Cystoid macular oedema (CMO)
- Epiretinal membrane
- Hypotony (Figs. 19.9 and 19.10)

The vitreous may become opaque because of the presence of cellular deposits, proteinaceous infiltration and degeneration of the gel structure. The inflammatory process can cause shrinkage of the gel which in the presence of vitreoretinal adhesion may produce either TRD or RRD [1, 4, 5]. In patients with intermediate uveitis, cystoid macular oedema may account for between 40% and 60% of eyes with poor vision [6, 7]. Ultimately phthisis bulbi from hypotony is the most severe endpoint from these inflammatory conditions [8]. It causes a catastrophic visual loss and even a cosmetically unacceptable eye, often in young patients.

Vitreous Opacification

Removal of the vitreous cells and debris in the vitreous gel may restore vision in patients with uveitis of the posterior segment [2, 9–12]. Intermediate uveitis may be complicated by vitreous haemorrhage that can be treated successfully by vitrectomy [13]. Many of these patients are young and have attached PHM, which will require removal but the PHM may be difficult to detach because of vitreoretinal adhesions. Postoperatively the eye may produce inflammation requiring systemic immunosuppressive cover over the perioperative period. Visual recovery is often limited because of the presence of optic atrophy or

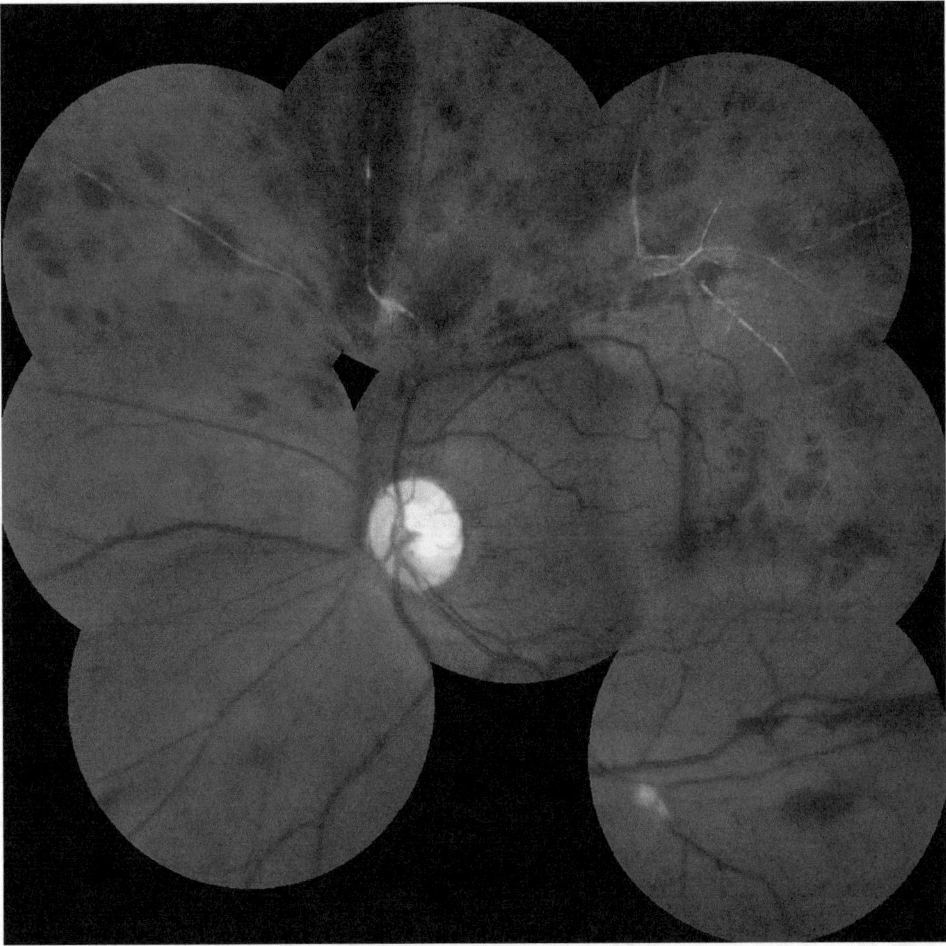

Fig. 19.4 This composite picture shows a pattern of Eales' disease. These patients can produce neovascularisation and vitreous haemorrhage

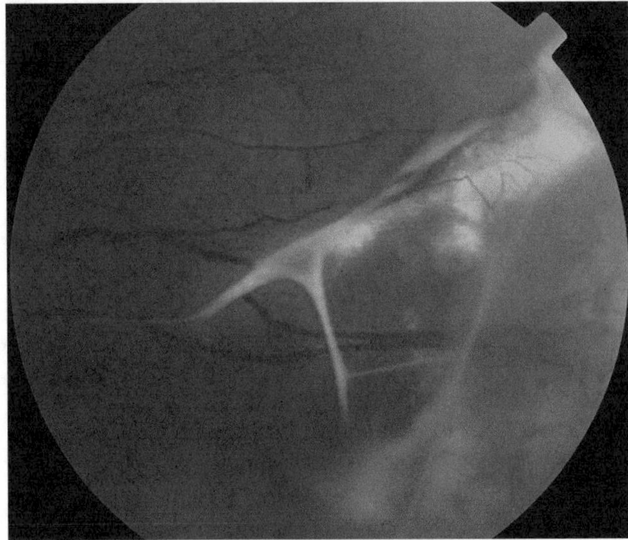

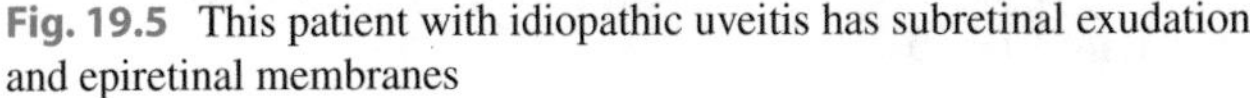

Fig. 19.5 This patient with idiopathic uveitis has subretinal exudation and epiretinal membranes

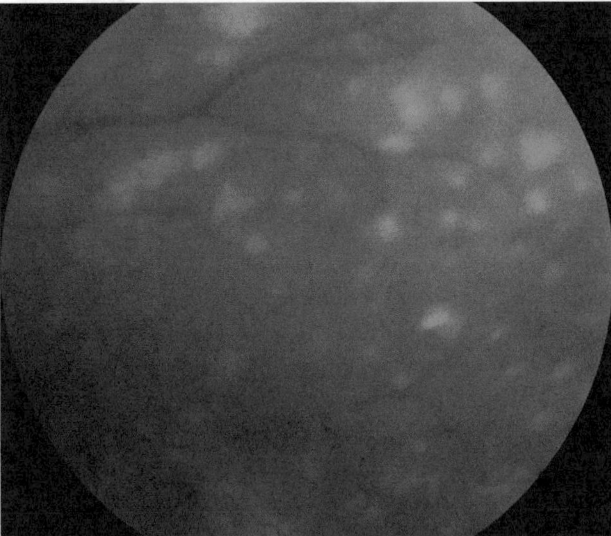

Fig. 19.6 Sympathetic uveitis is a rare cause characterised by white retinal spots, sometimes attributed to the pathological feature of Dalen Fuch's nodules

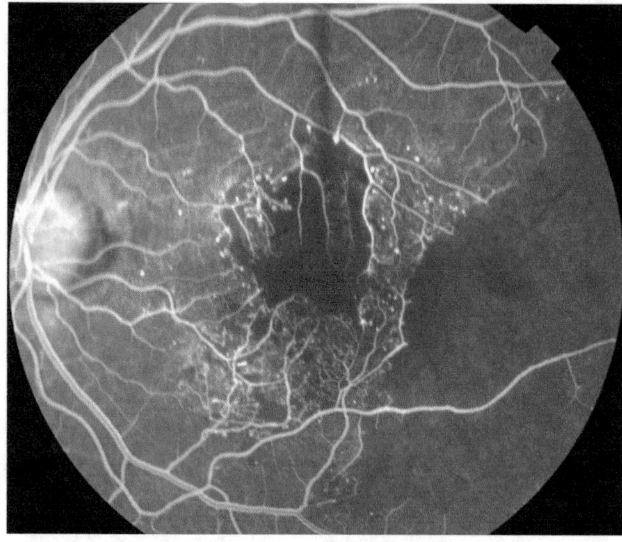

Fig. 19.7 Capillary drop out on fluorescein angiography in Eale's disease

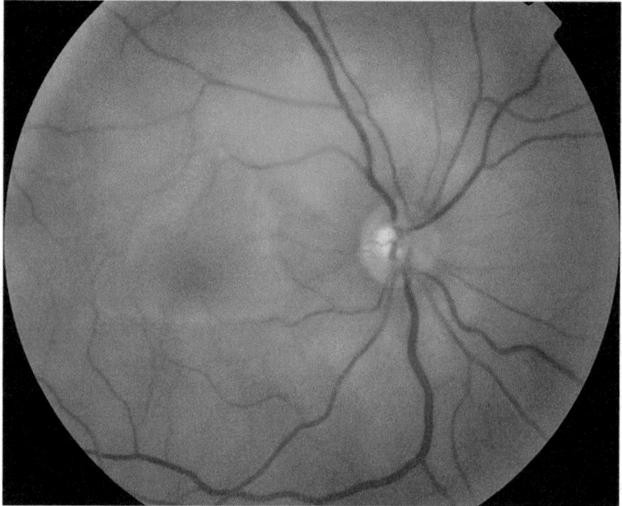

Fig. 19.8 A patient with exudative RD from Voyt–Koyanagi–Harada syndrome

retinal damage particularly from CMO [14, 15]. Some surgeons claim that removal of the gel reduces the ability of the eye to hold inflammatory mediators and thereby reduces the recurrence of inflammation in the long term. Evidence for this remains uncertain [4]. Others argue that improvement following surgery is a result of the removal of vitreous opacity rather than any influence on the inflammatory process [1]. Also, a reduction in medical treatment after surgery has been blamed for a rebound of inflammation 3–6 months later. Therefore, PPV is not recommended routinely in these patients but is reserved for the treatment of vitreoretinal complications.

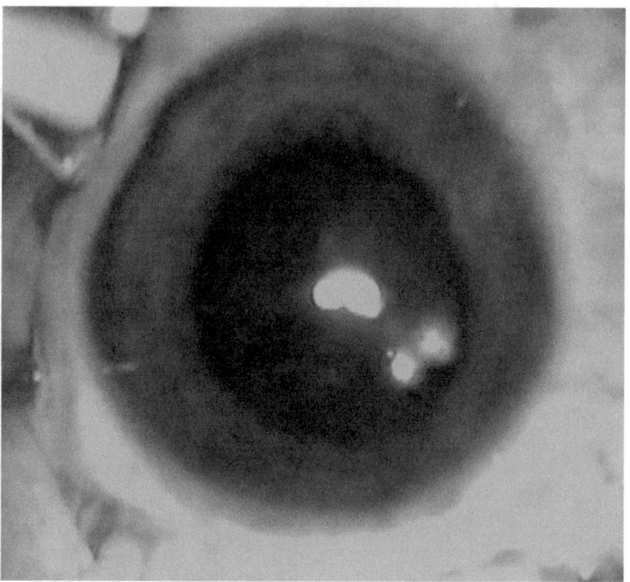

Fig. 19.9 Patients with uveitis vitreous with debris and cells can be adherent to the posterior lens surface obscuring the view for the surgery. With careful aspiration with the vitreous cutter, the vitreous can be teased off the posterior lens without damaging the posterior capsule

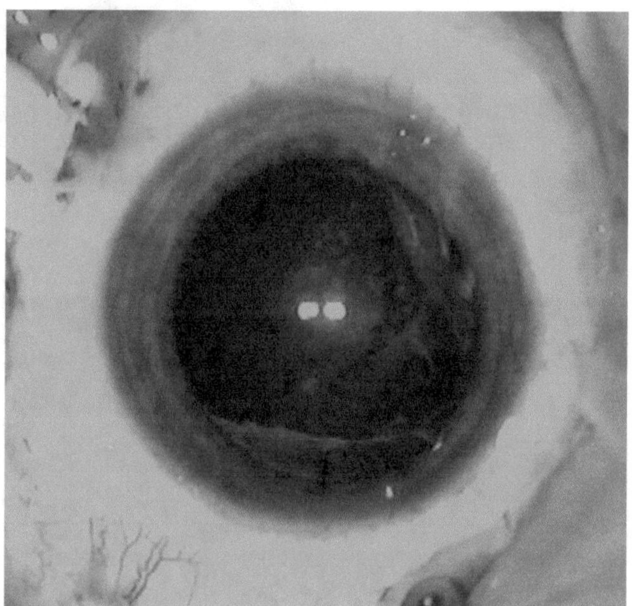

Fig. 19.10 The lens cleaned

Retinal vasculitis can produce ischemia and a neovascular response associated with vitreous haemorrhage. PPV can be used to relieve traction to prevent recurrent haemorrhage and clear the visual axis. Unlike diabetic retinopathy pan-retinal photocoagulation is not universally required (Figs. 19.11, 19.12, and 19.13).

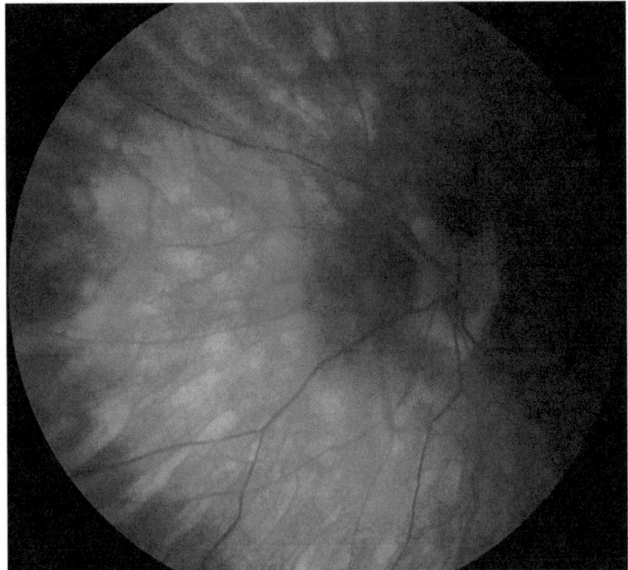

Fig. 19.11 Birdshot chorioretinopathy

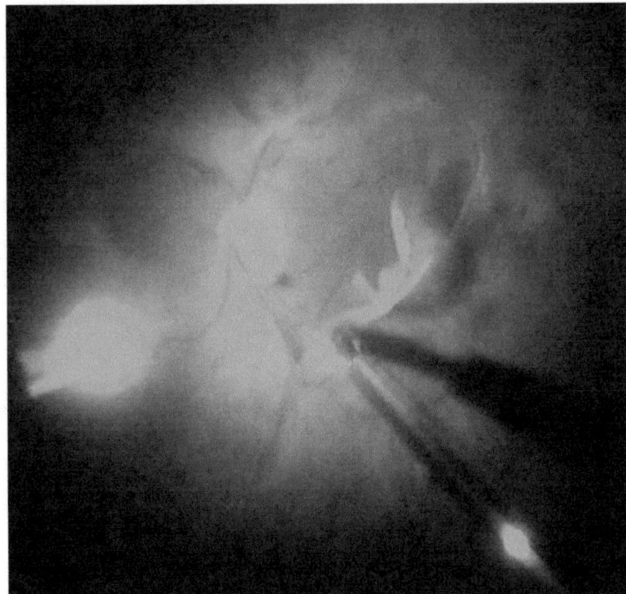

Fig. 19.12 In this patient with uveitis, a secondary epiretinal membrane has formed and has been removed during vitrectomy

Retinal Detachment

When TRD is associated with neovascularisation or fibrosis, delamination and dissection of the membranes are required. Vitreo-schisis, as seen in diabetic retinopathy (Chap. 9), may be present and must be recognised to allow appropriate dissection under the plane of the PHM to aid delamination.

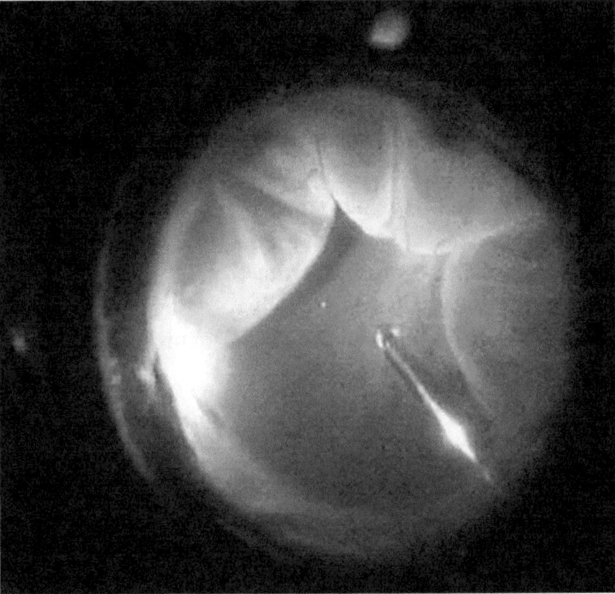

Fig. 19.13 In a patient with suspected exudative retinal detachment, heavies can be inserted onto the posterior pole and gradually expanded. If there are no retinal breaks, there is a route for the escape of subretinal fluid and the retina will bulge forward anteriorly in bullae around the top of the heavy liquids. If a retinal break is present, then sclera may be identified, and the subretinal fluid will spontaneously leave the subretinal space and the retinal detachment will resolve

Unfortunately, TRDs are often associated with severe subretinal exudation in uveitic eyes and visual recovery is often poor.

Rarely patients present with TRD without neovascularisation or preretinal fibrosis, a smooth elevation of the retina is seen. PPV and peeling of the PHM will suffice, allowing the retina to settle without the need to drain SRF.

RRD may occur from PVD formation and can be dealt with by routine means (see Chap. 6) whilst being aware of the possibility of exacerbation of the uveitis.

Exudative RD may be encountered and diagnosed by shifting fluid and the absence of retinal tears, traction and epiretinal fibrosis (despite a longstanding duration of retinal detachment) [16]. Beware that the patient does not have uveal effusion syndrome. If immunosuppressive therapy does not reattach the retina, PPV a retinotomy to drain the SRF or external drainage may help. During the surgery, the exudative nature of the retinal detachment can be confirmed by inserting heavy liquids onto the posterior retina. This will displace SRF anteriorly where it is trapped (because there is no retinal hole to allow drainage) and forms a tight ring bulla that overhangs the heavy liquid. Removal of the heavy liquid reveals a return of the retinal detachment to its previous configuration confirming no loss of SRF. Perform a small and peripheral retinotomy to drain SRF and laser the retinotomy. Alternatively bend a needle as for an external drain (see DACE procedure, Chap. 6), whilst viewing the retina internally via PPV, indent the sclera gently with the "heel" of the bend in the needle to locate its position. Locate the needle into an area of high SRF (fill the posterior pole with heavy liquid to create a ring bulla) then rotate the needle to insert the point through the sclera and choroid to commence drainage. With small gauge surgery, the needle can be inserted through the conjunctiva. Fill with long-acting gas or silicone oil. If the uveitis is then controlled, return of the retinal detachment is unlikely.

Cystoid Macular Oedema

Steroid injections or steroid implants into the vitreous cavity can reverse CMO in uveitis. However, the chronic nature of these conditions causes a return of the CMO after the steroid has been cleared from the eye [17]. Slow-release steroid implants or injections may overcome this difficulty and are now available. For example, slow-release dexamethasone pellets can be injected as an outpatient procedure; they have an effect for 3–6 months similar to intravitreal triamcinolone but appear to have less chance of an IOP rise [18, 19]. PPV has been performed to try to relieve traction on the macula to resolve cystoid macular oedema [7, 14, 20] because the vitreous is more often attached than not in patients with CMO [21]. Others have examined the severity of cystoid macular oedema and found both improvement [5, 22] and persistence of the complication following vitrectomy [23, 24]. Separating the response to vitrectomy from the natural history of the condition and from the effects of concomitant therapies is difficult because randomised studies have not been done. Suprachoroidal injections are theoretically possible and may provide a good space for a depot injection of steroid that might reduce secondary complications such as cataract and IOP elevation (Fig. 19.14).

Hypotony (Figs. 19.15, 19.16, 19.17, 19.18 and 19.19)

Hypotony occurs in these eyes because the ciliary body becomes involved in the uveitic process.

Causes of ciliary body failure:

- Tractional membranes
- Atrophy of ciliary processes
- Ciliary body detachment (Fig. 19.20)

Vitrectomy has been used to try and relieve traction on the ciliary body in hypotony [11]. Inspection of the ciliary body with dissection of any tractional membranes has been performed only in a few patients and is yet of uncertain worth especially as often the ciliary processes are atrophic and may be non-functional. Endoscopy can be used to inspect the ciliary body and to visualise membranectomy.

Insertion of hyaluronic to provide a temporary IOP rise has been employed. Silicone oil can be used for a more prolonged effect and to prevent severe shrinkage of the size of the eye if hypotony persists [25]. The long-term results of these interventions are unknown (Fig. 19.21). In general, hypotonous eyes are at risk of phthisis bulbi which once established is irreversible. A judgement of a pre-phthisical state can be made by the early presence of infolding of the posterior sclera or a shortening of the axial length. The opportunity should be taken to fill the globe with silicone oil to avoid further progression of shrinkage of the eye. Maintaining the globe will improve the chance of vision and better cosmesis. The hypotony will persist and there is a risk of corneal thickening and scarring in time. Keratoprosthesis can be considered in the late phases.

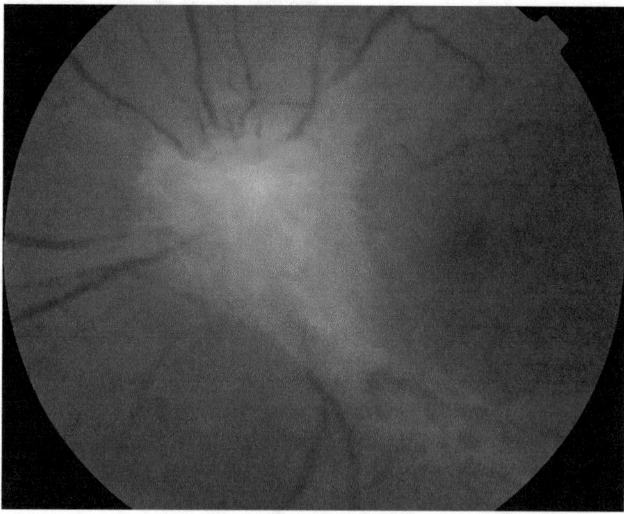

Fig. 19.14 A papillitis has stimulated an ERM which is wrinkling the fovea

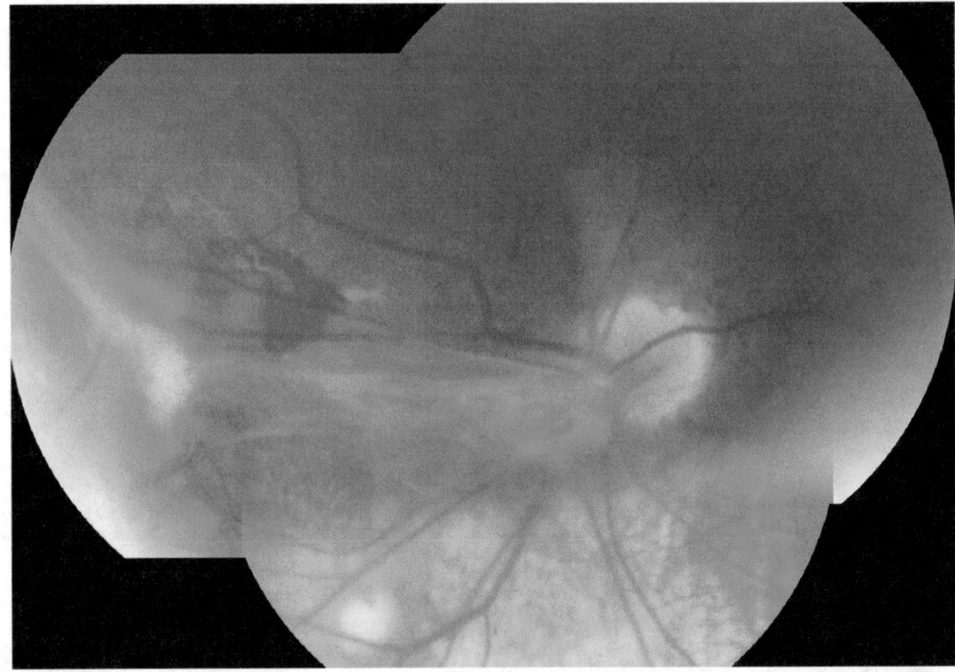

Fig. 19.15 A fold through the macula in a patient with severe panuveitis. The risk of putting the eye into hypotony must be considered before operating on any eye with panuveitis

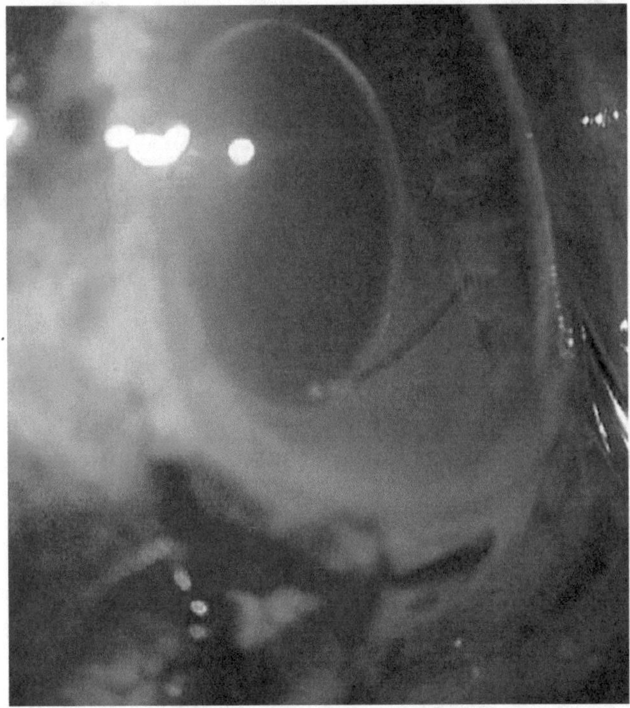

Fig. 19.16 Thin but relatively healthy ciliary processes

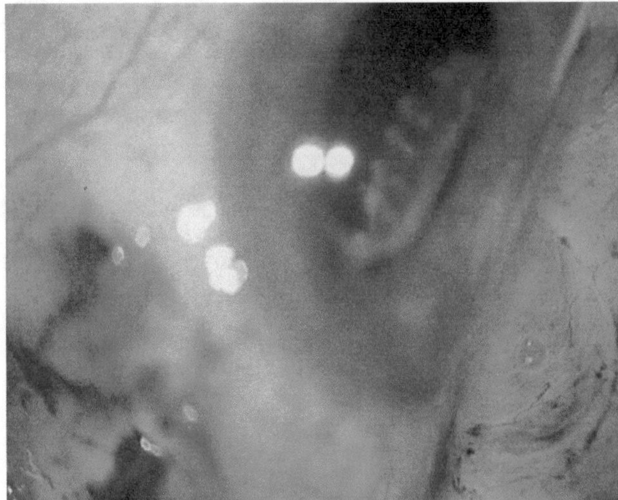

Fig. 19.17 Ciliary processes damaged by uveitis with white ridges

Drug	Mode of action	Typical adult maintenance dosage	Severe systemic complications
Prednisolone	Corticosteroid	1–15 mg	Peptic ulceration Myopathy Osteoporosis Adrenal suppression Cushing's syndrome
Azathioprine	Antiproliferative	1-3 mg/kg daily	Myelosuppression Especially those with low thiopurine methyltransferase activity
Mycophenolate mofetil	Antiproliferative	1 g twice daily	Leucopoenia Opportunistic infections
Methotrexate	Antimetabolite (inhibits dihydrofolate reductase)	7.5 mg weekly	Myelosuppression Mucositis Pneumonitis
Ciclosporin	Calcineurin inhibitor	5 mg/kg daily	Nephrotoxicity
Tacrolimus	Calcineurin inhibitor	Variable according to response	Neurotoxicity Cardiomyopathy
Infliximab	Tumour necrosis factor activity inhibition	3 mg/kg every 2 months by iv infusion	Infections Heart failure Hypersensitivity Blood disorders
Rituximab	Tumour necrosis factor activity inhibition	1 g every 2 weeks by iv infusion	Infections Heart failure Hypersensitivity Blood disorders
Etanercept	Tumour necrosis factor activity inhibition	25 mg twice weekly by subcutaneous injection	Infections Heart failure Hypersensitivity Blood disorders

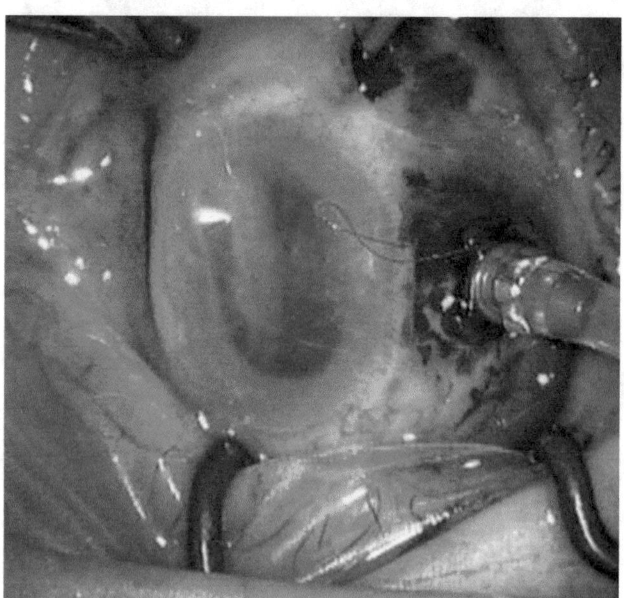

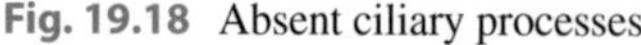

Fig. 19.18 Absent ciliary processes

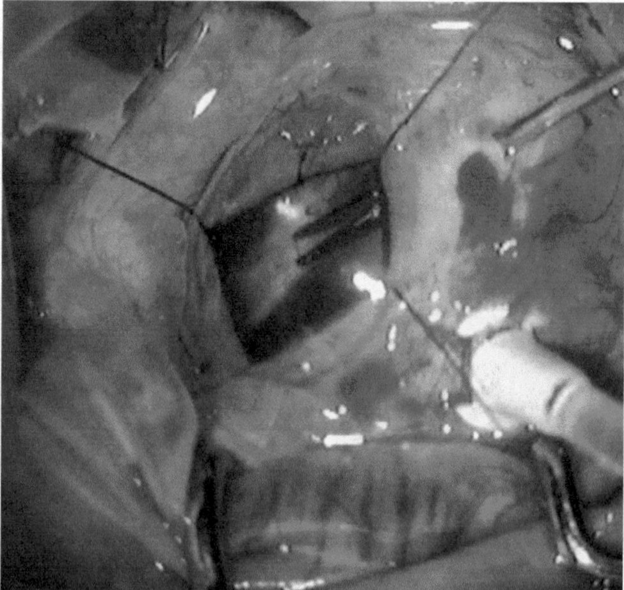

Fig. 19.19 Dense membranes on the ciliary body may detach the ciliry epithelium causing malfunction and hypotony

Diagnostic Confirmation

Uveitic syndromes may occasionally be difficult to discriminate from other causes of posterior infiltration such as infection and neoplasm. Polyclonal white cells are seen on cytology with a CD4/CD8 ratio of at least 4 [26]. A significant number of patients with uveitis do not have a definitive diagnosis. Only 66% of cases of anterior uveitis are associated with clinical and laboratory abnormalities which lead to a definitive diagnosis increasing to 85% in posterior uveitis [24]. Laboratory examination of the vitreous is particularly indicated when unusual or non-characteristic presentations occur.

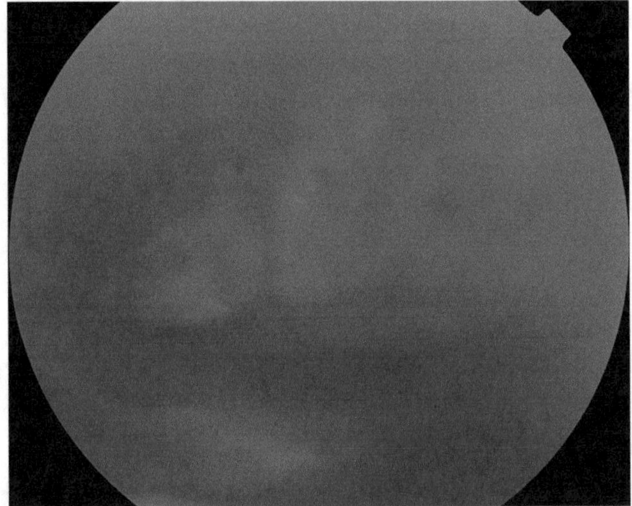

Fig. 19.20 The folds in the posterior layers of the eye are a precursor to phthisis in this patient with panuveitis. The surgeon may choose to fill the eye with silicone oil to retain a cosmetically acceptable globe size and shape, and vision of low grade

Biopsy of the vitreous by needle aspiration may be effective in postoperative endophthalmitis [27] where the vitreous is liquefied by the infection but may not be appropriate in non-infectious uveitis. Use of a vitreous cutter is recommended because of the greater incidence of vitreoretinal adhesion in uveitic patients increases the risk of retinal detachment or tear [14]. Many of these patients are young and likely to have non-syneretic vitreous gel increasing the likelihood of a "dry tap" with a needle. In some cases, vitrectomy is ideal; in addition to providing a vitreous sample, vitrectomy may allow visualisation of the fundus allowing characteristic features of the disease process to be recognised and hence revealing a supplementary diagnosis.

The Vitreous Biopsy

Use transconjunctival 23 or 25 gauge inserted at 4 mm form the corneal scleral limbus. (see Chap. 2).

A table of immune-suppressive agents that can be used in the treatment of uveitis.

Insert the cutter and visualise in the eye.

Maintain the IOP with a squint hook providing scleral indentation whilst employing the cutter to extract the vitreous to beyond the three-way tap (inserted on the first junction

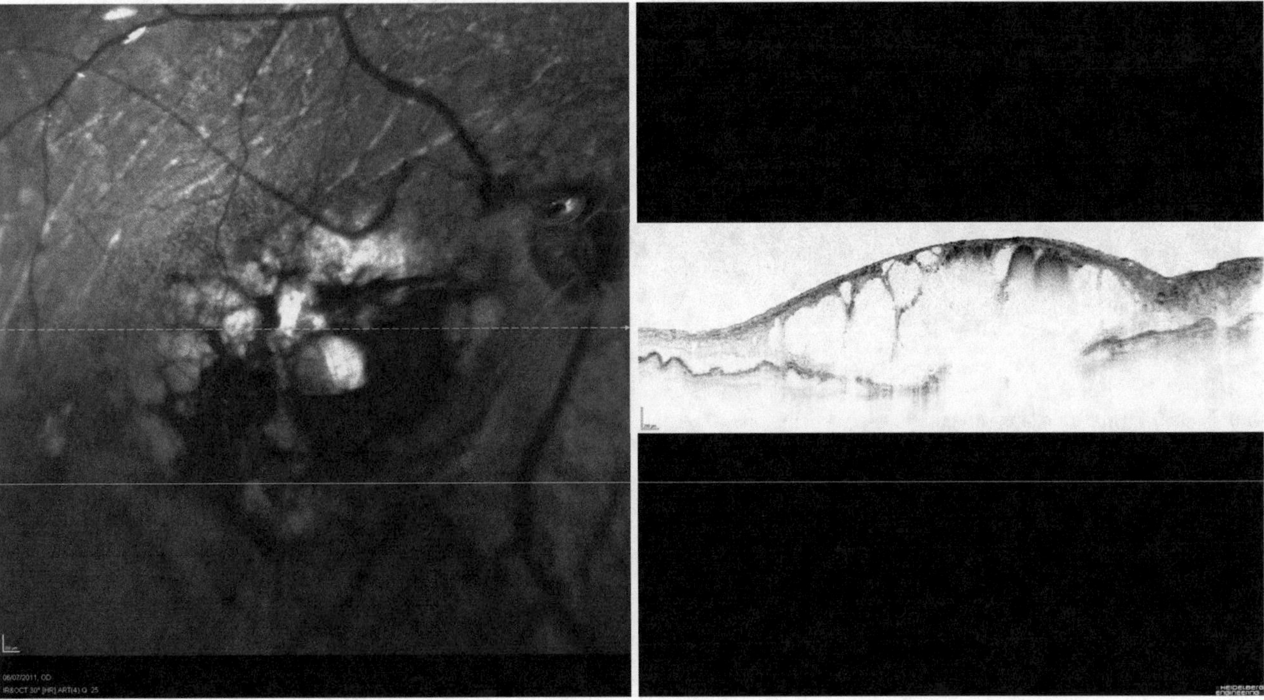

Fig. 19.21 A hypotonous eye is likely to have CMO

of the aspiration tubing), providing approximately 0.5 mls of vitreous.

Remove the cutter and re-inflate the eye with any intravitreal drug administration, e.g. antibiotics, whilst relieving the pressure on the squint hook.

Remove the sample from the tubing to send to the laboratory. Take an anterior chamber sample via a paracentesis as required.

Sampling at the Beginning of a PPV

If a small sample is required at the beginning of a PPV, the sample needs to be "dry", i.e. not diluted with the infusion fluid, therefore:

- Insert the infusion cannula but do not switch it on.
- Insert a superior trochar and remove the vitreous whilst applying pressure with the squint hook.
- Remove the cutter and extract the sample.
- Switch on the infusion and release the pressure with the squint hook.
- Continue the PPV.

At the end of the PPV after closing one sclerotomy and with the infusion switched off, insert any intravitreal injections, close the other sclerotomy and then remove the infusion cannula.

Special Situations

- If a large sample (2 mls) is required infuse the eye with heavy liquids which will fall to the back of the eye maintaining its IOP whilst allowing removal of the vitreous and a dry tap [28].
- For some conditions (e.g. candida and bacterial endophthalmitis for culturing, or lymphoma for cytometry) it is worth sending the "washings", vitreous diluted with infusion fluid in the vitrectomy equipment aspiration cassette, to the laboratory.
- Note if you are inserting gas or silicone oil and you want to use intravitreal drugs, insert the drugs into the vitreous cavity just before inserting the tamponade agent. This ensures that the drugs are of the correct dosage (diluted in 4–7 mls of fluid in the vitreous cavity). The concentration will remain the same in the thin layer of remaining fluid after fluid/oil or fluid/gas exchange (Table 19.1, Fig. 19.22).

Table 19.1 Adult Drug Dosages (these are guidelines only, the administration of the medications can vary in different institutions)

Disorder	Drug	Dosage	Route of administration
Candida endophthalmitis	Amphotericin B	0.005 mg in 0.1 ml	Intravitreal
	Fluconazole	200–400 mg/day 3 weeks	Oral
	Flucytosine (often combined with fluconazole to avoid resistance)	50–150 mg/kg/day divided doses (reduce in renal impairment)	Intravenous infusion
	Voriconazole	400 mg b.d. loading dose, 200 mg b.d.	Oral
CMV retinitis	Ganciclovir	1.5–2.0 mg/0.1 ml	Intravitreal
HSV and VZV acute retinal necrosis (treatment in the acute phase)	Foscarnet	2.4 mg/0.1 ml	Intravitreal
	Acyclovir	10 mg/kg t.d.s. For 10 days, monitor renal function	Intravenous infusion
	Valaciclovir	1 g t.d.s. for 10 days	Oral
HSV and VZV acute retinal necrosis (prevention of infection in the fellow eye)	Valaciclovir	300 mg t.d.s. for 3 months	Oral
Bacterial Endophthalmitis	Vancomycin Ceftazidime (used in combination)	2 mg/0.2 mls 2 mg/0.2 mls	Intravitreal
Intraocular inflammation or cystoid macular Oedema	Triamcinolone	2 mg/0.05 mls	Intravitreal
	Triamcinolone	40 mg	Sub-tenons
Lymphoma	Methotrexate	0.4 mg/0.16 mls	Intravitreal
Toxoplasmosis Chorioretinitis	Pyrimethamine Sulfadiazine Folinic acid Prednisolone (used in combination)	100 mg stat., then 25 mg b.d. for 3 weeks 1 g b.d. for 3 weeks (then 15 mg twice a week) 60 mg tapering, 10 mg every 5 days	Oral
	Clindamycin	300 mg q.d.s. for 3 weeks	Oral

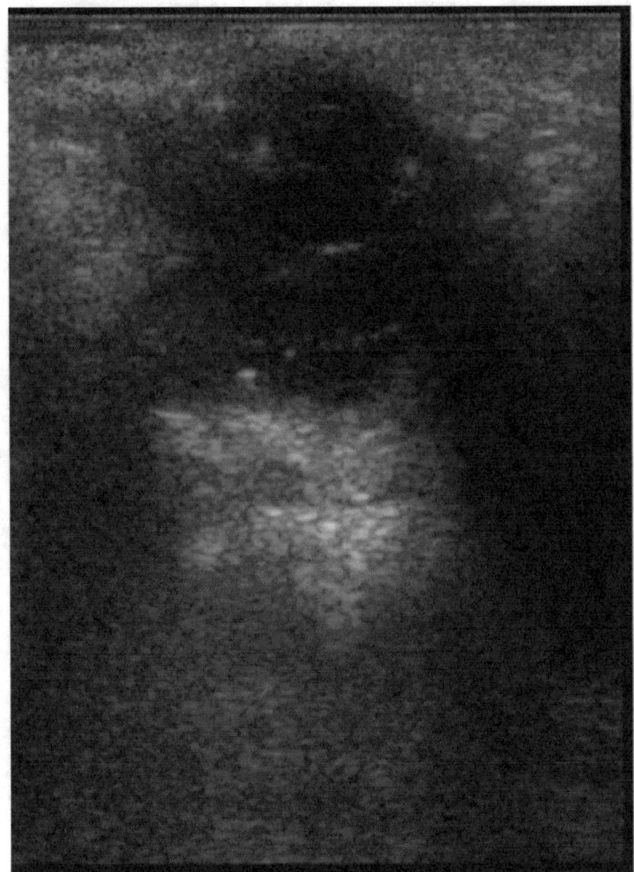

Fig. 19.22 An ultrasound of a patient with panuveitis with an intraocular pellet of slow-release steroid

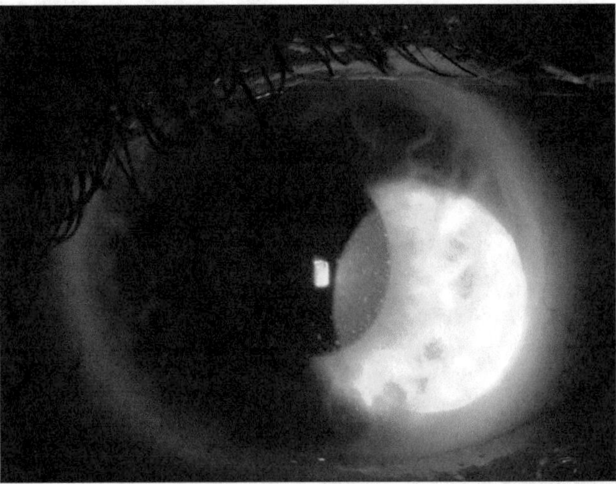

Fig. 19.23 Small "spidery" keratotic precipitates are often associated with virus-associated uveitis. In this patient, cytomegalovirus was detected on PCR analysis of an aqueous sample

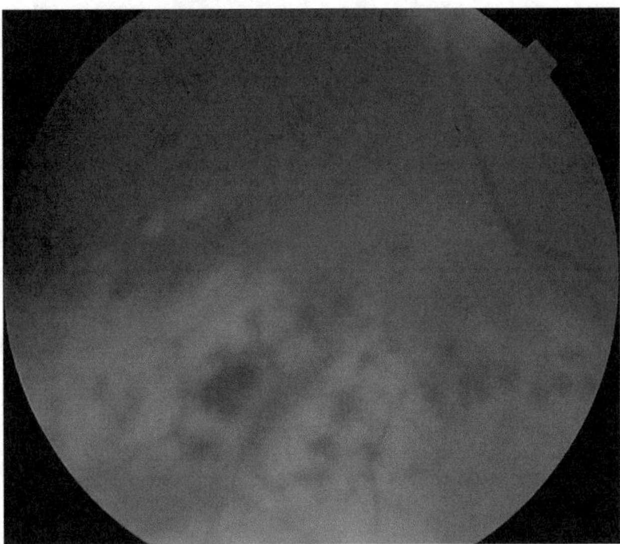

Fig. 19.24 The advancing edge of acute retinal necrosis is visible in this patient. Retinal detachments are extremely common in this condition

Acute Retinal Necrosis

Clinical Features (Figs. 19.23, 19.24, 19.25, 19.26, 19.27, 19.28, and 19.29)

Viral infections of the retina cause mixed arteritic and infiltrative retinitis. The causative viruses are common of the herpes simplex family [29].

Herpes simplex 1 is commoner in the young age group [30, 31].

These patients may have a history of cold sores.

Herpes zoster is commoner in the elderly [32–34] and can be associated with herpes zoster ophthalmicus [35] and chickenpox [36].

Herpes simplex 2 infections can also occur especially in children [30, 37, 38].

Epstein–Barr virus can rarely be detected but is often considered to be a coincidental finding [39].

Patients are generally not immune-compromised but herpes zoster is implicated in both ARN [39, 40] and progressive outer retinal necrosis in AIDs patients [41–46] and the immune-compromised.

There is a significant risk of bilateral disease [47, 48] with fellow eye involvement even years later [49] and long-term risk of encephalitis [50, 51].

The retina has the appearance of peripheral haemorrhage and infiltration, which spread posteriorly to involve the macula but the presentation has variable severity [51]. The retina may become moth-eaten and retinal detachment is common up to 50% [52]. In severe presentations, exudative retinal detachment can occur [53]. Patients have been described with giant retinal tears [54], retinal neovascularisation [55] and peripheral retinal pigment epithelial tears [56]. Proliferative vitreoretinopathy is common (Figs. 19.30, 19.31, and 19.32).

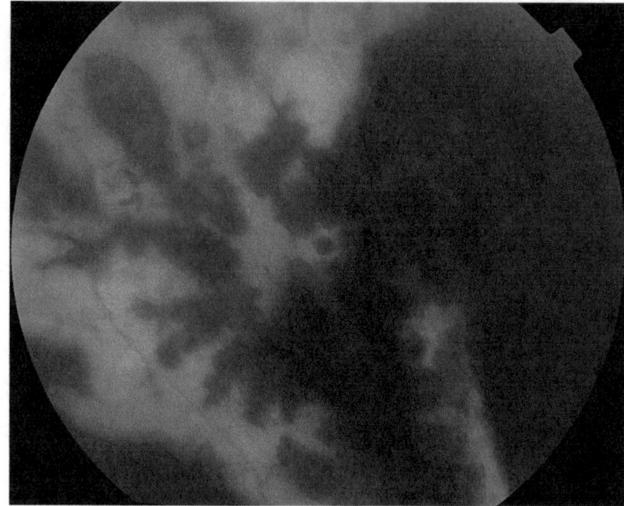

Fig. 19.25 Acute retinal necrosis is characterised by peripheral white lesions with a crenated edge advancing centrally sometimes with retinal haemorrhaging

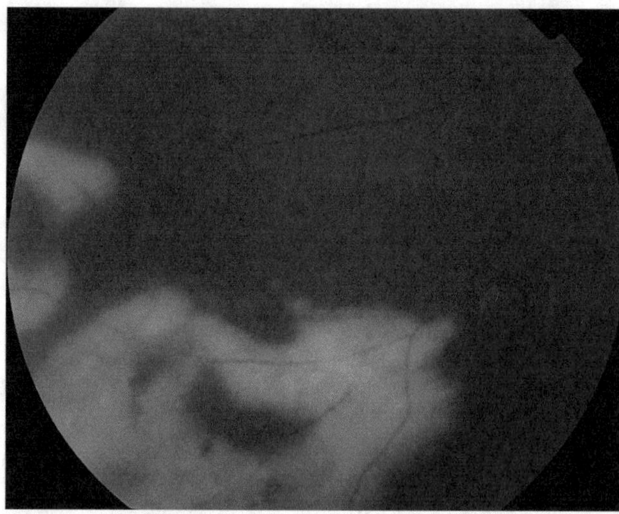

Fig. 19.27 ARN after commencement of steroid therapy

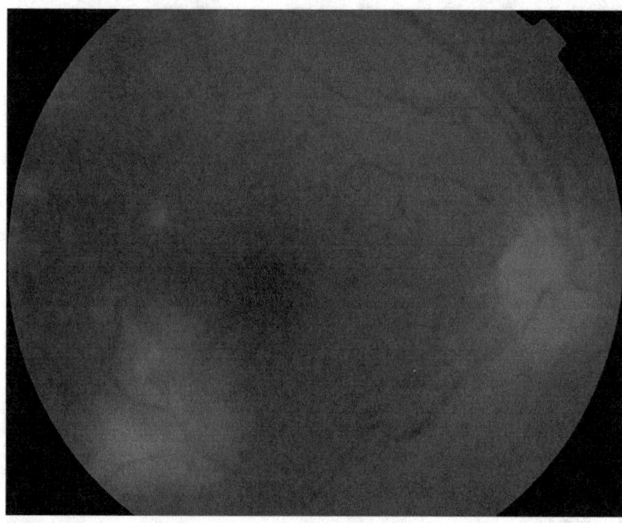

Fig. 19.26 When the infection reaches the optic nerve the vision drops severely

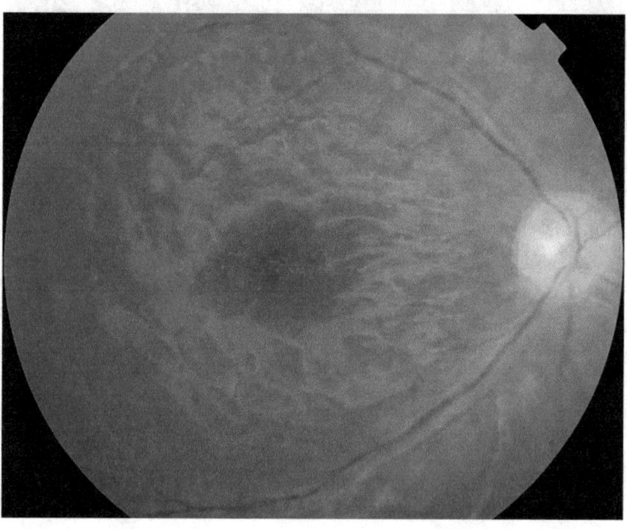

Fig. 19.28 A 5-year-old boy developed an atypical acute retinal necrosis without retinal infiltration but with retinal vasculitis in both eyes a few months after chickenpox. The vision was a perception of light in both eyes

Surgery (Table 19.2)

For Diagnosis (Fig. 19.33)

The clinical pattern can be useful in diagnosis, but vitreous biopsy is mandatory. A vitreous sample of 0.2 ml is usually sufficient to allow the detection of the virus on polymerase chain reaction (PCR) with a high yield of positive results of 60–80% [57, 58].

For Treatment

Systemic antiviral therapy is given over a period of months to try to prevent involvement of the second eye and encephalitis. Intravitreal antiviral, e.g. Foscarnet, can be inserted during biopsy [44, 59].

Management of retinal detachment requires PPV, gas, laser and buckle depending on the situation [59–62]. Insertion of silicone oil is usually necessary because a causative single break is frequently difficult to identify, large areas of the retina are thinned and damaged, and proliferative retinopathy is common [63]. Retinal attachment after multiple procedures is common (90%) but visual recovery is poor [60].

Performing a vitrectomy and silicone oil insertion prior to the development of retinal detachment has been tried in case series but is not yet of proven benefit.

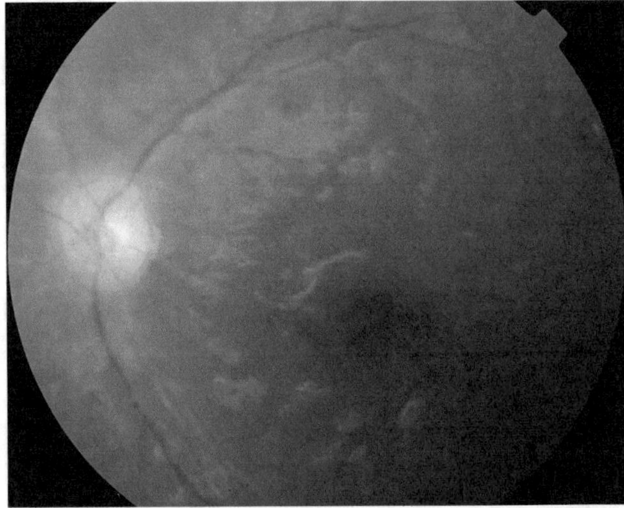

Fig. 19.29 The left eye

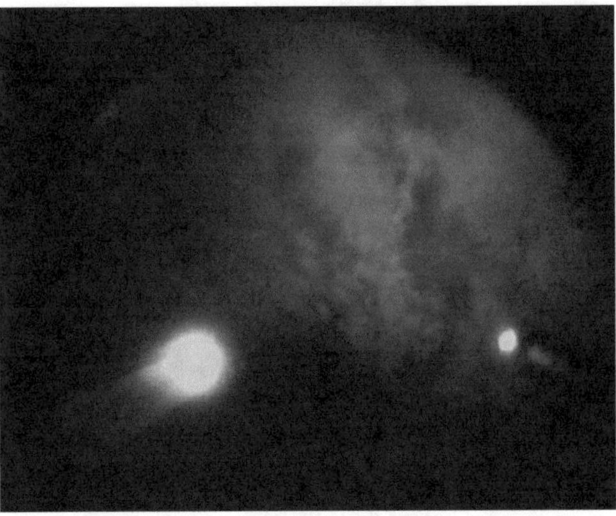

Fig. 19.31 In this patient, a retinal detachment has followed acute retinal necrosis. Sometimes discrete tears are identifiable, but often the retina is "moth eaten" and the exact location of breaks is difficult

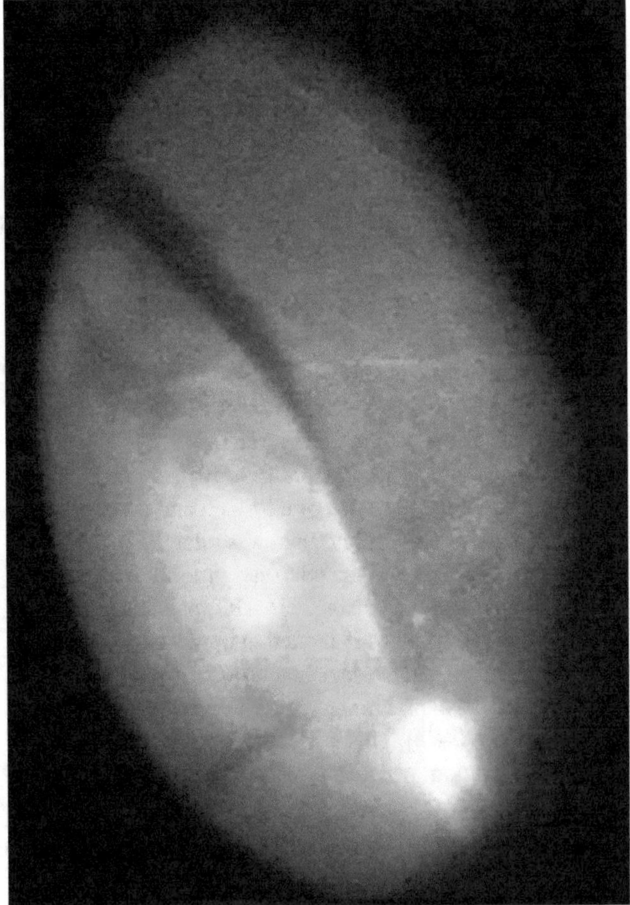

Fig. 19.30 A discrete edged large retinal break is seen on an indentation in this patient with acute retinal necrosis

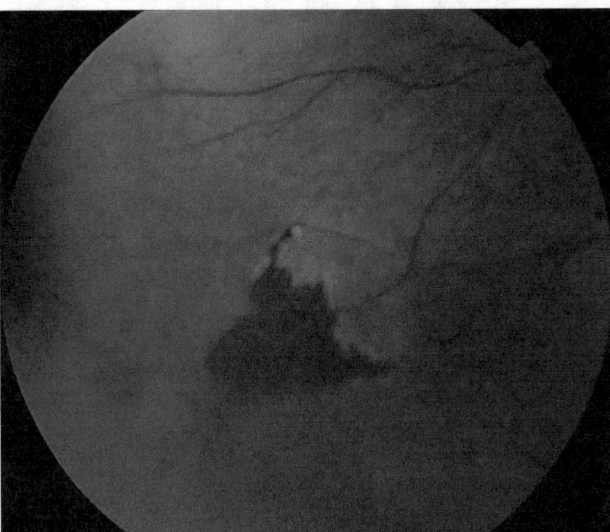

Fig. 19.32 Progressive outer retinal necrosis occurs in immunocompromised individuals with herpes simplex or zoster infection of the retina. Retinal tears and detachment are common

Table 19.2 Difficulty rating for surgery for ARN

Difficulty rating	High
Success rates	Low
Complication rates	Moderate
When to use in training	Late

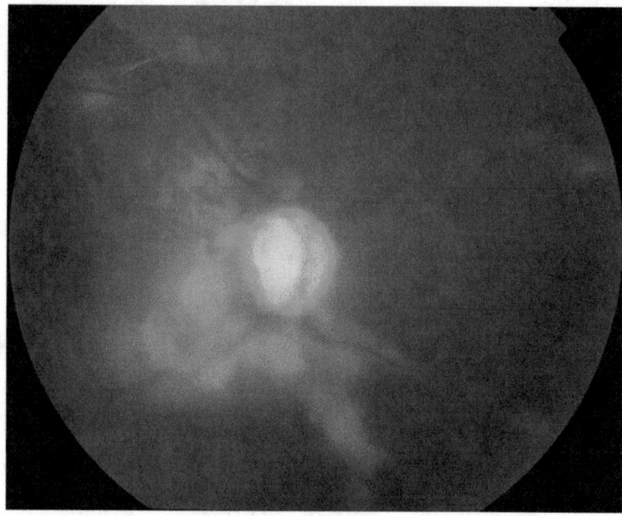

Fig. 19.33 Acute retinal necrosis after intravitreal steroid injection

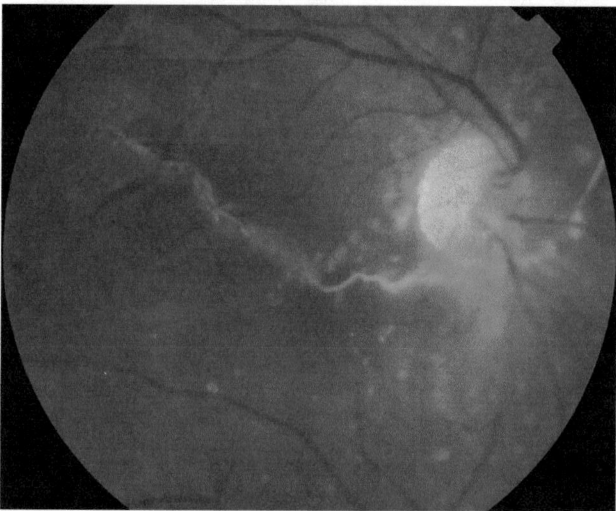

Fig. 19.34 This teenager suffered RRD after ARN, his retina is shown 4 years after the surgical repair reattached without silicone oil in situ with evidence of damage and a subretinal fibrous band

Visual Outcome (Figs. 19.34 and 19.35)

The prognosis for vision is poor in the affected eye; therefore, systemic therapy is essential to prevent involvement of the other eye (Fig. 19.36).

Cytomegalovirus Retinitis

Clinical Features (Fig. 19.37)

Cytomegalovirus (CMV) infects the retina in immunocompromised patients. Overwhelmingly these patients suffer from AIDs. Prior to highly active antiretroviral therapy (HAART) [64], 40% of AIDs patients developed CMV retinitis. Others requiring systemic immuno-suppression such as Wegener's granulomatosis or rheumatoid arthritis occasionally present [29, 65]. Classically in AIDs, the patient has a severe reduction in CD4 white blood cells to less than 50 cells/μL. With the introduction of HAART, control of viral load is much improved and consequently, CD4 counts are more often preserved. This has led to a large reduction in the numbers of new cases of retinitis which may only occur when there is a failure of or resistance to HAART [66–69]. Retinal detachment was a common complication of the retinitis before HAART (50% at 1 year after the development of retinitis [64, 70]), usually slow in onset because of the presence of a formed and attached vitreous gel in these young patients, and was bilateral in 70% [71]. Prior to HAART, this was linked to early mortality at approximately 6 months [72, 73]. Since HAART, patients with CMV retinitis have shown an 81% reduction in mortality [74] and a 60% reduction in retinal detachment [75]. Most with CMV retinitis will develop immune recovery uveitis which can reduce vision [76–78]. This is characterised by posterior segment inflammation which causes secondary complications such as cystoid macular oedema [73], vitreomacular traction [79], vitreous haemorrhage from retinal neovascularisation [80], and even activation of previously quiescent infections of the retina such as mycobacteria [81].

Note: Immune recovery uveitis is usually self-limiting causing only mild visual loss.

Increasingly, the control of the viral load is most important to the control of the retinitis by allowing cessation of anti CMV therapy as the CD4 count recovers [80].

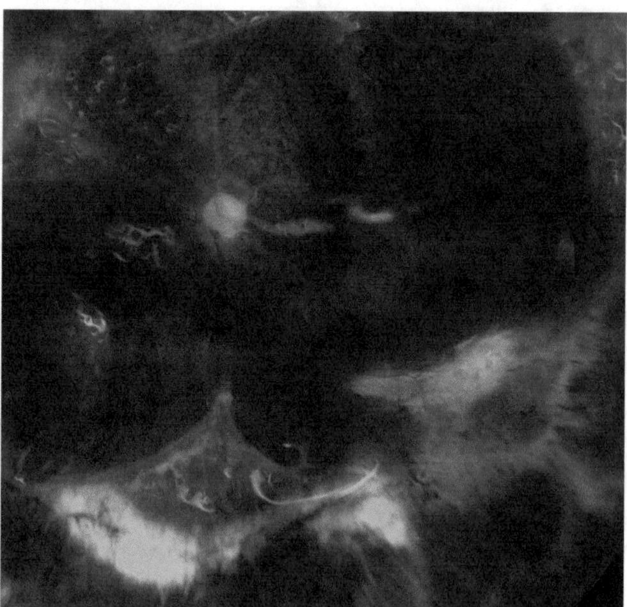

Fig. 19.35 Progressive outer retinal necrosis is shown postoperatively with oil in situ to retain a reattached retina with hand movements vision

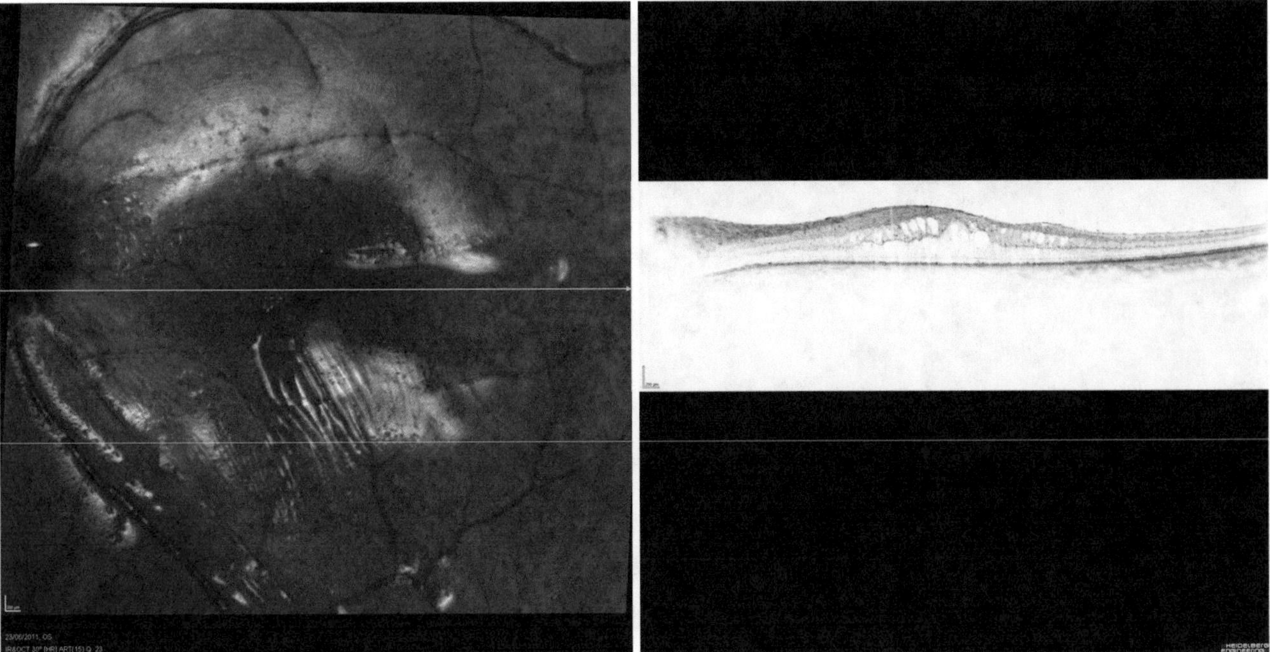

Fig. 19.36 Despite reattachment of the retina in this patient with ARN there is CMO of the macula

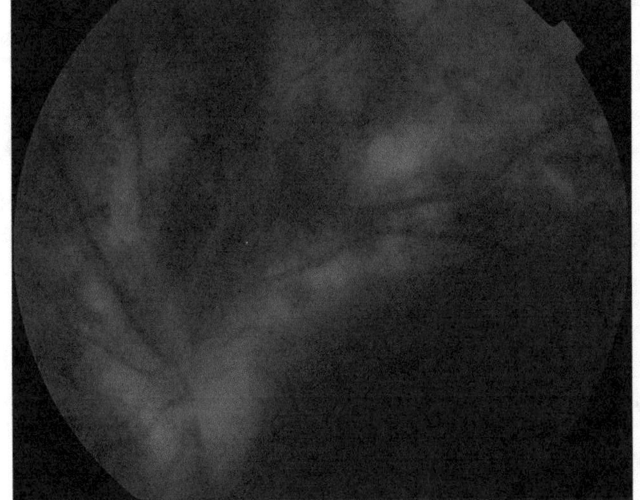

Fig. 19.37 CMV retinitis has become less common since the commencement of HAART therapy but may still be seen in immunocompromised individuals

Surgery (Table 19.3)

For Diagnosis

The retinal appearance is usually typical in the "at risk" patient with necrotising, haemorrhagic retinitis with a sharp demarcation between healthy and affected retina. A biopsy is required to allow targeted therapy. A vitreal biopsy of 0.2 mls is adequate for the detection of viral PCR for CMV.

Table 19.3 Difficulty rating for surgery for CMV retinitis

Difficulty rating	Moderate
Success rates	Moderate
Complication rates	Low
When to use in training	Middle

For Treatment (Figs. 19.38, 19.39 and 19.40)

Treatment of retinitis involves intravitreal antiviral drugs often in the form of a slow-release Ganciclovir implant. This contains 4.5 mg of Ganciclovir, is inserted into the pars plana at 4 mm from the corneoscleral limbus and may last up to 1 year. The implant provides local drug delivery bypassing the blood ocular barrier with low dosage whilst minimising systemic side effects. In approximately 12%, problems are encountered such as extrusion, vitreous haemorrhage or CMO [82, 83]. Endophthalmitis occurs in 0.4% [84].

Implants can be used in eyes with silicone oil insertion although the reduced aqueous layer means increased concentrations of the drug [85].

The clinical picture of retinal detachment has changed because of the use of HAART. Previously patients required PPV with silicone oil insertion without removal because of the inability to destroy the CMV infection and because the shortened life span restricted the development of oil-induced complications [72, 86–88]. Silicone oil has been used with and without inferior external buckle with similar success rates [89, 90]. Immune recovery means that retinitis is no longer progressive and the life span of patients is very much

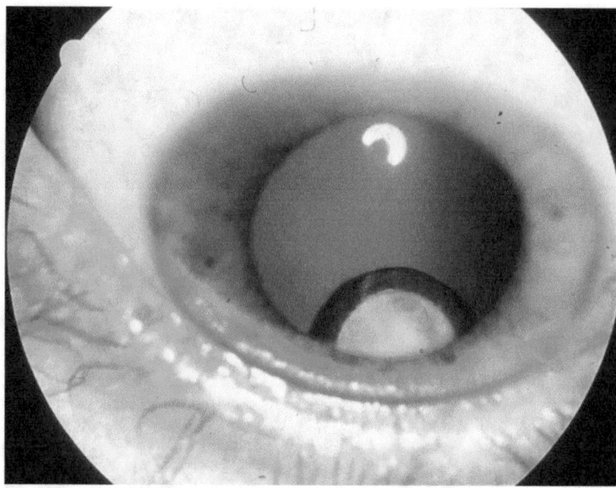

Fig. 19.38 A ganciclovir implant is visible in this eye with cytomegalovirus retinitis

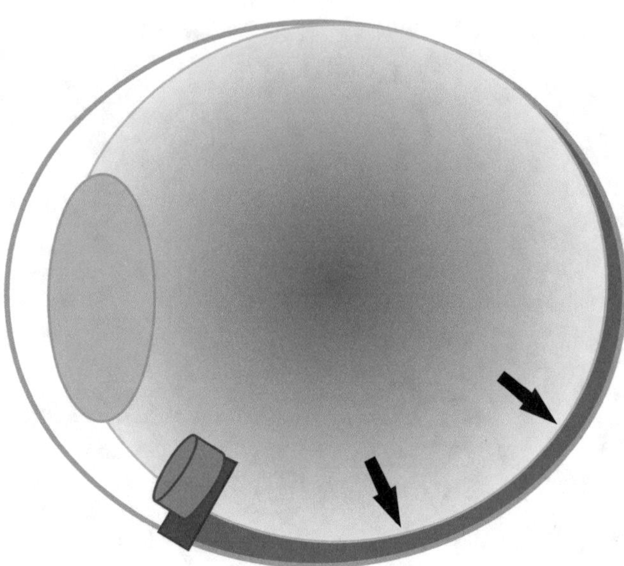

Fig. 19.39 Ganciclovir implants can be used in patients with silicone oil insertion. It is expected that there will be a higher concentration of the drug on the retina because of the thinner layer of the vitreous cavity aqueous fluid for the drug to dissolve in

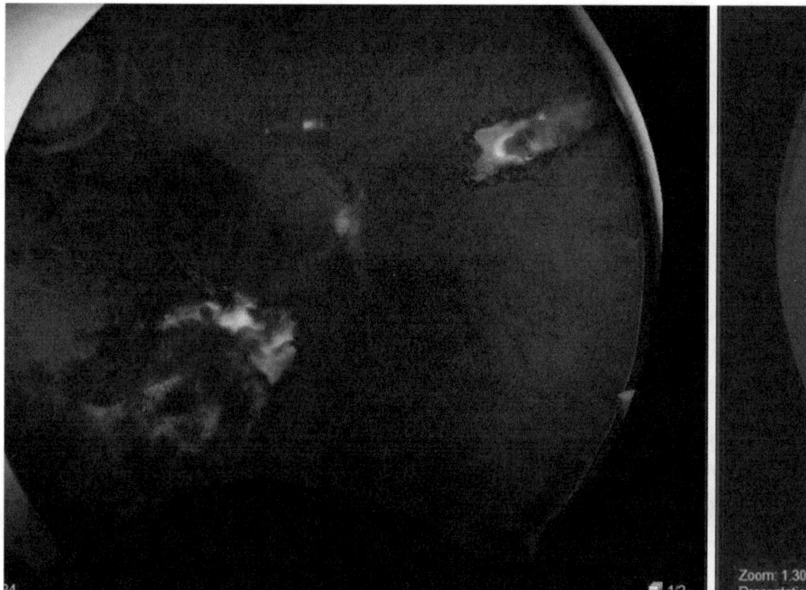

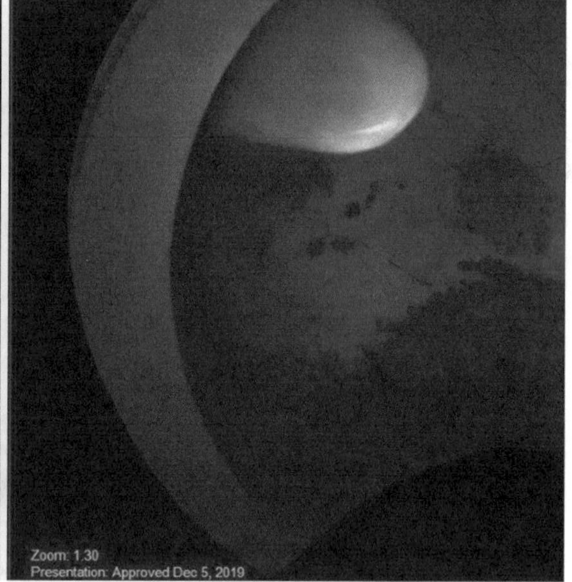

Fig. 19.40 A Ganciclovir implant 20 years after it was inserted

prolonged; therefore, surgery may be more successful with gas tamponade [91] or with silicone oil with later removal of the oil [92].

Attempts to restrict RRD formation or progression with prophylactic laser therapy around areas of retinitis had limited success [93–95] because the retinitis or retinal detachment would extend through the laser barrier.

Visual Outcome

If retinal detachment occurs the chance of visual recovery is better when the retina can be fixed with one operation [96] but good vision is only possible in approximately 50% [86] although this may have improved with HAART.

Fungal Endophthalmitis

Clinical Features (Figs. 19.41, 19.42, 19.43, 19.44, 19.45 and 19.46)

Fungal endophthalmitis (predominantly *candida albicans*) is usually seen in patients with intravenous long lines [97, 98],

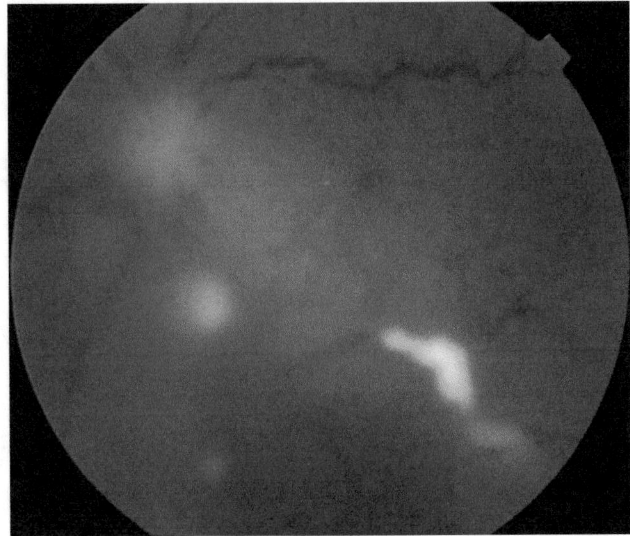

Fig. 19.41 Puffballs are seen in the mid vitreous in this patient's eye typical of candida endophthalmitis

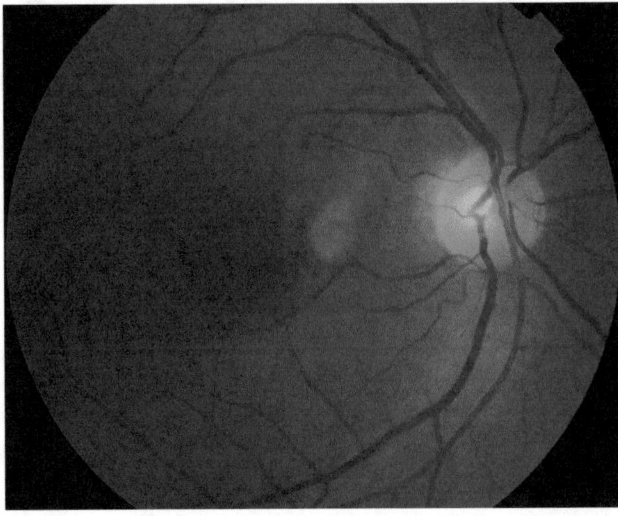

Fig. 19.43 An intravenous drug user has had candida endophthalmitis in both eyes with the right producing a secondary CNV which enlarged and in the left eye an ERM appeared which spontaneously separated towards the disc

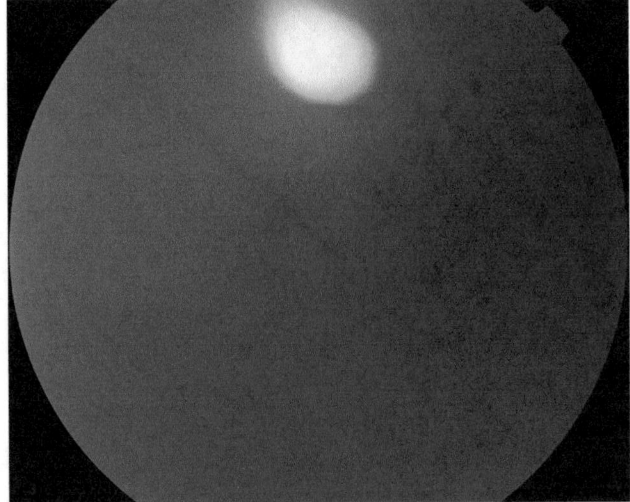

Fig. 19.42 A single focus of candida in the only functioning eye of an intravenous drug abuser. The patient was treated with systemic antifungals without a biopsy of the vitreous

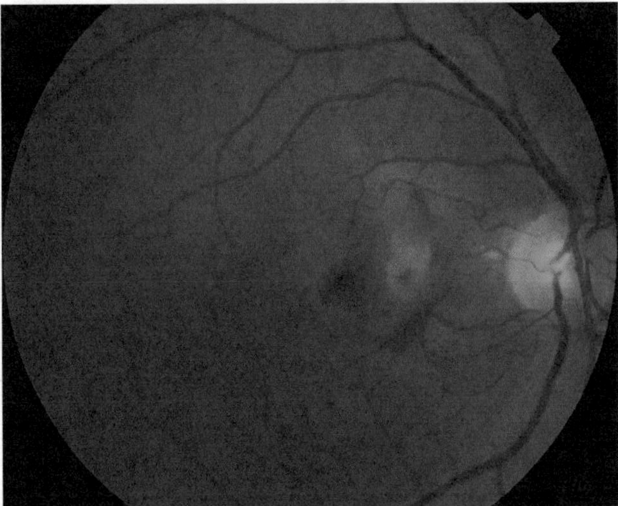

Fig. 19.44 Enlargement of the CNV

e.g. in intensive care units, or in patients with a history of intravenous drug abuse [99]. The presentation is slowly progressive endophthalmitis, sometimes bilateral [100], commencing with a white spot on the retina and then preretinal puffball infiltration often seen after a routine examination of the fundus in an asymptomatic patient [99, 101]. An intravenous line may have been used on only one occasion [102]. In heroin abuse, the patient presents with a reduction of vision after using acidic agents such as lemon juice (infected with candida) to dissolve brown heroin. Infections have been reported after gynaecological procedures [103, 104] toxic megacolon [105] and postpartum [106, 107]. Premature infants may also develop the infection [108–110]. Contaminated infusion fluid in cataract extraction may cause surgical outbreaks [111] and the infection can be introduced during penetrating injury [112]. Otherwise, the exogenous infection has been described in a hop grower [113].

The infection progresses to a more severe vitreal infiltration with "string of pearl" puffballs often with balls of white cells on the retina if the vitreous is detached. There may one or more foci of infiltration in the retina at the posterior pole. If untreated epiretinal membranes may form resulting in macular pucker [114]. Retinal detachment can occur, and phthisis bulbi result [111] (Figs. 19.47 and 19.48).

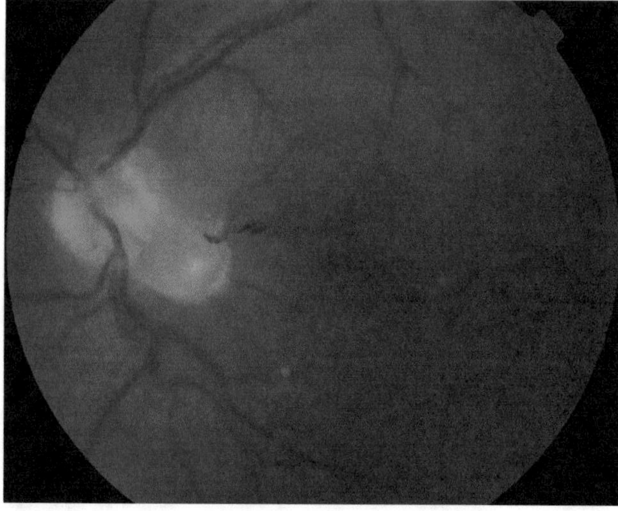

Fig. 19.45 A secondary ERM

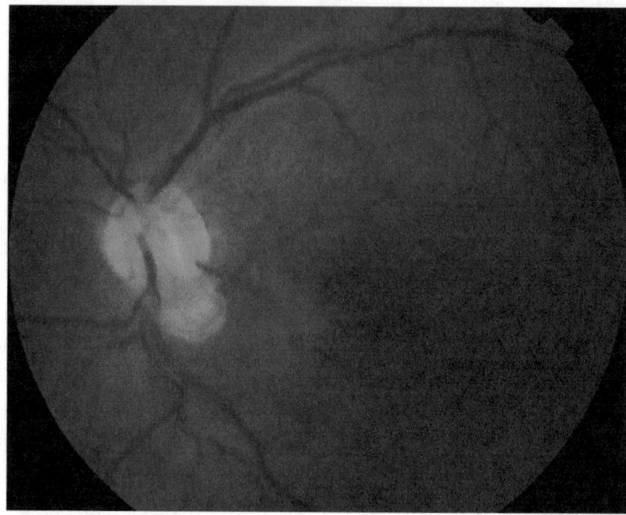

Fig. 19.46 This contracted towards the optic disc

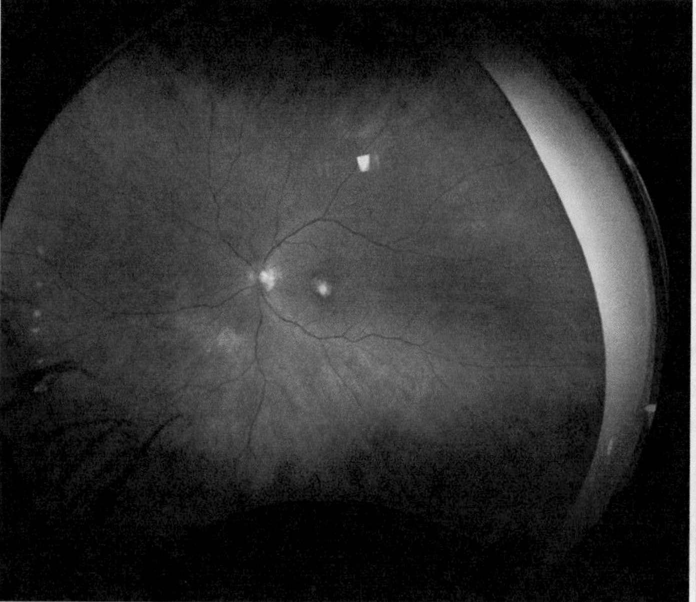

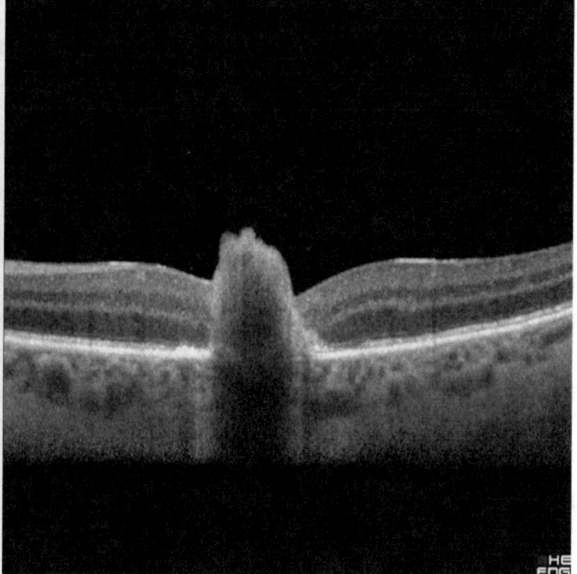

Fig. 19.47 A candidal infection has unfortunately damaged the fovea

Surgery (Table 19.4)

For Diagnosis

Often the clinical picture is so obvious that microbiological confirmation is only confirmatory. Fundoscopy screening of intensive care patients with candidemia can detect ocular involvement in a few per cent [115]. Pathologically the hyphae reside in the puffballs [116]. A vitreous biopsy may fail to identify the fungus because the hyphae are scanty in the vitreous. PPV with microbiological processing of the washings in the vitrectomy cassette usually yields the diagnosis, although PCR has also been advocated [117, 118]. The usual agent found is *candida albicans* and rarely others such as *candida krusei* [119] and others. Fifteen per cent of cases involve aspergillus whilst fusarium is rare [120] (Figs. 19.49, 19.50, 19.51 and Fig. 19.52).

For Treatment

The mainstay of therapy is systemic antifungal therapy [121]. This will easily deal with the early infection without the need for surgery and should be commenced immediately. More advanced infection with significant intravitreal infiltration requires PPV which, because of the poor viability of the fungus, in the eye will remove the local infection [122]. This

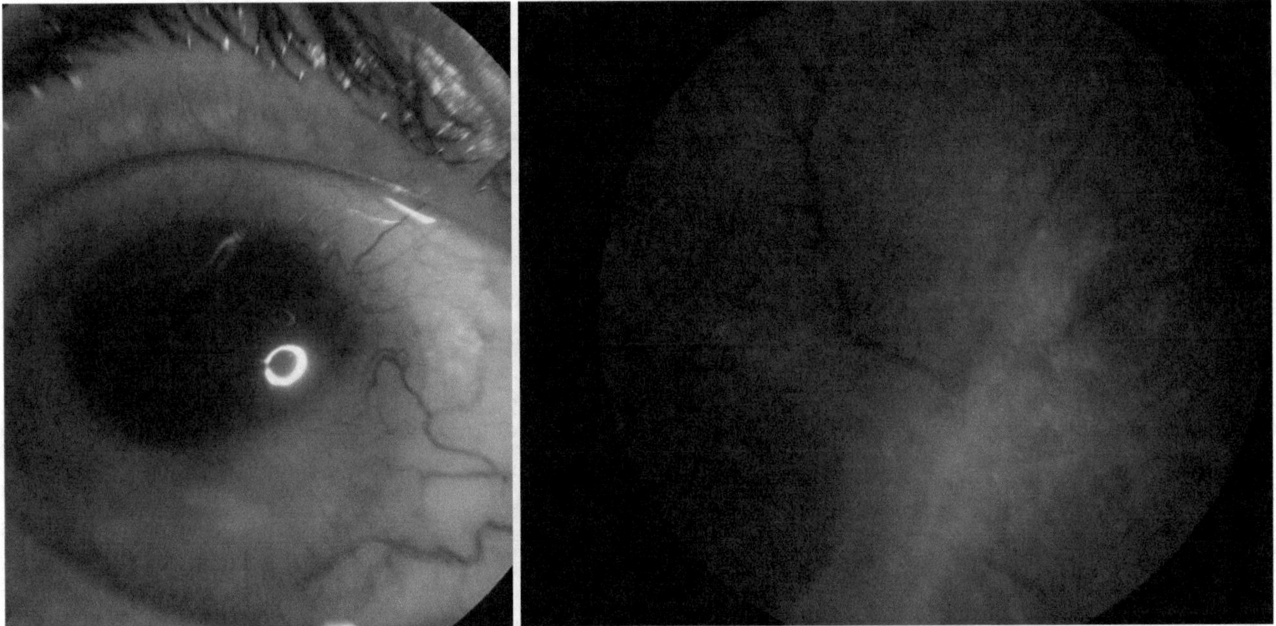

Fig. 19.48 A rare fungus (purpureocillium lilacinum) has caused endophthalmitis and preretinal membranes which finally lead to a funnel RRD

Table 19.4 Difficulty rating for PPV for candida endophthalmitis

Difficulty rating	Moderate
Success rates	High
Complication rates	Low
When to use in training	Middle

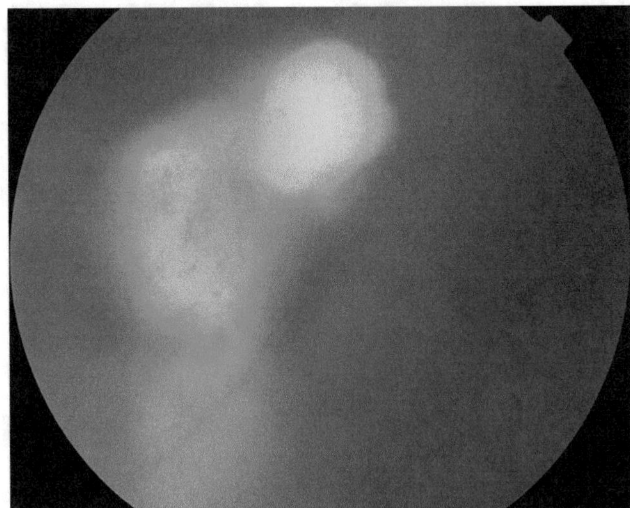

Fig. 19.49 This patient with leukaemia has developed fungal endophthalmitis from aspergillus

can be performed usually on the next available operating list assuming lists every 2–3 days. Intravitreal Amphotericin B is controversial because the eye will respond to systemic therapy and PPV alone [123]. After vitrectomy intravitreal

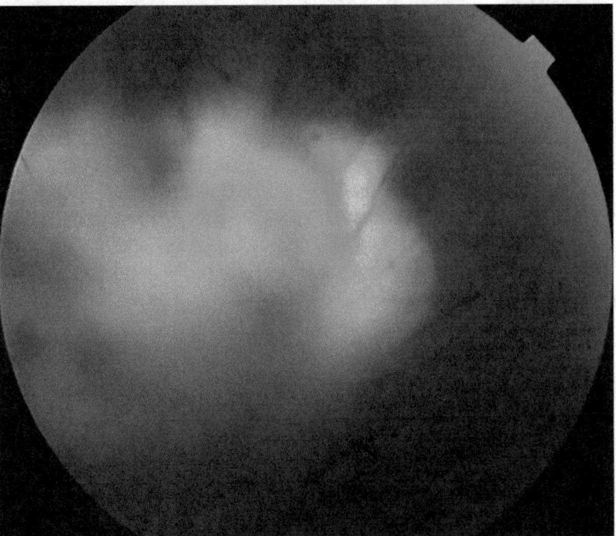

Fig. 19.50 The vitreous has been peeled from the retina in this patient with aspergillus in the eye revealing a deep retinal and choroidal infiltration

Amphotericin is cleared more quickly [124]. In general, Amphotericin is non-toxic; however, if used in too high a concentration, a panuveitis occurs which will settle without loss of vision (if the injection fluid looks yellow the Amphotericin is at too high a concentration) [125].

Perform a dry vitreous biopsy at the commencement of the surgery with the vitreous cutter. Many of these patients are young and therefore have an attached posterior hyaloid membrane (PHM). After core vitrectomy, the PHM should be separated from the retina. Any large focus of infiltration on the retina will usually detach the PHM without causing undue traction on the retina. Any residual white cells on the retinal surface can be aspirated. Secondary complications such as RRD or ERM can be dealt with by conventional methods.

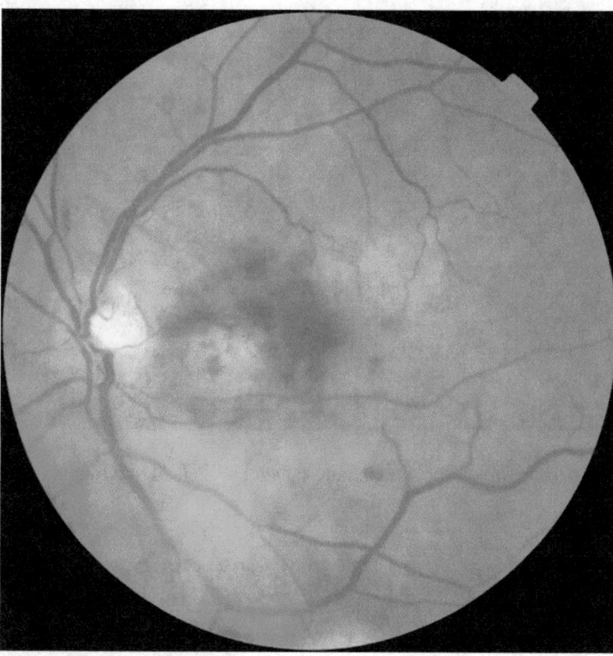

Fig. 19.51 This patient with acute myeloid leukaemia had multiple lesions in the skeletal muscles and the liver of probable fungal aetiology was on systemic antifungal therapy. He lost vision in both eyes the right with severe panuveitis and no fundal view and the left with a macular lesion as shown. He had right PPV and left vitreous biopsy with intravitreal Amphotericin in both eyes. Aspergillus was confirmed on culture. The left eye recovered 20/30 vision

Visual Outcome

Visual recovery depends on the severity of the infection and the location of any chorioretinal foci. In general, it is good if the infection is dealt with early. Late presentation or diagnosis is the main reason for poor visual outcome. Visual recovery with aspergillus or other fungi is usually poor (Fig. 19.53, 19.54 and 19.55)

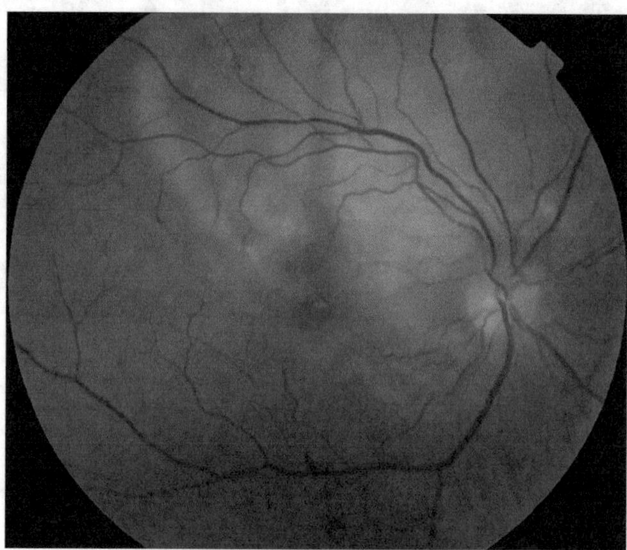

Fig. 19.53 This patient had acute leukaemia and lost vision from a suspected fungal choroiditis. A biopsy was performed to try to detect the pathogen. A shallow RRD occurred treated with silicone oil injection and subsequent removal. The infiltration settled on treatment with systemic antifungal therapy leaving an atrophic retina and RPE in the site of the infection

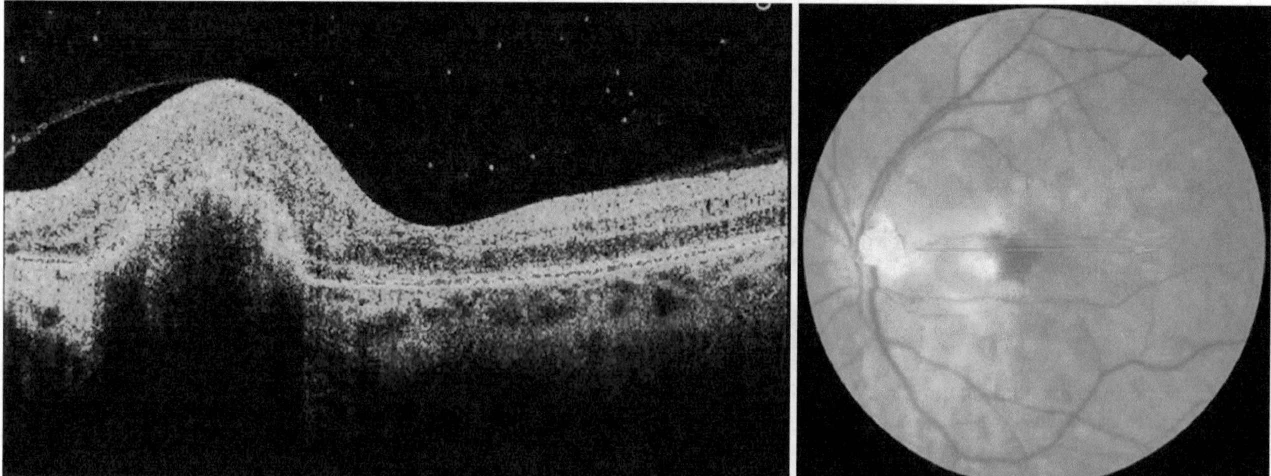

Fig. 19.52 A few months later the patient developed a secondary CNV on the scar. The CNV responded to intravitreal anti-VEGF injection retaining, 20/30 vision

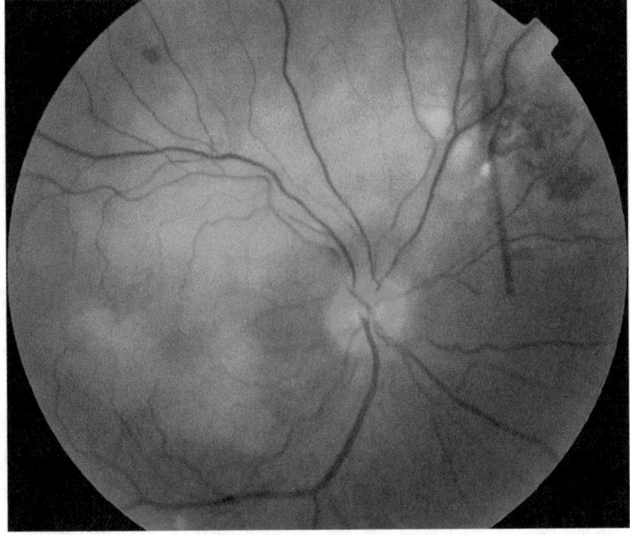

Fig. 19.54 Increase in the infected area

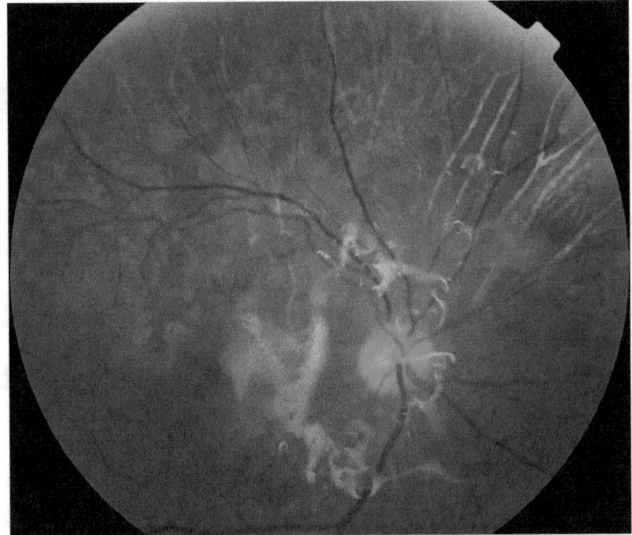

Fig. 19.55 After treatment and surgery

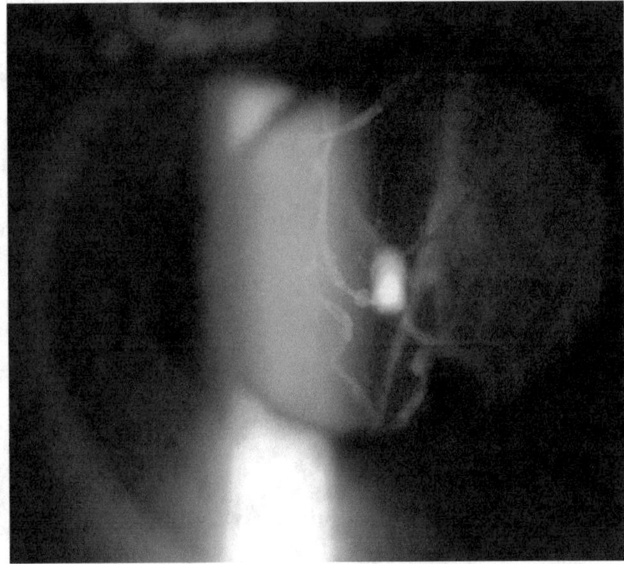

Fig. 19.56 Opacity in the vitreous is a common reason for PPV in patients with toxoplasmosis chorioretinitis

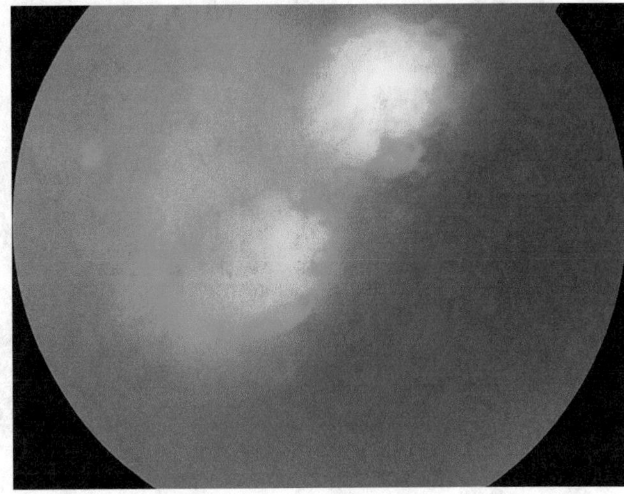

Fig. 19.57 A hazy vitreous with a toxoplasmosis scar

Other Infections

There are other less common presentations such as toxoplasmosis, (Figs. 19.56 and 19.57)which is associated with retinal detachments in approximately 6% of cases. Toxocara canis may be the cause of tractional retinal detachments in childhood. Tuberculosis produces a vasculitis similar to idiopathic vasculitis or Eales' disease, and can result in retinal detachment despite response to systemic therapy (Figs. 19.58, 19.59, 19.60, 19.61, 19.62, 19.63, 19.64, 19.65, 19.66, 19.67, 19.68 and 19.69, Table 19.5).

Causes of vitritis detectable by polymerase chain reaction (PCR).

- Herpes simplex virus 1 and 2 (HSV 1 and 2)
- Varicella zoster virus (VZV)
- Cytomegalovirus (CMV)
- Epstein–Barr virus (EBV)
- Borrelia burgdorferi
- Toxoplasma gondii
- *Mycobacterium tuberculosis*
- *Propionibacterium acnes*
- Whipple's disease

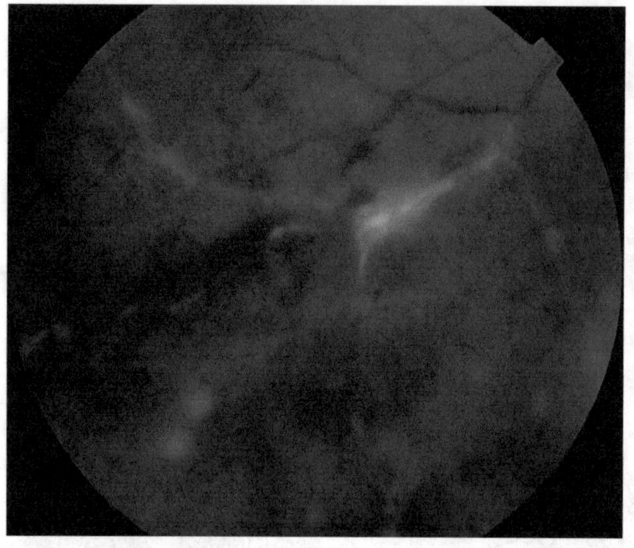

Fig. 19.58 A patient with tuberculous uveitis and a secondary vitreous haemorrhage

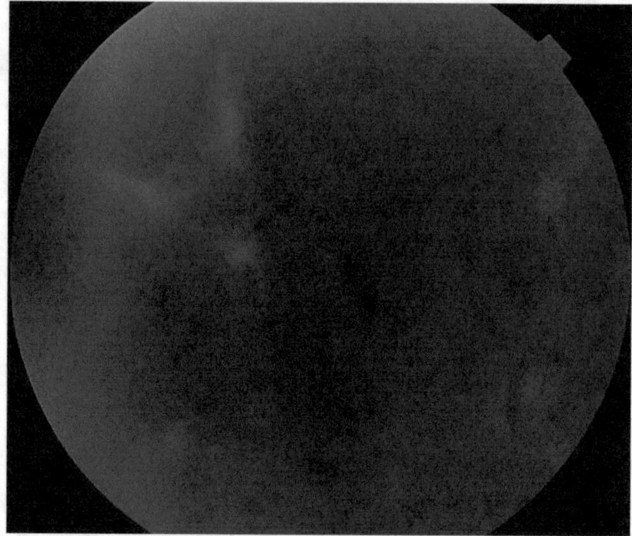

Fig. 19.59 Vitreous haemorrhage from TB uveitis

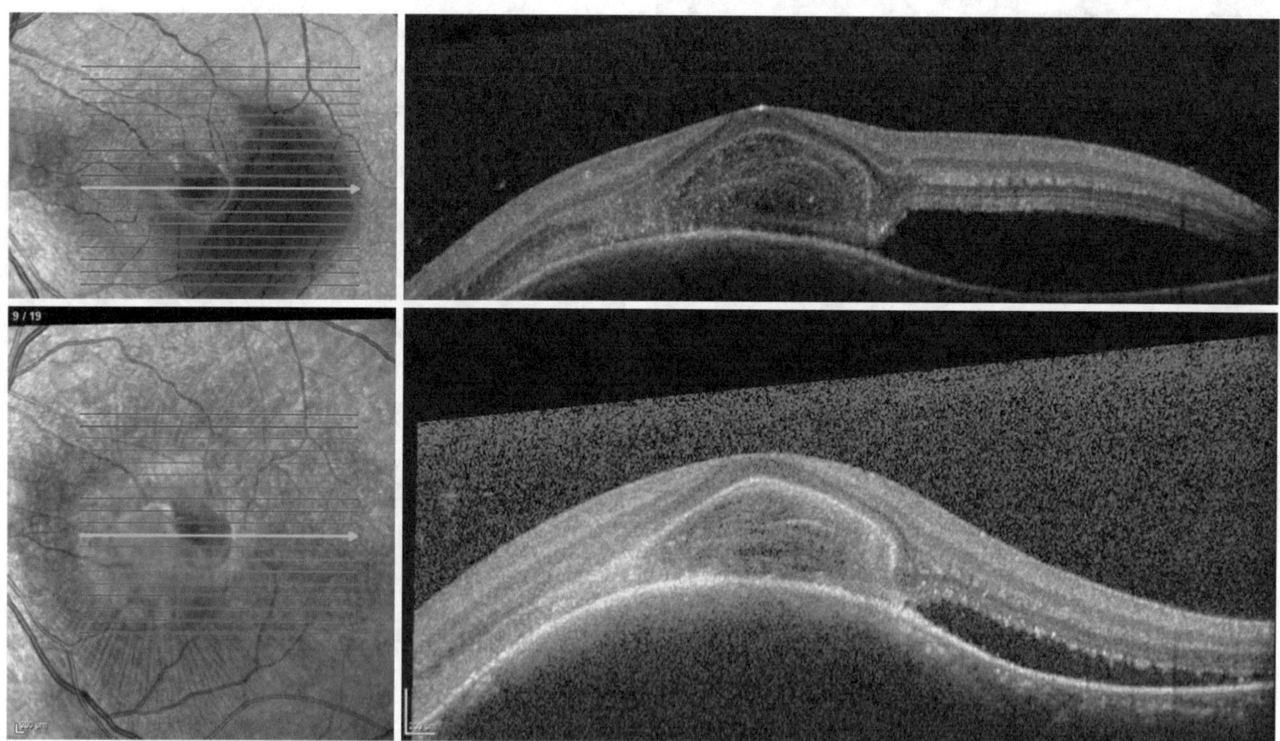

Fig. 19.60 Retinal elevation from Toxocara slowly resolves after treatment of inflammation

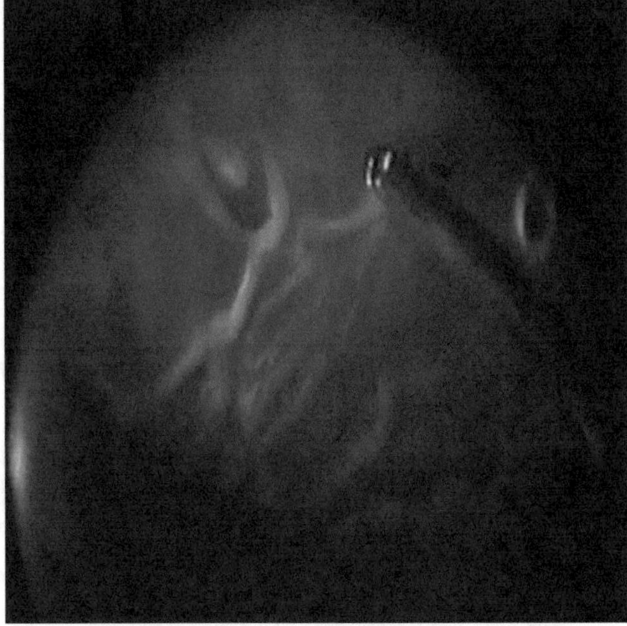

Fig. 19.61 This patient with tuberculosis and retinal vasculitis has developed a retinal tear and a retinal detachment

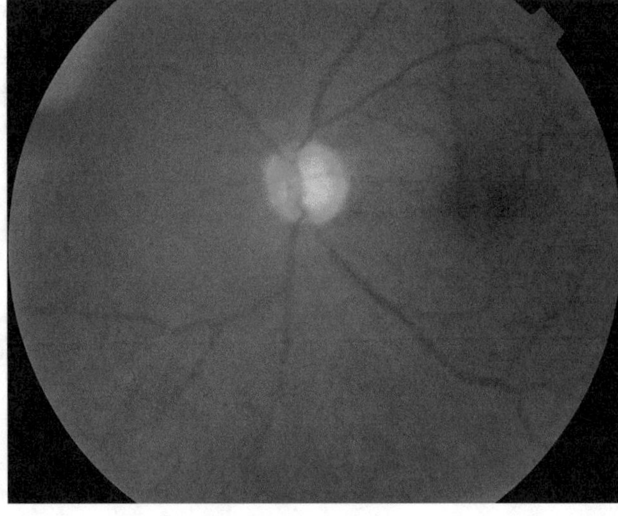

Fig. 19.63 The other eye after treatment

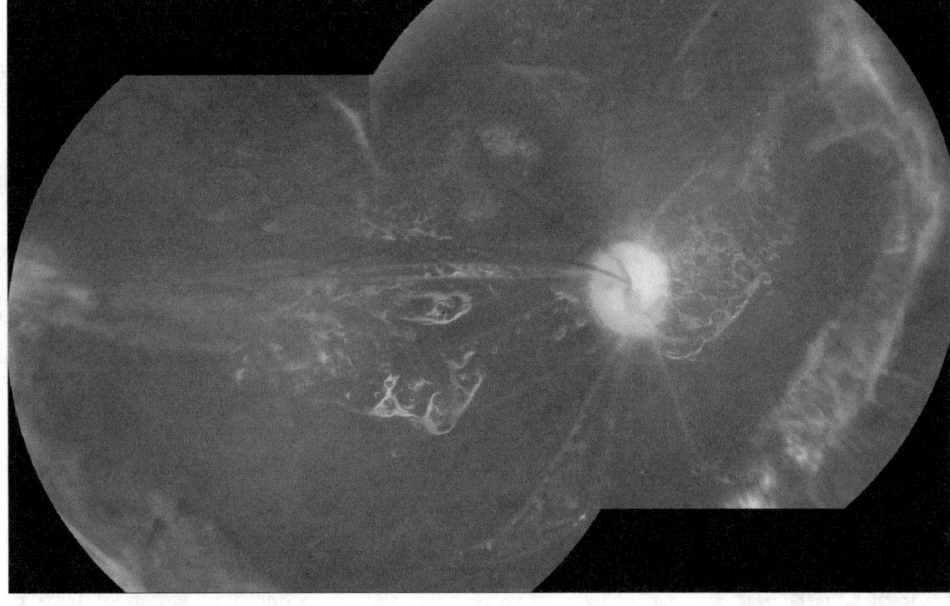

Fig. 19.62 This patient with tuberculosis retinitis and RRD required a PPV, 360-degree retinectomy and silicone oil insertion into the right eye and PPV and gas on the left with the visual recovery of counting fingers on the right and 20/30 left after systemic antitubercular therapy

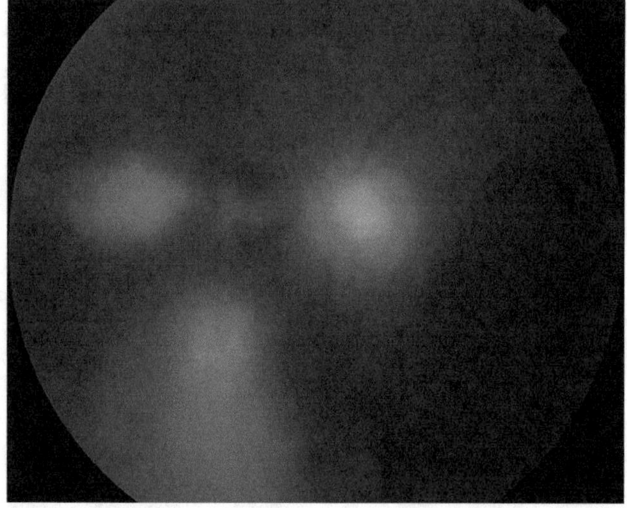

Fig. 19.64 Vitrectomy may be used to remove vitreous debris in ocular toxoplasmosis

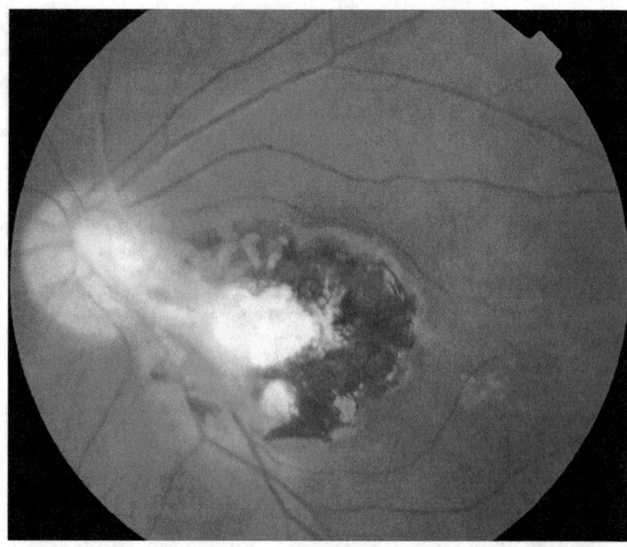

Fig. 19.66 The other eye

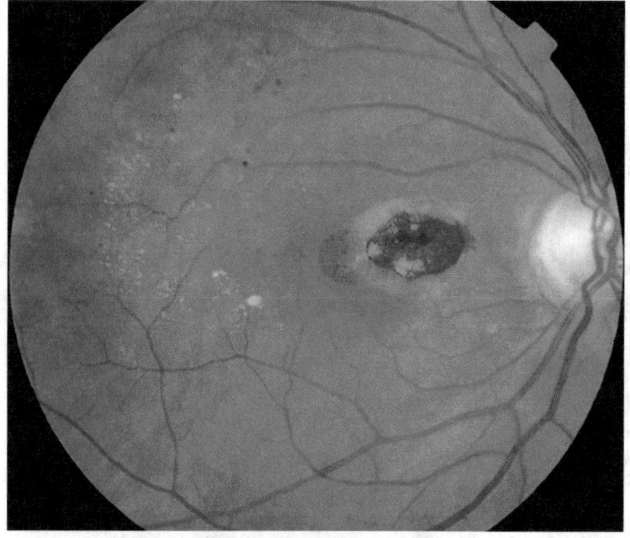

Fig. 19.65 This patient with congenital macular scars from toxoplasmosis developed a macular hole on the edge of the scar in the right eye which unfortunately did not close after surgery

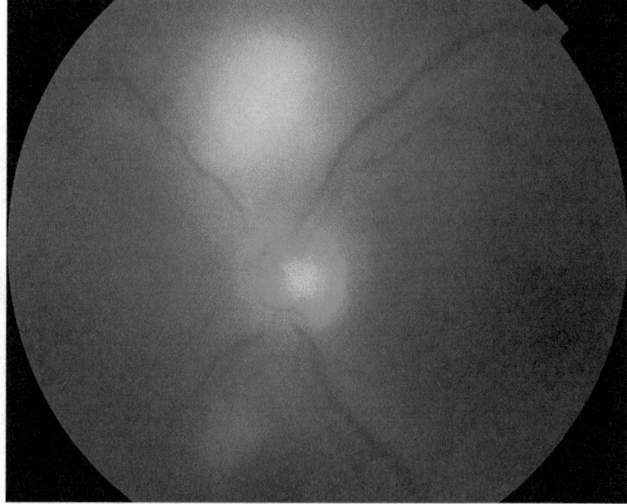

Fig. 19.67 This patient with posterior uveitis received an intravitreal steroid which caused an exacerbation of the uveitis, a diagnosis of toxoplasmosis was subsequently made on vitreal biopsy and PCR testing

Ocular Lymphoma

Clinical Features (Figs. 19.70, 19.71, 19.72 and 19.73)

Biopsy for neoplasia accounts for 14% of vitreous biopsies with 72% of these having ocular lymphoma [126].

Lymphoma in the eye presents in the elderly, often female and often bilaterally [127]. Ocular lymphoma should be considered in a patient with steroid-resistant posterior uveitis [128]. The clinical features however can be vague and varied with intravitreal white cells in a quiet eye, subretinal infiltration and occasional haemorrhagic retinal necrosis [129, 130]. Pseudo hypopyon can occur [131]. Fifty per cent of cases present because of ocular symptoms or signs, the remainder because of CNS involvement (20% of CNS lymphoma will affect the eye) [128, 132]. Usually a diffuse large cell B-cell lymphoma is found [133]. Epstein–Barr virus has been impli-

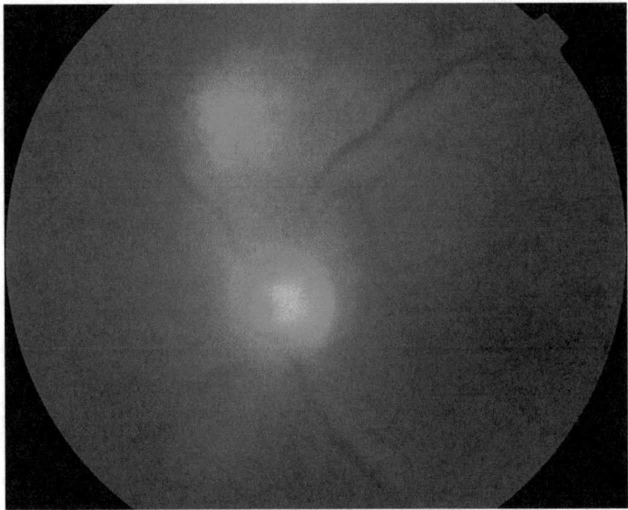

Fig. 19.68 After treatment of the toxoplasmosis, the inflammation began to subside

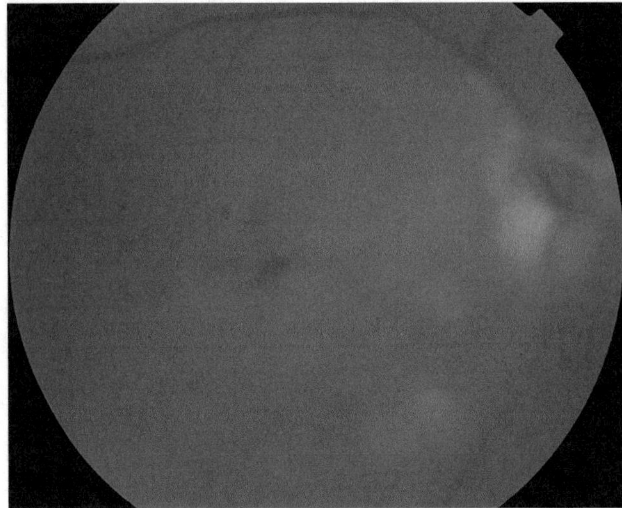

Fig. 19.69 Images are shown of a patient with tuberculous panuveitis. This patient developed bilateral RRD

Table 19.5 Cytology of the vitreous in infectious and non-infectious uveitis

Non-infectious uveitis	
Lymphoma	Atypical lymphocytes
Leukaemia	Atypical lymphoid cells
Metastatic tumour	Tumour cells
Melanoma	Tumour cells with melanin
Inflammatory uveitis	Inflammatory cells (plasma cells, lymphocytes, polymorphonuclear leucocytes, monocytes
Lens induced uveitis	Lens material, inflammatory multinucleate cells or phacolytic cells
Epithelial down growth	Fibroblasts
Amyloidosis	Acellular globules
Juvenile xanthogranuloma	Histiocytes, Touton giant cells
Infectious uveitis	
Bacteria	Bacteria, neutrophils
Mycobacteria	Acid-fast bacilli
Fungal	Yeast, hyphae, mononuclear cells
Toxoplasmosis	Tachyzoites
Toxocariasis	Eosinophilia, plasma cells, second-stage larvae
Acute retinal necrosis	Inflammatory cells
Viral infections	Mononuclear cells

cated in patients with AIDs, but biopsy samples are often positive for this virus without evidence of infection [134–136].

Investigation for systemic or intracerebral lymphoma is advised. Low-dose radiotherapy is very effective in reducing infiltration in these eyes [137] and systemic chemotherapy may be considered [129].

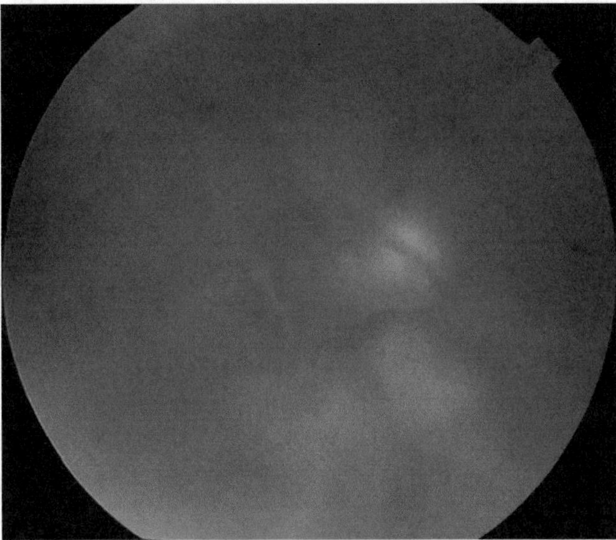

Fig. 19.70 This patient has intraocular lymphoma. This is often characterised by diffuse white cell infiltration in a non-specific manner. Clinically the diagnosis may be difficult to discriminate from other types of uveitis

Surgery (Table 19.6)

For Diagnosis (Fig. 19.74)

A vitreous biopsy should be taken but requires rapid processing of the sample [126, 138] because the lymphoma cells are fragile and barely viable. Often cytology fails to identify the cells and differentiation from inflammation is difficult. Immunotyping to identify monoclonal cell lines is useful to overcome the latter problem [139] (Fig. 19.75).

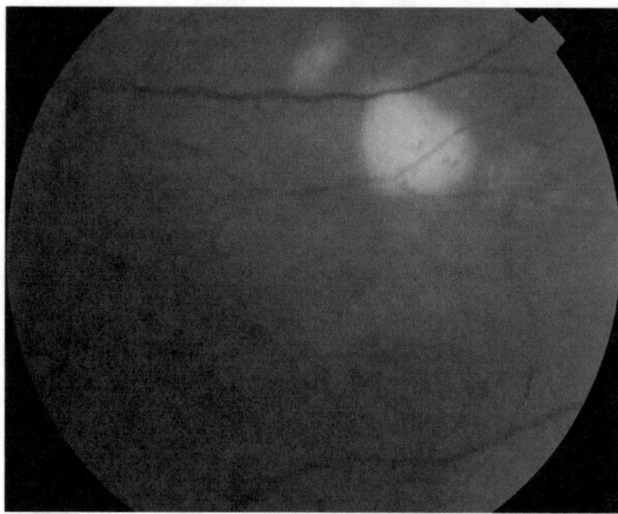

Fig. 19.71 Subretinal infiltrates are typical of intraocular lymphoma and can be biopsied to increase the yield from cytology

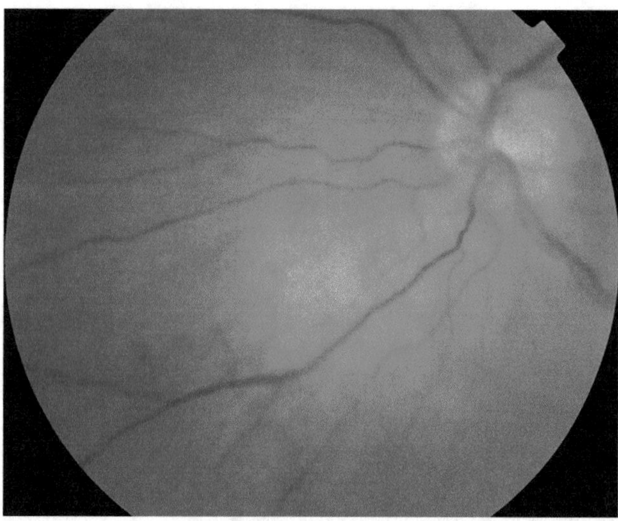

Fig. 19.72 A rare presentation of lymphoma with diffuse choroidal infiltration on fundoscopy and ultrasound

Chorioretinal Biopsy

Other options that have been employed include retinal biopsy [133] or aspiration of subretinal infiltrates [140]. These provide higher yields because the cells are more viable than those in the vitreous.

- Chose an area of the retina affected by infiltration approximately 2–3 disc diameters that is superior and midperipheral, away from large blood vessels.
- Surround the biopsy site with a confluent diode laser prior to excision (or if not available use endodiathermy burns) to close the choroidal blood vessels.
- Use vertical cutting scissors to cut through the centre of the burns incising both the choroid and retina.

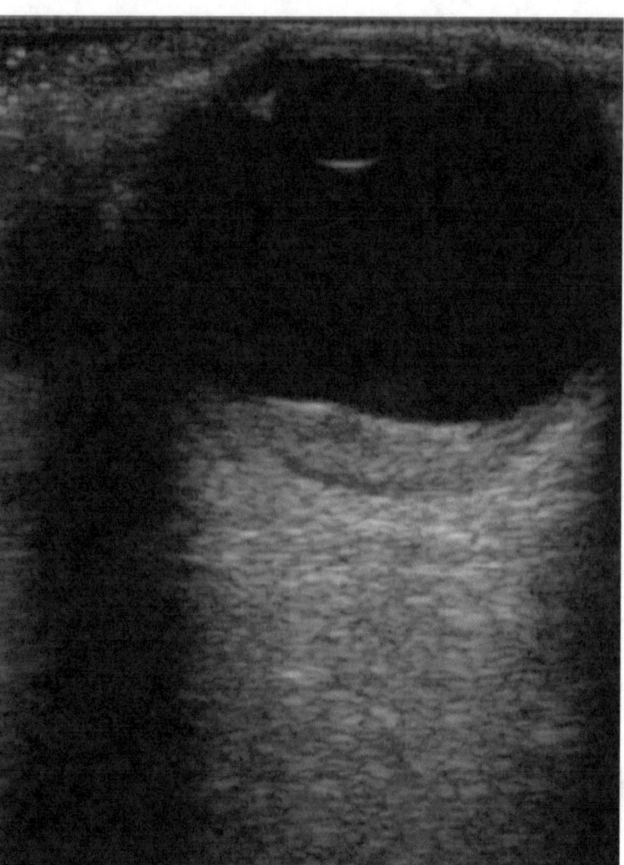

Fig. 19.73 The same patient's ultrasound demonstrating the degree of thickening

Table 19.6 Difficulty rating for PPV for ocular lymphoma

Difficulty rating	Moderate
Success rates	Moderate
Complication rates	Low
When to use in training	Middle

- Remove the block of tissue with forceps through an enlarged sclerotomy, you will need at least a 20-gauge sclerotomy. Take care, the choroid and retina can separate from each other during extraction. The retina is usually tough and is easily kept hold of, but the choroid can be washed away by fluid coming out of the sclerotomy. Inspect the tissue to check that you have both layers; search on the drape on the cheek of the patient if the pigmented choroid has been washed off!
- Laser around the site of excision.
- Insert long-acting gas to maintain a flat retina.

A chorioretinal biopsy is usually reserved for those eyes with poorer visual potential. Cells from a subretinal deposit can be aspirated through a small gauge cannula inserted via a retinotomy.

Intraocular Methothrexate may be inserted in resistant cases [141].

Samples should be examined by flow cytometry.

For Treatment

Surgery is performed for restoration of vision because the vitreous cells are reducing vitreal clarity. PPV can be used to clear the visual axis and is usually uneventful. Intravitreal Methotrexate may be injected to reduce the local response in the eye.

Visual Outcome and Survival

The prognosis for visual recovery is good. These lymphomas do not usually spread systemically. However, patients have a shortened life expectancy due to the development of intracerebral lymphoma resulting in poor survival for these patients of median 3 years [134] (Figs. 19.76 and 19.77).

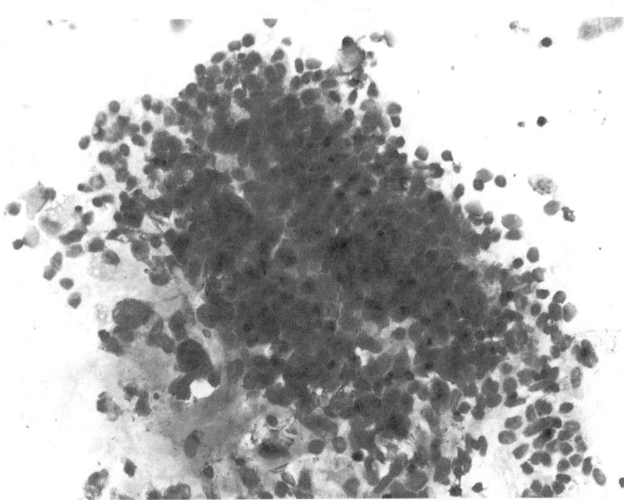

Fig. 19.74 Cytology can be performed but vitreous samples must be processed immediately to prevent loss of fragile lymphomatous cells

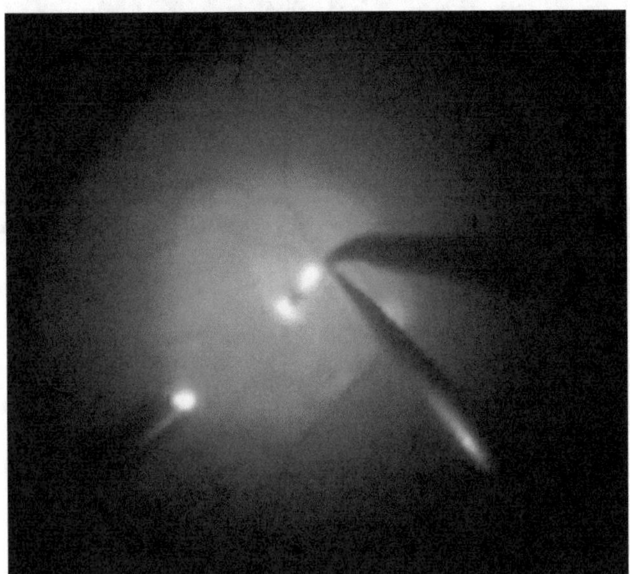

Fig. 19.75 Subretinal infiltrates in suspected ocular lymphoma are a good source of cells for diagnostic confirmation. These can be aspirated via a retinotomy

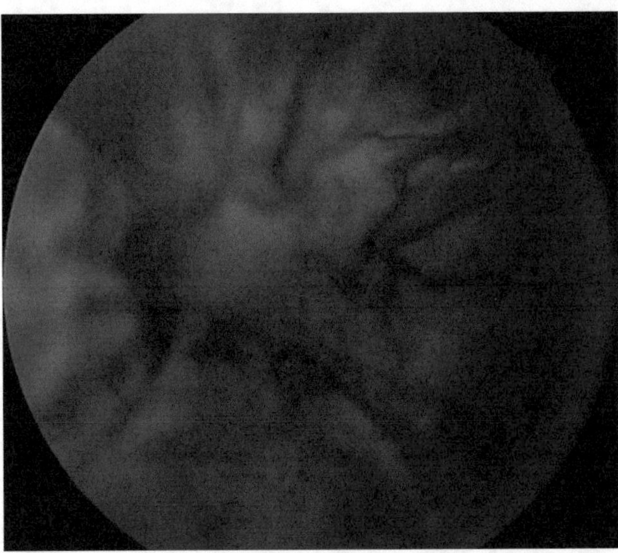

Fig. 19.76 An acute relapse of acute lymphocytic leukaemia in this patient was accompanied by exudative retinopathy

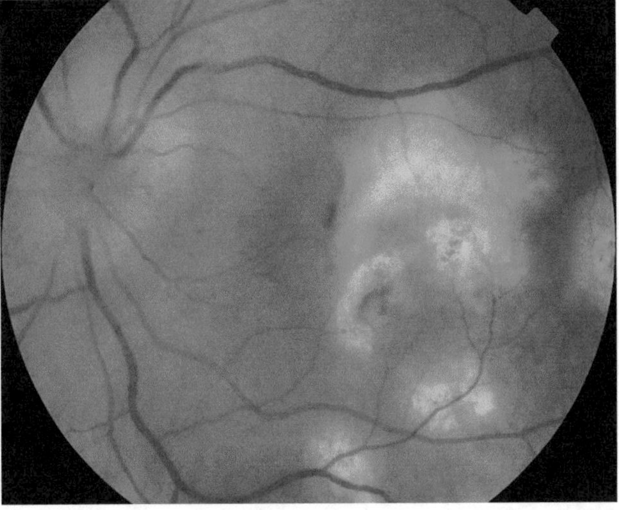

Fig. 19.77 In some patients, despite vitreous, retinal and choroidal biopsy, a definitive diagnosis is not reached. This patient had poor vision because of optic nerve involvement and had a CNV on the edge of scarring

Paraneoplastic Retinopathy

Patients with carcinoma or melanoma may present with severe loss of vision with a non-specific panuveitis [142]. Loss of vision occurs centrally with scotomas and photopsia. Antibodies to retinal proteins can be detected. Systemic workup and investigation is required if the source of the neoplasia is unknown. Suspect this rare diagnosis in a patient with diffuse non-specific retinal changes but a severe loss of vision (Fig. 19.78).

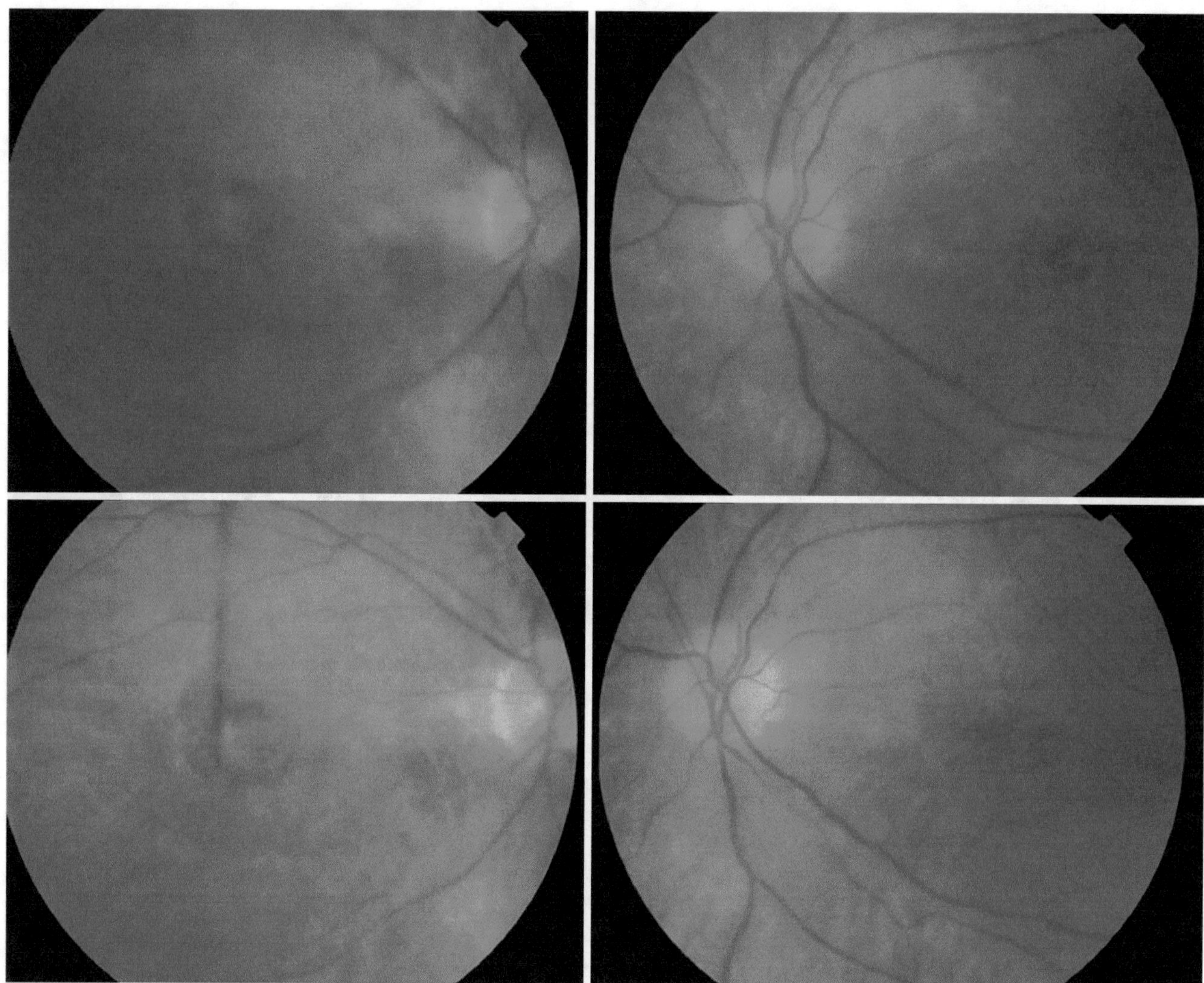

Fig. 19.78 A panuveitis with the development of macular changes and optic atrophy associated with the CRMP 5 gene and small cell carcinoma. A retinal biopsy was performed to try to aid the diagnosis

Summary

Vitreoretinal methods can be adapted to aid the diagnosis and treatment of a wide variety of uveitic, infectious and neoplastic conditions. All have their own hazards surgically and most often other specialities both ophthalmological and otherwise become involved in the care of the patient.

References

1. Mieler WF, Will BR, Lewis H, Aaberg TM. Vitrectomy in the management of peripheral uveitis. Ophthalmology. 1988;95(7):859–64.
2. Eckardt C, Bacskulin A. Vitrectomy in intermediate uveitis. Dev Ophthalmol. 1992;23:232–8.
3. Nolle B, Eckardt C. Vitrectomy in multifocal chorioretinitis. Ger J Ophthalmol. 1993;2(1):14–9.
4. Bovey EH, Herbort CP. Vitrectomy in the management of uveitis. Ocul Immunol Inflamm. 2000;8(4):285–91.
5. Heiligenhaus A, Bornfeld N, Foerster MH, Wessing A. Long-term results of pars plana vitrectomy in the management of complicated uveitis. Br J Ophthalmol. 1994;78(7):549–54.
6. Scott RA, Haynes RJ, Orr GM, Cooling RJ, Pavesio CE, Charteris DG. Vitreous surgery in the management of chronic endogenous posterior uveitis. Eye. 2003;17(2):221–7.
7. Dugel PU, Rao NA, Ozler S, Liggett PE, Smith RE. Pars plana vitrectomy for intraocular inflammation-related cystoid macular edema unresponsive to corticosteroids. A preliminary study. Ophthalmology. 1992;99(10):1535–41.
8. Kokame GT, de Leon MD, Tanji T. Serous retinal detachment and cystoid macular edema in hypotony maculopathy. Am J Ophthalmol. 2001;131(3):384–6.
9. Mieler WF, Aaberg TM. Vitreous surgery in the management of peripheral uveitis. Dev phthalmol. 1992;23:239–50.
10. Heimann K, Schmanke L, Brunner R, Amerian B. Pars plana vitrectomy in the treatment of chronic uveitis. Dev Ophthalmol. 1992;23:196–203.
11. Kaplan HJ. Surgical treatment of intermediate uveitis. Dev Ophthalmol. 1992;23:185–9.
12. Diamond JG, Kaplan HJ. Uveitis: effect of vitrectomy combined with lensectomy. Ophthalmology. 1979;86(7):1320–9.
13. Potter MJ, Myckatyn SO, Maberley AL, Lee AS. Vitrectomy for pars planitis complicated by vitreous hemorrhage: visual outcome and long-term follow-up. Am J Ophthalmol. 2001;131(4):514–5.
14. Verbraeken H. Therapeutic pars plana vitrectomy for chronic uveitis: a retrospective study of the long-term results. Graefes Arch Clin Exp Ophthalmol. 1996;234(5):288–93.
15. Waters FM, Goodall K, Jones NP, McLeod D. Vitrectomy for vitreous opacification in Fuchs' heterochromic uveitis. Eye. 2000;14(Pt 2):216–8.
16. Gaun S, Kurimoto Y, Komurasaki Y, Yoshimura N. Vitreous surgery for bilateral bullous retinal detachment in Vogt-Koyanagi-Harada syndrome. Ophthalmic Surg Lasers. 2002;33(6):508–10.
17. Antcliffe RJ, Spalton DJ, Stanford MR, Graham EM. Ffythche TJ, Marshall J. intravitreal triamcinolone for uveitic cystoid macular oedema: an optical coherence tomography study. Ophthalmology. 2001;108:765–2.
18. Haller JA, Bandello F, Belfort R Jr, Blumenkranz MS, Gillies M, Heier J, et al. Randomized, sham-controlled trial of dexamethasone intravitreal implant in patients with macular edema due to retinal vein occlusion. Ophthalmology. 117(6):1134–46. e3. S0161-6420(10)00311-8 [pii]. https://doi.org/10.1016/j.ophtha.2010.03.032.
19. Haller JA, Kuppermann BD, Blumenkranz MS, Williams GA, Weinberg DV, Chou C, et al. Randomized controlled trial of an intravitreous dexamethasone drug delivery system in patients with diabetic macular edema. Arch Ophthalmol. 128(3):289–96. 128/3/289 [pii]. https://doi.org/10.1001/archophthalmol.2010.21.
20. Aylward GW. The place of vitreoretinal surgery in the treatment of macular oedema. Doc Ophthalmol. 1999;97(3–4):433–8.
21. Davis JL, Chan CC, Nussenblatt RB. Diagnostic vitrectomy in intermediate uveitis. Dev Ophthalmol. 1992;23:120–32.
22. Tranos P, Scott R, Zambarakji H, Ayliffe W, Pavesio C, Charteris DG. The effect of pars plana vitrectomy on cystoid macular oedema associated with chronic uveitis: a randomised, controlled pilot study. Br J Ophthalmol. 2006;90(9):1107–10. doi: bjo.2006.092965 [pii]. https://doi.org/10.1136/bjo.2006.092965.
23. Diamond JG, Kaplan HJ. Lensectomy and vitrectomy for complicated cataract secondary to uveitis. Arch Ophthalmol. 1978;96(10):1798–804.
24. Priem H, Verbraeken H, De Laey JJ. Diagnostic problems in chronic vitreous inflammation. Graefes Arch Clin Exp Ophthalmol. 1993;231(8):453–6.
25. Morse LS, McCuen BW. The use of silicone oil in uveitis and hypotony. Retina. 1991;11(4):399–404.
26. Davis JL, Miller DM, Ruiz P. Diagnostic testing of vitrectomy specimens. Am J Ophthalmol. 2005;140(5):822–9. doi: S0002-9394(05)00611-2 [pii]. https://doi.org/10.1016/j.ajo.2005.05.032.
27. Han DP, Wisniewski SR, Kelsey SF, Doft BH, Barza M, Pavan PR. Microbiologic yields and complication rates of vitreous needle aspiration versus mechanized vitreous biopsy in the Endophthalmitis vitrectomy study. Retina. 1999;19(2):98–102.
28. Quiroz-Mercado H, Rivera-Sempertegui J, Macky TA, Navarro-Lopez P, Griselda-Alvarez L, Ibarra-Ponce N, et al. Performing vitreous biopsy by perfluorocarbon-perfused vitrectomy. Am J Ophthalmol. 2005;140(6):1161–3.
29. Akpek EK, Kent C, Jakobiec F, Caliendo AM, Foster CS. Bilateral acute retinal necrosis caused by cytomegalovirus in an immunocompromised patient. Am J Ophthalmol. 1999;127(1):93–5.
30. Rahhal FM, Siegel LM, Russak V, Wiley CA, Tedder DG, Weinberg A, et al. Clinicopathologic correlations in acute retinal necrosis caused by herpes simplex virus type 2. Arch Ophthalmol. 1996;114(11):1416–9.
31. Lewis ML, Culbertson WW, Post JD, Miller D, Kokame GT, Dix RD. Herpes simplex virus type 1. A cause of the acute retinal necrosis syndrome. Ophthalmology. 1989;96(6):875–8.
32. Freeman WR, Thomas EL, Rao NA, Pepose JS, Trousdale MD, Howes EL, et al. Demonstration of herpes group virus in acute retinal necrosis syndrome. Am J Ophthalmol. 1986;102(6):701–9.
33. Bali E, Huyghe P, Caspers L, Libert J. Vitrectomy and silicone oil in the treatment of acute endophthalmitis. Preliminary Results Bull Soc Belge Ophtalmol. 2003;288:9–14.
34. Zambarakji HJ, Obi AA, Mitchell SM. Successful treatment of varicella zoster virus retinitis with aggressive intravitreal and systemic antiviral therapy. Ocul Immunol Inflamm. 2002;10(1):41–6.
35. Nakanishi F, Takahashi H, Ohara K. Acute retinal necrosis following contralateral herpes zoster ophthalmicus. Jpn J Ophthalmol. 2000;44(5):561–4.
36. Culbertson WW, Brod RD, Flynn HW Jr, Taylor BC, Brod BA, Lightman DA, et al. Chickenpox-associated acute retinal necrosis syndrome. Ophthalmology. 1991;98(11):1641–5.
37. Markomichelakis NN, Zafirakis P, Karambogia-Karefillidi P, Drakoulis N, Vagiakou-Boudri E, Paterakis G, et al. Herpes simplex virus type 2: a cause of acute retinal necrosis syndrome. Ocul Immunol Inflamm. 2001;9(2):103–9.

38. Rappaport KD, Tang WM. Herpes simplex virus type 2 acute retinal necrosis in a patient with systemic lupus erythematosus. Retina. 2000;20(5):545–6.
39. Hershberger VS, Hutchins RK, Witte DP, Schneider S, Harris RE, McGonegle SJ. Epstein-Barr virus-related bilateral acute retinal necrosis in a patient with X-linked lymphoproliferative disorder. Arch Ophthalmol. 2003;121(7):1047–9.
40. Weinberg DV, Lyon AT. Repair of retinal detachments due to herpes varicella-zoster virus retinitis in patients with acquired immune deficiency syndrome. Ophthalmology. 1997;104(2):279–82.
41. Purdy KW, Heckenlively JR, Church JA, Keller MA. Progressive outer retinal necrosis caused by varicella-zoster virus in children with acquired immunodeficiency syndrome. Pediatr Infect Dis J. 2003;22(4):384–6.
42. Austin RB. Progressive outer retinal necrosis syndrome: a comprehensive review of its clinical presentation, relationship to immune system status, and management. Clin Eye Vis Care. 2000;12(3–4):119–29.
43. Moorthy RS, Weinberg DV, Teich SA, Berger BB, Minturn JT, Kumar S, et al. Management of varicella zoster virus retinitis in AIDS. Br J Ophthalmol. 1997;81(3):189–94.
44. Perez-Blazquez E, Traspas R, Mendez MI, Montero M. Intravitreal ganciclovir treatment in progressive outer retinal necrosis. Am J Ophthalmol. 1997;124(3):418–21.
45. Pavesio CE, Mitchell SM, Barton K, Schwartz SD, Towler HM, Lightman S. Progressive outer retinal necrosis (PORN) in AIDS patients: a different appearance of varicella-zoster retinitis. Eye. 1995;9(Pt 3):271–6.
46. Margolis TP, Lowder CY, Holland GN, Spaide RF, Logan AG, Weissman SS, et al. Varicella-zoster virus retinitis in patients with the acquired immunodeficiency syndrome. Am J Ophthalmol. 1991;112(2):119–31.
47. Ezra E, Pearson RV, Etchells DE, Gregor ZJ. Delayed fellow eye involvement in acute retinal necrosis syndrome. Am J Ophthalmol. 1995;120(1):115–7.
48. Martinez J, Lambert HM, Capone A, Sternberg P Jr, Aaberg TM, Lopez PF, et al. Delayed bilateral involvement in the acute retinal necrosis syndrome. Am J Ophthalmol. 1992;113(1):103–4.
49. Matsuo T, Nakayama T, Koyama T, Matsuo N. Mild type acute retinal necrosis syndrome involving both eyes at three-year interval. Jpn J Ophthalmol. 1987;31(3):455–60.
50. Ahmadieh H, Sajjadi SH, Azarmina M, Kalani H. Association of herpetic encephalitis with acute retinal necrosis syndrome. Ann Ophthalmol. 1991;23(6):215–9.
51. Bloom JN, Katz JI, Kaufman HE. Herpes simplex retinitis and encephalitis in an adult. Arch Ophthalmol. 1977;95(10):1798–9.
52. Carney MD, Peyman GA, Goldberg MF, Packo K, Pulido J, Nicholson D. Acute retinal necrosis. Retina. 1986;6(2):85–94.
53. Duker JS, Nielsen JC, Eagle RC Jr, Bosley TM, Granadier R, Benson WE. Rapidly progressive acute retinal necrosis secondary to herpes simplex virus, type 1. Ophthalmology. 1990;97(12):1638–43.
54. Topilow HW, Nussbaum JJ, Freeman HM, Dickersin GR, Szyfelbein W. Bilateral acute retinal necrosis. Clinical and ultrastructural study. Arch Ophthalmol. 1982;100(12):1901–8.
55. Wang CL, Kaplan HJ, Waldrep JC, Pulliam M. Retinal neovascularization associated with acute retinal necrosis. Retina. 1983;3(4):249–52.
56. Fox GM, Blumenkranz M. Giant retinal pigment epithelial tears in acute retinal necrosis. Am J Ophthalmol. 1993;116(3):302–6.
57. Gerling J, Neumann-Haefelin D, Seuffert HM, Schrader W, Hansen LL. Diagnosis and management of the acute retinal necrosis syndrome. Ger J Ophthalmol. 1992;1(6):388–93.
58. Verbraeken H, Libert J. Vitrectomy in non-haemorrhagic hazy vitreous. Bull Soc Belge Ophtalmol. 1995;258:47–62.
59. Immonen I, Laatikainen L, Linnanvuori K. Acute retinal necrosis syndrome treated with vitrectomy and intravenous acyclovir. Acta Ophthalmol(Copenh). 1989;67(1):106–8.
60. McDonald HR, Lewis H, Kreiger AE, Sidikaro Y, Heckenlively J. Surgical management of retinal detachment associated with the acute retinal necrosis syndrome. Br J Ophthalmol. 1991;75(8):455–8.
61. Blumenkranz M, Clarkson J, Culbertson WW, Flynn HW, Lewis ML, Young GM. Visual results and complications after retinal reattachment in the acute retinal necrosis syndrome. The influence of operative technique. Retina. 1989;9(3):170–4.
62. Blumenkranz M, Clarkson J, Culbertson WW, Flynn HW, Lewis ML, Young GA. Vitrectomy for retinal detachment associated with acute retinal necrosis. Am J Ophthalmol. 1988;106(4):426–9.
63. Ahmadieh H, Soheilian M, Azarmina M, Dehghan MH, Mashayekhi A. Surgical management of retinal detachment secondary to acute retinal necrosis: clinical features, surgical techniques, and long-term results. Jpn J Ophthalmol. 2003;47(5):484–91.
64. Jabs DA. Ocular manifestations of HIV infection. Trans Am Ophthalmol Soc. 1995;93:623–83.
65. Fraenkel G, Ross B, Wong HC. Cytomegalovirus retinitis in a patient with rheumatoid arthritis being treated with combination immunosuppressive therapy. Retina. 1995;15(2):169–70.
66. Uphold CR, Smith MF, Bender BS. Failure of a prospective trial to detect cytomegalovirus retinitis after initiation of highly active antiretroviral therapy. AIDS Patient Care STDS. 1998;12(12):907–12.
67. Mitchell SM, Membrey WL, Youle MS, Obi A, Worrell S, Gazzard BG. Cytomegalovirus retinitis after the initiation of highly active antiretroviral therapy: a 2 year prospective study. Br J Ophthalmol. 1999;83(6):652–5.
68. Mocroft A, Katlama C, Johnson AM, Pradier C, Antunes F, Mulcahy F, et al. AIDS across Europe, 1994–98: the EuroSIDA study. Lancet. 2000;356(9226):291–6.
69. Jalali S, Reed JB, Mizoguchi M, Flynn N, Gordon J, Morse LS. Effect of highly active antiretroviral therapy on the incidence of HIV-related cytomegalovirus retinitis and retinal detachment. AIDS Patient Care STDS. 2000;14(7):343–6.
70. Jabs DA, Enger C, Haller J, de Bustros S. Retinal detachments in patients with cytomegalovirus retinitis. Arch Ophthalmol. 1991;109(6):794–9.
71. Sidikaro Y, Silver L, Holland GN, Kreiger AE. Rhegmatogenous retinal detachments in patients with AIDS and necrotizing retinal infections. Ophthalmology. 1991;98(2):129–35.
72. Dugel PU, Liggett PE, Lee MB, Ziogas A, Forster DJ, Smith RE, et al. Repair of retinal detachment caused by cytomegalovirus retinitis in patients with the acquired immunodeficiency syndrome. Am J Ophthalmol. 1991;112(3):235–42.
73. Irvine AR, Lonn L, Schwartz D, Zarbin M, Ballesteros F, Kroll S. Retinal detachment in AIDS: long-term results after repair with silicone oil. Br J Ophthalmol. 1997;81(3):180–3.
74. Kempen JH, Jabs DA, Wilson LA, Dunn JP, West SK, Tonascia J. Mortality risk for patients with cytomegalovirus retinitis and acquired immune deficiency syndrome. Clin Infect Dis. 2003;37(10):1365–73.
75. Kempen JH, Jabs DA, Dunn JP, West SK, Tonascia J. Retinal detachment risk in cytomegalovirus retinitis related to the acquired immunodeficiency syndrome. Arch Ophthalmol. 2001;119(1):33–40.
76. Holbrook JT, Jabs DA, Weinberg DV, Lewis RA, Davis MD, Friedberg D. Visual loss in patients with cytomegalovirus retinitis and acquired immunodeficiency syndrome before widespread availability of highly active antiretroviral therapy. Arch Ophthalmol. 2003;121(1):99–107.

77. Arevalo JF, Mendoza AJ, Ferretti Y. Immune recovery uveitis in AIDS patients with cytomegalovirus retinitis treated with highly active antiretroviral therapy in Venezuela. Retina. 2003;23(4):495–502.
78. Song MK, Azen SP, Buley A, Torriani F, Cheng L, Chaidhawangul S, et al. Effect of anti-cytomegalovirus therapy on the incidence of immune recovery uveitis in AIDS patients with healed cytomegalovirus retinitis. Am J Ophthalmol. 2003;136(4):696–702.
79. Canzano JC, Reed JB, Morse LS. Vitreomacular traction syndrome following highly active antiretroviral therapy in AIDS patients with cytomegalovirus retinitis. Retina. 1998;18(5):443–7.
80. Wright ME, Suzman DL, Csaky KG, Masur H, Polis MA, Robinson MR. Extensive retinal neovascularization as a late finding in human immunodeficiency virus-infected patients with immune recovery uveitis. Clin Infect Dis. 2003;36(8):1063–6.
81. Zamir E, Hudson H, Ober RR, Kumar SK, Wang RC, Read RW, et al. Massive mycobacterial choroiditis during highly active antiretroviral therapy: another immune-recovery uveitis? Ophthalmology. 2002;109(11):2144–8.
82. Lim JI, Wolitz RA, Dowling AH, Bloom HR, Irvine AR, Schwartz DM. Visual and anatomic outcomes associated with posterior segment complications after ganciclovir implant procedures in patients with AIDS and cytomegalovirus retinitis. Am J Ophthalmol. 1999;127(3):288–93.
83. Guembel HO, Krieglsteiner S, Rosenkranz C, Hattenbach LO, Koch FH, Ohrloff C. Complications after implantation of intraocular devices in patients with cytomegalovirus retinitis. Graefes Arch Clin Exp Ophthalmol. 1999;237(10):824–9.
84. Shane TS, Martin DF. Endophthalmitis after ganciclovir implant in patients with AIDS and cytomegalovirus retinitis. Am J Ophthalmol. 2003;136(4):649–54.
85. Martidis A, Danis RP, Ciulla TA. Treating cytomegalovirus retinitis-related retinal detachment by combining silicone oil tamponade and ganciclovir implant. Ophthalmic Surg Lasers. 2002;33(2):135–9.
86. Azen SP, Scott IU, Flynn HW Jr, Lai MY, Topping TM, Benati L, et al. Silicone oil in the repair of complex retinal detachments. A prospective observational multicenter study. Ophthalmology. 1998;105(9):1587–97.
87. Lim JI, Enger C, Haller JA, Campochiaro PA, Meredith TA, de Bustros S, et al. Improved visual results after surgical repair of cytomegalovirus-related retinal detachments. Ophthalmology. 1994;101(2):264–9.
88. Regillo CD, Vander JF, Duker JS, Fischer DH, Belmont JB, Kleiner R. Repair of retinitis-related retinal detachments with silicone oil in patients with acquired immunodeficiency syndrome. Am J Ophthalmol. 1992;113(1):21–7.
89. Nasemann JE, Mutsch A, Wiltfang R, Klauss V. Early pars plana vitrectomy without buckling procedure in cytomegalovirus retinitis-induced retinal detachment. Retina. 1995;15(2):111–6.
90. Garcia RF, Flores-Aguilar M, Quiceno JI, Capparelli EV, Munguia D, Kuppermann BD, et al. Results of rhegmatogenous retinal detachment repair in cytomegalovirus retinitis with and without scleral buckling. Ophthalmology. 1995;102(2):236–45.
91. Canzano JC, Morse LS, Wendel RT. Surgical repair of cytomegalovirus-related retinal detachment without silicone oil in patients with AIDS. Retina. 1999;19(4):274–80.
92. Schaller UC, MacDonald JC, Mueller AJ, Karavellas MP, Klauss V, Scheider A, et al. Removal of silicone oil with vision improvement after rhegmatogenous retinal detachment following CMV retinitis in patients with AIDS. Retina. 1999;19(6):495–8.
93. Althaus C, Loeffler KU, Schimkat M, Hudde T, Sundmacher R. Prophylactic argon laser coagulation for rhegmatogenous retinal detachment in AIDS patients with cytomegalovirus retinitis. Graefes Arch Clin Exp Ophthalmol. 1998;236(5):359–64.
94. Davis JL, Hummer J, Feuer WJ. Laser photocoagulation for retinal detachments and retinal tears in cytomegalovirus retinitis. Ophthalmology. 1997;104(12):2053–60.
95. Freeman WR, Quiceno JI, Crapotta JA, Listhaus A, Munguia D, Aguilar MF. Surgical repair of rhegmatogenous retinal detachment in immunosuppressed patients with cytomegalovirus retinitis. Ophthalmology. 1992;99(3):466–74.
96. Scott IU, Flynn HW, Lai M, Chang S, Azen SP. First operation anatomic success and other predictors of postoperative vision after complex retinal detachment repair with vitrectomy and silicone oil tamponade. Am J Ophthalmol. 2000;130(6):745–50.
97. Graham E, Chignell AH, Eykyn S. Candida endophthalmitis: a complication of prolonged intravenous therapy and antibiotic treatment. J Infect. 1986;13(2):167–73.
98. Jackson TL, Eykyn SJ, Graham EM, Stanford MR. Endogenous bacterial endophthalmitis: a 17-year prospective series and review of 267 reported cases. Surv Ophthalmol. 2003;48(4):403–23.
99. Aguilar GL, Blumenkrantz MS, Egbert PR, McCulley JP. Candida endophthalmitis after intravenous drug abuse. Arch Ophthalmol. 1979;97(1):96–100.
100. Wong VK, Tasman W, Eagle RC Jr, Rodriguez A. Bilateral *Candida parapsilosis* endophthalmitis. Arch Ophthalmol. 1997;115(5):670–2.
101. Chignell AH. Endogenous candida endophthalmitis. J R Soc Med. 1992;85(12):721–4.
102. Gupta A, Gupta V, Dogra MR, Chakrabarti A, Ray P, Ram J, et al. Fungal endophthalmitis after a single intravenous administration of presumably contaminated dextrose infusion fluid. Retina. 2000;20(3):262–8.
103. Chang TS, Chen WC, Chen HS, Lee HW. Endogenous Candida endophthalmitis after two consecutive procedures of suction dilatation and curettage. Chang Gung Med J. 2002;25(11):778–82.
104. Chen SJ, Chung YM, Liu JH. Endogenous Candida endophthalmitis after induced abortion. Am J Ophthalmol. 1998;125(6):873–5.
105. Henderson T, Irfan S. Bilateral endogenous Candida endophthalmitis and chorioretinitis following toxic megacolon. Eye. 1996;10(Pt 6):755–7.
106. Tsai CC, Chen SJ, Chung YM, Yu KW, Hsu WM. Postpartum endogenous Candida endophthalmitis. J Formos Med Assoc. 2002;101(6):432–6.
107. Cantrill HL, Rodman WP, Ramsay RC, Knobloch WH. Postpartum Candida endophthalmitis. JAMA. 1980;243(11):1163–5.
108. Gago LC, Capone A Jr, Trese MT. Bilateral presumed endogenous candida endophthalmitis and stage 3 retinopathy of prematurity. Am J Ophthalmol. 2002;134(4):611–3.
109. Stern JH, Calvano C, Simon JW. Recurrent endogenous candidal endophthalmitis in a premature infant. JAAPOS. 2001;5(1):50–1.
110. Annable WL, Kachmer ML, DiMarco M, DeSantis D. Long-term follow-up of Candida endophthalmitis in the premature infant. J Pediatr Ophthalmol Strabismus. 1990;27(2):103–6.
111. Sasoh M, Uji Y, Arima M, Sawada T, Doi M, Fukui R. Retinal detachment due to breaks in pars plicata of ciliary body after endogenous fungal endophthalmitis. Jpn J Ophthalmol. 1993;37(1):93–9.
112. Peyman GA, Vastine DW, Diamond JG. Vitrectomy in exogenous Candida endophthalmitis. Albrecht Von Graefes Arch Klin Exp Ophthalmol. 1975;197(1):55–9.
113. Mackiewicz J, Haszcz D, Zagorski Z. Exogenous Candida endophthalmitis in a hop grower--a case report. Ann Agric Environ Med. 2000;7(2):131–2.
114. McDonald HR, de Bustros S, Sipperley JO. Vitrectomy for epiretinal membrane with Candida chorioretinitis. Ophthalmology. 1990;97(4):466–9.
115. Rodriques-Adrian LJ, King RT, Tamayo-Derat LG, Miller JW, Gargia CA, Rex JH. Retinal lesions as clues to disseminated

bactgerial and candidal infections: frequency, natural history, and aetiology. Medicine (Baltimore). 2003;82(3):187–202.
116. Ohnishi Y, Tawara A, Murata T, Sakamoto T, Arakawa T, Ishibashi T. Postmortem findings two weeks after oral treatment for metastatic Candida endophthalmitis with fluconazole. Ophthalmologica. 1999;213(5):341–4.
117. Hidalgo JA, Alangaden GJ, Eliott D, Akins RA, Puklin J, Abrams G, et al. Fungal endophthalmitis diagnosis by detection of *Candida albicans* DNA in intraocular fluid by use of a species-specific polymerase chain reaction assay. J Infect Dis. 2000;181(3):1198–201.
118. Jaeger EE, Carroll NM, Choudhury S, Dunlop AA, Towler HM, Matheson MM, et al. Rapid detection and identification of Candida, Aspergillus, and Fusarium species in ocular samples using nested PCR. J Clin Microbiol. 2000;38(8):2902–8.
119. McQuillen DP, Zingman BS, Meunier F, Levitz SM. Invasive infections due to *Candida krusei*: report of ten cases of fungemia that include three cases of endophthalmitis. Clin Infect Dis. 1992;14(2):472–8.
120. Essman TF, Flynn HW Jr, Smiddy WE, Brod RD, Murray TG, Davis JL, et al. Treatment outcomes in a 10-year study of endogenous fungal endophthalmitis. Ophthalmic Surg Lasers. 1997;28(3):185–94.
121. Christmas NJ, Smiddy WE. Vitrectomy and systemic fluconazole for treatment of endogenous fungal endophthalmitis. Ophthalmic Surg Lasers. 1996;27(12):1012–8.
122. Barrie T. The place of elective vitrectomy in the management of patients with Candida endophthalmitis. Graefes Arch Clin Exp Ophthalmol. 1987;225(2):107–13.
123. Brod RD, Flynn HW Jr, Clarkson JG, Pflugfelder SC, Culbertson WW, Miller D. Endogenous Candida endophthalmitis. Management without intravenous amphotericin B. Ophthalmology. 1990;97(5):666–72.
124. Doft BH, Weiskopf J, Nilsson-Ehle I, Wingard LB Jr. Amphotericin clearance in vitrectomized versus nonvitrectomized eyes. Ophthalmology. 1985;92(11):1601–5.
125. Payne JF, Keenum DG, Sternberg P Jr, Thliveris A, Kala A, Olsen TW. Concentrated intravitreal amphotericin B in fungal endophthalmitis. Arch Ophthalmol. 128(12):1546–50. 128/12/1546 [pii]. https://doi.org/10.1001/archophthalmol.2010.305.
126. Verbraeken HE, Hanssens M, Priem H, Lafaut BA, De Laey JJ. Ocular non-Hodgkin's lymphoma: a clinical study of nine cases. Br J Ophthalmol. 1997;81(1):31–6.
127. Palexas GN, Green WR, Goldberg MF, Ding Y. Diagnostic pars plana vitrectomy report of a 21-year retrospective study. Trans Am Ophthalmol Soc. 1995;93:281–308.
128. Peterson K, Gordon KB, Heinemann MH, Deangelis LM. The clinical spectrum of ocular lymphoma. Cancer. 1993;72(3):843–9.
129. Akpek EK, Ahmed I, Hochberg FH, Soheilian M, Dryja TP, Jakobiec FA, et al. Intraocular-central nervous system lymphoma: clinical features, diagnosis, and outcomes. Ophthalmology. 1999;106(9):1805–10.
130. Ridley ME, McDonald HR, Sternberg P Jr, Blumenkranz MS, Zarbin MA, Schachat AP. Retinal manifestations of ocular lymphoma (reticulum cell sarcoma). Ophthalmology. 1992;99(7):1153–60.
131. Lobo A, Larkin G, Clark BJ, Towler HM, Lightman S. Pseudohypopyon as the presenting feature in B-cell and T-cell intraocular lymphoma. Clin Experiment Ophthalmol. 2003;31(2):155–8.
132. Herrlinger U. Primary CNS lymphoma: findings outside the brain. J Neurooncol. 1999;43(3):227–30.
133. Coupland SE, Bechrakis NE, Anastassiou G, Foerster AM, Heiligenhaus A, Pleyer U, et al. Evaluation of vitrectomy specimens and chorioretinal biopsies in the diagnosis of primary intraocular lymphoma in patients with masquerade syndrome. Graefes Arch Clin Exp Ophthalmol. 2003;241(10):860–70.
134. Batara JF, Grossman SA. Primary central nervous system lymphomas. Curr Opin Neurol. 2003;16(6):671–5.
135. Rivero ME, Kuppermann BD, Wiley CA, Garcia CR, Smith MD, Dreilinger A, et al. Acquired immunodeficiency syndrome-related intraocular B-cell lymphoma. Arch Ophthalmol. 1999;117(5):616–22.
136. Mittra RA, Pulido JS, Hanson GA, Kajdacsy-Balla A, Brummitt CF. Primary ocular Epstein-Barr virus-associated non-Hodgkin's lymphoma in a patient with AIDS: a clinicopathologic report. Retina. 1999;19(1):45–50.
137. Margolis L, Fraser R, Lichter A, Char DH. The role of radiation therapy in the management of ocular reticulum cell sarcoma. Cancer. 1980;45(4):688–92.
138. Whitcup SM, de Smet MD, Rubin BI, Palestine AG, Martin DF, Burnier M Jr, et al. Intraocular lymphoma. Clinical and histopathologic diagnosis. Ophthalmology. 1993;100(9):1399–406.
139. Davis JL, Viciana AL, Ruiz P. Diagnosis of intraocular lymphoma by flow cytometry. Am J Ophthalmol. 1997;124(3):362–72.
140. Ciulla TA, Pesavento RD, Yoo S. Subretinal aspiration biopsy of ocular lymphoma. Am J Ophthalmol. 1997;123(3):420–2.
141. Valluri S, Moorthy RS, Khan A, Rao NA. Combination treatment of intraocular lymphoma. Retina. 1995;15(2):125–9.
142. Lu Y, Jia L, He S, Hurley MC, Leys MJ, Jayasundera T, et al. Melanoma-associated retinopathy: a paraneoplastic autoimmune complication. Arch Ophthalmol. 2009;127(12):1572–80. doi: 127/12/1572 [pii]. https://doi.org/10.1001/archophthalmol.2009.311.

Pathological High Myopia

20

Contents

Introduction

Pathological high myopia (PHM) can be defined as extreme myopia of more than −10 D with chorioretinal atrophy and posterior staphyloma. It presents its own set of problems:

- Macular schisis
- Macular hole
- Rhegmatogenous retinal detachment
- Choroidal neovascular membrane
- Spontaneous choroidal haemorrhage
- Myopic maculopathy
- Dome-shaped maculopathy

The patterns of presentation of these often have different clinical features to routine vitreoretinal disorders. Surgery often must be adapted to the specifics of the PHM eye. The condition is likely to be a multifactorial genetic condition with alteration in the collagen of the eye. Myopia, in general, is on the increase as lifestyles become more indoor and vision more utilised for close work. There are racial differences in prevalence with the condition more common in oriental patients. This may also affect response to and outcomes of surgery (Figs. 20.1, 20.2, 20.3 and 20.4)

Myopic Macular Schisis

PHM eyes seem to continue to elongate with age. The presence of a staphyloma and continued growth of the eye causes tension to arise between the stiff ILM and the posterior progression of the sclera. The ILM is unable to stretch into the staphyloma causing the macula retina to be thickened into schisis. The patient experiences a slow reduction in vision over months. If a progressive drop in vision and thickening of the retina is detected, surgery can be performed.

Perform PPV and remove the ILM. This allows the more elastic retina to settle into the staphyloma and allow the vision to improve. There is a risk of macular hole production as the retina stretches back into the coloboma. For this reason, some surgeons leave a collaret of ILM around the fovea. No gas is required. Be careful of vitreous schisis. It is therefore extremely useful to determine if the vitreous is detached preop by OCT or to check for vitreous remaining on the ret-

T. H. Williamson, *Vitreoretinal Surgery*, https://doi.org/10.1007/978-3-030-68769-4_20

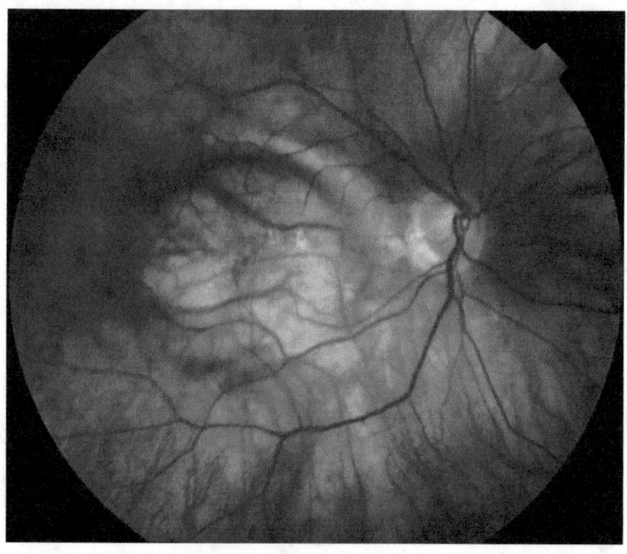

Fig. 20.1 In highly myopic patients with posterior staphyloma, posterior RRD from breaks in the macula can occur

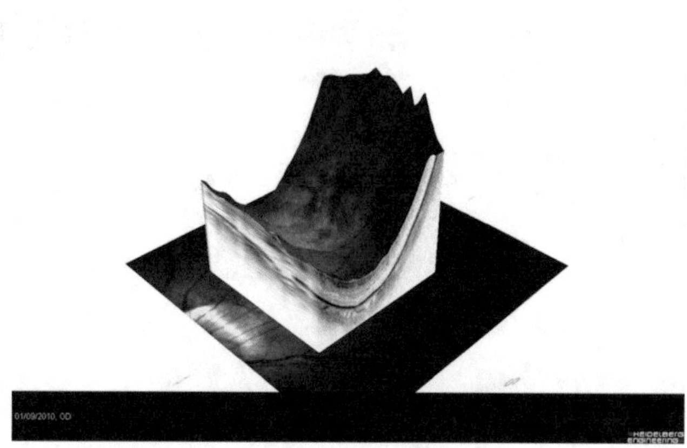

Fig. 20.2 A composite OCT picture showing the steep curvature of a myopic staphyloma

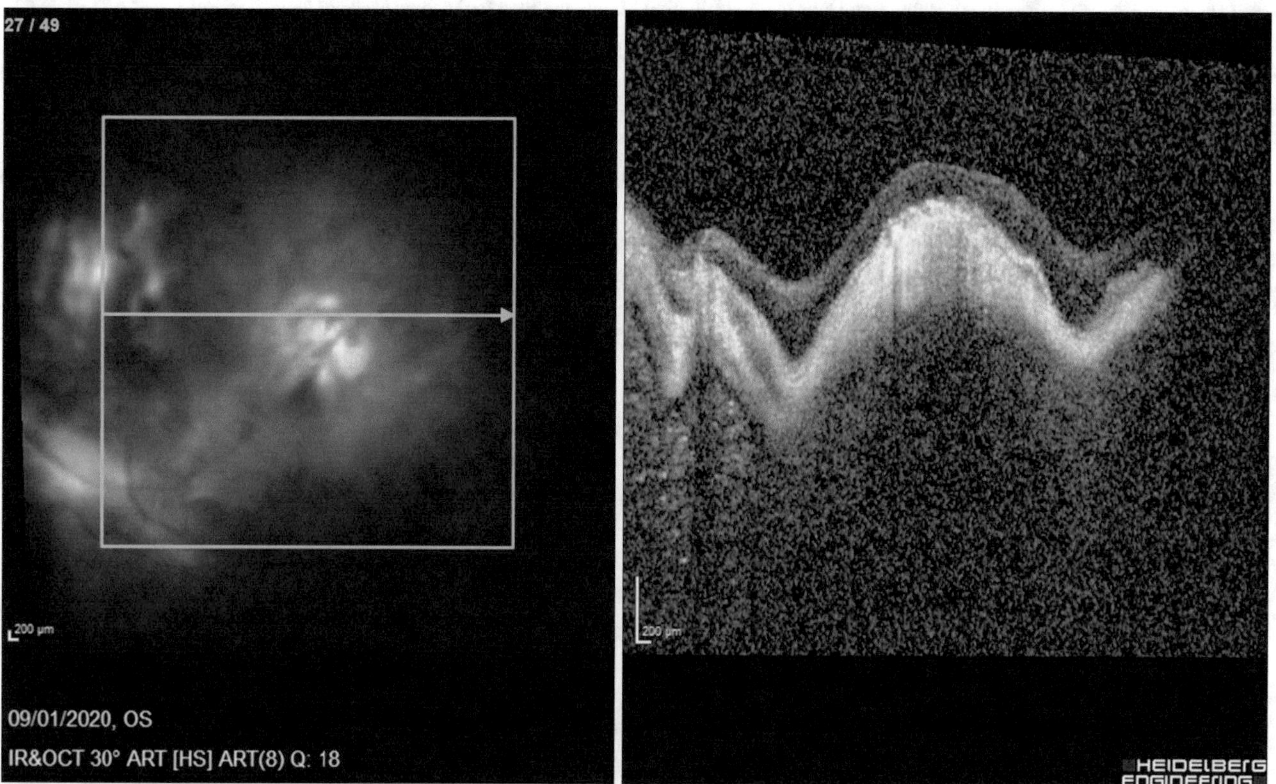

Fig. 20.3 Extreme high myopia

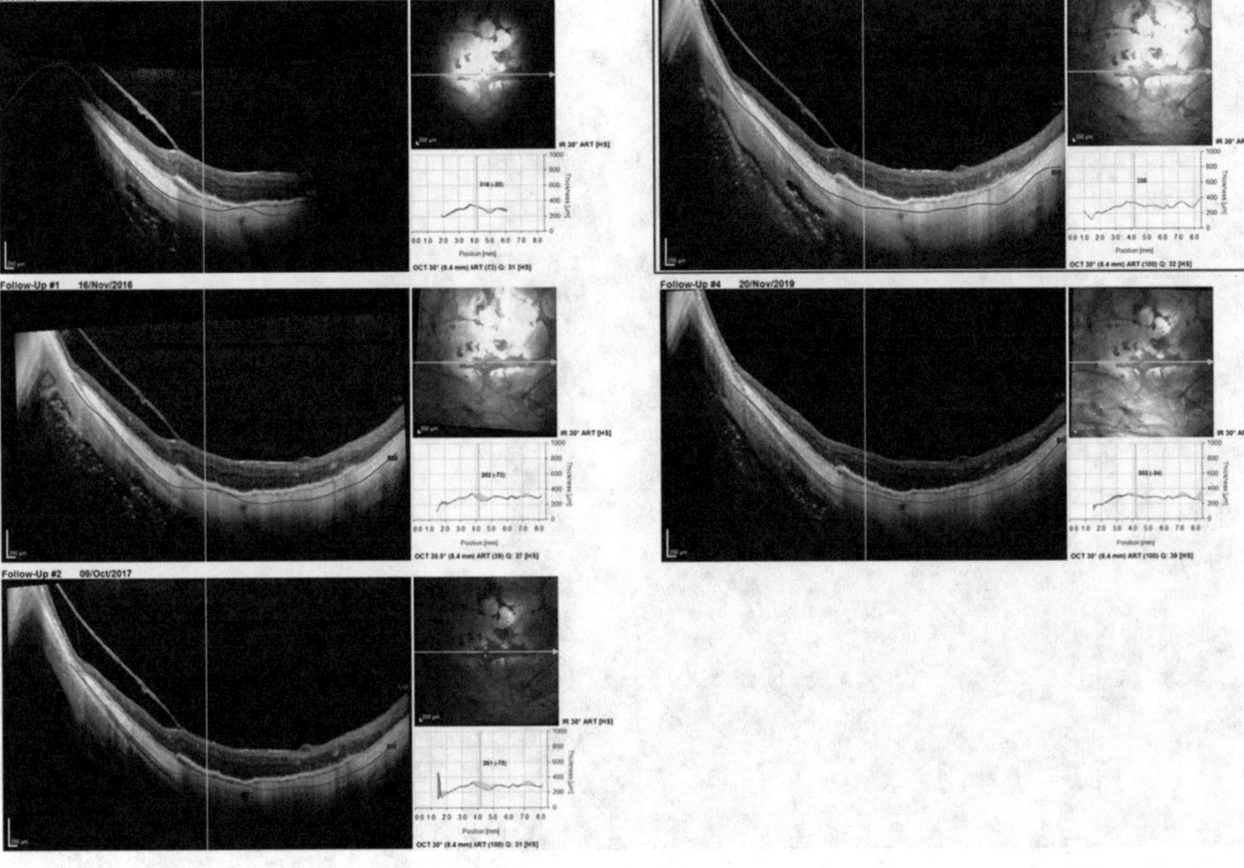

Fig. 20.4 Spontaneous separation of vitreal traction in a high myope

ina during surgery. Many surgeons favour Triamcinolone particles, injected at the time of surgery, to detect residual vitreous. Some patients will develop ERM in addition, if so, treat with PPV, peel of the ERM and ILM peel. Leave a collaret of ILM around the fovea to avoid creating a macular hole (Figs. 20.5, 20.6, 20.7 and 20.8)

Myopic Macular Hole

Sometimes the schisis will progress to a macular hole. The hole may allow SRF to enter and proceed to an RRD; however, the hole may enlarge without RRD. Surgery is performed as in a macular hole with ILM peel but an ILM flap is recommended as the holes are more difficult to close. Visual recovery may be less due to chorioretinal atrophy. Again watch out for vitreoschisis (Figs. 20.9 and 20.10).

Success Rates

These vary from geographical locations with higher success rates in oriental populations than European. Hole closure rates vary from 25 to 50% although the hole can be flattened and remain open [1, 2].

Surgical Pearl

Retracting Door Internal Limiting Membrane Flap for Myopic Macular Holes

The retracting door ILM flap represents part of the armamentarium of surgical options to close macular holes [3]. For successful retraction of the flap, it should be based temporal to the fovea, which would allow the flap to retract tempo-

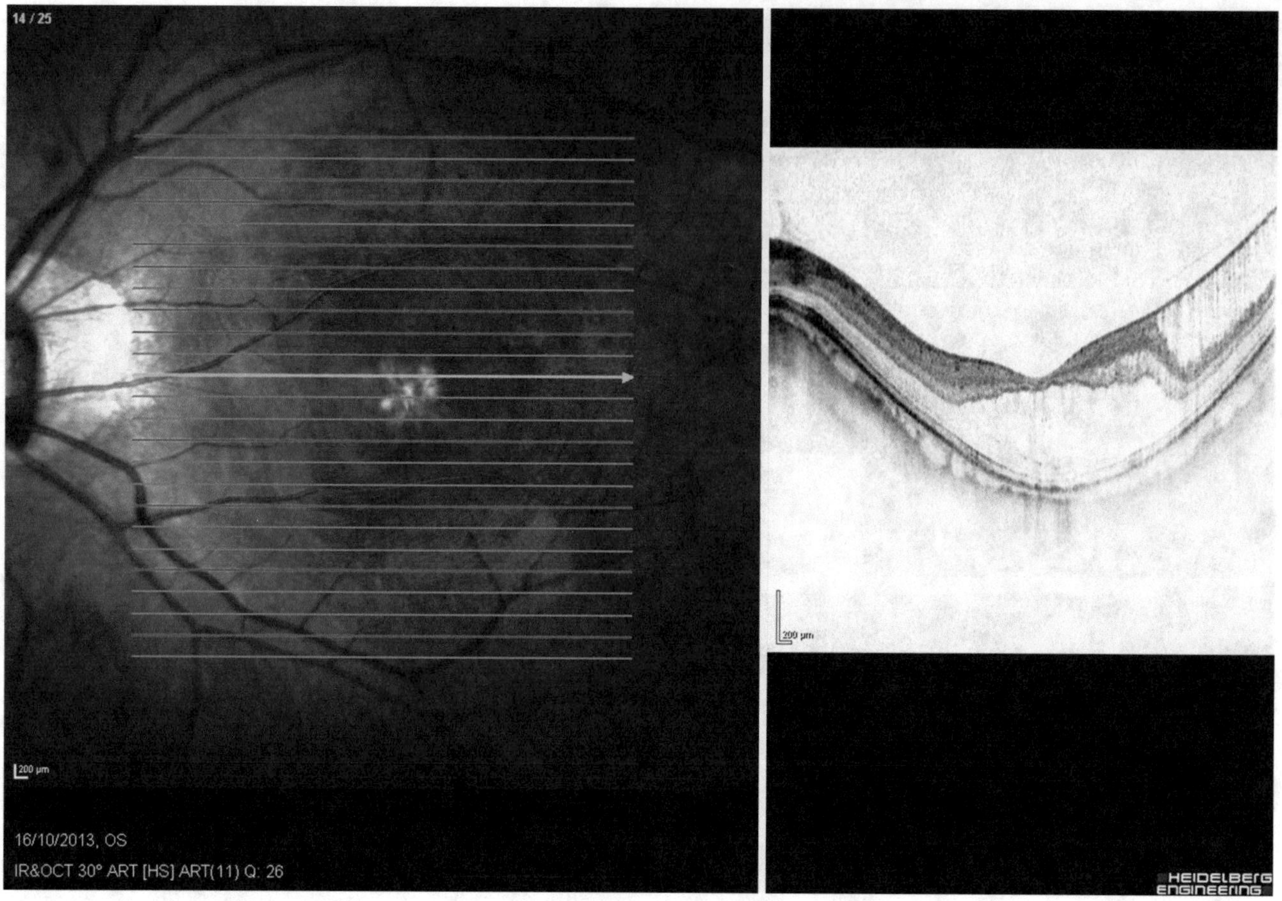

Fig. 20.5 Myopic schitic retina from traction

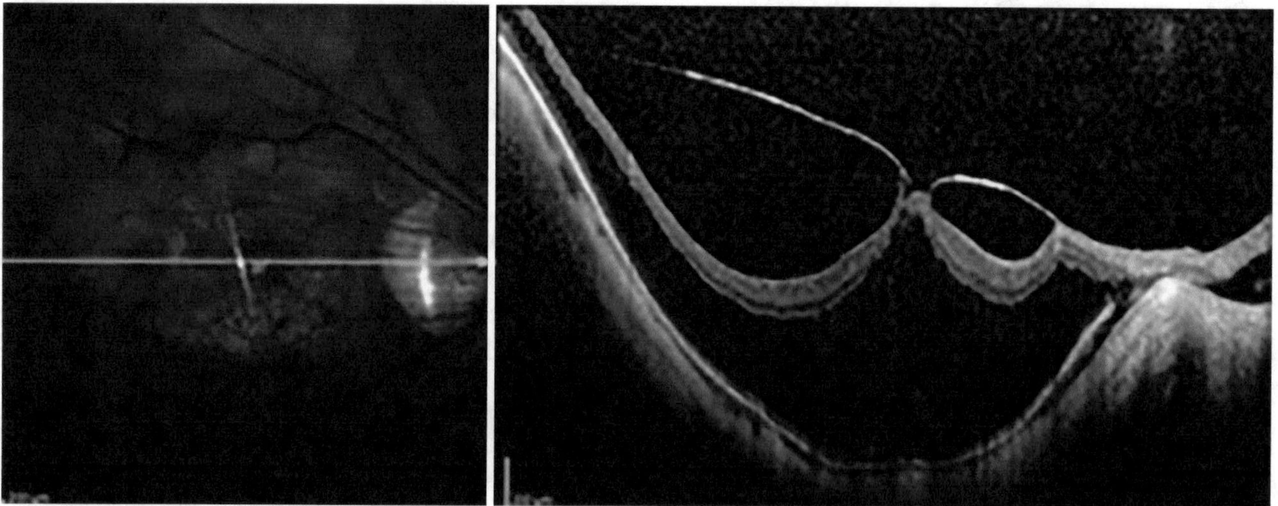

Fig. 20.6 Myopic VMT with outer retinal SRF

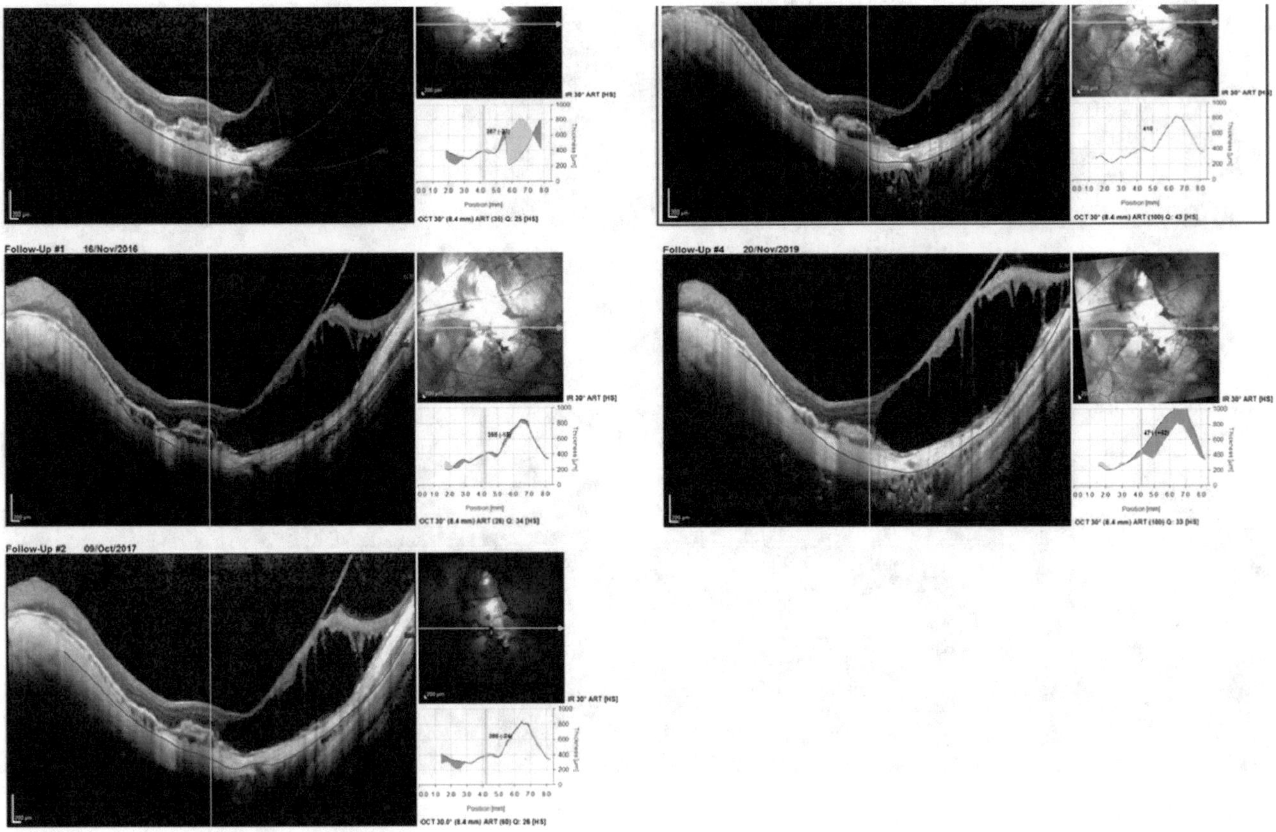

Fig. 20.7 Progressive myopic macular schisis. This may need surgery with ILM peel to reverse the schisis. There is a risk of creating a macular hole but by leaving an ILM flap this may be avoided. Patients can experience improvement in vision after myopic macular schisis vitrectomy

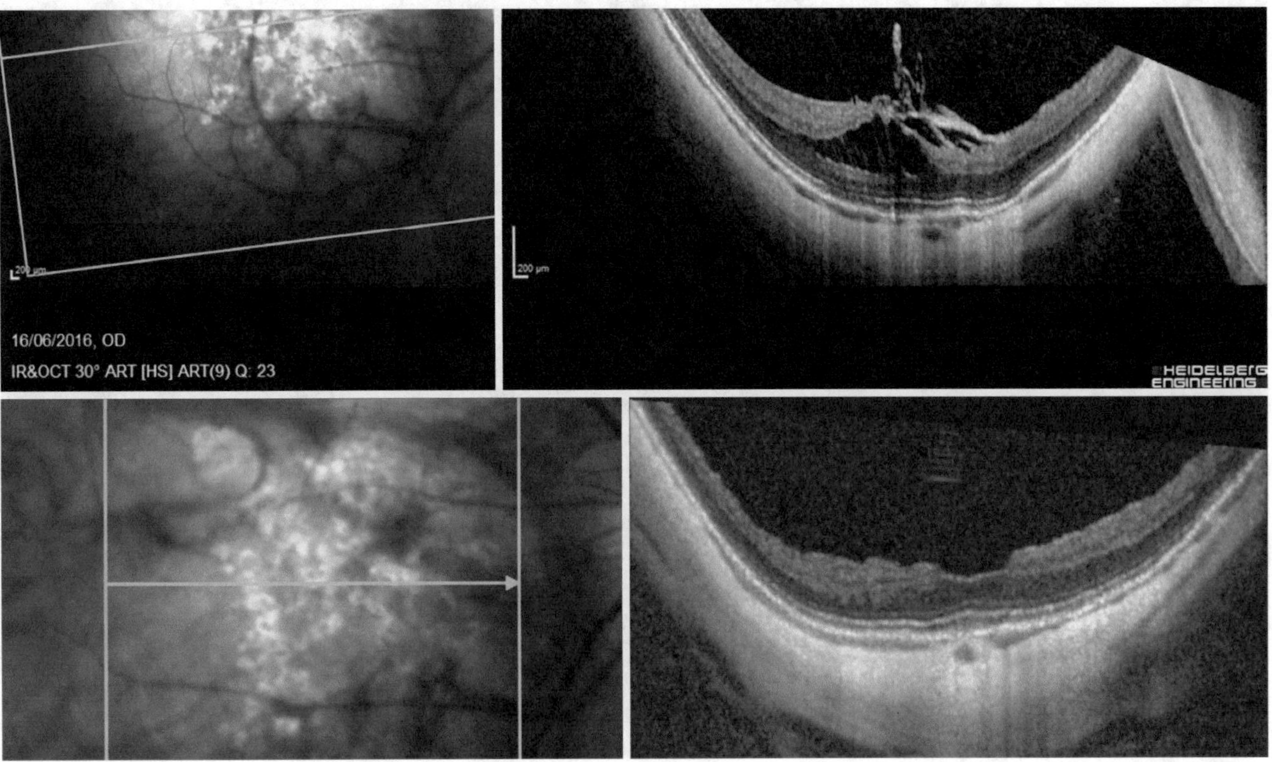

Fig. 20.8 Pathological myopia with ERM and ILM peel

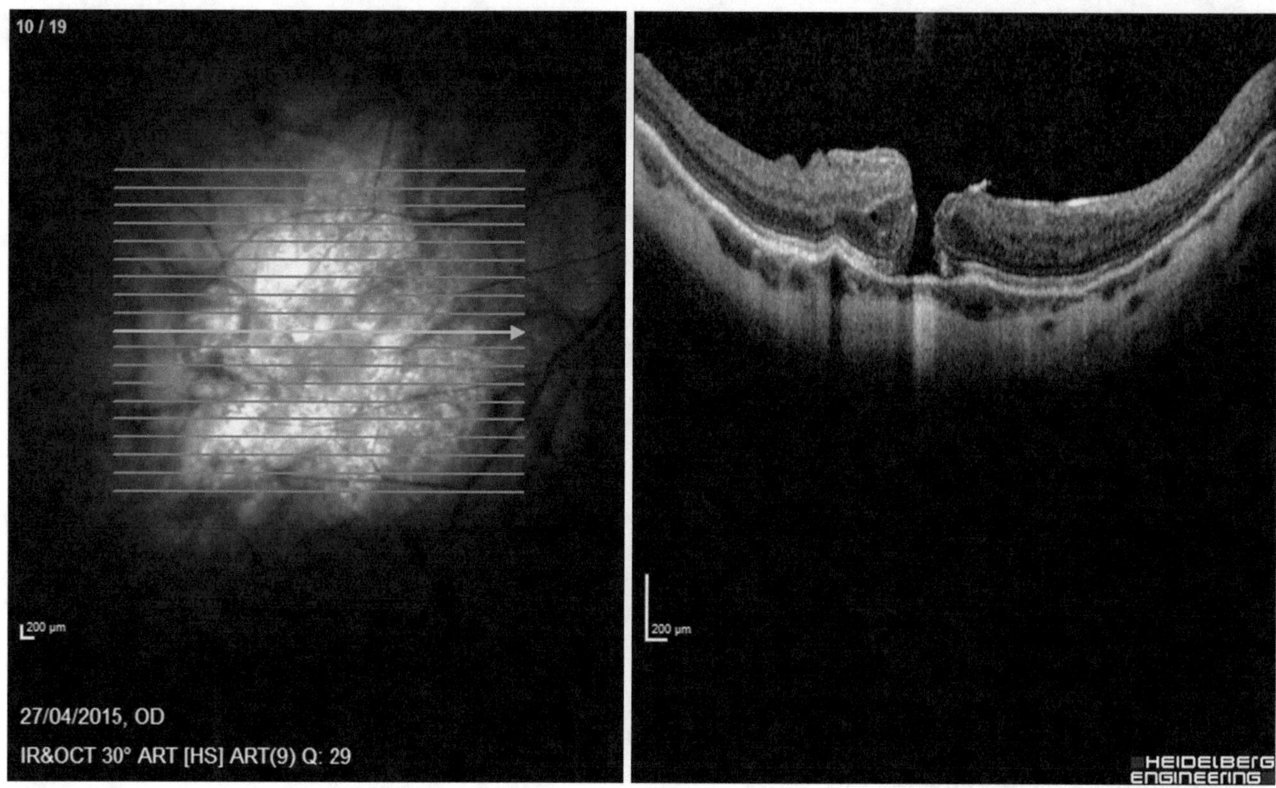

Fig. 20.9 A macular hole in a high myope

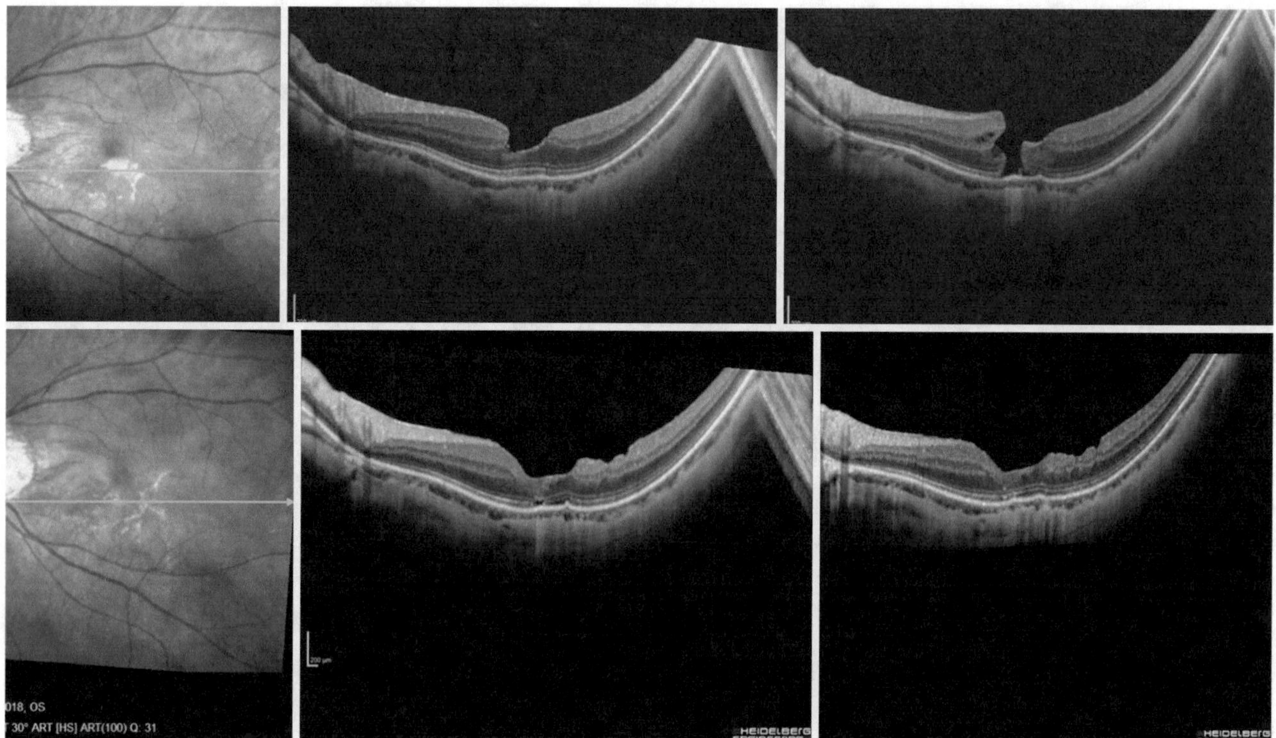

Fig. 20.10 Development of a myopic macular hole and closure by PPV, gas and ILM peel

rally, while the retina moves nasally under gas so holes would close [4]. This retraction is more in myopic holes due to the release of the increased tangential traction providing more retraction of the flap to help close macular holes.

For successful retraction, one should attempt at developing one intact flap without any radial cuts through the flap. Here are some tips to achieve such flap:

1. After staining the ILM, use the flex loop and extend it slightly out for better control.
2. Start developing the ILM edge superior, inferior, and nasal to the fovea. You can start close to the disc nasally and may reach close to arcades or at least halfway between fovea and arcades superiorly and inferiorly.
3. Do not peel ILM yet, just work your way with the flex loop to just develop those edges as if you are drawing the flap. This allows the flap when you start peeling to stay as one unit without any radial lines, since the force exerted with the loop with be transmitted through those lines of least resistance you created.
4. One can then peel that flap all the way temporally as far temporal to fovea as possible, if one can keep it as one flap. I like using the flex loop again for this step as it is more controlled. If forceps are used, one may exert more traction on one side of the flap, which may cause radial cuts that will lessen the retraction to close the hole. Additionally, you should not grasp with the forceps the folded part of the flap that is in contact with the retina when peeling, as this can easily amputate or damage the flap, but always grasp the flap at the free edge already created on the nasal side close to the disc.
5. Once the flap is peeled all the way temporally, use the loop to bring it back in place over the hole. Slow fluid air exchange close to the disc will keep the flap in place covering the hole.

Tamer H. Mahmoud, Beaumont Neuroscience Center Building, Royal Oak, Michigan, USA.

Rhegmatogenous Retinal Detachment

Clinical Features

Breaks in the macula in emmetropic eyes do not usually cause retinal detachment (e.g. senile macular holes) (Figs. 20.11 and 20.12). In highly myopic eyes, posterior breaks, especially at the macula or nasal to the optic disc, often associated with areas of chorioretinal atrophy and with posterior staphylomas will often cause retinal detachment. The detachment usually remains at the posterior pole occasionally extending anteriorly if peripheral breaks are also present. The internal limiting membrane (ILM), vitreoschisis and partial vitreous separation [5] around the hole may be implicated in the pathogenesis of the retinal detachment because surgical removal of residual vitreous cortex and ILM during vitrectomy facilitates retinal reattachment, the retina remaining flat even if the hole is open postoperatively and untreated by retinopexy [6]. Histopathology shows a fibro cellular component in the ILM in these cases [7, 8]. During follow-up, 8.5% develop RRD in their fellow eyes in 5 years [9]. In addition, the retina of the macula may become schitic or even dome shaped without a retinal break but with an associated drop in vision. If followed these eyes can develop macular SRF or macular hole [10] and the staphylomas progress [11] (Figs. 20.13, 20.14, 20.15, 20.16 and 20.17).

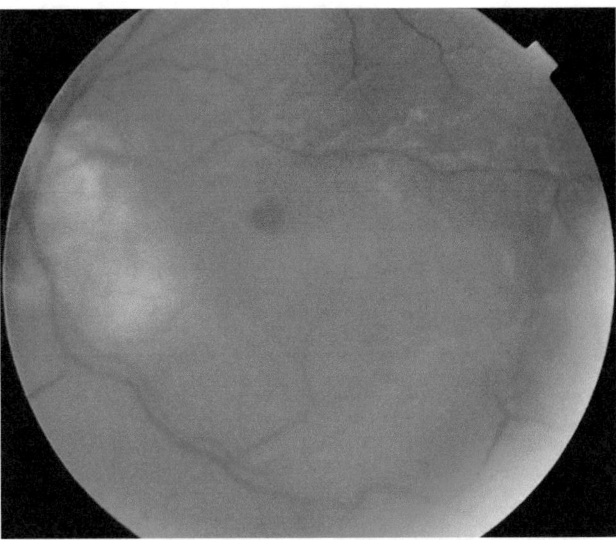

Fig. 20.11 A shallow retinal detachment in the posterior pole is seen in a high myope who has a foveal hole inducing retinal detachment

Surgery (Table 20.3)

Additional surgical steps

1. Search the posterior pole for the break.
2. Stain the macula with brilliant blue or intravitreal triamcinolone acetonide.
3. Peel the vitreous cortex/ILM complex.
4. Insert air.
5. Exchange for long-acting gas.

Although gas injection and PPV alone can reattach these retinae [12], removal of the internal limiting membrane and residual vitreous cortex during PPV appears to increase the likelihood of success. A successful search for the macular retinal break is helpful. If this is found it reassures the surgeon that there is unlikely to be a peripheral break to explain

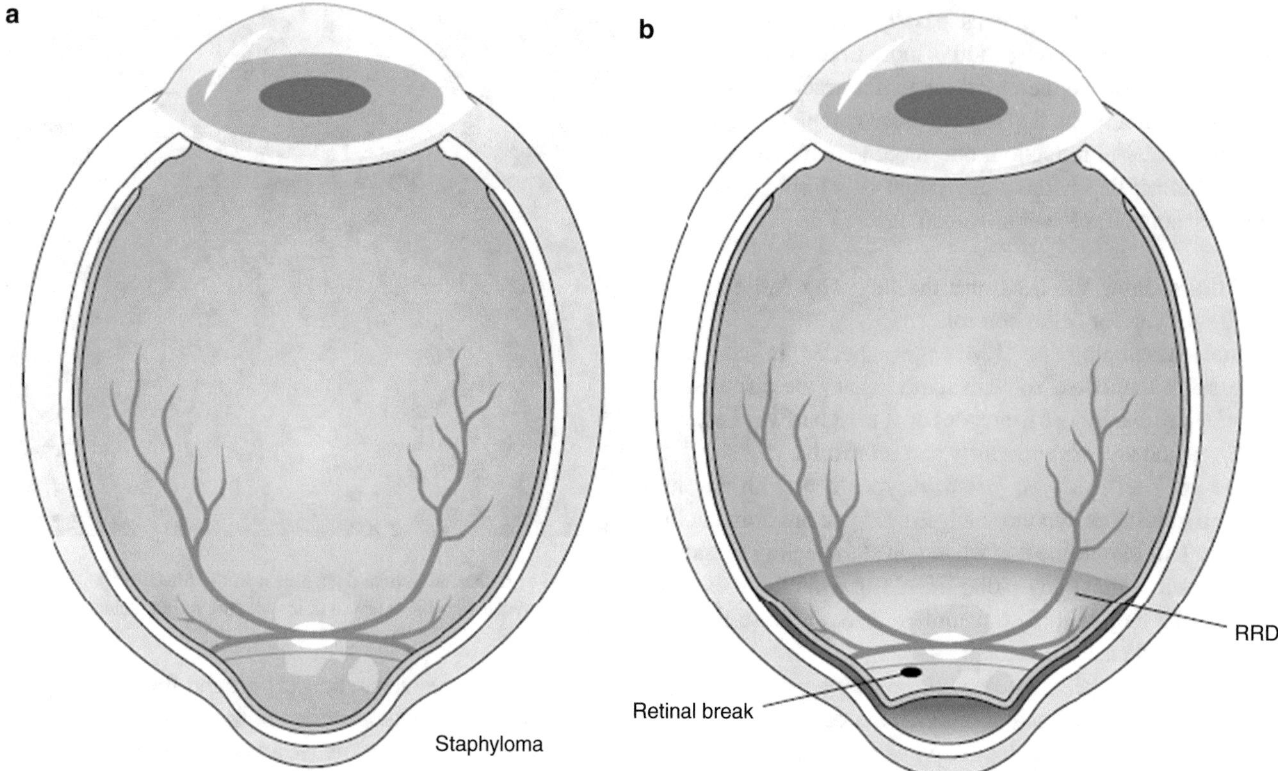

Fig. 20.12 Posterior staphyloma in myopic eyes seems to be involved in the mechanism of myopic macular hole retinal detachment (**a**). A retinal break in the staphyloma allows the SRF to accumulate (**b**)

the findings. The atrophic breaks in these patients are not easy to find, check the fovea and the edge of any chorioretinal atrophy, e.g. peripapillary atrophy. Use a flute needle to gently aspirate over the macular retina (not the fovea) to see if you can cause the hole to pout but be aware that with the excessive aspiration you can produce a hole (especially in the fovea) with this method. The periphery should also be searched. Apply either Triamcinolone acetonide [13] or brilliant blue to the macular area. These allow visualisation of the ILM and cortex for peeling and removal with forceps [14–17]. Insert long-acting gas such as perfluoro propane (Figs. 20.18, 20.19 and 20.20).

Note: Retinopexy is not required for myopic macular breaks.

Macular retinoschisis without a retinal break has also been treated in this way [17–20] but may run the risk of creating a foveal hole in some patients. A scleral buckle can be placed to produce a macular plombage to flatten the retina as an alternative to PPV [21, 22]. Posterior pole buckles have also been used to slow the progression of myopia [23]. Another method used has been the insertion of an amniotic membrane [24, 25] (Figs. 20.21 and 20.22).

Success Rates

Retinal reattachment rates are improved by the use of ILM peeling [26]. Expect primary success rates with a gas of 75% or so with a final success of 85% [2, 27].

Spontaneous Suprachoroidal Haemorrhage

Highly myopic eyes have occasionally been described with a spontaneous presentation of Scheme [28]. Thankfully the thin sclera of these eye seems to allow more rapid resolution of SCH. SCH has been described particularly in those patients on systemic antithrombotic therapy [29, 30].

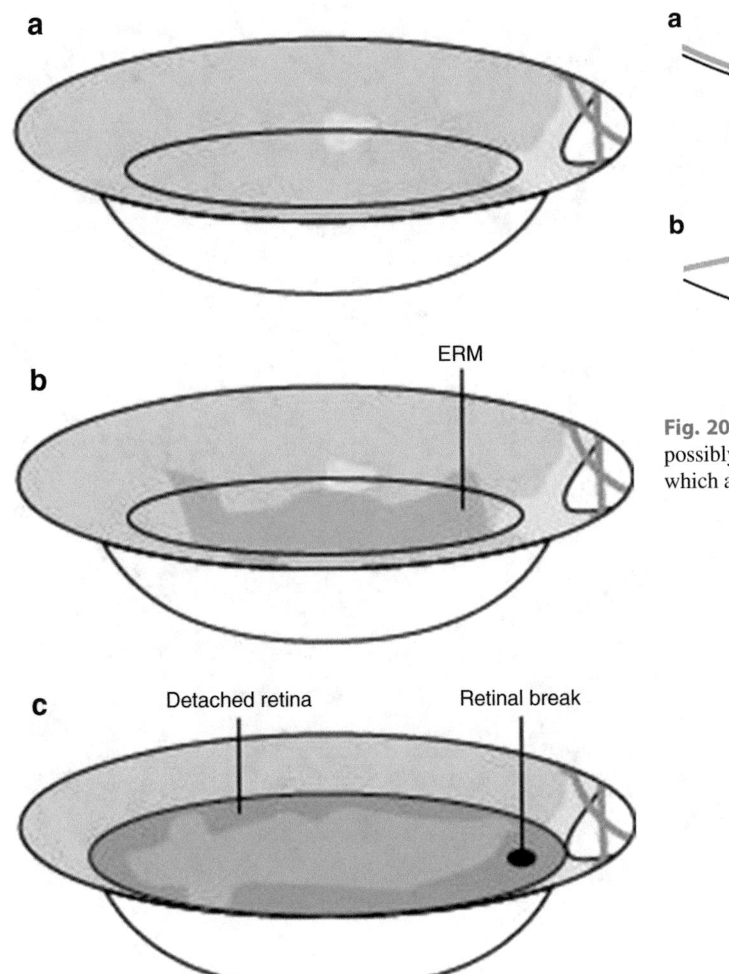

Fig. 20.13 The macula of a myopic patient with a macular hole retinal detachment is characterised by a membrane (consisting of ILM and vitreous cortex) on the macular surface (**a** and **b**). Once a break appears SRF appears (**c**). Peeling this membrane during PPV followed by insertion of gas is enough to achieve successful retinal reattachment of the retina. Traction of the membrane causes the retina to split into a schisis followed by retinal break formation and retinal detachment

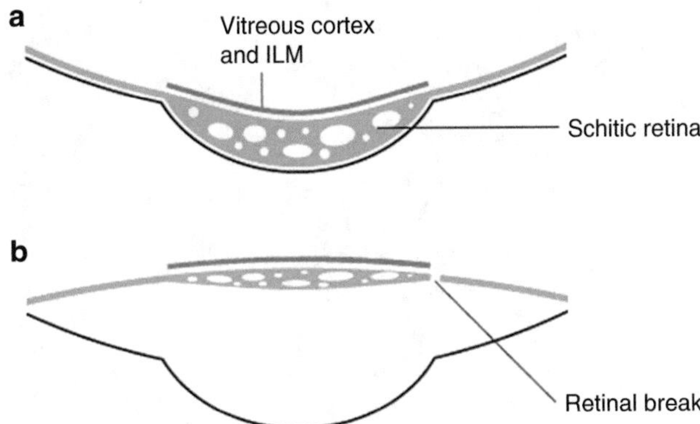

Fig. 20.14 A cross-section to illustrate the macular retinoschisis (**a**) possibly created by preretinal membranes in a posterior staphyloma which after retinal hole formation allows retinal detachment (**b**)

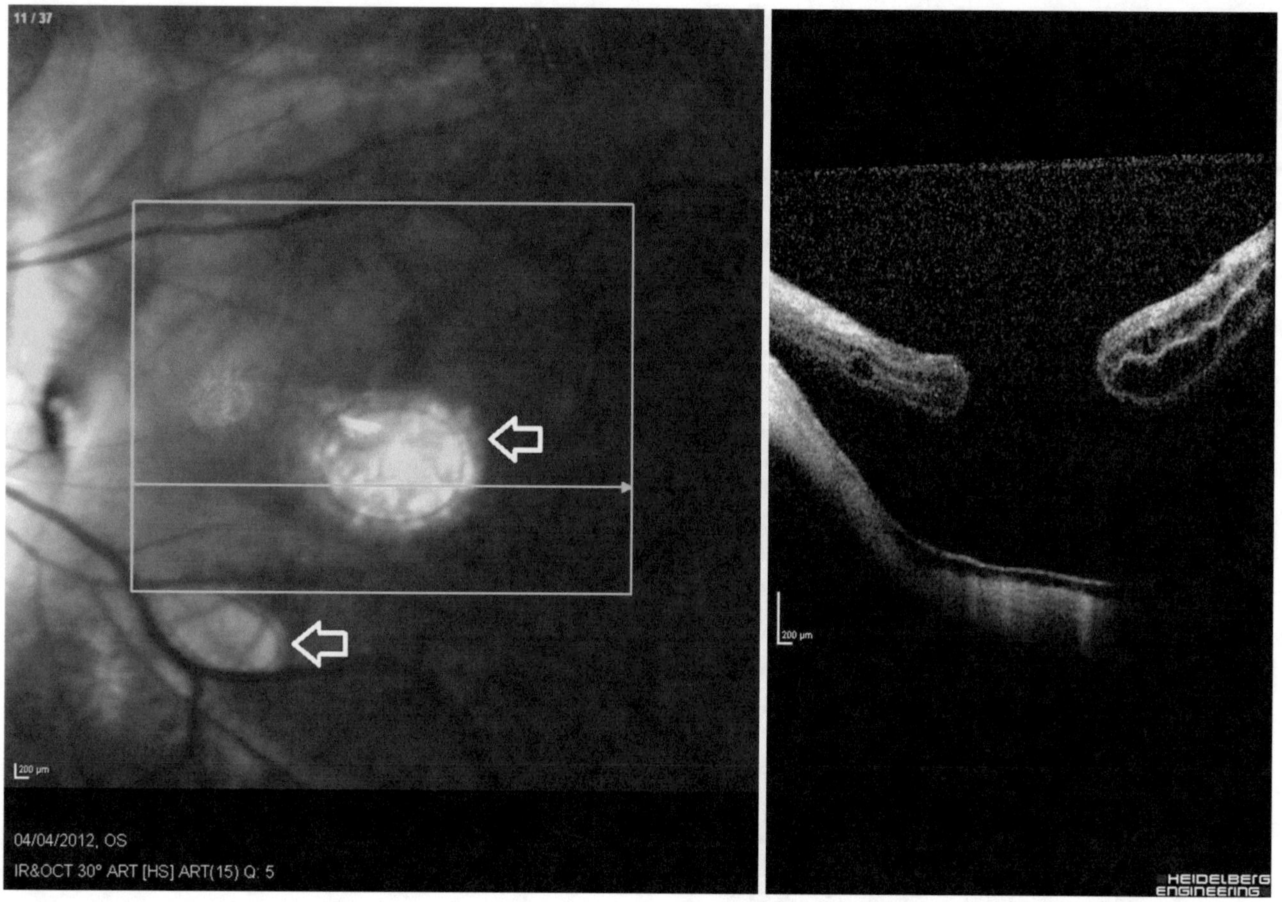

Fig. 20.15 A pathological high myope with RRD from two retinal holes

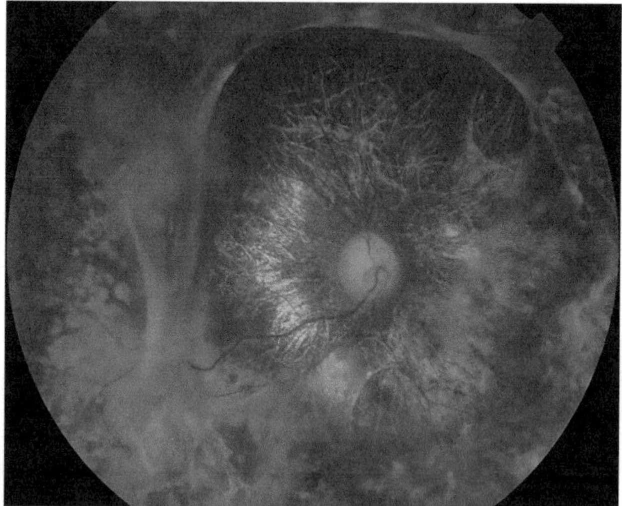

Fig. 20.16 This patient had a PPV 10 years ago but the posterior layer of the vitreoschisis seen in these patients was not removed and has developed into an ERM with traction over the years

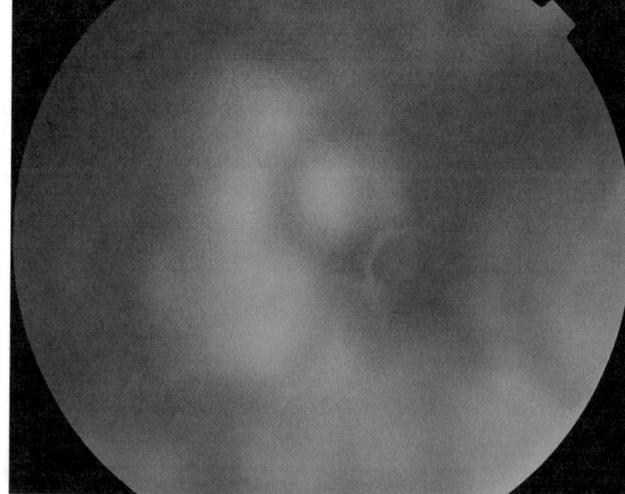

Fig. 20.17 A surgeon has performed PPV in a high myope for symptomatic floaters but has missed a vitreoschisis. Consequently, the patient presented with a PVD (the Weiss ring is visible in the image) and RRD a year after the PPV

Table 20.3 Difficulty rating for PPV for myopic macular RRD

Difficulty rating	High
Success rates	Low
Complication rates	Medium
When to use in training	Late

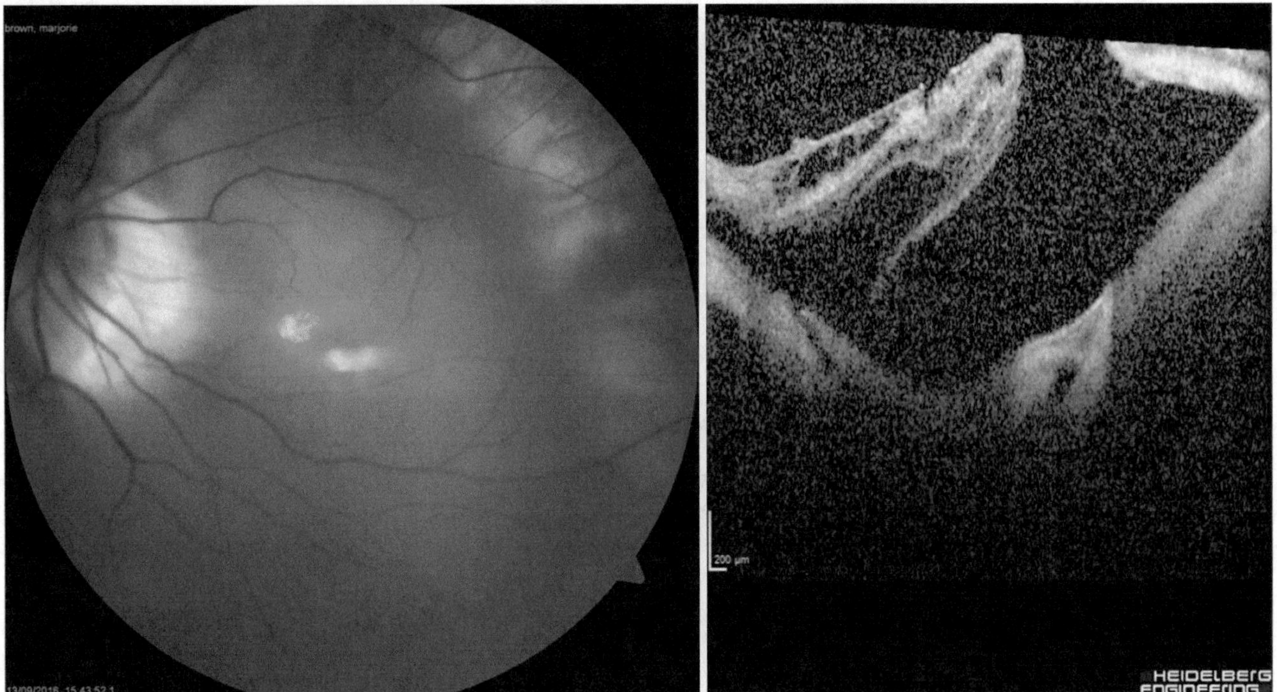

Fig. 20.18 A myopic macular hole RRD

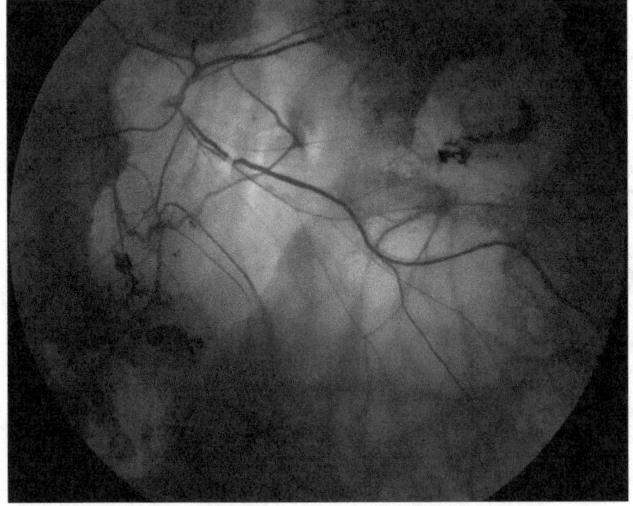

Fig. 20.19 An RRD in a pathologically highly myopic eye

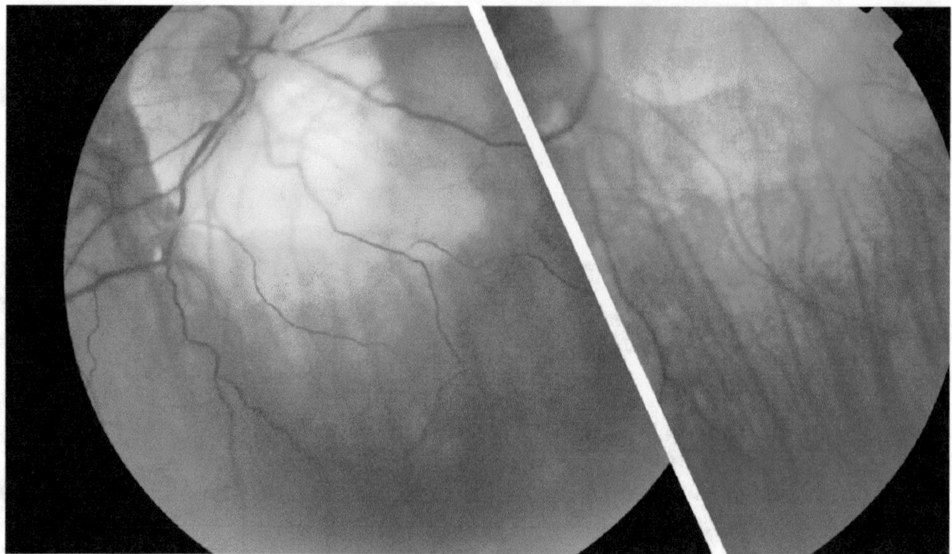

Fig. 20.20 This myopic RRD spontaneously resolved. This is a rare occurrence and the mechanism is unknown

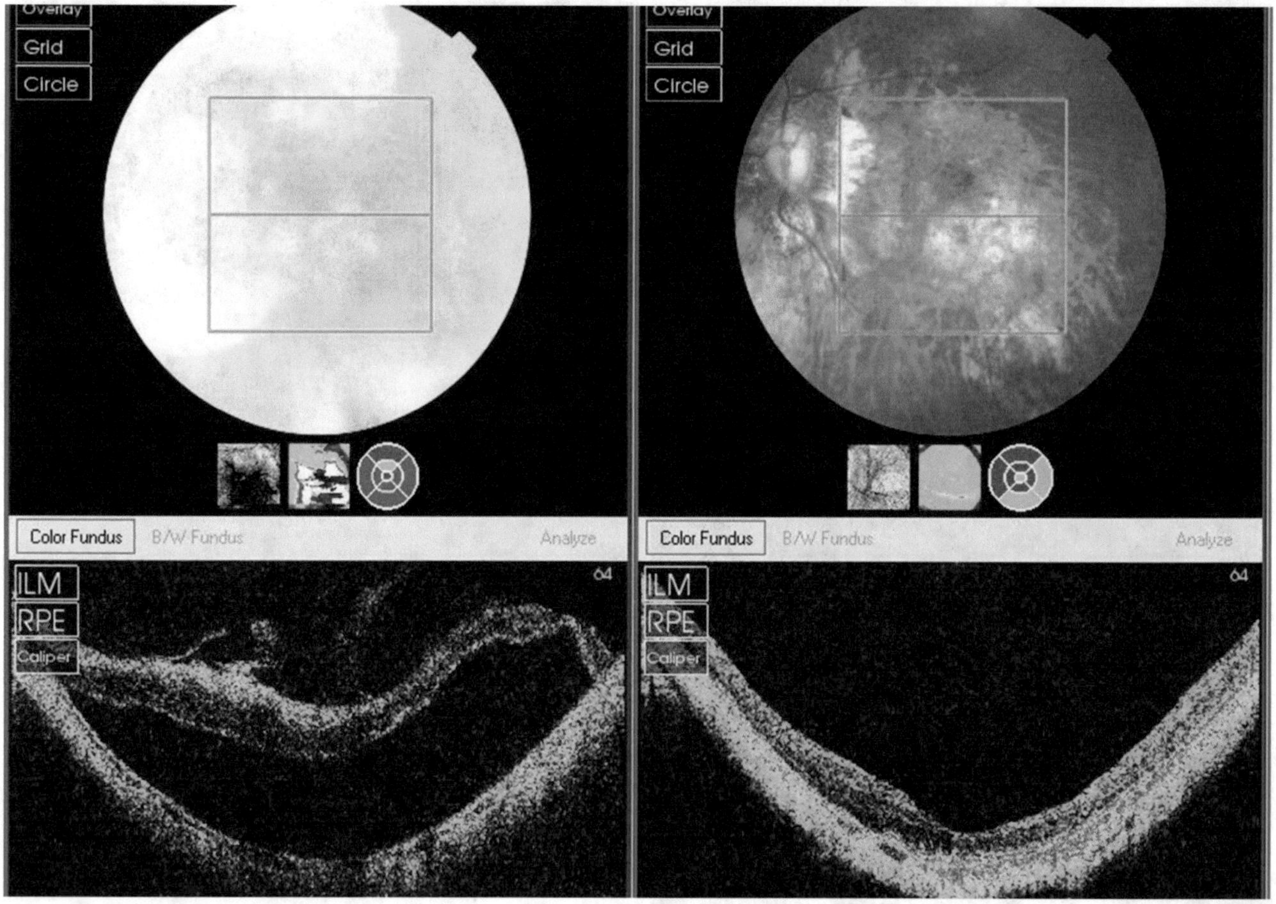

Fig. 20.21 Preoperative (left) and postoperative (right) OCTs of the macula of a high myope with a staphylomatous eye, in whom the ILM and residual vitreous remnants have been removed

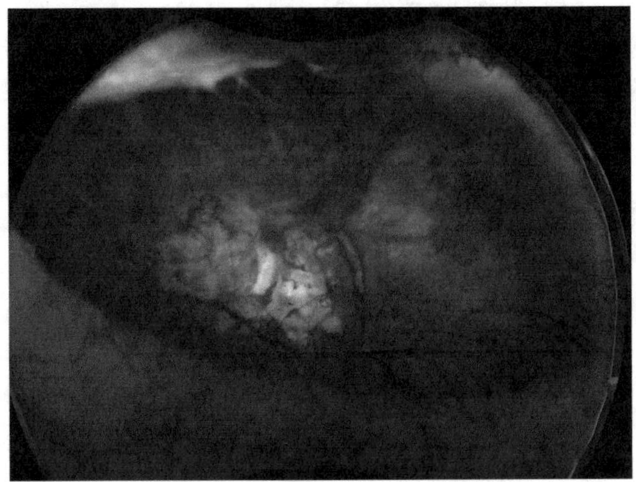

Fig. 20.22 Subretinal haemorrhage in a myopic eye

References

1. Laviers H, Li JO, Grabowska A, Charles SJ, Charteris D, Haynes RJ, et al. The management of macular hole retinal detachment and macular retinoschisis in pathological myopia; a UK collaborative study. Eye (Lond). 2018;32(11):1743–51. https://doi.org/10.1038/s41433-018-0166-4.
2. Kakinoki M, Araki T, Iwasaki M, Ueda T, Sano H, Hirano Y, et al. Surgical outcomes of Vitrectomy for macular hole retinal detachment in highly myopic eyes: a multicenter study. Ophthalmol Retina. 2019;3(10):874–8. https://doi.org/10.1016/j.oret.2019.04.026.
3. Finn AP, Mahmoud TH. Internal limiting membrane retracting door for myopic macular holes. Retina. 2019;39(Suppl 1):S92–S4. https://doi.org/10.1097/IAE.0000000000001787.
4. Akahori T, Iwase T, Yamamoto K, Ra E, Kawano K, Ito Y, et al. Macular displacement after Vitrectomy in eyes with idiopathic macular hole determined by optical coherence tomography angiography. Am J Ophthalmol. 2018;189:111–21. https://doi.org/10.1016/j.ajo.2018.02.021.
5. Matsumura N, Ikuno Y, Tano Y. Posterior vitreous detachment and macular hole formation in myopic foveoschisis. Am J Ophthalmol. 2004;138(6):1071–3.
6. Ikuno Y, Sayanagi K, Oshima T, Gomi F, Kusaka S, Kamei M, et al. Optical coherence tomographic findings of macular holes and retinal detachment after vitrectomy in highly myopic eyes. Am J Ophthalmol. 2003;136(3):477–81.
7. Bando H, Ikuno Y, Choi JS, Tano Y, Yamanaka I, Ishibashi T. Ultrastructure of internal limiting membrane in myopic foveoschisis. Am J Ophthalmol. 2005;139(1):197–9.
8. Sakaguchi H, Ikuno Y, Choi JS, Ohji M, Tano T. Multiple components of epiretinal tissues detected by triamcinolone and indocyanine green in macular hole and retinal detachment as a result of high myopia. Am J Ophthalmol. 2004;138(6):1079–81.
9. Oie Y, Emi K. Incidence of fellow eye retinal detachment resulting from macular hole. Am J Ophthalmol. 2007;143(2):203–5. doi: S0002-9394(06)01098-1 [pii]. https://doi.org/10.1016/j.ajo.2006.09.044.
10. Shimada N, Ohno-Matsui K, Baba T, Futagami S, Tokoro T, Mochizuki M. Natural course of macular retinoschisis in highly myopic eyes without macular hole or retinal detachment. Am J Ophthalmol. 2006;142(3):497–500. doi: S0002-9394(06)00432-6 [pii]. https://doi.org/10.1016/j.ajo.2006.03.048.
11. Hsiang HW, Ohno-Matsui K, Shimada N, Hayashi K, Moriyama M, Yoshida T, et al. Clinical characteristics of posterior staphyloma in eyes with pathologic myopia. Am J Ophthalmol. 2008;146(1):102–10. doi: S0002-9394(08)00183-9 [pii]. https://doi.org/10.1016/j.ajo.2008.03.010.
12. Blankenship GW, Ibanez-Langlois S. Treatment of myopic macular hole and detachment. Intravitreal Gas Exchange Ophthalmology. 1987;94(4):333–6.
13. Yamamoto N, Ozaki N, Murakami K. Triamcinolone acetonide facilitates removal of the epiretinal membrane and separation of the residual vitreous cortex in highly myopic eyes with retinal detachment due to a macular hole. Ophthalmologica. 2004;218(4):248–56.
14. Uemoto R, Yamamoto S, Tsukahara I, Takeuchi S. Efficacy of internal limiting membrane removal for retinal detachments resulting from a myopic macular hole. Retina. 2004;24(4):560–6.
15. Kadonosono K, Yazama F, Itoh N, Uchio E, Nakamura S, Akura J, et al. Treatment of retinal detachment resulting from myopic macular hole with internal limiting membrane removal. Am J Ophthalmol. 2001;131(2):203–7.
16. Kwok AK, Lai TY. Internal limiting membrane removal in macular hole surgery for severely myopic eyes: a case-control study. Br J Ophthalmol. 2003;87(7):885–9.
17. Kuhn F. Internal limiting membrane removal for macular detachment in highly myopic eyes. Am J Ophthalmol. 2003;135(4):547–9.
18. Ikuno Y, Sayanagi K, Ohji M, Kamei M, Gomi F, Harino S, et al. Vitrectomy and internal limiting membrane peeling for myopic foveoschisis. Am J Ophthalmol. 2004;137(4):719–24.
19. Kobayashi H, Kishi S. Vitreous surgery for highly myopic eyes with foveal detachment and retinoschisis. Ophthalmology. 2003;110(9):1702–7.
20. Kanda S, Uemura A, Sakamoto Y, Kita H. Vitrectomy with internal limiting membrane peeling for macular retinoschisis and retinal detachment without macular hole in highly myopic eyes. Am J Ophthalmol. 2003;136(1):177–80.
21. Baba T, Tanaka S, Maesawa A, Teramatsu T, Noda Y, Yamamoto S. Scleral buckling with macular plombe for eyes with myopic macular retinoschisis and retinal detachment without macular hole. Am J Ophthalmol. 2006;142(3):483–7. doi: S0002-9394(06)00543-5 [pii]. https://doi.org/10.1016/j.ajo.2006.04.046.
22. Alkabes M, Mateo C. Macular buckle technique in myopic traction maculopathy: a 16-year review of the literature and a comparison with vitreous surgery. Graefes Arch Clin Exp Ophthalmol. 2018;256(5):863–77. https://doi.org/10.1007/s00417-018-3947-3.
23. Ward B, Tarutta EP, Mayer MJ. The efficacy and safety of posterior pole buckles in the control of progressive high myopia. Eye (Lond). 2009;23(12):2169–74. doi: eye2008433 [pii]. https://doi.org/10.1038/eye.2008.433.
24. Caporossi T, Pacini B, De Angelis L, Barca F, Peiretti E, Rizzo S. Human amniotic membrane to close recurrent, high myopic macular holes in pathologic myopia with axial length of >/=30 mm. Retina. 2019; https://doi.org/10.1097/IAE.0000000000002699.
25. Caporossi T, De Angelis L, Pacini B, Tartaro R, Finocchio L, Barca F, et al. A human amniotic membrane plug to manage high myopic macular hole associated with retinal detachment. Acta Ophthalmol. 2020;98(2):e252–e25. https://doi.org/10.1111/aos.14174. Epub 2019 Jul 18

26. Gao X, Guo J, Meng X, Wang J, Peng X, Ikuno Y. A meta-analysis of vitrectomy with or without internal limiting membrane peeling for macular hole retinal detachment in the highly myopic eyes. BMC Ophthalmol. 2016;16:87. https://doi.org/10.1186/s12886-016-0266-5.
27. Lim LS, Tsai A, Wong D, Wong E, Yeo I, Loh BK, et al. Prognostic factor analysis of vitrectomy for retinal detachment associated with myopic macular holes. Ophthalmology. 2014;121(1):305–10. https://doi.org/10.1016/j.ophtha.2013.08.033.
28. Chak M, Williamson TH. Spontaneous suprachoroidal haemorrhage associated with high myopia and aspirin. Eye (Lond). 2003;17(4):525–7. https://doi.org/10.1038/sj.eye.6700388.
29. Masri I, Smith JM, Wride NK, Ghosh S. A rare case of acute angle closure due to spontaneous suprachoroidal haemorrhage secondary to loss of anti-coagulation control: a case report. BMC Ophthalmol. 2018;18(Suppl 1):224. https://doi.org/10.1186/s12886-018-0857-4.
30. Chandra A, Barsam A, Hugkulstone C. A spontaneous suprachoroidal haemorrhage: a case report. Cases J. 2009;2:185. https://doi.org/10.1186/1757-1626-2-185.

21 Miscellaneous Conditions

Contents

T. H. Williamson, *Vitreoretinal Surgery*, https://doi.org/10.1007/978-3-030-68769-4_21

Vitrectomy for Vitreous Opacities

Symptomatic vitreous floaters are common. In most circumstances, patients find the nuisance of floaters tolerable; however, there are some eyes that have considerable debris, and some patients who require clarity of the vision, e.g. musicians, find reading music difficult when floaters are present. A hazy vitreous is associated with reduced contrast sensitivity [1–6]. In conditions in which this is already reduced, e.g. multifocal lens implantation, vitreous debris can have an additive effect.

Common causes of persistent floaters

- Posterior vitreous detachment
- Vitreous syneresis, e.g. high myopia
- Resolved vitreous haemorrhage
- Uveitis
- Asteroid hyalosis
- Silicone oil emulsion

Make sure that the symptoms are consistent with floaters and not scotoma, see Chap. 4. It is reassuring to detect vitreous opacities on ophthalmoscopy before offering surgery. Watch out for previously undiagnosed conditions such as intermediate uveitis.

Be aware that the vitreous is often not detached. It is helpful to determine if the vitreous is detached, in which case the surgery is highly likely to be safe. Ultrasound can be used to look for gross detachment. More commonly use OCT (high resolution) to look for an optically empty space above the optic nerve and macula. This indicates the absence of vitreous and PVD.

Vitreous attachment will be seen on OCT as a hazy diffuse opacity overlying the retina or nerve. There may be micro-separation of the vitreous from the macula. In the presence of an attached vitreous, the surgeon may expect an increase in the chance of complications such as retinal tear formation, macular ERM or hole formation, and vitreous haemorrhage, or more likelihood for gas insertion.

Overall complications have been described in 1–2%. Phakic patients should expect early cataract formation. In patients over 5 years of age combined, Phaco IOL and PPV should be considered.

Patients are, however, incredibly pleased to have no floaters or vitreous opacity after successful surgery. Careful preparation of the expectations of the patient and communication of the risks of surgery is particularly important pre-operatively.

Warn the patient about the possible need for an air or gas bubble after surgery. The patient may still experience an occasional cell in the vitreous cavity seen as a small dark round opacity. Cataract development is common, and therefore there is the need for multiple surgeries, however, retaining 3–4 mm of vitreous behind the lens may delay the onset of lens opacity [7]. Patients are often happy with the surgical result of vitrectomy for floaters with better overall vision and loss of the focal effects of the degenerated vitreous (Figs. 21.1, 21.2, 21.3 and 21.4)

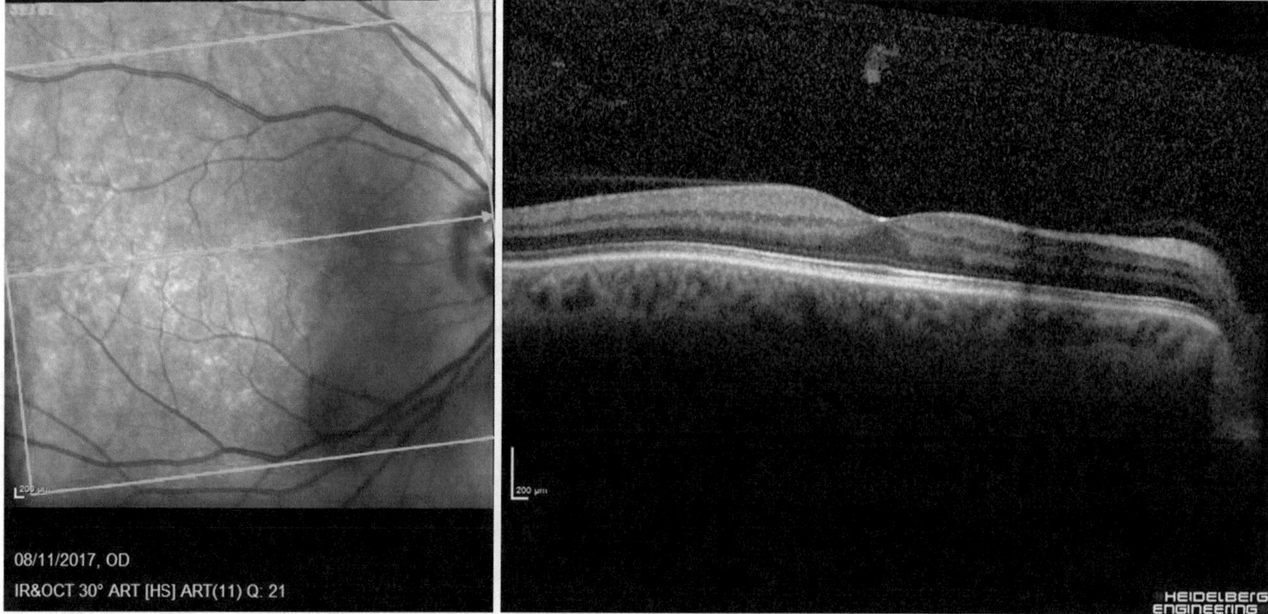

Fig. 21.1 A premacular opacity in vitreous syneresis which may be symptomatic

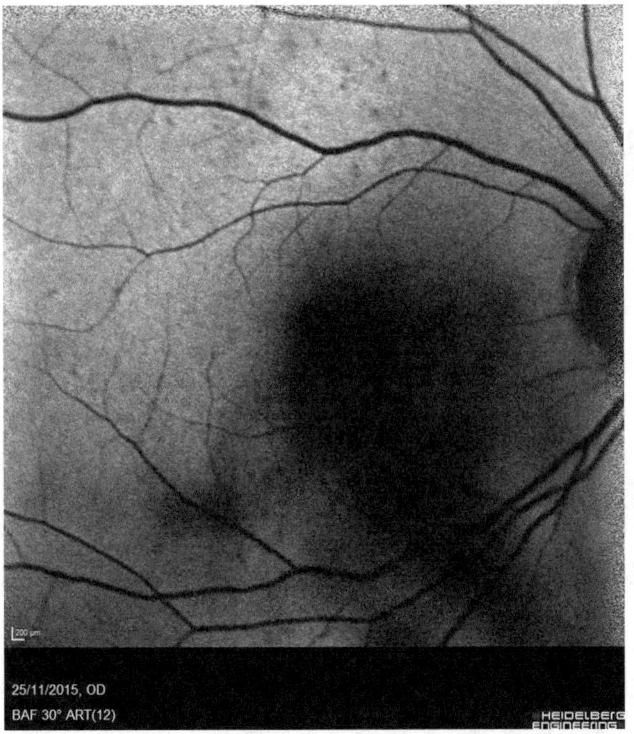

Fig. 21.2 Vitreous opacities are obscuring the view of the retina

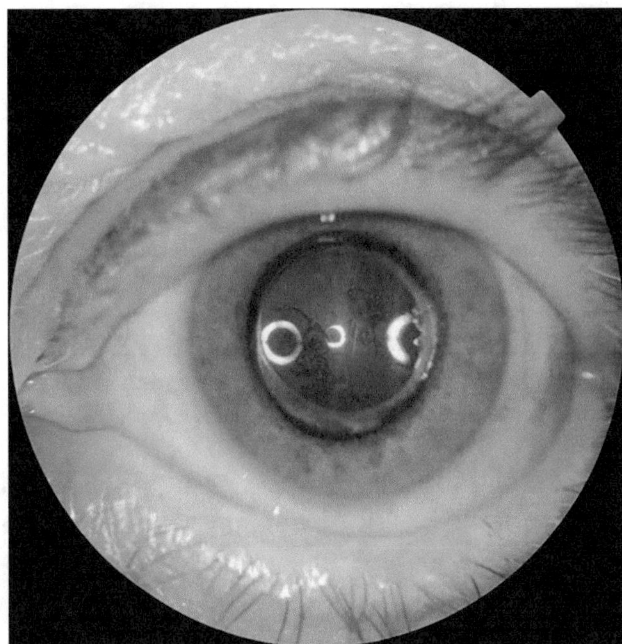

Fig. 21.3 Anterior vitreous opacities

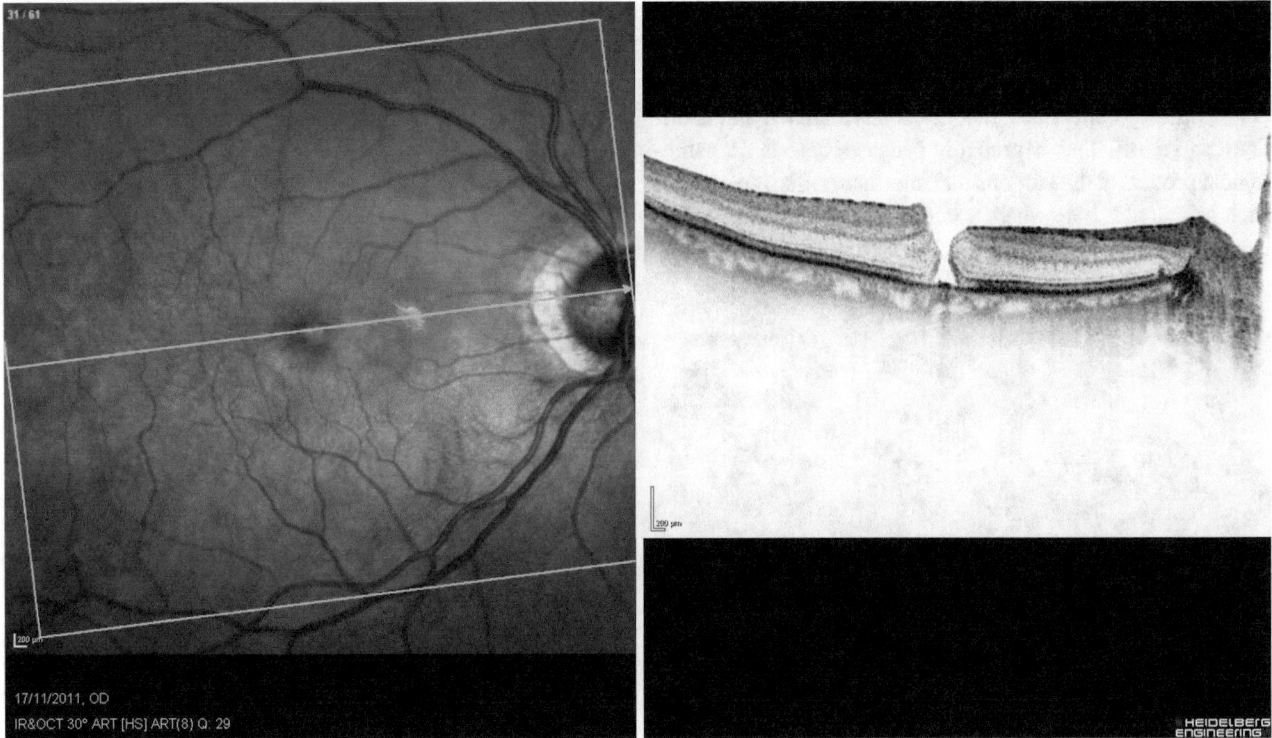

Fig. 21.4 This patient, who was a surgeon, had PPV for vitreous floaters from syneresis and developed a macular hole after the surgery, which required further surgery

Vitreous Anomalies

Persistent Hyperplastic Primary Vitreous

The most frequent severe developmental anomaly in the vitreous is persistent hyperplastic primary vitreous, which usually presents in infancy as a microphthalmic strabismic eye with leukocoria. Pupil dilatation may demonstrate dragging of the ciliary processes towards a central plaque of fibrovascular tissue, which invades the lens posteriorly and ultimately causes a complete cataract and secondary angle closure glaucoma. Using vitrectomy techniques, the anomaly can be removed but with little visual recovery [8].

Asteroid Hyalosis (Fig. 21.5)

Asteroid hyalosis is a specific form of gel degeneration in which globules of calcium soaps (hydroxyl apatite, calcium, and phosphate) aggregate on vitreous fibrils and move with the gel on eye movement [9]. It has been found in 2% of autopsy specimens [10] with increased prevalence with increasing age and the presence of PVD. The process of formation may be like lithiasis, stone formation in the body.

Dense, asteroid bodies may preclude ophthalmoscopic visualisation of the retina, though they rarely impair the patient's vision. They are not associated with any systemic condition and their aetiology is unknown.

Occasionally vitrectomy is required to improve vision [11–13] in my experience, the vitreous is attached and is difficult to get off. This is probably because there is no pathological process at the vitreoretinal interface, unlike conditions such as macular hole where a micro-vitreoretinal separation is present.

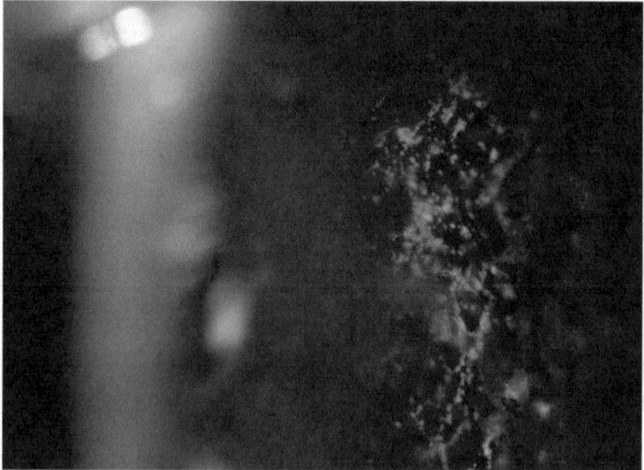

Fig. 21.5 Asteroid hyalosis in the anterior vitreous

Amyloidosis

Amyloidosis of the vitreous is a rare condition usually associated with primary or familial (dominantly inherited) forms of amyloidosis. Proteinaceous material, probably derived from the retinal circulation, becomes coated on the collagenous framework of the gel bilaterally to produce a "glass-wool" opacification; associated cellular invasion is conspicuous by its absence [14–18]. Vitrectomy may be used to clear opacities.

Retinal Haemangioma and Telangiectasia

Coats Disease

This is a rare non-hereditary condition classically of juvenile males and unilateral, however, it has a varied presentation. The description has been used for many exudative telangiectatic retinal presentations. The role of surgery is uncertain. External drainage of exudative retinal detachment, scleral buckling, injection of anti-VEGF and laser retinal ablation have been used [19–22] (Figs. 21.6, 21.7, 21.8, 21.9, 21.10, 21.11, 21.12, 21.13, 21.14, 21.15, 21.16 and 21.17)

Von Hippel–Lindau

Retinal angioma (retinal capillary haemangioma) can occur as a solitary lesion not associated with systemic disease or as

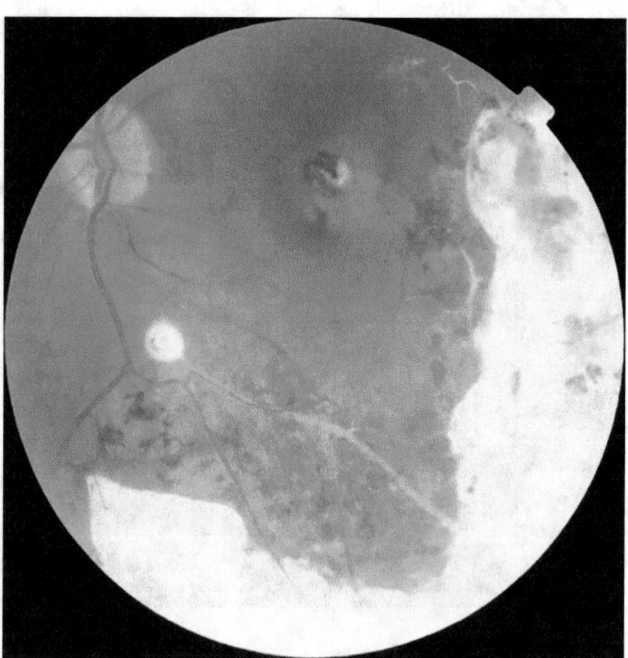

Fig. 21.6 Exudation from Coats disease

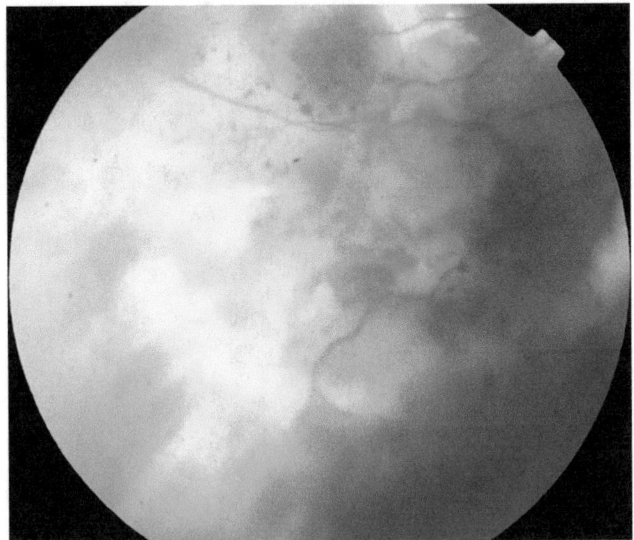

Fig. 21.7 A peripheral lesion in Coats disease

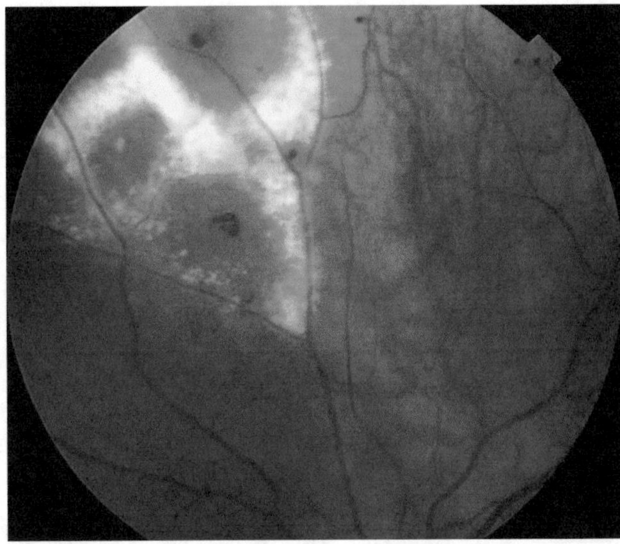

Fig. 21.9 A patient with Coats disease with the progression of exudation over 3 years in their third decade

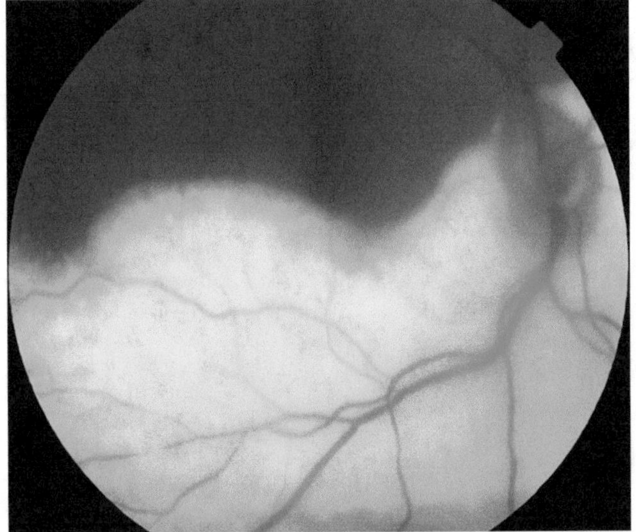

Fig. 21.8 Extension of exudate into the macula in Coats disease

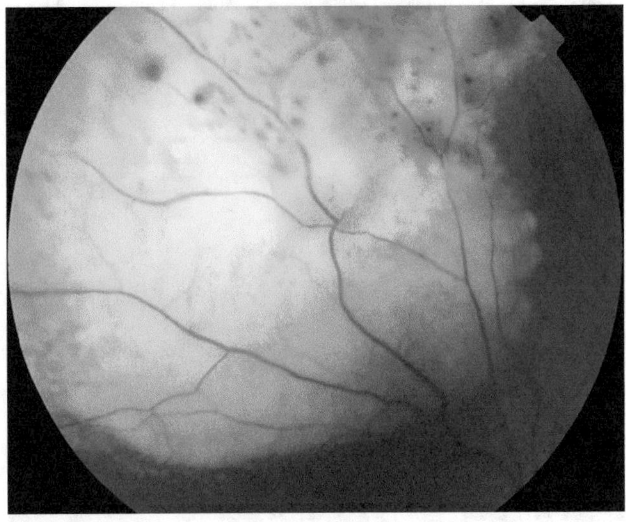

Fig. 21.10 Progression of the exudation

multiple lesions in Von Hippel–Lindau disease (VHL). In the former, the mean age at presentation (36 years) is older than in Von Hippel–Lindau (17 years) [23, 24]. Most tumours are located in the superotemporal quadrant in the retinal mid periphery [25]. 17% of angiomas in VHL occur on the optic nerve [26]. New tumours are rare in patients without VHL. Isolated retinal angiomas have been described after RRD surgery [27].

In VHL a mean of four tumours are seen per eye, and new lesions tend to occur before the age of 47 years. In VHL extraocular lesions occur as:

1. Central nervous system haemangioma
2. Renal cyst, renal carcinoma
3. Pancreatic cysts and adenoma, pancreatic islet cell tumours
4. Pheochromocytoma
5. Endolymphatic sac tumour of the inner ear
6. Cystadenoma of the epididymis and broad ligament

Retinal angiomas may cause vitreous haemorrhage, tractional, exudative, or rhegmatogenous retinal detachment, and macular pucker or hole [28–33]. Treatment may involve

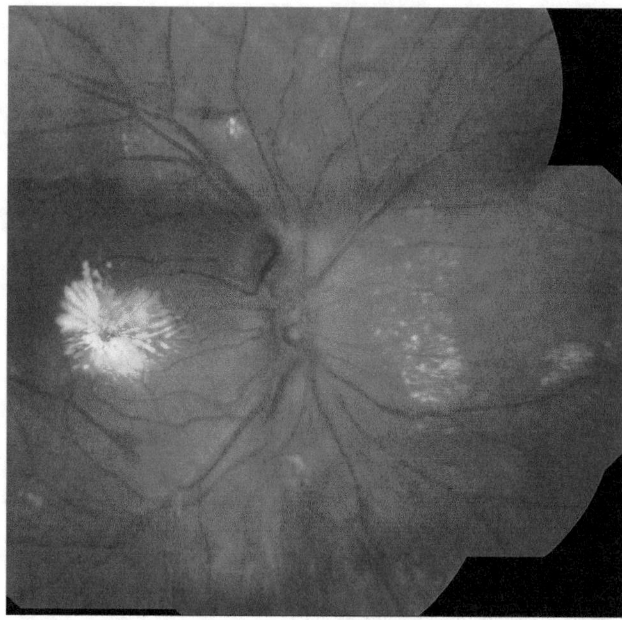

Fig. 21.11 There is a spectrum of retinal vascular anomalies which may affect the eye, including Coats disease, isolated angiomas and Von Hippel–Lindau. In this young patient, there is an angioma on the disc causing macular swelling. There is no effective way of treating optic nerve disease. FFA confirms leakage

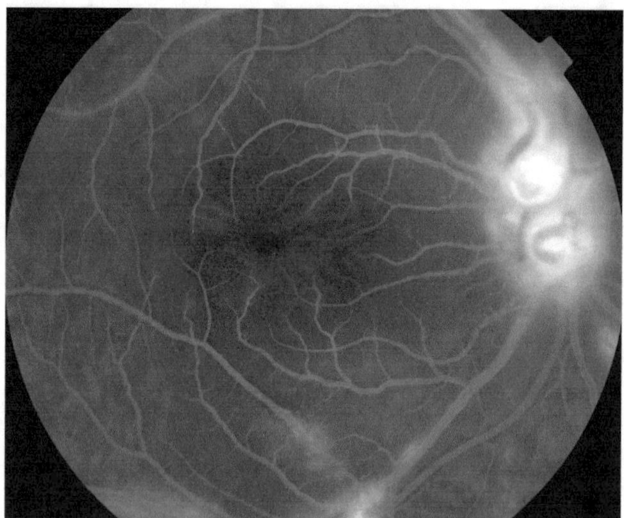

Fig. 21.12 FFA of the angioma

1. Observation
2. Laser photocoagulation of angiomas smaller than 1.5 mm
3. Cryotherapy to larger lesions
4. Vitrectomy surgery for the complications such as vitreous haemorrhage, retinal detachment and macular pucker [26, 34]

Unfortunately, PVR formation is common, making surgery hazardous.

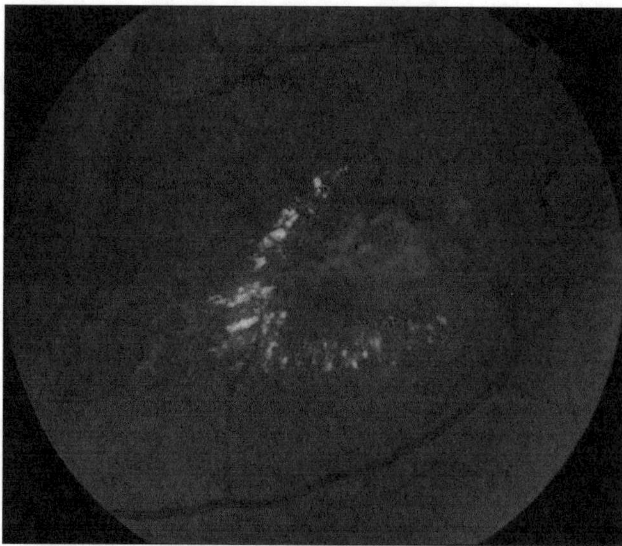

Fig. 21.13 A small angioma in Von Hippel–Lindau. These angiomata can produce devastating problems within the retina, such as exudative retinal detachment, vitreous haemorrhage and subretinal and intraretinal exudation

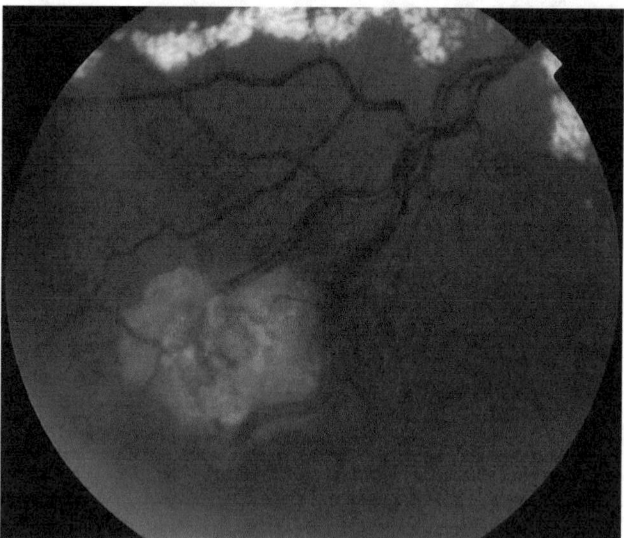

Fig. 21.14 A large angioma in VHL

External beam radiotherapy has been tried where other treatments have failed to regress the lesions [35], but as yet an appropriate therapeutic option is not available for optic nerve lesions [36] (Figs. 21.18, 21.19, 21.20, 21.21, 21.22, 21.23, 21.24, 21.25, 21.26 and 21.27).

Familial Exudative Vitreoretinopathy

This is a group of hereditary conditions characterised by abnormal peripheral retinal angiogenesis like ROP [37].

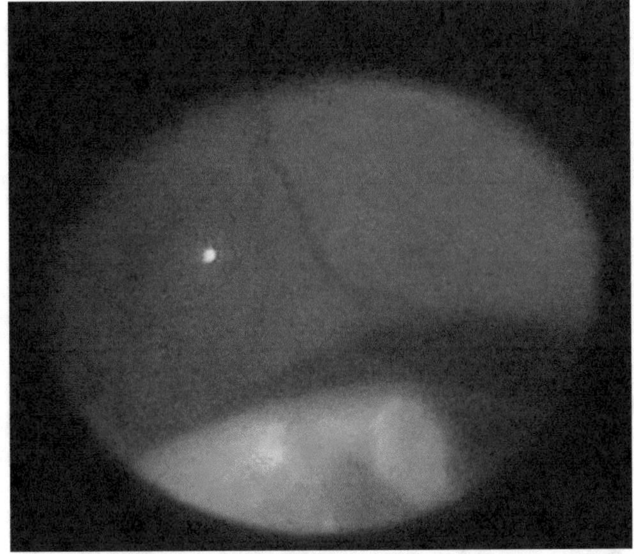

Fig. 21.15 A peripheral angioma seen on indentation

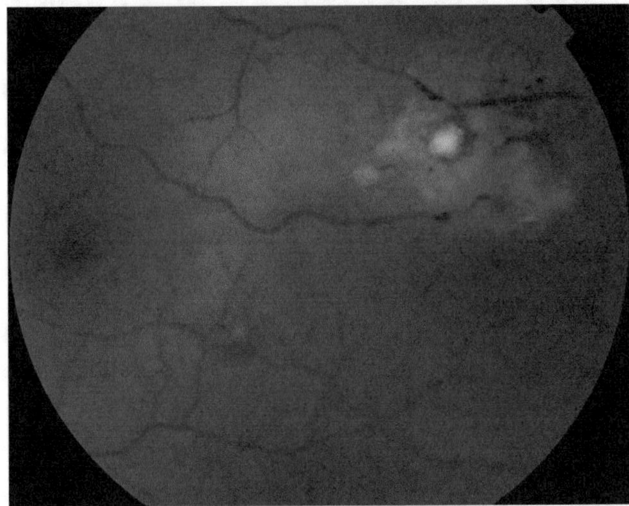

Fig. 21.16 An occluded retinal angioma in VHL

Clinical Signs

- Avascular peripheral retina
- Retinal telangiectasia
- Arteriovenous shunts
- Dragged retinal vessels and macula
- Retinal (falciform) folds
- Neovascularisation
- Subretinal exudation
- Retinal detachments
- Persistent fetal vasculature

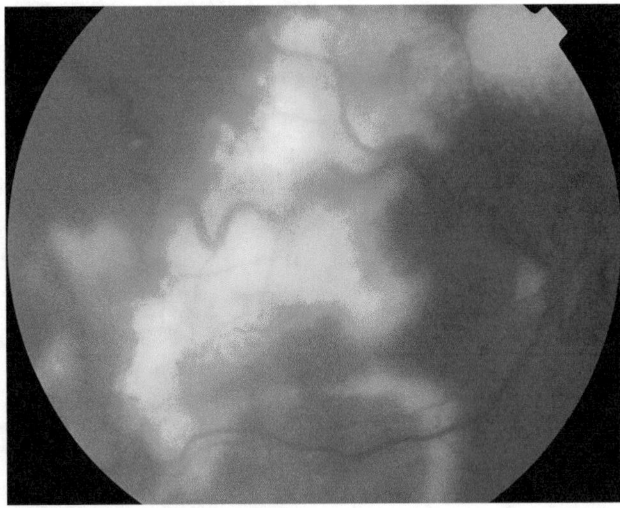

Fig. 21.17 An exudative retinal detachment in VHL

Vitreoretinal Presentations

- Retinal detachment
- Vitreous haemorrhage
- Epiretinal membrane

In general, l caution is required before operating on these patients as the retina is prone to PVR formation. If surgery can be performed externally, then this should be utilised [38]. If you are required to perform PPV, it is important to avoid retinal breaks. Apply laser to ischaemic areas of the retina. Take care in an eye with a dragged macula that you know where the fovea is and do not mistake the macula for nasal retina. (Figs. 21.28, 21.29, 21.30 and 21.31)

Optic Disc Anomalies

Various optic disc anomalies are associated with retinal elevation.

Optic Disc Pits and Optic Disc Coloboma (Figs. 21.32, 21.33, 21.34, 21.35, 21.36, 21.37, 21.38, 21.39, 21.40, 21.41 and 21.42)

The source of the intraretinal and subretinal fluid remains a mystery in these conditions, with theories postulated that the fluid arises from the disc, perhaps leaking from the subarachnoid space or from a defect in the surface of the disc allowing vitreous fluid to enter. Certainly, it is usually impossible to

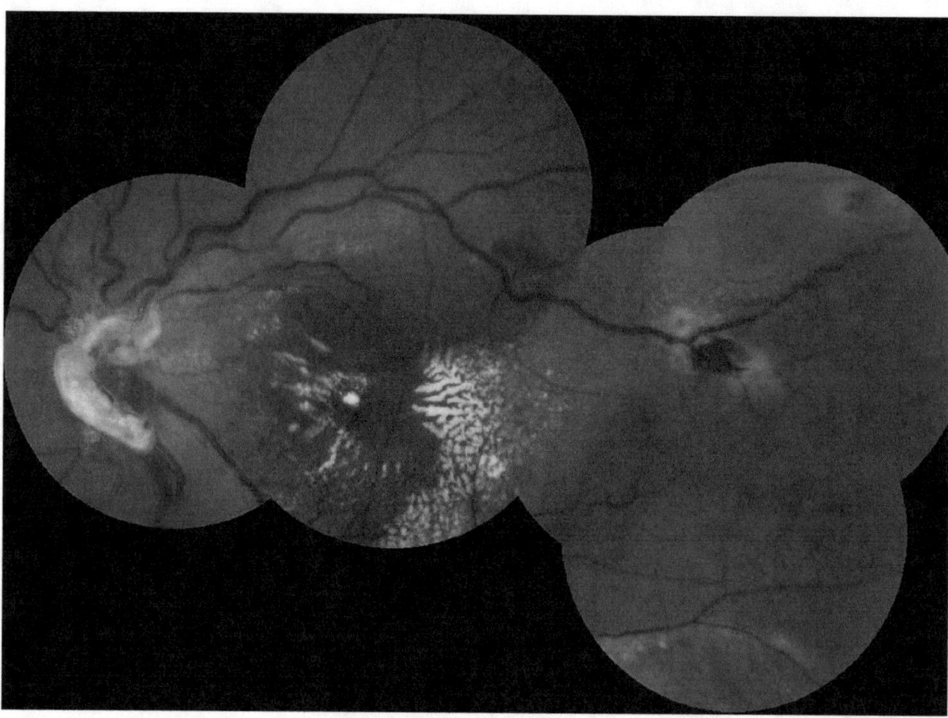

Fig. 21.18 A composite picture showing treated lesions, macular exudation, and an optic nerve head angioma

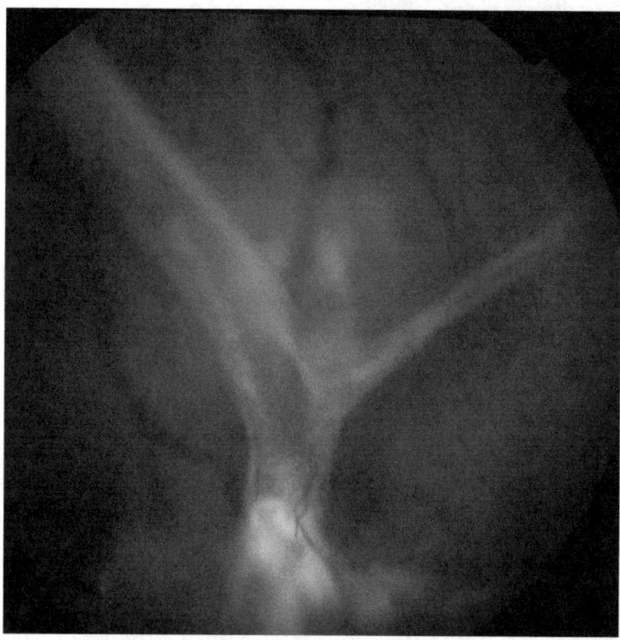

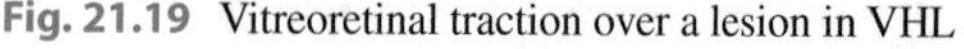

Fig. 21.19 Vitreoretinal traction over a lesion in VHL

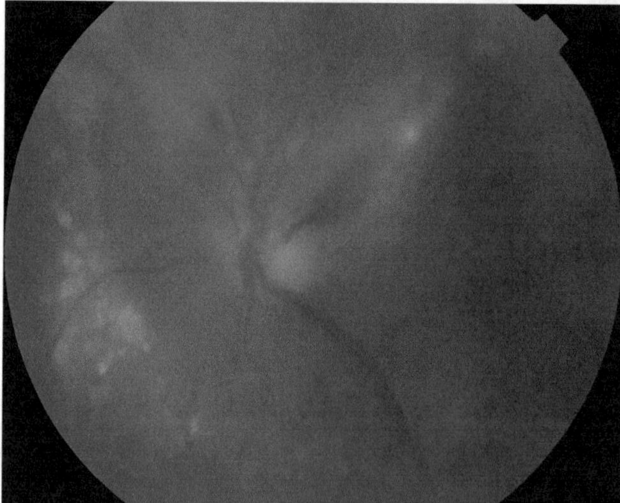

Fig. 21.20 This patient had 16 procedures on his eyes for the retinal complications of Von Hippel–Lindau, which included rhegmatogenous retinal detachment, exudative retinal detachment, PVR, and cystoid macular oedema. Only the eye shown retained a useful vision of 20/120 but with untreatable peripapillary angiomas

detect a retinal break. The retinal elevation appears to consist of a multi-layered schisis of the retina [39, 40].

Therapy is controversial with peripapillary laser applied to try to block any channels for the dispersion of fluid into the macula. Both pneumatic retinopexy and vitrectomy and gas have been used to oppose the peripapillary retina to allow the laser to seal and to disperse macular fluid [41, 42]. Others have used vitrectomy and gas without laser with slow resolution of the RD [43]; however, spontaneous resolution may also occur.

I perform PPV, laser to the RPE at the edge of the optic disc. The retina does not need to be flat during the laser application; indeed its elevation helps prevent damage to the overlying nerve fibres. Apply the laser only to the area with elevated retina with minimal blanching of the retina. Insert 30% perfluoro propane.

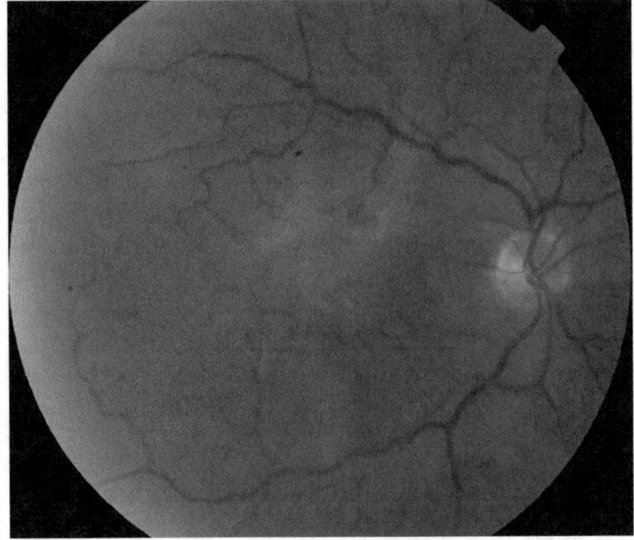

Fig. 21.21 Parafoveal telangiectasia causing an ERM

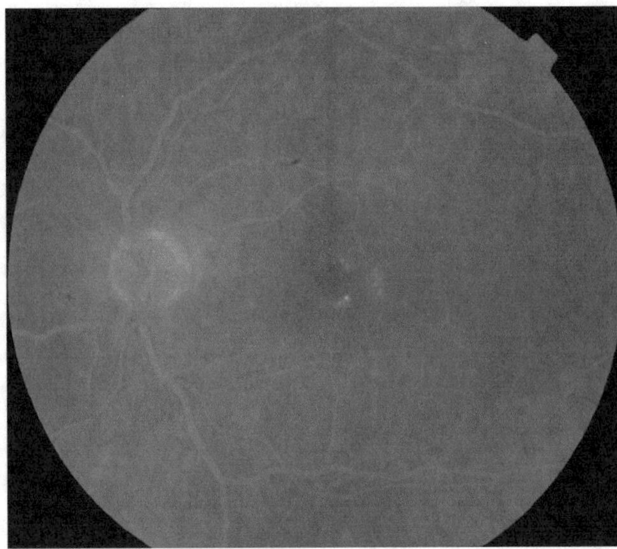

Fig. 21.22 FFA of parafoveal telangiectasia causing an ERM. Macular holes secondary to MacTel do not do well with surgery

Fig. 21.23 Multiple leaking telangiectasia sometimes called Leber's miliary aneurysms

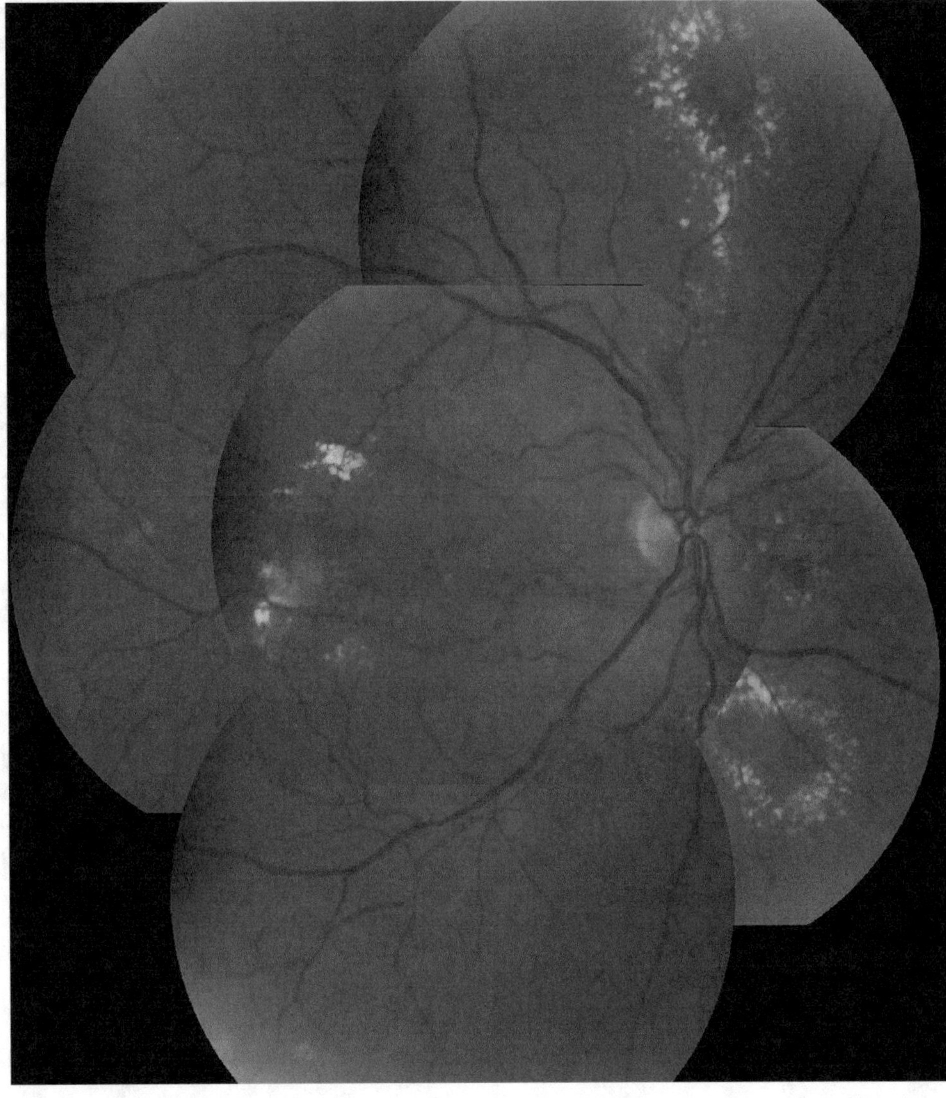

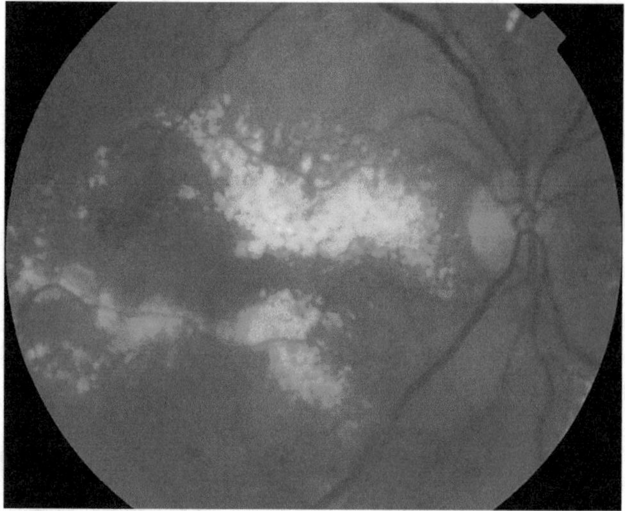

Fig. 21.24 Macular leakage

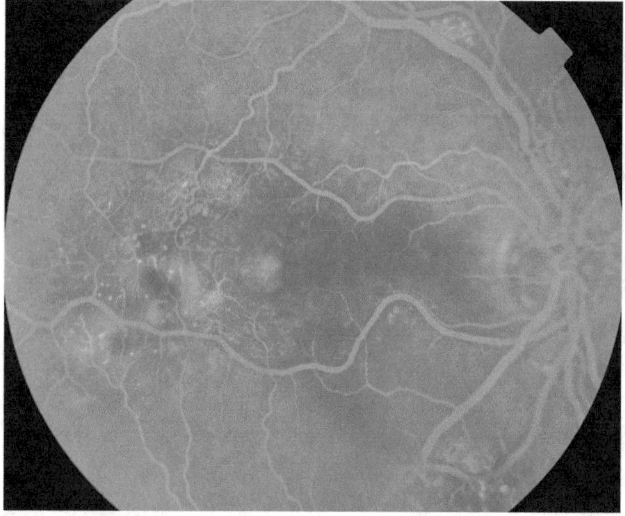

Fig. 21.25 FFA showing vascular abnormalities

Warn the patient that the resolution of the retinal elevation may take 9 months postoperatively.

An additional step is to insert an ILM flap into the pit or coloboma. This is alleged to induce more rapid resolution of the fluid. The ILM can be taken from the arcades and pulled towards the optic disc leaving it attached to the retina at the edge of the disc. The ILM can then be folded into the defect.

I have seen one case in whom I inserted an ILM fap. The flap dislocated, and the patient described a floater for 9 months. The macular schisis persisted. At 9 months, the floater disappeared, and the flap could now be seen in the pit. The schisis had now resolved.

Other methods include ILM peel, inner retinal fenestration, and tissues used to "plug" the hole are amniotic membrane and sclera [44, 45] (Figs. 21.43, 21.44 and 21.45).

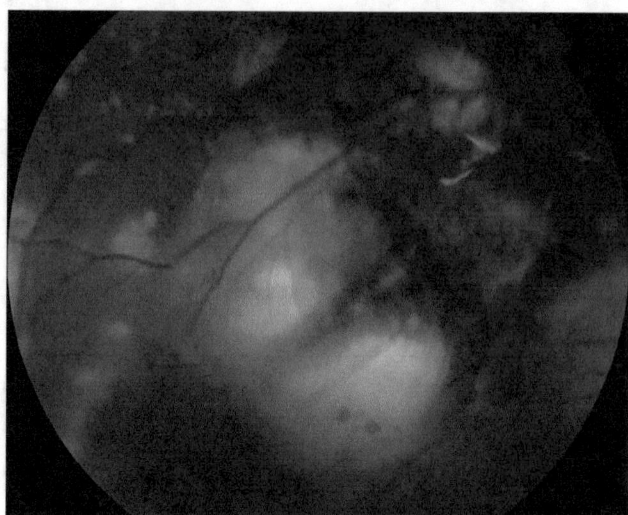

Fig. 21.26 Familial exudative vitreoretinopathy presents with a dragged disc and retinal telangiectasia. Occasionally RRD occurs but with a high chance of PVR as with most retinal telangiectatic disease

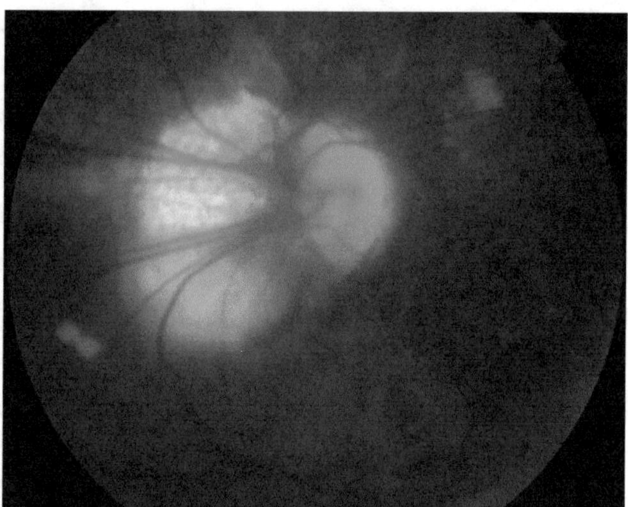

Fig. 21.27 The retina is dragged over the disc in this patient with FEVR, the macula is on the right of the disc in this right eye. The surgeon can be fooled during surgery into thinking that the macula is on the left, running the risk that the macula will not be appropriately protected from surgical manoeuvres

Some patients may be suffering from renal coloboma syndrome with renal hypoplasia and a mutation of the PAX2 gene and therefore renal investigations may be advisable [46] (Figs. 21.41, 21.44, 21.46, 21.47, 21.48, 21.49, 21.50, 21.51, 21.52, 21.53, 21.54, 21.55).

Morning Glory Syndrome (Fig. 21.56)

This severe optic disc anomaly can be associated with posterior polar retinal detachment in as many as 35% of patients

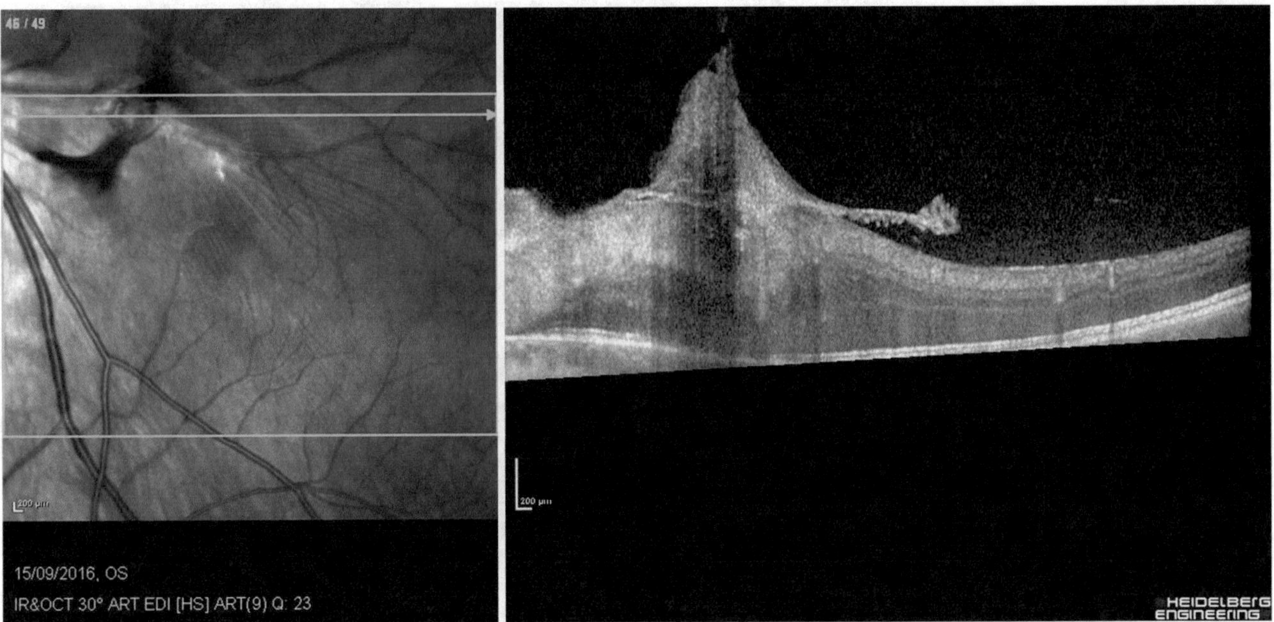

Fig. 21.28 An ERM in FEVR is disrupting the central vision

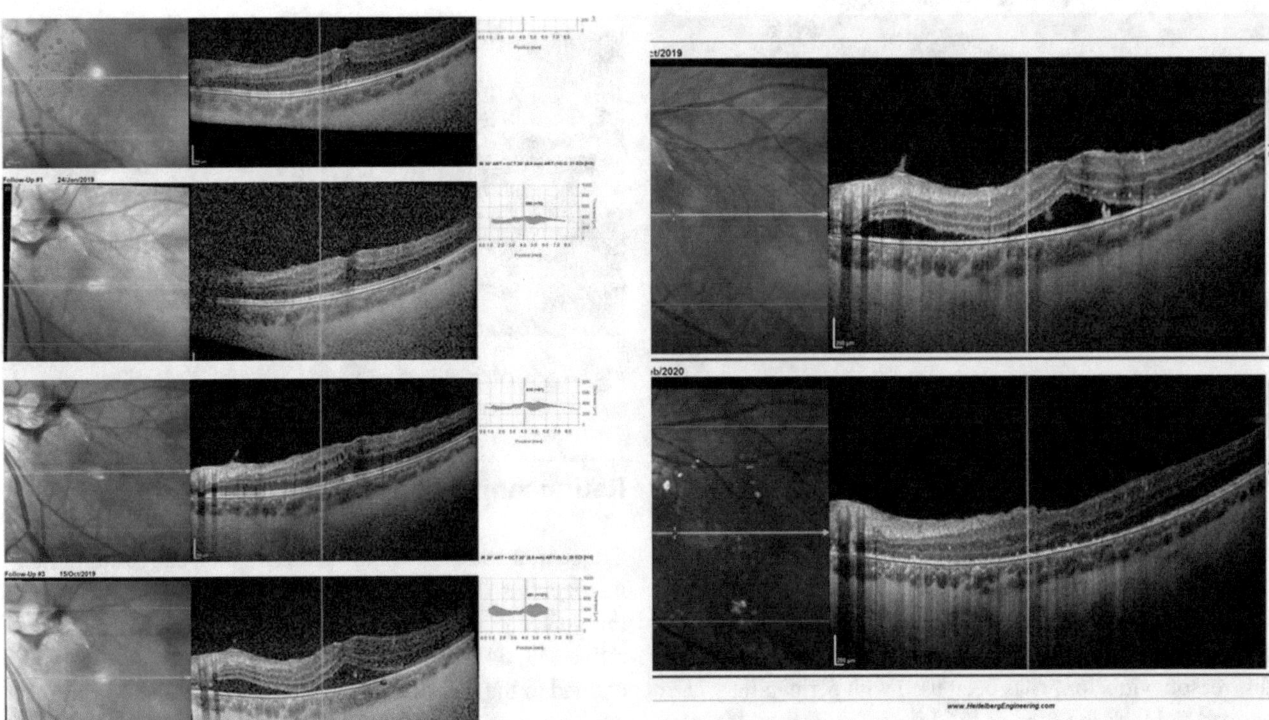

Fig. 21.29 The ERM caused gradual progression to serous elevation of the macula but thankfully responded to surgery with PPV and peel with great care not to create any retinal breaks

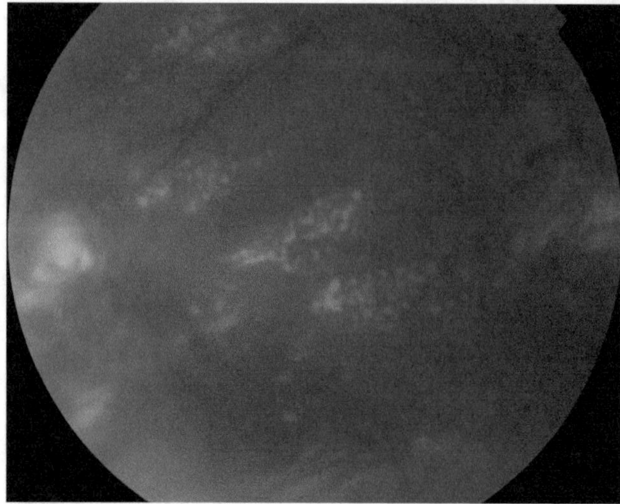

Fig. 21.30 Retinal detachment in FEVR treated by 360 encircling band

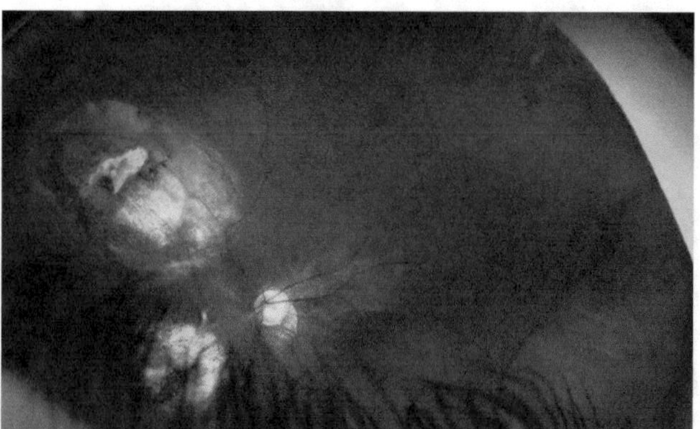

Fig. 21.31 An eye with FEVR

[47]. (Fig. 21.57) Often vision is poor because of the disc abnormality. A communication has been described between the subarachnoid space [48] and the subretinal space (metrizamide cisternography has shown dye migration into the SRF). Patients have been treated by optic nerve sheath fenestration, where a window of dura is removed from the optic nerve, with the resolution of the RD [49]. More commonly, a hole on the optic nerve head has been blamed for the passage of fluid form the vitreous cavity to the subretinal space. For this reason, vitrectomy has been used with peripapillary laser applied to block the flow of fluid and with internal tamponade. Such a communication has been demonstrated by the complication of subretinal oil or gas occurring post operatively in these cases [50] (Fig. 21.58, 21.59, 21.60 and 21.61).

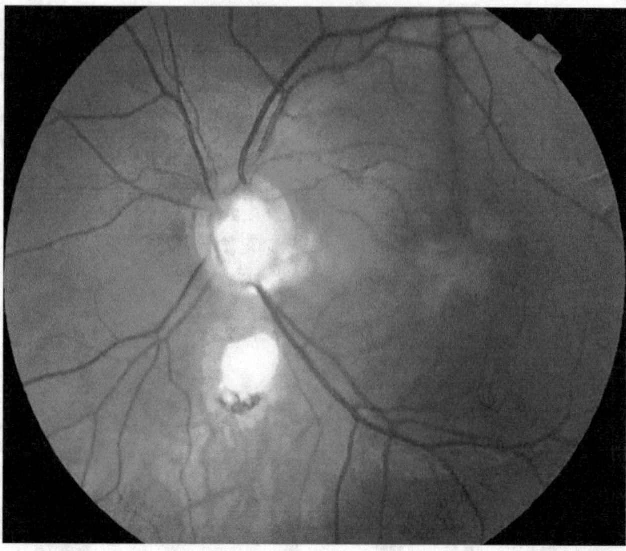

Fig. 21.32 An optic disc coloboma causing a macular retinoschisis. OCT shows a retinoschisis post operatively after pneumatic displacement by pneumatic retinopexy with SF6 gas and peripapillary laser application. The OCT demonstrates closure of the schisis around the peripapillary area and reduction in the height of the schisis associated with visual improvement to 20/30

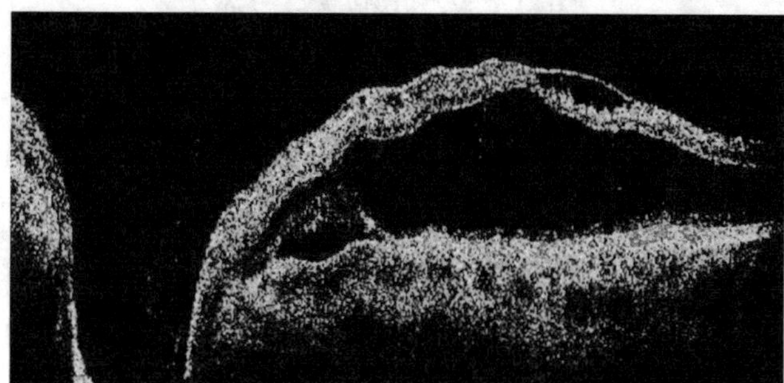

Fig. 21.33 OCT of the macular schisis

Retinochoroidal Coloboma (Fig. 21.62)

Congenital coloboma of the posterior pole can result in rhegmatogenous retinal detachment from breaks on the edge of the defect [51]., in the coloboma [52] or in the peripheral retina [53, 54]. For breaks in the coloboma, laser should be applied to the edge of the coloboma but take care if the laser must be applied to the disc margin as visual loss can occur [55]. Internal tamponade with or without a scleral buckle can be used. Cyanoacrylate retinopexy has been used to seal breaks in the coloboma [56].

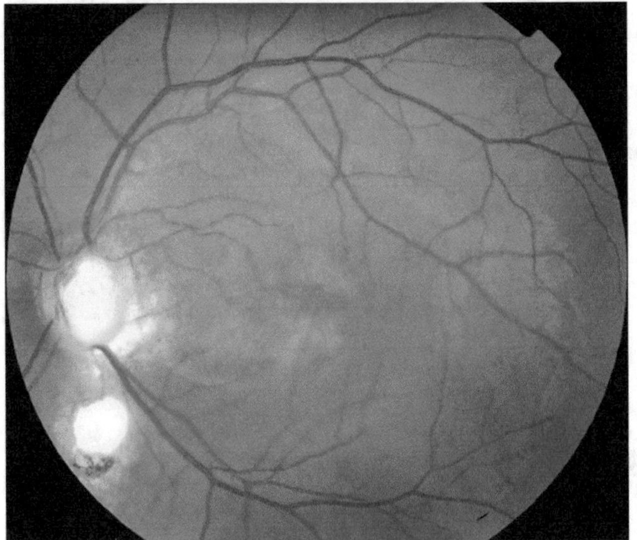

Fig. 21.34 The macula after surgery

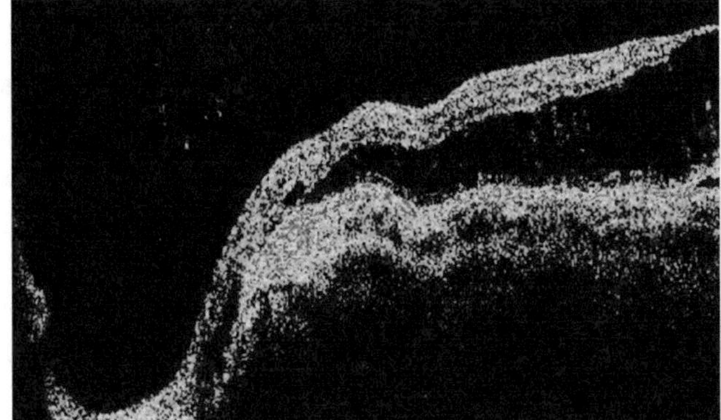

Fig. 21.35 OCT shows reduction in the schisis

Marfan's Syndrome (Figs. 21.63, 21.64, 21.65 and 21.66)

Marfan's syndrome is a connective tissue disorder that affects the skeleton, lungs, eyes, heart, and blood vessels. The disease is characterised by unusually long limbs (arm span longer than the patient's height) and long fingers, especially the middle phalanx. Marfan's syndrome is an autosomal dominant disorder and has been linked to the FBN1 gene on chromosome 15; this encodes a protein called fibrillin, essential for the formation of elastic fibres.

These patients present in two ways with ocular problems, with dislocated or subluxated crystalline lenses, or with RRD associated with their high myopia. Bilaterality of RRD is high at 70% [57], with tears varying from small breaks to

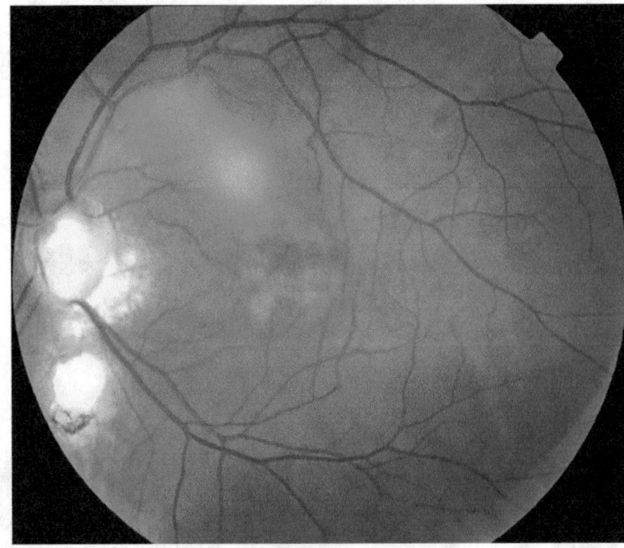

Fig. 21.36 Three years later, the patient has a flat fovea

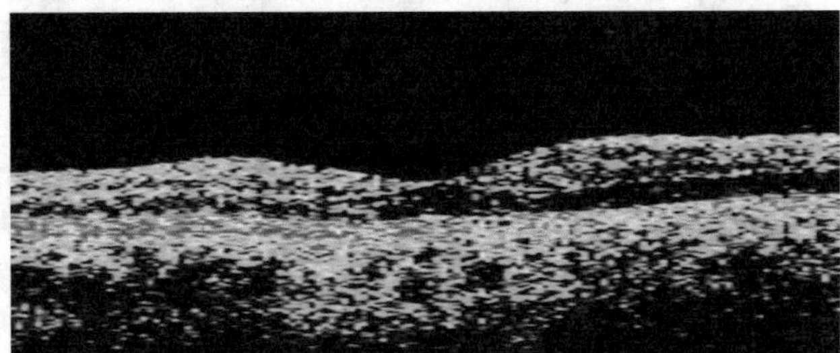

Fig. 21.37 OCT of the fovea

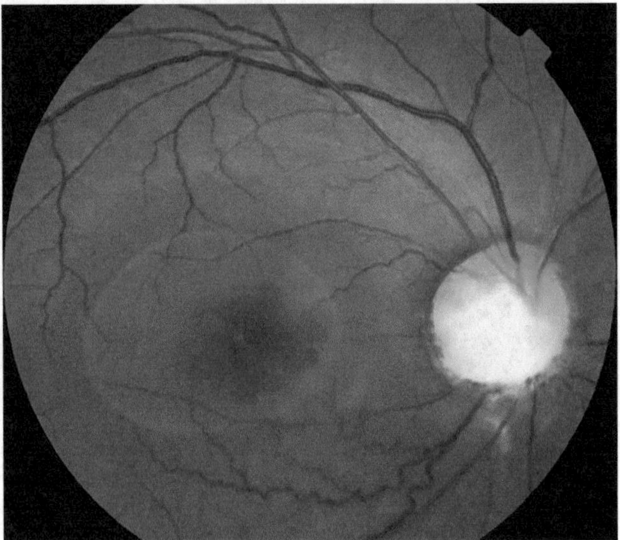

Fig. 21.38 Serous elevation probably with retinoschisis on OCT occurs in patients with optic pit

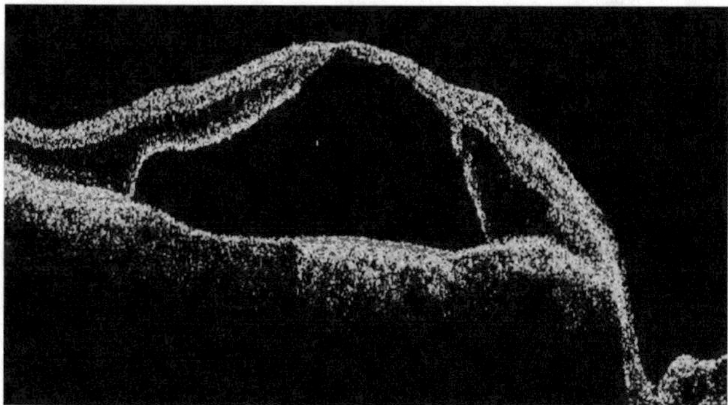

Fig. 21.39 OCT of the macular elevation

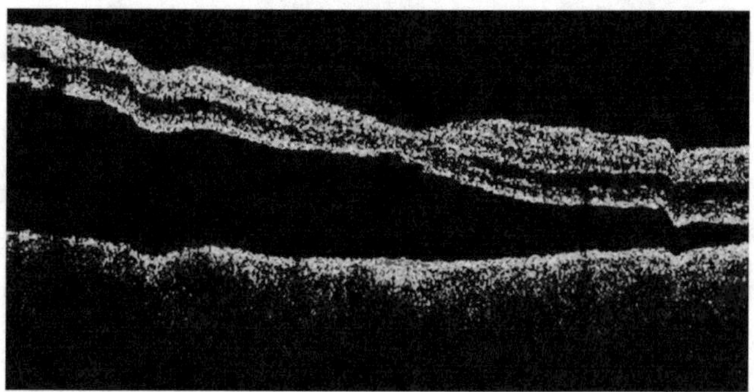

Fig. 21.40 Fluid has been displaced inferiorly by gas injection

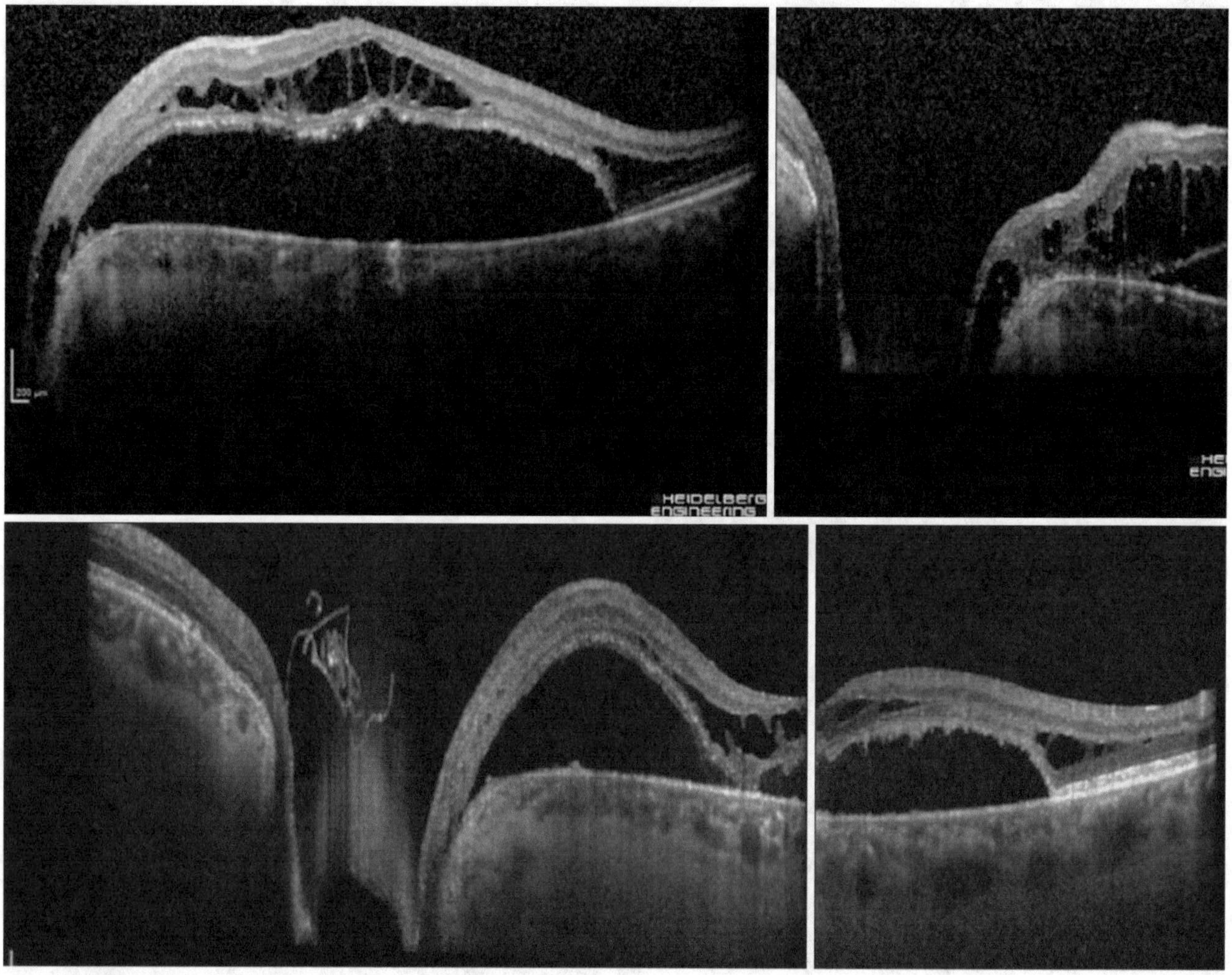

Fig. 21.41 A patient with recurrent macular schisis from the optic pit and a chorioretinal coloboma. Treated by ILM flap, which dislocated. Once the flap re-entered the optic pit spontaneously, the schisis began to resolve

giant retinal tears [58]. Dislocated lenses can be observed until these become problematic, with the edge of the lens interfering with the visual axis.

The lenses usually require removal by vitreolensectomy [59], often at a young age. Lens implantation is problematic in that sutured sulcus lenses are prone to problems such as suture erosion, vitreous haemorrhage, lens tilt and dislocation in the long term [60, 61]. Therefore, leaving the eye aphakic may be appropriate with contact lens usage. Fully dislocated lenses may be left in situ if asymptomatic but there is a risk of lens-

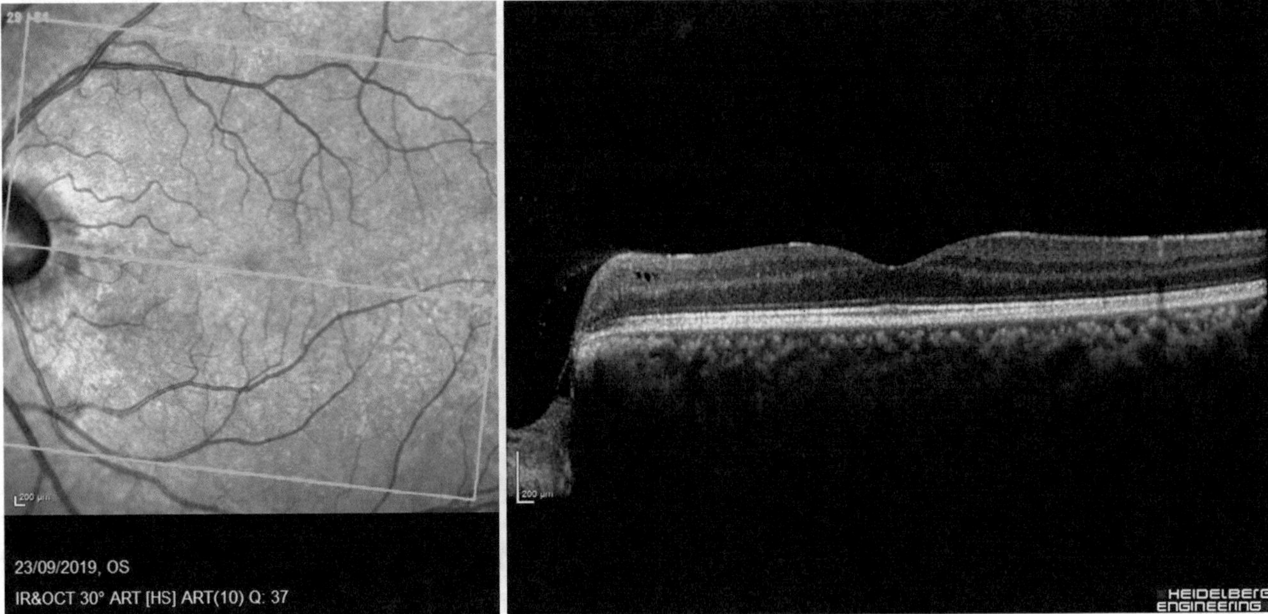

Fig. 21.42 Exceedingly early changes with an optic pit

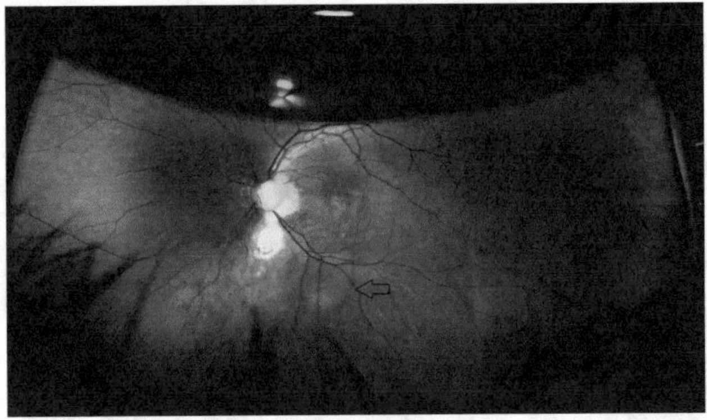

Fig. 21.43 A wide-angle view of an eye with gas insertion for optic pit maculopathy. The patient also has a chorioretinal coloboma. Note the displacement of retinal fluid inferiorly (arrow)

induced uveitis or glaucoma [62] or lens dislocation into the anterior chamber. See management of aphakia for other alternative lens implantation methods [63] (Fig. 21.67).

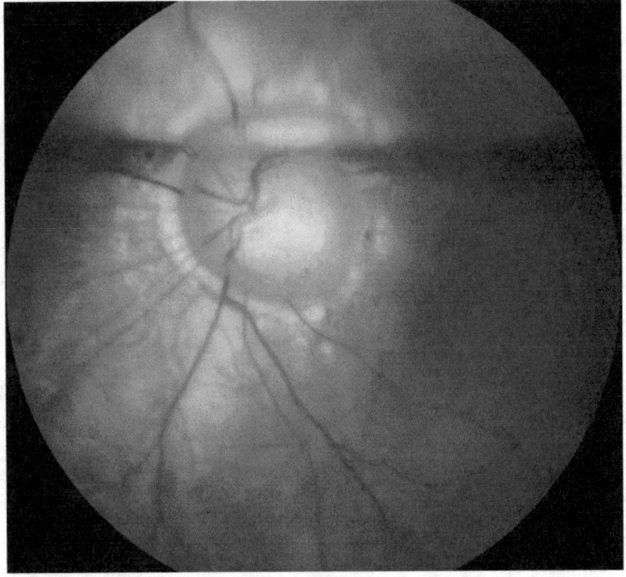

Fig. 21.44 A macular schisis from an optic nerve coloboma has been treated with peripapillary laser and gas

Retinopathy of Prematurity

Prematurity of birth is defined as less than 32 weeks' gestation and birth weight of less than 1500 g, but especially less than 1250 grams. Premature infants may progress to severe tractional retinal detachment and vitreous haemorrhage from neovascularisation arising between vascularized and nonvascularized retina. ROP is categorised by the lowest zone and the highest stage observed in each eye.

Zones	
Zone 1	The centre of zone 1 is the optic nerve. The zone extends twice the distance from the optic nerve to the macula in a circle.
Zone 2	Is a circle surrounding the zone 1 circle with the nasal ora serrata as its nasal border.
Zone 3	Is the crescent that the circle of zone 2 did not encompass temporally.

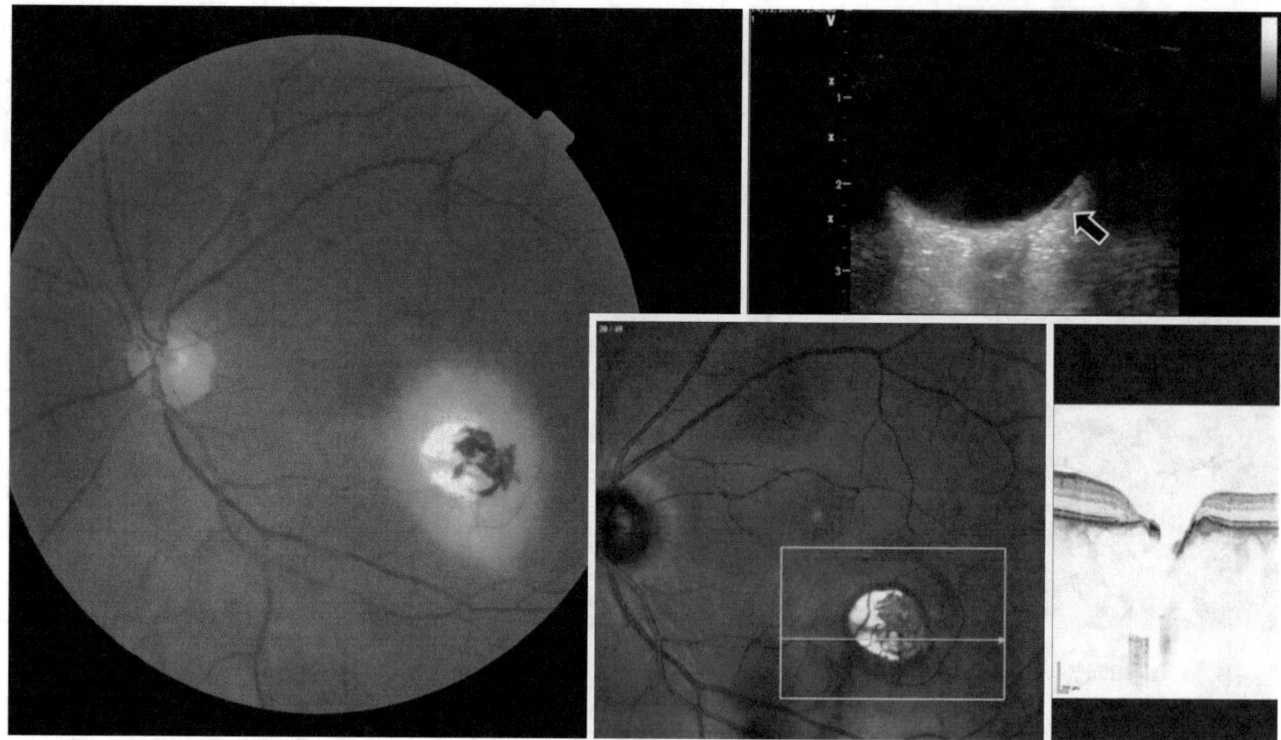

Fig. 21.45 A coloboma has a communication with a small orbital cyst. Larger more disruptive cysts may be seen

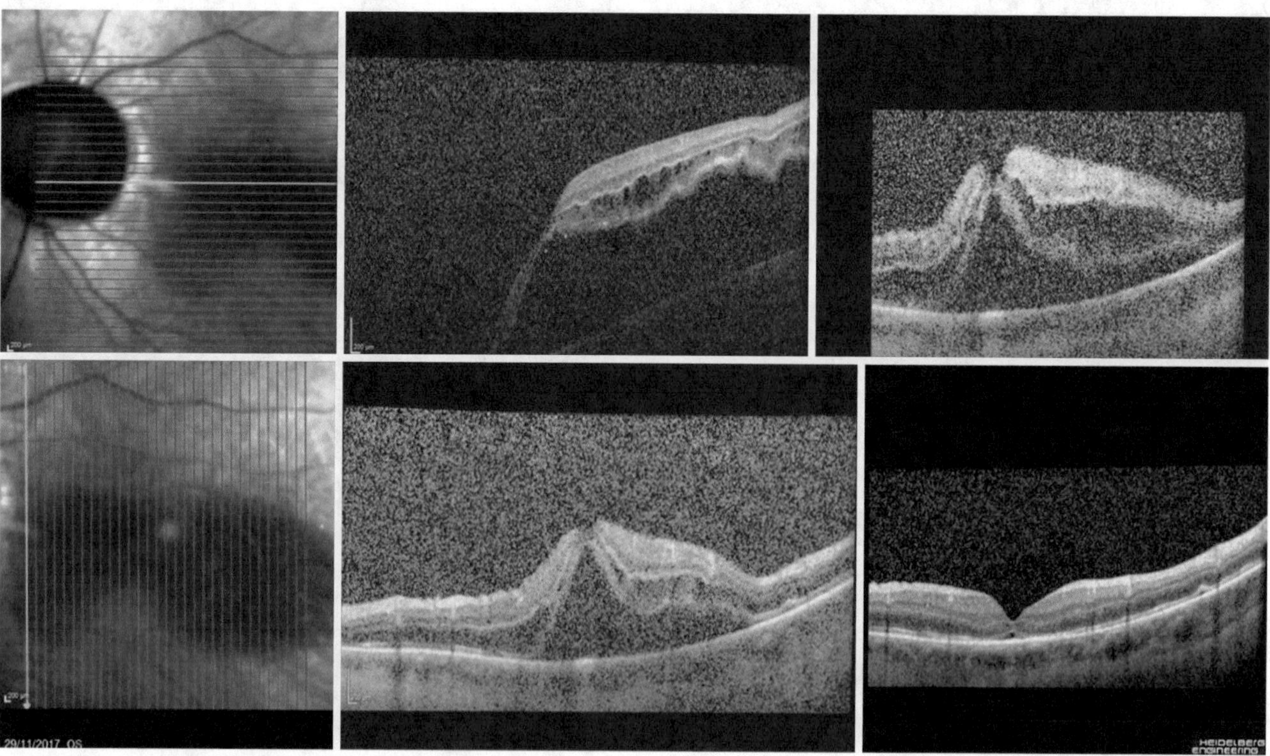

Fig. 21.46 Resolution of macular SRF in a patient with optic nerve coloboma after vitrectomy, peripapillary laser, ILM flaps in the coloboma and gas

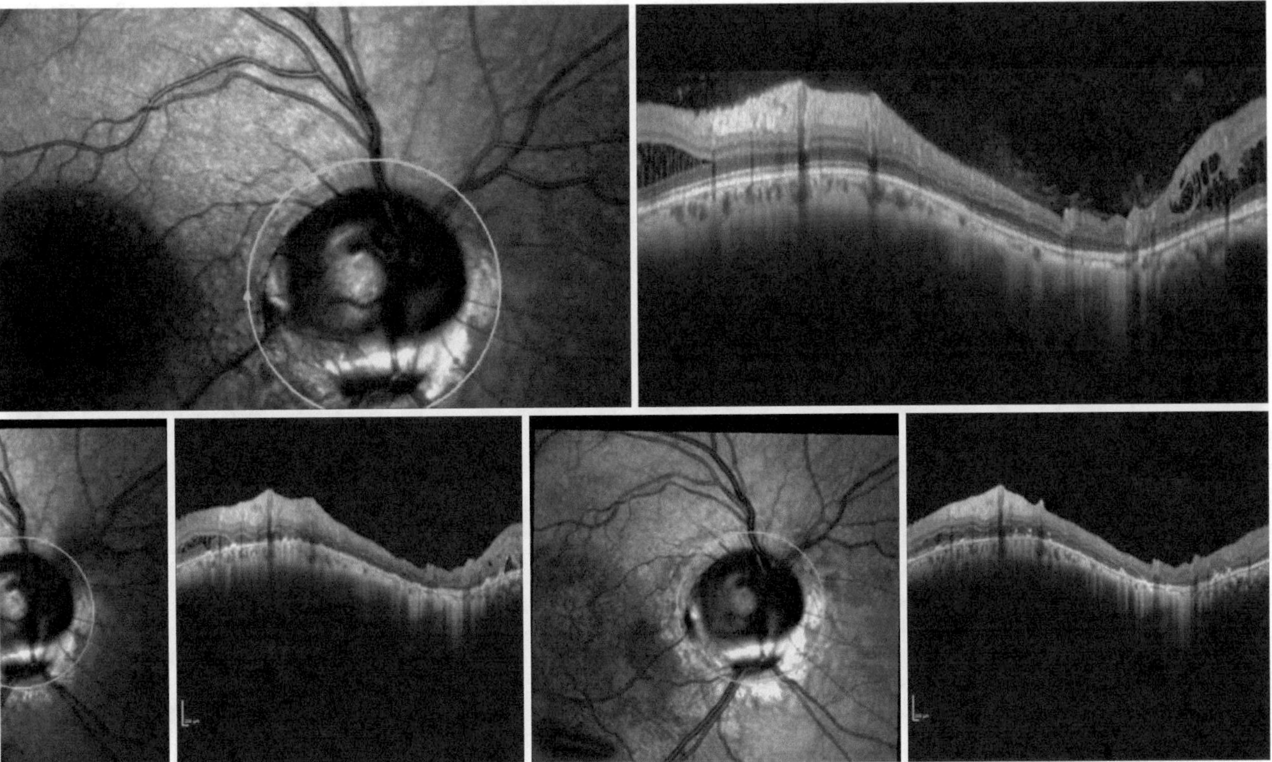

Fig. 21.47 An optic disc coloboma with optic nerve scans after surgery

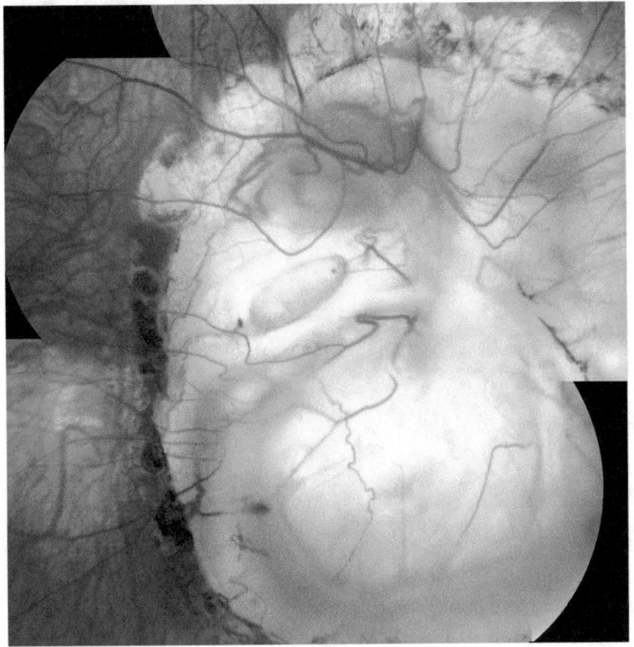

Fig. 21.48 A 14 year old patient with CHARGE syndrome (coloboma of the eye, heart defects, atresia of the nasal choanae, retardation of growth, genito-urinary abnormalities, ear abnormalities and deafness) presented with RRD from the right coloboma, which was successfully treated with laser to the edge of the coloboma and 2 months silicone oil tamponade then removal of the oil, retaining 20/120 vision. A postoperative view is shown with laser scars in the right eye

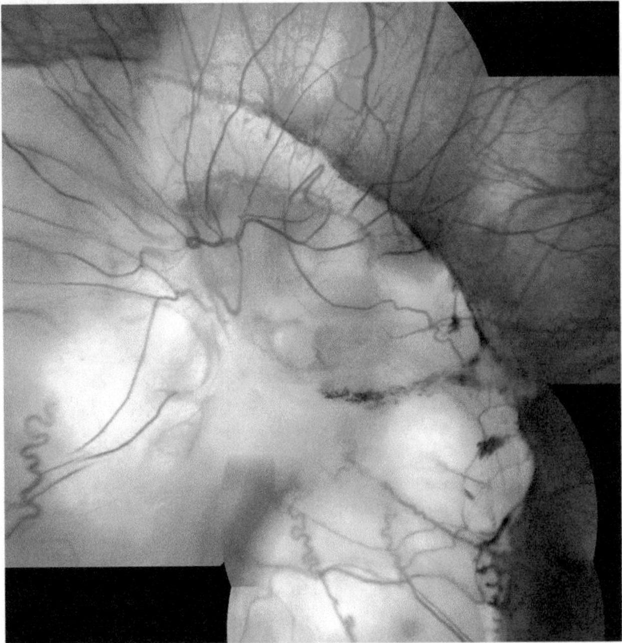

Fig. 21.49 The other eye

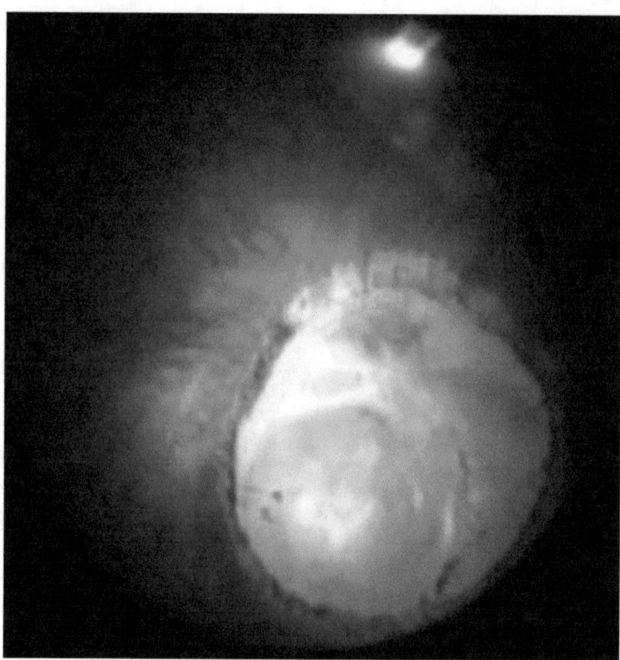

Fig. 21.50 A peroperative view of coloboma in CHARGE syndrome

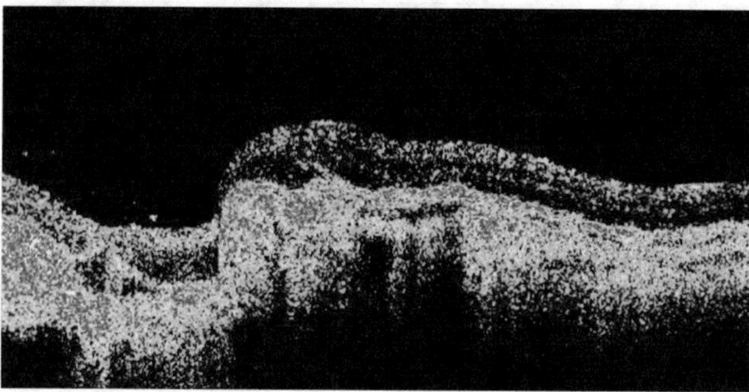

Fig. 21.51 An OCT of the edge of the coloboma in a patient with CHARGE syndrome. Note the sudden posterior displacement of the tissues with some evidence of membranes in the coloboma

Stages	
Stage 0	Characterised by immature retinal vasculature. No clear demarcation of vascularized and non-vascularised retina is present.
Stage 1	A fine, thin demarcation line can be seen between the vascular and avascular regions.
Stage 2	A broad, thick ridge exists between the vascular and the avascular retina.
Stage 3	Neovascularization is present on the ridge, on the posterior surface of the ridge or anteriorly toward the vitreous cavity.
Stage 4	A subtotal retinal detachment is present, beginning at the ridge.
Stage 4A	Does not involve the fovea.
Stage 4B	Involves the fovea.
Stage 5	This stage is a total retinal detachment in the shape of a funnel.
Stage 5A	An open funnel.
Stage 5B	A closed funnel.

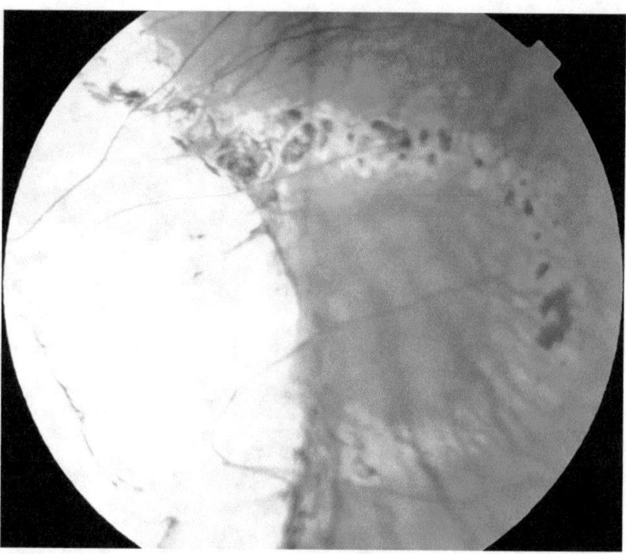

Fig. 21.52 Retinal adhesion from laser photocoagulation to prevent the spread of SRF can be employed in selected cases. This can only be used successfully in eyes in which there is very gradual fluid accumulation (tiny break or formed attached vitreous) or little momentum in the SRF to lift the adherent edge (shallow SRF or low volume of SRF). It has been used successfully in this patient with CHARGE who has a shallow "blister" of SRF leaking under the retina on the edge of the coloboma, thereby avoiding more invasive surgery in this complex case

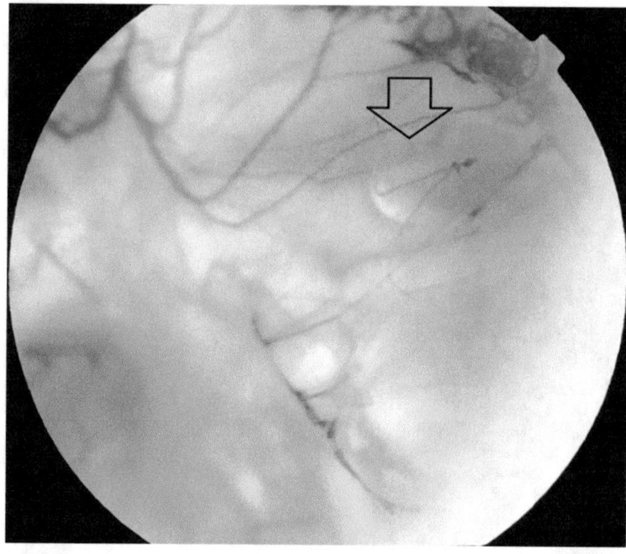

Fig. 21.53 A droplet of oil can be seen under the retina in the coloboma suggesting a communication from the vitreous cavity and the subretinal space postoperatively

Plus disease is defined as dilation and tortuosity of the peripheral retinal vessels, iris vascular engorgement, pupillary rigidity, and vitreous haze (Fig. 21.68).

Vitrectomy methods have been used for the more severe grades of retinopathy, stages 4A to 5B. Although there are reports of patients with better vision, up to 20/25 [64, 65], most successful anatomical outcomes result in "fixing and

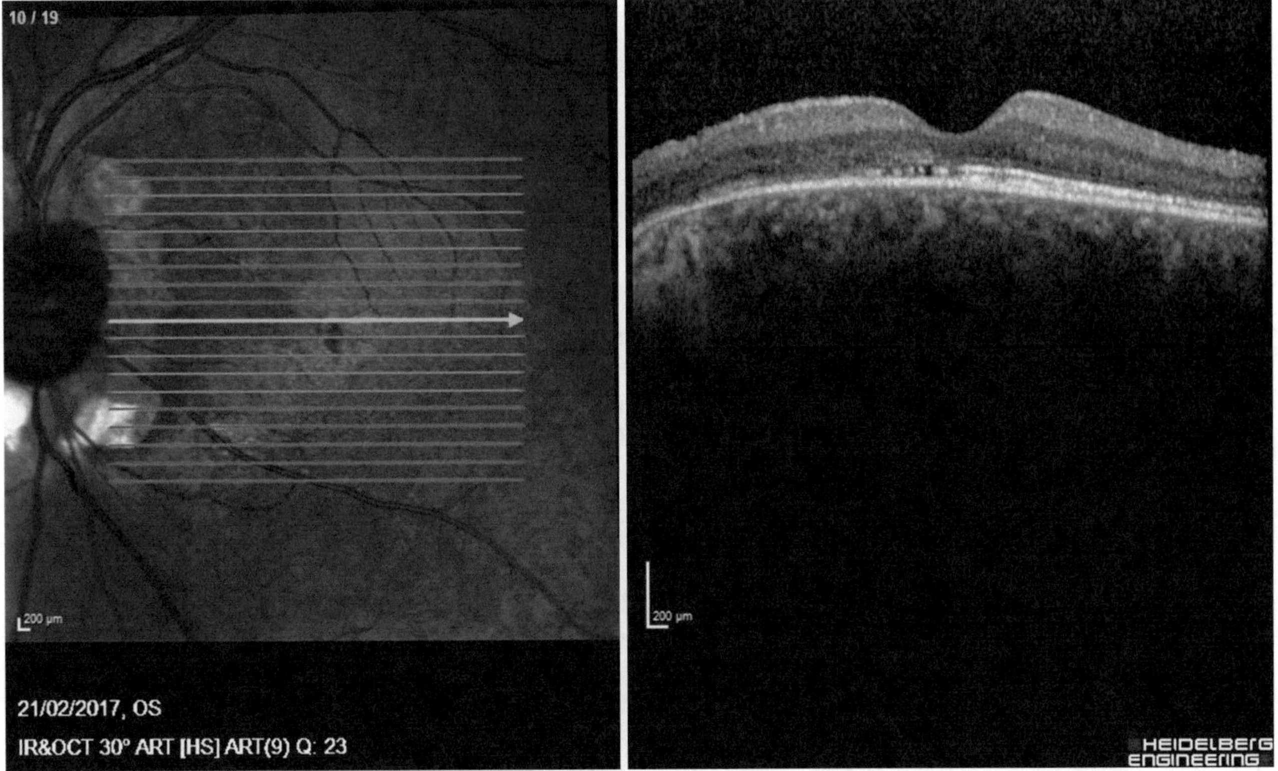

Fig. 21.54 A patient with CHARGE and an optic nerve coloboma with macular schisis treated by PPV, gas, and peripapillary laser

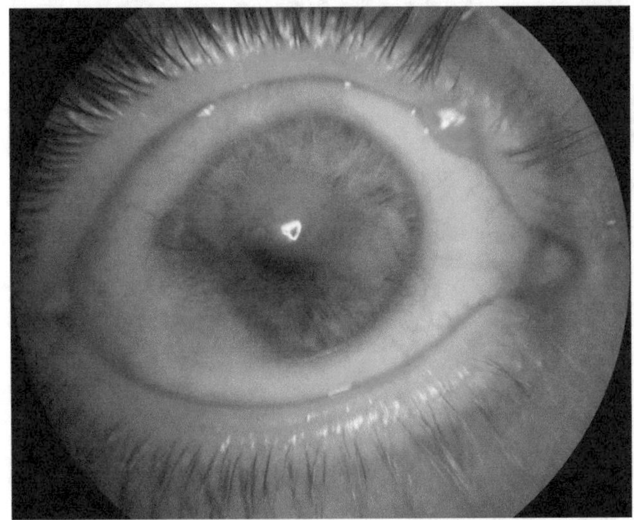

Fig. 21.55 Dermoids can be rarely associated with optic nerve coloboma in Encephalocraniocutaneous Lipomatosis

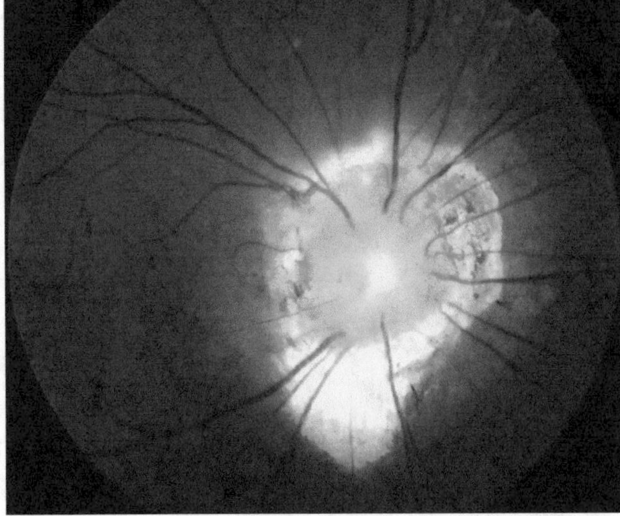

Fig. 21.56 A morning glory disc is shown, which can be associated with retinal detachment

following" acuities [66–69]. Electrophysiology has tended to confirm poor retinal function [70]. In this eventuality, functional blindness is highly likely even with surgical intervention. Initially, scleral buckling [71–73] was used, then vitrectomy was combined with lensectomy [74, 75] because of the small size of the eye and the lack of a pars plana. More recently, lens sparing techniques have been described [76–78]. Plus disease appears to be associated with a poorer chance of success [79]. It has been questioned whether patients who receive vitrectomy do any better than those who have not been operated upon [80]. PPV for stage 5 ROP achieves a flat macula in only 28–45% [81, 82].

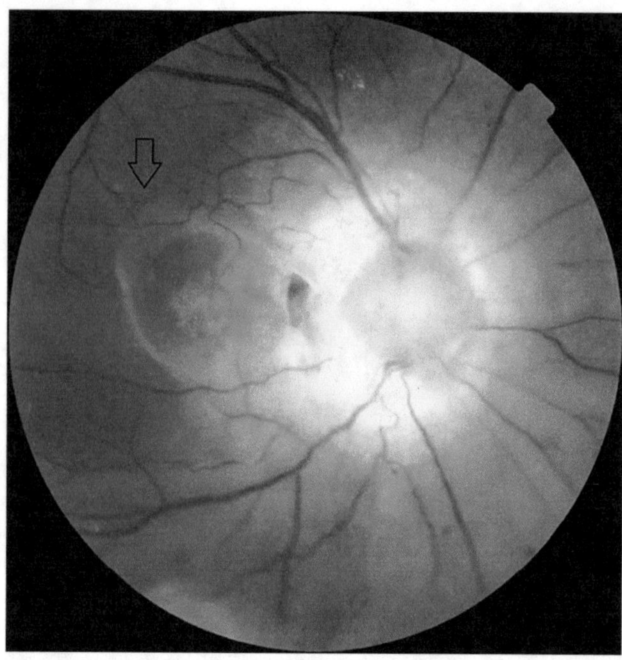

Fig. 21.57 A patient with morning glory optic nerve with a retinal elevation (arrow indicated superior edge) extending up through the fovea probably from leakage through the optic nerve head. Note the foveal pigment near the edge of the morning glory defect

Adults who suffered ROP in infancy may present in adulthood with RRD related to myopia or early PVD RRD occurs in early adulthood mean 23 years, and bilaterality is common [83]. Lattice degeneration is commonly seen [84] and tractional retinal detachments may appear. The retinas can be successfully repaired, although with a higher chance of multiple procedures of 23–50% [85–87] with final success rates of approximately 83%.

Surgical Pearl

Elevating the Hyaloid in Paediatric Rhegmatogenous Retinal Detachment

Completely disinserting the hyaloid from the surface of the retina is key to successfully repairing a rhegmatogenous retinal detachment (RRD) in the paediatric population. This act diminishes the potential contraction of hyaloid remnants and, thereby, decreases the chance of developing PVR, which is extremely high in this patient population. For a variety of reasons, complete removal of the hyaloid from the retinal surface is challenging in children. In healthy younger patients, who may have a traumatic RRD, the vitreous is very

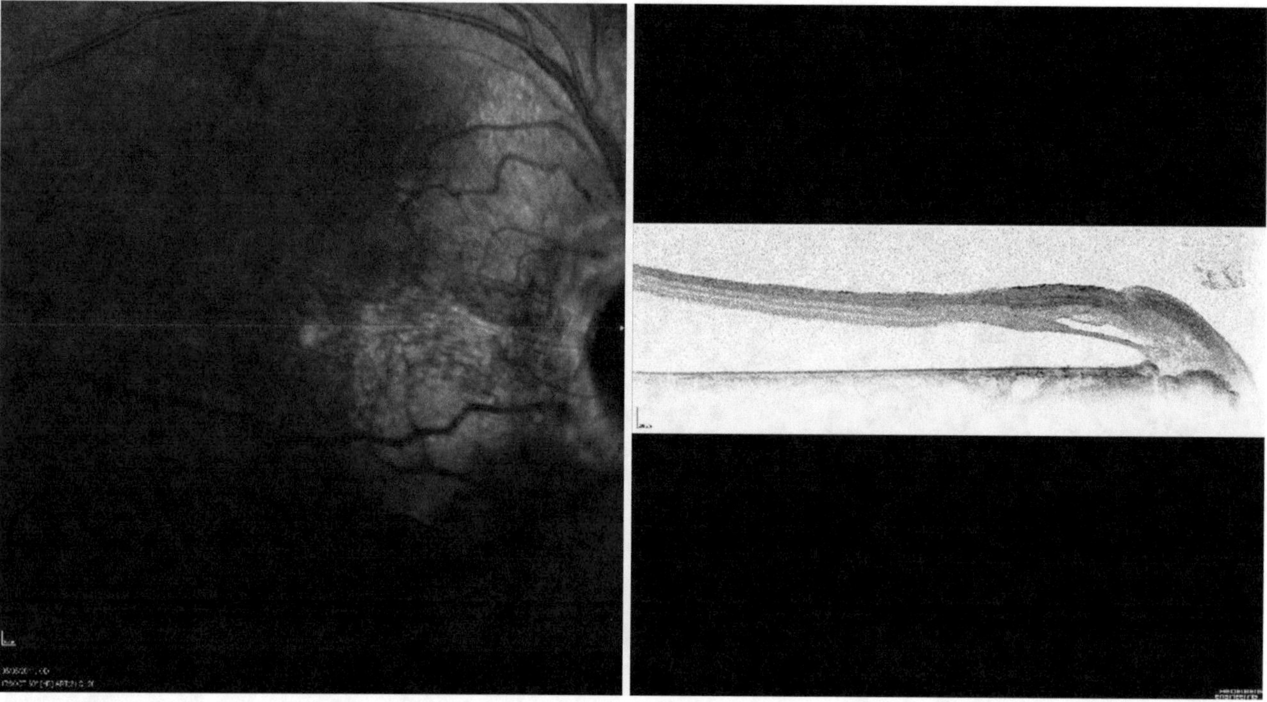

Fig. 21.58 An OCT of retinal elevation in a patient with morning glory syndrome

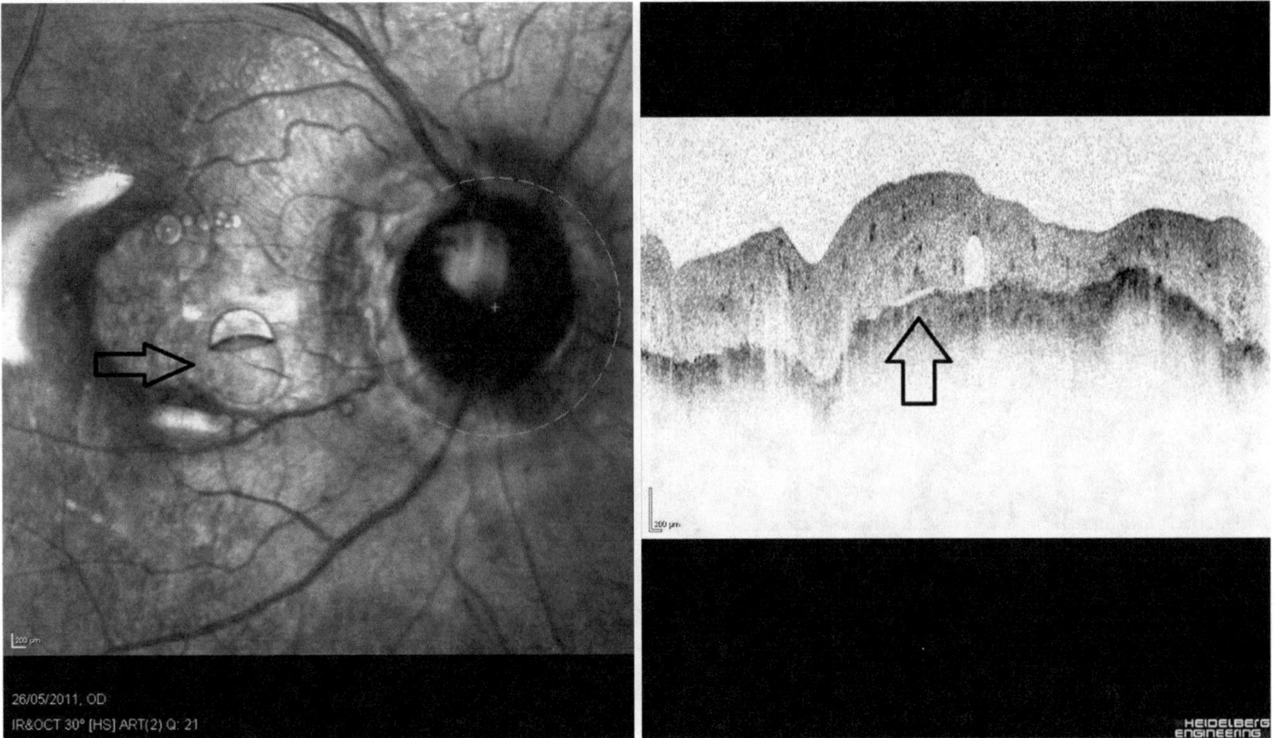

Fig. 21.59 Subretinal oil and heavy liquid can be seen in this patient with morning glory syndrome horizontal arrow. The vertical arrow may indicate a persistent communication with the optic nerve and the retina on the nasal side despite laser application

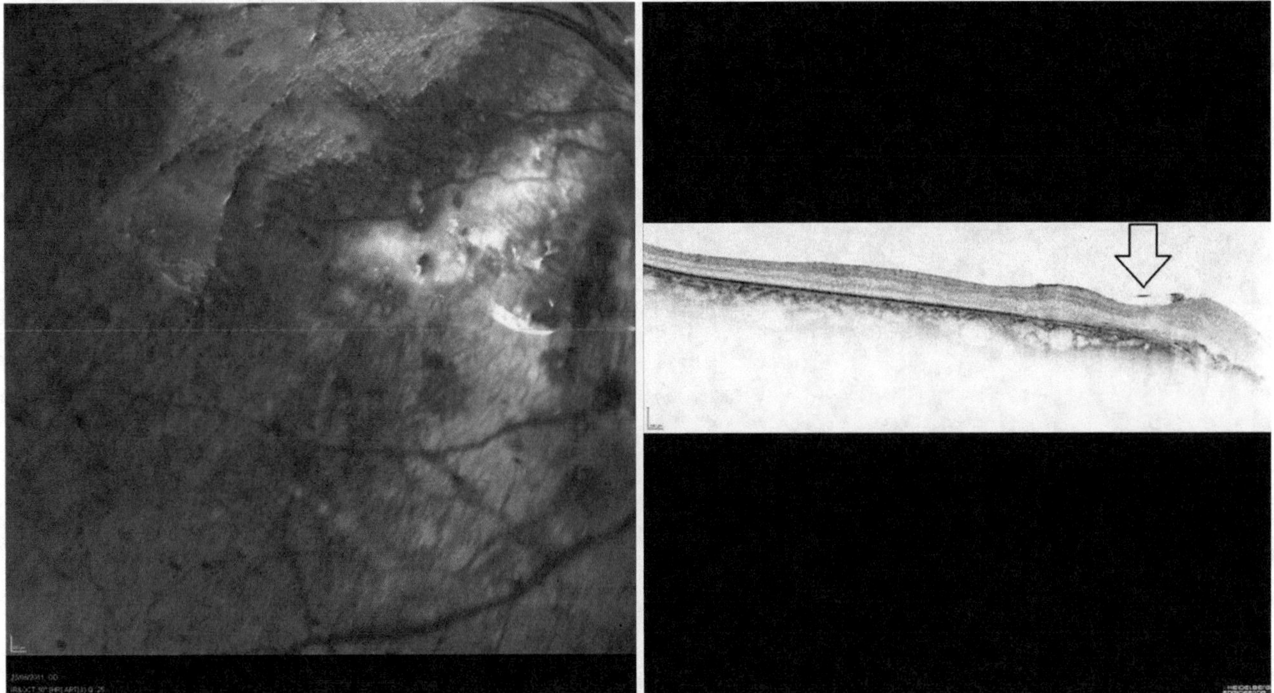

Fig. 21.60 Finally, the fovea is flattened under silicone oil after the removal of the subretinal oil and heavy liquid. Note the fovea is on the edge of the optic disc (arrow)

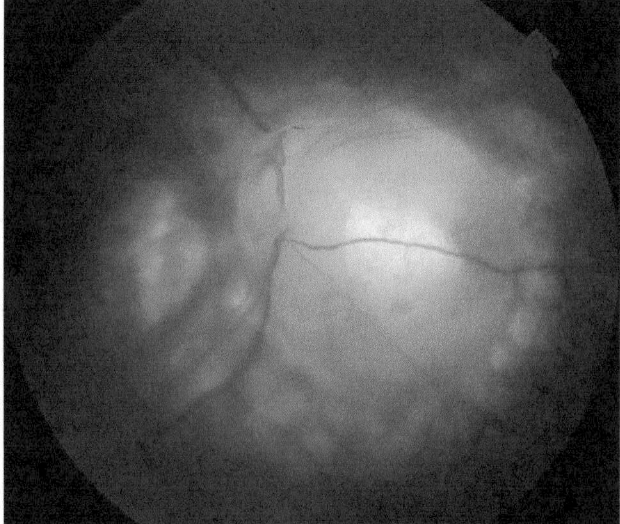

Fig. 21.61 Optic disc anomalies associated with retinal detachment have been shown to develop subretinal oil or gas, possibly through communication through the optic disc. Subretinal oil was demonstrated in this patient with an optic disc anomaly

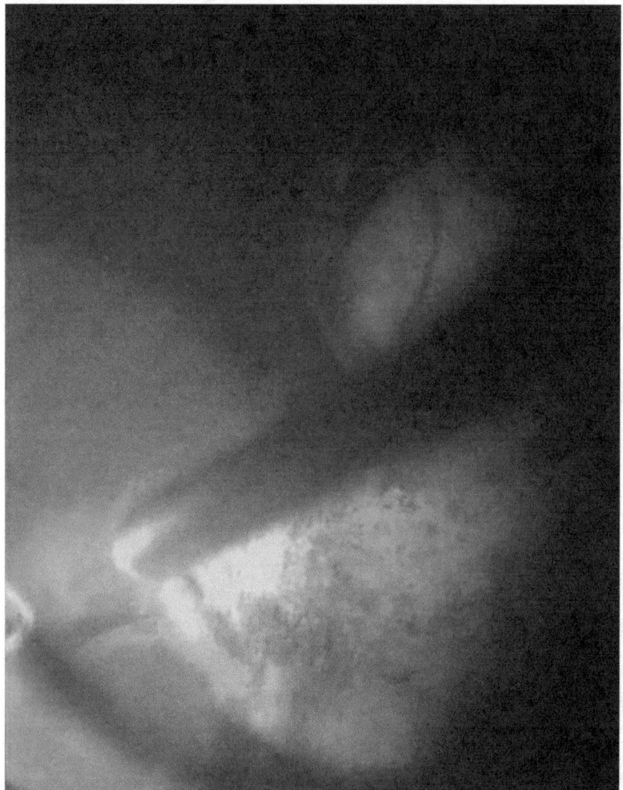

Fig. 21.62 A retinal detachment in a patient with retinochoroidal coloboma in this case with a tear between the coloboma and the ora serrata which responded to PPV and inferior indent

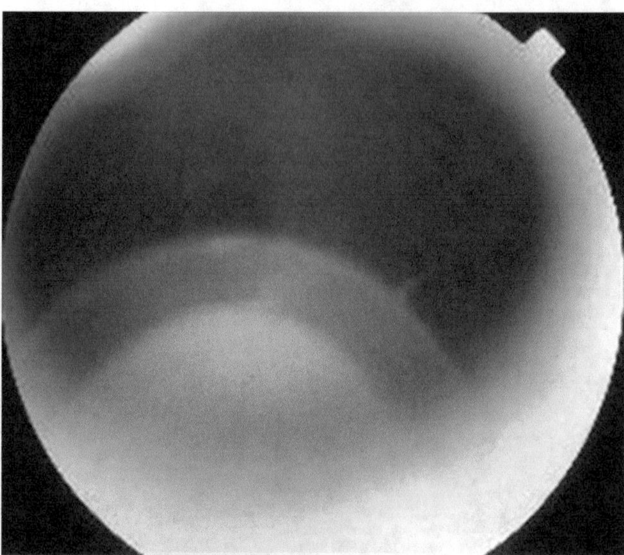

Fig. 21.63 A crystalline lens has dislocated into the posterior segment. A demarcation between the dense nuclear sclerosis and a clearer cortical lens material can be seen with some residual zonular fibres

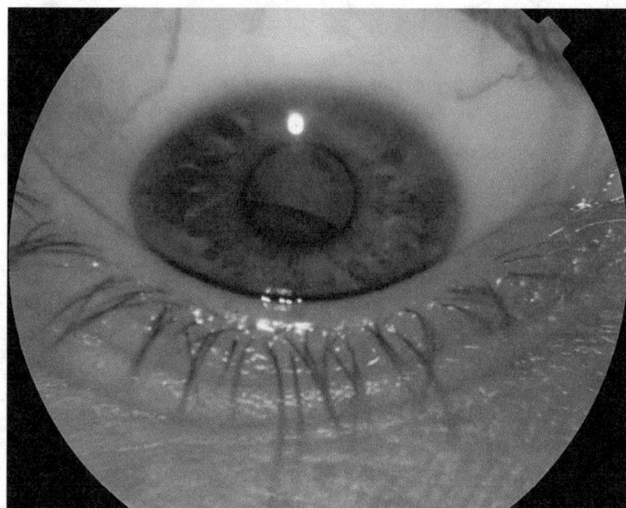

Fig. 21.64 A subluxed lens in a patient with Marfan's syndrome

well formed, and the hyaloid is very adherent to the retina. In eyes that may have more vitreous syneresis, such as Stickler's syndrome, the hyaloid will split giving the surgeon the false impression that the hyaloid was successfully disinserted. Furthermore, many children with RRDs have underlying genetic conditions, which further complicates surgery by presenting atypical vitreous behaviour and more cellular interactions between the vitreous and the retina.

For successful disinsertion of the hyaloid there are a few tricks that may be helpful:

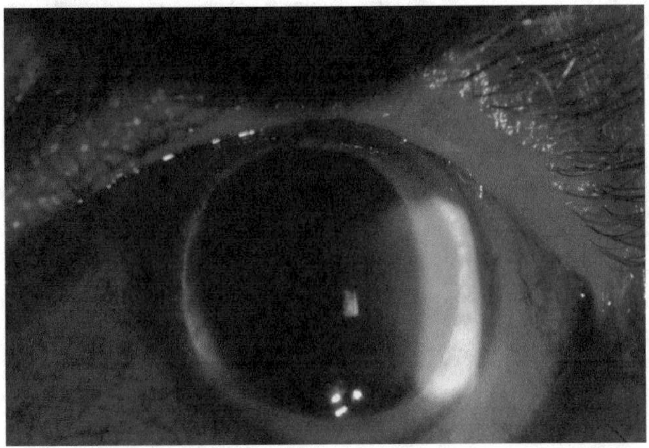

Fig. 21.65 This patient with Marfan's syndrome has a dislocated lens that has entered the anterior chamber, causing pupil block glaucoma, the iris is behind the equator of the lens. Lying the patient prone and massaging the eye allowed the lens to drop into the posterior segment with later PPV and removal of the lens

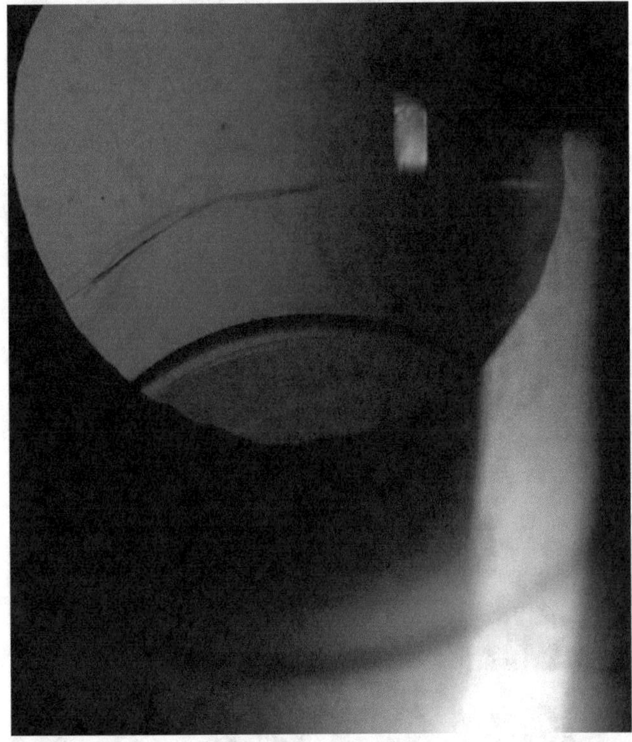

Fig. 21.66 A dislocated IOL in a patient with Marfan's syndrome

1. After removing as much vitreous as possible use a stain or triamcinolone to visualise the vitreous and hyaloid remnants.
2. Use an instrument to elevate sticky adherent hyaloid off the retina. A flex loop, Tano scraper, or MVR blade can all be employed in this move. The safest place to do this usually in the papillo-macular bundle where the macular bursa can be entered, and fluid dynamics aid in dissecting the hyaloid away from the retina.
3. Once it is felt that the hyaloid removal is complete, peel a small area of ILM. In doing so, the last sheet of split hyaloid often comes off with the ILM.
4. Use a "third" hand to help with the hyaloid dissection. A small bubble of perfluorocarbon liquid in the posterior pole acts to elevate the edge of the hyaloid while protecting the retina from the mechanical stress of pulling on the hyaloid-retina junction. Sequentially lift the hyaloid and add more perfluorocarbon to "walk" the hyaloid out to the periphery.
5. When available (such as cases where vitreomacular traction can be demonstrated), preoperative treatment with ocriplasmin is very helpful in degrading the tight adhesion of the hyaloid to the retina and significantly decreases the mechanical stress of using extrusion to elevate the hyaloid.

Kimberly Drenser, Beaumont Hospital, Royal Oak, Michigan, USA

Uveal Effusion Syndrome

Clinical Features (Figs. 21.69, 21.70, 21.71, 21.72 and Fig. 21.73)

The uveal effusion syndrome is an unusual condition often mistaken for either a rhegmatogenous detachment complicated by choroidal detachment or a "ring melanoma" of the anterior choroid. It is characterised by deep ciliochoroidal detachments, mottling of pigment epithelium (leopard spots) and serous retinal detachment, which exhibits marked "shifting fluid" (movement of subretinal fluid with gravity). Eyes may be nan ophthalmic or hypermetropic. Spontaneous resolution may occur over a period of months. The sclera is typically thickened, and it is thought fluid egress is restricted [88] (Table 21.1, Figs. 21.74 and 21.75).

Surgery

Deep sclerectomy of large patches of sclera between the extraocular muscles is effective in reversing the exudation in most patients [89]. Incise the sclera to 90% depth and excise as large a patch as possible in two quadrants. Decompression of the vortex veins, in addition, has been described but appears not to be necessary. In addition, some surgeons penetrate the sclera to create a fistula into the suprachoroidal space. Nan ophthalmic eyes are less likely to respond to surgery (Fig. 21.76).

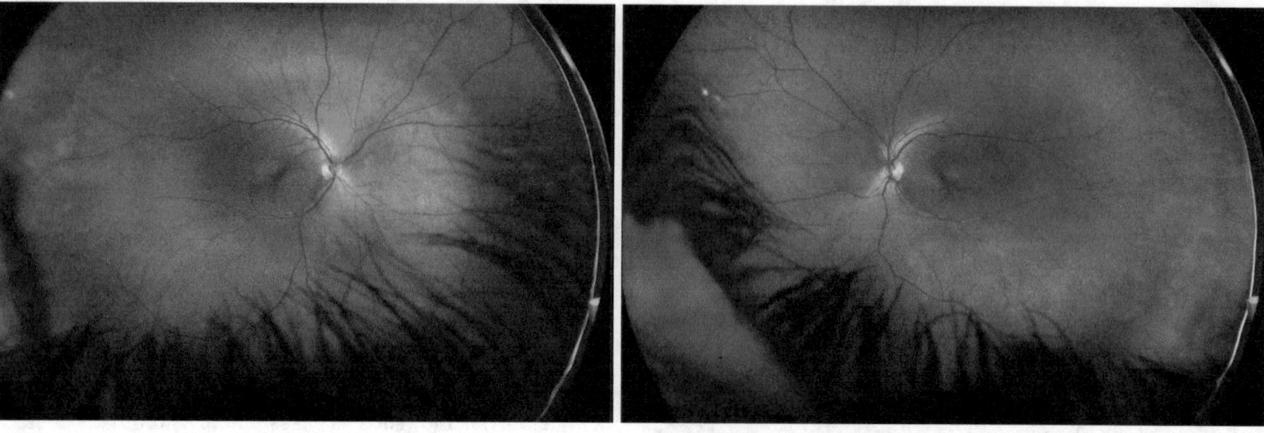

Fig. 21.67 The retinas of a patient with Marfan's syndrome. Although the eyes are myopic and at increased risk of RRD, there are often no specific retinal features

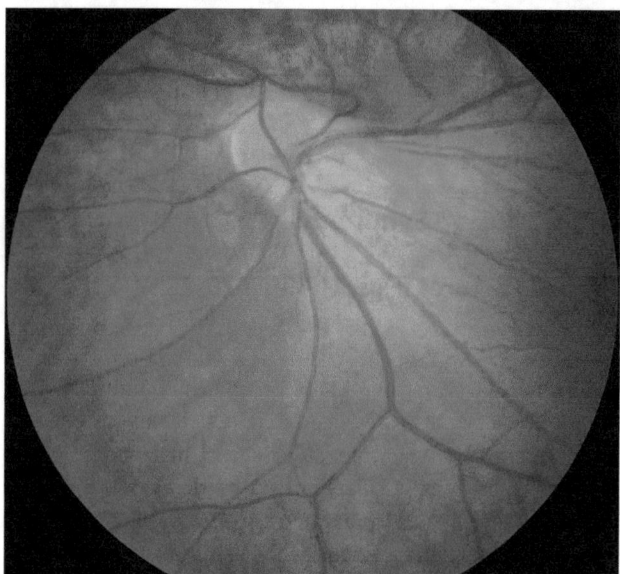

Fig. 21.68 A dragged disc in ROP

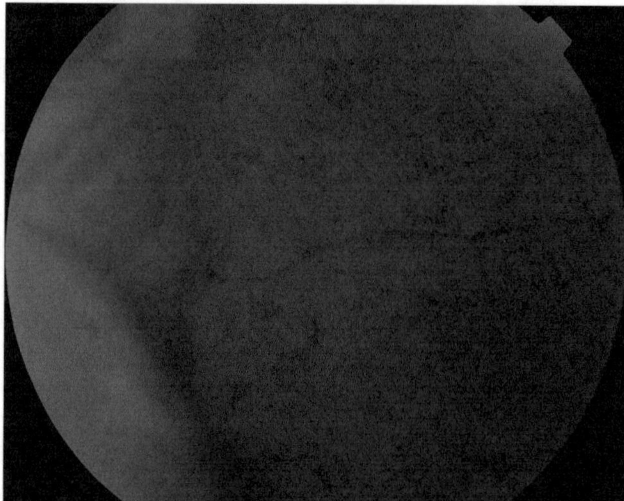

Fig. 21.69 Choroidal elevation in uveal effusion syndrome

Terson's Syndrome

Patients with subarachnoid haemorrhage from intracerebral aneurysms may develop intraocular bleeds [90–98] and have been described in as much as 20%. Histopathology has shown haemorrhage in the vitreous, subhyaloid space, sub-ILM, within the retina, in the optic nerve and the optic nerve sheath. Secondary complications such as macular hole have been seen [99]. The hyaloid is often attached during surgery, sub-ILM blood can be evacuated, but the retina may suffer damage from the blood or from subretinal or intraretinal bleeds.

The sub-ILM blood may be toxic to the retina if left too long. A high rate of entry site breaks has been reported after PPV surgery [95] (Fig. 21.77).

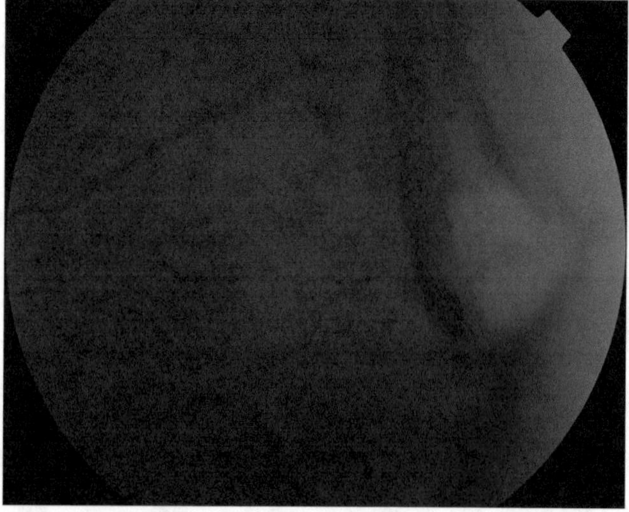

Fig. 21.70 Choroidal effusion

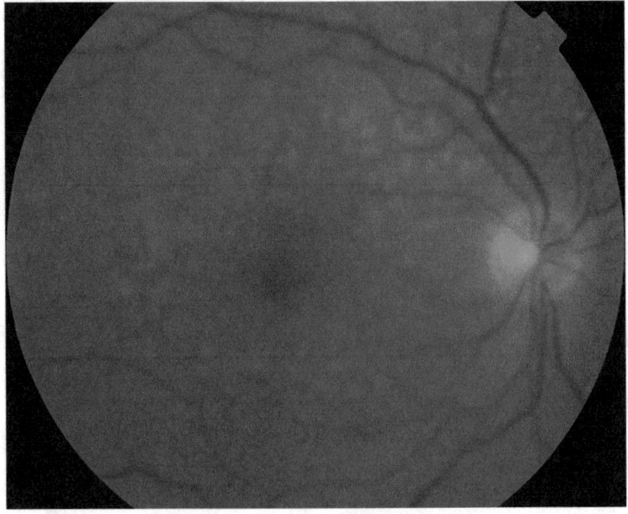

Fig. 21.71 Macular changes in uveal effusion syndrome

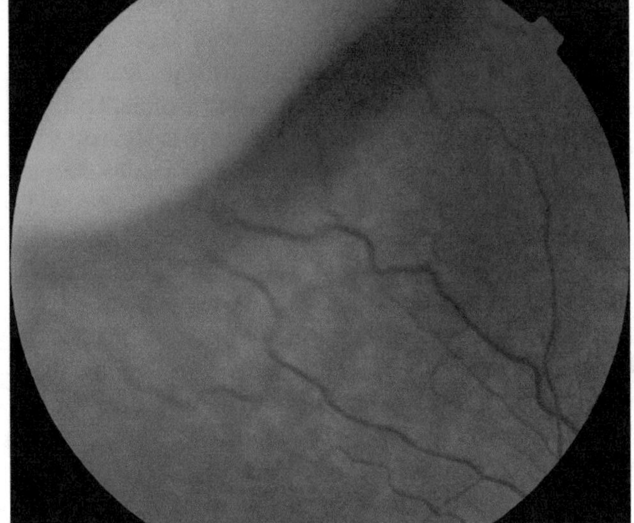

Fig. 21.72 This patient has an exudative retinal detachment from uveal effusion syndrome

Intraocular Tumours

Rarely intraocular tumours such as choroidal malignant melanoma and metastases will present with vitreous haemorrhage or serous retinal elevation [100, 101]. Vitreous biopsy without vitrectomy using a 25G cutter has been described [102–104]. Vitrectomy with endoresection of the tumour is used in specialised centres for selected cases [105–108]. The vitrectomy surgeon may be called upon to deal with various complications of treatment of melanoma, including ERM, macular hole, vitreous haemorrhage and retinal detachment [109–116]. A para-neoplastic effect may severely reduce retinal function bilaterally [117] (Figs. 21.78 and 21.79)

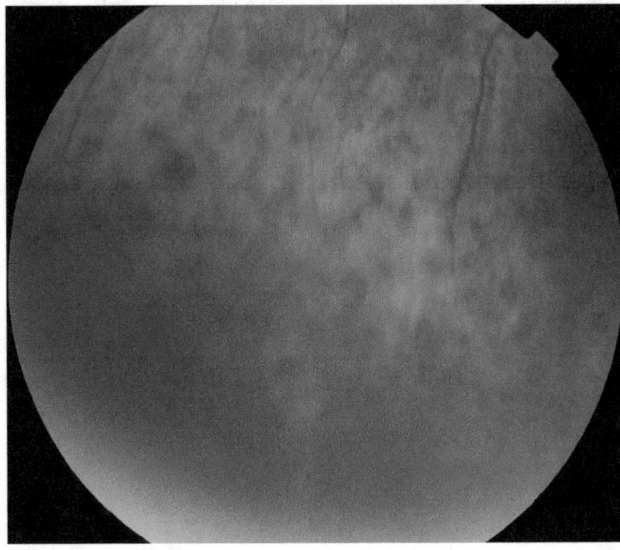

Fig. 21.73 Typical leopard spots in a patient with uveal effusion syndrome

Table 21.1 Causes of exudative retinal detachment

Exudative Retinal Detachment, common causes	
Uveal effusion syndrome	
Coat's disease	
Central serous retinopathy	
Dominant exudative vitreoretinopathy	
Idiopathic telangiectasia	
Scleritis	Wegener's granulomatosis Rheumatoid arthritis
Endophthalmitis/cellulitis	
Uveitis	Vogt Koyanagi-Harada syndrome Acute multifocal posterior pigment epitheliopathy
Vasculitis	
Tumours	Malignant melanoma Metastases Haemangioma Von Hippel–Lindau syndrome
Vasculopathic	Toxaemia of pregnancy Hypertensive retinopathy Ocular ischaemia
Surgery/laser	

Disseminated Intravascular Coagulation (Fig. 21.80)

This severe presentation after septicaemia, involving widespread intravascular coagulation resulting in loss of clotting factors, is associated with multiorgan vascular occlusion and haemorrhage. In the eye, it has been associated with choroidal infarction and vitreous haemorrhage with retinal damage and proliferative vitreoretinopathy [118] (Fig. 21.81).

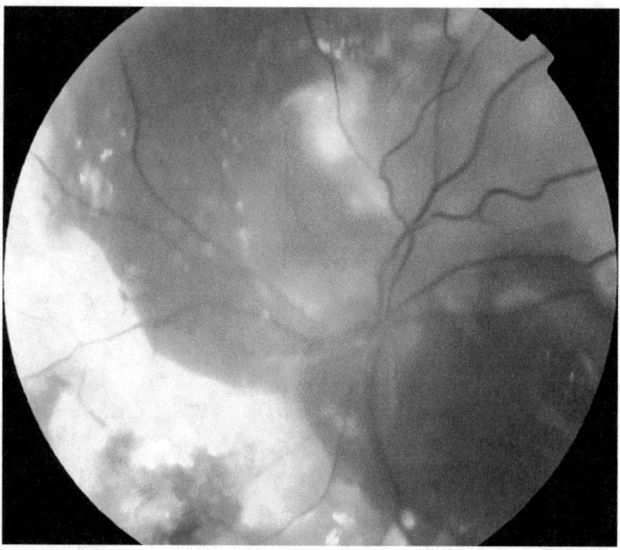

Fig. 21.74 Coat's disease in an 8-year-old boy with counting fingers vision. In general, with unilateral Coat's disease treatments are not worthwhile as the other eye is good, and any intervention may disturb the anatomy of the eye producing cosmetic problems

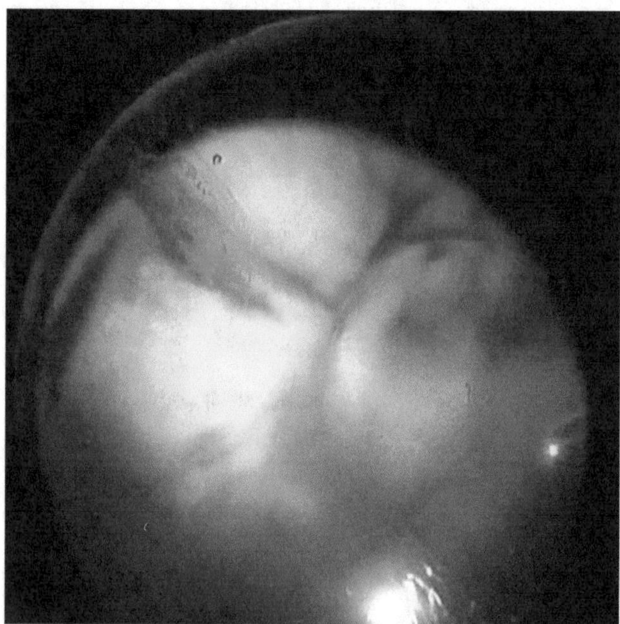

Fig. 21.75 Familial exudative vitreoretinopathy may present with vitreous haemorrhage or exudative retinal detachment

Hypotony and Pre-Phthisis Bulbi

Some patients will have hypotony because of RRD and repair of the RD will reverse the hypotony. Anterior surgery may create a cyclodialysis cleft which results in low IOP and repair of this by stitching the ciliary body back onto the sclera will increase the IOP (Fig. 21.82).

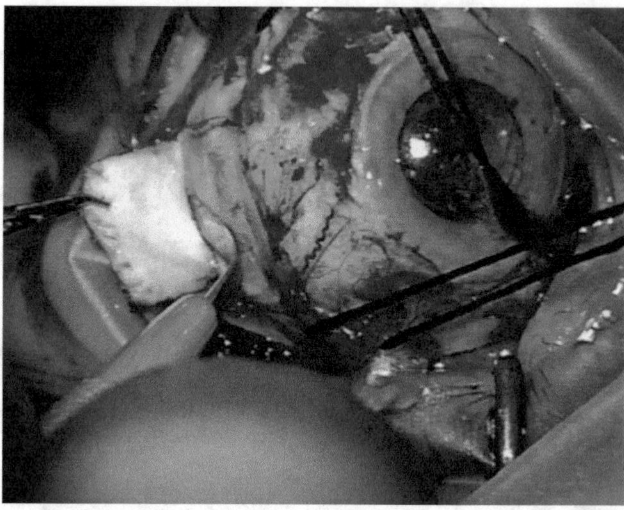

Fig. 21.76 A deep sclerotomy has been created as deep as possible in uveal effusion syndrome

Others will have complex ocular conditions such as chronic uveitis, trauma, or failed posterior segment surgery, which may lead to hypotony and eventually phthisis bulbi for which re-establishment of the IOP is not possible. There is a period that may last months when the eye is shrinking, but irreversible phthisis has not occurred. This can be detected by shortening the axial length and early infolding of the sclera. This is a window of opportunity to fill the eye with silicone oil to act as a spacer to prevent further shrinkage and to maintain vision. Often this will need to be combined with ambitious anterior segment surgery such as the Boston Keratoprosthesis (BKP) [119, 120]. Care for the BKP requires considerable commitment from the patient but surprisingly good vision can be obtained (Fig. 21.83).

Even with successful surgery, the patient will still have hypotony and will suffer hypotony-related cystoid macular oedema. Persistent retinal detachment may resolve as the sclera shrinks slightly onto the oil.

Retinal Prosthesis

Retinal electrodes are being designed and trailed in patients with retinitis pigmentosa. As yet a definitive design has not been established, but early systems have shown encouraging results for levels of vision, e.g. 16 pixels [121, 122].

Summary

The rarity of some of these conditions means that exact patterns of clinical care have not been well defined. It is up to the surgeon to develop experience over the years and to use

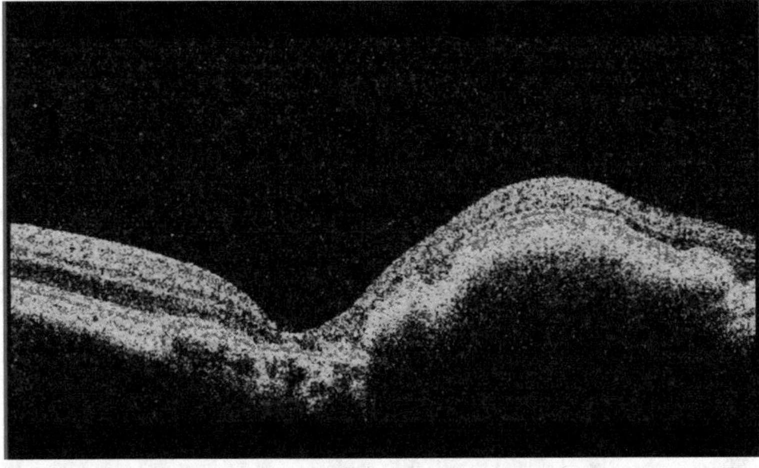
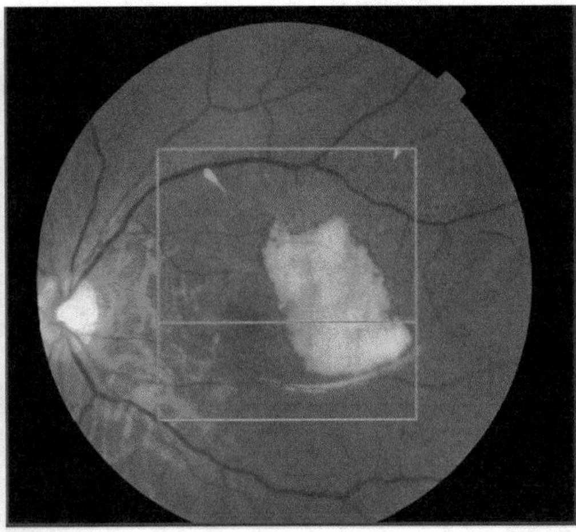

Fig. 21.77 This patient was found to have a subretinal haemorrhage adjacent to the fovea after removal of vitreous haemorrhage from Terson's syndrome. The vision remained at 20/120 despite retraction of the subretinal haemorrhage from the fovea

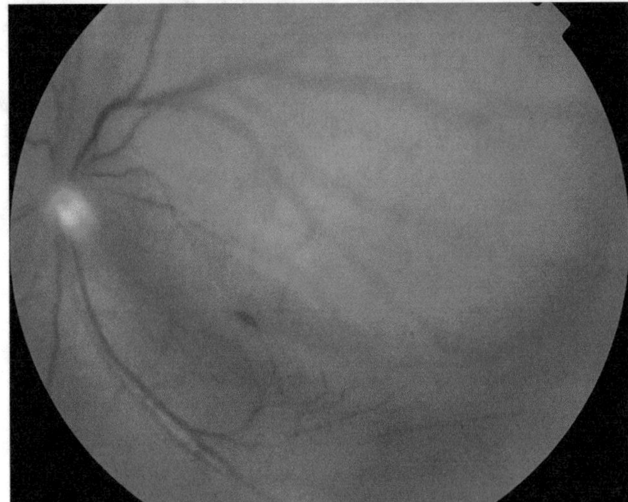

Fig. 21.78 Serous elevation secondary to a choroidal mass

this to best manage these patients. Use the principles applied to the commoner conditions as a guide but be aware there are differences in the rarer conditions in how they will respond to surgery.

Condition and referral

Condition	Characteristics	Referral	Why
Symptomatic PVD	Symptoms less than 6 weeks	Immediate	Risk of retinal breaks
	Symptoms more than 6 weeks	Routine	Risk of retinal breaks leading to RRD is low
RRD with PVD	Macula on	Immediate	Prevent macula detaching
	Macula off less 1–3 days	Immediate	Best results with prompt surgery
	Macula off less 4–7 days	1–3 days	Macula should recover well
	Macula off 1–2 weeks	1 week	Macula should recover well
	Macula off 2–6 weeks	1–2 weeks	Macula will show moderate recovery
	Macula off >6 weeks	2–3 weeks	Macula unlikely to recover well
RRD without PVD		1 week	Slow progression
Macular hole	Duration <12 months	Refer 1 month	Good surgical results
	Duration >12 months	Discuss poor prognosis and refer if requested	Poor surgical results
Macular pucker	Duration <24 months	Refer routinely	Good surgical results
	Duration >24 months	Discuss poor prognosis and refer if requested	Poor surgical results
Trauma	Rupture	1–2 weeks	After primary repair and antibiotics
	Penetrating	1–2 weeks	After primary repair and antibiotics
	Penetrating with IOFB	Immediate	For antibiotics then IOFB removal
	Contusion	1–2 weeks	Depends on retinal complication
Dropped nucleus	All	1 week	Control IOP and inflammation
Complicated cataract Operation		Routine referral for assessment	Risk of RRD

Condition	Characteristics	Referral	Why
Diabetic	Vitreous haemorrhage with PRP	Routine referral	
	Tractional RD with PRP	Routine referral	
	Vitreous haemorrhage without PRP	2–3 weeks	
	Tractional RD without PRP	2–3 weeks	
	Combined RRD /TRD	1 week	
Non-diabetic vitreous haemorrhage	PVD	Immediate	
	No PVD	2–3 weeks	
	Subretinal blood	1–3 days	

This table is a guide to the urgency of referral to a vitreoretinal service, it is assumed that access to the service is approximately 6–8 weeks for a routine appointment. The referral patterns are generalisations only and there will be circumstances where more urgent referral is required for a particular patient. In addition, local services should be consulted for their referral criteria and recommendations.

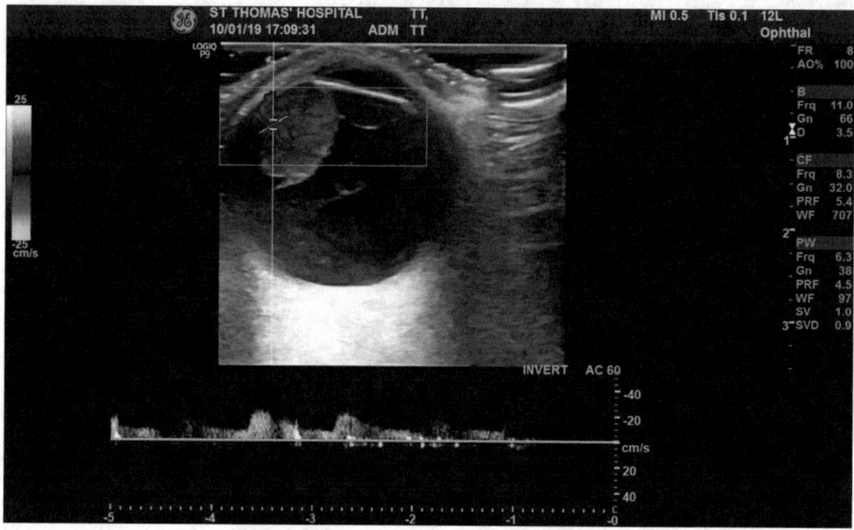

Fig. 21.79 A tumour circulation in a choroidal melanoma

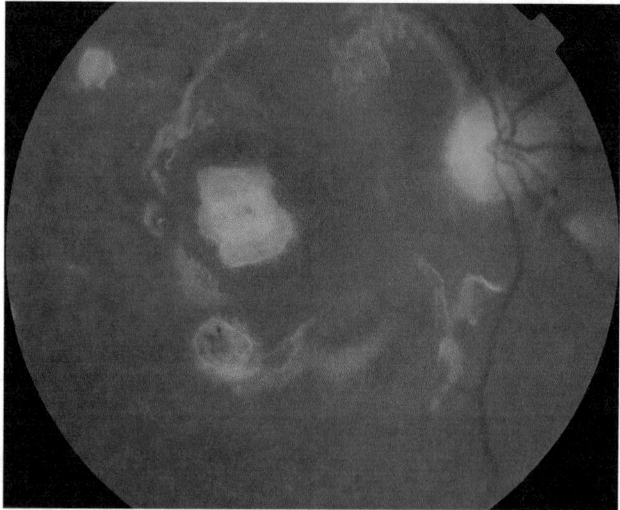

Fig. 21.80 A patient with disseminated intravascular coagulation and severe haemorrhage 6 years after surgery with a large macular hole and silicone oil in situ

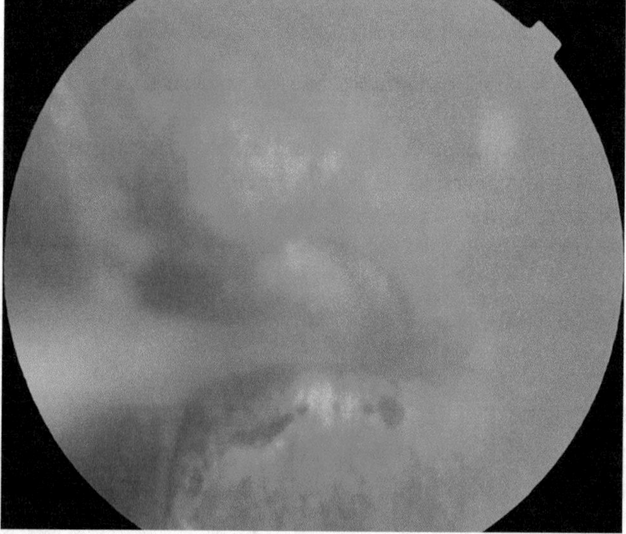

Fig. 21.81 This patient had a cataract removed in infancy to reveal a posterior persistent hyaloid artery which was a membrane from the optic disc to the back of the lens. There was dragging of peripheral ciliary pigment epithelium into the membrane at its anterior end

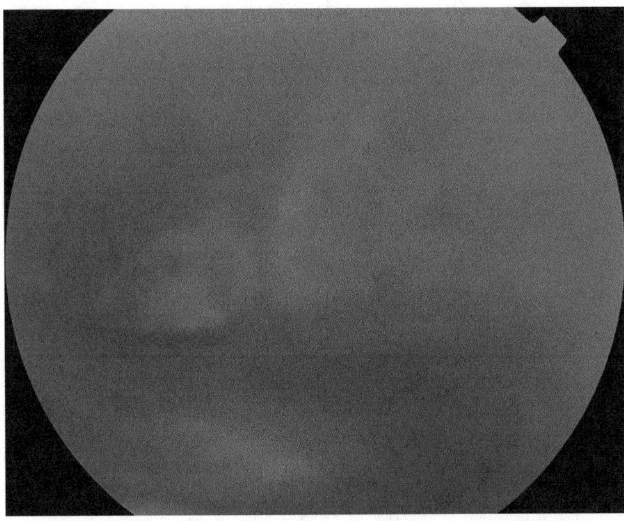

Fig. 21.82 The folds in the posterior layers of the eye are a precursor to phthisis in this patient with panuveitis. The surgeon may choose to fill the eye with silicone oil to retain a cosmetically acceptable globe size and shape, and vision of low grade

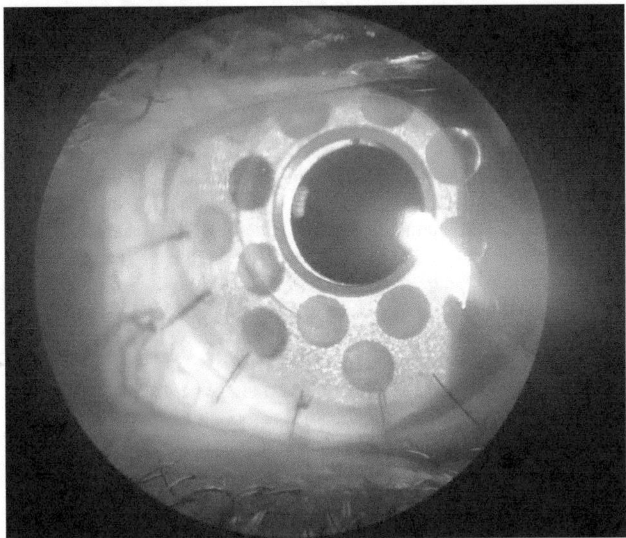

Fig. 21.83 A Boston Keratoprosthesis used to restore the anterior segment in a patient with pre-phthisis

References

1. Sebag J, Yee KMP, Nguyen JH, Nguyen-Cuu J. Long-term safety and efficacy of limited Vitrectomy for vision degrading Vitreopathy resulting from vitreous floaters. Ophthalmol Retina. 2018;2(9):881–7. https://doi.org/10.1016/j.oret.2018.03.011.
2. Milston R, Madigan MC, Sebag J. Vitreous floaters: etiology, diagnostics, and management. Surv Ophthalmol. 2016;61(2):211–27. https://doi.org/10.1016/j.survophthal.2015.11.008.
3. Mamou J, Wa CA, Yee KM, Silverman RH, Ketterling JA, Sadun AA, et al. Ultrasound-based quantification of vitreous floaters correlates with contrast sensitivity and quality of life. Invest Ophthalmol Vis Sci. 2015;56(3):1611–7. https://doi.org/10.1167/iovs.14-15414.
4. Sebag J, Yee KM, Wa CA, Huang LC, Sadun AA. Vitrectomy for floaters: prospective efficacy analyses and retrospective safety profile. Retina. 2014;34(6):1062–8. https://doi.org/10.1097/IAE.0000000000000065.
5. Wa C, Sebag J. Safety of vitrectomy for floaters. Am J Ophthalmol. 2011;152(6):1077.; author reply 8. https://doi.org/10.1016/j.ajo.2011.09.003.
6. Sebag J. Floaters and the quality of life. Am J Ophthalmol. 2011;152(1):3–4. e1. https://doi.org/10.1016/j.ajo.2011.02.015.
7. Yee KMP, Tan S, Lesnik Oberstein SY, Filas B, Nguyen JH, Nguyen-Cuu J, et al. Incidence of cataract surgery after Vitrectomy for vitreous opacities. Ophthalmol Retina. 2017;1(2):154–7. https://doi.org/10.1016/j.oret.2016.11.012.
8. Laatikainen L, Tarkkanen A. Microsurgery of persistent hyperplastic primary vitreous. Ophthalmologica. 1982;185(4):193–8.
9. Winkler J, Lunsdorf H. Ultrastructure and composition of asteroid bodies. Invest Ophthalmol Vis Sci. 2001;42(5):902–7.
10. Fawzi AA, Vo B, Kriwanek R, Ramkumar HL, Cha C, Carts A, et al. Asteroid hyalosis in an autopsy population: the University of California at Los Angeles (UCLA) experience. Arch Ophthalmol. 2005;123(4):486–90.
11. Parnes RE, Zakov ZN, Novak MA, Rice TA. Vitrectomy in patients with decreased visual acuity secondary to asteroid hyalosis. Am J Ophthalmol. 1998;125(5):703–4.
12. Feist RM, Morris RE, Witherspoon CD, Blair NP, Ticho BH, White MF Jr. Vitrectomy in asteroid hyalosis. Retina. 1990;10(3):173–7.
13. Renaldo DP. Pars plana vitrectomy for asteroid hyalosis. Retina. 1981;1(3):252–4.
14. Tamez H, Patel S, Agarwal A. Ocular Amyloidosis. Ophthalmology. 2017;124(9):1367. https://doi.org/10.1016/j.ophtha.2017.02.029.
15. Venkatesh P, Selvan H, Singh SB, Gupta D, Kashyap S, Temkar S, et al. Vitreous amyloidosis: ocular, systemic, and genetic insights. Ophthalmology. 2017;124(7):1014–22. https://doi.org/10.1016/j.ophtha.2017.03.011.
16. Schweitzer K, Ehmann D, Garcia R, Alport E. Oculoleptomeningeal amyloidosis in 3 individuals with the transthyretin variant Tyr69His. Can J Ophthalmol. 2009;44(3):317–9. doi: i09-023 [pii]. https://doi.org/10.3129/i09-023.
17. Gregory ME, Carey M, Hawkins PN, Banerjee S, Gillmore JD. Characterisation and management of vitreous and nerve amyloid in familial amyloid polyneuropathy due to variant transthyretin, Phe33Val. Br J Ophthalmol. 2008;92(1):34–5. 142. doi: 92/1/34 [pii]. https://doi.org/10.1136/bjo.2007.124123.
18. Koga T, Ando E, Hirata A, Fukushima M, Kimura A, Ando Y, et al. Vitreous opacities and outcome of vitreous surgery in patients with familial amyloidotic polyneuropathy. Am J Ophthalmol. 2003;135(2):188–93.
19. Li AS, Capone A Jr, Trese MT, Sears JE, Kychenthal A, De la Huerta I, et al. Long-term outcomes of Total exudative retinal detachments in stage 3B coats disease. Ophthalmology. 2018;125(6):887–93. https://doi.org/10.1016/j.ophtha.2017.12.010.
20. Yadav NK, Vasudha K, Gupta K, Shetty KB. Vitrectomy for epiretinal membrane secondary to treatment for juvenile Coats' disease. Eye (Lond). 2013;27(2):278–80. doi: eye2012275 [pii]. https://doi.org/10.1038/eye.2012.275.
21. Schmidt-Erfurth U, Lucke K. Vitreoretinal surgery in advanced Coat's disease. Ger J Ophthalmol. 1995;4(1):32–6.
22. Yoshizumi MO, Kreiger AE, Lewis H, Foxman B, Hakakha BA. Vitrectomy techniques in late-stage Coats'-like exudative retinal detachment. Doc Ophthalmol. 1995;90(4):387–94.
23. Singh AD, Nouri M, Shields CL, Shields JA, Smith AF. Retinal capillary hemangioma: a comparison of sporadic cases and cases

associated with von Hippel-Lindau disease. Ophthalmology. 2001;108(10):1907–11.
24. Singh A, Shields J, Shields C. Solitary retinal capillary hemangioma: hereditary (von Hippel-Lindau disease) or nonhereditary? Arch Ophthalmol. 2001;119(2):232–4.
25. Singh AD, Shields CL, Shields JA. von Hippel-Lindau Disease. Surv Ophthalmol. 2001;46(2):117–42.
26. Singh AD, Nouri M, Shields CL, Shields JA, Perez N. Treatment of retinal capillary hemangioma. Ophthalmology. 2002;109(10):1799–806.
27. Gray RH, Gregor ZJ. Acquired peripheral retinal telangiectasia after retinal surgery. Retina. 1994;14(1):10–3.
28. Inoue M, Yamazaki K, Shinoda K, Ishida S, Shinoda H, Noda K, et al. A clinicopathologic case report on macular hole associated with von Hippel-Lindau disease: a novel ultrastructural finding of wormlike, wavy tangles of filaments. Graefes Arch Clin Exp Ophthalmol. 2004;242(10):881–6.
29. Schwartz PL, Fastenberg DM, Shakin JL. Management of macular puckers associated with retinal angiomas. Ophthalmic Surg. 1990;21(8):550–6.
30. Laatikainen L, Immonen I, Summanen P. Peripheral retinal angioma like lesion and macular pucker. Am J Ophthalmol. 1989;108(5):563–6.
31. Ferguson A, Singh J. Total exudative detachment as a first presentation of von Hippel Lindau disease. Br J Ophthalmol. 2002;86(6):701–2.
32. Loewenstein JI. Bilateral macular holes in von Hippel-Lindau disease. Arch Ophthalmol. 1995;113(2):143–4.
33. Machemer R, Williams JM Sr. Pathogenesis and therapy of traction detachment in various retinal vascular diseases. Am J Ophthalmol. 1988;105(2):170–81.
34. Raju B, Majji AB, Jalali S. von Hippel angioma in south Indian subjects--a clinical study. Retina. 2003;23(5):670–4.
35. Raja D, Benz MS, Murray TG, Escalona-Benz EM, Markoe A. Salvage external beam radiotherapy of retinal capillary hemangiomas secondary to von Hippel-Lindau disease: visual and anatomic outcomes. Ophthalmology. 2004;111(1):150–3.
36. Garcia-Arumi J, Sararols LH, Cavero L, Escalada F, Corcostegui BF. Therapeutic options for capillary papillary hemangiomas. Ophthalmology. 2000;107(1):48–54.
37. Kashani AH, Brown KT, Chang E, Drenser KA, Capone A, Trese MT. Diversity of retinal vascular anomalies in patients with familial exudative vitreoretinopathy. Ophthalmology. 2014;121(11):2220–7. https://doi.org/10.1016/j.ophtha.2014.05.029.
38. Katagiri S, Yokoi T, Yoshida-Uemura T, Nishina S, Azuma N. Characteristics of retinal breaks and surgical outcomes in Rhegmatogenous retinal detachment in familial exudative Vitreoretinopathy. Ophthalmol Retina. 2018;2(7):720–5. https://doi.org/10.1016/j.oret.2017.11.003.
39. Steel DHW, Suleman J, Murphy DC, Song A, Dodds S, Rees J. Optic disc pit Maculopathy: a two-year Nationwide prospective population-based study. Ophthalmology. 2018;125(11):1757–64. https://doi.org/10.1016/j.ophtha.2018.05.009.
40. Steel DH, Williamson TH, Laidlaw DA, Sharma P, Matthews C, Rees J, et al. Extent and location of Intraretinal and subretinal fluid as prognostic factors for the outcome of patients with optic disk pit Maculopathy. Retina. 2016;36(1):110–8. https://doi.org/10.1097/IAE.0000000000000658.
41. Garcia-Arumi J, Guraya BC, Espax AB, Castillo VM, Ramsay LS, Motta RM. Optical coherence tomography in optic pit maculopathy managed with vitrectomy-laser-gas. Graefes Arch Clin Exp Ophthalmol. 2004;242(10):819–26.
42. Lincoff H, Kreissig I. Optical coherence tomography of pneumatic displacement of optic disc pit maculopathy. Br J Ophthalmol. 1998;82(4):367–72.
43. Hirakata A, Okada AA, Hida T. Long-term results of vitrectomy without laser treatment for macular detachment associated with an optic disc pit. Ophthalmology. 2005;112(8):1430–5.
44. Rizzo S, Caporossi T, Pacini B, De Angelis L, De Vitto ML, Gainsanti F. Management of Optic Disk pit-associated Macular Detachment with human amniotic membrane patch. Retina. 2020; https://doi.org/10.1097/IAE.0000000000002753.
45. Zheng A, Singh RP, Lavine JA. Surgical options and outcomes in the treatment of optic pit Maculopathy: a meta-analysis and systematic review. Ophthalmol Retina. 2019; https://doi.org/10.1016/j.oret.2019.10.011.
46. Dureau P, Ttie-Bitach T, Salomon R, Bettembourg O, Amiel J, Uteza Y, et al. Renal coloboma syndrome. Ophthalmology. 2001;108(10):1912–6.
47. Haik BG, Greenstein SH, Smith ME, Abramson DH, Ellsworth RM. Retinal detachment in the morning glory anomaly. Ophthalmology. 1984;91(12):1638–47.
48. Chang S, Haik BG, Ellsworth RM, St LL, Berrocal JA. Treatment of total retinal detachment in morning glory syndrome. Am J Ophthalmol. 1984;97(5):596–600.
49. Irvine AR, Crawford JB, Sullivan JH. The pathogenesis of retinal detachment with morning glory disc and optic pit. Retina. 1986;6(3):146–50.
50. Coll GE, Chang S, Flynn TE, Brown GC. Communication between the subretinal space and the vitreous cavity in the morning glory syndrome. Graefes Arch Clin Exp Ophthalmol. 1995;233(7):441–3.
51. Steahly LP. Retinochoroidal coloboma: varieties of clinical presentations. Ann Ophthalmol. 1990;22(1):9–14.
52. Corcostegui B, Guell JL, Garcia-Arumi J. Surgical treatment of retinal detachment in the choroidal colobomas. Retina. 1992;12(3):237–41.
53. Gopal L, Kini MM, Badrinath SS, Sharma T. Management of retinal detachment with choroidal coloboma. Ophthalmology. 1991;98(11):1622–7.
54. Gopal L, Badrinath SS, Sharma T, Parikh SN, Biswas J. Pattern of retinal breaks and retinal detachments in eyes with choroidal coloboma. Ophthalmology. 1995;102(8):1212–7.
55. McDonald HR, Lewis H, Brown G, Sipperley JO. Vitreous surgery for retinal detachment associated with choroidal coloboma. Arch Ophthalmol. 1991;109(10):1399–402.
56. Hotta K, Hirakata A, Hida T. The management of retinal detachments associated with choroidal colobomas by vitrectomy with cyanoacrylate retinopexy. Jpn J Ophthalmol. 1998;42(4):323–6.
57. Abboud EB. Retinal detachment surgery in Marfan's syndrome. Retina. 1998;18(5):405–9.
58. Dotrelova D, Karel I, Clupkova E. Retinal detachment in Marfan's syndrome. Characteristics and surgical results. Retina. 1997;17(5):390–6.
59. Hubbard AD, Charteris DG, Cooling RJ. Vitreolensectomy in Marfan's syndrome. Eye. 1998;12(Pt 3a):412–6.
60. Bading G, Hillenkamp J, Sachs HG, Gabel VP, Framme C. Long-term safety and functional outcome of combined pars plana vitrectomy and scleral-fixated sutured posterior chamber lens implantation. Am J Ophthalmol. 2007;144(3):371–7. doi: S0002-9394(07)00480-1 [pii]. https://doi.org/10.1016/j.ajo.2007.05.014.
61. Johnston RL, Charteris DG, Horgan SE, Cooling RJ. Combined pars plana vitrectomy and sutured posterior chamber implant. Arch Ophthalmol. 2000;118(7):905–10.
62. Abourizk N, Ishaq AM, Arora T, Briones JC, Kaldany A, Aiello LM, et al. Ocular surgery in patients with diabetic nephropathy. Diabetes Care. 1980;3(4):530–2.
63. Hirashima DE, Soriano ES, Meirelles RL, Alberti GN, Nose W. Outcomes of iris-claw anterior chamber versus iris-fixated

foldable intraocular lens in subluxated lens secondary to Marfan syndrome. Ophthalmology. 2010;117(8):1479–85. https://doi.org/10.1016/j.ophtha.2009.12.043.

64. Nudleman E, Robinson J, Rao P, Drenser KA, Capone A, Trese MT. Long-term outcomes on lens clarity after lens-sparing vitrectomy for retinopathy of prematurity. Ophthalmology. 2015;122(4):755–9. https://doi.org/10.1016/j.ophtha.2014.11.004.
65. Fuchino Y, Hayashi H, Kono T, Ohshima K. Long-term follow up of visual acuity in eyes with stage 5 retinopathy of prematurity after closed vitrectomy. Am J Ophthalmol. 1995;120(3):308–16.
66. Capone A Jr, Trese MT. Lens-sparing vitreous surgery for tractional stage 4A retinopathy of prematurity retinal detachments. Ophthalmology. 2001;108(11):2068–70.
67. Chong LP, Machemer R, de Juan E. Vitrectomy for advanced stages of retinopathy of prematurity. Am J Ophthalmol. 1986;102(6):710–6.
68. Seaber JH, Machemer R, Eliott D, Buckley EG. deJuan E, Martin DF. Long-term visual results of children after initially successful vitrectomy for stage V retinopathy of prematurity. Ophthalmology. 1995;102(2):199–204.
69. Trese MT, Droste PJ. Long-term postoperative results of a consecutive series of stages 4 and 5 retinopathy of prematurity. Ophthalmology. 1998;105(6):992–7.
70. Cherry TA, Lambert SR, Capone A Jr. Electroretinographic findings in stage 5 retinopathy of prematurity after retinal reattachment. Retina. 1995;15(1):21–4.
71. Machemer R. Late traction detachment in retinopathy of prematurity or ROP-like cases. Graefes Arch Clin Exp Ophthalmol. 1993;231(7):389–94.
72. Ricci B, Santo A, Ricci F, Minicucci G, Molle F. Scleral buckling surgery in stage 4 retinopathy of prematurity. Graefes Arch Clin Exp Ophthalmol. 1996;234(Suppl 1):S38–41.
73. Topilow HW, Ackerman AL, Wang FM. The treatment of advanced retinopathy of prematurity by cryotherapy and scleral buckling surgery. Ophthalmology. 1985;92(3):379–87.
74. Machemer R. Closed vitrectomy for severe retrolental fibroplasia in the infant. Ophthalmology. 1983;90(5):436–41.
75. Mintz-Hittner HA, O'Malley RE, Kretzer FL. Long-term form identification vision after early, closed, lensectomy-vitrectomy for stage 5 retinopathy of prematurity. Ophthalmology. 1997;104(3):454–9.
76. Prenner JL, Capone A Jr, Trese MT. Visual outcomes after lens-sparing vitrectomy for stage 4A retinopathy of prematurity. Ophthalmology. 2004;111(12):2271–3.
77. Ferrone PJ, Harrison C, Trese MT. Lens clarity after lens-sparing vitrectomy in a pediatric population. Ophthalmology. 1997;104(2):273–8.
78. Lakhanpal RR, Sun RL, Albini TA, Holz ER. Anatomic success rate after 3-port lens-sparing vitrectomy in stage 4A or 4B retinopathy of prematurity. Ophthalmology. 2005;112(9):1569–73.
79. Hartnett ME. Features associated with surgical outcome in patients with stages 4 and 5 retinopathy of prematurity. Retina. 2003;23(3):322–9.
80. Quinn GE, Dobson V, Barr CC, Davis BR, Flynn JT, Palmer EA, et al. Visual acuity in infants after vitrectomy for severe retinopathy of prematurity. Ophthalmology. 1991;98(1):5–13.
81. Lakhanpal RR, Sun RL, Albini TA, Holz ER. Anatomical success rate after primary three-port lens-sparing vitrectomy in stage 5 retinopathy of prematurity. Retina. 2006;26(7):724–8. https://doi.org/10.1097/01.iae.0000244274.95963.1e. 00006982-200609000-00002 [pii]
82. Cusick M, Charles MK, Agron E, Sangiovanni JP, Ferris FL 3rd, Charles S. Anatomical and visual results of vitreoretinal surgery for stage 5 retinopathy of prematurity. Retina. 2006;26(7):729–35. https://doi.org/10.1097/01.iae.0000244268.21514.f7. 00006982-200609000-00003 [pii]
83. Terasaki H, Hirose T. Late-onset retinal detachment associated with regressed retinopathy of prematurity. Jpn J Ophthalmol. 2003;47(5):492–7.
84. Tasman W. Late complications of retrolental fibroplasia. Ophthalmology. 1979;86(10):1724–40.
85. Kaiser RS, Trese MT, Williams GA, Cox MS Jr. Adult retinopathy of prematurity: outcomes of rhegmatogenous retinal detachments and retinal tears. Ophthalmology. 2001;108(9):1647–53.
86. Sneed SR, Pulido JS, Blodi CF, Clarkson JG, Flynn HW Jr, Mieler WF. Surgical management of late-onset retinal detachments associated with regressed retinopathy of prematurity. Ophthalmology. 1990;97(2):179–83.
87. Tufail A, Singh AJ, Haynes RJ, Dodd CR, McLeod D, Charteris DG. Late onset vitreoretinal complications of regressed retinopathy of prematurity. Br J Ophthalmol. 2004;88(2):243–6.
88. Jackson TL, Hussain A, Morley AM, Sullivan PM, Hodgetts A, El-Osta A, et al. Scleral hydraulic conductivity and macromolecular diffusion in patients with uveal effusion syndrome. Invest Ophthalmol Vis Sci. 2008;49(11):5033–40. doi: iovs.08-1980 [pii]. https://doi.org/10.1167/iovs.08-1980.
89. Schneiderman TE, Johnson MW. A new approach to the surgical management of idiopathic uveal effusion syndrome. Am J Ophthalmol. 1997;123(2):262–3.
90. Terson A. De l'hemorrhagie dans le corp vitre au cours de l'hemorrhagie cerebrale. Clin Ophthalmol. 1900;6:309–12.
91. van Rens GH, Bos PJ, van Dalen JT. Vitrectomy in two cases of bilateral Terson syndrome. Doc Ophthalmol. 1983;56(1–2):155–9.
92. Weingeist TA, Goldman EJ, Folk JC, Packer AJ, Ossoinig KC. Terson's syndrome. Clinicopathologic Correlations Ophthalmology. 1986;93(11):1435–42.
93. Schultz PN, Sobol WM, Weingeist TA. Long-term visual outcome in Terson syndrome. Ophthalmology. 1991;98(12):1814–9.
94. Kuhn F, Morris R, Witherspoon CD, Mester V. Terson syndrome. Results of vitrectomy and the significance of vitreous hemorrhage in patients with subarachnoid hemorrhage. Ophthalmology. 1998;105(3):472–7.
95. Murjaneh S, Hale JE, Mishra S, Ling RH, Simcock PR. Terson's syndrome: surgical outcome in relation to entry site pathology. Br J Ophthalmol. 2006;90(4):512–3. doi: 90/4/512 [pii]. https://doi.org/10.1136/bjo.2005.080325.
96. Garweg JG, Koerner F. Outcome indicators for vitrectomy in Terson syndrome. Acta Ophthalmol. 2009;87(2):222–6. doi: AOS1200 [pii]. https://doi.org/10.1111/j.1755-3768.2008.01200.x.
97. Narayanan R, Taylor SC, Nayaka A, Deshpande R, St Aubin D, Hrisomalos FN, et al. Visual outcomes after Vitrectomy for Terson syndrome secondary to traumatic brain injury. Ophthalmology. 2017;124(1):118–22. https://doi.org/10.1016/j.ophtha.2016.09.009.
98. Skevas C, Czorlich P, Knospe V, Stemplewitz B, Richard G, Westphal M, et al. Terson's syndrome--rate and surgical approach in patients with subarachnoid hemorrhage: a prospective interdisciplinary study. Ophthalmology. 2014;121(8):1628–33. https://doi.org/10.1016/j.ophtha.2014.02.015.
99. Rubowitz A, Desai U. Nontraumatic macular holes associated with Terson syndrome. Retina. 2006;26(2):230–2. doi: 00006982-200602000-00022 [pii]
100. Kielar RA. Choroidal melanoma appearing as vitreous hemorrhage. Ann Ophthalmol. 1982;14(5):461–4.
101. Gibran SK, Kapoor KG. Management of exudative retinal detachment in choroidal melanoma. Clin Exp Ophthalmol. 2009;37(7):654–9. doi: CEO2127 [pii]. https://doi.org/10.1111/j.1442-9071.2009.02127.x.

102. Reddy DM, Mason LB, Mason JO 3rd, Crosson JN, Yunker JJ. Vitrectomy and Vitrector port needle biopsy of Choroidal melanoma for gene expression profile testing immediately before brachytherapy. Ophthalmology. 2017;124(9):1377–82. https://doi.org/10.1016/j.ophtha.2017.03.053.
103. Bagger M, Tebering JF, Kiilgaard JF. The ocular consequences and applicability of minimally invasive 25-gauge Transvitreal Retinochoroidal biopsy. Ophthalmology. 2013; https://doi.org/10.1016/j.ophtha.2013.07.043.
104. Sen J, Groenewald C, Hiscott PS, Smith PA, Damato BE. Transretinal choroidal tumor biopsy with a 25-gauge vitrector. Ophthalmology. 2006;113(6):1028–31. doi: S0161-6420(06)00332-0 [pii]. https://doi.org/10.1016/j.ophtha.2006.02.048.
105. Reichstein D, Karan K. Endoresection utilizing pars plana vitrectomy for benign and malignant intraocular tumors. Curr Opin Ophthalmol. 2019;30(3):151–8. https://doi.org/10.1097/icu.0000000000000561.
106. Caminal JM, Mejia K, Masuet-Aumadell C, Arias L, Piulats JM, Gutierrez C, et al. Endoresection versus iodine-125 plaque brachytherapy for the treatment of choroidal melanoma. Am J Ophthalmol. 2013;156(2):334–42. e1. https://doi.org/10.1016/j.ajo.2013.03.036.
107. Karkhaneh R, Chams H, Amoli FA, Riazi-Esfahani M, Ahmadabadi MN, Mansouri MR, et al. Long-term surgical outcome of posterior choroidal melanoma treated by endoresection. Retina. 2007;27(7):908–14. https://doi.org/10.1097/IAE.0b013e31802fa2db. 00006982-200709000-00016 [pii]
108. Damato B, Groenewald C, McGalliard J, Wong D. Endoresection of choroidal melanoma. Br J Ophthalmol. 1998;82(3):213–8.
109. Grixti A, Angi M, Damato BE, Jmor F, Konstantinidis L, Groenewald C, et al. Vitreoretinal surgery for complications of choroidal tumor biopsy. Ophthalmology. 2014;121(12):2482–8. https://doi.org/10.1016/j.ophtha.2014.06.029.
110. Bansal AS, Bianciotto CG, Maguire JI, Regillo CD, Shields JA, Shields CL. Safety of pars plana vitrectomy in eyes with plaque-irradiated posterior uveal melanoma. Arch Ophthalmol. 2012;130(10):1285–90. doi: 1377724 [pii]. https://doi.org/10.1001/archophthalmol.2012.2391.
111. Bianciotto C, Shields CL, Pirondini C, Mashayekhi A, Furuta M, Shields JA. Proliferative radiation retinopathy after plaque radiotherapy for uveal melanoma. Ophthalmology. 2010;117(5):1005–12. https://doi.org/10.1016/j.ophtha.2009.10.015.
112. Mashayekhi A, Shields CL, Lee SC, Marr BP, Shields JA. Retinal break and rhegmatogenous retinal detachment after transpupillary thermotherapy as primary or adjunct treatment of choroidal melanoma. Retina. 2008;28(2):274–81. https://doi.org/10.1097/IAE.0b013e318145abe8. 00006982-200802000-00011 [pii]
113. Foster WJ, Harbour JW, Holekamp NM, Shah GK, Thomas MA. Pars plana vitrectomy in eyes containing a treated posterior uveal melanoma. Am J Ophthalmol. 2003;136(3):471–6.
114. Balestrazzi A, Blasi MA, Scupola TA, Balestrazzi TE. Retinal detachment due to macular hole after transpupillary thermotherapy of choroidal melanoma. Retina. 2001;21(4):384–5.
115. Haimovici R, Mukai S, Schachat AP, Haynie GD, Thomas MA, Meredith TA, et al. Rhegmatogenous retinal detachment in eyes with uveal melanoma. Retina. 1996;16(6):488–96.
116. Laqua H, Volcker HE. Pars plana vitrectomy in eyes with malignant melanoma. Graefes Arch Clin Exp Ophthalmol. 1983;220(6):279–84.
117. Lu Y, Jia L, He S, Hurley MC, Leys MJ, Jayasundera T, et al. Melanoma-associated retinopathy: a paraneoplastic autoimmune complication. Arch Ophthalmol. 2009;127(12):1572–80. doi: 127/12/1572 [pii]. https://doi.org/10.1001/archophthalmol.2009.311.
118. Lewis K, Herbert EN, Williamson TH. Severe ocular involvement in disseminated intravascular coagulation complicating meningococcaemia. Graefes Arch Clin Exp Ophthalmol. 2005;243(10):1069–70.
119. Perez VL, Leung EH, Berrocal AM, Albini TA, Parel JM, Amescua G, et al. Impact of Total pars Plana Vitrectomy on postoperative complications in Aphakic, snap-on, type 1 Boston Keratoprosthesis. Ophthalmology. 2017;124(10):1504–9. https://doi.org/10.1016/j.ophtha.2017.04.016.
120. Harissi-Dagher M, Durr GM, Biernacki K, Sebag M, Rheaume MA. Pars plana vitrectomy through the Boston Keratoprosthesis type 1. Eye (Lond). 2013;27(6):767–9. https://doi.org/10.1038/eye.2013.58.
121. Yanai D, Weiland JD, Mahadevappa M, Greenberg RJ, Fine I, Humayun MS. Visual performance using a retinal prosthesis in three subjects with retinitis pigmentosa. Am J Ophthalmol. 2007;143(5):820–7. doi: S0002-9394(07)00067-0 [pii]. https://doi.org/10.1016/j.ajo.2007.01.027.
122. Roessler G, Laube T, Brockmann C, Kirschkamp T, Mazinani B, Goertz M, et al. Implantation and explantation of a wireless epiretinal retina implant device: observations during the EPIRET3 prospective clinical trial. Invest Ophthalmol Vis Sci. 2009;50(6):3003–8. doi: iovs.08-2752 [pii]. https://doi.org/10.1167/iovs.08-2752.

Glossary of Abbreviations

AC	anterior chamber	anterior portion of the eye
ARMD	age-related macular degeneration	
ARN	acute retinal necrosis	viral retinal infection
BRVO	branch retinal vein occlusion	blockage of a retinal venule
CME	cystoid macular oedema	intraretinal fluid accumulation in the macula
CNV	choroidal neovascular membrane	a fibrovascular proliferation under the neuroretina
CRVO	central retinal vein occlusion	blockage of the retinal vein in the optic nerve
C3F8	carbon tetrafluoride	gas for retinal tamponade
C2F6	Hexafluoroethane	long acting gas
DACE	drainage air cryotherapy and explant	external procedure for retinal reattachment
ERM	epiretinal membrane	membrane on the surface of the retina
EUA	examination under anaesthetic	examining the eye with general anaesthesia
GRT	giant retinal tear	more than 90° retinal break
HRVO	hemiretinal vein occlusion	partial blockage of the retinal vein in the optic nerve
ILM	internal limiting membrane	a normally occurring anatomical membrane on the inner retina
ICG	indocyanine green	dye used in macular surgery
IOFB	intraocular foreign body	extraneous material in the eye usually secondary to trauma
IOL	intraocular lens implant	lens device for cataract surgery
IOP	intraocular pressure	pressure of the globe of the eye
NVD	neovascularisation of the disc	abnormal blood vessel formation at the optic nerve head
NVE	neovascularisation elsewhere	abnormal blood vessel formation on the retina
OCT	optical coherence tomography	laser method for examining the macula
PIC	punctate inner choroidopathy	
PCR	polymerase chain reaction	method for detection of viruses in vitreous samples
POAG	primary open-angle glaucoma	
POHS	presumed ocular histoplasmosis syndrome	
PORN	progressive outer retinal necrosis	viral infection of the outer retinal layers
PPV	pars plana vitrectomy	surgical removal of the vitreous gel
PRP	panretinal photocoagulation	laser therapy for retinal neovascularisation
PVD	posterior vitreous detachment	separation of the vitreous from the surface of the inner retina
PVR	proliferative vitreoretinopathy	fibrous tissue deposition on the retina in rhegmatogenous retinal detachment
RAPD	relative afferent papillary defect	measure of optic nerve function
RRD	rhegmatogenous retinal detachment	retinal elevation from retinal breaks
RPE	retinal pigment epithelium	outer layer of the retina
SRF	subretinal fluid	fluid between detached neuroretina and the retinal pigment epithelium
SRNVM	subretinal neovascular membrane	a fibrovascular proliferation under the neuroretina
SF6	sulphur hexafluoride	gas for retinal tamponade
TRD	tractional retinal detachment	retinal elevation from contraction of fibrous or neovascular tissue
VH	vitreous hemorrhage	bleeding into the vitreous gel
VA	visual acuity	central vision measure
YAG	Yttrium aluminium garnet	surgical laser

Others

CF	counting fingers
CVA	cerebrovascular accident
DM	diabetes mellitus
FH	family history
HBP	high blood pressure
HM	hand movements
LA	local anaesthesia
LP	light perception
MI	myocardial infarction
NS	nuclear sclerosis
NLP	no light perception
PSC	posterior subcapsular
RTA	road traffic accident
Snellen PH	visual acuity with pinhole or best corrected

T. H. Williamson, *Vitreoretinal Surgery*, https://doi.org/10.1007/978-3-030-68769-4

Appendix

Useful Formulae and Rules

Cryotherapy

- **The Joule–Thomson Effect** arises because real gases (non-ideal) exhibit molecular interactions. Each gas has a threshold temperature below which it cools when expanded and can drain energy from the surrounding environment causing it to cool down. At room temperature, nitrogen and oxygen cool on expansion whereas helium, for example, warms.

Fluids (i.e. Both Gases and Liquids)

- **Surface Tension**. The forces present on the surface of a liquid and a gas, produced by intermolecular bonds, which must be overcome to break the surface of the liquid in the air.
  - The surface tension in surgery is used to keep the gas as one bubble, e.g. avoiding the separation off of a bubble that might pass through a retinal break.
  - An air or gas bubble in the eye has a flattened inferior aspect because the gravitational force of the liquid under the bubble, combined with the high buoyancy of the gas, is high enough to overcome the surface tension of the gas bubble (which without gravitational forces would create a sphere), thus causing the bubble to flatten rather than achieve a sphere. Similarly, the forces acting on the bubble are enough to overcome the surface tension to cause the bubble to conform to the shape of the eye superiorly. This causes a large surface area in contact with the retina superiorly but a gap in contact inferiorly (Fig. A.1).
  - As the bubble becomes smaller the balance of gravitational forces relative to surface tension is changed. If a bubble separates off, it remains so because the surface tension effects overcome the gravitational effects of the fluid and the fluid remains between the bubbles separating them; therefore, multiple separate bubbles appear just before the bubble disperses.

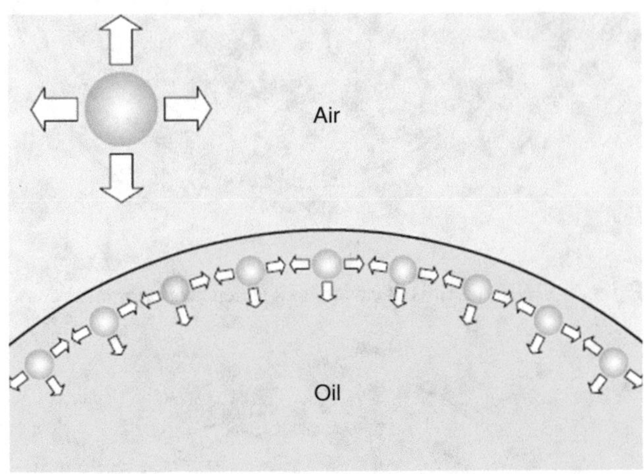

Fig. A.1 The intermolecular attractions are shown around the molecules in a liquid (e.g. oil) in contact with another liquid or a gas (e.g. air). Within the liquid each molecule is pulled equally in all directions by neighbouring liquid molecules top left, resulting in a net force of zero. At the surface of the liquid, the molecules are more attracted to other molecules inside the liquid than outside in the gas, producing an overall force inwards. The liquid would like to be a sphere but is usually distorted by other forces, e.g. gravitational

- **Interfacial Tension.** As above but between two liquids.
  - The interfacial tension in surgery is used to keep a liquid as one bubble, e.g. avoiding the separation off of a bubble that might pass through a retinal break. The interfacial tension of silicone oil (being less than the surface tension of a gas) may be overcome if a retinal tear is under high tension, e.g. proliferative vitreoretinopathy, causing the silicone oil to pass through a tear into the subretinal space.
  - A silicone oil bubble in the eye has a nearly spherical shape because the gravitational forces of the liquid *around* the bubble, which is quite weakly buoyant, are not enough to overcome the interfacial tension of the oil bubble thus giving the natural spherical form. As there is a sphere within a sphere there is much less surface area in contact with the retina than with gas (in practice with a maximal fill of oil, probably in contact from the horizontal meridian upwards) (Figs. A.2, A.3 and A.4).

T. H. Williamson, *Vitreoretinal Surgery*, https://doi.org/10.1007/978-3-030-68769-4

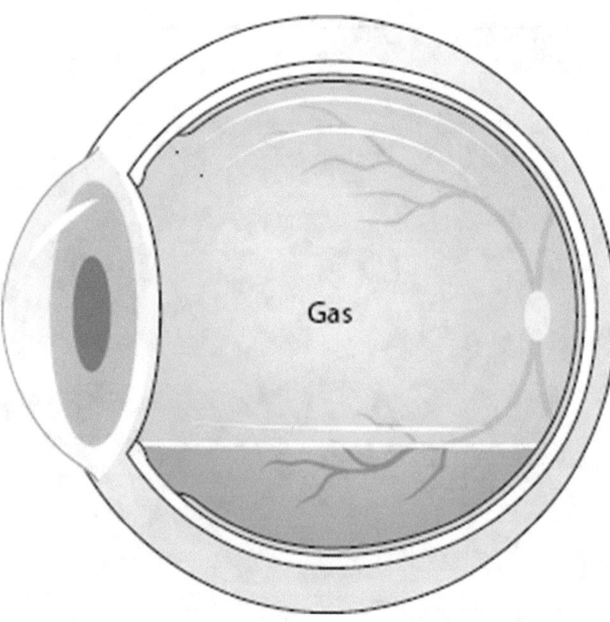

Fig. A.2 Gas in the vitreous cavity has a flattened inferior meniscus

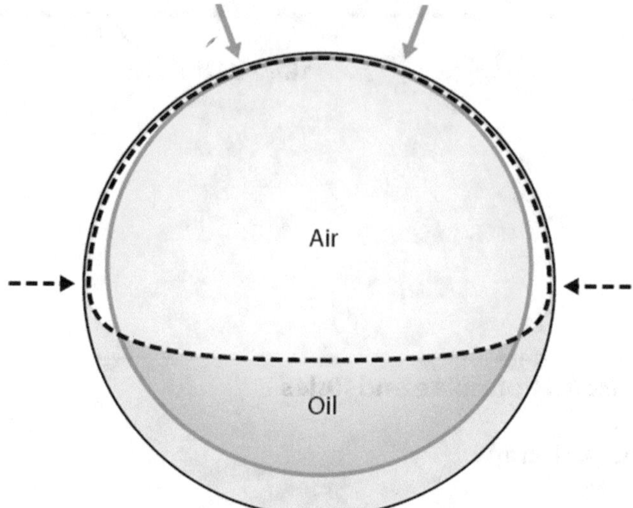

Fig. A.4 Even a large bubble of a fluid that takes up a spheroidal shape (e.g. oil) within a sphere (the eye) has a small contact area on the inside of the sphere (grey line and arrows) whereas a smaller bubble of distortable fluid (e.g. air) with a flat meniscus will have a large contact area (black dashed lines)

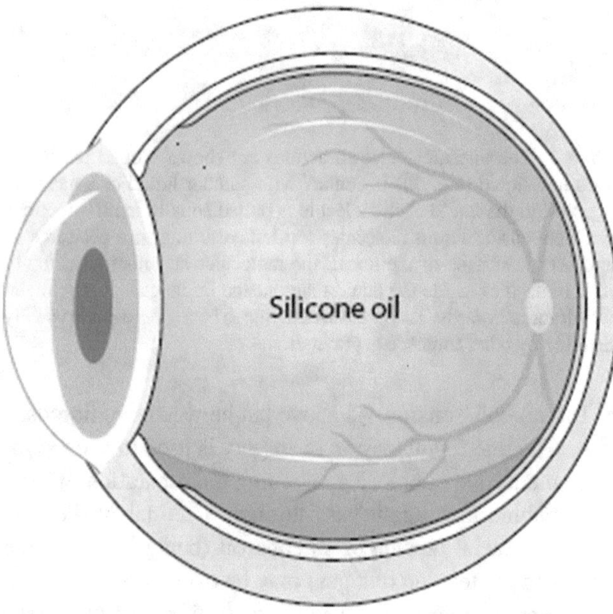

Fig. A.3 Silicone oil in the vitreous cavity has a more spherical inferior meniscus

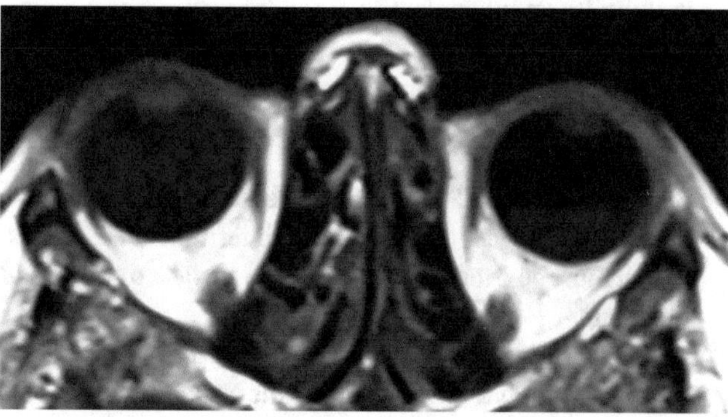

Fig. A.5 Notice the gas in the vitreous cavity visible on MRI with the patient face up. There is a flattened inferior meniscus

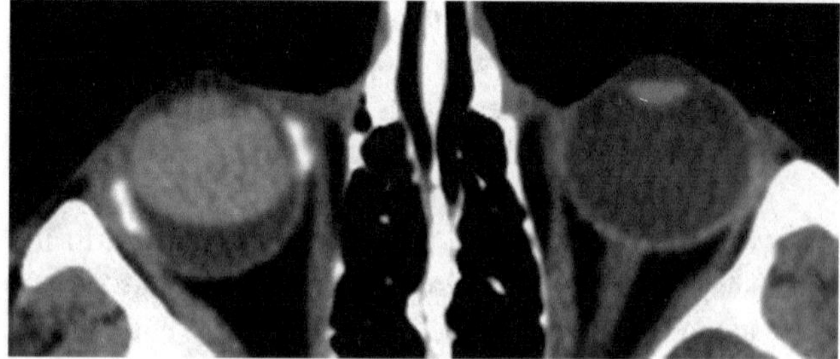

Fig. A.6 Oil has a spherical inferior profile (CT scan patient face up)

Gases (Figs. A.5 and A.6)

- **Gases are compressible.**
- **Fick's Diffusion equation** states that the rate of diffusion of a gas through a thin membrane is increased by: the concentration differential; area of the membrane; the diffusivity of the gas and reduced by the thickness of the membrane. This equation explains the longevity of some gases, e.g. perfluoro propane, in the eye, and why these can expand (Fig. A.7).

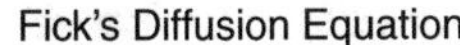

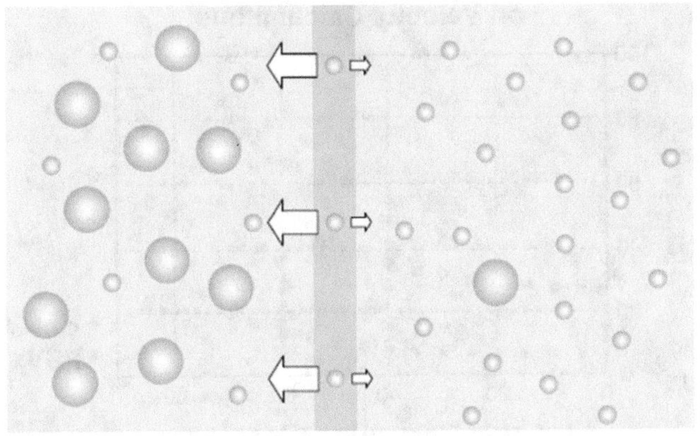

Fig. A.7 The large molecule gas has low diffusivity and passes across the membrane slowly. The small molecule gas moves rapidly across the membrane. Therefore, initially the gas bubble on the left expands in relation to the gas bubble on the right

$$F = -D(c2 - c1) / x$$

F = rate of passage of the gas
D = diffusivity of the gas
$c2–c1$ = gas concentration difference across the membrane
x = thickness of thin membrane

- **Boyle's law** states that, at a constant temperature, the volume of a given mass of gas varies inversely with pressure.

Liquids

- Liquids are not compressible for practical purposes.
- Infusion Heights When calculating infusion bottle heights in vitrectomy surgery use:

$$14 \text{ mm} H_2O = 1 \text{ mmHg}$$

- Bernoulli's Principle states that as the speed of moving liquid increases, the pressure within the liquid decreases. This principle may be the reason that a retinal break flattens onto an indent in non-drain retinal detachment surgery.

$$\text{Pressure} \times \text{velocity} = k$$

- **Blood Flow rate** = Blood Velocity x Cross-sectional Area of the Blood Vessel.
- **Laplace's Law for pressure in a tube radius (*r*).**

$$\text{Transmural Pressure} = \frac{\text{Wall Tension}}{r}$$

And a sphere

$$\text{Transmural Pressure} = \frac{2 \times \text{Wall Tension}}{r}$$

This demonstrates that the larger the fluid-filled cavity for the same pressure the higher the tension on the wall. Theoretically, a highly myopic eye is more vulnerable to wall rupture for the same pressure.

- Hagan–Poiseuille Law

$$\text{Volume Flow Rate}(Q) = \frac{\pi d^4 (\text{Pa} - \text{Pb})}{L8n}$$

d = diameter of the tube
Pa–Pb = pressure difference between ends
L = length of the tube
n = viscosity

Higher pressure is required to make highly viscous materials such as silicone oil to pass through a tube. Five thousand millipascal seconds oil is, therefore, more difficult to remove through a small hole or tube than 1000 mPas oil.

- Emulsion (Fig. A.8)

This is a complex interaction of otherwise immiscible substances such as oil and water to create small droplets of one in the other. In the eye silicone oil emulsion in aqueous (water) is probably facilitated by the presence of proteins in the aque-

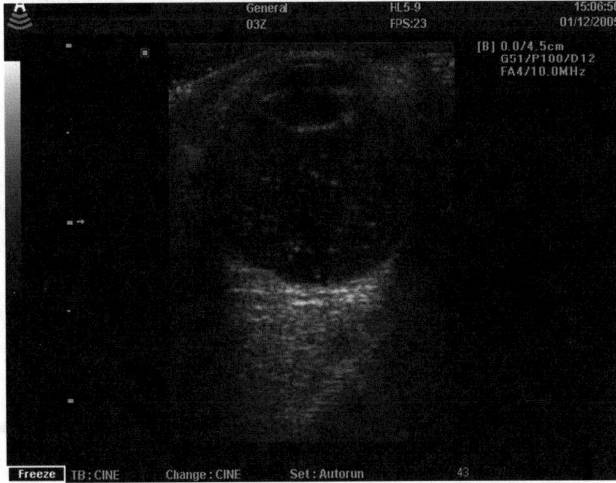

Fig. A.8 Emulsified droplets of oil are visible in the vitreous cavity of this patient on ultrasound

ous and the mechanical action of eye movements on the surface of the oil bubble. The protein is acting as an emulsifier.

The **Bancroft rule** applies, that is the emulsifiers and emulsifying particles tend to promote dispersion of the phase in which they do not dissolve very well.

The protein dissolves better in water than in oil and so tends to facilitate oil-in-water emulsions (that is, it promotes the dispersion of oil droplets throughout a continuous phase of water).

- **Reynold's Number**. This is an empirical number to calculate the likelihood of turbulence in a fluid. The thin layer of fluid between the retina and a silicone oil bubble is unlikely to allow the development of eddies (turbulence) which may be a factor for the effect of oil in retaining the attachment of in inferior retinectomy despite the fact that the oil is not in contact with the retinectomy edge.

$$R = \frac{P2rV}{N}$$

R = Reynold's number
P = pressure
r = radius of a tube
n = viscosity of the fluid
V = velocity of the fluid

- **Vapour pressure** is the pressure exerted above a liquid by its own vapour. If a liquid has a high characteristic vapour pressure, then the liquid is more likely to evaporate.
- **Pascal's Principle** Pressure is transmitted undiminished in an enclosed static fluid. Therefore, a blow to the front of the eye allows damage to the retina at the back of the eye.

Ultrasound (Fig. A.9)

- **Velocity of sound in 1000 mPas silicone oil** = 986 m/s. An ultrasound of the eye with oil in situ appears to show an enlarged eye because the sound waves are slowed down and take longer to return to the transducer. The increased delay is falsely interpreted as from increased distance.
- **Meldrum's formula** adjusts the axial length calculated by an ultrasound scan for the presence of 1000 mPas silicone oil:

$$\text{Axial length}(\text{mm}) = \text{length of}(\text{anterior chamber} + \text{lens}) + (0.63 \times \text{vitreous length}) + \text{the retro– silicone space}$$

- **Doppler Equation**

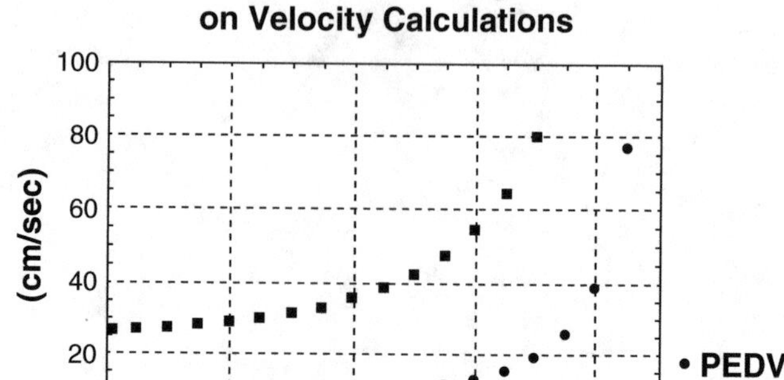

Fig. A.9 The effect of the angle of incidence of the Doppler beam on the velocity measurements is shown. At high angles the effect on the measurements is high

$$V\,\text{flow} = \frac{V\,\text{sound} \times \Delta\,\text{Frequency}}{2\,F\,\text{out}\cos A}$$

V flow = fluid velocity
V sound = velocity of sound
Δ Frequency = change in frequency
F out = Transmit frequency
A = angle of incidence of the Doppler beam to the direction of flow (should be small)

Diffusion and Viscosity

Viscosity of vitreous 5–2000 cP (aqueous 1 cP)

- Inversely related to the diffusion of a molecule
  - Fick's law
    Diffusion flux (J) = D/Concentration gradient (dc/dx)
  - Stokes–Einstein
    Diffusion Coefficient (D) = $RT/6\pi nrN$
- D = Diffusion coefficient
- R = Molar gas constant
- T = temperature in Kelvins
- n = viscosity of the medium
- r = radius of the diffusing molecule
- N = Avogadro's number

Visual Acuity

$$\textbf{LogMar} = \log 10(\text{denominator VA} / \text{numerator VA})$$

Conversion chart for Snellen to LogMar [1–3].

Snellen in feet		LogMar	Snellen in Metres	
20	10	−0.30103	6	3
20	20	0	6	6
20	30	0.176091	6	9
20	40	0.30103	6	12
20	50	0.39794	6	15
20	60	0.477121	6	18
20	70	0.544068	6	21
20	80	0.60206	6	24
20	90	0.653213	6	27
20	100	0.69897	6	30
20	110	0.740363	6	33
20	120	0.778151	6	36
20	130	0.812913	6	39
20	140	0.845098	6	42
20	150	0.875061	6	45
20	160	0.90309	6	48
20	170	0.929419	6	51
20	180	0.954243	6	54
20	190	0.977724	6	57
20	200	1	6	60
20	210	1.021189	6	63
20	220	1.041393	6	66
20	230	1.060698	6	69
20	240	1.079181	6	72
20	250	1.09691	6	75
20	260	1.113943	6	78
20	270	1.130334	6	81
20	280	1.146128	6	84
20	290	1.161368	6	87
20	300	1.176091	6	90
20	400	1.30103	6	120
20	500	1.39794	6	150
20	600	1.477121	6	180
20	700	1.544068	6	210
20	800	1.60206	6	240
20	900	1.653213	6	270
Counting fingers		1.85		
Hand movements		2.3		
Perception of light		2.6		
No perception of light		2.9		

Diffusion

Fick's law

$$\text{Diffusion flux}\left(J\right)=D/c1-c2$$

Stokes–Einstein

$$\text{Diffusion Coefficient}\left(D\right)=RT/6\pi\mu rN$$

c = concentration
R = molar gas constant
T = temperature
μ = viscosity
r = radius of the molecule
N = Avogadro's number [4, 5]
Convection and permeability
Darcy's law

$$v_{\text{Fluid}}=-\left(K/\mu_{\text{Fluid}}\right)P$$

v_{Fluid} = velocity of the fluid
K = hydraulic conductivity
μ_{Fluid} = viscosity of the fluid
P = gradient of pressure
Starling's law
Hydrostatic and osmotic gradients in balance

$$P-Q=O$$

Drop in interstitial pressure may contribute to CMO.

References

1. Holladay JT. Proper method for calculating average visual acuity. J Refract Surg. 1997;13(4):388–91.
2. Lange C, Feltgen N, Junker B, Schulze-Bonsel K, Bach M. Resolving the clinical acuity categories "hand motion" and "counting fingers" using the Freiburg visual acuity test (FrACT). Graefes Arch Clin Exp Ophthalmol. 2009;247(1):137–42. https://doi.org/10.1007/s00417-008-0926-0.
3. Schulze-Bonsel K, Feltgen N, Burau H, Hansen L, Bach M. Visual acuities "hand motion" and "counting fingers" can be quantified with the freiburg visual acuity test. Invest Ophthalmol Vis Sci. 2006;47(3):1236–40. https://doi.org/10.1167/iovs.05-0981.
4. Stefansson E. Physiology of vitreous surgery. Graefes Arch Clin Exp Ophthalmol. 2009;247(2):147–63. https://doi.org/10.1007/s00417-008-0980-7.
5. Barton KA, Shui YB, Petrash JM, Beebe DC. Comment on: the stokes-Einstein equation and the physiological effects of vitreous surgery. Acta Ophthalmol Scand. 2007;85(3):339–40. https://doi.org/10.1111/j.1600-0420.2007.00902.x.

Printed in the United States
by Baker & Taylor Publisher Services